Gene Therapy

Gene Therapy

Therapeutic Mechanisms and Strategies

edited by

Nancy Smyth Templeton

Baylor College of Medicine
Houston, Texas

Danilo D. Lasic

Liposome Consultations
Newark, California

MARCEL DEKKER

MARCEL DEKKER, INC. NEW YORK • BASEL

ISBN: 0-8247-7665-8

This book is printed on acid-free paper.

Headquarters
Marcel Dekker, Inc.
270 Madison Avenue, New York, NY 10016
tel: 212-696-9000; fax: 212-685-4540

Eastern Hemisphere Distribution
Marcel Dekker AG
Hutgasse 4, Postfach 812, CH-4001 Basel, Switzerland
tel: 41-61-261-8482; fax: 41-61-261-8896

World Wide Web
http://www.dekker.com

The publisher offers discounts on this book when ordered in bulk quantities. For more information, write to Special Sales/Professional Marketing at the headquarters address above.

Current printing (last digit):
10 9 8 7 6 5 4 3 2 1

PRINTED IN THE UNITED STATES OF AMERICA

To our friend and colleague
Michael Strauss

Foreword

The promise of being able to manipulate human genetic material in order to treat diseases has long been a hope for patients with heretofore untreatable diseases, as well as a goal for scientists and an anticipated new tool in the physician's medicine bag. However, lest we forget, Edward Jenner in 1798 pioneered the then unheralded use of cowpox as a vaccine to prevent smallpox. Today we know that specific immunity to a virus similar to smallpox was induced in the persons who were vaccinated, and that from a global perspective, the practice, if not the knowledge of altering the gene structure of humans has proceeded for 200 years. In fact, the United States has a broad-based public policy that such vaccinations represent good public health practice, and the list of vaccines required for infants and children continues to grow. Thus, the modern hope stems from an older proven idea.

However, vaccines have been less successful in preventing or treating diseases of noninfectious origin. In this volume you will find an astonishing variety of potential strategies to treat and prevent genetic diseases, cancer, and metabolic, neurological, and other therapeutically resistant disorders. You will find that the original theories about using viruses as natural messengers of genes have been greatly augmented by novel collaborations among chemists, biochemists—engineers, physicists, and others to provide a wonderfully synergistic, dare one say, holistic—approach to specified genetic therapies. Chemical approaches to soap films lead to liposomes with plasmids. Highly technical engineering leads to a gun to drive genes directly through the cell wall. Molecular biologists who know how to reengineer any sequence to whatever is needed work with leading virologists who can pull from their freezers viral tools once used mostly as reagents to form the most intriguing of therapeutic agents.

Going once more back to see the future, how did this happen? An apocryphal theory that I have on occasion put forward is that the United States had a ''secret'' 40-year bond, one that began in 1957 with the launch of the Russian-developed satellite Sputnik. Massive public investment in education, engineering, medical specialties, and other struggling disciplines led to a dizzying array of breakthroughs: large-scale successful vaccination programs, solid-state electronics, the Internet, the broadening of the National Institutes of Health, and progress in new chemistry, physics and biology, and biotechnology. Medical specialties proliferated, and chemical and biological advances led to immunosuppression making it possible for human organs to be transplanted. The first wave of biotechnology yielded new products that could stimulate growth of red and white cells, while products formerly produced from animals were now made synthetically in bacterial, animal, and human cells. With the Internet has come the democratization of knowledge so that patients are as knowledgeable about diseases as many physicians, and are beginning to ask the hard question of ''why not for me?'' Like any good 40-year bond that matures, it is time to pick the fruits of that investment and reinvest in the future, a future that must deliver on the excitement and promise of the past 40 years.

Indeed, what you will glimpse in this volume is the beginning of the reinvestment, and a knowledgeable public will be able to encourage, as well as judge, how its reinvestment is progressing. Unlike any other field of pharmaceutical and biological product production, gene therapy has always been open to the scrutiny of the public, as detailed in the chapter on regulatory aspects of gene therapy. This public scrutiny has not always focused strictly on science, but it has the distinctly American flavor of allowing everyone to participate, particularly public policy makers, ethicists, and patients. In that sense it places the public, who paid for that initial 40-year bond, in the position in which they can, will, and should shape the public policy of how to further the potential of gene therapy as a reality.

To end this brief foreword, let us focus on the word ''reality.'' At this writing, no gene therapy product has been approved by the FDA as safe and effective for any disease. It is the hope that that will happen in the future. How near that future is, depends on all of us—the public, the FDA, the NIH, industry—to work, debate, and negotiate toward this goal in the new millennium. I am honored by the request of the publisher and editors to provide this brief introduction, and I am pleased that many of the chapters are written not just by outstanding scientists but also by groups conducting clinical trials regulated by the FDA. The authors are representative of the large arena of gene therapy participants, and as such they and others are moving the field forward in a professional, collegial, and rigorous manner. It is my hope that the authors consider the FDA to be a partner in these efforts.

Philip D. Noguchi, M.D.
Director
Division of Cellular and Gene Therapies
Center for Biologics Evaluation and Research
Food and Drug Administration
Rockville, Maryland

Preface

These are exciting times for everyone involved in gene therapy as it evolves into a mature scientific field. Much progress has been made since its inception in the early 1970s. As you will read in this text, many hurdles remain that must be overcome in order for gene therapy to be used routinely as a therapeutic in the clinic. However, the current problems should not be taken as deterrents or barriers to future work or as reasons to abandon gene therapy for the treatment of disease. These hurdles should be embraced as challenges that can be overcome with greater knowledge and research efforts. The authors of this text have provided thoughtful insights into the challenges that must be met in specific applications of gene therapy.

Medicine has passed through several revolutions in its history. In early times, the healing power of some plants was discovered. Later, primitive surgery and immobilization of broken bones had been achieved. In the last centuries developments included anesthesia, vaccination, blood transfusion, surgery, and antibiotics. Most recently, major improvements have included novel imaging methods, microsurgery, lasers, organ transplantation, drug libraries based on combinatorial chemistry and high-throughput screening, and the emerging field of gene therapy discussed in this monograph.

The origin of many diseases is defective genes. For example, cells can overexpress certain proteins or produce nonfunctional proteins leading to uncontrolled cell division. The goal of gene therapy is to produce normal gene products or, alternatively, to turn off, silence, or down-regulate genes encoding undesirable gene products. The first approach requires the delivery of an appropriate cDNA encoding a gene product into the nuclei of the target cells, while protein synthesis can be prevented by antisense oligonucleotides and/or ribozymes that destroy the ability of target mRNAs to be translated. Successful gene therapy requires the knowledge of the molecular origin of the disease and the ability to synthesize wild-type gene products at appropriate levels in the target cells.

Following the ground-breaking 1950s, the first concepts of gene transfection and its use in therapy emerged in the 1960s. The obstacles were immense and, although the concept was proven, the first promising results surfaced only in the 1990s. In nature, only viruses and sperm cells are able to transfect their genetic material into appropriate cells in the human body. While the former mechanism is accompanied by severe unwanted side effects, the latter operates in highly specialized conditions. Obviously, man must design new gene delivery systems. Three basic strategies have appeared, including mechanical methods (direct injection, gene gun, electroporation), chemical methods (the complexation of plasmids with cations, polymers, or liposomes), and biological approaches (redesigned, semiartificial viruses).

Increased understanding of the genetic origins of many diseases has provided therapeutically interesting results with biological end-points as discussed in the present volume. Furthermore, developments in recombinant DNA technology have produced large-scale preparation of high-expression plasmids and gene delivery vehicles. The field of gene therapy is extremely multidisciplinary, consisting of researchers in life sciences, molecular biologists, biochemists, physiologists, and many other investigators who track the origin of diseases and determine the functionality of various proteins. Scientists involved in recombinant DNA technology are constructing and manufacturing plasmids, and virologists are modifying viruses. Chemists are synthesizing new polymers and lipids, and physicists are studying the structure of various DNA-carrier constructs. Pharmacologists, toxicologists, and physicians analyze the results of gene therapeutics in preclinical models and clinical trials.

Because the field of gene therapy is so broad, researchers have found it difficult to be familiar with all the different multidisciplinary aspects. Although several books exist, they cover the field mainly from rather specialized perspectives. The need for a more inclusive treatment, as well as the rapid advances resulting in important new developments, was the reason for assembling this book. We have organized the volume in several parts so that all aspects would be covered comprehensively by leading experts. An additional goal was to assemble a concise and up-to-date book that could be used by students as a textbook. Therefore, we asked the contributors to broaden introductions in order to provide sufficient fundamental information to allow easy learning and understanding.

The authors have provided knowledge covering broad topics in their areas of expertise and have gone well beyond discussion of their focused research efforts. The primary goal of this book is to provide students, scientists, and other interested readers with a broad knowledge of all aspects and tools available in the field of gene therapy. We welcome your comments and criticisms for use in the preparation of future editions. We hope to provide frequent updates that will include additional volumes to cover other topics in depth. This volume is designed to encompass the most widely used vehicles for the delivery of nucleic acids, including viral and nonviral systems, and discussions of the major disease targets for gene therapy. All chapters and illustrations are composed so that readers from diverse disciplines can understand the topics presented.

We wish to thank all the individuals who were not able to contribute to this edition but provided much useful advice, including Drs. Flossie Wong-Staal, Didier Trono, Theodore Friedmann, Imi Kovesdi, Fred Ledley, and others.

Nancy Smyth Templeton
Danilo D. Lasic

Contents

Contributors

Kurosh Ameri Department of Pathology Medical School, The University of Sheffield, Sheffield, England

W. French Anderson Gene Therapy Laboratories, Keck School of Medicine at the University of Southern California, Los Angeles, California

Jean-Paul Behr Laboratoire de Chimie Génétique, CNRS–URA 1386, Illkirch, France

C. Frank Bennett Antisense Research, Isis Pharmaceuticals, Inc., Carlsbad, California

Helen M. Blau Department of Molecular Pharmacology, Stanford University School of Medicine, Stanford, California

Ulrike Blömer Department of Neurosurgery, Medical School Hannover, Hannover, Germany

David M. Bodine Laboratory of Gene Transfer, National Human Genome Research Institute, National Institutes of Health, Bethesda, Maryland

Richard C. Boucher Cystic Fibrosis Research Center, University of North Carolina at Chapel Hill, Chapel Hill, North Carolina

Karsten Brand Molecular Cell Biology, Department of Biology, Humboldt-University Berlin, Berlin-Buch, Germany

Madeline Butler Department of Pharmacology, Isis Pharmaceuticals, Inc., Carlsbad, California

Paula M. Cannon Gene Therapy Laboratories, Keck School of Medicine at the University of Southern California, Los Angeles, California

Barrie J. Carter Research and Development, Targeted Genetics Corporation, Seattle, Washington

P. Dan Cook Department of Medicinal Chemistry, Isis Pharmaceuticals, Inc., Carlsbad, California

Ronald G. Crystal Institute of Medicine and Division of Pulmonary and Critical Care Medicine, Weill Medical College of Cornell University, New York, New York

Pieter Cullis Inex Pharmaceuticals Corporation, Burnaby, British Columbia, Canada

Barbara Demeneix Laboratoire de Physiologie Générale et Comparée, CNRS–UMR 8572, Muséum National d'Historie Naturelle, Paris, France

Hemant Deshmukh Drug Delivery Research and Pharmaceutical Development, Isis Pharmaceuticals, Inc., Carlsbad, California

Ralph Dornburg Center for Human Virology, The Dorrance H. Hamilton Labs, Thomas Jefferson University, Philadelphia, Pennsylvania

Thomas W. Dubensky, Jr. Vaccines and Gene Therapy, Chiron Corporation, Emeryville, California

Victor J. Dzau Department of Medicine, Brigham and Women's Hospital, and Harvard Medical School, Boston, Massachusetts

Afshin Ehsan Department of Medicine, Brigham and Women's Hospital, and Harvard Medical School, Boston, Massachusetts

Dwaine F. Emerich Department of Neuroscience, Alkermes, Inc., Cambridge, Massachusetts

David J. Fink Department of Neurology and Molecular Genetics and Biochemistry, University of Pittsburgh School of Medicine, Pittsburgh, Pennsylvania

F. H. Gage Laboratory of Genetics, The Salk Institute for Biological Studies, La Jolla, California

Richard S. Geary Pharmacokinetics and Drug Metabolism, Isis Pharmaceuticals, Inc., Carlsbad, California

Joseph C. Glorioso, III Department of Molecular Genetics and Biochemistry, University of Pittsburgh School of Medicine, Pittsburgh, Pennsylvania

William F. Goins Department of Molecular Genetics and Biochemistry, University of Pittsburgh School of Medicine, Pittsburgh, Pennsylvania

Michael M. Gottesman Laboratory of Cell Biology, National Cancer Institute, National Institutes of Health, Bethesda, Maryland

D. Goula Laboratoire de Physiologie Générale et Comparée, CNRS–UMR 8572, Muséum National d'Historie Naturelle, Paris, France

Roger W. Graham Inex Pharmaceuticals Corporation, Burnaby, British Columbia, Canada

Neil R. Hackett Belfer Gene Therapy Core Facility, Weill Medical College of Cornell University, New York, New York

Peter Hafkemeyer* Laboratory of Cell Biology, National Cancer Institute, National Institutes of Health, Bethesda, Maryland

Greg Hardee Drug Delivery Research and Pharmaceutical Development, Isis Pharmaceuticals, Inc., Carlsbad, California

* *Current affiliation*: University Hospital Freiburg, Freiburg, Germany.

Cary O. Harding Department of Pediatrics, University of Wisconsin–Madison, Madison, Wisconsin

Ulrich R. Hengge Department of Dermatology, Venerology, and Allergology, University of Essen, Essen, Germany

Mitchell E. Horwitz Laboratory of Host Defenses, National Institute of Allergy and Infectious Diseases, National Institutes of Health, Bethesda, Maryland

Christine A. Hrycyna Laboratory of Cell Biology, National Cancer Institute, National Institutes of Health, Bethesda, Maryland

Larry G. Johnson Cystic Fibrosis Research Center and Department of Medicine, University of North Carolina at Chapel Hill, Chapel Hill, North Carolina

Douglas J. Jolly Center for Gene Therapy, Chiron Corporation, San Diego, California

Paul A. Khavari VA Palo Alto Healthcare System, Palo Alto, and Department of Dermatology and Molecular Pharmacology, Stanford University School of Medicine, Stanford, California

Jong J. Kim Merck Research Laboratories, Merck & Company, West Point, Pennsylvania

Danilo D. Lasic Liposome Consultations, Newark, California

Caroline Lee* Laboratory of Cell Biology, National Cancer Institute, National Institutes of Health, Bethesda, Maryland

Arthur A. Levin Toxicology and Pharmacokinetics, Isis Pharmaceuticals, Inc., Carlsbad, California

Thomas Licht† Laboratory of Molecular Biology, National Cancer Institute, National Institutes of Health, Bethesda, Maryland

Ian MacLachlan Inex Pharmaceuticals Corporation, Burnaby, British Columbia, Canada

Harry L. Malech Laboratory of Host Defenses, National Institute of Allergy and Infectious Diseases, National Institutes of Health, Bethesda, Maryland

Michael J. Mann Brigham and Women's Hospital, and Harvard Medical School, Boston, Massachusetts

Rahul Mehta Drug Delivery Research and Pharmaceutical Development, Isis Pharmaceuticals, Inc., Carlsbad, California

Lynn Milich Center for Genetic and Cellular Therapies, Duke University Medical Center, Durham, North Carolina

Andra E. Miller Division of Cellular and Gene Therapies, Center for Biologics, Evaluation and Review, Food and Drug Administration, Rockville, Maryland

Bert W. O'Malley, Jr. Department of Otolaryngology–Head and Neck Surgery, The University of Maryland School of Medicine, Baltimore, Maryland

Clare R. Ozawa Department of Molecular Pharmacology, Stanford University School of Medicine, Stanford, California

---

Current affiliation:
* National University of Singapore, Singapore.
† Technical University of Munich, Munich, Germany.

V. A. Parsegian Laboratory of Physical and Structural Biology, National Institute of Child Health and Human Development, National Institutes of Health, Bethesda, Maryland

Ira Pastan Laboratory of Molecular Biology, National Cancer Institute, National Institutes of Health, Bethesda, Maryland

Rudolf Podgornik Department of Physics, University of Ljubljana, Ljubljana, Slovenia, and Laboratory of Physical and Structural Biology, National Institute of Child Health and Human Development, National Institutes of Health, Bethesda, Maryland

John M. Polo Vaccines and Gene Therapy, Chiron Corporation, Emeryville, California

Roger J. Pomerantz Division of Infectious Diseases, Department of Medicine, Center for Human Virology, Thomas Jefferson University, Philadelphia, Pennsylvania

Elizabeth Razee CytoTherapeutics, Inc., Lincoln, Rhode Island

Dirk Schadendorf Clinical Cooperation Unit for Dermatooncology, Department of Dermatology, University of Mannheim, Mannheim, Germany

Tzipora Shoshani-Kupitz* Laboratory of Cell Biology, National Cancer Institute, National Institutes of Health, Bethesda, Maryland

Stephanie L. Simek Division of Cellular and Gene Therapies, Center for Biologics, Evaluation and Review, Food and Drug Administration, Rockville, Maryland

Matthew L. Springer Department of Molecular Pharmacology, Stanford University School of Medicine, Stanford, California

Michael Strauss† Molecular Cell Biology, Department of Biology, Humboldt-University Berlin, Berlin-Buch, Germany

Helmut H. Strey Department of Polymer Science and Engineering, University of Massachusetts, Amherst, Massachussetts

Bruce A. Sullenger Department of Surgery, Duke University Medical Center, Durham, North Carolina

Nancy Smyth Templeton Center for Cell and Gene Therapy, Baylor College of Medicine, Houston, Texas

Ching-Leou Teng Drug Delivery Research and Pharmaceutical Development, Isis Pharmaceuticals, Inc., Carlsbad, California

Lloyd Tillman Drug Delivery Research and Pharmaceutical Development, Isis Pharmaceuticals, Inc., Carlsbad, California

I. M. Verma Laboratory of Genetics, The Salk Institute for Biological Studies, La Jolla, California

Ernst Wagner Cancer Vaccines, Boehringer Ingelheim Austria, Vienna, Austria

David B. Weiner Department of Pathology, University of Pennsylvania, Philadelphia, Pennsylvania

* *Current affiliation*: QBI Enterprises Ltd., Nes Ziona, Israel.
† Deceased.

Darren Wolfe Department of Molecular Genetics and Biochemistry, University of Pittsburgh School of Medicine, Pittsburgh, Pennsylvania

Jon A. Wolff Department of Pediatrics, University of Wisconsin–Madison, Madison, Wisconsin

Gerhard Wolff Laboratory for Gene Therapy, Theragen AG, Biomedical Research Campus, Berlin-Buch, Germany

Yi Zhou Laboratory of Molecular Biology, National Cancer Institute, National Institutes of Health, Bethesda, Maryland

S. M. Zou Laboratoire de Chimie Génétique, CNRS–URA 1386, Illkirch, France

Gene Therapy

1

Retroviral Vectors for Gene Therapy

Paula M. Cannon and W. French Anderson
Keck School of Medicine at the University of Southern California, Los Angeles, California

I. INTRODUCTION

Gene therapy aims to treat both genetic and infectious diseases by the introduction of new genetic material into the appropriate cells in the body (1). In the simplest case of a defective gene causing disease, addition of the new gene will restore function. Alternatively, the new genetic material can be designed to selectively kill a tumor cell, to induce an immune response, or to protectively ''immunize'' a cell against an incoming pathogen. Nontherapeutic uses of gene therapy include gene marking, which has proved especially useful in identifying the sources of recurring malignancies in autologous bone marrow transplant patients. These potential applications of gene therapy are described in Scheme 1.

The first approved gene therapy clinical protocol began in September 1990, using retroviral vectors to introduce copies of the adenosine deaminase (ADA) gene into T cells from a patient with ADA deficiency (2). Nine years later, more than 300 clinical protocols have been approved worldwide incorporating more than 3000 patients. Most of these trials use viral vectors, and more than 60% use retroviral vectors. This chapter will explore the features of retroviral vectors that make them so versatile for gene therapy and will highlight both their current limitations and potential improvements.

II. RETROVIRAL VECTORS

Retroviruses can efficiently carry out gene transfer to many cell types and can stably integrate their genomes into a host cell chromosome, thereby producing the possibility of long-term gene expression. To date, the most common vectors used in clinical gene therapy protocols have been based on the murine leukemia virus (MuLV), and a variety of packaging systems to enclose the vector genome within viral particles have been developed (reviewed in Ref. 3). The vectors themselves have all of the viral genes removed, are fully replication defective, and can accept up to approximately 6–8 kb of exogenous DNA. These current vector

1. Gene replacement/augmentation
   Especially suited to single gene defects and discrete populations of target cells e.g., ADA deficiency, cystic fibrosis.
2. Suicide/toxic genes
   To eliminate certain cells e.g., HSV thymidine kinase for cancer cells.
3. Protective genes
   Expression of the gene product renders the cell resistant to viral attack in particular e.g., intracellular antibodies, antisense constructs for HIV gene therapy.
4. Immune stimulation
   To stimulate the host's immune system, in particular to cancer cells e.g., HLA genes, immune stimulatory cytokines.
5. Cell marking
   For autologous bone marrow transplantation in cancer therapy e.g., neomycin.

Scheme 1

systems seem to pose minimal risk to patients, and to date there have been no reports of toxicity or long-term problems associated with their use.

A. Retroviral Life Cycle

Fundamental to the utility of retroviral vectors are the particular characteristics of the retroviral life cycle, illustrated in Figure 1. The initial steps of the life cycle, from binding of the virus to a target cell through integration of its genetic material into that cell's genome, do not require the de novo synthesis of any viral proteins. Accordingly, a retroviral particle can be used as a vector to deliver genetic material without the requirement for any viral protein synthesis or infectious particle production.

The retroviral genome codes for three basic polyproteins (Figure 2) produced by alternate splicing of the RNA transcript, which are further processed into their component proteins. The *gag* gene products produce the protein core of the viral particle, which encapsidates two copies of the linear RNA genome. Also associated with the viral core are the products of the *pol* gene, the enzymes involved in particle maturation (protease) and DNA metabolism (reverse transcriptase and integrase). The *env* gene product is a glycoprotein that is anchored in the plasma membrane of the host cell. It is therefore incorporated into the lipid envelope that surrounds the retroviral particle as a result of its budding from a host cell. The budding process does not kill the host cell, which allows for the establishment of stable producer cell lines that continuously release retroviral vector particles.

A retrovirus binds to a new host cell by virtue of the interaction of the Env glycoprotein with an appropriate

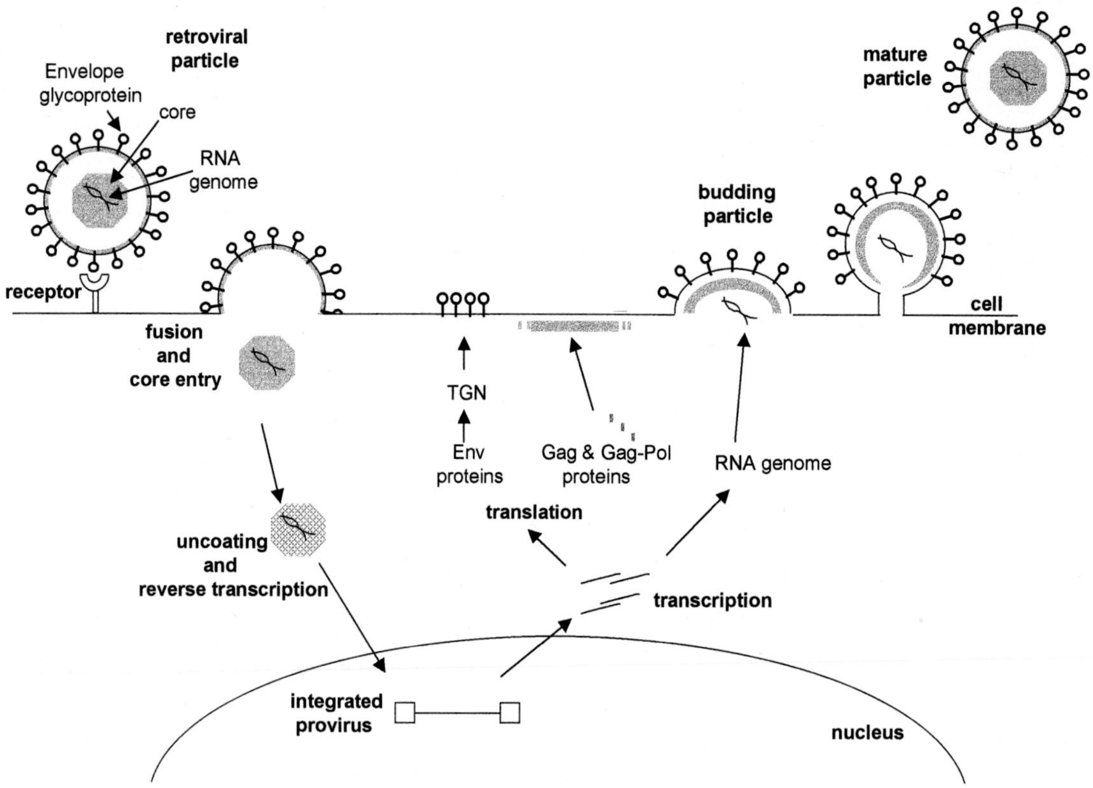

Figure 1 Retroviral life cycle: Retroviral infection is initiated by binding of the envelope glycoprotein embedded in the outer lipid membrane of the retrovirus to a specific cell surface receptor. This interaction triggers fusion between the viral and host cell membranes and releases the viral core into the cytoplasm of the cell. The viral RNA genome is transcribed into a DNA copy by the viral reverse transcriptase protein and is integrated into the host cell chromosome by the action of the integrase protein. The inserted provirus is flanked by complete copies of the LTR sequence (shown as boxes), resulting from the reverse transcription process. The 5′ LTR drives transcription of the retroviral genome, which gives rise to RNAs that code for the viral proteins (Gag, Pol, and Env) as well as the viral genome. Gag and Gag-Pol proteins assemble as viral core particles at the plasma membrane and package the viral RNA genome. The particles bud from the surface of the cell, taking with them a lipid envelope derived from the host plasma membrane containing the Env glycoprotein. TGN, Trans-Golgi network.

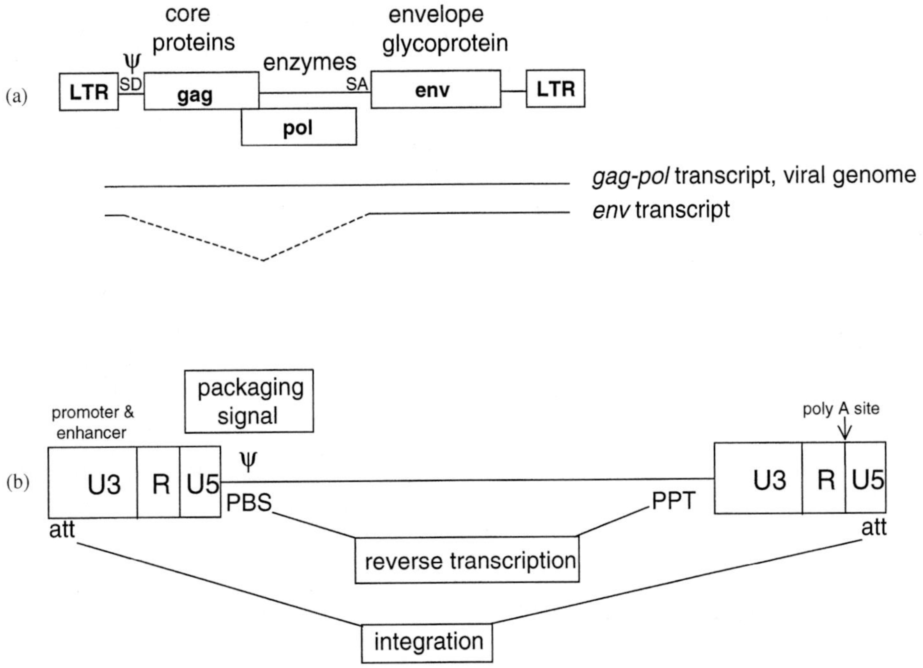

Figure 2 (a) Retroviral proteins: The LTR sequences contain promoter (5′) and polyadenylation (3′) sequences and produce full-length and spliced transcripts. These code for three major polyproteins; Gag and Gag-Pol are translated from the full-length transcript and Env is translated from the spliced transcript. The full-length transcript also serves as the RNA genome. SD, Splice donor; SA, splice acceptor. (b) RNA sequences: The LTRs consist of three regions, designated U3, R, and U5. The promoter and enhancer sequences are active in the 5′ LTR only and are located in the U3 region, while the polyadenylation site in the 3′ LTR defines the R/U5 boundary. The primer binding site (PBS) and polypurine tract (PPT) are important for the process of reverse transcription, while the *att* sequences at the ends of the LTRs are necessary for integration. At the 5′ region of the genome is a packaging signal (Ψ) that is necessary for the incorporation of the genome into viral particles.

cellular receptor. This interaction triggers a series of events that ultimately lead to the fusion of the lipid envelope surrounding the virus with the target cell membrane. Entry of the retroviral core into the cell allows the reverse transcriptase enzyme to copy the viral RNA genome into a double-stranded DNA provirus, which is then randomly inserted into a host chromosome through the action of the integrase protein. Certain sequences in the RNA genome are essential for packaging, reverse transcription, and integration to occur and are highlighted in Figure 2.

B. Basic Components of Retroviral Vectors

The simplest type of vector system comprises a packaging construct that provides all the viral proteins in *trans* but is not itself packaged because of a deletion in the packaging signal (Ψ) at the 5′ end of the genome and a vector genome that codes for no viral proteins but retains all of the necessary RNA regions for packaging, reverse transcription, and integration (4). This basic principle of vector design is illustrated in Figure 3. The gene to be delivered is cloned into the vector genome construct and typically utilizes the 5′ LTR promoter to drive its subsequent expression. When both the vector and packaging constructs are present in a producer cell, retroviral vector particles are released that are capable of delivering the vector genome with its inserted gene. This process of gene delivery is referred to as transduction. Such strategies have been applied to derive vector systems from several different types of retroviruses, including the murine and avian oncoviruses (4,5), human and nonhuman lentiviruses (see Section V.B), and human foamy viruses (6).

C. Recent Improvements

The basic arrangement described above is functional but unsatisfactory in several ways. In particular, the sequence overlap that remains between the vector and packaging components means that there is a very high risk of recombination occurring that could recreate an infectious replication-competent retrovirus (RCR) (7). The overlap exists

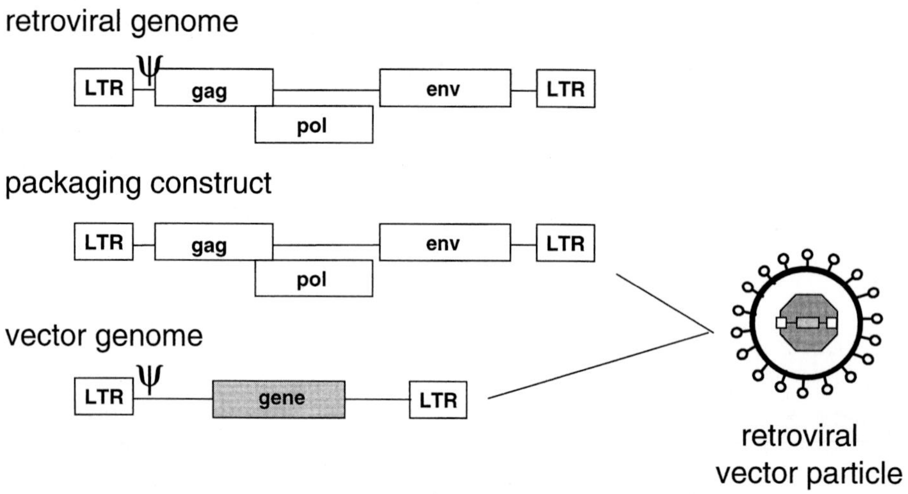

Figure 3 Basic retroviral vector design: The packaging construct provides all of the viral proteins in *trans* to the vector genome, which codes for no viral proteins but retains all of the necessary *cis* elements. The deletion of the packaging signal (Ψ) from the packaging construct prevents its incorporation into viral particles.

largely because extensive sequences of the *gag* gene are retained in the vector to enhance the efficiency of packaging (8), although Gag protein expression is prevented by mutation. In addition, the LTRs are frequently retained in the packaging construct to provide both promoter and polyadenylation sequences. Finally, as most of the early MuLV-based packaging cell lines were established in murine NIH 3T3 cells, the possibility also exists for RCR generation through recombination between vector constructs and endogenous MuLV-like sequences present in the mouse genome.

In order to minimize the risk of RCR production, an improvement in vector design was to split the packaging components, placing the *gag-pol* and *env* genes onto separate plasmids that could be introduced separately into the packaging cell (9,10) (Figure 4a). The risk of recombination has been further reduced by the use of heterologous Env proteins that have no homology with the parental virus but are able to be incorporated into the viral particle (a process referred to as pseudotyping) and the use of nonmurine producer cell lines. Finally, it has now been shown for MuLV vectors that the *gag* sequences can be removed from the vector genome without significant loss of packaging efficiency (11).

The problem of the LTR overlap that exists between the vector components has been solved through the use of heterologous promoters and polyadenylation signals in the packaging constructs. This can also have the advantage of enhancing titer (12), because the MuLV LTR promoter will not always drive high-level gene expression in nonmurine producer cell lines. In the vector itself, the LTR sequences can also be significantly deleted. Heterologous promoters, frequently the CMV immediate-early promoter, have been used to replace the 5′ U3 promoter, which is possible because the U3 sequences in the retroviral vector are derived from the 3′LTR. Even the 3′U3 sequences can be significantly deleted, as is the case with self-inactivating or SIN vectors, as long as the sequences necessary for recognition by the integrase protein are retained (13). These features are summarized in Figure 4b.

Improvements have also been made in the titer [number of colony-forming units (cfu) per mL] achieved by retroviral vectors. In stable producer cell lines, titer has been maximized by linking expression of the Gag-Pol and Env components to selectable markers to facilitate screening for high titer producer cells (14) and nonmurine cell lines have been exploited to produce the vectors. Titers have also been boosted through the development of transient expression systems, which are capable of producing very high titers during a brief and very active burst of activity in the transfected cell. In general, these systems rely on the use of a highly transfectable cell line, such as 293T cells, combined with strategies to maximize the production of the individual components through the use of the strong CMV promoter and treatment with the transcription enhancer sodium butyrate (12). We have recently shown that titers can be further improved by the inclusion of the adenovirus VAI gene to enhance translation (A. Lin and P. M. Cannon, unpublished data). The combination of these various approaches makes possible the routine production of

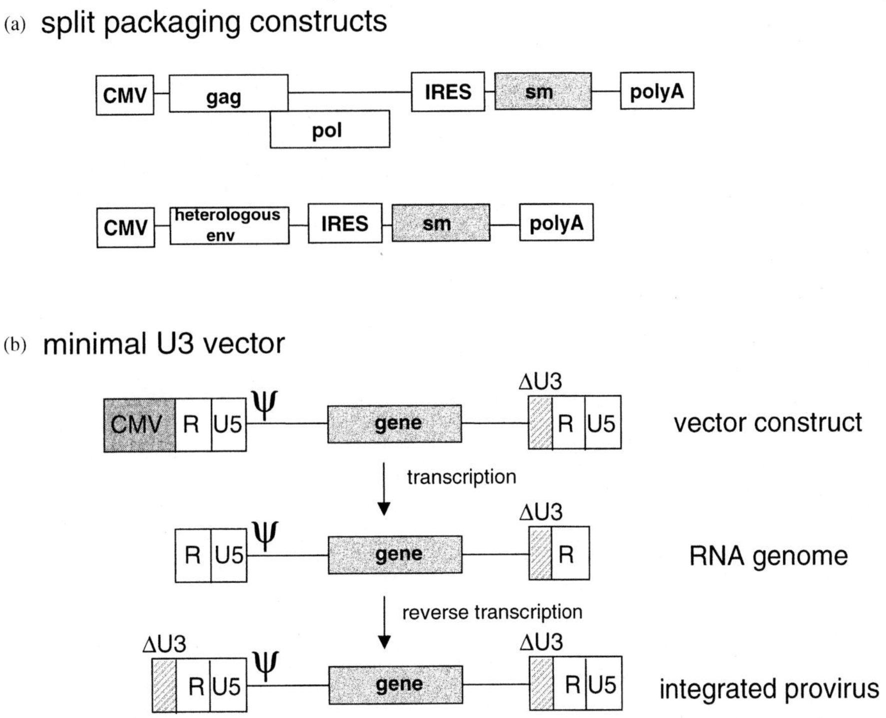

Figure 4 Improvements in vector design: (a) Packaging construct: The Gag-Pol and Env proteins are separated onto two different plasmids, and safety is further increased by the use of heterologous envelope proteins. Expression is maximized from the packaging construct through the use of a non-LTR promoter (CMV) and linkage to a selectable marker (sm). (b) Vector construct: The U3 sequences are replaced at the 5′ LTR and minimized in the 3′ LTR. Following reverse transcription, the deleted U3 sequences (ΔU3) are copied into both the 5′ and 3′ LTRs of the provirus. The 5′ LTR therefore has greatly reduced promoter activity. This is the basis of self-inactivating (SIN) vectors.

vector supernatants in the laboratory with titers in excess of 10^7 cfu/mL. Whether such transient production systems will ever be useful for large-scale production is uncertain because of potential difficulties in the scale-up and vector characterization procedures.

Although currently preferred for large-scale vector production, the use of stable producer cell lines precludes the use of cytotoxic components. These include both the therapeutic gene product itself and also components of the vector system. A notable example is the vesicular stomatitis virus G protein (VSV-G), which is an extremely useful fusion protein for producing pseudotyped retroviral vectors with a very broad host range (15) but is unfortunately very toxic to its host cell. One way around this problem is to use transient systems as described above (16), but an alternate strategy is to regulate gene expression through use of an inducible promoter. In particular, the tetracycline-regulated Tet system (17) has proved popular for regulating the expression of VSV-G (18), where its production is suppressed in the producer cell line by the addition of tetracycline to the culture and activated by the subsequent removal of the antibiotic just before harvesting the vectors. In this way, the cells can be grown to an optimum density before the toxic fusion protein is expressed. However, although such cell lines are appropriate for laboratory-scale preparation, it is not clear if such a system will be sufficiently stable for industrial production.

As stated in the introduction, retroviral vectors are currently the most commonly used gene-delivery vehicle in human gene therapy protocols. This is partly for historical reasons; vectors derived from MuLV were the first real vector system to be established, and a relatively large amount of information about the performance of such vectors in patients is available. However, their most attractive feature, their ability to integrate into target cells, can have a downside as well as being advantageous. In the following two sections, we will review the key properties of retroviral vectors that have made them such attractive gene-delivery vehicles and also point out their current limitations and the steps being taken to introduce improvements.

III. ADVANTAGES OF RETROVIRAL VECTORS

A. Defective Vectors

Retroviral vectors represent a truly defective vector system; none of the viral proteins need to be expressed in the target cell for efficient gene transfer to occur and can simply be provided in *trans* in the producer cell. In addition, no de novo viral protein synthesis is needed to maintain or repair the integrated provirus. This has implications for long-term gene expression in the transduced cells because even a low-level production of viral proteins will increase the likelihood of an unwanted immune response being triggered against the transduced cells (in addition to any immune response that may be mounted against the transgene itself). Such vector antigenicity is largely responsible for the transient nature of the gene expression seen with current adenoviral vectors, although the problem is being aggressively pursued through the development of ''gutless'' adenoviral vectors.

B. Vector Integration

A major advantage of retroviral vectors is that they integrate into the host cell chromosomes. The only other vector system that allows efficient integration is based on adeno-associated virus, reviewed elsewhere in this book. A great deal is known about the process of retroviral integration, which is carried out by the viral integrase protein. Integrase recognizes sequences at the ends of the LTRs of the DNA provirus (the *att* sites Fig. 2), and inserts the provirus more or less randomly into the host genome, although some sequence preferences have been reported (19).

The ability of vectors to integrate is a two-edged sword. On the one hand, it allows for the possibility of stable long-term gene expression, with the integrated provirus being passed on to all daughter cells. However, the possibility of insertion into a nonfavorable site also exists, which could both influence the ability of the vector to drive gene expression and also interfere with the normal functioning of nearby host genes. Retroviruses were first identified on the basis of their ability to cause oncogenic transformation, and the possibility of insertional mutagenesis is of concern. This is discussed in greater detail in Section VI. B.

One possible way around these negative aspects would be to engineer the integrase protein to direct integration only into certain preselected regions of the host cell genome. The rationale for such an approach is based on the integration site preference exhibited by the related integrase protein of the yeast transposable element, Ty3, which preferentially integrates upstream of Pol III promoters (20). Furthermore, chimeras between the integrase proteins of Ty3 and MuLV have been shown to be functional, although no redirection of MuLV integration has yet been demonstrated (21).

In a different approach, site-specific integration is being attempted through engineering of the retroviral integrase protein to contain additional DNA targeting domains that will direct the integration complex to specific sites. Some specificity of site selection has been demonstrated in vitro for chimeras containing DNA binding zinc finger proteins, (22) but the ability to redirect integration in vivo has not yet been demonstrated.

C. Modularity of Components

The three basic components of the retroviral vector—the core and its enzymes, the envelope protein, and the vector genome itself—can be viewed as discrete components that in some cases can be ''mixed and matched'' for custom applications. This flexibility enables the exploitation of the natural variations in the host ranges of different viruses and in some cases may allow transduction of a cell that is resistant to standard vector combinations. The clearest example is in the use of different envelope proteins to pseudotype the vectors. For example, when compared to MuLV vectors containing the amphotropic MuLV Env protein, pseudotyping with VSV-G, RD114, or GaLV Env proteins enhances the transduction of primary human hematopoietic cells (23–25).

In addition, different core and vector components can also be used. The combination of GaLV cores with MuLV or GaLV vector genomes has been reported to enhance the transduction of certain human cell lines (26), and hybrid genomes (27) and cores (28) between MuLV and lentiviruses have been constructed which may offer new properties. Finally, the LTRs can also be manipulated to improve gene expression in certain cell types. The MPSV LTR has been used in place of the related MuLV LTR to provide enhanced gene expression in ES and embryonic stem cells (29), and the enhancer elements of the LTR can be replaced with more specific sequences in order to optimize gene expression from the LTR in a given host cell (see Section IV).

D. Flexibility of Gene Expression Strategies

The 5′ retroviral LTR is itself a promoter and the simplest vector design uses the LTR to drive transgene expression (30) (Fig. 5). In addition, the use of heterologous promoters placed internally within the retroviral transcription unit increases the flexibility of gene expression, because constitutive, inducible, or tissue specific promoters can be included. Expression of more than one transgene can be achieved through the use of both the LTR and an internal

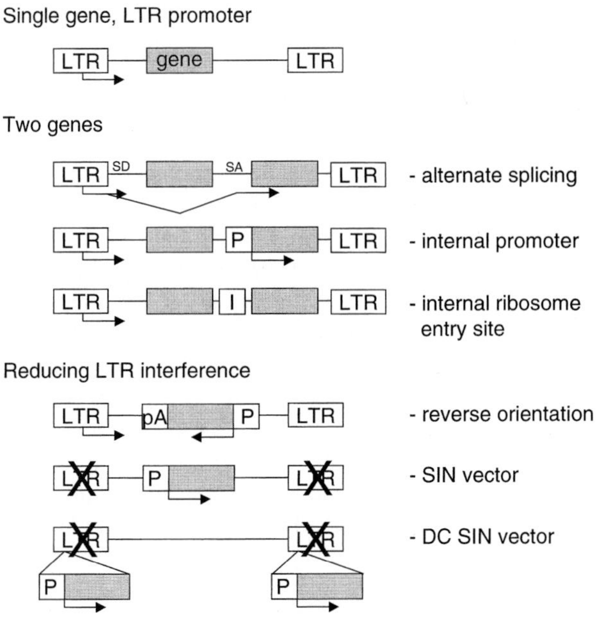

Figure 5 Gene expression from retroviral vectors: Strategies to drive expression of one or two genes and to minimize interference by the 5′ LTR promoter. SD, Splice donor; SA, splice acceptor; P, promoter; I, internal ribosome entry site; pA, polyA sequences; SIN, self-inactivating; DC, double copy.

promoter or by exploiting the differential splicing of the vector that occurs when the major splice acceptor site upstream of the *env* gene is retained (31). In addition, the expression of the two genes can be linked by the use of an internal ribosome entry site (IRES) (32). The transcriptional activity of the LTR can in some cases be a problem, interfering with the activity of internal promoters (promoter interference) (33). These problems can be reduced by the use of SIN vectors. The level of gene expression can also be increased through the use of double copy (DC) vectors (34). Here, the therapeutic gene and its promoter are inserted into the 3′ LTR itself, with the result that after reverse transcription two copies of this expression cassette are created in the provirus.

IV. CURRENT LIMITATIONS OF RETROVIRAL VECTORS

Investigators face several problems in developing retroviral vectors that will be clinically effective. First, the vector genomes themselves have limited capacity for insertion of foreign sequences, based on the packaging constraints imposed by the viral core proteins; MuLV-based vectors cannot greatly exceed the 8.3 kb size of the MuLV genome. The stability of the engineered vectors can also be a concern. The presence of two copies of the vector genome in a viral particle and the process of reverse transcription both contribute to a relatively high level of rearrangement and instability, which is also influenced by the nature of the inserted sequences. The retroviral life cycle and the process of reverse transcription preclude the use of intron-containing sequences in a vector unless the gene is inserted in reverse orientation in the vector, and even with a cDNA copy of a gene, cryptic splice sites can become apparent when the gene is placed inside the retroviral vector.

Major improvements are also required in the overall efficiency of delivery of retroviral vectors. This will involve both the Env-directed entry process and overcoming any postentry blocks to transduction that might occur, including the ability to transduce nondividing cells. Once delivered to a target cell, improvements will be needed in the ability of the vectors to sustain gene expression in the long term and for the therapeutic gene and its controlling sequences to respond to appropriate stimuli—be they natural developmental or physiological signals or regulatory drugs administered to the patient. Finally, cost-effective ways to manufacture the vector and at high enough titers will be required, with appropriate assurances of safety.

Specific issues related to the transduction of nondividing cells are dealt with in Section V.B. and manufacturing and safety concerns are discussed in Section VI. Below, we review current attempts to improve the specificity of gene delivery with retroviral vectors and the strategies designed to improve gene expression from those vectors.

A. Obtaining Efficient and Specific Gene Delivery

An ideal retroviral vector is one that could specifically home in on its target cell in the body and limit its transduction to only that type of cell. This would allow the in vivo delivery of the vector and greatly facilitate the clinical procedure for gene therapy. The entry of a retrovirus into a cell is determined in large part by the properties of its envelope glycoprotein and the specificity of the interaction of that protein with its receptor. To some extent these restrictions can be circumvented by the use of heterologous fusion proteins to pseudotype the vector particles. However, other host range restrictions also exist, including several postentry blocks to transduction. An obvious example of this is the requirement for nuclear membrane breakdown for MuLV entry to the nucleus, but other less well-characterized resistance mechanisms are also present in some cells. For example, certain human cell lines that were poorly transduced by MuLV-based vectors were shown to be more susceptible to transduction by vectors based on GaLV (26). In addition, the LTR promoter can also be considered a determinant of tropism, and if gene expression is to be driven from that promoter, then its function in a particular cell type will also be an important consideration.

Current clinical protocols for retroviral vectors primarily use an ex vivo approach. As many of the cells to be transduced by the vectors express a high level of the natural amphotropic MuLV receptor and are actively dividing at the time of exposure to the vector (either naturally or as a result of culturing conditions), they will therefore be transduced by MuLV vectors pseudotyped by the amphotropic MuLV Env. An important exception at present are the primitive hematopoietic stem cells (HSC), which are reported to have a low level of amphotropic receptor and are poorly transducible (35). However the use of the GaLV and VSV-G pseudotypes has gone some way towards enhancing transduction, as has the use of lentiviral vectors (36) (see Section V).

Pseudotyping with natural viral fusion proteins that interact with different cell surface receptors, such as the amphotropic, xenotropic, polytropic, and 10A1 MuLV Env proteins and the GaLV and VSV-G proteins, may provide enhanced transduction of a particular cell type ex vivo, but these are all still broad host range proteins that do not provide much specificity. This therefore limits the ability of such vectors to be useful in vivo, because introducing the vectors systemically would result in the particles binding to the majority of cells that they encountered and being diluted out before reaching their target cells. The problem can be quantitated. The human body contains approximately 5×10^{13} cells. Using concentrated stocks of retroviral vectors pseudotyped with VSV-G (which have been reported to give titers of up to 10^9 per mL) and infusing 100 mL of such a vector into a patient would result in the delivery of about 10^{11} active vector particles. Even if every vector particle were 100% efficient, only 1 cell in 500 could possibly be transduced, and this scenario does not take into account the sequestering of the vectors into the first tissue that they come into contact with (typically the lungs) or the inactivation of particles in vivo by both innate immunity and more specific humoral responses. In addition, there will very likely be detrimental side effects resulting from the delivery of the vector to nontarget tissues as a result of the broad host range of the vector. An important step towards the in vivo use of retroviral vectors will clearly be the development of retroviral particles that can preferentially bind to and transduce their target cells and can be manufactured at a high titer.

Efforts to target specific cell types have concentrated mainly on the engineering of natural retroviral envelope proteins, in particular the rodent cell–specific ecotropic Moloney MuLV protein (reviewed in 37,38). Retroviral Env proteins exist as an oligomeric complex (in the case of MuLV Env, probably a trimer) comprising two subunits: the surface (SU) protein that contains the receptor recognition domain and the transmembrane (TM) protein that anchors the complex in the retroviral envelope (Fig. 6). The binding of SU to a specific cell surface receptor is thought to trigger conformational changes in SU and the associated TM protein that result in the exposure of a hydrophobic stretch of amino acids at the N terminus of TM, the fusion peptide, and the subsequent fusion between viral and host cell membranes (Fig. 6b). The challenge of engineering Env has been to redirect binding of the SU moiety to an heterologous cell surface molecule, while retaining the ability of such an interaction to recapitulate the natural postbinding events that lead to fusion. This has proved a daunting task, and despite early optimism in the field there have now been numerous reports of failure of targeting strategies with MuLV Env proteins (37–40), although the Env protein of spleen necrosis virus appears to be more amenable to engineering (41).

Two broad approaches have been taken to produce targeted envelope proteins (Fig. 7). First, the natural receptor-binding domain of the SU protein can be replaced with a ligand or single chain antibody designed to bind to a specific cell surface molecule on the target cell. A whole range of receptors have been targeted in this way, but the difficulty remains that even when specific binding can be obtained between the engineered vector and the target cell receptor, the subsequent fusion event is not triggered and gene transfer is correspondingly low (39,40). It is apparent that engineering the receptor-binding domain of SU to redirect binding while maintaining the ability of the envelope protein to carry out fusion will require a better understanding of the structure/function relationships within the envelope protein complex. The recently available three-dimensional structure of the receptor-binding domain of the murine ecotropic (Friend strain) SU protein (42), coupled with structure/function studies to delineate the various domains in MuLV Env and to understand the pathway of signal transmission within the Env protein complex (43,44), should allow a more rational approach to engineering the Env protein in the future.

In a second broad approach to Env targeting that could be called "tethering," the interaction with the native receptor is maintained so that entry occurs through the natural route, but the vectors are concentrated on certain cell types or at certain sites by the presence of an additional binding moiety. The insertion of a collagen binding ligand into the ecotropic MuLV Env protein, for example, did not perturb the ability of the protein to transduce rodent cells but did allow an effective concentration of the vector at sites of

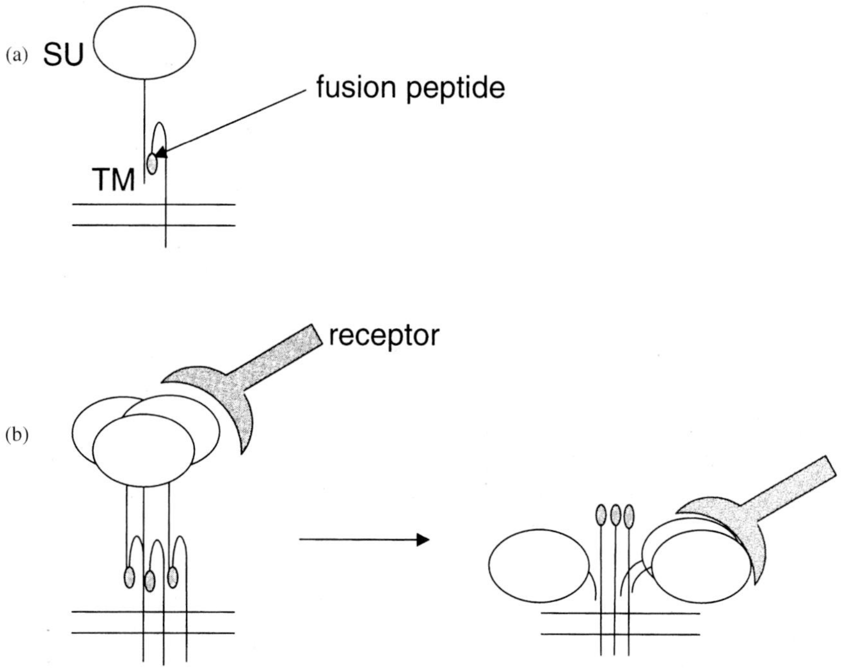

Figure 6 Retroviral Env protein: (a) The Env protein consists of two noncovalently linked subunits—the SU protein that contains the residues that interact with the receptor and the membrane-anchored TM protein that promotes the fusion of viral and host cell membranes. At the N terminus of TM is a stretch of hydrophobic amino acids called the fusion peptide. (b) The retroviral Env protein is oligomeric, and MuLV Env probably exists as a trimer. Following binding to its receptor, the Env complex is thought to undergo conformational changes that result in the exposure of the fusion peptide, enabling it to interact with the host cell membrane and trigger the fusion process.

collagen deposition (45). Such a strategy may have utility in directing vectors to areas of injury, for example, in the cardiovascular system after angioplasty.

A different strategy to concentrate vectors on cells expressing the EGF receptor has been reported, which uses a chimeric MuLV Env protein where the natural receptor binding site is initially blocked by an EGF moiety (46). Following binding to the EGF receptor-expressing cells, the EGF ligand is removed by the action of a protease (envisioned to be present on the cell surface and which can therefore be made cell specific). This cleavage event frees the Env protein to interact with its natural receptor and to subsequently enter the cells. Such a strategy seems particularly suited to cancer cell targeting. Finally, ''bridging constructs'' have been described for the ASLV Env protein that combine an EGF targeting domain with the extracellular domain of the ASLV receptor (47). This hybrid protein binds to ASLV Env pseudotyped particles and thereby ''bridges'' them to target cells expressing the EGF receptor. The interaction of the soluble receptor fragment with the Env protein also triggers the normal fusion process, thereby allowing entry of the vector to the specific target cells in the absence of the natural receptor.

B. Sustaining and Regulating Gene Expression

Assuming that efficient gene-transfer strategies can be developed, the next issue to be addressed is how to maintain an appropriate level of gene expression. With their ability to integrate into host cell chromosomes and therefore be passed on to daughter cells, retroviral vectors are an attractive delivery system when lifelong gene expression is required. However, maintaining gene expression from an integrated provirus has proved problematic in the past. This is perhaps the largest shortcoming of all present vector systems. Since sustaining gene expression in the target cell is not just a problem facing retroviruses, much of the following discussion will apply to gene transfer vectors of all types.

Several factors are involved in maintaining the stable expression of genes after their transfer, which can be

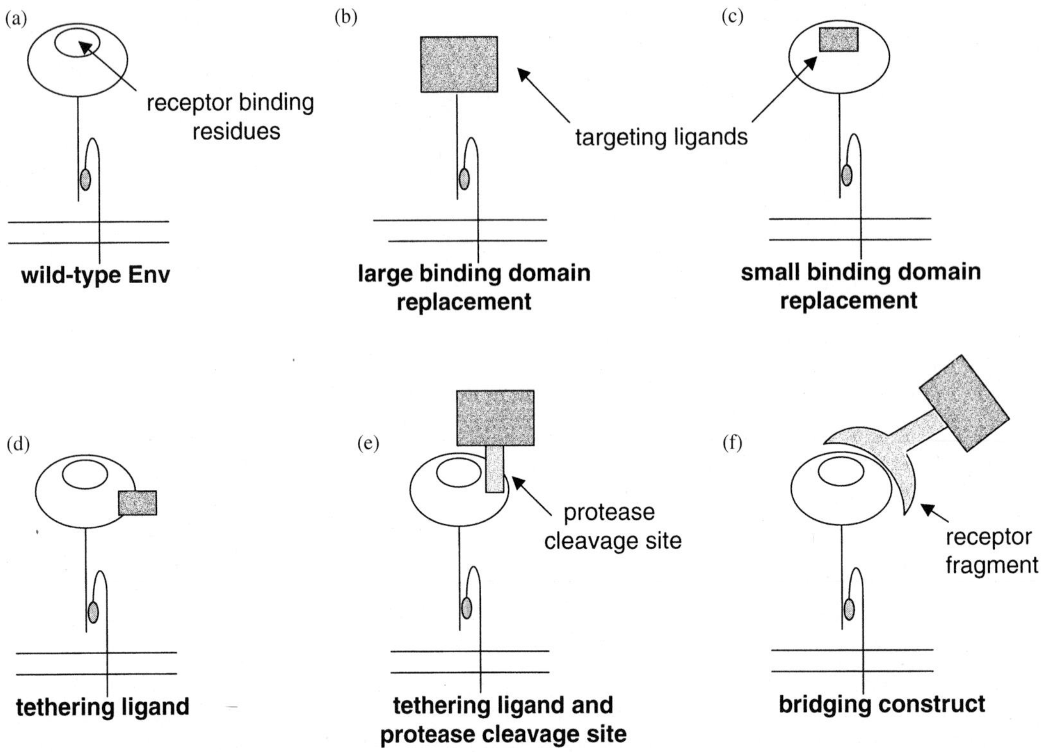

Figure 7 Targeted Env proteins: (a) Wild-type Env protein. (b, c) Targeting to heterologous receptors: The interaction with the natural receptor is replaced by a heterologous binding ligand, either a small peptide or scFv insert, or the whole of the receptor-binding domain of SU is replaced with a binding moiety. (d, e) Tethering strategies: The natural receptor binding site is retained, but the vectors are concentrated on target cells by the action of a binding ligand. In some cases (e) the targeting ligand obscures the natural receptor-binding site, which is only revealed after the binding ligand has been removed, for example, by proteolytic cleavage. (f) Bridging strategy: A chimeric protein comprising a soluble receptor and a targeting ligand binds the vector to target cells. The soluble receptor activates the Env protein, allowing fusion to occur with a cell that does not express the natural receptor.

broadly divided into two categories. The first set concern the activity of the promoter and regulatory sequences themselves. Depending on the site of integration of the vector, host mechanisms may suppress (or inappropriately activate) expression from a promoter, and even if gene expression is initially high it is frequently not sustained long term. There is a tendency for the cell to recognize foreign promoters (particularly viral promoters like SV40 and CMV) and inactivate them, for example, by methylation, and the retroviral LTR promoter is subject to suppression, particularly in embryonic cells, although strategies have been developed to reduce this problem (29).

The second mechanism that causes loss of gene activity is due to the fact that even if gene expression remains active, the transduced cell often loses viability. The body can recognize as foreign a therapeutic gene product and can mount an immune response that will eventually eliminate the gene-engineered cells. Even a normal human protein appears abnormal to an immune system that has never been exposed to it.

The problems identified with the use of constitutive viral promoters in vectors have led to recent attempts to use more authentic regulatory sequences to direct gene expression. The use of a gene's own promoter and regulatory sequences may provide more stable long-term gene expression than can be obtained with current viral promoters, but identifying all the necessary components can be difficult. As an extreme case, the regulatory sequences involved in β-globin expression are spread over nearly 100 kb, and because a retroviral vector can only accommodate 6–8 kb, the minimal functional regulatory sequences need to be identified.

Alternatively, certain key elements can be included in the LTR region to provide a measure of cell specific expression, as has been demonstrated by the insertion of a minimal tyrosinase promoter into the MuLV U3 region that results in melanoma-specific gene expression (48). The use of cell specific gene expression can also be considered an alternative or supplemental approach to targeting, for even if the entry of a vector cannot be restricted to the desired target cell population, its subsequent gene expression could. Finally, the use of authentic genomic elements in retroviral vectors also holds promise for improving gene-expression strategies. Chromosome remodeling sequences such as scaffold attachment regions (49), locus control regions, and insulator sequences may allow stable gene expression whatever the integration site of the vector and, in addition, isolate the effects of the transcriptional unit in the vector from any deleterious effects on downstream host genes.

An additional factor that can influence gene expression is the environment of the host cell being used to express the therapeutic gene. Even when natural regulatory elements are used, they may not function out of context in a different cellular environment. For example, the insulin enhancer/promoter still cannot direct regulated expression of that protein when expressed in fibroblasts. This highlights further the need to develop vectors that are capable of gene transfer to specific cell types.

Although in some gene-therapy scenarios, low levels of essentially unregulated expression may be appropriate (e.g., hemophilia, ADA deficiency); for other situations, regulatable gene expression will be desirable. Many of our important genes are not expressed at the same level all the time but respond to physiological signals within the body. One approach will be to use regulatory sequences that respond to the body's own physiological signals in the vector, so that the therapeutic gene will function in the same way as normal endogenous genes. However, if knowledge of such signals and the corresponding DNA sequences is insufficient to attempt such a strategy, alternate synthetic gene-regulation systems could be used where drugs could be administered to control gene expression, such as with the Tet system (50).

V. DIVIDING AND NONDIVIDING CELLULAR TARGETS

MuLV, and the vectors derived from it, are only able to infect dividing cells. This is because the preintegration nucleoprotein complex is unable to cross an intact nuclear membrane. In contrast, the prototypical lentivirus HIV-1 has been shown capable of nuclear import even when an intact membrane exists, and HIV-1–derived vectors are therefore able to transduce nondividing cells (51). This property of HIV vectors makes them particularly attractive candidates for gene therapy when the target cell is nondividing and stable integration of the transgene is required. However, as outlined below, the restricted tropism of MuLV for dividing cells can also be used to advantage, limiting transduction to dividing cells such as tumor cells.

A. Tropism for Dividing Cells in Cancer Gene Therapy

The selectivity of MuLV for dividing cells is being exploited in a phase III clinical trial currently underway to test the efficacy of a suicide gene-therapy approach to treating glioblastoma multiforma, a malignant brain tumor (52). The rationale is to insert a gene capable of killing cells into the tumor while protecting the normal brain cells. The vector contains the herpes simplex thymidine kinase (TK) gene, which is able to phosphorylate the drug ganciclovir, resulting in a toxic derivative that is incorporated into DNA. The vector is produced in situ in the residual tumor and peritumor areas, following surgical resection of the tumor, by the injection of a mouse producer cell line that generates the retroviral particles. Although both tumor cells and healthy cells in the area of a growing brain tumor could potentially be transduced, only the tumor cells themselves and the vasculature supplying blood to the tumor are considered likely targets because they will be actively dividing. Tumor killing is achieved by giving the drug ganciclovir to the patient; the TK enzyme converts this to a toxic nucleotide that is incorporated into the DNA of the tumor cells, killing them.

B. Lentiviral Vectors Transduce Nondividing Cells

There are many situations where one would want to insert a therapeutic gene into normal nondividing cells. In vivo, only certain blood cells and the cells lining the GI system are continually in division, so the majority of potential target cells in the human body are nondividing. Lentiviruses such as HIV-1 are able to infect nondividing cells, and the demonstration that HIV vectors could also transduce such cells has been an exciting development in retroviral vector technology (51). The mechanism whereby HIV can infect nondividing cells remains somewhat controversial, but there appears to be more than one mechanism involved in making the HIV preintegration complex karyophilic (53–55). Attempts to transfer into murine retroviral vectors the specific signals from the HIV virus that allow transduction of nondividing cells have not been successful (28), indicating the complexity of the process.

Vectors constructed from lentiviruses, and HIV in particular, raise safety concerns because of the possibility of a pathogenic RCR arising by recombination. Recently constructed HIV-based vectors contain just 25% of the HIV genome and do not express any proteins. Furthermore, non-

HIV envelope proteins such as VSV-G are used to pseudotype the vectors. The safety of such systems is constantly being improved, for example, by the development of CMV-driven SIN vectors (56) or minimal packaging constructs with all of the non-essential genes removed (57). Much is known about the pathogenicity of HIV, and the removal of these genes from a vector would, in theory, produce a crippled RCR, even if one did arise. Finally, vector systems based on nonprimate lentiviruses such as FIV are also being developed (58).

VI. RETROVIRAL VECTORS AS PHARMACEUTICALS

A. Manufacturing Considerations

Although any consideration of how pharmaceutical companies would be able to manufacture gene-therapy vectors was an irrelevant concern a decade ago, it has now become a real issue. Retroviral vectors are biological agents that can only be made by living cells, and such systems are not easy for carrying out good manufacturing practice (GMP) and quality assurance/quality control (QA/QC) assays. Furthermore, the large-scale production of retroviral vectors requires the establishment of producer cell lines that maintain a stable arrangement of vector sequences and sufficiently high vector production levels during the procedure. In addition, the subsequent purification of vectors from the supernatant of producer cells is a relatively cumbersome procedure, and some loss of titer is inevitable. For vectors pseudotyped with the amphotropic MuLV Env, much of the loss of activity is due to the relative lability of the Env protein (the two subunits are noncovalently attached and can dissociate under conditions of shear stress). In part, this problem could be countered by the use of a single polypeptide fusion protein such as VSV-G, although the inherent cytotoxicity of this protein makes the use of stable producer cell lines difficult (see Section II.C).

B. Safety Considerations

One of the major concerns arising from the use of retroviral vectors is the possibility that an RCR could arise during the manufacturing process (59). Such a virus could result from recombination between the vector and packaging components in the producer cells, even with the newer split packaging cell lines (60), or be due to the acquisition of sequences from endogenous retroviruses. Essentially all mammalian cells have their own endogenous retroviruses that could potentially recombine with the vector to produce a new and possibly pathogenic RCR, and many of these endogenous viruses are still unknown. Although any cell line is suspect, the use of primate or human cells as packaging cells raises the greatest safety concerns in this regard. There is no way to predict the pathogenicity of such potential recombinants, although it would be naive to assume that nonnatural combinations of viral components will not be infectious. For example, it has been demonstrated that if the use of an SIV-based vector pseudotyped with the amphotropic MuLV Env protein gave rise to an RCR, such a chimeric virus could indeed replicate in vivo in monkeys (61).

Another safety consideration when using retroviral vectors arises from their ability to integrate randomly into host cell DNA. It is possible that a vector may insert itself into a tumor suppressor gene, thereby increasing the propensity for the cell to become cancerous. The only example of unintentional tumor production in a retroviral gene-transfer experiment in large animals occurred when three cases of lymphoma were reported among 10 rhesus monkeys that had received myeloablative irradiation and then been transplanted with hematopoietic stem cells that had been exposed to a large number of RCR together with the experimental vector. Subsequent analyses revealed that the cancers resulted from integration of an RCR (not of the retroviral vector), were clonal events, and developed only after long periods (6–7 months) of retroviremia (62,63).

The subjects of RCR production, safety, and potential tumor induction were extensively analyzed in a report to the NIH RAC and FDA (64). The report concluded that current QA/QC procedures required by FDA made it exceedingly unlikely that any patient could receive sufficient RCR to produce either a retroviremia or a malignancy. However, the manufacturing and testing processes required to ensure this degree of safety are complex and expensive.

C. In Vivo Use

A major goal of present research in retroviral vector development is the production of a gene therapy vector that could be injected directly into the body. Such in vivo use poses additional problems that must be considered. For example, mouse packaging cells produce retroviral vectors that are rapidly destroyed by human complement, markedly reducing their half-life in vivo and the overall efficiency of gene transfer. The major component of this sensitivity arises from the presence of unique sugar groups on the glycoproteins produced in the murine packaging cells (65). However, such an acute problem can be overcome by the use of other, including human, producer cell lines (66). A humoral immune response developing against the retroviral vector particle may also be a concern, at least for any repeat administrations, although the problem of preexisting immunity that is seen with adenoviral vectors should not occur with most current retroviral vector systems.

VII. CLINICAL TRIALS

A. Strategies for Gene Delivery in Clinical Applications

There are three categories of somatic cell gene therapy (Scheme 2). The first and most common is ex vivo, where cells are removed from the body, incubated with a vector, and then returned to the body. This procedure is usually done with blood cells because they are the easiest to remove and return. The second category is in situ, where the vector or a producer cell line is placed directly into the tissues to be transduced. Examples of this include direct injection into tumors or delivery of vectors into the bronchi for cystic fibrosis therapy. The third category is in vivo, where a vector would be injected directly into the blood stream but subsequent transduction (or expression) would be restricted to a limited cell population. At present, there are no clinical examples of this third category, but if gene therapy is to fulfill its promise as a therapeutic option, in vivo injectable vectors must be developed.

B. Summary of Current Clinical Trials

At present there are more than 300 approved clinical protocols worldwide. Detailed information is available on the 272 protocols that had been approved in the United States as of the end of 1998, of which the majority are based on retroviral vectors. The original ADA deficiency gene therapy trial (2) was started in 1990, giving gene-corrected autologous T lymphocytes to two girls suffering from this disease. ADA deficiency is a rare genetic disorder that produces severe immunodeficiency in children. Patient 1 (A. D.) received a total of 11 infusions, the last being in the summer of 1992. Her total T-cell level and her level of transduced Toolls have remained essentially constant since then. Both she and patient 2 (C. C.) continue to receive PEG-ADA treatment in addition to their gene-therapy treatments. Although both girls retain gene-engineered T lymphocytes in their circulation, no final conclusion can be drawn as to the relative roles of PEG-ADA and gene therapy in their excellent clinical course.

Only one phase III clinical trial using retroviral vectors is currently underway, sponsored by Genetic Therapy Inc./Novartis. The trial is for the treatment of glioblastoma multiforma, based on the in situ production of an amphotropic retroviral vector expressing TK from a mouse producer cell line (52). The producer cells are inoculated into the residual tumor and surrounding areas following tumor resection, and after 7 days the patient is treated with ganciclovir. In theory the tumor cells that have been transduced with the vector containing the TK gene will phosphorylate the ganciclovir, producing a toxic phosphorylated derivative that blocks the DNA synthetic machinery and kills the cells. The phase III trial includes a total of more than 40 centers in North America and Europe and is scheduled to enroll a total of 250 patients.

Several phase II trials are also underway testing retroviral vectors as ''vaccines.'' Viagen/Chiron has completed a phase II trial of about 200 patients over 2 years in which a retroviral vector encoding the *env* and *rev* gene segments of HIV-1 was injected intramuscularly to induce anti-HIV CTL responses as a treatment for AIDS (67). Unfortunately, efficacy measurements in this trial were not possible because of the advent of triple drug therapy, but no evidence of toxicity was seen.

1. Ex vivo
   Cells are removed from body, incubated with vector and engineered cells are then returned e.g., T lymphocytes for anti-HIV therapy.
2. In situ
   Vector or producer cells are placed directly into the tissues to be transduced e.g., TK vectors in brain tumors.
3. In vivo
   Vector would be directly injected into the bloodstream and would home in on its target cells (no examples yet).

Scheme 2

VIII. CONCLUSIONS AND FUTURE PROSPECTS

As stated in the introduction, retroviral vectors are currently the most commonly used gene-delivery vehicle in human gene-therapy protocols. The simplicity of their design, their broad host range and their ability to integrate into a cell's genome are responsible for their popularity. Although the potential for RCR formation remains a concern, even with the latest vectors, assays are in place to detect such recombinants and guidelines for the production of clinical grade vectors are established. Retroviral vectors are simple vectors to manipulate and produce, albeit at lower titers than some other vector systems, notably adenovirus vectors. Their broad tissue tropism and the ability to vary this feature through the use of different pseudotypes has resulted as a wide range of potential target tissues in patients. In the future, the development of cell-targeted vectors will further enhance the utility of these vectors, and the use of lentiviral vectors may overcome some of the current limitations seen with MuLV-based vectors.

REFERENCES

1. Anderson WF. Human gene therapy. Nature 1998; 392: 25–30.
2. Blaese RM, Culver KW, Miller AD, Carter CS, Fleisher T, Clerici M, Shearer G, Chang L, Chiang Y, Tolstoshev P, Greenblatt JJ, Rosenberg SA, Klein H, Berger M, Mullen CA, Ramsey WJ, Muul L, Morgan RA, Anderson WF. T lymphocyte-directed gene therapy for ADA-SCID: initial trial results after 4 years. Science 1995; 270:475–480.
3. Miller AD. Development and applications of retroviral vectors. In: Coffin JM, Hughes SH, Varmus HE, eds. Retroviruses. New York: CSHL Press, 1997.
4. Mann R, Mulligan RC, Baltimore D. Construction of a retrovirus packaging mutant and its use to produce helper-free defective retrovirus. Cell 1983; 33:153–159.
5. Watanabe S, Temin HM. Construction of a helper cell line for avian reticuloendotheliosis virus cloning vectors. Mol Cell Biol 1983; 3:2241–2249.
6. Russell DW, Miller AD. Foamy virus vectors. J Virol 1996; 70:217–222.
7. Muenchau DD, Freeman SM, Cornetta K, Zwiebel JA, Anderson WF. Analysis of retroviral packaging lines for generation of replication-competent virus. Virology 1990; 176: 262–265.
8. Bender MA, Palmer TD, Gelinas RE, Miller AD. Evidence that the packaging signal of Moloney murine leukemia virus extends into the gag region. J Virol 1987; 61:1639–1646.
9. Danos O, Mulligan RC. Safe and efficient generation of recombinant retroviruses with amphotropic and ecotropic host ranges. Proc Natl Acad Sci 1988; 85:6460–6464.
10. Markowitz D, Goff S, Bank A. A safe packaging line for gene transfer: separating viral genes on two different plasmids. J Virol 1988; 62:1120–1124.
11. Kim SH, Yu SS, Park JS, Robbins PD, An CS, Kim S. Construction of retroviral vectors with improved safety, gene expression, and versatility. J Virol 1998; 72: 994–1004.
12. Soneoka Y, Cannon PM, Ramsdale EE, Griffiths JC, Romano G, Kingsman SM, Kingsman AJ. A transient three-plasmid expression system for the production of high titer retroviral vectors. Nucleic Acids Res 1995; 25:628–633.
13. Yu SF, von Ruden T, Kantoff PW, Garber C, Seiberg M, Ruther U, Anderson WF, Wagner EF, Gilboa E. Self-inactivating retroviral vectors designed for transfer of whole genes into mammalian cells. Proc Natl Acad Sci 1986; 83: 3194–3198.
14. Cosset FL, Takeuchi Y, Battini JL, Weiss RA, Collins MK. High-titer packaging cells producing recombinant retroviruses resistant to human serum. J Virol 1995; 69: 7430–7436.
15. Burns JC, Friedmann T, Driever W, Burrascano M, Yee JK. Vesicular stomatitis virus G glycoprotein pseudotyped retroviral vectors: concentration to very high titer and efficient gene transfer into mammalian and nonmammalian cells. Proc Natl Acad Sci 1993; 90:8033–8037.
16. Yee JK, Miyanohara A, LaPorte P, Bouic K, Burns JC, Friedmann T. A general method for the generatino of high-titer, pantropic retroviral vectors: highly efficient infection of primary hepatocytes. Proc Natl Acad Sci 1994; 91: 9564–9568.
17. Gossen M, Bujard H. Tight control of gene expression in mammalian cells by tetracycline-responsive promoters. Proc Natl Acad Sci 1992; 89:5547–5551.
18. Yang Y, Vanin EF, Whitt MA, Fornerod M, Zwart R, Schneiderman RD, Grosveld G, Nienhuis AW. Inducible, high-level production of infectious murine leukemia retroviral vector particles pseudotyped with vesicular stomatitis virus G envelope protein. Human Gene Ther 1995; 6: 1203–1213.
19. Carteau S, Hoffmann C, Bushman F. Chromosome structure and human immunodeficiency virus type 1 cDNA integration: centromeric alphoid repeats are a disfavored target. J Virol 1998; 72:4005–4014.
20. Kirchner J, Connolly CM, Sandmeyer SB. Requirement of RNA polymerase III transcription factors for in vitro position-specific integration of a retroviruslike element. Science 1995; 267:1488–1491.
21. Dildine SL, Respess J, Jolly D, Sandmeyer SB. A chimeric Ty3/Moloney murine leukemia virus integrase protein is active in vivo. J Virol 1998; 72:4297–4307.
22. Bushman FD, Miller MD. Tethering human immunodeficiency virus type 1 preintegration complexes to target DNA promotes integration at nearby sites. J Virol 1997; 71: 458–464.
23. von Kalle C, Kiem HP, Goehle S, Darovsky B, Heimfeld S, Torok-Storb B, Storb R, Schuening FG. Increased gene transfer into human hematopoietic progenitor cells by extended in vitro exposure to a pseudotyped retroviral vector. Blood 1994; 84:2890–2897.
24. Porter CD, Collins MK, Tailor CS, Parkar MH, Cosset FL, Weiss RA, Takeuchi Y. Comparison of efficiency of infection of human gene therapy target cells via four different retroviral receptors. Human Gene Ther 1996; 20:913–919.
25. Sharma S, Cantwell M, Kipps TJ, Friedmann T. Efficient infection of a human T-cell line and of human primary peripheral blood leukocytes with a pseudotyped retrovirus vector. Proc Natl Acad Sci USA 1996; 93:11842–11847.
26. Eglitis MA, Schneiderman RD, Rice PM, Eiden MV. Evaluation of retroviral vectors based on the gibbon ape leukemia virus. Gene Ther 1995; 2:486–492.
27. Cannon PM, Kim N, Kingsman SM, Kingsman AJ. Murine leukemia virus-based Tat-inducible long terminal repeat replacement vectors: a new system for anti-human immunodeficiency virus gene therapy. J Virol 1996; 70:8234–8240.
28. Deminie CA, Emerman M. Functional exchange of an oncoretrovirus and a lentivirus matrix protein. J Virol 1994; 68:4442–4449.

29. Challita PM, Skelton D, el-Khoueiry A, Yu XJ, Weinberg K, Kohn DB. Multiple modifications in cis elements of the long terminal repeat of retroviral vectors lead to increased expression and decreased DNA methylation in embryonic carcinoma cells. J Virol 1995; 69:748–755.
30. Cepko CL, Roberts BE, Mulligan RC. 1984. Construction and applications of a highly transmissible murine retrovirus shuttle vector. Cell 1984; 37:1053–1062.
31. Korman AJ, Frantz JD, Strominger JL, Mulligan RC. Expression of human class II major histocompatibility complex antigens using retrovirus vectors. Proc Natl Acad Sci 1987; 84:2150–2154.
32. Adam MA, Ramesh N, Miller AD, Osborne WRA. Internal initiation of translation in retroviral vectors carrying picornavirus 5″ nontranslated regions. J Virol 1991; 65: 4985–4990.
33. Emerman M, Temin HM. Genes with promoters in retrovirus vectors can be independently suppressed by an epigenetic mechanism. Cell 1984; 39:449–467.
34. Adam MA, Osborne WR, Miller AD. R-region cDNA inserts in retroviral vectors are compatible with virus replication and high level protein synthesis from the insert. Human Gene Ther 1995; 6:1169–1176.
35. Orlic D, Girard LJ, Jordan CT, Anderson SM, Cline AP, Bodine DM. The level of mRNA encoding the amphotropic retrovirus receptor in mouse and human hematopoietic stem cells is low and correlates with the efficiency of retrovirus transduction. Proc Natl Acad Sci USA 1996; 93: 11097–11102.
36. Uchida N, Sutton RE, Friera AM, He D, Reitsma MJ, Chang WC, Veres G, Scollay R, Weissman IL. HIV, but not murine leukemia virus, vectors mediate high efficiency gene transfer into freshly isolated G0/G1 human hematopoietic stem cells. Proc Natl Acad Sci USA 1998; 95:11939–11944.
37. Schnierle BS, Groner B. Retroviral targeted delivery. Gene Ther 1996; 3:1069–1073.
38. Cosset FL, Russell SJ. Targeting retrovirus entry. Gene Ther 1996; 3:946–956.
39. Benedict CA, Tun RY, Rubinstein DB, Guillaume T, Cannon PM, Anderson WF. Targeting retroviral vectors to CD34-expressing cells: binding to CD34 does not catalyze virus-cell fusion. Human Gene Ther 1999; 10:545–557.
40. Zhao Y, Zhu L, Lee S, Li L, Chang E, Soong NW, Douer D, Anderson WF. Identification of the block in targeted retroviral-mediated gene transfer. Proc Natl Acad Sci USA 1999; 96:4005–4010.
41. Jiang A, Chu TH, Nocken F, Cichutek K, Dornburg R. Cell-type-specific gene transfer into human cells with retroviral vectors that display single-chain antibodies. J Virol 1998; 72:10148–10156.
42. Fass D, Davey RA, Hamson CA, Kim PS, Cunningham JM, Berger JM. Structure of a murine leukemia virus receptor-binding glycoprotein at 2.0 angstrom resolution. Science 1997; 277:1662–1666.
43. Zhao, Y, Lee S, Anderson WF. Functional interactions between monomers of the retroviral envelope protein complex. J Virol 1997; 71:6967–6972.
44. Zhao Y, Zhu L, Benedict C, Chen D, Anderson WF, Cannon PM. Functional domains in retroviral transmembrane protein. J Virol 1998; 72:5392–5398.
45. Hall FL, Gordon EM, Wu L, Zhu NL, Skotzko MJ, Starnes VA, Anderson WF. Targeting retroviral vectors to vascular lesions by genetic engineering of the MoMuLV gp70 envelope protein. Human Gene Ther 1997; 8:2183–2192.
46. Nilson BH, Morling FJ, Cosset FL, Russell SJ. Targeting of retroviral vectors through protease-substrate interactions. Gene Ther 1996; 3:28–286.
47. Snitkovsky S, Young JA. Cell-specific viral targeting mediated by a soluble retroviral receptor-ligand fusion protein. Proc Natl Acad Sci USA 1998; 95:7063–7068.
48. Vile RG, Hart IR. Use of tissue-specific expression of the herpes simplex virus thymidine kinase gene to inhibit growth of established murine melanomas following direct intratumoral injection of DNA. Cancer Res 1993; 53: 3860–3864.
49. Agarwal M, Austin TW, Morel F, Chen J, Bohnlein E, Plavec I. Scaffold attachment region-mediated enhancement of retroviral vector expression in primary T cells. J Virol 1998; 72:3720–3728.
50. Rendahl KG, Leff SE, Otten GR, Spratt SK, Bohl D, Van Roey M, Donahue BA, Cohen LK, Mandel RJ, Danos O, Snyder RO. Regulation of gene expression in vivo following transduction by two separate rAAV vectors. Nat Biotechnol 1998; 16:757–761.
51. Naldini L, Blomer U, Gallay P, Ory D, Mulligan R, Gage FH, Verma IM, Trono D. In vivo gene delivery and stable transduction of nondividing cells by a lentiviral vector. Science 1996; 272:263–267.
52. Ram Z, Culver KW, Oshiro EM, Viola JJ, DeVroom HL, Otto E, Long Z, Chiang Y, McGarrity GJ, Muul LM, Katz D, Blaese RM, Oldfield EH. Therapy of malignant brain tumors by intratumoral implantation of retroviral vector-producing cells. Nat Med 1997; 3:1354–1361.
53. Bukrinsky MI, Haggerty S, Dempsey MP, Sharova N, Adzhubel A, Spitz L, Lewis P, Goldfarb D, Emerman M, Stevenson M. A nuclear localization signal within HIV-1 matrix protein that governs infection of non-dividing cells. Nature 1993; 365:666–669.
54. Gallay P, Hope T, Chin D, Trono D. HIV-1 infection of nondividing cells through the recognition of integrase by the importin/karyopherin pathway. Proc Natl Acad Sci USA 1997; 94:9825–9830.
55. Heinzinger NK, Bukinsky MI, Haggerty SA, Ragland AM, Kewalramani V, Lee MA, Gendelman HE, Ratner L, Stevenson M, Emerman M. The Vpr protein of human immunodeficiency virus type 1 influences nuclear localization of viral nucleic acids in nondividing host cells. Proc Natl Acad Sci USA 1994; 91:7311–7315.
56. Zufferey R, Dull T, Mandel RJ, Bukovsky A, Quiroz D, Naldini L, Trono D. Self-inactivating lentivirus vector for safe and efficient in vivo gene delivery. J Virol 1998; 72: 9873–9880.
57. Zufferey R, Nagy D, Mandel RJ, Naldini L, Trono D. Multiply attenuated lentiviral vector achieves efficient gene delivery in vivo. Nat Biotechnol 1997; 15:871–875.

58. Poeschla EM, Wong-Staal F, Looney DJ. Efficient transduction of nondividing human cells by feline immunodeficiency virus lentiviral vectors. Nat Med 1998; 4:354–357.
59. Otto E, Jones-Trower A, Vanin EF, Stambaugh K, Mueller SN, Anderson WF, McGarrity GJ. Characterization of a replication-competent retrovirus resulting from recombination of packaging and vector sequences. Human Gene Ther 1994; 5:567–575.
60. Chong H, Vile RG. Replication-competent retrovirus produced by a 'split function' third generation amphotropic packaging cell line. Gene Ther 1996; 3:624–629.
61. Reiprich S, Gundlach BR, Fleckenstein B, Uberla K. Replication-competent chimeric lenti-oncovirus with expanded host cell tropism. J Virol 1997; 71:3328–3331.
62. Donahue RE, Kessler SW, Bodine D, McDonagh K, Dunbar C, Goodman S, Agricola B, Byrne E, Raffeld M, Moen R, Bacher J, Zsebo KM, Nienhuis AW. Helper virus induced T cell lymphoma in nonhuman primates after retroviral mediated gene transfer. J Exp Med 1992; 176:1125–1135.
63. Vanin EF, Kaloss M, Broscius C, Nienhuis AW. Characterization of replication-competent retroviruses from nonhuman primates with virus-induced T-cell lymphomas and observations regarding the mechanism of oncogenesis. J Virol 1994; 68:4241–4250.
64. Anderson WF, McGarrity GJ, Moen RC. Report to the NIH Recombinant DNA Advisory Committee on murine replication-competent retrovirus (RCR) assays (February 17, 1993). Human Gene Ther 1993; 4:311–321.
65. Rother RP, Fodor WL, Springhorn JP, Birks CW, Setter E, Sandrin MS, Squinto SP, Rollins SA. A novel mechanism of retrovirus inactivation in human serum mediated by anti-α-galactosyl natural antibody. J Exp Med 1995; 182: 1345–1355.
66. Takeuchi Y, Cosset FL, Lachmann PJ, Okada H, Weiss RA, Collines MK. Type C retrovirus inactivation by human complement is determined by both the viral genome and the producer cell. J Virol 1994; 68:8001–8007.
67. Haubrich R, McCutchan JA, Holdredge R, Heiner L, Merritt J, Merchant B. An open label, phase I/II clinical trial to evaluate the safety and biological activity of HIV-IT (V) (HIV-1IIIBenv/rev retroviral vector) in HIV-1-infected subjects. Human Gene Ther 1995; 6:941–955.

2

Adenovirus Vectors for Gene Therapy

Neil R. Hackett and Ronald G. Crystal
Weill Medical College of Cornell University, New York, New York

I. INTRODUCTION

The emergence of recombinant DNA as a tool to study medicine quickly promulgated the concept of cloned genes as therapeutics. As originally conceived, the concept of gene therapy was to simply to introduce a wild-type copy of a deficient gene into cells to restore function in trans (1–5). Viewed in this way, the technical challenge was to efficiently deliver the gene to the appropriate cell and have it expressed for sufficient time, or readminister as often as needed, for the therapeutic application. Adenovirus gene-transfer vectors offer one strategy to achieve this. The focus on adenoviruses (Ad) for gene transfer was based on basic research establishing the biology of Ad and the knowledge that Ad efficiently delivers the viral genome to the target cells (1). Importantly, Ad are not oncogenic in humans, the genomes of common Ad are completely defined, the Ad genome can be easily modified, and recombinant Ad can be readily produced in large quantities and highly concentrated without modifying the ability of the virus to infect cells (1,3).

In retrospect, the original goal of using Ad as simple delivery systems to permanently complement genetic defects seems naive. Whereas Ad gene-transfer vectors can achieve robust expression of the transgene in many target organs, expression of the transgene is limited in time, resulting from a complex combination of innate and adaptive immune host defenses against the virus (6–11). In this context, Ad vectors in their present form are useful in applications where transient (days to weeks) expression is sufficient to have the desired therapeutic effect. For applications where persistent expression is required to achieve a therapeutic goal, there are still many challenges before Ad vectors will be successful. In this chapter we will summarize the biology of Ad, the construction and use of first-generation Ad vectors, the current status of advanced forms of Ad vectors, clinical applications of Ad vectors, and the future prospects of using Ad in gene-transfer applications.

II. BIOLOGY OF ADENOVIRUSES

Human Ad are a group of double-stranded DNA viruses that infect a variety of vertebrate hosts including rodents, chickens, and nonhuman primates (reviewed in Ref. 12). Human Ad have been isolated from several sources including the upper respiratory tracts of military recruits with respiratory infections, adenoids, conjunctiva, and the stool of infants with diarrhea. As with other viruses, there is an immune response to Ad infection, which includes the production of neutralizing antibodies, defined as antibodies that prevent Ad infection in vitro. Neutralizing sera have been used to distinguish 49 different adenovirus serotypes (12). These are divided into six subgroups according to rather arbitrary criteria of ability to transform rodent cells, pattern of hemagglutination, and GC content of the DNA (see Table 1). In the context of gene therapy, serotypes 5 and 2 of the subgroup C have been used almost exclusively because the most is known about the structure and biology of these serotypes and there are convenient biological reagents available to produce recombinant subgroup C Ad gene-transfer vectors in large quantities.

A. Pathology

Adenoviruses are associated with an number of disorders, most of which are mild (Table 1). The pathology is primar-

Table 1 Representative Serotypes and Pathology of Different Subgroups of Adenoviruses

	Subgroup					
	A	B	C	D	E	F
Representative serotypes	12,31	3,7	2,5	9,17,30	4	4,041
Cryptic enteritis	X					
Acute respiratory infections		X			X	
Hemorrhagic cystitis		X				
Pharyngitis		X	X			
Pneumonia		X	X			
Keratoconjunctivitis				X		
Diarrhea						X

ily from inflammation and loss of infected epithelial cells (13). Viruses of subgroups A and F are associated primarily with gastrointestinal infections. Although Ad account for only a small percentage of diarrhea cases, 50% of children develop antibodies against enteric adenoviruses by age 4 (14). Viruses of subgroups B and C cause various respiratory infections as outbreaks either in confined groups (such as military recruits) or in children. In children, respiratory symptoms associated with subgroups B and C may be associated with conjunctival infections. The hallmark of viruses of subgroup D are conjunctival infection. Subgroup E has only one member (Ad4), which is closely related to types 3 and 7 of subgroup B (15). The known predilection of subgroup C for the respiratory tract helped propel the initial uses of Ad gene therapy for the treatment of cystic fibrosis and thus the focus on serotypes 2 and 5.

B. Structure

Adenovirus consists of an icosohedral protein capsid of approximately 70–100 nm diameter and, within that capsid, a single copy of a double stranded DNA molecule of length approximately 36,000 bp (Fig. 1) (reviewed in Ref. 16). In the context of gene therapy, the fiber, penton base, and hexon are the most important capsid proteins. The 20 triangular faces of the viral capsid are built from hexon, the major capsid protein. The 240 hexon capsomeres in the capsid are trimers comprising three copies of the 105 kDa hexon subunit, with each trimer interacting with six others in a pseudo-equivalent fashion. The three-dimensional structure of hexon (17) shows that the homotrimer has loops, which project out from the capsid surface. Capsid proteins VI, VIII, and IX are associated with hexon, and their role is to stabilize the capsid structure. The 12 vertices are made up of the penton capsomere, a complex of five copies of the penton base, and three copies of fiber. Each penton capsomere interacts with five hexon capsomeres, one from each of the five faces that converge at the vertex.

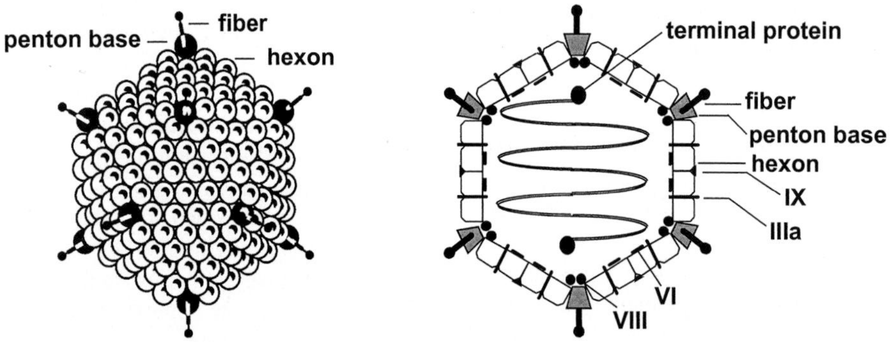

Figure 1 Structure of the adenovirus capsid. Shown (left) is a three-dimensional representation and (right) a simplified cross section of the capsid showing the deployment of the capsid proteins and Ad genome. The capsid is a icosahedron with 20 faces and 12 vertices. The faces are composed of hexons, each comprised of trimers of the hexon protein. The hexons are trapezoid-shaped, with three loops on top, extending from the face of the capsid. The loops represent the variable regions that differ among serotypes and are the major epitopes for neutralizing antibodies. Proteins IX and VIII are associated with the hexon and are thought to stabilize the capsid. The vertices are composed of a fiber and penton base. The fiber has three domains: the base, which interacts with penton, the shaft, and the knob. The knob interacts with a high-affinity receptor on the target cell, and the shaft holds the virus away from the surface of the cell, depending on the length of the shaft. The penton base interacts with the hexon and the fiber and contains epitopes that interact with integrins on the cell surface. The 36 kb double-stranded DNA genome is wrapped around capsid core protein VII, and the terminal protein is attached to the two 5′ ends of the Ad genome. (Adapted from Ref. 16.)

The fiber protein projects outward from the penton base. The DNA is wrapped in the histone-like core protein VII, and there is a terminal protein attached to the 5′ end of each strand of the DNA.

Neutralizing antibodies are directed primarily against epitopes located on the loops of the hexon. This is expected, because the loops project from the surface of the virus where they are accessible to antibodies. When the primary structures of the capsids of different serotypes are compared, related Ad differ most in these loops, suggesting that the selective pressures applied by the immune system result in the emergence of mutations in the external hexon loops (18).

The fiber protein is a trimer consisting of three domains: the base, the shaft, and the knob. The N-terminal base domain interacts with the penton base. The shaft includes an extended domain consisting of variable numbers of a 15-amino-acid pseudorepeat. The number of repeats, and therefore the length of the shaft, varies between 23 copies for the group A viruses and 6 copies for the subgroup B viruses. The distal C-terminal domain of the fiber protein, referred to as the ''knob,'' interacts with the high-affinity receptor on the surface of the target cell. The high-affinity receptor for adenoviruses, except those of subgroup B (19), is referred to as ''CAR'' (corsackie virus-adenovirus receptor), reflecting the fact that the B coxsackie viruses and most serotypes of Ad share the same receptor (20). CAR is a single membrane-spanning protein with two extracellular immunoglobulin-like domains. Apart from acting as a virus receptor, the function of CAR is unknown.

The penton base at the vertex of the Ad capsid interacts with hexons of the five faces that meet at that vertex and with the fiber that projects from it. A sequence motif on the penton base is involved in internalization of the virus after high-affinity CAR-fiber interaction. In serotypes 2 and 5, the amino acid motif arginine-glycine-aspartate (RGD) interacts with $\alpha_V\beta_3$ and $\alpha_V\beta_5$ integrins of the cell surface, and this interaction is essential for efficient internalization.

For adenovirus type 5, the most commonly used Ad for gene-transfer vectors, the complete 35,935 bp DNA sequence is known. For convenient reference, the genome is divided into 100 equally spaced map units. A detailed transcription map at various time points postinfection is used to divide the genome into interspersed early (E) and late (L) regions (Fig. 2) (reviewed in Ref. 16). There is considerable transcriptional overlap among the genes, making manipulation of some areas of the genome difficult. Each of the five early genes is comprised of a complex transcription unit with alternative sites for transcription initiation, termination, and splicing. The E1A and E1B genes are transcribed rightwards at the left-hand end of the genome close to the DNA replication origin and packaging signal. The E4 region is transcribed leftward at the right-hand end of the genome. Distal to the E1 and E4 regions are the termini of the DNA, which are inverted copies of the same sequence. Replication of the ends of the DNA is achieved by the attachment of terminal protein to the 5′ end of the DNA, which acts as a primer to initiate unidirectional replication. This terminal protein is one of the components of the E2 transcriptional unit, which is transcribed leftward commencing at map unit 75. The remaining early transcription unit is the E3 gene, which is transcribed rightward commencing at map unit 77. The five late genes are expressed after the beginning of DNA replication and encode the viral structural proteins. These late transcripts are all transcribed rightward originating from map unit 17 and contain the same three-part leader sequence before alternate splicing generates different mature mRNAs.

C. Viral Replication

The Ad viral life cycle is understood best for subgroup C, which is another factor in the choice of Ad5 and 2 as gene-therapy vectors (Fig. 3). The knob of the fiber protein binds to the CAR receptor followed by an interaction of the RGD sequence in the penton base with cell surface $\alpha_V\beta_3$ or $\alpha_V\beta_5$ integrins (21). Excess soluble integrins inhibit Ad internalization but not binding, suggesting that penton base-integrin interaction is instrumental in internalization (22). Ad modified with deletion of the RGD motif replicate effectively in vitro so the penton base-integrin interaction is likely related to efficiency of Ad infection but is not essential (23). The Ad enters the cell by endocytosis into clathrin-coated pits, a process that can be blocked by dynamin inhibitors (24). After endocytosis, Ad is very rapidly released into the cytoplasm prior to extensive endosome fusion (25). The virus proceeds rapidly to the nucleus, probably actively transported on microtubules, and then binds to the surface of the nucleus near the nuclear pore (25–28). Using fluorescent viruses, this process has been shown to be efficient and rapid, with $>90\%$ of Ad5 delivered to the nucleus within 1 hour (25). At the nuclear membrane, the DNA and terminal protein are internalized by an unknown mechanism and are assembled into the nuclear scaffold for active transcription.

With wild-type Ad, the viral E1A gene is transcribed immediately after infection (16). After alternate splicing, the E1 mRNAs are translated into the two E1A proteins essential for transcription of other early viral mRNAs. E1A proteins promote the expression of cellular genes needed for DNA replication by interacting with the retinoblastoma susceptibility protein (Rb), which normally suppresses entry into the S phase of the cell cycle by complexing with

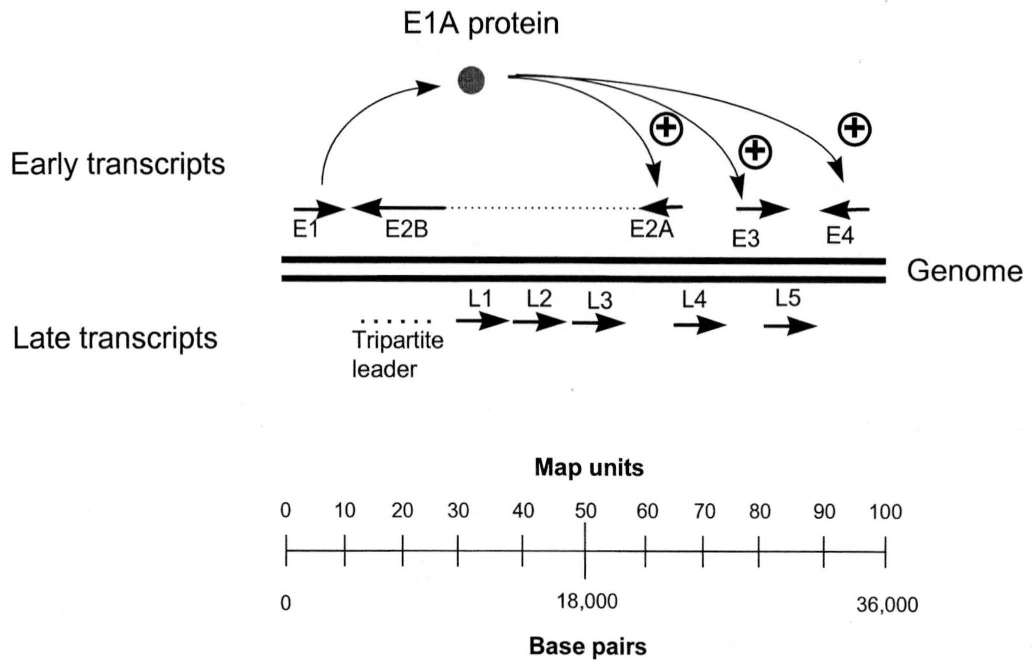

Figure 2 Structure and transcription of the major genes of the adenovirus type 5 genome. Schematic summary of the transcription of adenovirus during lytic infection. The genome is represented as two parallel lines and is divided by the scale shown on top into 100 map units (1 map unit = 360 bp). There are nine major complex transcription units divided into early (above the genome) and late transcripts (below). The four early transcripts are produced before the commencement of DNA replication and specify regulatory proteins and proteins required for DNA replication. Upon initial infection of a cell, the E1A protein is produced from transcripts in the E1 region. E1A is a major regulatory factor required for transcription of E1B, E2, E3, and E4. In replication-deficient adenovirus vectors, the E1 region is deleted. Proteins coded by the E2 and E4 regions are required for late gene transcription. The E3 region codes for proteins that help the virus evade host defenses. All late transcripts rightwards originate at the same point and are produced by alternate splicing. The tripartite leader sequence is present at the 5′ end of all late transcripts. The L3 region specifies hexon, the L5 region specifies fiber, and the L2 region specifies penton.

the host transcription factor E2F. E1A also interacts with a number of cellular transcriptional factors to promote the assembly of complexes that promote transcription of other early adenoviral genes. Among the important downstream products induced by E1A is the product of the E1B gene, which blocks the apoptotic pathway through interaction with p53 long enough for a productive viral infection. The E1B 55 kDa protein also complexes with the ORF6 protein from the E4 region to modulate expression of the viral late genes, which begin to be expressed around 6 hours postinfection. At that time, DNA replication begins and the transcription of late genes commences, providing the capsid components that assemble into mature virions (16). The new virions are assembled in the nucleus, necessitating transport of capsid proteins into the nucleus. As the viral infection proceeds, the integrity and viability of the cells decrease, but the mechanism of viral release from the cell is not understood.

In the context of gene therapy, the E3 region is important because it encodes immunosuppressive functions that work through two mechanisms. The E3 gp19 kDa protein prevents major histocompatibility complex class II–mediated antigen presentation on the cell surface, thereby inhibiting the differentiation of cytotoxic T lymphocytes directed against viral antigens (29). The E3 14.7 kDa and E3 10.4 kDa proteins inhibit apoptosis of infected cells initiated by fas/fas ligand and/or tumor necrosis factor (30). The promoter for the E3 region requires E1 products, and thus in $E1^-$ deleted Ad vectors the presence or absence of the E3 region is not relevant (see below).

Transcripts from the E2 region specify the three nonhost proteins directly involved in DNA replication: the DNA polymerase, the single-stranded DNA binding protein (ssDBP), and the preterminal protein (16). Like other viruses, adenovirus has developed a specific strategy for the faithful replication of the ends of its DNA. The last 103

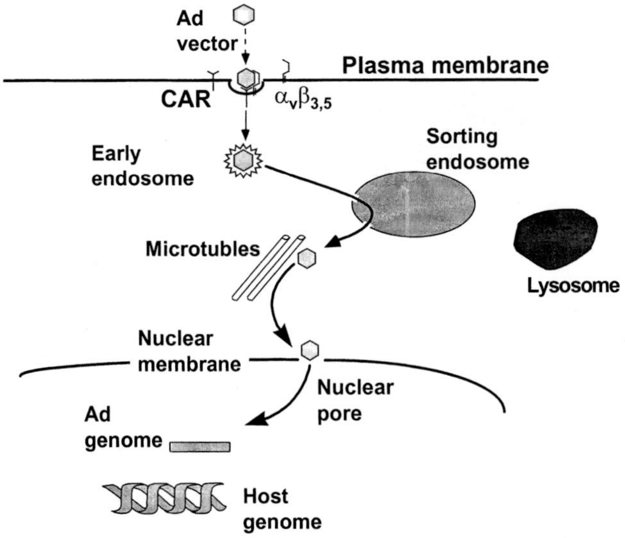

Figure 3 Trafficking of adenovirus from membrane to nucleus. The initial contact between the virus and cell is mediated by the knob of fiber and the CAR (coxsackie virus, adenovirus receptor). This allows the secondary interaction between the penton and $\alpha_V\beta_3$ or $\alpha_V\beta_5$ integrins, which is required for internalization. The initial internalization is via coated pits, which give rise to coated vesicles. After a very short interval, prior to fusion of early endosomes into sorting endosomes, a conformational change in the viral capsid allows escape of the virus into the cytoplasm. Microtubules carry the virus towards the nucleus. The whole capsid attaches to the outside of the nucleus, but only the DNA and terminal protein are inserted into the nucleus itself, where they are assembled onto the nuclear matrix to allow transcription. (Courtesy of P. Leopold, Weill Medical College of Cornell University.)

base pairs at both ends of the genome consist of inverted copies of the identical sequence. The terminal protein binds covalently to the 5′ end and acts as a primer for DNA synthesis by the adenoviral DNA polymerase of the leading strand starting at either end. DNA polymerase proceeds by a strand-displacement mechanism, creating a duplex and a displaced strand that is sequestered by the ssDBP and has terminal protein attached to one end. Base pairing of the ends of the single strand creates a panhandle structure with ends identical to those of the duplex. Reformation of duplex from the single-stranded form occurs by the same mechanism, with the Ad polymerase initiating at the terminal protein and displacing the ssDBP. Interestingly, the viral genomes undergoing replication are at a different location from those being transcribed (31). DNA is packaged into capsids as directed by a DNA sequence close to the left-hand end of the virus. The efficiency of packaging depends on the length of DNA; genomes greater than 105% or less than 95% of the normal length propagate much less efficiently (32).

The E4 region plays important roles in the viral life cycle by promoting the selective expression of viral genes at the expense of cellular genes. For example, the E4-ORF3 and ORF6 proteins inhibit the transport of transcripts of cellular genes from nucleus to cytoplasm while promoting the transport of late viral transcripts. The E4 region is therefore essential for viral gene expression and subsequent viral replication.

III. CONSTRUCTION AND USE OF FIRST GENERATION ADENOVIRUS VECTORS

A. Construction

Although the pathology associated with wild-type adenovirus infections is generally mild, there is a potential risk of using $E1^+$ Ad for gene transfer in that the inflammatory host responses to Ad infection may alter organ function. There is also the possibility of overwhelming infection if Ad replication is allowed to progress when there are deficiencies in the host defense system. Since the E1A products are essential for expression of other early and late genes and for DNA replication, the most direct approach to eliminating replication is to delete the E1A genes. To produce $E1^-$ Ad vectors, the classic approach is to transfect the recombinant $E1^-$ Ad vector genome into the human embryonic kidney cell line 293, a cell line originally established by transforming primary cells with Ad5 (33–35). The 293 cells contain approximately 11 map units of the Ad5 genome, originating at the left-hand end (36,37).

One example of a so-called first-generation adenovirus vector expresses the human cystic fibrosis transmembrane conductance regulator (CFTR) cDNA under control of the constitutively highly active cytomegalovirus immediate/early promoter (CMV) (Fig. 4) (38). A polyadenylation site is located following the cDNA, and the whole expression cassette in a right-to-left orientation replaces the E1A and part of the E1B genes. Since the expression cassette is 5601 bp in length while the E1 deletion is 2970 bp, it is necessary to delete part of the E3 region in order to construct the vector. Since the E3 region is nonessential in vitro, this deletion does not affect propagation of the replication-deficient virus in 293 cells. However, for some therapeutic genes, if the extra space is not necessary, the E3 region can be retained. As described above, without E1 function, the E3 promoter does not function, and thus loss of E3 genes is not relevant.

To make a first-generation Ad vector, two DNA components are necessary: the left end containing the expression

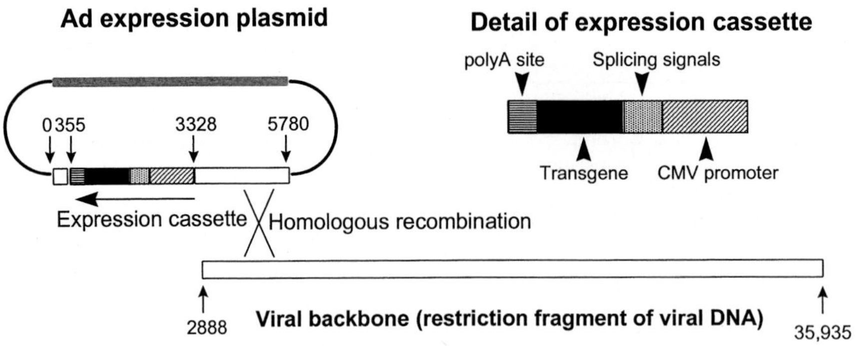

Figure 4 Construction of first generation E1$^-$, E3$^-$ Ad by homologous recombination in human embryonic kidney 293 cells. The transgene is cloned into an expression cassette, typically consisting of a strong viral promoter such as the CMV immediate/early promoter/enhancer, an artificial intron with splicing signals, and the cDNA for the transgene followed by a polyadenylation/transcriptional stop site. This expression cassette is cloned into the deleted E1A/E1B (nucleotides 355–3328) region of a plasmid containing approximately 15 map units from the left-hand end of the Ad genome. The signals needed for DNA replication and packaging are located in the first 355 nt of the Ad genome. The region from 3328 to 5780 allows homologous recombination between the Ad expression plasmid and the backbone, which consists of map units 9 through 100 with the E3 deletion. The backbone can originate from a genomic clone propagated in *E. coli* or can be purified from Ad DNA after appropriate restriction digestion. These two plasmids are cotransfected into 293 cells, and a homologous recombination event results in the E1$^-$ E3$^-$ Ad vector.

cassette and the right end containing the majority of the Ad genome (Fig. 4) (39). The two fragments are fused by homologous recombination after cotransfection into 293 cells. The left end is a plasmid vector containing the terminal repeat and replication origin of the virus and the expression cassette in the E1 region. The right end is the Ad backbone (either a plasmid or DNA purified from restriction enzyme digests of the viral DNA). The two fragments partially overlap, allowing homologous recombination in the 293 cells to create a full-length virus that is then able to replicate with the E1 helper function from the 293 cells.

Once made, a new vector is plaque purified repeatedly in 293 cells (to remove any contaminating wild-type virus) and is then propagated to produce the required amounts of the vector. Under standard laboratory conditions, it is possible to produce up to 2×10^{13} viral particles from 50 150-mm cell culture plates (about 10^9 293 cells). The recombinant Ad is easily purified from cell lysates on equilibrium cesium chloride density gradients. After purification, the vector is assayed for infectivity by plaquing efficiency on 293 cells, the presence of contaminating replication competent Ad (RCA) by the plaquing efficiency on A549 cells (an E1$^-$ cell line) (40), and the activity of the transgene (using whatever assay is relevant). Titer on 293 cells gives the titer in plaque-forming units (pfu) per mL. This has historically been the activity unit used to standardize doses for experimental animals and patients. However, it has become evident that the pfu is an arbitrary, poorly reproducible measurement, and thus most laboratories now use particle units (pu) as the dosing unit, based on the premise that highly purified viruses made by a standard protocol represent a uniform population of potentially infectious units. The particle count is calculated from the absorbance at 260 nm using the formula $1A_{260} = 1.25 \times 10^{12}$ particles/mL and is typically 10–100 times the titer in pfu (41).

B. In Vitro Studies

The methods outlined above have been used to make a large number of first-generation E1$^-$E3$^-$ adenoviral vectors. Among the most widely used are those that express readily monitored reporter genes such as β-galactosidase, luciferase, chloramphenicol acetyl transferase (CAT), and green fluorescent protein (GFP). As a control, viruses with the same promoter driving expression of no transgene (AdNull) are used.

Using the reporter gene Ad vectors, many studies have examined the ease of gene transfer to different primary cells and cell lines. Some primary epithelial cells are easily infected by wild-type adenovirus type 5 and, as expected, are easily transfected by adenoviral vectors. In contrast, primary menenchymal cells, macrophages (42), and B cells (43,44) are more difficult to infect, and only very high multiplicities of infection in concentrated cell suspensions are effective. The discovery that CAR is the adenoviral receptor partially accounts for the relative ease of infection. There are several studies in which the overexpression of

CAR was shown to be sufficient to make an otherwise refractory cell line susceptible to gene transfer by Ad (45,46). But integrins and postinternalization factors must also affect the efficiency of gene transfer.

A large number of cancer cell lines have been shown to be susceptible to gene transfer including cells derived from hepatoma (47–49), glioblastoma (50), myeloma (51,52), melanoma (53,54), prostate (55), and ovarian cancer (56,57). On the other hand, lymphoma cell lines (51) are resistant to infection. Studies in which cells are infected in vitro are instructive in indicating which cell types and therefore diseases might be candidates for adenoviral gene therapy. It is difficult to evaluate if studies with reporter genes show that therapeutic levels of proteins are achievable in any cell type due to the use of Ad vectors with different promoters, reporter genes, multiplicities of infection, and times of exposure.

In cells infected in vitro with E1-deleted, replication-deficient adenovirus vectors, a low level of transcription of early and late genes (58,59) as well as a small amount of DNA synthesis (60) can be detected. The reason for this is not entirely understood but is hypothesized to result from E1-like activities in the target cell that support expression of Ad genes. In dividing cells there would also be a high level of E2F, which would support adenoviral transcription. However, measurements of viral load in cultures suggest that this does not translate into the production of infectious viral particles in the absence of contaminating wild-type adenovirus. While cells may continue to divide after infection, the absolute level of vector does not increase or decrease even if the amount of vector per cell does decrease to the point when a small minority of cells are infected. Based on this evidence, the Ad genome is likely to remain episomal and is not integrated into the cellular genome, although this is difficult to prove because it is very hard to detect integrated DNA at a very low frequency.

C. In Vivo Studies and Tissue Specificity of Gene Transfer

The feasibility of Ad vector-mediated gene transfer in vitro posed the question of the efficiency of this vector system in vivo. Since Ad gene-transfer vectors are made from human adenoviruses, there was no a priori reason to believe they would infect rodents or other model animals. Some early studies (34,35,61,62) used cotton rats, since this species had been shown previously to be permissive for replication of human adenoviruses (13). For example, intratracheal administration of a replication-deficient virus expressing the reporter gene β-galactosidase to cotton rats resulted in expression of β-galactosidase in the airway epithelium (63). Numerous other animals have been used to demonstrate efficient adenovirus vector-mediated gene transfer, including rats, mice, pigs, rabbits, and nonhuman primates. From these studies, a number of general conclusions can be drawn. Importantly, many tissues can be infected based on the route of administration. As expected from the tropism of Ad5, the transgene delivered to the respiratory epithelium is readily expressed after intranasal or intratracheal administration. But intravenous injection into rodents results primarily in transgene expression in the liver and spleen (8,64). It is not known if the hepatocytes or hepatic endothelium account for this tropism, since surprisingly, the preference for liver does not correspond to the distribution of the CAR receptor among organs (20). Direct injection into the peritoneum (65), kidney (66,67), pancreas (68), cerebral spinal fluid (69), skeletal muscle (64,70,71), brain (72,73), cardiac muscle (74,75), the coronary artery (76), and many other tissues results in local expression of the transgene. But the absolute efficiency of gene transfer and expression and leakage to other organs has seldom been calculated, and it is often unclear if therapeutic levels of transgene expression can be achieved.

D. Host Responses

Another important concept that emerged from in vivo studies in experimental animals was the short duration of transgene expression mediated by Ad vectors. Typically, transgene expression levels peak in 1–7 days and decline rapidly to undetectable levels by 2–4 weeks (Fig. 5). This is true for most routes of administration with the exception of direct injection into a few immunoprivileged tissues such as brain (77–79). Interestingly, the delivery of Ad vector expressing α_1-antitrypsin to mice results in rapid clearance in the CH3/J strain, while expression persists for several months in C57BL/6J strain (80). Immediately upon administration, the innate immune system serves to eliminate a large amount of vector. Using viral DNA levels as a means to monitor viral clearance from the liver, approximately 90% of an intravenous bolus cleared after 24 hours (11). Similar kinetics are seen in immunodeficient mice. Inhibitors of the reticulo-endothelium system reduce this early loss of vector, suggesting that macrophages are responsible for early vector clearance (81).

It is known that infection by wild-type human adenoviruses results in a strong immune response in experimental animals and humans. It is not clear whether replication-deficient gene-therapy vectors would have the same effect since the net expression of viral genes would be so much lower and the tissues involved would be different from those involved in natural infections. In practice, both cellular and humoral immune responses are observed in rodents

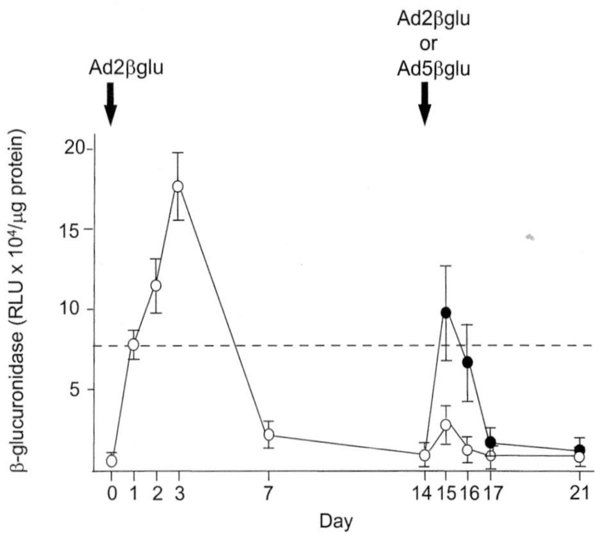

Figure 5 Quantification of β-glucuronidase expression in the lung over time following repeat administration of the same serotype vector or a vector from an alternate serotype. β-Glucuronidase expression in the lung after initial intratracheal administration of Ad2βglu (10^{11} particles) followed 14 days later by intratracheal administration of either the same vector (Ad2βglu, 10^9 pfu, ○), or a vector of the alternate serotype (Ad5βglu, 10^9 pfu, ●). (From Ref. 96.)

after intratracheal (6,82), intravenous (8,83), and intraperitoneal (7,84) administration. Antibodies against various adenoviral proteins including hexon are induced, which can be detected by Western blotting and neutralizing assays. Cytotoxic T-lymphocyte (CTL) responses are also observed. The CTL are assumed, but not proven in all cases, to eliminate cells infected by the vector in vivo. When a transgene is used that is foreign to the host, CTL and antibodies are usually, but not always, detected against the transgene (9,10,59).

These observations lead to the hypothesis that the immune response is essential for the elimination of adenoviral vectors. The availability of immune-deficient mice provides a way to test this hypothesis. In many studies, the persistence of vector and transgene expression has been shown to be much longer in immunodeficient mice (11,85,86). Practically, it also suggested ways in which a partial transient deficiency in the immune system might be exploited to prolong the expression of a therapeutic gene.

Conventional immunosuppressants such as corticosteroids (87), cyclosporine (88–90), and FK506 (58,91) have been used to reduce anti-Ad immune responses and increase the duration of transgene expression in experimental animals. The danger of applying this to human subjects is that opportunistic infections or infection from contaminating wild-type adenovirus may result. But greater persistence of Ad vectors can also be achieved via simultaneous systemic administration of molecules such as antibodies against CD40 (92,93) ligand and CTLA4Ig (91,94), which block interaction between T cells and antigen-presenting cells. These immunomoduilators could be used locally, possibly coexpressed on the same adenovirus as the therapeutic gene, to give more specific immunosupression.

The humoral and cellular responses also evoke immunological memory, which prevents effective gene expression following subsequent administration of the same vector (Fig. 5). Neutralizing antibodies sequester the readministered vector before it infects cells and cause its immune clearance. Thus, the barriers to readministration of a second vector should be serotype specific, a concept that has been proven in experimental studies (Fig. 5) (95,96). Cellular immune system memory can also eliminate any readministered vectors that escape neutralization and infect host cells. The determinants of the cellular immune response are more conserved between serotype, and a second vector of different serotype is eliminated faster from immune animals than from naive animals (Fig. 5).

IV. IMPROVED ADENOVIRUS VECTORS

Two salient points emerge from the data discussed above. The first is that only some cells and tissues can be efficiently infected by adenovirus vectors. The second is that there is a strong immune response against adenoviral vectors, which results in elimination of cells infected by the vector and the inability to achieve effective gene transfer and expression following readministration of the same vector. A number of approaches are being developed that might mitigate these problems.

A. Elimination of Replication-Competent Adenovirus

Adenoviral vectors are produced in the 293 cell line that provide in trans the E1 functions that render them conditionally replication competent, permitting vector growth. The difficulty with this approach to propagating vectors is that there is the possibility of homologous recombination between the replication-deficient vector and the chromosomal copy of the Ad5 genome (Fig. 6). This inevitably occurs at a low frequency resulting in the production of $E1^+$, $E3^-$ replication-competent adenovirus (RCA). Once formed, RCA will outgrow the replication-deficient gene therapy vector in vitro. To minimize the production of RCA, Ad are plaque purified several times on 293 cells and exhaustively tested for the presence of RCA, which is

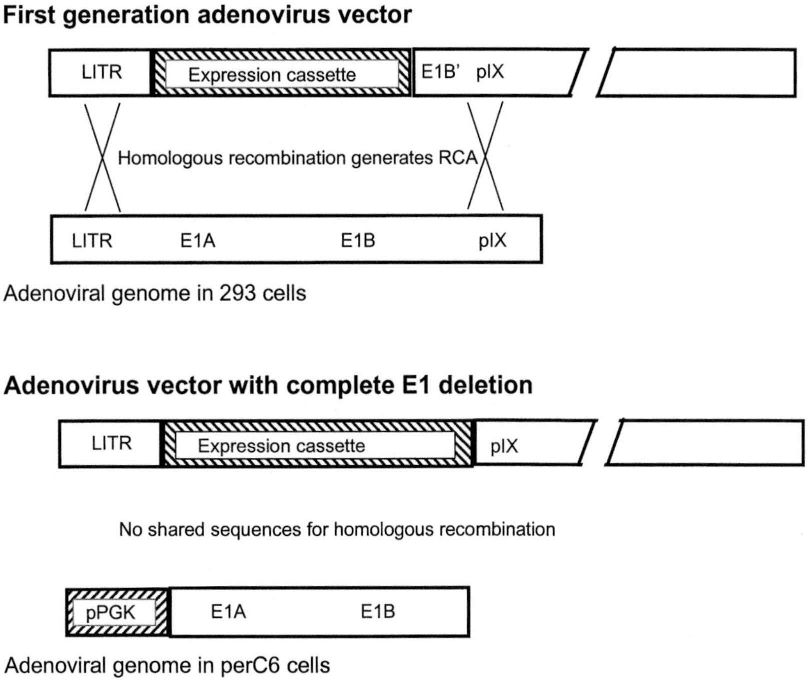

Figure 6 Production of replication competent adenovirus by homologous recombination between Ad vector and genome of 293 cells. The 293 cell line (open rectangle) contains nucleotides 1 through 4344 from adenovirus type 5 including the left inverted terminal repeat (LITR), the E1A and E1B genes, and the adjacent protein IX gene (pIX). The E1 deletion in most first-generation vectors (top rectangle) stretches from nucleotide 355 through 3328, which is replaced by the expression cassette for the therapeutic gene. Therefore, two homologous recombination events (crossed line) can occur, which restore the E1 region and give a replication-competent (albeit $E3^-$) virus. In the second example, the extent of the E1 deletion in the vector has been extended to encompass all of the E1A and E1B genes. At the same time, the E1A and E1B genes in the complementing cell line [i.e., perC6 cells (139)] have no flanking sequence and expression is driven by the phosphoglycerol kinase promoter. As a result there is no homology at either end and only two illegitimate recombination events can result in the production of RCA. As a result the frequency is very low.

readily detected on the basis of its ability to form plaques on E1-negative cell lines such as the human lung epithelial cell line A549 (40). For clinical studies, adenoviral vectors should be uncontaminated by RCA (level < 1 RCA per dose). However, the preparation of Ad vector of this quality is difficult, and most in vivo animal and in vitro studies are done with preps of uncharacterized levels of RCA that are probably >1 RCA per 10^8 particles.

To reduce RCA production, two approaches can be used: reduce the size of the trans-complementing E1 region in the cell line or increase the size of the E1 deletion in the vector. Several cell lines have been developed that have less of the Ad genome (compared to 293 cells), while retaining the ability to supply the E1A and E1B functions in trans and the high productivity of the 293 cell line (Table 2). The E1 deletion in the first-generation clinical vectors was smaller than optimal, retaining 31% of the 3′ end of the E1B gene. Deleting this sequence in conjunction with cell lines that express E1A/B from nonadenoviral promoter allows production of adenoviruses in circumstances where there is no overlap between the cellular sequence and the vector (Fig. 6). In these cell lines, RCA is virtually eliminated since it can only arise through two illegitimate recombination events, an occurrence that is very rare.

B. Vectors with Additional Early Gene Deletions

First-generation Ad vectors permit limited Ad gene expression and DNA replication, which probably contributes to the immune response against the vector. In addition, the possibility of making RCA during propagation is a potentially dangerous feature. By making additional mutations or deletions in the Ad genome, both of these problems can be avoided. One implementation is to make an $E1^-$ vector with an E2A mutation that renders the vector replication

Table 2 Adenovirus Deletions and Complementing Cell Lines

Cell line (Genotype)	Deletions complemented	Comments	Refs.
293 (E1A/B+)	E1-	Human embryonic kidney cells transformed by nucleotides 1–4344 of Ad5	141
911 (E1A/B+)	E1-	Human embryonic retinoblast cells containing nucleotides 79–5789 of Ad5. Enhanced plaquing efficiency over 293	142
perC6 (E1A/B+)	E1-	Nucleotides 459–3510 of Ad5 driven by phosphoglycerate kinase promoter; reduced production of RCA compared to 911 and 293	139
293-E4 (E1A/B+, E4+)	E1-, E4-	293 derivative with E4 gene expression driven by mouse alpha-inhibin promoter	143
293-ORF6 (E1A/B+, E4(ORF6)+)	E1-, E4-	293 derivative expressing E4-ORF6 from metallothionein promoter	99
IGRP2 (E1A/B+, E4(ORF6/7)+)	E1-, E4-	293 derivative with ORF 6 and 7 of E4 driven by MMTV-LTR promoter	144
VK2-20 & VK10-9 (E1A/B+, pIX+ E4+)	E1-, E4-, pIX-	293 derivative expressing E4 and pIX from MMTV-LTR or metallothionein promoters allows larger genes to be inserted in E1 region	145
293 (E1A/B+, pTP+)	E1-, TP-	293 derivative expressing terminal protein inducible by tetracycline	146
293 (E1A/B+, pTP+, pol+)	E1-, TP-, pol-	293 derivative expressing both terminal protein and DNA polymerase	145,147
293-C2 (E1+, E2A+)	E1-, E2A-	293 derivative with 5.9 kb fragment of Ad5 containing E2a region	148
AE1-2a (E1A/B+, E2A+)	E1-, E2A-	Lung epidermal carcinoma line A549 derivative transformed by E1 and E2A gene under glucocorticoid responsive promoters	60
293-Cre (E1A/B+, Cre+)	All viral genes (with lox containing helper)	293 derivative expressing cre recombinase, which excises packaging signal from helper virus	106,107,109

incompetent at 37°C (97). Such temperature-sensitive vectors can be propagated at 32°C but cannot replicate in the mammalian host at 37°C even if E1-like activities were present. Further, if homologous recombination in 293 cells during production results in a E1+ viral genome, the ability to replicate in a mammalian host is not restored. In vivo studies show that this defect reduces the inflammatory response following vector administration and permits larger transgene expression (98). However, the temperature-sensitive mutation is unstable and partially replication competent at 37°C.

Other mutations in early genes have been utilized in Ad vectors, including partial and complete E2 and E4 deletions. Both of these genes are essential for viral replication and therefore necessitate the production of cell lines that complement both the E2 or E4 deletion as well as the E1 deletion. In general, this has been achieved using 293 cells transfected with the appropriate E2 or E4 gene driven by an inducible promoter (Table 2). In a typical example, E4-deleted vectors were constructed in a cell line which expressed the E4 OFR6 behind an inducible metallothionine promoter (99). Cell lines of this type are more difficult to work with than 293 cells, and the efficiency of vector production is often lower. Data on whether additional genomic deletions result in a blunted immune response and whether this translates into longer persistence of transgene expression are inconsistent. Some studies are complicated by the immune response to the foreign transgene as well as to the vector and by the tendency of the commonly used CMV promoter to be inactivated over time without vector elimination. For example, one report (100) indicates that a complete E4 deletion has no effect on the time course of gene expression in immunocompetent animals after administration to lung or liver. This is at variance with another report (83) showing that E4 deletion results in a reduced immune response and longer transgene expression. The details of vector construction, route of administration, dose, and genotype of the recipient are critical to the efficacy of

E4 (and other) deletion(s). It is likely that studies in humans will be necessary to determine if additional genomic deletions have an impact on the duration of expression of the therapeutic gene and whether this translates into a significant clinical impact.

C. E3 Restored Vectors

The E3 region encodes genes that repress host response to infection by both reducing antigen presentation on the cell surface and protecting infected cells against tumor necrosis factor-α (TNF) and/or fas/fasL-mediated apoptosis. E3 is deleted in most adenovirus vectors to make room for the transgene within the length constraints of packaging. Arguing that E3 expression might increase persistence of vectors, several groups have sought to restore one or more E3 functions. In mice, expression of the E3gp19K protein has been shown to reduce MHC class I expression in vitro (101) and reduce cytotoxic T lymphocyte levels in vivo (102), but there are contradictory results as to whether this translates into prolonged persistence (101,103). On the other hand, two studies have shown that the whole E3 region does in fact prolong vector persistence in vivo. This is true whether the E3 region is expressed from an exogenous promoter in the E1 region (104) or expressed from its own promoter in the normal position (105). Since E1 function is required for E3 expression, the latter result is surprising and may indicate that a low level of E3 expression is sufficient to prolong persistence. As with other modifications of the viral backbone, the critical question is if the expression of $E3^+$ vectors would be longer in humans when administered in the route intended for therapy. This has not yet been answered.

D. Helper-Dependent Vectors

On the premise that any adenoviral gene expression would cause an immune response, some investigators have developed methods to eliminate all the adenovirus genes from the vector. In fact, the size constraints imposed by some large genes such as dystrophin require that most of the Ad genome be deleted simply to make space for the therapeutic gene and promoter. But deletion of all adenovirus genes requires that those functions be provided in trans for vector production. This is achieved by using helper viruses that are deficient in packaging. In an early implementation, a helper virus with defective packaging signals was used, which is packaged into virion with much lower efficiency than the therapeutic virus, which has two intact packaging signals. By this method, a mixed lysate is formed with two viruses that differ in size and therefore can be separated on cesium chloride equilibrium density gradients (5).

A refinement of this technology utilizes the lox/Cre system to negatively select for helper virus in a coinfection of helper and helper-dependent virus vectors (106–109). In the lox/Cre system, the DNA recombinase Cre from bacteriophage lambda efficiently mediates recombination between lox sites; thus sequences between two lox sites in the same orientation are deleted. A helper virus called psi5 has been engineered that has lox sites flanking the packaging signal so that Cre recombinase excises the packaging signal and prevents packaging of the genome. The psi5 vector propagates normally in 293 cells but packages inefficiently in 293 derivatives expressing the Cre recombinase. Coinfection of psi5 and helper-dependent vector results primarily in packaging of the helper-dependent vector using proteins specified by the psi5 genome.

The utility of helper-dependent vectors is not yet established. The efficiency of gene transfer in vitro is comparable to first-generation vectors. The data in vivo is limited but suggests a considerably longer duration of transgene expression compared to first-generation vectors (108,110). According to one report (110), a helper-dependent vector expressing the human α_1-antitrypsin cDNA can be administered to immunocompetent mice and result in prolonged gene expression with little decline over 10 months. But in that study expression from a first-generation vector declined by only 10-fold over the same time period, which differs from the data reported by other groups. In contrast (107), a helper-dependent vector with a smaller genomic deletion was eliminated even faster after intravenous administration to mice than a first-generation vector. The difference between these two observations may rest in the retention of the E4 gene in the latter case or possibly in the size of the overall genome.

E. Sero-Switch Vectors

The induction of neutralizing antibodies is presumably one of the barriers against successful readministration of the same Ad gene-transfer vector. In experimental animals, this has been observed for intravenous (111), intratracheal (74,112), and intraperitoneal (65) administration where the vector is exposed to antibodies prior to contact with the tissue. Effective readministration of the same vector has also been demonstrated to not be possible using direct tissue injection (113).

Since prior infection by one Ad does not protect against infection by a different serotype (96), using different serotypes of gene therapy vector should allow readministration of the same transgene. Extensive testing of this concept is difficult because existing vectors are only of serotypes 2 and 5 since the E1 functions of these two viruses can be efficiently complemented by the 293 cell line. For example

(Fig. 5), when rats were administered intratracheally with Ad of serotype 2 expressing β-glucuronidase, there was expression, which peaked at 3 days and declined to undetectable levels by 14 days. Readministration of the same vector resulted in a very low level of gene expression due to the immune response to the first vector administration. A second administration of a vector expressing the same transgene but of serotype 5 resulted in a level of gene expression at day 1 comparable to that seen in a naive rat. The decline to baseline was faster than in naive animals, probably due to the elimination of infected cells by the cellular immune system using epitopes conserved between serotypes 2 and 5 (96).

These data posed the question as to which epitopes are responsible for preventing readministration of the same serotype. Vectors have been constructed with the capsid of serotype 5 but with the fiber gene of serotype 7a (114). Fortunately, the fiber protein from serotype 7a interacts with the penton base of serotype 5 allowing the assembly of serotype 7a/5 chimeric capsids In vivo experiments show that the fiber switch from 5 to 7a does not facilitate readministration, suggesting that the immune response to fiber is not the barrier that prevents readministration of the same serotype (114). This is consistent with the concept that the primary humoral immune response is directed to the external loops of the hexon protein. Vectors have been constructed in which the hexon gene of Ad5 has been replaced by that of Ad serotype 2 (115). Even though the level of serological cross-reaction between the pure Ad5 capsid and the variant with hexon from Ad2 was low, the hexon switch did not allow successful readministration in vivo. This illustrates the importance of other arms of the immune system and the diversity of epitopes that are involved in immune response to gene-therapy vectors.

It is not clear if sero-switching is a viable strategy for long-term gene therapy. First, the difficulty of making efficient complementing cell lines for viruses of different subgroups is considerable. Second, the delivery of a therapeutic gene to the target tissue and its subsequent expression would not necessarily be the same among serotypes. Finally, even if this could be achieved, the therapeutic advantage of expressing the transgene once for a few days rather than several times for a few days might not be all that great in terms of genetic disease, where persistent gene therapy is needed.

F. Vectors with Modified Tropism

The specificity of adenoviral infections in vitro is dictated by the presence of the CAR receptor and integrins. The role of these receptors in vivo is less certain since the cell types to which a vector is exposed becomes a critical issue. Since a majority of vector administered intravenously in rodents is found in the liver, gene therapy for other tissues requires a delivery system to the target. For lung epithelium, intratracheal administration is feasible. Direct injection is possible in some other applications, for example, into the myocardium or directly into a tumor. But vector that is inadvertently injected into capillaries or drains into the circulation through the lymphatic system will find its way to the liver. Alternatively, there are cells types such as B cells that are very difficult to infect with type 5 Ad vectors. These considerations raise questions about whether vectors can be retargeted to cells or tissues of interest, or at least if the expression of the transgene could be limited to that tissue.

Many vectors use the CMV immediate/early promoter/enhancer, which was chosen on the basis that it directs a high level of transgene expression and is expressed in most tissues studied. But many times, expression in a specific tissue or cell type is more desirable and expression in other tissues might be toxic. Therefore, the promoters of genes specific to a cell type have sometimes been used for specific applications (116–119). For example, carcinoembryonic antigen (CEA) and α-fetoprotein (AFP) are tumor-specific antigens that are not expressed by normal cells. When a therapeutic gene is expressed from an Ad vector with a AFP promoter, expression should be confined to specific tumor cells expressing AFP and not normal cells. Kaneko et al. (117) have shown this theory to be correct and have further demonstrated that the expected selectivity is maintained in vivo. In this context, the vector Av1AFPTK1 [expressing thymidine kinase from herpes simplex virus (HSV-TK) from the AFP promoter] can prevent tumor growth in gancyclovir-treated nude mice implanted with a AFP-expressing tumor cell line but not in identical mice implanted with a control (non–AFP-expressing) tumor cell line. By contrast, the vector Av1TK1, which expresses HSV-TK from the Rous sarcoma virus promoter, protects gancyclovir-treated nude mice no matter which cell line is used to transduce the tumor.

Alternatively, modifications of the fiber/high affinity receptor interaction or the penton/integrin interaction might be used to modify tissue tropism. In this context, the seroswitch vectors described above (114,115) as well as capsid chimeras with part of the Ad3 fiber (120–122) or the fiber gene from Ad17 (123) might be more effective in certain tissues since, a priori, serotypes of different wild-type adenoviruses with different known pathologies should target different tissues. The initial choice of Ad5 as a vector for gene therapy rested partially on its tropism for airway epithelium, which was also the intended target for gene therapy in cystic fibrosis, the first disease treated with adenoviral vectors in humans (124).

Some groups have taken the approach of directly screening for serotypes that replicate preferentially in brain or lung epithelium. In both cases, wild-type strains were screened for efficient replication and certain subgroup D viruses, including serotype 17, were identified to replicate more efficiently. On this basis, a serotype 2 virus with the fiber from Ad17 was constructed and used to study infection of various cell types in vitro. This hybrid is much more efficient at gene transfer to human umbilical vein endothelial cells, neurons, glioma cell lines, and lung epithelial cells than the pure Ad2 gene transfer vector (123). However, it is sufficiently proficient in infecting 293 cells that it can still be propagated and titered for production purposes. It is not known if this translates into better gene transfer efficiency in vivo.

A number of other approaches to modifying tropism have been identified. For example, the fiber protein can tolerate some manipulation without impairing virus production. The determination of the three-dimensional structure of fiber assists in the identification of domains where insertions might be tolerated without grossly affecting structure. An early modification to fiber was the addition of an oligolysine motif to the N terminal of the fiber protein, giving the virus an affinity for polyanions such as heparin sulfate (125). This profoundly affects the cells types that can be infected in vitro, allowing cells lacking CAR, such as vascular smooth muscle cells and B cells, to be infected. It has also been shown that this oligolysine addition allows for more efficient gene transfer to smooth muscle cells in vivo. Additional manipulations (summarized in Table 3) have been described to modify the tropism of Ad vectors. The interaction of integrin and penton base has been modified both by elimination of the RGD motif in penton base (23) and by its replacement by the LDV motif, which should promote interaction with $\alpha_4\beta_1$ integrins, characteristic of B cells (23). Modest changes in specificity can be obtained in this way. In addition, the RGD motif has been added to the knob of fiber, resulting in a greatly enhanced infection of a number of CAR-deficient cell types such as primary human fibroblasts and ovarian cancer cells (45,126).

Bispecific antibodies have been used as a reagent to direct Ad towards particular cell types (127–129). For example, using a bispecific antibody conjugate with one arm

Table 3 Examples of Retargeting of Adenovirus Gene-Transfer Vectors

Modification	Target	Rationale	Refs.
Ad5(fiber7a)	Cells expressing Ad7 high affinity receptors	Replace whole of Ad5 fiber by that of Ad7a (subgroup B)	114
Penton LDV	Lymphocytes, monocytes	Replace RGD $\alpha_v\beta_5$-binding motif in penton base by LDV, which interacts with $\alpha_4\beta_1$ integrin	23
Conjugations to anti-Ad Fabs	Tumor cells	Conjugate ligands (e.g., FGF, folate) to Fab fragments specific to fiber; bind to vector before delivery to cells bearing cognate receptor	149,150
Bifunctional antibody	Tumor cells	Retarget to EGFR-expressing cells; bind virus with bispecific antibody against EGFR and Ad fiber	127
Bifunctional antibody	Smooth muscle cells, endothelium	Create vector with penton modified to express defined epitope (Ad-FLAG); use bi-specific antibody vs. FLAG and α_v integrin (or E selectin) to target cells expressing α_v integrin (or E selectin)	128
Bispecific antibody (antiCD3)	T cells	Use AdFLAG vector and bispecific antibody (AntiFLAG, antiCD3) to target CD3+ T cells	129
Oligolysine	Cells with surface heparin sulfate	Add seven lysine residues to C-terminus of fiber	125
Fiber RGD	Cells expressing $\alpha_v\beta_3$ and $\alpha_v\beta_5$ integrins	Add RGD integrin binding motif to knob of fiber	45,126
Ad5(fiber 17)	Endothelium, lung epithelium, brain	Replace fiber gene of Ad2 vector with that of Ad17 (subgroup D)	123
Ad5/9 (short shaft)	Melanoma, glioma, smooth muscle cells	Place knob of Ad9 on shaft of Ad5 after 8 repeats	151

EGFR: Epidermal growth factor receptor.

binding the Ad fiber and the other binding the epidermal growth factor (EGF) receptor (127), is was possible to increase the specificity of Ad vectors towards glioma cell lines with low levels of CAR but high levels of the EGF receptor.

V. APPLICATIONS

Before commencing human clinical studies, batches of virus must be produced under FDA current good manufacturing practice (cGMP) conditions and subjected to testing. One of the primary foci of such testing was to prove there is no replication-competent adenovirus in the preparations. While it is possible to make small batches of virus free of RCA sufficient for small phase I trials on a few patients, making enough for large clinical studies or marketing is a significant challenge. If the frequency of homologous recombination to make RCA is estimated as 1 in 10^{12}, then making batches of 10^{15} particles essentially free of RCA is a major hurdle. This has been the driving force behind the production of cell lines less likely to produce RCA than the 293 cells. In addition, issues of reproducibility in large-scale production, formulation, and distribution will need to be solved before more extensive use of Ad vectors might become possible.

Human clinical studies also require prior say studies in experimental animals. The design of toxicity studies is complicated by the life cycle of human adenoviruses, which renders them replication competent only in human cells. When they infect rodent cells, the life cycle is aborted before DNA replication commences. Therefore, the complications of contaminating RCA, or RCA generated by recombination with endogenous adenoviruses, cannot be predicted in rodent studies. In addition, some serotypes of Ad are actually oncogenic in rodents but not in humans.

Data on models of disease in experimental animals provided sufficient basis to proceed to adenovirus vector-mediated gene transfer in humans. A number of small phase I/II trials have been commenced for various indications (Table 4): Most of the early studies were directed at cystic fibrosis, but about three quarters of protocols use either a pro-drug activation strategy or anti-oncogenes in attempts to treat cancers. There is one protocol to study metabolic disease (ornithine transcarbamoylase deficiency), three protocols to use adenoviruses for angiogenesis, and two protocols to study gene therapy in normal subjects.

The most significant observation in the clinical studies to date is that at doses compatible with therapy there have been no serious side effects attributable to the transgene or vector. Although the numbers of patients involved in each study is small, there are now hundreds of patients who have received adenovirus gene therapy. In addition to showing safety, several studies have shown that there is also effective delivery of the vector to the patient and subsequent expression of the therapeutic gene. Demonstrations of actual therapeutic benefit have been more elusive, and none of the anecdotal reports of clinical benefit have yet received careful, placebo-controlled testing.

A. Pulmonary

When gene therapy is conceived as the addition of a good copy of a defective gene, it is natural that the initial focus would be on genetic diseases such as cystic fibrosis. As described above, the feasibility of intratracheal administration to the lung was demonstrated in animals and the first clinical trial of an adenovirus vector was to the lung of CF patients (124). The initial study was a dose-escalating safety study in which vector was administered to the bronchi in 20 mL of fluid. It became clear that this volume was not well tolerated, and so subsequent studies used smaller volumes or a spray of aerosolized vector into the bronchi. The relative accessibility of the site of administration allows that samples of respiratory epithelium can be recovered by bronchial brushing and the presence of vector and therapeutic gene expression can be assessed repetitively. By sensitive quantitative PCR methods, the expression of the CFTR gene delivered by the vector is seen at the site of administration at vector doses of $\geq 5 \times 10^8$ pfu. The level of vector-derived CFTR mRNA is approximately 5% of the level of expression of the endogenous CFTR gene, which is believed to be sufficient for therapeutic effect. However, this level of expression is only achieved for a period of a few days, and expression rapidly declines to baseline by 30 days (130). Interestingly, the administration of the vector to the airway does not lead to a significant immune response against adenovirus reflected in either neutralizing antibodies or adenovirus-specific T-cell proliferation.

Since the initial safety of vectors expressing CFTR was demonstrated, a study with repetitive administration has been completed. The important result of this study is that expression is reduced or eliminated in subsequent administrations as expected from the data from experimental animals, presumably from the immune response to the first dose (130).

B. Metabolic

To date, only one study of adenoviral vectors for metabolic disease has begun. This is not surprising since the animal data suggests only a short time of expression of genes delivered by Ad vectors to the liver; i.e., this therapy, if successful, would only be applicable to acute metabolic crises. Ornithine transcarbamylase (OTC) deficiency is a recessive metabolic disorder of nitrogen metabolism. A $E1^-$, $E4^-$ deleted adenovirus vector ex-

Table 4 Clinical Studies with Adenovirus Gene Transfer Vectors[a]

Category	Indication	Transgene	Therapeutic strategy	Route of administration	Investigator
Cancer	Mesothelioma	HSV-TK	Local pro-drug activation	Intrapleural	S. Albelda
	B7.1	Renal cell carcinoma	Immunotherapy	Subcutaneous	S. J. Antonia
	Squamous cell carcinoma (head and neck)	p53	Growth suppressor gene	Intratumor	R. Beau
	Hepatocellular carcinoma	p53	Growth suppressor gene	Intratumor	C. Belani
	Prostate cancer	p53	Growth suppressor gene	Intratumor	A. Belldegrun
	Neuroblastoma	IL-2	Immunotherapy	Subcutaneous	L. Bowman
	Neuroblastoma	IL-2	Immunotherapy	Subcutaneous	M. Brenner
	Squamous cell carcinoma (head and neck)	p53	Growth suppressor gene	Intratumor	G. Clayman
	Hepatic metastases	Cytosine deaminase	Local pro-drug activation	Intratumor	R. Crystal
	Ovarian cancer	Anti-erbB-2 single chain antibody	Immunotherapy	Intraperitoneal	D. Curiel
	Non-small cell lung cancer	GM-CSF	Immunostimulation	Subcutaneous	G. Dranoff
	Melanoma	GM-CSF	Immunostimulation	Subcutaneous	G. Dranoff
	Squamous cell carcinoma (head and neck)	p53	Growth suppressor gene	Intratumor	R. Dreicer
	MART-1	Melanoma	Immunotherapy	Intradermal or intravenous	J. S. Economou
	CNS cancer	HSV-TK	Local pro-drug activation	Intratumor	S. Eck
	Prostate cancer	HSV-TK	Local pro-drug activation	Intratumor	T. A. Gardner
	CNS malignancy	HSV-TK	Local pro-drug activation	Intratumor	R. Grossman
	Prostate cancer	HSV-TK	Local pro-drug activation	Intratumor	S. Hall and S. Woo
	Prostate cancer	HSV-TK	Local pro-drug activation	Intratumor	D. Kadmon
	Ovarian cancer	HSV-TK	Local pro-drug activation	Intraperitoneal	D. Kieback
	Chronic lymphocytic leukemia	CD154	Immunotherapy	Autologous cells	T. Kipps
	Malignant glioma	p53	Growth suppressor gene	Intratumor	F. F. Lang
	Glioblastoma	HSV-TK	Local pro-drug activation	Intratumor	F. Lieberman
	Prostate cancer	p53	Growth suppressor gene	Intratumor	C. Logothetis
	Breast cancer	p53	Growth suppressor gene	Subcutaneous	M. Mehren
	Melanoma	HSV-TK	Local pro-drug activation	Intratumor	J. C. Morris
	Ovarian cancer	p53	Growth suppressor gene	Intraperitoneal	C. Y. Muller
	Squamous cell carcinoma (head and neck)	HSV-TK	Local pro-drug activation	Intratumor	B. O'Malley
	Prostate cancer	E1B	Cytolytic adenovirus	Intratumor	J. Simons
	Breast cancer	B7.1	Immunotherapy	Intratumor	L. Schuchter
	Non–small-cell lung cancer	p53	Growth suppressor gene	Intratumor	S. Swisher
	Non–small-cell lung cancer	p53	Growth suppressor gene	Intratumor	J. Roth
	Melanoma	GM-CSF	Immunotherapy	Intradermal and subcutaneous	T. Suzuki
	Hepatic metastasis	HSV-TK	Local pro-drug activation	Intratumor	M. Sung
	Bladder cancer	Retinoblastoma	Growth suppressor gene	Intravesical	E. Small
	Prostate cancer	HSV-TK	Local pro-drug activation	Intratumor	P. Scardino
	Non–small-cell lung cancer	HSV-TK	Local pro-drug activation	Intratumor	W. Rom and S. Woo
	Melanoma	MART-1	Immunotherapy	Subcutaneous	S. Rosenberg
	Hepatic metastases	p53	Growth suppressor gene	Hepatic artery	A. Venook
	Ovarian cancer	p53	Growth suppressor gene	Intraperitoneal	J. K. Wolf
Cardiovascular	Cardiac artery disease	VEGF	Angiogenesis	Intramyocardial	R. Crystal
	Peripheral vascular disease	VEGF121	Angiogenesis	Intramuscular	R. Crystal
	Coronary artery disease	VEGF121	Angiogenesis	Intramyocardial	R. Crystal
	Cardiac artery disease	FGF-4	Angiogenesis	Intracoronary	J. Lee

Table 4 (Continued)

Category	Indication	Transgene	Therapeutic strategy	Route of administration	Investigator
Genetic disease	Cystic fibrosis	CFTR	Genetic defect	Intranasal	R. Boucher
	Cystic fibrosis	CFTR	Genetic defect	Airway instillation	R. Crystal
	Cystic fibrosis	CFTR	Genetic defect	Intrabronchial aerosol	R. Crystal
	Cystic fibrosis	CFTR	Genetic defect	Aerosol to airways	H. Dorkin
	Cystic fibrosis	CFTR	Genetic defect	Instillation to airways	H. Dorkin
	Cystic fibrosis	CFTR	Genetic defect	Intrasinus	M. Welsh
	Cystic fibrosis	CFTR	Genetic defect	Intranasal	M. Welsh
	Cystic fibrosis	CFTR	Genetic defect	Intranasal/Airways	R. Wilmott
	Cystic fibrosis	CFTR	Genetic defect	Airway instillation	J. Wilson
Metabolic	Ornithine transcarbamylase deficiency	Ornithine transcarbamylase	Genetic defect	Autologous blood cells	M. Batshaw
Normal	Normal subjects	Cytosine deaminase	Measure immune parameters	Intradermal	R. Crystal
	Normal subjects	Cytosine deaminase	Measure immune parameters	Intratracheal	R. Crystal

[a] Trials that have been submitted to the NIH recombinant DNA advisory committee as of February 1999.
CFTR: Cystic fibrosis transmembrane regulator; HSV-TK: herpes simplex virus-thymidine kinase; GM-CSF: granulocyte-macrophage colony-stimulating factor; erbB-2: truncated EGF receptor oncogene; MART-1: melanoma-specific antigen; VEGF121: 121 amino acid form of vascular endothelial growth factor; FGF4: fibroblast growth factor-4; CD154: CD40 ligand, T-cell costimulatory molecules.

pressing the cDNA for OTC was constructed and administered by the intrahepatic route to adults with partial OTC deficiency and safety parameters and the efficiency of gene transfer are currently being assessed. A report of a death in this trial at high doses ($>10^{13}$ particle units, intrahepatic route) suggests that the maximum safe dose is below this level.

C. Oncologic

Due to the unknown safety profile of adenovirus vectors, it was generally easier to design the early human trials for life-threatening disease. A number of approaches were devised to target cancer; 39 out of 56 trials listed are directed towards malignant disease (Table 4). Three basic approaches can be identified: local pro-drug activation, tumor suppressor genes, and immunotherapy.

One of the first strategies of human gene therapy for cancer was to locally deliver novel enzymes that metabolize prodrugs into the active chemotherapy agent. The general concept of these studies is that local activation of the prodrug in the tumor will concentrate the active agent in the tumor, thus limiting the systemic toxicity from the active drug. Two genes have been used in human clinical trials: the herpes simplex virus thymidine kinase gene (HSV-TK) and the *E. coli* cytosine deaminase (CD) gene. The HSV-TK protein activates the prodrug gancyclovir to gancyclovir monophosphate, an inhibitor of DNA polymerase. For CD, the prodrug is 5-fluorocytosine, which is activated by CD into the active chemotherapeutic agent 5-fluorouracil. For both agents and activating enzymes, a theoretical benefit is the bystander effect in which active drug would be excreted from the infected cells to kill the neighboring cells of the tumor. Thus, it is not essential to infect every cell of the tumor with the adenovirus vector.

Currently active protocols apply the prodrug strategy to many types of cancer, including prostate cancer, central nervous system (CNS) malignancies, ovarian cancer, mesothelioma, hepatic metastases of colon cancer, and squamous cell carcinoma of the head and neck (Table 4). Most studies involve phase I/II studies with intratumoral injection of escalating doses of vector prior to chemotherapy with the prodrug and subsequent scheduled surgery. Tumor removal provides samples for analysis of vector levels, expression of the therapeutic gene, and activation of prodrug and histological studies for cell death and inflammation. The primary endpoint of these studies is safety, which has been established in some cases.

Tumor supressor genes have also been used in human clinical studies: p53 (for ovarian cancer, prostate cancer, squamous cancer of the head and neck, breast cancer, non–small-cell lung cancer, hepatic carcinoma and hepatic metastases), retinoblastoma susceptibility gene (for bladder cancer) and anti-erbB-2 single-chain antibodies (for ovarian cancer) (Table 4). The concept is that tumor cells have defective tumor supressor genes that cannot limit cell division, but restoration of the wild-type gene will limit cell division. The theoretical limitation of using antiproliferative genes for tumor therapy is that they will only inhibit proliferation of the cell they infect and have no *cis* effect on neighboring cells. The trial designs are generally similar to those for the prodrug strategy.

A novel antiproliferative approach has been used in human studies using conditionally replication-competent viruses (131). As described above, the E1B gene is essential for viral replication by protecting adenovirus-infected cells from apoptosis, and its mode of action is through interaction with p53. It follows that E1B function would only be effective in p53-positive cells, but not in p53-deficient tumor cells, therefore, the absence of E1B results in p53-dependent apoptosis and no viral replication in normal cells, but replication can occur in p53-negative cells. In this context, E1A-positive, E1B-negative viruses have been demonstrated in animal models to show selective cytolytic effects against tumors. The same viruses have been used in phase I and phase II studies of human ovarian cancers, pancreatic cancer, and head and neck cancer with direct intratumoral injection in conjunction with chemotherapy. These studies are now being extended to phase III testing.

A third general approach to adenovirus gene therapy for cancers has used immunostimulatory genes (Table 4). Several different genes have been used in human studies, including CD40 ligand for chronic lymphocytic leukemia, granulocyte-macrophage colony-stimulating factor for melanoma and non–small-cell lung cancer, interleukin-2 for neuroblastoma, MART-1 (a melanoma-specific antigen) and B7 (CD80) for melanoma. The concept of immunostimulatory gene therapy is to promote the natural immune surveillance and elimination of tumors that express abnormal antigens by giving a general boost to the cellular immune system (e.g., with IL-2) or a with a tumor-specific antigen (e.g., MART-1).

D. Cardiovascular

With the observation that there is only short-term gene expression from Ad vectors, the question arose as to which medical applications might benefit from transient expression of a therapeutic gene. The general area of tissue repair and engineering emerged as a good candidate where secreted growth factors would initiate the desired cascade of tissue remodeling, which, once initiated, would not require the continuous presence of the therapeutic gene. For example, expression of vascular endothelial growth factor (VEGF) after injection of a Ad vector expressing VEGF into rat retroperitoneal fat pad is brief, reverting to baseline after 10 days (Fig. 7). In contrast, the VEGF protein induces an angiogenic response that persists long after the stimulus has disappeared.

Three tissue-remodeling protocols have reached phase I clinical studies using VEGF or fibroblast growth factor 4 for therapeutic angiogenesis. The growth of new blood vessels in the ischemic heart is a particularly significant potential application due to the large patient population (74,132).

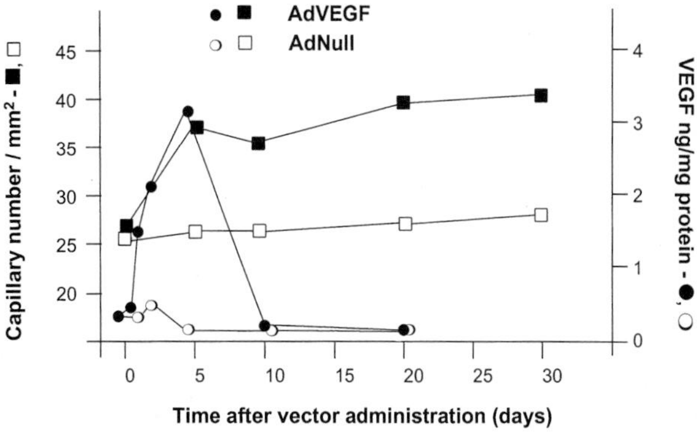

Figure 7 Time course of gene expression and anatomical response after administration of Ad expressing vascular endothelial growth factor (VEGF). The retroperitoneal fat pad of rats was injected with 5×10^8 pfu of either AdVEGF (a first-generation $E1^-E3^-$ vector expressing the 165-amino-acid form of human VEGF, solid symbols) or the control vector expressing no transgene (AdNull, open symbols). At intervals, animals were anesthetized, a laporatomy performed, and the fat pad photographed. The number of vessels crossing a circle of 1 cm diameter centered on the injection site were measured (left axis—□, ■). The fat pad was also homogenized and the level of VEGF determined by ELISA (right axis—○, ●). (From Ref. 140.)

E. Normals

The early Ad gene therapy trials demonstrated that, while effective gene transfer could be achieved, persistence of expression is clearly a problem for Ad vectors. While there was clearly an immune response to the vector and possibly the transgene itself, the biology of that response is not well understood. Animal models, particularly those involving inbred mice, have limited utility in predicting the immune response in humans. To assess the human host response to Ad vectors, two trials with normal subjects are ongoing using intradermal or intratracheal administration of an Ad vector expressing the *E. coli* cytosine deaminase (CD) gene. The intent of these trials is to describe the immune response in humans to an $E1^-$, $E3^-$ Ad vector to provide a background to assess more advanced vectors on a rational basis.

VI. FUTURE PROSPECTS

A. Decreasing Vector Elimination

A number of approaches have been developed that should reduce the immune response to Ad vectors, prolong transgene expression, and enhance the efficiency of readministration. The basic hypothesis is that by reducing adenoviral gene expression, there should be a decrease in the host response to the vector and an increase in persistence. This is observed in some experimental animal models but not others. The basic problem posed by these data is whether prolonged persistence and reduced host response will be observed in humans with an administration route compatible with treatment. The only way to answer this question will be to perform the appropriate clinical studies in humans.

The limitations of Ad have prompted some investigators to make hybrids that exploit the wide range of cell types infected by Ad but allow persistence using features of other viruses such as retroviruses (133–135). For example, retroviruses can be produced in situ by coinfection of cells by two Ad vectors (134). The first Ad contains the expression cassette for the therapeutic gene flanked by the retrovirus terminal repeats with the necessary *cis* sequences for packaging, all of this being transcribed from a CMV promoter. The second Ad expresses the *trans* factors (pol/gag/env) required for assembly of infectious retroviral particles, which will then infect the neighboring cells and result in long-term gene therapy. The use of such hybrids has been demonstrated both in vitro and in vivo but does not overcome the need of retroviral vectors for dividing cells, a limitation that might be overcome by making Ad/lentivirus hybrids or Ad/adenoassociated virus hybrids (136,137).

Phage display technology has provided an approach to selecting a peptide sequence with desirable binding properties. This has been exploited in selecting phages that target different tissues after intravenous injection, presumably through interacting with the endothelium of that tissue. It is likely that these peptide motifs can be incorporated into the knob of the adenovirus fiber to facilitate targeting of adenovirus vectors to a desired tissue. This requires that the knob-modified vector be able to propagate in 293 cells, but strategies have been developed to over-come this production hurdle (120,138).

B. Applications for Transient Gene Therapy

The technical innovations described above are at best laboratory proofs that will require extensive animal studies before clinical testing. But the clinical data to date suggest that success with currently available Ad vectors is possible in applications where transient expression might be sufficient. For example, studies of therapeutic angiogenesis for coronary artery disease described above are a prototype of this type of application. Medical indications like cancer, infectious disease, and tissue remodeling (angiogenesis, recovery from surgery, stroke, or injury) are areas in which development might be most appropriate. On the other hand, metabolic and genetic disease, auto-immune disease, and other chronic conditions would seem to need substantial advances in adenoviral vector design or more likely some kind of hybrid vector before they become treatable on a persistent basis. Importantly, the knowledge of the cellular and host response to Ad infection in humans is still quite rudimentary and will need to be described in much greater detail before more rational approaches to prolonging expression can be devised.

ACKNOWLEDGMENTS

We thank N. Mohamed for help with this manuscript. These studies were supported, in part, by the NIH PO1 HL51746, PO1 HL59312, HL 57318; the Will Rogers Memorial Fund, Los Angeles, CA; Cystic Fibrosis Foundation, Bethesda, MD; and Gen Vec, Inc., Rockville, MD.

REFERENCES

1. Brody SI, Crystal RG. Adenovirus-mediated in vivo gene transfer. Ann NY Acad Sci 1994; 716:90–101.
2. O'Neal WK, Beaudet AL. Somatic gene therapy for cystic fibrosis. Hum Mol Genet 1994; 3:1497–1502.
3. Ali M, Lemoine NR, Ring CJ. The use of DNA viruses as vectors for gene therapy. Gene Ther 1994; 1:367–384.
4. Mitani K, Clemens PR, Moseley AB, Caskey CT. Gene transfer therapy for heritable disease: cell and expression targeting. Philos Trans R Soc Lond B Biol Sci 1993; 339: 217–224.
5. Mitani K, Graham FL, Caskey CT, Kochanek S. Rescue, propagation, and partial purification of a helper virus-dependent adenovirus vector. Proc Natl Acad Sci USA 1995; 92:3854–3858.
6. Chirmule N, Hughes JV, Gao GP, Raper SE, Wilson JM. Role of E4 in eliciting CD4 T-cell and B-cell responses to adenovirus vectors delivered to murine and nonhuman primate lungs. J Virol 1998; 72:6138–6145.
7. Molnar-Kimber KL, Sterman DH, Chang M, Kang EH, ElBash M, Lanuti M, Elshami A, Gelfand K, Wilson JM, Kaiser LR, Albelda SM. Impact of preexisting and induced humoral and cellular immune responses in an adenovirus-based gene therapy phase I clinical trial for localized mesothelioma. Human Gene Ther 1998; 9:2121–2133.
8. Peeters MJ, Patijn GA, Lieber A, Meuse L, Kay MA. Adenovirus-mediated hepatic gene transfer in mice: comparison of intravascular and biliary administration. Human Gene Ther 1996; 7:1693–1699.
9. Song W, Kong HL, Traktman P, Crystal RG. Cytotoxic T lymphocyte responses to proteins encoded by heterologous transgenes transferred in vivo by adenoviral vectors. Human Gene Ther 1997; 8:1207–1217.
10. Tripathy SK, Black HB, Goldwasser E, Leiden JM. Immune responses to transgene-encoded proteins limit the

stability of gene expression after injection of replication-defective adenovirus vectors. Nat Med 1996; 2:545–550.
11. Worgall S, Wolff G, Falck-Pedersen E, Crystal RG. Innate immune mechanisms dominate elimination of adenoviral vectors following in vivo administration. Human Gene Ther 1997; 8:37–44.
12. Horwitz MS. In: Fields BN, Knipe DM, Howley PM, eds. Fields Virology. Philadelphia: Lippincott-Raven 1996: 2149.
13. Ginsberg HS, Prince GA. The molecular basis of adenovirus pathogenesis. Infect Agents Dis 1994; 3:1–8.
14. Shinozaki T, Araki K, Ushijima H, Fujii R, Eshita Y. Use of Graham 293 cells in suspension for isolating enteric adenoviruses from the stools of patients with acute gastroenteritis. J Infect Dis 1987; 156:246.
15. Bailey A, Mautner V. Phylogenetic relationships among adenovirus serotypes. Virology 1994; 205:438–452.
16. Shenk T. In: Fields BN, Knipe DM, Howley PM, eds. Fields Virology. Philadelphia: Lippincott-Raven, 1996: 2111.
17. Athappilly FK, Murali R, Rux JJ, Cai Z, Burnett RM. The refined crystal structure of hexon, the major coat protein of adenovirus type 2, at 2.9 A resolution. J Mol Biol 1994; 242:430–455
18. Crawford-Miksza L, Schnurr DP. Analysis of 15 adenovirus hexon proteins reveals the location and structure of seven hypervariable regions containing serotype-specific residues. J Virol 1996; 70:1836–1844.
19. Roelvink PW, Lizonova A, Lee JG, Li Y, Bergelson JM, Finberg RW, Brough DE, Kovesdi I, Wickham TJ. The coxsackievirus-adenovirus receptor protein can function as a cellular attachment protein for adenovirus serotypes from subgroups A, C, D, E, and F. J Virol 1998; 72: 7909–7915.
20. Bergelson JM, Cunningham JA, Droguett G, Kurt-Jones EA, Krithivas A, Hong JS, Horwitz MS, Crowell RL, Finberg RW. Isolation of a common receptor for coxsackie B viruses and adenoviruses 2 and 5. Science 1997; 275: 1320–1323.
21. Mathias P, Wickham T, Moore M, Nemerow G. Multiple adenovirus serotypes use alpha v integrins for infection. J Virol 1994; 68:6811–6814.
22. Wickham TJ, Filardo EJ, Cheresh DA, Nemerow GR. Integrin $\alpha_V\beta_5$ selectively promotes adenovirus mediated cell membrane permeabilization. J Cell Biol 1994; 127: 257–264.
23. Wickham TJ, Carrion ME, Kovesdi I. Targeting of adenovirus penton base to new receptors through replacement of its RGD motif with other receptor-specific peptide motifs. Gene Ther 1995; 2:750–756.
24. Wang K, Huang S, Kapoor-Munshi A, Nemerow G. Adenovirus internalization and infection require dynamin. J Virol 1998; 72:3455–3458.
25. Leopold PL, Ferris B, Grinberg I, Worgall S, Hackett NR, Crystal RG. Fluorescent virions: dynamic tracking of the pathway of adenoviral gene transfer vectors in living cells. Hum Gene Ther 1998; 9:367–378.
26. Greber UF, Suomalainen M, Stidwill RP, Boucke K, Ebersold MW, Helenius A. The role of the nuclear pore complex in adenovirus DNA entry. EMBO J 1997; 16: 5998–6007.
27. Miyazawa N, Leopold PL, Hackett NR, Ferris B, Worgall S, Falck-Pedersen E, Crystal RG. Fiber swap between adenovirus subgroups B and C alters intracellular trafficking of adenovirus gene transfer vectors. J Virol 1999; 73: 6056–6065.
28. Wisnivesky J, Rempel S, Ramalingam R, Leopold PL, Crystal RG. Characterization of in vitro interaction between adenovirus and purified nuclei. American Society of Gene Therapy, 1st Annual Meeting, Seattle, Washington, May 28–31, 1998.
29. Wold WS, Tollefson AE, Hermiston TW. E3 transcription unit of adenovirus. Curr Top Microbiol Immunol 1995; 199:237–274.
30. Shisler J, Yang C, Walter B, Ware CF, Gooding LR. The adenovirus E3-10.4K/14.5K complex mediates loss of cell surface Fas (CD95) and resistance to Fas-induced apoptosis. J Virol 1997; 71:8299–8306.
31. Puvion-Dutilleul F, Puvion E. Sites of transcription of adenovirus type 5 genomes in relation to early viral DNA replication in infected HeLa cells. A high resolution in situ hybridization and autoradiographical study. Biol Cell 1991; 71:135–147.
32. Alemany R, Dai Y, Lou YC, Sethi E, Prokopenko E, Josephs SF, Zhang WW. Complementation of helper-dependent adenoviral vectors: size effects and titer fluctuations. J Virol Methods 1997; 68:147–159.
33. Graham FL, Prevec L. Methods for construction of adenovirus vectors. Mol Biotechmol 1995; 3:207–220.
34. Rosenfeld MA, Siegfried W, Yoshimura K, Yoneyama K, Fukayama M, Stier LE, Paakko PK, Gilardi P, Stratford-Perricaudet LD, Perricaudet M, Jallat S, Pavirani A, Lecocq J-P, Crystal RG. Adenovirus-mediated transfer of a recombinant α1-antitrypsin gene to the lung epithelium in vivo. Science 1991; 252:431–434.
35. Rosenfeld MA, Yoshimura K, Trapnell BC, Yoneyama K, Rosenthal ER, Dalemans W, Fukayama M, Bargon J, Stier LE, Stratford-Perricaudet L, Perricaudet M, Guggino WB, Pavirani A, Lecocq J-P, Crystal RG. In vivo transfer of the human cystic fibrosis transmembrane conductance regulator gene to the airway epithelium. Cell 1992; 68: 143–155.
36. Louis N, Evelegh C, Graham FL. Cloning and sequencing of the cellular-viral junctions from the human adenovirus type 5 transformed 293 cell line. Virology 1997; 233: 423–429.
37. Graham FL, Smiley J, Russell WC, Nairn R. Characteristics of a human cell line transformed by DNA from human adenovirus type 5. J Gen Virol 1977; 36:59–74.
38. Rosenfeld MA, Rosenfeld SJ, Danel C, Banks TC, Crystal RG. Increasing expression of the normal human CFTR cDNA in cystic fibrosis epithelial cells results in a progressive increase in the level of CFTR protein expression, but a limit on the level of cAMP-stimulated chloride secretion. Human Gene Ther 1994; 5:1121–1129.

39. Bett AJ, Haddara W, Prevec L, Graham FL. An efficient and flexible system for construction of adenovirus vectors with insertions or deletions in early regions 1 and 3. Proc Natl Acad Sci USA 1994; 91:8802–8806.
40. Hehir KM, Armentano D, Cardoza LM, Choquette TL, Berthelette PB, White GA, Couture LA, Everton MB, Keegan J, Martin JM, Pratt DA, Smith MP, Smith AE, Wadsworth SC. Molecular characterization of replication-competent variants of adenovirus vectors and genome modifications to prevent their occurrence. J Virol 1996; 70:8459–8467.
41. Mittereder N, March KL, Trapnell BC. Evaluation of the concentration and bioactivity of adenovirus vectors for gene therapy. J Virol 1996; 70:7498–7509.
42. Foxwell B, Browne K, Bonderson J, Clarke C, de Martin R, Brennan F, Feldmann M. Efficient adenoviral infection with IκB alpha reveals that macrophage tumor necrosis factor alpha production in rheumatoid arthritis is NF-κB dependent. Proc Natl Acad Sci USA 1998; 95:8211–8215.
43. Cantwell MJ, Sharma S, Friedmann T, Kipps TJ. Adenovirus vector infection of chronic lymphocytic leukemia B cells. Blood 1996; 88:4676–4683.
44. Leon RP, Hedlund T, Meech SJ, Li S, Schaack J, Hunger SP, Duke RC, De Gregori J. Adenoviral-mediated gene transfer in lymphocytes. Proc Natl Acad Sci USA 1998; 95:13159–13164.
45. Hidaka C, Milano E, Leopold PL, Bergelson JM, Hackett NR, Finberg RW, Wickham TJ, Kovesdi I, Roelvink P, Crystal RG. CAR-dependent and CAR-independent pathways of adenovirus vector-mediated gene transfer and expression in human fibroblasts. J Clin Invest 1999; 103: 579–587.
46. Kaner RJ, Worgall S, Leopold PL, Stolze E, Milano E, Hidaka C, Ramalingam R, Hackett NR, Singh R, Bergelson J, Finberg R, Falck-Pedersen E, Crystal RG. Modification of the genetic program of human alveolar macrophages by adenovirus vectors in vitro is feasible but inefficient, limited in part by the low level of expression of the coxsackie/adenovirus receptor. Am J Respir Cell Mol Biol 1999; 20:361–370.
47. Arbuthnot PB, Bralet MP, Le Jossic C, Dedieu JF, Perricaudet M, Brechot C, Ferry N. In vitro and in vivo hepatoma cell-specific expression of a gene transfered with an adenoviral vector. Hum Gene Ther 1996; 7:1503–1514.
48. Huang H, Chen SH, Kosai K, Finegold MJ, Woo SL. Gene therapy for hepatocellular carcinoma: long-term remission of primary and metastatic tumors in mice by interleukin-2 gene therapy in vivo. Gene Ther 1996; 3:980–987.
49. Kanai F, Lan KH, Shiratori Y, Tanaka T, Ohashi M, Okudaira T, Yoshida Y, Wakimoto H, Hamada H, Nakabayashi H, Tamaoki T, Omata M. In vivo gene therapy for alpha-fetoprotein-producing hepatocellular carcinoma by adenovirus-mediated transfer of cytosine deaminase gene. Cancer Res 1997; 57:461–465.
50. Kock H, Harris MP, Anderson SC, Machemer T, Hancock W, Sutjipto S, Wills KN, Gregory RJ, Shepard HM, Westphal M, Maneval DC. Adenovirus-mediated p53 gene transfer suppresses growth of human glioblastoma cells in vitro and in vivo. Int J Cancer 1996; 67:808–815.
51. Prince HM, Dessureault S, Gallinger S, Krajden M, Sutherland DR, Addison C, Zhang Y, Graham FL, Stewart AK. Efficient adenovirus-mediated gene expression in malignant human plasma cells: relative lymphoid cell resistance. Exp Hematol 1998; 26:27–36.
52. Wattel E, Vanrumbeke M, Abina MA, Cambier N, Preudhomme C, Haddada H, Fenaux P. Differential efficacy of adenoviral mediated gene transfer into cells from hematological cell lines and fresh hematological malignancies. Leukemia 1996; 10:171–174.
53. Bonnekoh B, Greenhalgh DA, Bundman DS, Eckhardt JN, Longley MA, Chen SH, Woo SL, Roop DR. Inhibition of melanoma growth by adenoviral-mediated HSV thymidine kinase gene transfer in vivo. J Invest Dermatol 1995; 104: 313–317.
54. Zatloukal K, Schneeberger A, Berger M, Koszik F, Schmidt W, Wagner E, Cotten M, Buschle M, Maass G, Stingl G. Genetic modification of cells by receptor-mediated adenovirus-augmented gene delivery: a new approach for immunotherapy of cancer. Verh Dtsch Ges Pathol 1994; 78:171–176.
55. Hall SJ, Mutchnik SE, Chen SH, Woo SL, Thompson TC. Adenovirus-mediated herpes simplex virus thymidine kinase gene and ganciclovir therapy leads to systemic activity against spontaneous and induced metastasis in an orthotopic mouse model of prostate cancer. Int J Cancer 1997; 70:183–187.
56. Behbakht K, Benjamin I, Chiu HC, Eck SL, Van Deerlin PG, Rubin SC, Boyd J. Adenovirus-mediated gene therapy of ovarian cancer in a mouse model. Am J Obstet Gynecol 1996; 175:1260–1265.
57. Tong XW, Block A, Chen SH, Woo SL, Kieback DG. Adenovirus-mediated thymidine kinase gene transduction in human epithelial ovarian cancer cell lines followed by exposure to ganciclovir. Anticancer Res 1996; 16: 1611–1617.
58. Christ M, Lusky M, Stoeckel F, Dreyer D, Dieterle A, Michou AI, Pavirani A, Mehtali M. Gene therapy with recombinant adenovirus vectors: evaluation of the host immune response. Immunol Lett 1997; 57:19–25.
59. Gao GP, Yang Y, Wilson JM. Biology of adenovirus vectors with E1 and E4 deletions for liver-directed gene therapy. J Virol 1996; 70:8934–8943.
60. Gorziglia MI, Kadan MJ, Yei S, Lim J, Lee GM, Luthra R, Trapnell BC. Elimination of both E1 and E2 from adenovirus vectors further improves prospects for in vivo human gene therapy. J Virol 1996; 70:4173–4178.
61. Yei S, Mittereder N, Wert S, Whitsett JA, Wilmott RW, Trapnell BC. In vivo evaluation of the safety of adenovirus-mediated transfer of the human cystic fibrosis transmembrane conductance regulator cDNA to the lung. Human Gene Ther 1994; 5:731–744.
62. Zabner J, Petersen DM, Puga AP, Graham SM, Couture LA, Keyes LD, Lukason MJ, St George JA, Gregory RJ,

Smith AE. Safety and efficacy of repetitive adenovirus-mediated transfer of CFTR cDNA to airway epithelia of primates and cotton rats. Nat Genet 1994; 6:75–83.

63. Mastrangeli A, Danel C, Rosenfeld MA, Stratford-Perricaudet L, Perricaudet M, Pavirani A, Lecocq JP, Crystal RG. Diversity of airway epithelial cell targets for in vivo recombinant adenovirus-mediated gene transfer. J Clin Invest 1993; 91:225–234.
64. Huard J, Lochmuller H, Acsadi G, Jani A, Massie B, Karpati G. The route of administration is a major determinant of the transduction efficiency of rat tissues by adenoviral recombinants. Gene Ther 1995; 2:107–115.
65. Setoguchi Y, Jaffe HA, Chu CS, Crystal RG. Intraperitoneal in vivo gene therapy to deliver α1-antitrypsin to the systemic circulation. Am J Respir Cell Mol Biol 1994; 10: 369–377.
66. Heikkila P, Parpala T, Lukkarinen O, Weber M, Tryggvason K. Engineering tissue-specific expression of a recombinant adenovirus: selective transgene transcription in the pancreas using the amylase promoter. J Surg Res 1997; 72:155–161.
67. Zhu G, Nicolson AG, Cowley BD, Rosen S, Sukhatme VP. Adenovirus-mediated gene transfer into kidney glomeruli using an ex vivo and in vivo kidney perfusion system—first steps towards gene therapy of Alport syndrome. Gene Ther 1996; 3:21–27.
68. Raper SE, Dematteo RP. Adenovirus-mediated in vivo gene transfer and expression in normal rat pancreas. Pancreas 1996; 12:401–410.
69. Bajocchi G, Feldman SH, Crystal RG, Mastrangeli A. Direct in vivo gene transfer to ependymal cells in the central nervous system using recombinant adenovirus vectors. Nat Genet 1993; 3:229–234.
70. Marmary Y, Parlow AF, Goldsmith CM, He X, Wellner RB, Satomura K, Kriete MF, Robey PG, Nieman LK, Baum BJ. Construction and in vivo efficacy of a replication-deficient recombinant adenovirus encoding murine growth hormone. Endocrinology 1999; 140:260–265.
71. Xing Z, Ohkawara Y, Jordana M, Graham FL, Gauldie J. Adenoviral vector-mediated interleukin-10 expression in vivo: intramuscular gene transfer inhibits cytokine responses in endotoxemia. Gene Ther 1997; 4:140–149.
72. Barkats M, Bilang-Bleuel A, Buc-Caron MH, Castel-Barthe MN, Corti O, Finiels F, Horellou P, Revah F, Sabate O, Mallet J. Adenovirus in the brain: recent advances of gene therapy for neurodegenerative diseases. Prog Neurobiol 1998; 55:333–341.
73. Ross BD, Kim B, Davidson BL. Assessment of ganciclovir toxicity to experimental intracranial gliomas following recombinant adenoviral-mediated transfer of the herpes simplex virus thymidine kinase gene by magnetic resonance imaging and proton magnetic resonance spectroscopy. Clin Cancer Res 1995; 1:651–657.
74. Mack CA, Patel SR, Schwarz EA, Zanzonico P, Hahn RT, Ilercil A, Devereux RB, Goldsmith SJ, Christian TF, Sanborn TA, Kovesdi I, Hackett N, Isom OW, Crystal RG, Rosengart TK. Biologic bypass with the use of adenovirus-mediated gene transfer of the complementary deoxyribonucleic acid for vascular endothelial growth factor 121 improves myocardial perfusion and function in the ischemic porcine heart. J Thorac Cardiovasc Surg 1998; 115: 168–176.
75. Muhlhauser J, Merrill MJ, Pili R, Maeda H, Bacic M, Bewig B, Passaniti A, Edwards NA, Crystal RG, Capogrossi MC. VEGF165 expressed by a replication-deficient recombinant adenovirus vector induces angiogenesis in vivo. Circ Res 1995; 77:1077–1086.
76. French BA, Mazur W, Ali NM, Geske RS, Finnigan JP, Rodgers GP, Roberts R, Raizner AE. Percutaneous transluminal in vivo gene transfer by recombinant adenovirus in normal porcine coronary arteries, atherosclerotic arteries, and two models of coronary restenosis. Circulation 1994; 90:2402–2413.
77. Byrnes AP, MacLaren RE, Charlton HM. Immunological instability of persistent adenovirus vectors in the brain: peripheral exposure to vector leads to renewed inflammation, reduced gene expression, and demyelination. J Neurosci 1996; 16:3045–3055.
78. Di Polo A, Aigner LJ, Dunn RJ, Bray GM, Aguayo AJ. Prolonged delivery of brain-derived neurotrophic factor by adenovirus-infected Muller cells temporarily rescues injured retinal ganglion cells. Proc Natl Acad Sci USA 1998; 95:3978–3983.
79. Parr MJ, Wen PY, Schaub M, Khoury SJ, Sayegh MH, Fine HA. Immune parameters affecting adenoviral vector gene therapy in the brain. J Neurovirol 1998; 4:194–203.
80. Morral N, O'Neal W, Zhou H, Langston C, Beaudet A. Immune responses to reporter proteins and high viral dose limit duration of expression with adenoviral vectors: comparison of E2a wild type and E2a deleted vectors. Human Gene Ther 1997; 8:1275–1286.
81. Worgall S, Leopold PL, Wolff G, Ferris B, Van Roijen N, Crystal RG. Role of alveolar macrophages in rapid elimination of adenovirus vectors administered to the epithelial surface of the respiratory tract. Human Gene Ther 1997; 8:1675–1684.
82. Yang Y, Su Q, Wilson JM. Role of viral antigens in destructive cellular immune responses to adenovirus vector-transduced cells in mouse lungs. J Virol 1996; 70: 7209–7212.
83. Gao GP, Yang Y, Wilson JM. Biology of adenovirus vectors with E1 and E4 deletions for liver-directed gene therapy. J Virol 1996; 70:8934–8943.
84. Setoguchi Y, Jaffe HA, Chu CS, Crystal RG. Intraperitoneal in vivo gene therapy to deliver alpha 1-antitrypsin to the systemic circulation. Am J Respir Cell Mol Biol 1994; 10:369–377.
85. Dai Y, Schwarz EM, Gu D, Zhang WW, Sarvetnick N, Verma IM. Cellular and humoral immune responses to adenoviral vectors containing factor IX gene: tolerization of factor IX and vector antigens allows for long-term expression. Proc Natl Acad Sci USA 1995; 92:1401–1405.

86. Michou AI, Santoro L, Christ M, Julliard V, Pavirani A, Mehtali M. Adenovirus-mediated gene transfer: influence of transgene, mouse strain and type of immune response on persistence of transgene expression. Gene Ther 1997; 4:473–482.
87. Sullivan DE, Dash S, Du H, Hiramatsu N, Aydin F, Kolls J, Blanchard J, Baskin G, Gerber MA. Liver-directed gene transfer in non-human primates. Human Gene Ther 1997; 8:1195–1206.
88. Cassivi SD, Liu M, Boehler A, Tanswell AK, Slutsky AS, Keshavjee S, Todd STRJ. Transgene expression after adenovirus-mediated retransfection of rat lungs is increased and prolonged by transplant immunosuppression. J Thorac Cardiovasc Surg 1999; 117:1–7.
89. Elshami AA, Kucharczuk JC, Sterman DH, Smythe WR, Hwang HC, Amin KM, Litzky LA, Albelda SM, Kaiser LR. The role of immunosuppression in the efficacy of cancer gene therapy using adenovirus transfer of the herpes simplex thymidine kinase gene. Ann Surg 1995; 222: 298–307.
90. Geddes BJ, Harding TC, Hughes DS, Byrnes AP, Lightman SL, Conde G, Uney JB. Persistent transgene expression in the hypothalamus following stereotaxic delivery of a recombinant adenovirus: suppression of the immune response with cyclosporin. Endocrinology 1996; 137:5166–5169.
91. Guibinga GH, Lochmuller H, Massie B, Nalbantoglu J, Karpati G, Petrof BJ. Combinatorial blockade of calcineurin and CD28 signaling facilitates primary and secondary therapeutic gene transfer by adenovirus vectors in dystrophic (MDX) mouse muscles. J Virol 1998; 72: 4601–4609.
92. Scaria A, St George JA, Gregory RJ, Noelle RJ, Wadsworth SC, Smith AE, Kaplan JM. Antibody to CD40 ligand inhibits both humoral and cellular immune responses to adenoviral vectors and facilitates repeated administration to mouse airway. Gene Ther 1997; 4:611–617.
93. Yang Y, Su Q, Grewal IS, Schilz R, Flavell RA, Wilson JM. Transient subversion of CD40 ligand function diminishes immune responses to adenovirus vectors in mouse liver and lung tissues. J Virol 1996; 70:6370–6377.
94. Jooss K, Turka LA, Wilson JM. Blunting of immune responses to adenoviral vectors in mouse liver and lung with CTLA4Ig. Gene Ther 1998; 5:309–319.
95. Kass-Eisler A, Leinwand L, Gall J, Bloom B, Falck-Pedersen E. Circumventing the immune response to adenovirus-mediated gene therapy. Gene Ther 1996; 3:154–162.
96. Mack CA, Song WR, Carpenter H, Wickham TJ, Kovesdi I, Harvey BG, Magovern CJ, Isom OW, Rosengart T, Falck-Pedersen E, Hackett NR, Crystal RG, Mastrangeli A. Circumvention of anti-adenovirus neutralizing immunity by administration of an adenoviral vector of an alternate serotype. Human Gene Ther 1997; 8:99–109.
97. Yang Y, Nunes FA, Berencsi K, Gonczol E, Engelhardt JF, Wilson JM. Inactivation of E2a in recombinant adenoviruses improves the prospect for gene therapy in cystic fibrosis. Nat Genet 1994; 7:362–369.
98. Engelhardt JF, Ye X, Doranz B, Wilson JM. Ablation of E2A in recombinant adenoviruses improves transgene persistence and decreases inflammatory response in mouse liver. Proc Natl Acad Sci USA 1994; 91:6196–6200.
99. Brough DE, Lizonova A, Hsu C, Kulesa VA, Kovesdi I. A gene transfer vector-cell line system for complete functional complementation of adenovirus early regions E1 and E4. J Virol 1996; 70:6497–6501.
100. Brough DE, Hsu C, Kulesa VA, Lee GM, Cantolupo LJ, Lizonova A, Kovesdi I. Activation of transgene expression by early region 4 is responsible for a high level of persistent transgene expression from adenovirus vectors in vivo. J Virol 1997; 71:9206–9213.
101. Schowalter DB, Tubb JC, Liu M, Wilson CB, Kay MA. Heterologous expression of adenovirus E3-gp19K in an E1a-deleted adenovirus vector inhibits MHC I expression in vitro, but does not prolong transgene expression in vivo. Gene Ther 1997; 4:351–360.
102. Lee MG, Abina MA, Haddada H, Perricaudet M. The constitutive expression of the immunomodulatory gp19k protein in E1-, E3-adenoviral vectors strongly reduces the host cytotoxic T cell response against the vector. Gene Ther 1995; 2:256–262.
103. Bruder JT, Jie T, McVey DL, Kovesdi I. Expression of gp19K increases the persistence of transgene expression from an adenovirus vector in the mouse lung and liver. J Virol 1997; 71:7623–7628.
104. Ilan Y, Droguett G, Chowdhury NR, Li Y, Sengupta K, Thummala NR, Davidson A, Chowdhury JR, Horwitz MS. Insertion of the adenoviral E3 region into a recombinant viral vector prevents antiviral humoral and cellular immune responses and permits long-term gene expression. Proc Natl Acad Sci USA 1997; 94:2587–2592.
105. Poller W, Schneider-Rasp S, Liebert U, Merklein F, Thalheimer P, Haack A, Schwaab R, Schmitt C, Brackmann HH. Stabilization of transgene expression by incorporation of E3 region genes into an adenoviral factor IX vector and by transient anti-CD4 treatment of the host. Gene Ther 1996; 3:521–530.
106. Hardy S, Kitamura M, Harris-Stansil T, Dai Y, Phipps ML. Construction of adenovirus vectors through Cre-lox recombination. J Virol 1997; 71:1842–1849.
107. Lieber A, He CY, Kirillova I, Kay MA. Recombinant adenoviruses with large deletions generated by Cre-mediated excision exhibit different biological properties compared with first-generation vectors in vitro and in vivo. J Virol 1996; 70:8944–8960.
108. Morsy MA, Gu M, Motzel S, Zhao J, Lin J, Su Q, Allen H, Franlin L, Parks RJ, Graham FL, Kochanek S, Bett AJ, Caskey CT. An adenoviral vector deleted for all viral coding sequences results in enhanced safety and extended expression of a leptin transgene. Proc Natl Acad Sci USA 1998; 95:7866–7871.
109. Parks RJ, Chen L, Anton M, Sankar U, Rudnicki MA, Graham FL. A helper-dependent adenovirus vector system: removal of helper virus by Cre-mediated excision of

the viral packaging signal. Proc Natl Acad Sci USA 1996; 93:13565–13570.

110. Schiedner G, Morral N, Parks RJ, Wu Y, Koopmans SC, Langston C, Graham FL, Beaudet AL, Kochanek S. Genomic DNA transfer with a high-capacity adenovirus vector results in improved in vivo gene expression and decreased toxicity. Nat Genet 1998; 18:180–183.
111. Smith TA, White BD, Gardner JM, Kaleko M, McClelland A. Transient immunosuppression permits successful repetitive intravenous administration of an adenovirus vector. Gene Ther 1996; 3:496–502.
112. Dong JY, Wang D, Van Ginkel FW, Pascual DW, Frizzell RA. Systematic analysis of repeated gene delivery into animal lungs with a recombinant adenovirus vector. Hum Gene Ther 1996; 7:319–331.
113. Kagami H, Atkinson JC, Michalek SM, Handelman B, Yu S, Baum BJ, O'Connell B. Repetitive adenovirus administration to the parotid gland: role of immunological barriers and induction of oral tolerance. Hum Gene Ther 1998; 9: 305–313.
114. Gall J, Kass-Eisler A, Leinwand L, Falck-Pedersen E. Adenovirus type 5 and 7 capsid chimera: fiber replacement alters receptor tropism without affecting primary immune neutralization epitopes. J Virol 1996; 70:2116–2123.
115. Gall JG, Crystal RG, Falck-Pedersen E. Construction and characterization of hexon-chimeric adenoviruses: specification of adenovirus serotype. J Virol 1998; 72: 10260–10264.
116. Dematteo RP, McClane SJ, Fisher K, Yeh H, Chu G, Burke C, Raper SE. Engineering tissue-specific expression of a recombinant adenovirus: selective transgene transcription in the pancreas using the amylase promoter. J Surg Res 1997; 72:155–161.
117. Kaneko S, Hallenbeck P, Kotani T, Nakabayashi H, McGarrity G, Tamaoki T, Anderson WF, Chiang YL. Adenovirus-mediated gene therapy of hepatocellular carcinoma using cancer-specific gene expression. Cancer Res 1995; 55:5283–5287.
118. Rothmann T, Katus HA, Hartong R, Perricaudet M, Franz WM. Heart muscle-specific gene expression using replication defective recombinant adenovirus. Gene Ther 1996; 3:919–926.
119. Larochelle N, Lochmuller H, Zhao J, Jani A, Hallauer P, Hastings KE, Massie B, Prescott S, Petrof BJ, Karpati G, Nalbantoglu J. Efficient muscle-specific transgene expression after adenovirus-mediated gene transfer in mice using a 1.35 kb muscle creatine kinase promoter/enhancer. Gene Ther 1997; 4:465–472.
120. Douglas JT and Curiel DT. Strategies to accomplish targeted gene delivery to muscle cells employing tropism-modified adenoviral vectors. Neuromuscul Disord 1997; 7:284–298.
121. Krasnykh VN, Mikheeva GV, Douglas JT, Curiel DT. Generation of recombinant adenovirus vectors with modified fibers for altering viral tropism. J Virol 1996; 70: 6839–6846.
122. Stevenson SC, Rollence M, Marshall-Neff J, McClelland A. Selective targeting of human cells by a chimeric adenovirus vector containing a modified fiber protein. J Virol 1997; 71:4782–4790.
123. Chillon M, Bosch A, Zabner J, Law L, Armentano D, Welsh MJ, Davidson BL. Group D adenoviruses infect primary central nervous system cells more efficiently than those from group C. J Virol 1999; 73:2537–2540.
124. Crystal RG, McElvaney NG, Rosenfeld MA, Chu CS, Mastrangeli A, Hay JG, Brody SL, Jaffe HA, Eissa NT, Danel C. Administration of an adenovirus containing the human CFTR cDNA to the respiratory tract of individuals with cystic fibrosis. Nat Genet 1994; 8:42–51.
125. Wickham TJ, Roelvink PW, Brough DE, Kovesdi I. Adenovirus targeted to heparan-containing receptors increases its gene delivery efficiency to multiple cell types. Nat Biotechnol 1996; 14:1570–1573.
126. Dmitriev I, Krasnykh V, Miller CR, Wang M, Kashentseva E, Mikheeva G, Belousova N, Curiel DT. An adenovirus vector with genetically modified fibers demonstrates expanded tropism via utilization of a coxsackievirus and adenovirus receptor-independent cell entry mechanism. J Virol 1998; 72:9706–9713.
127. Miller CR, Buchsbaum DJ, Reynolds PN, Douglas JT, Gillespie GY, Mayo MS, Raben D, Curiel DT. Differential susceptibility of primary and established human glioma cells to adenovirus infection: targeting via the epidermal growth factor receptor achieves fiber receptor-independent gene transfer. Cancer Res 1998; 58:5738–5748.
128. Wickham TJ, Segal DM, Roelvink PW, Carrion ME, Lizonova A, Lee GM, Kovesdi I. Targeted adenovirus gene transfer to endothelial and smooth muscle cells by using bispecific antibodies. J Virol 1996; 70:6831–6838.
129. Wickham TJ, Lee GM, Titus JA, Sconocchia G, Bakacs T, Kovesdi I, Segal DM. Targeted adenovirus-mediated gene delivery to T cells via CD3. J Virol 1997; 71: 7663–7669.
130. Harvey B-G, Worgall S, Bialos B, Ramirez M, Crystal RG. Humoral anti-Ad5 immune responses after lung administration of first generation Ad vectors to normals and individuals with cystic fibrosis. Pediatr Pulmonol 1999; Suppl 19:225.
131. Heise C, Sampson-Johannes A, Williams A, McCormick F, Von Hoff DD, Kim DH. ONYX-015, an E1B gene-attenuated adenovirus, causes tumor-specific cytolysis and antitumoral efficacy that can be augmented by standard chemotherapeutic agents. Nat Med 1997; 3:639–645.
132. Giordano FJ, Ping P, McKirnan MD, Nozaki S, De Maria AN, Dillmann WH, Mathieu-Costello O, Hammond HK. Intracoronary gene transfer of fibroblast growth factor-5 increases blood flow and contractile function in an ischemic region of the heart. Nat Med 1996; 2:534–539.
133. Bilbao G, Feng M, Rancourt C, Jackson WHJ, Curiel DT. Adenoviral/retrovial vector chimeras: a novel strategy to achieve high-efficiency stable transduction in vivo. FASEB J 1997; 11:624–634.

134. Feng M, Jackson WHJ, Goldman CK, Rancourt C, Wang M, Dusing SK, Siegal G, Curiel DT. Stable in vivo gene transduction via a novel adenoviral/retroviral chimeric vector. Nat Biotechnol 1997; 15:866–870.
135. Ramsey WJ, Caplen NJ, Li Q, Higginbotham JN, Shah M, Blaese RM. Adenovirus vectors as transcomplementing templates for the production of replication defective retroviral vectors. Biochem Biophys Res Commun 1998; 246:912–919.
136. Fisher KJ, Kelley WM, Burda JF, Wilson JM. A novel adenovirus-adeno-associated virus hybrid vector that displays efficient rescue and delivery of the AAV genome. Human Gene Ther 1996; 7:2079–2087.
137. Gao GP, Qu G, Faust LZ, Engdahl RK, Xiao W, Hughes JV, Zoltick PW, Wilson JM. High-titer adeno-associated viral vectors from a Rep/Cap cell line and hybrid shuttle virus. Human Gene Ther 1998; 9:2353–2362.
138. Legrand V, Spehner D, Schlesinger Y, Settelen N, Pavirani A, Mehtali M. Fiberless recombinant adenoviruses: virus maturation and infectivity in the absence of fiber. J Virol 1999; 73:907–919.
139. Fallaux FJ, Bout A, van dV, I, van den Wollenberg DJ, Hehir KM, Keegan J, Auger C, Cramer SJ, van Ormondt H, van der Eb AJ, Valerio D, Hoeben RC. New helper cells and matched early region 1-deleted adenovirus vectors prevent generation of replication-competent adenoviruses. Human Gene Ther 1998; 9:1909–1917.
140. Magovern CJ, Mack CA, Zhang J, Rosengart TK, Isom OW, Crystal RG. Regional angiogenesis induced in nonischemic tissue by an adenoviral vector expressing vascular endothelial growth factor. Human Gene Ther 1997; 8: 215–227.
141. Graham FL, Smiley J, Russell WC, Naim R. Characteristics of a human cell line transformed by DNA from human adenovirus type 5. J Gen Virol 1997; 36:59–74.
142. Fallaux FJ, Kranenburg O, Cramer SJ, Houweling A, van Ormondt H, Hoeben RC, van der Eb AJ. Characterization of 911: a new helper cell line for the titration and propagation of early region 1-deleted adenoviral vectors. Human Gene Ther 1996; 7:215–222.
143. Wang Q, Jia XC, Finer MH. A packaging cell line for propagation of recombinant adenovirus vectors containing two lethal gene-region deletions. Gene Ther 1995; 2: 775–783.
144. Yeh P, Dedieu JF, Orsini C, Vigne E, Denefle P, Perricaudet M. Efficient dual transcomplementation of adenovirus E1 and E4 regions from a 293-derived cell line expressing a minimal E4 functional unit. J Virol 1996; 70: 559–565.
145. Krougliak V and Graham FL. Development of cell lines capable of complementing E1, E4, and protein IX defective adenovirus type 5 mutants. Human Gene Ther 1995; 6: 1575–1586.
146. Langer SJ and Schaack J. 293 cell lines that inducibly express high levels of adenovirus type 5 precursor terminal protein. Virology 1996; 221:172–179.
147. Amalfitano A and Chamberlain JS. Isolation and characterization of packaging cell lines that coexpress the adenovirus E1, DNA polymerase, and preterminal proteins: implications for gene therapy. Gene Ther 1997; 4:258–263.
148. Zhou H, O'Neal W, Morral N, Beaudet AL. Development of a complementing cell line and a system for construction of adenovirus vectors with E1 and E2a deleted. J Virol 1996; 70:7030–7038.
149. Goldman CK, Rogers BE, Douglas JT, Sosnowski BA, Ying W, Siegal GP, Baird A, Campain JA, Curiel DT. Targeted gene delivery to Kaposi's sarcoma cells via the fibroblast growth factor receptor. Cancer Res 1997; 57: 1447–1451.
150. Rogers BE, Douglas JT, Ahlem C, Buchsbaum DJ, Frincke J, Curiel DT. Use of a novel cross-linking method to modify adenovirus tropism. Gene Ther 1997; 4:1387–1392.
151. Roelvink PW, Kovesdi I, Wickham TJ. Comparative analysis of adenovirus fiber-cell interaction: adenovirus type 2 (Ad2) and Ad9 utilize the same cellular fiber receptor but use different binding strategies for attachment. J Virol 1996; 70:7614–7621.

3

Adeno-Associated Virus and Adeno-Associated Virus Vectors for Gene Delivery

Barrie J. Carter
Targeted Genetics Corporation, Seattle, Washington

I. ADENO-ASSOCIATED VIRUS VECTORS

Adeno-associated virus (AAV) vectors have a number of advantageous properties as gene-delivery vehicles. The parental virus does not cause disease, the vectors can readily transduce both dividing or nondividing cells and can persist essentially for the lifetime of the cell. AAV vectors contain no viral genes, and they do not elicit host cellular immune responses and appear not to induce inflammatory responses. The primary host response that might impact use of AAV vectors is a neutralizing antibody response. Thus, AAV vectors can mediate impressive long-term gene expression in vivo. Consequently these vectors may be used for gene therapy by delivering the vector only infrequently and any host antibody response to the AAV capsid protein may be less inhibitory. AAV vectors are the smallest and most chemically defined particulate gene-delivery system, and they may eventually be classified as well-characterized biologics for therapeutic applications. The main limitations of AAV vectors are the limited payload capacity of about 4.5 kb and, until recently, the lack of good producer systems that could generate high titer virus.

Production of AAV vectors has improved and progress has been made both by increasing the specific productivity of producer cells and by designing systems that can be scaled for commercial production. There have been significant advances in upstream production of AAV as well as advances in downstream purification. AAV particles are hardy and resistant to robust handling, which facilitates purification and concentration. Previously, this was achieved by banding in CsCl, but more pharmaceutically relevant procedures such as chromatography are now being developed. Clinical applications of AAV vectors are beginning to be developed and clinical trials in cystic fibrosis (CF) patients are ongoing (1,2). Clinical trials for additional applications such as factor IX deficiency (hemophilia B) may be launched soon.

I will not attempt to provide an exhaustive collection of references on development of AAV vectors but will discuss the several key advances in the last several years including improvements in vector production, studies on the applications for persistent gene expression, and early approaches to regulation of gene expression. I will also provide some historical comment on early studies on AAV since these very interesting and seminal studies are often overlooked in current reviews. General reviews of AAV may be found in Refs. 3 and 4. Extensive discussions on the background and applications of AAV vectors are available (7–10), and a recent cataloging of work with AAV vectors is provided in other references (11–13).

II. ADENO-ASSOCIATED VIRUS

A. AAV Virus Biology

1. AAV Discovery

Adeno-associated virus is a small, DNA-containing virus that belongs to the family Parvoviridae within the genus *Dependovirus.* AAV was first observed during analysis of adenovirus preparations by electron microscopy and was mistakenly thought to represent subunits of adenovirus. However, AAV was repeatedly observed as a contaminant of laboratory preparations of adenovirus and was recognized as a virus that was different from adenovirus but was dependent upon adenovirus for its replication (14,15). This explained the serendipitous contamination of adenovirus preparations with AAV. It is worth noting that AAV has been a frequent contaminant of laboratory strains of adenovirus, and many of the standard stocks of adenovirus were originally laid down before AAV was recognized. Thus, standard archival stocks of adenovirus cannot be assumed to be free of AAV unless specifically tested.

2. Epidemiology

Soon after the discovery of AAV in laboratory stocks of adenoviruses, it was isolated from humans. AAV has not been associated with the cause of any disease but has been isolated from humans, generally in association with an infection by adenovirus (16). There are at least five defined serotypes of AAV. In the United States, most of the population over age 10 is seropositive for AAV2 and AAV3. A signal epidemiological study of AAV was carried out in a population of children in an orphanage in Washington, DC. In this population, seroconversion to AAV was observed in young children during the course of an adenovirus infection. In infected individuals, the virus is shed in body fluids including sputum and stool. AAV appears to be transmitted primarily in nursery populations in conjunction with the helper adenovirus and thus appears to be replication defective also in its natural human host. It is noteworthy that the early epidemiological studies also analyzed neutralizing antibody responses to AAV in humans. The existence of neutralizing antibody did not prevent reinfection of humans by AAV but did prevent shedding of the virus (16). This is significant for use of AAV as a gene-delivery vector (17).

3. Mode of Cell Entry and Host Tropism

AAV appears to have a broad host range and different AAV serotypes grow in vitro in many human cells and a variety of simian and rodent cell lines if a helper virus with the appropriate host range is also present. This indicated that any cellular receptor for AAV was likely to be relatively common on many cell types. AAV also infects various animal species, and human isolates of AAV will grow in mice or monkeys if the appropriate mouse or monkey adenovirus is also present. However, recent in vivo studies with AAV vectors suggested that some tissues or cell types may be more readily transduced than others, and these observations may reflect differences in receptors that mediate AAV entry.

Recent experiments have provided insight into the mechanism of AAV entry into cells. First it was demonstrated (18) that AAV particles can bind to cells via heparin sulfate proteoglycans (HSPG) in a manner such that binding and infection could be competed in a dose-dependent fashion by soluble heparin. Cell lines that did not produce HSPG were significantly impaired for AAV binding and infection. Additional studies suggest that cellular entry of AAV is more complex and requires also a co-receptor for efficient internalization. Two possible co-receptors for AAV were identified. One co-receptor (19) appears to be $\alpha_V\beta_5$ integrin and the other (20) is the human fibroblast growth factor receptor 1 (FGFR1). These observations will be important in developing gene-therapy applications and may be important in indicating possible differences in the ability of cells of varying tissue specificity to be transduced by AAV vectors.

Variations in the presence or concentration of the AAV co-receptors may have an impact on the transduction efficiency of hematopoietic stem cells (CD34+) cells from different donors (21), and this may help to resolve the question as to whether AAV can infect such cells. It is of interest that the $\alpha_V\beta_5$ integrin co-receptor, which is used for a similar purpose by adenovirus types 2 and 5, is preferentially located in airway epithelial cells in the more distal cells of the conducting airway (22). This may be important for use of an AAV gene therapy for cystic fibrosis since the distal airway is the region of the lung most impacted by the disease. It is also noteworthy that FGFR is expressed in most tissues but is of highest abundance in skeletal muscle and neuroblasts and glioblasts in the brain, and these two organs appear to be excellent targets for AAV transduction.

The existence of more than one co-receptor suggests that AAV may have multiple mechanisms for cell entry, and there is already some evidence to support this concept (23). AAV was able to transduce polarized airway epithelial cells more efficiently via the basolateral surface than the apical surface, and this difference correlated with the relative abundance of HSPG. UV irradiation decreased basolateral transduction, and this was associated with decreased HSPG, whereas the same treatment increased apical transduction but did not increase apical HSPG. Rather, apical endocytosis of AAV apeared to be enhanced through an independent mechanism.

Cell entry may also be impacted by the route of delivery. AAV vectors can transduce airway cells when delivered directly to the lung or muscle and brain cells when delivered directly to these organs. However, when delivered intravenously by tail vein injection in mice (24), the vector preferentially accumulated in the liver, and this may reflect both the presence of a much more porous vasculature in the liver and also the small size of the AAV particles. The small size of the AAV particle also may be of advantage in passing through the basal lamina pores in muscle, thus accessing a larger number of myoblasts and myotubes.

4. Biology of AAV Life Cycle

AAV is a defective parvovirus that grows only in cells in which certain functions are provided by a coinfecting helper virus, which is generally an adenovirus or a herpesvirus (4). AAV has both a broad host range and wide cell and tissue specificity and replicates in many cell lines of human, simian, or rodent origin provided an appropriate helper virus is present. Accumulating evidence from in vivo studies with AAV vectors indicates that there may be some limitations to AAV tissue specificity or at least some significant differences in efficiency of transduction of different tissues and organs. Some of the limitations to AAV cell specificity may reflect the receptor and co-receptors apparently utilized by AAV for entry into cells as already discussed. A second set of parameters that may impact AAV tissue and organ specificity reflect both the permissivity of cells for AAV and the nature of the helper function provided by helper viruses (40).

The most central event required for efficient function of AAV as a gene delivery vehicle is the need to convert the incoming single-stranded DNA genome to a double-stranded molecule to permit transcription and gene expression. This process is termed single-strand conversion or metabolic activation (26), and the rate at which it occurs depends largely on the physiological state of the cell, but the process may be accelerated by treatment of the cell with genotoxic agents or by certain helper virus functions.

Infection of cells by AAV in the absence of helper functions results in persistence of AAV as a latent provirus integrated into the host cell genome. In such cell lines, the integrated AAV genome may be rescued and replicated to yield a burst of infectious progeny AAV particles if the cells are superinfected with a helper virus such as adenovirus. In cultured cells, AAV exhibits a high preference for integration at a specific region, the AAVS1 site, on human chromosome 19. The efficiency and specificity of this process is mediated by the AAV *rep* gene and therefore *rep*-deleted AAV vectors do not retain specificity for integration into the chromosome 19 region (27–29).

B. AAV Molecular Biology

1. Particle Structure

AAV is a nonenveloped particle about 20 nm in diameter with icosahedral symmetry that is stable to heat, mild proteolytic digestion, and nonionic detergents. The AAV particle is comprised of a protein coat, containing the three capsid proteins VP1, VP2, and VP3, which encloses a linear single-stranded DNA genome having a molecular weight of 1.5×10^6. The VP1, VP2, and VP3 proteins are present in the viral capsid in the ratio of 1:1:8. The DNA represents 25% by mass of the particle, which therefore exhibits a high buoyant density (1.41 g/cm^3) in cesium chloride. The relative stability of the AAV particle is an important property since it can withstand robust purification procedures, and this should facilitate scaled-up production of AAV vectors.

Several serotypes of AAV have been distinguished. AAV1, AAV2, AAV3, and AAV4 have extensive DNA homology and significant serological overlap, but AAV5 is somewhat less related. AAV2 and 3 are the most frequently isolated from humans, whereas AAV5 has been isolated from humans only once. AAV4 is a simian isolate that does not infect humans. AAV1 originally may have been isolated as a simian virus.

A novel feature of AAV is that although each particle contains only one single-stranded genome, strands of either complementary sense, ''plus'' or ''minus'' strands, are packaged into individual particles. Equal numbers of AAV particles contain either a plus or minus strand, both of which are equally infectious, and AAV displays single-hit kinetics.

When DNA is extracted from AAV particles, the plus and minus strands anneal to generate duplex molecules of 3.0×10^6 molecular weight. This posed an early conundrum as noted by Crawford and colleagues (30), who showed on the basis of a careful physical characterization of AAV particles that each particle appeared to contain only DNA of 1.5×10^6 molecular weight yet yielded a 3.0×10^6 molecular weight duplex DNA after extraction from the particles. They suggested that the only way to reconcile this puzzle was to propose that individual plus and minus strands must be packaged into individual particles.

An elegant proof of the Crawford conundrum was provided by Rose and colleagues (31), who took advantage of the fact that BUdR-substituted DNA has a higher density, as compared to unsubstituted DNA, when banded to equilibrium in CsCl density gradients. They made two preparations of AAV particles, one of which had thymidine substituted by bromodeoxyuridine. Extraction of DNA from the two preparations separately gave duplex DNA that banded at the heavy density of the substituted DNA or the light density of the unsubstituted DNA. In contrast, when the two preparations of particles were mixed prior to extraction of DNA, the analysis of the duplex DNA obtained upon extraction also showed components with intermediate density formed by individual strands from substituted or unsubstituted particles that had annealed during extraction. This constituted formal proof of the novel DNA strand segregation exhibited by AAV during packaging of its DNA.

2. AAV Genome Structure

The AAV DNA genome is 4681 nucleotides long with one copy of the 145-nucleotide ITR (inverted terminal repeat) at each end and a unique sequence region of 4391 nucleotides that contains two main open reading frames for the *rep* and *cap* genes (Fig. 1). The unique region contains three transcription promoters—p_5, p_{19}, and p_{40}—that are used to express the *rep* and *cap* genes. The ITR sequences are required in *cis* to provide functional origins of replication (*ori*) as well as signals for encapsidation, integration into the cell genome, and rescue from either host cell chromosomes or recombinant plasmids.

The *rep* gene is transcribed from two promoters, p_5 and p_{19}, to generate two families of transcripts and two families of rep proteins (Fig. 1). In addition, splicing of these mRNAs leads to at least two different carboxyl-terminal regions in the rep proteins. The capsid gene is expressed from transcripts from the p_{40} promoter, which accumulate as two 2.3 kb mRNAs that are alternately spliced. The majority 2.3 kb transcript codes for the VP3 protein initiated from a consensus AUG initiation codon, but at about a 10-fold lower frequency translation of this transcript also occurs slightly upstream at a nonconsensus ACG initiation codon to yield VP2. The minority 2.3 kb mRNA is spliced using an alternate 3′ donor site that is 30 nucleotides upstream of the donor site used in the majority transcript. This has the effect of retaining 30 additional nucleotides in the minority transcript, which includes an AUG codon that is used to initiate translation of VP1. Thus, VP1 and VP2 have the same polypeptide sequence as VP3 but have additional amino terminal sequences. This elegant arrangement results in generation of VP1, VP2, and VP3 in ratios of about 1 : 1 : 8, which is the same as the ratio of these proteins in the viral particle.

3. AAV Replication

In a productive infection (6,33), the infecting parental AAV single-strand genome is converted to a parental duplex replicating form (RF) by a self-priming mechanism, which takes advantage of the ability of the ITR to form a hairpin structure (Fig. 2). This process is performed by a cellular DNA polymerase and occurs in the absence of helper virus, but it may be enhanced by helper virus. The parental RF molecule is then amplified to form a large pool of progeny RF molecules in a process that requires both the helper functions and the AAV *rep* gene products, Rep78 and Rep68. AAV RF genomes are a mixture of head-to-head or tail-to-tail multimers or concatemers and are precursors to progeny single-strand (SS) DNA genomes that are packaged into preformed empty AAV capsids.

The kinetics of AAV replication and assembly have been investigated (33,34). When human HeLa or 293 cells

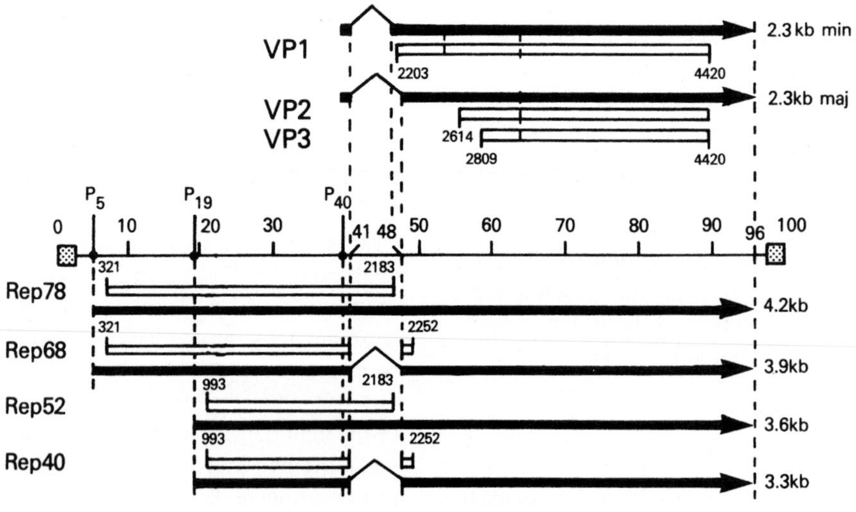

Figure 1 Structure of the AAV 2 genome. The AAV2 genome is shown as a single bar with a 100 map unit scale (1 map unit is approximately 47 nucleotides). Stippled boxes indicate inverted terminal repeats (ITRs, replication origins) and solid circles indicate transcription promoters (p_5, p_{19}, p_{40}). The polyA site is at map position 96. RNAs from AAV promoters are shown as heavy arrows with introns indicated by the caret. The coding regions for the four rep proteins (Rep78, Rep68, Rep52, Rep40) and for the viral capsid proteins (VP1, VP2, and VP3) are shown with open boxes, and the numbers indicate the locations of initiation and termination codons. (From Ref. 32.)

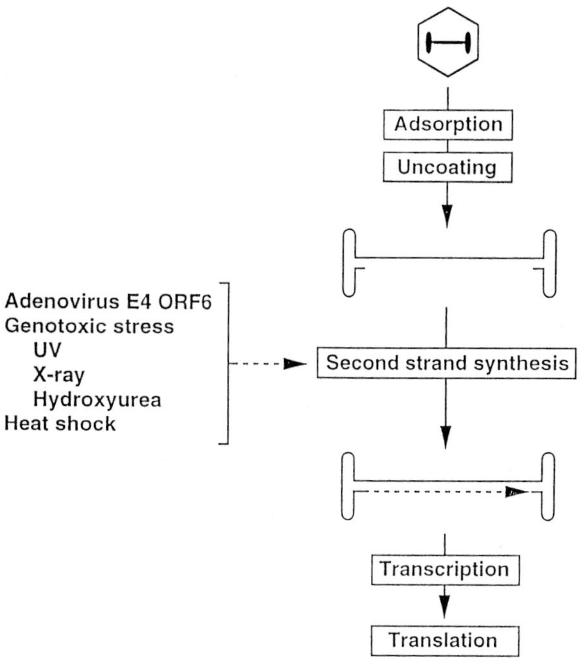

Figure 2 Metabolic pathway of AAV genomes in cells. Adsorption and entry of AAV is independent of helper virus functions. Conversion of the infecting single-strand genome to a duplex structure (or parental RF) through the process of metabolic activation (second strand synthesis) can occur independently of helper virus. This process may be enhanced by infection with helper adenovirus genes such as E4orf6 or by other metabolic insults including genotoxic stress or heat shock. Treatments that enhance metabolic activation may enhance gene expression from the vector template. The single strand and duplex strands are drawn to show the ITR in the base-paired hairpin conformation, which allows self-priming of replication to form a duplex template using cellular DNA polymerases. For further details see text. (From Ref. 85.)

are simultaneously infected with AAV and adenovirus there are three phases of the growth cycle. In the first 8–10 hours, the cell becomes permissive for AAV replication as a result of expression of the adenovirus genes. During this period, the infecting AAV genome is converted to the initial parental duplex RF DNA by self-priming from the terminal base-paired 3′ hydroxyl group provided by the ability of the ITR to form a self-paired hairpin. This initial generation of a duplex genome also provides a template for transcription and expression of AAV proteins.

In the second phase, from about 10–20 hours after infection, the bulk of the AAV rep and cap proteins are synthesized and accumulate. Also during this period, there is a large amplification of duplex AAV RF genomes, and this includes both monomeric and concatemeric RF species. It is important to note that the concatemer RF species that are produced during this phase of AAV replication are head-to-head or tail-to-tail concatemers, which follows directly from use of the terminal hairpin as a base-paired replication origin.

By about 16–20 hours, the amount of RF DNA becomes constant, but single-strand progeny molecules, synthesized by a strand-displacement replication mechanism, begin to accumulate and are packaged into preformed capsids. This initiates the third phase of AAV growth in which, between 16–30 hours, there is a rapid accumulation of mature, infectious AAV particles. Kinetic analysis (34) showed that during this third phase, the single-strand progeny DNA is packaged into preformed capsids in a process that involves the single-strand genome becoming associated with an empty capsid very soon after, or simultaneously with, its synthesis. This is followed by a slower process that occurs over several hours in which the DNA and the associated capsid are converted into a mature, fully infectious AAV particle. There is an intermediate state in which the DNA and capsid are associated in a complex that is not stable and which has an extended conformation such that the DNA is accessible to degradation by DNAse. This intermediate complex has a sedimentation coefficient between 60S and 110S. In contrast, empty AAV particles sediment at 60S and mature, infectious AAV particles sediment at 110S. The DNA genomes in mature infectious AAV particles are completely resistant to attack by DNAse, and this is used as a diagnostic criterion for AAV vectors. The particle titer of AAV vectors is generally measured as the number of DNAse-resistant particles.

The rep proteins perform important biochemical functions (6). Rep68 and Rep78 bind to the ITR and are site-specific, strand-specific endonucleases that cleave the hairpin in an RF molecule at the site that is the 5′ terminus of the mature strand. In addition, these proteins contain an ATP-binding site, which is important for the enzymatic activity but not for binding to the ITR. Further, Rep78 and Rep68 have both DNA and RNA helicase activity. These rep proteins also regulate transcription (6,9,11). Rep78 is a negative auto-regulator of the p_5 promoter (i.e., of its own synthesis) but is an activator of the p_{40} promoter to enhance capsid protein production. Rep52 and Rep40 have none of the enzymatic activities of the larger rep proteins and do not bind to the ITR but do function in assembly of mature particles. Also, the smaller rep proteins are antirepressors and block the negative auto-regulation of p_5 by Rep78 (35).

The AAV growth cycle is highly coordinated with respect to expression of rep and cap proteins and the relationship between replication and assembly (34,35). Any vector-production process that mimics this must necessarily provide the rep and cap functions by complementation and may therefore decrease the efficiency of this highly regulated process. More importantly, as the process becomes less efficient, fewer of the particles may mature to fully infectious particles and unstable, immature particles may be more predominant. This may account for various observations that some vector-production systems lead to generation of AAV vector particles that are unstable, particularly if banded in CsCl buoyant density gradients.

It is noteworthy that the production of AAV is highly efficient and AAV has one of the largest burst sizes of any virus. Thus, following infection of cells with AAV and adenovirus as helper, the burst size of AAV may be well in excess of 100,000 particles per cell (8). This is important in developing vector-production systems because it implies that a high yield of AAV vector particles per cell theoretically is attainable. Attaining high specific productivity is of crucial importance in developing scaled-up production because the ability to obtain maximum yields ideally requires both high specific productivity (yield of particles per cell) or large biomass (total number of cells). Maximizing the specific productivity may avoid unnecessary increases in biomass.

4. AAV Genetics

The cloning of infectious AAV genomes in bacterial plasmids facilitated a molecular genetic analysis of AAV. These studies showed that the *rep* and *cap* genes are required in *trans* to provide functions for replication and encapsidation of viral genomes, respectively, and that the ITR is required in *cis* (6,9,32). Mutations in the ITR have an Ori phenotype and cannot be complemented in *trans.*

The *rep* gene is expressed as family of four proteins—Rep78, Rep68, Rep52, and Rep40—that comprise a common internal region sequence but differ in their amino- and carboxy-terminal regions. Mutations that affect the Rep78 and Rep68 proteins have a Rep phenotype and are deficient for both the bulk replication and amplification of duplex RF molecules and for accumulation of single-strand, progeny genomes. A mutation that affected only the Rep52 and Rep40 proteins showed an Ssd phenotype in which duplex RF replication occurred normally but no single-strand progeny DNA accumulated. This appears to be directly related to the phenotype of mutations in the VP1 protein and shows that the Rep52 and Rep40 proteins are not required directly for AAV DNA replication but are required for assembly of particles in order to package DNA into the preformed capsid.

The *cap* gene encodes the proteins VP1, VP2, and VP3 that share a common overlapping sequence but VP1 and VP2 contain additional amino-terminal sequence. All three proteins are required for capsid production. Mutations that affect VP2 or VP3 have a Cap phenotype and block capsid assembly and prevent any accumulation of single-strand DNA. This indicates that VP3 and VP2 are primarily responsible for forming the capsid and that single-strand DNA does not accumulate unless it can be packaged into capsids. Mutations that affect only the VP1 protein, in the amino terminus of that protein, do not prevent accumulation of capsids and permit accumulation of single-strand DNA. However, there are no infectious AAV particles generated and this phenotype has been described as either Inf or Lip (low-infectivity particles).

These genetic studies together with additional biochemical studies show that Rep68 and Rep78 are required for replication, that VP2 and VP3 are required to form the capsid and that Rep52 and Rep40 appear to act in concert together with VP1 to encapsidate the DNA and stabilize the particles (6,8).

The rep proteins exhibit several pleiotropic regulatory activities including positive and negative regulation of AAV genes and expression from some heterologous promoters as well as inhibitory effects on the host cell. Because of the inhibitory effects of expression of *rep* on cell growth, expression of rep protein in stable cell lines was difficult to achieve and this delayed development of AAV packaging cell lines (36). For this reason, various approaches to AAV vector production employed transient transfection of cells with AAV vector plasmids and complementing rep-cap plasmids. However, even in these transfection systems, the closely coordinated regulation of *rep* and *cap* gene expression and the interactions of the three AAV promoters (35) are important considerations in optimizing vector production.

C. AAV Latency

1. History

In the course of a U.S. government screening program to assess human cell lines for suitability for vaccine production, it was observed on several occasions that infection of primary cultures of human embryonic kidney cells with adenovirus resulted in rescue of infectious AAV even though in the absence of adenovirus lysates of the cultures could not be shown to contain infectious AAV particles. This suggested that some cultures may have carried a latent form of AAV. This was tested directly (37) by infecting a human cell line, Detroit 6, with AAV at a high multiplicity of infection and passaging the cell cultures until no infectious AAV genomes were present, which required at least 10 cell passages. Following this, superinfection of the cultures with adenovirus resulted in rescue of infectious AAV.

2. Structure of Latent Virus

Analysis of cells carrying latent AAV showed that they contained a relatively low number of AAV genomes that were integrated into the host cell chromosome mostly as tandem repeats. This provided an important demonstration of a way in which AAV can survive in cells if conditions are not permissive for replication. Early studies of cells stably transduced with AAV vectors also showed that most stable copies in the cell existed as tandem repeats with a head-to-tail conformation (38). Analysis of chromosomal flanking sequences showed that for wild-type AAV a significant proportion of these integration events occur in a defined region (39). When wild-type AAV infects human cell lines in culture up to 50–70% of these integration events occur at a region know as the AAVS1 site on the q arm of chromosome 19. It remains to be determined if the remainder of the integration events occur at other specific sites or are completely random.

3. Mechanism of Persistence and Integration

Both the specificity and efficiency of AAV integration appear to be mediated by the AAV Rep protein, which binds to the ITR and to a site in the AAVS1 site on human chromosome 19 (27). AAV vectors that contain no AAV *rep* coding sequences have reduced efficiency and specificity for integration at the chromosome 19 site (28,29). In general, the integrated AAV genome is present at a relatively low copy number but exists as a tandem head-to-tail repeat (38). Additional analysis indicated that AAV vectors may be able to persist in a low copy, quasi-episomal state. This evidence came from fluorescent in situ hybridization (FISH) analysis of cell lines transduced with AAV vectors, which carried a low number of copies of an AAV vector as determined by Southern hybridization or FISH analysis of interphase nuclei but in which FISH analysis of metaphase chromosomes showed a reduced proportion of the cells carrying all the copies at a metaphase chromosomal site (28). These studies were performed on cells in culture, and it is noteworthy that no naturally occurring, latent AAV genomes have been described in humans or any other animal species. It is more difficult to examine integration of AAV or AAV vectors after infection of cells in vivo, but this may be approached in studies of prolonged AAV vector persistence in animal models.

A number of studies have now shown that AAV can persist for extended periods of time when administered in vivo (40–43). The predominant form of the persisting vector genomes appears to be multimeric structures, which are predominantly head-to-tail concatemers (43,45–48). Whether any replication of the AAV genome is required for integration was unclear from previous analysis of AAV vector transduced cells (38). However, the recent evidence that there is a generation of episomal head-to-tail concatemers (40–43), particularly following in vivo delivery, suggests that these structures are potential precursors of integrated genomes and that they may be generated by replication. This process occurs for rep-deleted AAV vectors so it presumably does not require rep expression and any replication must be mediated by cellular DNA polymerases. The mechanism of AAV integration is not resolved, but it was hypothesized (29,49) that integration may be mediated by a circular intermediate. Interestingly, circularization might also facilitate rolling circle replication that would be predicted to generate head-to-tail concatemers rather than the head-to-head or tail-to-tail concatemer RFs that result from AAV DNA replication involving initiation from the self-priming ITR. Some initial evidence for formation of circular duplex intermediates of AAV genomes has been reported (50,51). These observations suggest a generally consistent model in which AAV or AAV vectors may be able to persist in either an integrated or episomal state.

4. Targeted Integration

Although AAV vectors that do not contain the rep gene do not integrate at the AAVS1 site with any frequency, they can be directed to integrate at the chromosome 19 site by supplying the rep gene in *trans*. For instance, a plasmid containing an AAV vector comprised of a reporter gene between the AAV ITRs and having a rep gene also in the plasmid, but outside the ITRs resulted in integration of the AAV ITR vector cassette into the chromosomal site at 19q in human 293 cells in vitro (52). Also, a baculovirus vector that contained an AAV reporter gene vector and separately contained an AAV rep gene was able to direct integration of the AAV vector into the AAVS1 site in human 293 cells (53). Similarly, co-transduction of an epithelial tumor cell line (HeLa) or a hepatoma cell line (HepG2) with two hybrid Ad/AAV viruses, one carrying an AAV vector and the other expressing the *rep* gene, resulted in integration of the AAV vector into the AAVS1 site (54).

In another application, an AAV vector was used to examine the ability of sequences in AAV vectors to mediate homologous recombination with chromosomal sequences. It was demonstrated that AAV vectors could mediate homologous recombination at specific chromosomal sites at frequencies of 1/100,000 to 1/200 (55). In several human cell lines, an integrated hygromycin-resistance gene or the HPRT gene could be targeted by homologous recombination at low frequency.

D. AAV Permissivity

1. Helper Functions Provided by Other Viruses

The precise mechanism of the helper function provided by adenovirus or other helper viruses has not been clearly defined. These helper functions may be complex but relatively indirect in that they probably affect cellular physiology rather than provide proteins that specifically interact with the AAV-replication system. Studies with adenovirus (25) have clearly defined that only a limited set of adenovirus genes are required, and these comprise the early genes E1A, E1B, E2A, E4orf6 and the VA RNA. The primary role of E1A is to transcriptionally activate the other adenovirus genes, but it may also transcriptionally activate the AAV p5 promoter. E1B and the E4orf 6 protein of adenovirus interact to form a complex, and this may be important to mRNA transport. The E2A gene of adenovirus has a complex function because it is a single-strand DNA-binding protein that is directly involved in adenovirus replication, but it also has an important role in regulating adenovirus gene expression. The role of E2A for AAV appears not to be a DNA-replication function but to involve enhancement of AAV gene expression and particularly expression of AAV capsid protein. The VA RNA is also important in maximizing the level of AAV gene expression.

2. Alternate Pathways to Permissivity

The concept that the helper virus renders the cell permissive by enhancing AAV replication in an indirect way is consistent with the evidence that helper virus genes do not appear to provide enzymatic functions required for AAV DNA replication and that these functions are provided by AAV rep protein and the cellular DNA replication apparatus (25). This is also consistent with the observations that in certain cells lines, particularly if they are transformed with an oncogene, helper-independent replication of AAV DNA can occur if the cells are also treated with genotoxic reagents such as ultraviolet or x-irradiation of with hydroxyurea (56–58). In these circumstances, a small proportion of the cells can be rendered permissive for AAV replication, but the level of replication production of infectious AAV was very low.

3. Replication or Persistence

Two distinguishable phases of the AAV life cycle occur in permissive or nonpermissive cells, respectively. In either case the infecting single strand is converted to a duplex structure. However, in permissive cells in the presence of helper virus, this genome then appears to follow the pathway of bulk replication using the self-priming property of the ITR to yield a large pool of head-to-head and tail-to-tail RF molecules and ultimately a large burst of progeny particles. In nonpermissive cells in the absence of helper, these genomes follow a pathway that leads to generation of head-to-tail concatemers, which persist as episomes or become integrated into the host cell chromosome. In this nonpermissive state there are two important parameters, which may have different consequences for AAV or AAV vectors. In either case there is no helper function provided by another virus. However, for wild-type AAV, the *rep* gene is present and therefore may be expressed. This may explain why AAV integrates efficiently into the chromosome 19. For a vector, the *rep* gene is not present, and thus vectors may progress through the integration pathway more slowly and integrate less efficiently. This model is supported by a direct comparison of the metabolic fates of wild-type AAV and AAV vector genomes after infection in the absence of helper virus. Wild-type AAV was converted more rapidly and efficiently to head-to-tail concatemers than an AAV vector (T. Quinton, B. Carter, and C. Lynch, personal communication).

The precise mechanism by which the physiological state of the host cell effects the integration of AAV or conversion from SS to duplex, and thus expression from AAV vectors, remains unresolved. There is accumulating evidence that the single-strand genome may be converted to either linear duplexes or circular duplex molecules (50). The linear duplexes may be precursors of either the head-to-head and tail-to-tail RF concatemers seen in normal AAV replication or the head-to-tail concatemers that appear to be an intermediate in the integration pathway. The circular duplexes appear to be candidate precursors of the head-to-tail concatemers and also may be precursors of the integrated genomes. How the circularization event occurs is unknown, but the adenovirus E4orf6 gene promotes circularization whereas the adenovirus E2A gene promotes RF concatemers (59). Thus, AAV vectors can provide long-term expression in vivo in nondividing or slowly proliferating cells, and the dominant persistent species that accumulates over time is the head-tail concatemer. Whether this species is integrated or remains as a high molecular weight episome remains to be determined.

III. AAV VECTORS

A. Design of AAV Vectors

The ability to generate AAV vectors was facilitated by the observation that molecular cloning of double-strand AAV DNA into bacterial plasmids (8) followed by transfection into helper virus–infected mammalian cells resulted in rescue and replication of the AAV genome free of any plasmid sequence to yield a burst of infectious AAV particles. This rescue may occur by a mechanism analogous to that used in rescue of a latent provirus after superinfection of cells with adenovirus.

The general principles of AAV vector construction (6,8,9) are based upon modifying the molecular clones by substituting the AAV coding sequence with foreign DNA to generate a vector plasmid. In the vector, only the *cis*-

acting ITR sequences must be retained intact. The vector plasmid is introduced into producer cells, which are also rendered permissive by an appropriate helper virus such as adenovirus. In order to achieve replication and encapsidation of the vector genome into AAV particles, the vector plasmid must be complemented for the *trans*-acting AAV *rep* and *cap* functions that were deleted in construction of the vector plasmid. AAV vector particles can be purified and concentrated from lysates of such producer cells.

The AAV capsid has three important effects for AAV vectors. There is a limit of about 5 kb of DNA that can be packaged in an AAV vector particle. This places constraints on expression of very large cDNAs and may also affect the ability to include regulatory control sequences in the vector. The capsid also interacts with the AAV receptor and co-receptors and thus mediates cell entry. The capsid may also induce humoral immune responses that could limit delivery of AAV vectors for some applications.

Except for the limitation on packaging size and the requirements for ITRs, there are no obvious limitations on the design of gene cassettes in AAV vectors. The ITR can function as a transcription promoter (60) but does not interfere with other promoters. Tissue-specific promoters appear to retain specificity (61,62), and a number of other regulated expression systems have now been used successfully in AAV vectors. Introns function and may enhance expression, and more than one promoter and gene cassette can be inserted in the same vector. Importantly, transcription from AAV does not seem to be susceptible to in vivo silencing (43,44,63).

B. Production of AAV Vectors

There are several challenges in production of AAV vectors. It is likely that use of AAV vectors in human gene-therapy applications may require doses of at least 10^{10} or several orders of magnitude higher. However, the cytostatic properties of the AAV rep protein presented an obstacle to generation of packaging cell lines for AAV. Consequently, AAV vector production initially was based on transfection of a vector plasmid and a second plasmid, to provide complementing *rep* and *cap* functions, into adenovirus-infected cells, usually the transformed human 293 cell line. Initial vector production systems had low specific productivity and yielded a mixture of AAV vector particles and adenovirus particles (6,8). Furthermore, recombination between the vector plasmid and complementing plasmids generates wild-type AAV (AAV), pseudo wild-type or replication-competent AAV (rcAAV), or other recombinant AAV species (64,65).

There were several important issues to be addressed for improved AAV vector production. First, specific productivity needed to be improved. Second, removal of adenovirus is an important safety issue for clinical use of AAV vectors. Third, the presence of AAV or rcAAV may alter the properties or efficiency of AAV vectors and therefore is undesirable. Fourth, DNA transfection is less desirable for scale-up for commercial production. Fifth, purification of AAV by centrifugation, such as in density gradients of CsCl, may not completely remove adenovirus and is unwieldy for commercial manufacturing. Recent developments in both upstream production and downstream purification of AAV have addressed these general issues in several ways.

1. Complementation Systems

Three approaches have been taken with respect to upstream production of AAV vectors. First, in the two plasmid transfection systems various modifications have been made to the complementing rep-cap plasmid in an attempt to enhance specific productivity and to decrease production of rcAAV. One group suggested that expression of rep and cap proteins may be limiting (66), but two other studies (67,68) suggested that cap proteins were limiting due to downregulation by increased production of rep. A packaging plasmid which has the Rep78/69 expression downregulated by changing the initiation codon AUG to ACG was reported to give higher cap expression and higher yields of vector particles (68).

Early work showed that the only adenovirus genes required for full helper function were E1, E2A, E4, and VA, and transfection of the latter three genes into cells that contain the E1 genes, such as 293 cells, could provide full permissivity for AAV (25). Two groups (69,70) therefore replaced infectious adenovirus as the helper with a plasmid containing only the adenovirus E2A, E4, and VA genes, which, together with the E1A genes supplied by 293 cells, provided a complete helper function in the absence of adenovirus production. Another group (71) used a plasmid containing nearly all of the adenovirus genome except the E1 region, but this yielded infectious adenovirus, probably by recombination with the E1 region in the cell. All of these systems require transfection with three plasmids for vector, rep-cap, and adenovirus helper function, respectively. In contrast, Grimm et al. (72) combined all of the three adenovirus genes and the rep-cap genes into a single plasmid. In general, all of these approaches increased vector productivity compared to earlier systems such as pAAV/Ad (73), and productivities of at least 10^4 particles per cell have been reported. Nevertheless, these approaches still require DNA transfection and may be unwieldy for scale-up production.

A third approach is to generate cell lines that contain the *rep* and *cap* complementing systems or the vector genome or both. If transfection is to be avoided, the cells must still be infected by a helper virus, adenovirus, but this can be removed by advances in downstream purification processes. Cell lines containing AAV vectors in an EBV-episomal plasmid were described in which transfection with a packaging plasmid and infection with adenovirus could yield vector (74). However, it may be difficult to ensure the stability of vectors contained in an episomal plasmid. In contrast, rescue of vector from a producer line having the vector stably integrated was demonstrated by transfecting a *rep-cap* helper plasmid and infecting with adenovirus (75).

Stable cell lines containing a *rep* gene capable of generating functional *rep* protein were constructed by Yang et al. (36), who replaced the p_5 promoter with a heterologous promoter. Clark et al. (76) generated cell lines containing the *rep* and *cap* gene cassettes but deleted for AAV ITRs. Infection of the packaging cells with adenovirus activated *rep* and *cap* gene expression. Furthermore, the vector plasmid could be stably incorporated into the packaging cells to yield AAV vector producer cell lines that need only be infected with adenovirus to generate vector (76). Producer cell lines may provide a scalable AAV vector production system that does not require manufacture of DNA and may reduce generation of rcAAV.

A modification of the packaging cell method was reported (77) in which a similar cell line with a *rep-cap* gene cassette is infected first with one adenovirus to render the cells permissive and to provide the E1 gene function and then with a second E1-deleted adenovirus that contains the AAV ITR vector cassette. A possible advantage of this approach is that the same packaging cell line can be used for production of different AAV vectors by changing the Ad/AAV hybrid virus but a disadvantage is the need to use two different adenoviruses

Another packaging cell system was described (78) in which the packaging cell contains both a *rep-cap* cassette and the AAV ITR vector cassette and both cassettes are attached to an SV40 replication origin. Also in the cells is a SV T-antigen gene, which is under control of the *tet*-regulated system such that addition of doxycycline induces T-antigen that in turn results in amplification of the *rep-cap* and the vector cassettes. Subsequent infection of the cells with adenovirus renders them permissive for vector production.

Two groups examined the use of herpes simplex virus (HSV) in production of AAV vectors by generating two types of HSV/AAV hybrid viruses. One approach (79) utilizes an HSV/AAV hybrid virus in which the AAV *rep-cap* genes, under control of their native promoters, were inserted into the HSV genome. This HSV/AAV *rep-cap* virus could generate AAV vector when infected into cells lines along with a transfected AAV vector plasmid or into cell lines carrying an AAV vector provirus. Alternatively, an HSV/AAV hybrid virus was constructed by inserting an AAV ITR vector cassette between HSV genome replication origins and then packaging this construct into an HSV particle using an HSV amplicon system (80). These HSV/AAV vector hybrids were infectious for neural cells, and gene expression from the AAV vector was maintained over 2 weeks even though the HSV genome sequences were lost from the vector. Presumably, the AAV ITR cassette was amplified after infection. When the AAV *rep* gene was included within the hybrid HSV/AAV genome out outside the AAV ITRs, there was a modest effect in prolonging gene expression. The biological properties and fate of these HSV/AAV hybrid genomes after infection of cells is complex and not yet well understood.

2. Replication Competent or Wild-Type AAV

Wild-type AAV is not a human pathogen but generation of wild-type or rcAAV needs to be avoided for several reasons. The presence of wild-type AAV in vector preparations may result in expression of *rep* and *cap* genes that could increase the likelihood of vector mobilization following a helper virus infection in the patient, increase the likelihood immune responses to capsid protein, and cause significant alterations in the biology of the vector because of the pleiotropic effect of rep protein.

The earliest AAV vectors (6,8) were produced by cotransfection with helper plasmids that had overlapping homology with the vector, and this generated vector particles contaminated with wild-type AAV due to homologous recombination. Reduction of the overlapping AAV sequence homology between the vector and helper plasmids reduced, but did not eliminate, generation of wild-type AAV. In the widely used pAAV/Ad packaging system of Samulski et al. (73), overlapping homology is almost eliminated between the two plasmids but there is still generation of wild-type AAV at significant levels (64,75).

Flotte et al. (75) described a combination of vector plasmid and packaging plasmid in which the AAV region containing the P_5 promoter was not present in either plasmid. This prevented generation of wt AAV but some pseudo-wild-type AAV (rcAAV) was generated at very low frequency by nonhomologous recombination (64). This nonhomologous recombination was decreased to undetectable levels in a packaging system (split-gene packaging) carrying *rep* and *cap* genes in separate cassettes (64). This split-gene system would require three or four recombination events to generate rcAAV.

It is likely that all transfection systems may have a propensity to generate rcAAV or other recombinants of AAV because it not possible to eliminate nonhomologous recombination in transfected DNA, especially in view of the very large genome numbers that are normally introduced into transfected cells. Thus, packaging systems in which transfection is avoided may help to reduce the frequency of such recombination.

Standardized assays to analyze and evaluate such rcAAV or recombinant species in AAV vector preparations have not yet been developed and universally accepted. However, to detect replication-competent species, an assay that employs two cycles of amplification by replication and then a sensitive readout such as hybridization (rather than rep or cap immunoassays) will likely be required. Further, the availability of cells line providing *rep* and *cap* complementing functions will allow evaluation of such recombinant species without having to add wild-type AAV. This will facilitate detection of species that are only very poorly replication competent.

3. Purification

Historically, AAV was purified by proteolytic digestion of cell lysates in the presence of detergents followed by banding in CsCl gradients to concentrate and purify the particles and separate adenovirus particles. This remains the basis of most vector-purification schemes but for scale-up, procedures such as centrifugation in CsCl gradients are cumbersome and unacceptable for commercial production. Tamayose et al. (81) reported the use of sulfonated-cellulose column chromatography to purify AAV vectors. An alternative procedure using affinity chromatography with an antibody that recognizes assembled AAV particles and not free AAV capsid protein was described (72). Another approach that may be useful for smaller-scale purification (S. Zolotukhin, N. Muzyczka, B. Byrne, C. Summerford, and R. Samulski, personal communication) employs centrifugation through a discontinuous gradient of iodoxanol, followed by affinity purification on a heparinized support matrix and HPLC chromotography. Chromatographic procedures in general will be more acceptable for the biopharmaceutical manufacturing that will be required for full development of AAV vectors as therapeutic entities.

C. Properties of AAV Vectors

1. In Vitro Studies

AAV vectors have been extensively studied by transduction of cells grown in vitro (9,11). In general, AAV vectors can provide expression of a transduced gene in many types of cells and cell lines. The efficiency of this transduction may depend on whether the cells are stable, transformed cell lines, or primary cultures and whether the cells are stationary or dividing (82–84). There are no fully defined general rules, but two factors appear to be important. One factor determining transduction efficiency is metabolic activation (single-strand conversion), which tends to occur more quickly in dividing cells (85,86). A second factor is the AAV genome persistence. As noted above, vectors deleted for *rep* may integrate nonspecifically and with low efficiency. Thus, in cells that are rapidly dividing in culture, AAV vectors may give very efficient transient transduction but then may be rapidly diluted out as cell division proceeds.

In quiescent cell cultures, the transduction may depend upon the longer time required for conversion of single strands to duplexes. This process presumably requires cellular DNA polymerase and can be enhanced by procedures that stimulate DNA synthesis (Fig. 1) including DNA-damaging agents such UV or gamma irradiation, genotoxic agents such as hydroxyurea, topoisomerase inhibitor drugs such as topoisomerase inhibitor, or the adenovirus E4 Orf6 gene (85–87). While it is likely that some of the stimulatory effects of these agents do reflect enhancement of single-strand conversion, some reevaluation of these studies may be required. It is probable that in several of these studies the results were impacted by amplification of double-strand templates in the presence of *rep* expressed by contaminating wild-type AAV that also was present in the vector stocks (88,89). In spite of these observations, it appears that for in vivo applications these treatments are not required because in nondividing cells there is time for generation of double-strand templates to occur. Also, many in vivo gene therapy targets comprise nondividing or slowly turning-over differentiated cells, and these are very good targets for AAV transduction and long-term expression. (see below).

As with many other gene-delivery vectors, in vitro assays are useful to study vector design and transduction mechanisms but are not predictable for behavior in vivo (63). In vitro studies also have been useful for demonstrating biological efficacy of the vector. For instance, human airway epithelial cells from cystic fibrosis patients grown in vitro and transduced with an AAV vector expressing the CFTR cDNA were functionally corrected for their electrophysiological defect in chloride channel function (60). Most studies with AAV vectors are now focused on direct in vivo delivery.

2. In Vivo Studies

AAV vectors have proven remarkably efficient for long-term gene expression in vivo. Most of these in vivo studies have addressed differentiated target cells, which are either slowly proliferating or postmitotic and nondividing, and these types of cells may be the best targets for AAV gene therapy. AAV vectors expressed the human CFTR cDNA in the airway epithelium of rabbits (Fig. 3) and rhesus macaques for at least 6 months (40,90). Direct stereotactic

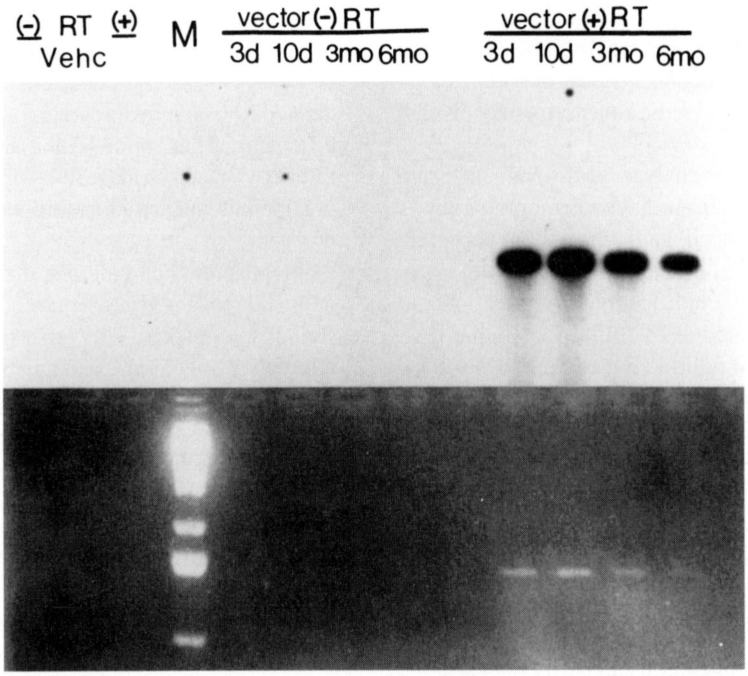

Figure 3 Expression of mRNA from an AAV-CFTR vector persists for 6 months after instillation into rabbit lungs. The AAV-CFTR vector was instilled into the right lower lobe of the lungs of New Zealand white rabbits. RNA was extracted at 3 days, 10 days, 3 months, and 6 months after instillation of the vector and analyzed by RT PCR in the presence (+) or absence (−) of reverse transcriptase followed by gel electrophoresis and ethidium bromide staining (bottom panel) and southern blotting (top panel). CFTR expression is demonstrated by the amplified fragment. Control lanes (Vehc) include RNAs from a lung homogenate from an animal treated only with vehicle from which there is no signal either in the presence or absence of reverse transcriptase. The duplicates of each sample that were assayed without reverse transcriptase demonstrate the completeness of vector DNA digestion. (From Ref. 40.)

injection into the rodent or nonhuman primate brain of AAV vectors expressing reporter genes or tyrosine hydroxylase can mediate gene expression for at least 3–6 months (42,91). Prolonged expression of reporter genes for up to 18 months was achieved in immunocompetent mice by direct intramuscular injection of AAV vectors (43). Delivery of AAV vectors expressing a clotting factor IX cDNA in mice by tail vein or portal vein injection led to factor IX expression for up to a year (47,92). Prolonged persistence of a therapeutic level of human erythropoietin (huEpo) was achieved by intramuscular injection of an AAV huEpo vector (44). Subcutaneous injection into the eye can mediate robust, persistent expression in the retinal pigment cells (62).

Some in vitro experiments, as noted above, indicated that conversion of SS to duplex could be enhanced by a variety of treatments that damage DNA. However, this has not proven necessary in most in vivo studies. Indeed, when this was tested in delivery to mouse liver or brain, expression was not greatly improved and the phenomenon was dependent on the presence of wild-type AAV (88). However, it is important to avoid wild-type AAV in vector preparations because it may drastically impact transduction and provide misleading conclusions. In one study, contaminating wild-type AAV prevented transduction by AAV vectors in rabbit lungs (89).

The in vivo studies show that the conversion of SS DNA to duplex transcription clearly occurs and that robust and therapeutic levels of gene expression can be obtained. In some of these studies, and particularly in muscle, expression rises over the first several weeks and then is maintained at a constant level. This reflects both the slow process of conversion to duplex genomes and then to concatemeric structures. In rhesus macaques, an AAV CFTR vector was present 3 months after instillation in the lung and appeared to be a dimeric concatemer (41). In muscle or liver after several weeks, high molecular weight head-to-tail concatemers are formed (47,48). These observations reflect the mechanism of the AAV persistence pathway discussed above. In the in vivo studies, it has been difficult to rigorously demonstrate if any of the persistent form of the AAV vector is actually integrated or remains as a high molecular weight episome.

3. Regulated Gene Expression in AAV Vectors

For some applications it may be very important to obtain precise regulation of gene expression from AAV vectors. This may be particularly important if the level of gene expression continues to rise for a considerable period of time. For instance, expression in the muscle may continue to increase for up to 2 months (63). For certain therapeutic applications this may present an important issue in establishing a drug dose, and it is likely that the level of the therapeutic gene product will need to be closely regulated. Ideally, this may be achieved by a tissue-specific promoter or a promoter that responds to a relevant physiological signal, but this type of gene regulation has not yet been established in AAV vectors. However, two groups have examined the regulation of expression from AAV vectors using a promoter regulated by an exogenously administered drug. In each case this required simultaneous transduction with two AAV vectors.

In one study (93), mice were injected intramuscularly with one AAV vector expressing an inducible murine erythropoietin gene and a second AAV vector containing a transcriptional activator that was regulated by tetracycline. Expression was maintained over 18 weeks by administration of tetracycline, and no humoral response to the transcriptional activator was observed. In a similar study (94) the first AAV vector expressed two domains of a chimeric transcriptional activator and the second AAV vector expressed erythropoietin from a promoter activated in response to the chimeric transcriptional activator. Formation of the two domains of the transcriptional activator into a functional complex was mediated by binding of an exogenously administered drug, rapamycin. Again, this system functioned to regulate Epo when administered intramuscularly to mice, and there did not appear to be an inhibitory humoral immune response. Unfortunately, this system failed in rhesus macaques where after several months an inhibitory immune response was mounted against the transcription activator, and this is likely to limit the application of such systems.

In all of the in vivo studies thus far with AAV vectors in rodent, rabbit, or rhesus macaques, there has been no evidence of inflammatory or cytokine-mediated responses and little evidence of cellular immune responses. There is only relatively preliminary information on the likelihood of generation of humoral antibody responses to the AAV capsid protein, and more extensive studies will be required to assess whether induction of neutralizing antibody responses will pose any limitations to AAV vectors.

In one study in which two AAV vectors expressing as reporter genes either the bacterial protein LacZ or the human alkaline phosphatase gene were successively administered to lungs of rabbits, expression from the second administered vector was impaired, which was ascribed to a neutralizing antibody response (95). Similar studies in mice also implied that neutralizing antibodies impaired readministration of AAV vectors but that this could be partially or completely overcome by transient immunosupression with anti-CD40 ligand antibodies or soluble CTLA4-immunoglobin at the time of the initial vector administration (89,96). The interpretation of such studies is complicated by the expression of foreign reporter proteins that may represent confounding variables. For instance, in another study (17) up to three successive administrations of AAV vectors to rabbit lungs over a 20-week period did not prevent gene expression from the third delivery of vector. Furthermore, transient immunosuppression at the time of vector delivery may not be an attractive option for therapeutic use of AAV or any other gene-delivery vectors. This will most likely require studies in humans to determine if the various animal models such as rodents or rabbits are predictive for the immune response to AAV vectors in humans and whether such immune responses will pose any limitations to their therapeutic application.

In some studies, such as of intramuscular delivery in mice, there has also been no immune response to an expressed foreign reporter gene such as the bacterial gene LacZ, and it was been suggested that AAV may a poor adjuvant and may not readily infect professional antigen presenting cells in muscle (97). However, an AAV vector expressing the herpes simplex virus type2 gB protein was delivered intramuscularly into mice and elicited both MHC Class I restricted CTL responses against the gB protein and anti-gB antibodies (98).

The toxicity of AAV vectors has been most extensively tested by delivery of AAV CFTR vector particles directly to the lung in rabbits and nonhuman primates. In rabbits (40) the vector persisted and expressed for at least 6 months, but no short-term or long-term toxicity was observed and there was no indication of T-cell infiltration or inflammatory responses. In rhesus macaques (90) AAV CFTR vector particles were delivered directly to one lobe of a lung and also persisted and expressed for at least 6 months. No toxicities were observed by pulmonary function testing, by radiological examination, analysis of blood gases and cell counts and differential in broncho-alveolar lavage or by gross morphological examination or histopathological examination or organ tissues. There was minimal spread of the vector to organs outside of the lung and no vector in gonads and no toxicity noted in any organ. Studies in rhesus macaques were also performed to determine if the AAV-CFTR vector could possibly be shed or rescued from a treated individual (41). AAV-CFTR particles were delivered to the lower right lobe of the lung, and a high dose of adenovirus and wild-type AAV particles were administered to the nose of the animals. These studies indicated that the vector was not readily rescued and suggested that the probability of vector shedding and transmission to others is likely to be low.

D. AAV Vector Applications

AAV vectors are now being developed for therapeutic applications. On the basis of extensive preclinical studies performed in rabbits and nonhuman primates, an AAV vector expressing the CFTR cDNA has been introduced into clinical trials in cystic fibrosis patients. These are the first clinical trials with an AAV vector (26). AAV vectors expressing factor IX provided at least partial therapeutic correction of factor IX deficiency in dogs and soon may be introduced into clinical trials in patients with hemophilia B. Also, AAV vectors have been used in an animal model to deliver a ribozyme to inhibit an autosomal dominant gene in the retina, and these vectors are now being developed for treatment of ophthalmic diseases such as diabetic retinopathy and macular degeneration. Other possible clinical applications suggested by current studies include CNS defects (42,91) such as Parkinson's disease. Whether AAV vectors can be used for cancer targets to ablate tumors using a suicide gene such as herpesvirus thymidine kinase or prodrugs (11) needs careful consideration because the propensity of AAV to transduce nondividing cells might result in serious consequences in nontumor cells.

1. Cystic Fibrosis

Cystic fibrosis (CF) is a lethal autosomal recessive disease, which is caused by a mutation in the cystic fibrosis transmembrane conductance regulator (CFTR) gene. The CFTR protein is a chloride ion channel generally expressed in epithelial cells and a defect in this protein leads to complex biochemical changes in several organs including lung and often the exocrine pancreas. In the lung there is a decreased mucociliary clearance, increased bacterial colonization, and a chronic neutrophil-dominated inflammatory response, which leads to progressive destruction of tissue in the conducting airways. The usual cause of morbidity and eventual mortality in CF patients is progressive loss of lung function. Thus, the goal of a gene therapy for CF is to deliver the CFTR cDNA into the epithelial cells in the conducting airways of the lung.

An AAV vector expressing the CFTR cDNA has been introduced into clinical trials in CF patients by delivery of the vector to the lung and the nasal epithelium (1) and in addition into the maxillary sinus (2). Although the lung is the target for a therapeutic gene therapy for CF, delivery to the maxillary sinus is a novel approach in an attempt to obtain an early indication of the potential of the AAV CFTR vector. The maxillary sinuses of CF patients exhibit chronic inflammation and bacterial colonization, which is reflective of some aspects of the CF disease in the lung. In addition, in CF patients who have undergone surgical bilateral anstrostomy, the maxillary sinus is accessible to instillation of vectors and for sampling and biopsy. In an initial trial, 15 sinuses of CF patients were treated with increasing doses of the AAV-CFTR vector (2). Biopsy of the sinuses followed by DNA PCR indicated that there was dose-dependent delivery of the vector and that the vector genomes persisted in the sinus for at least 70 days after instillation. In epithelial cell surfaces of CF patients, the transmembrane potential is hyperpolarized compared to normal patients because of the absence of a functional CFTR chloride channel. Analysis of the transmembrane potential difference across the epithelial surface of the treated sinuses indicated that at the higher doses of vector there was some reversal of the electrophysiological defect. This constitutes presumptive evidence of expression of the CFTR protein from the delivered vector.

2. Hemophilia

Hemophilia B is a severe X-linked recessive disease that results from mutations in the blood coagulation factor IX, and the absence of functional factor IX leads to severe bleeding diathesis. Delivery of factor IX protein at levels of 1% of the normal level (50 ng/mL) can decrease the risk of spontaneous bleeding into joints and soft tissues and lowers the risk of fatal intracranial bleeding. However, the protein has a very short half-life, and this has stimulated interest in developing gene-therapy approaches in which the factor IX protein may be produced more persistently. AAV vectors appear to be well suited for such an application, and several groups have provided evidence that factor IX protein can be expressed for prolonged periods in both murine and canine models after delivery of factor IX vectors to either the liver by portal vein injection or by intramuscular injection (46,47,99–101). In general, the levels of expression have indicated that at least a partial correction of the defect in both murine and canine disease models can be achieved and suggest that accumulation of therapeutic amounts of factor IX may be achievable in humans. One caution is that most of these studies have determined the levels of functional factor IX in serum using the whole blood clotting time (WBCT) assay, which is an unreliable assay, rather than activated partial thromboplastin time (APT), which may be a more reliable measure.

AAV vector delivery of the human factor IX gene into either immunodeficient or immunocompetent mice by portal vein injection into liver resulted in prolonged expression of factor IX for up to 36 weeks at levels of 250–2000 ng/mL in serum, which is equivalent to about one fifth of the normal human level (47). Similar delivery of human factor IX in hemophiliac dogs resulted in expression of factor IX at about 1% of normal canine levels, an absence of inhibitors, and sustained partial correction of WBCT for at least 8 months (99). In another study by Herzog et al. (46), intramuscular injection of an AAV human factor IX vector in mice led to prolonged expression in immunodeficient mice of about 350 ng/mL for at least 6 months, but in immunocompetent mice there was generation of inhibitory antibody. These same investigators (100) subsequently showed that in hemophiliac dogs, intramuscular injection of high doses of the AAV-canine factor IX achieved expression for over 17 months and demonstrated a stable, dose-dependent partial correction of the WBCT, and at the highest dose there was a partial correction of APT. Finally, in another study (101) intramuscular injection of an AAV human factor IX vector also led to a transient reduction of WBCT in the first week, but this was rapidly lost as the animals developed anti-factor IX antibody.

3. Ophthalmic Disease

Other recent studies illustrate the possible applications of AAV vectors to ophthalmic disease (62,102–104). For instance, photoreceptor cells in rodent models can readily be transduced by injection into the subretinal space of AAV vectors containing a reporter gene expressed from a rod opsin transcription promoter (62). Gene delivery was extremely efficient, with nearly 100% transduction of the subretinal area that was targeted, which represented about 10–20% of the entire retina, with expression continuing for at least 10 weeks. In a further study, this approach was used to demonstrate phenotypic correction of an ophthalmic disease model of autosomal dominant retinitis pigmentosa (102). Twelve percent of Americans with the blinding disease autosomal retinitis pigmentosa (ADRP) carry an autosomal dominant P23H mutation in their rhodopsin gene, and a similar transgenic rat model of this disease is available. Delivery with an AAV vector of a ribozyme targeted at this mutation in the rodent model protected photoreceptors from death and resulted in significantly slowing the degenerative disease for 3 months (102).

IV. SUMMARY

The work summarized in this chapter illustrates the increasingly rapid progress that is now being made in developing therapeutic applications of AAV vectors. One group initiated clinical testing of AAV vectors for CF, and this has been extremely important in establishing the regulatory environment for AAV vectors. As more groups have extended investigations to additional in vivo models, the potential utility of AAV vectors as therapeutic gene-delivery vehicles has gained more widespread interest. The development of more sophisticated production systems for AAV vectors has enhanced both the quantity and quality of vectors that can be produced. It is likely that in the next few years there will be a significant increase in testing of AAV vectors for additional therapeutic applications.

REFERENCES

1. Flotte TR, Carter BJ, Conrad CK, Guggino WB, Reynolds TC, Rosenstein BJ, Taylor G, Walden S, Wetzel R. A phase I study of an adeno-associated virus-CFTR gene vector in adult CF patients with mild lung disease. Hum. Gene Ther 1996; 7:1145–1159.
2. Wagner J A, Messner AH, Moran ML, Daifuku R, Kouyama K, Desch JK, Manley S, Norbash AM, Conrad CK, Friborg A, Reynolds T, Guggino WB, Moss RB, Carter BJ, Wine JJ, Flotte TR, Gardner P. Safety and biological efficacy of an adeno-associated virus vector-cystic fibrosis transmembrane regulator (AAV-CFTR) in the cystic fibrosis maxillary sinus. Laryngoscope 1999; 109:266–274.
3. Carter BJ. The growth cycle of adeno-associated virus. In: Tjissen P, ed. Handbook of Parvoviruses. Boca Raton, FL: CRC Press, 1989:155–168.
4. Berns KI. In: Fields BN, Knipe DM, et al., eds. Virology. New York: Raven Press, 1990:1743–1764.
5. Carter BJ. Parvoviruses as vectors. In: Tjissen P, ed. Handbook of Parvoviruses. Boca Raton, FL: CRC Press, 1989: 155–168.
6. Muzyczka N. Use of adeno-associated virus as a generalized transduction vector in mammalian cells. Current Topics Microbiol Immunol 1992; 158:97–129.
7. Berns KI., Giraud C. Adeno-associated virus (AAV) vectors in gene therapy. Current Topics Microbiol Immunol 1996; 218:1–144.
8. Carter BJ. Adeno-associated virus vectors. Current Opinion Biotechnol 1992; 3:533–539.
9. Flotte TR, Carter BJ. Adeno-associated virus vectors for gene therapy. Gene Ther 1995; 2:357–362.
10. Kotin RM. Prospects for the use of adeno-associated virus as a vector for human gene therapy. Human Gene Ther 1994; 5:793–801.
11. Hallek M, Girod A, Braun-Flaco M, Clemens-Martin W, Bogedin C, Horer M. Recombinant adeno-associated virus vectors. Curr Res Mol Therapeut 1998; 1:417–430.
12. Rabinowitz JE, Samulski R. Adeno-associated virus expression systems for gene transfer. Curr Opin Biotechnol 1998; 9:470–475.
13. Summerford C, Samulski RJ. Adeno-associated viral vectors for gene therapy. Biogenic Amines 1998; 14:451–475.
14. Atchison RW, Casto BC, Hammon McD. Adenovirus-associated defective virus particles Science 1965; 149: 754–756.

15. Hoggan MD, Blacklow NR, Rowe WP. Studies of small DNA viruses found in various adenovirus preparations: physical, biological and immunological characteristics. Proc Natl Acad Sci USA 1966; 55:1467–1472.
16. Blacklow NR. Adeno-associated viruses of human. In: Pattison JR, ed. Parvoviruses and Human Disease. Boca Raton, FL: CRC Press, 1988:165–174.
17. Beck, SE, Jones L, Chesnut K, Reynolds T, Flotte T, Guggino WB. Repeat airway delivery of AAV vectors results in gene expression and expression. Pediatr Pulmonol 1998; 17:262–263.
18. Summerford C, Samulski RJ. Membrane-associated heparan sulfate proteoglycan is a receptor for adeno-associated virus type 2 virions. J Virol 1998; 72:1438–1445.
19. Summerford C, Bartlett JS, Samulski RJ. $\alpha_V\beta_5$ integrin: a co-receptor for adeno-associated virus type 2 infection. Nat Med 1999; 5:78–82.
20. Qing K, Mah C, Hansen J, Zhou S, Dwarki V, Srivastava A. Human fibroblast growth factor receptor 1 is a co-receptor for infection by adeno-associated virus 2. Nature Med 1999; 5:71–77.
21. Mah C, Qing K, Hansen J, Khuntirat B, Yoder MC, Srivastava A. Gene transfer with adeno-associated virus 2 vectors: the growth factor receptor connection. Gene Ther Mol Biol 1999; in press.
22. Goldman M, Su Q, Wilson JM. Gradient of RGD-dependent entry of adenoviral vector in nasal and intrapulmonary epithelia: implications for gene therapy of cystic fibrosis. Gene Ther 1996; 3:811–818.
23. Duan D, Yue Y, Yan Y, McCray PB, Engelhardt JF. Polarity influences the efficiency of recombinant adeno-associated virus infection in differentiated airway epithelia. Human Gene Ther 1998; 9:2761–2776.
24. Ponnazhagan S, Mukherjee P, Yoder MC, Wang X-S, Zhou SZ, Kaplan J, Wadsworth S, Srivastava A. Adeno-associated virus type 2-mediated gene transfer in vivo: organ-tropism and expression of transduced sequences in mice. Gene 1997; 190:203–210.
25. Carter BJ. Adeno-associated virus helper functions. In: Tjissen P, ed. Handbook of Parvoviruses. Boca Raton, FL: CRC Press, 1990:255–282.
26. Carter BJ. The promise of adeno-associated virus vectors. Nature Biotechnol 1996; 14:1725–1726.
27. Weitzman MD, Kyostio SRM, Kotin RM, Owens RA. Adeno-associated virus (AAV) Rep proteins mediate complex formation between AAV DNA and its integration site in human DNA. Proc Natl Acad Sci USA 1994; 91: 5808–5812.
28. Kearns WG, Afione SA, Fulmer SB, Pang MG, Erikson D, Egan L, Landrum MJ, Flotte TR, Cutting GR. Recombinant adeno-associated virus (AAV-CFTR) vectors do not integrate in a site-specific fashion in an immortalized epithelial cell line. Gene Ther 1996; 3:748–755.
29. Linden RM, Ward P, Giraud C, Winocour E, Berns KI. Site-specific integration by adeno-associated virus. Proc Natl Acad Sci USA 1996; 93:11288–11294.
30. Crawford LV, Follett, EAC, Burdon MG, McGeoch DJ. The DNA of a minute virus of mice. J Gen Virol 1969; 4:37–48.
31. Rose JA, Berns KI, Hoggan MD, Koczot FJ. Evidence for a single-stranded adenovirus-associated virus genome: formation of a DNA density hybrid upon release of viral DNA. Proc Natl Acad Sci USA 1969; 64:863–869.
32. Smuda JW, Carter BJ. Adeno-associated viruses having nonsense mutations in the capsid gene: growth in mammalian cells having an inducible amber suppressor. Virology 1991; 184:310–318.
33. Carter BJ, Mendelson E, Trempe, JP. AAV DNA replication, integration and genetics. In: Tjissen P, ed. Handbook of Parvoviruses. Boca Raton, FL: CRC Press, 1989: 169–226.
34. Redemann B, Mendelson E, Carter BJ. Adeno-associated virus rep protein synthesis during productive infection. J Virol 1998; 63:873–882.
35. Perriera DJ, McCarty D, Muzyczka, N. The adeno-associated virus (AAV) rep protein acts as both a repressor and an activator to regulate AAV transcription during a productive infection. J Virol 1997; 71:1079–1088.
36. Yang Q, Chen F, Trempe JP. Characterization of cell lines that inducibly express the adeno-associated virus Rep proteins. J Virol 1994; 68:4847–4856.
37. Hoggan MD, Thomas GF, Johnson FB. Continuous carriage of adenovirus-associated virus genome in cell culture in the absence of helper adenovirus. Proceedings of the Fourth Lepetit Colloqium. Amsterdam: North Holland, 1972:41–47.
38. McLaughlin SK, Collis P, Hermonat PL, Muzyczka N. Adeno-associated virus general transduction vectors: analysis of proviral structure. J Virol 1988; 62:1963–1973.
39. Kotin RM, Siniscalco M, Samulski RJ, Zhu XD, Hunter L, Laughlin CA, McLaughlin S, Muzyczka N, Rocchi M, Berns KI. Site-specific integration by adeno-associated virus. Proc Natl Acad Sci USA 1990; 87:2211–2215.
40. Flotte IR, Afione SA, Solow R, McGrath SA, Conrad C, Zeitlin PL, Guggino WB Carter BJ. In vivo delivery of adeno-associated vectors expressing the cystic fibrosis transmembrane conductance regulator to the airway epithelium. Proc Natl Acad Sci USA 1993; 93:10163–10617.
41. Afione SA, Conrad CK, Kearns WG, Chunduru S, Adams R, Reynolds TC, Guggino WB, Cutting GR, Carter BJ, Flotte TR. In vivo model of adeno-associated virus vector persistence and rescue. J Virol 1996; 70:3235–3241.
42. Kaplitt MG, Leone P, Samulski RJ, Xiao X, Pfaff D, O'Malley KL, During M. Long-term gene expression and phenotypic connection using adeno-associated virus vectors in the mammalian brain. Nature Genetics 1994; 8: 148–154.
43. Xiao X, Li J, Samulski RJ. Efficient long-term gene transfer into muscle tissue of immunocompetent mice by adeno-associated virus vector. J Virol 1996; 70:8098–8108.
44. Kessler PD, Podsakoff GM, Chen X, McQuiston SA, Colosi PC, Matelis LA, Kurtzman GJ, Byrne B. Gene delivery

to skeletal muscle results in sustained expression and systemic delivery of a therapeutic protein. Proc Natl Acad Sci USA 1996; 93:14082–14087.
45. Fisher KJ, Jooss K, Alston J, Yang Y, Haecker SH, High K, Pathak R, Raper S, Wilson LM. Recombinant adeno-associated virus vectors for muscle directed gene therapy. Nature Med 1997; 8:306–312.
46. Herzog RW, Hagstrom JN, Kung S-H, Tai SJ, Wilson JM, Fisher KJ, High KA. Stable gene transfer and expression of human blood coagulation factor IX after intramuscular injection of recombinant adeno-associated virus. Proc Natl Acad Sci USA 1997; 94:5804–5809.
47. Snyder RO, Spratt SK, Lagarde C, Bohl C, Kaspar B, Sloan B, Cohen LK, Danos O. Efficient and stable adeno-associated virus-mediated transduction of the skeletal muscle of adult immunocompetent mice. Human Gene Ther 1997; 8:1891–1900.
48. Miao CH, Snyder RO, Schowalter DB, Patijn GA, Donahue B, Winther B, Kay MA. The kinetics of rAAV integration into the liver. Nature Genetics 1998; 19:13–14.
49. McKeon C, Samulski RJ. NIDDK Workshop on AAV vectors: gene transfer into quiescent cells. Human Gene Ther 1996; 7:1615–1619.
50. Duan D, Sharma P, Yang J, Yue Y, Dudus L, Zhang Y, Fisher KJ, Engelhardt JF. Circular intermediates of recombinant adeno-associated virus have defined structural characteristics responsible for long-term episomal persistence in muscle tissue. J Virol 1998; 72:8568–8577.
51. Vincent-Lacaze N, Snyder RO, Gluzman R, Bohl D, Lagarde C, Danos O. Structure of adeno-associated virus vector DNA following transduction of the skeletal muscle. J Virol 1999; 73:1949–1955.
52. Surosky RT, Urabe M, Godwin SG, McQuiston SA, Kurtzman GJ, Ozawa K, Natsoulis G. Adeno-associated virus rep proteins target DNA sequences to a unique locus in the human genome. J Virol 1997; 71:7951–7959.
53. Palombo F, Monciotti A, Recchia A, Cortese R, Ciliberto G, La Monica N. Site-specific integration in mammalian cells mediated by a new hybrid baculovirus-adeno-associated virus vector. J Virol 1998; 72:5025–5034.
54. Recchia A, Parks RJ, Lamartina S, Toniatti C, Pieroni L, Palombo F, Ciliberto G, Graham FL, Cortese R, La Monica N. Site-specific integration mediated by a hybrid adenovirus/adeno-associated virus vector. Proc Natl Acad Sci USA 1999; 96:2615–2620.
55. Russell, DW, Hirata RK. Human gene targeting by viral vectors. Nature Genetics 1998; 18:325–330.
56. Yakobson B, Koch T, Winocour E. Replication of adeno-associated virus in synchronized cells without the addition of helper virus. J Virol 1987; 61:972–981.
57. Yakobson B, Hrynko TA, Peak MJ, Winocour E. Replication of adeno-associated virus in cells irradiated with UV light at 254 nm. J Virol 1988; 63:1023–1030.
58. Bantel-Schaal U, zur Hausen H. Adeno-associated viruses inhibit SV40 DNA amplification and replication of herpes simplex virus in SV40-transformed hamster cells. Virology 1988; 164:64–74.
59. Duan D, Sharma P, Dudus L, Zhang Y, Sanlioglu S, Yan Z, Yue Y, Ye Y, Lester R, Yang J, Fisher KJ, Engelhardt JF. Formation of adeno-associated virus circular genomes is differentially regulated by adenovirus E4 orf6 and E2A gene expression. J Virol 1999; 73:161–169.
60. Flotte TR, Zeitlin PL, Solow, Afione S, Owens RA, Markakis D, Drumm M, Guggino WB, Carter BJ. Expression of the cystic fibrosis transmembrane conductance regulator from a novel adeno-associated virus promoter. J Biol Chem 1993; 268:3781–3790.
61. Peel AL, Zolotukhin S, Schrimsher GW, Muzyczka N, Reier PJ. Efficient transduction of green fluorescent protein in spinal cord neurons using adeno-associated virus vectors containing cell type-specific promoters. Gene Ther 1997; 4:16–24.
62. Flannery JG, Zolotukhin S, Vaquero MI, LaVail MM, Muzyczka N, Hauswirth WW. Efficient photoreceptor-targeted gene expression in vivo by recombinant adeno-associated virus. Proc Natl Acad Sci USA 1997; 94: 6916–6921.
63. Song S, Morgan M, Ellis T, Poirier A, Chesnut K, Wang J, Brantly M, Muzyczka N, Byrne BJ, Atkinson M, Flotte TR. Sustained secretion of human alpha-1 antitrypsin from murine muscle transduced with adeno-associated virus vectors. Proc Natl Acad Sci USA 1998; 95:14384–14388.
64. Allen JA, Debelak DJ, Reynolds TC, Miller AD. Identification and elimination of replication-competent adeno-associated virus (AAV) that can arise by non-homologous recombination during AAV vector production. J Virol 1997; 71:6816–6822.
65. Wang XS, Khuntirat B, Qing K, Ponnazhagan S, Kube DM, Zhou S, Dwarki VJ, Srivastava A. Characterization of wild-type adeno-associated virus type 2-like particles generated during recombinant viral vector production and strategies for their elimination. J Virol 1998; 72: 5472–5480.
66. Fan P-D, Dong J-Y. Replication of rep-cap genes is essential or the high-efficiency production of recombinant AAV. Human Gene Ther 1997; 8:87–98.
67. Vincent K, Piraino ST, Wadsworth SC. Analysis of recombinant adeno-associated virus packaging and requirements for rep and cap gene products. J Virol 1997; 71: 1897–1905.
68. Li J, Samulski RJ, Xiao X. Role for highly regulated rep gene expression in adeno-associated virus vector production. J Virol 1997; 71:5236–5243.
69. Xiao X, Li J, Samulski RJ: Production of high-titer recombinant adeno-associated virus vectors in the absence of helper adenovirus. J Virol 1998; 72:2224–2232.
70. Matushita T, Elliger S, Elliger C, Podskaoff G, Villareal L, Kurtzman GJ, Iwaki Y, Colosi P. Adeno-associated virus vectors can be efficiently produced without helper virus. Gene Ther 1998; 5:938–945.
71. Salvetti AS, Oreve S, Chadeuf G, Favre D, Cherel Y, Champion-Arnaud P, David-Ameline J, Mouillier P. Factors influencing recombinant adeno-associated virus production. Human Gene Ther 1998; 9:695–706.

72. Grimm D, Kern A, Rittnet K, Kleinschmidt JA. Novel tools for production and purification of recombinant adeno-associated virus vectors. Human Gene Ther 1998; 9:2745–2760.
73. Samulski RJ, Chang LS, Shenk TE. Helper-free stocks of recombinant adeno-associated viruses: normal integration does not require viral gene expression. J Virol 1989; 63: 3822–3828.
74. Lebkowski JS, McNally MA, Okarma TB: Production of recombinant adeno-associated virus vectors. U.S. Patent 5,173,414. 1992.
75. Flotte TR, Barrazza-Ortiz X, Solow R, Afione SA, Carter BJ, Guggino WB. An improved system for packaging recombinant adeno-associated virus vectors capable of in vivo transduction. Gene Ther 1995; 2:39–47.
76. Clark KR, Voulgaropoulou F, Fraley DM, Johnson PR. Cell lines for the production of recombinant adeno-associated virus. Human Gene Ther 1995; 6:1329–1341.
77. Gao G-P, Qu G, Faust LZ, Engdahl RK, Xiao W, Hughes JV, Zoltick PW, Wilson JM. High-titer adeno-associated viral vectors from a rep/cap cell line and hybrid shuttle virus. Human Gene Ther 1998; 9:2353–2362.
78. Inoue I, Russell DW. Packaging cells based on inducible gene amplification for the production of adeno-associated virus vectors. J Virol 1998; 72:7024–7031.
79. Conway JE, Zolotukhin S, Muzyczka N, Hayward GS, Byrne BJ. Recombinant adeno-associated virus type 2 replication and packaging is entirely supported by a herpes simplex virus type 1 amplicon expressing rep and cap. J Virol 1997; 71:8780–8789.
80. Johnston KM, Jacoby D, Pechan PA, Fraefel C, Borghesani P, Schuback D, Dunn RJ, Smith FI, Breakfield O. HSV/AAV hybrid amplicaon vectors extend transgene expression in human glioma cells. Human Gene Ther 1997; 8:359–370.
81. Tamayose K, Hirai Y, Shimada T. A new strategy for large-scale preparation of high titer recombinant adeno-associated virus vectors by using packaging cell lines and sulfonated cellulose column chromatography. Human Gene Ther 1996; 7:507–513.
82. Russell DW, Alexander IE, Miller AD. Adeno-associated virus vectors preferentially transduce cells in S phase. Proc Natl Acad Sci USA 1994; 91:8915–8919.
83. Flotte TR, Afione SA, Zeitlin PL. Adeno-associated virus vector gene expression occurs in nondividing cells in the anbsence of vector DNA integration. Am J Respir Cell Mol Biol 1994; 11:517–521.
84. Podsakoff G, Wong KK, Chatterjee S. Efficient gene transfer into nondividing cells by adeno-associated virus based vectors. J Virol 1994; 68:5656–5666.
85. Ferrari FK. Samulski T, Shenk T, Samulski RJ. Second-strand synthesis is a rate limiting step for efficient transduction by recombinant adeno-associated virus vectors. J Virol 1996; 70:3227–3234.
86. Fisher KJ, Gao GP, Weitzman MD, DeMatteo R, Burda JF, Wilson JM. Transduction with recombinant adeno-associated virus vectors for gene therapy is limited by leading strand synthesis. J Virol 1996; 70:520–532.
87. Russell DW, Alexander IE, Miller AD. DNA synthesis and topoisomerase inhibitors increase transduction by adeno-associated virus vectors. J Virol 1995; 92:5719–5723.
88. Koerberl DD, Alexander IE, Halbert CL, Russell DW, Miller AD. Persistent expression of human clotting factor IX from mouse liver after intravenous injection of AAV vectors. Proc Natl Acad Sci USA 1997; 94:1426–1431.
89. Halbert CL, Standaert TA, Wilson CB, Miller AD. Successful readministration of adeno-associated virus vectors to the mouse lung requires transient immunosuppression during initial exposure. J. Virol 1998; 72:9795–9805.
90. Conrad CK, Allen SS, Afione SA, Reynolds TC, Beck SE, Fee-Maki M, Barrazza-Ortiz X, Adams R, Askin FB, Carter BJ, Guggino WB, Flotte TR. Safety of single-dose administration of an adeno-associated virus (AAV-CFTR) vector in the primate lung. Gene Ther 1996; 3:658–668.
91. Xiao X, Li J, McCown TJ, Samulski RJ. Gene transfer by adeno-associated virus vectors into the central nervous system. Exp Neurol 1997; 144:113–124.
92. Snyder RO, Miao CH, Patijn GA, Spratt SK, Danos O, Nagy D, Gown AM, Winther B, Meuse L, Cohen LK, Thompson AR, Kay MA. Persistent and therapeutic concentrations of human factor IX in mice after hepatic gene transfer of recombinant AAV vectors. Nature Genetics 1997; 116:270–275.
93. Rendahl KG, Leff SE, Otten GR, Spratt SK, Bohl D, van Roey M, Donahue B, Cohen LK, mandel RJ, Danos O, Snyder RO. Regulation of gene expression in vivo following transduction by two separate rAAV vectors. Nature Biotechnol 1998; 16:757–761.
94. Ye X, Rivera, Zoltick P, Cerasoli F, Schnell MA, Gao GP, Hughes JV, Gilman M, Wilson JM. Regulated delivery of therapeutic proteins after in vivo somatic cell gene transfer. Science 1999; 283:88–91.
95. Halbert CL, Standaert TA, Aitken ML, Alexander IE, Russell DW, Miller AD. Transduction by adeno-associated virus vectors in the rabbit airway: efficiency, persistence and readministration. J Virol 1997; 71:5932–5941.
96. Manning WC, Zhou S, Bland MP, Escobedo JA, Dwarki V. Transient immunosuppression allows transgene expression following readministration of adeno-associated virus vectors. Human Gene Ther 1998; 9:477–485.
97. Jooss K, Yang Y, Fisher KJ, Wilson JM. Transduction of dendritic cells by DNA viral vectors directs the immune response to transgene products in muscle fibers. J Virol 1998; 72:4212–4223.
98. Manning WC, Paliard X, Zhou S, Bland MP, Lee AY, Hong K, Walker CM, Escobedo JA, Dwarki V. Genetic immunization with adeno-associated virus vectors expressing herpes simplex type2 glycoproteins B and D. J Virol 1997; 71:7960–7962.

99. Snyder RO, Miao C, Meuse L, Tubb J, Donahue BA, Lin H-F, Stafford, DW, Patel S, Thompson AR, Nichols T, Read MS, Bellinger DA, Brinkhous KM, Kay MA. Correction of hemophilia B in canine and murine models using recombinant adeno-associated vectors. Nature Med 1999; 5:64–69.

100. Herzog RW, Yang EY, Couto LB, Hagstrom JN, Elwell D, Fields PA, Burton M, BNellinger DA, Read MS, Brinkhous KM, Podsakoff GM, Nichols TC, Kurtzman GJ, High KA. Long-term correction of canine hemophilia by gene transfer of blood coagulation factor IX mediated by adeno-associated viral vector. Nature Med 1999; 5: 56–63.

101. Monahan PE, Samulski RJ, Tazelar J, Xiao X, Nichols TC, Bellinger DA, Read MS, Walsh CE. Direct intramuscular injection with recombinant AAV vectors resulyts in sustained expression in a dog model of hemophilia. Gene Ther 1998; 5:40–49.

102. Lewin AS, Drenser KA, Hauswirth WW, Nishikawa S, Yasumura D, Flannery JG, LaVail MM. Ribozyme rescue of photoreceptor cells in transgenic model of autosomal dominant retinitis pigmentosa. Nature Med 1998; 4: 967–971.

103. Guy J, Qi X, Hauswirth WW. Adeno-associated viral-mediated catalase expression suppresses optic neuritis in experimental allergic encephalomyelitis. Proc Natl Acad Sci USA 1998; 95:13847–13852.

104. Jomary C, Vincent KA, Grist J, Neal MJ, Jones SE. Rescue of photoreceptor function by AAV-mediated gene transfer in a mouse model of inherited retinal degeneration. Gene Ther 1997; 4:683–690.

4

Ex Vivo Gene Therapy Using Myoblasts and Regulatable Retroviral Vectors

Clare R. Ozawa, Matthew L. Springer, and Helen M. Blau
Stanford University School of Medicine, Stanford, California

I. INTRODUCTION: SKELETAL MUSCLE AS A TARGET TISSUE FOR GENE THERAPY

Human gene therapy—clinical treatments aimed at introducing or repairing genes to provide long-term correction for a defect caused by acquired or inherited disease—has been rapidly shuttled from a realm of theory and speculation into one of impending reality. The first approved protocol for human somatic gene therapy entered clinical trials in 1990 (1); the number of clinical trials worldwide has since burgeoned into the hundreds. Although gene therapy is still in its infancy and has yet to overcome a variety of pitfalls and problems, significant progress has been made. In this chapter we discuss some advances in developing efficient means of gene delivery and in regulating gene expression to achieve pulsatile protein delivery when desired and to avoid toxic levels. Although many of the features of muscle described below make it ideally suited for adenoviral, adeno-associated viral (AAV), lentiviral, and naked DNA delivery, the primary focus of this review will be ex vivo gene delivery. To date, ex vivo myoblast-mediated gene delivery surpasses most other methods leading to long-term physiological levels of therapeutic proteins in the circulation. Moreover, problematic immunological effects currently associated with most other methods are avoided with autologous myoblast-mediated delivery.

Of the many preclinical studies past and present, a number of approaches have employed skeletal muscle for delivery of genes in attempts to treat muscle disorders and other types of diseases. Skeletal muscle has been a target of special interest for gene therapy because of inherent properties that set it apart from other tissue types. Among its advantages is the fact that it is a very well-studied and understood tissue. This knowledge is invaluable for engineering strategies of gene delivery and assessing and controlling therapeutic protein expression. Skeletal muscle comprises a large percentage of the total body mass and thus is easily accessible to gene delivery. Mature, differentiated myofibers are relatively long-lived, providing a lasting substrate for the stable expression of recombinant genes. Myoblasts that are purified and genetically engineered in tissue culture can be reinjected and will then enter host fibers where they are nurtured, properly innervated, and in close proximity to the blood. The multinucleate nature of muscle cells facilitates delivery of two or more different vectors encoding products that can meet inside the cell. This is particularly advantageous for vectors with limited capacity, such as AAV, or for introducing gene regulatory systems (see below). Moreover, although rich in contractile apparatus and not obviously suited for secretion, genetically altered skeletal muscle tissue has proven to be a surprisingly efficient factory for the production and delivery of recombinant proteins to the circulation, allowing for the treatment of a broad array of muscle and nonmuscle disorders where cell type–specific expression is not required.

In addition to the ex vivo gene transfer approach, an in vivo method of gene delivery to muscle is currently being tested and developed. In the in vivo approach, a vector harboring a copy of a corrected gene or encoding a product that can remedy a patient's defect is introduced directly into the muscle tissue of the patient. The vector employed may be either viral or nonviral in nature. Viral vectors that have been examined for their ability to transduce nondividing cells characteristic of muscle tissues include adenovirus, AAV, lentivirus, and herpes simplex type-1 virus (2–4). While promising, in vivo approaches utilizing viral vectors face several challenges, such as immune reactions elicited against viral elements (2,3). Although the most persistent expression has been seen with AAV (5–9), small capacity limits cDNA size, and difficulties in achieving adequate viral titers necessary for clinical trials have yet to be overcome. New generations of viral vectors characterized by more efficient production, lower immunogenicity, and more stable expression are currently being developed that may prove to be powerful tools for muscle-mediated gene therapy.

Nonviral in vivo approaches for gene delivery to skeletal muscle center on intramuscular injection of plasmid DNA vectors. In the early 1990s, studies by Wolff and coworkers demonstrated that direct injection of naked plasmid DNA directly into the muscle tissues of mice led to transfection of skeletal myocytes and persistence of expression for at least 19 months in vivo (10,11). Naked plasmid DNA has also been shown to be taken up and expressed by cardiac muscle (12–14). Plasmid vectors have a number of advantages for muscle-based gene therapy and efforts to improve the efficiency of delivery appear warranted. These include simplicity of preparation and introduction into the host and the ability to be produced and stored in large quantities. In addition, the vectors are nonviral and are unlikely to be transmitted to other tissues. They also do not integrate into the genomes of host cells, precluding the risk of cancer by activation of a neighboring oncogene. Because achieving high levels of transgene expression using this approach has been problematic, direct plasmid DNA injection has been applied mostly to applications where only very low levels of transgene expression are required. One such application is in using intramuscular injection of plasmid DNA for vaccination purposes (15–18). Plasmids encoding antigenic proteins may be used to generate host antibodies specific to the antigen; since only small amounts of antigen are needed to elicit an immune response, plasmid vectors are well suited for this purpose. Recently, new progress has been made in developing methods for attaining stable, high-level gene expression using plasmid vectors. These include modifying DNA sequences within plasmids to enhance transcriptional efficiency of the vector (19) and combining plasmid DNA injection with the delivery of electric pulses to increase efficiency of myofiber transfection (20,21). While promising, these methods require further study and development before they can be effectively applied to the therapeutic realm.

Cell-mediated or ex vivo gene delivery may provide a method of drug delivery for the treatment of a wide range of diseases (22). Skeletal muscle cells can be maintained as either proliferating or differentiating cells. The proliferative cells, known as myoblasts, are mononucleate muscle progenitors capable of fusing with each other to form new muscle fibers or with preexisting myofibers (Fig. 1). Myoblasts can be readily isolated from muscle and expanded in cell culture. In vitro, they may be genetically engineered and extensively characterized and then reimplanted back

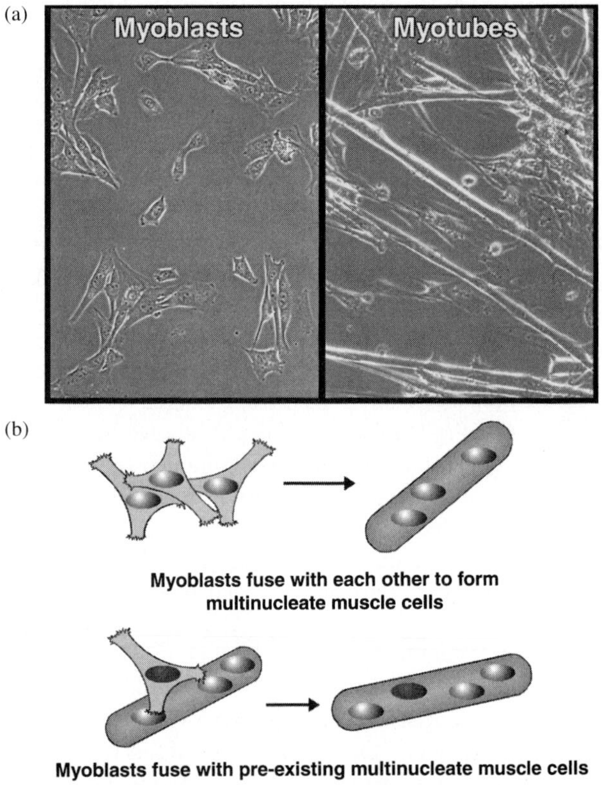

Figure 1 Myoblasts fuse to form multinucleate muscle cells. (a) Myoblasts are mononucleate muscle progenitor cells that can be isolated from muscle tissue and grown in cell culture (left). When provided with appropriate growth conditions, myoblasts fuse with each other in culture to form long, cylindrical, multinucleate myotubes (right). (b) Myoblasts can either fuse with each other to form new muscle cells or they can fuse with preexisting muscle cells. Myoblasts of one genotype (shown with a dark gray nucleus) can fuse with multinucleate muscle cells of another genotype (light gray nucleus), thus delivering new genetic information to the preexisting muscle cell.

into muscle, where they stably fuse with myofibers (Figure 1). This unique property of skeletal muscle tissue has allowed for the development of myoblast-mediated gene transfer (23–25). Although the ex vivo approach of gene transfer to muscle is currently more cumbersome and costly than the in vivo approach, it provides certain advantages not offered by in vivo methods. Genetically altered myoblasts may be fully characterized in vitro before in vivo injection to ensure secretion of recombinant products of correct size and function at physiologically useful levels. In addition, isolated myoblasts are engineered outside of the body with retroviruses, a process that generally assures that only the proper cell type is transduced. In contrast, introduction of viral or nonviral vectors directly into muscle could theoretically lead to inadvertent low-level transduction of cells other than those being targeted, for example, cells of the germline. Finally, recent studies suggest that a major limitation to ex vivo gene delivery—the requirement that syngeneic myoblasts isolated from one patient be reinjected into that same patient to avoid rejection of cells by the immune system—may be overcome. Encapsulation of myoblasts overrides the requirement for a ''tailor-made'' therapy, allowing allogeneic cells that are invisible to the immune system to be used. Myoblasts appear advantageous over other cell types for this purpose because they do not overgrow and die within capsules, but instead differentiate and persist (26–28). Although this procedure prevents myoblasts from fusing into preexisting muscle, it theoretically allows universal donor cells to be derived from muscles of a single patient and implanted at ectopic sites in different patients for delivery of diverse products. All of these advantages make ex vivo gene delivery via myoblasts a promising candidate for human gene therapy in the future. The remainder of this chapter will focus on ex vivo gene delivery to skeletal muscle.

II. DEVELOPMENT OF EX VIVO GENE DELIVERY BY MYOBLAST TRANSPLANTATION

A. Evidence for Myogenic Precursor Cells: Myoblasts

Skeletal muscle comprises approximately 10% of the total human body mass and is highly accessible to manipulation. A typical striated mature skeletal muscle cell, known as a myofiber, is large (1–40 mm in length and 10–50 μm wide), cylindrical, and multinucleated (as many as 100 nuclei per cell). Myofibers contain many nuclei because they are formed during development by the fusion of mononucleated precursor cells known as myoblasts. Myoblasts persist in mature muscle tissue as satellite cells, which can be viewed by electron microscopy as being ''wedged'' between the plasma membrane of the myofiber and the surrounding extracellular matrix (29) (Fig. 2). These cells can continue to fuse to neighboring myofibers in mature muscle, aiding in new muscle formation during regeneration following injury (30).

Interest in myoblasts as vehicles for gene delivery arose from studies of muscle cell biology and development. Studies of pattern formation in skeletal muscle showed that myoblasts are greatly influenced by extrinsic factors and become integrated into existing muscle fibers. Mammalian skeletal muscle is composed of a complex pattern of myofibers. Fiber types differ in their rate of contraction (fast

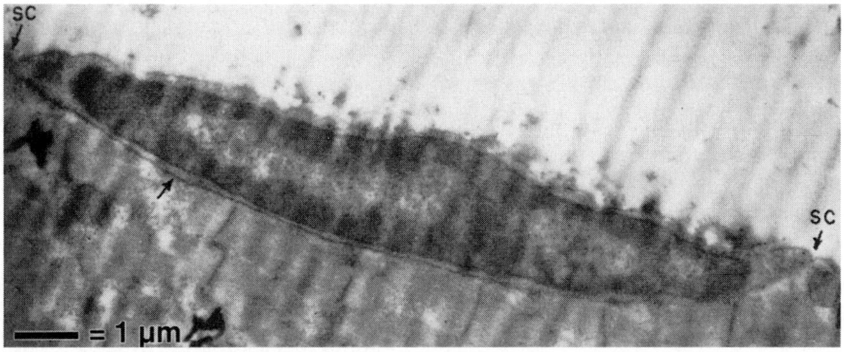

Figure 2 Satellite cell viewed by electron microscopy. Electron micrograph of a satellite cell in frog skeletal muscle, seen in longitudinal view. Extreme poles of the cell are indicated (sc). The arrow marks where the plasma membrane of the satellite cell is juxtaposed with that of the muscle fiber. (Reproduced from The Journal of Biophysical and Biochemical Cytology, 1961, vol. 9, p. 495 by copyright permission of The Rockefeller University Press.)

and slow), determined in part by the ratio of fast and slow myosin heavy-chain (MyHC) isoforms contained in each fiber (31). Although both fiber types occur in all skeletal muscles, the ratio of the two classes differs between muscles and even in different regions of a single muscle (32). Whereas lineage and myoblast-intrinsic properties play a role in muscle fiber patterning, as shown by the finding that myoblasts expressing different slow isoforms are characteristic of different developmental stages (33), a number of experiments suggest that the environment is important in the generation and maintenance of that pattern (34). During early development of human limb muscle when multiple fiber types are forming, virtually all myoblasts, irrespective of the stage of development from which they are taken, give rise to clones expressing slow MyHC upon differentiation in culture. This is seen to be true even when myoblasts are taken from muscle at midgestation, when only 3% of fibers in vivo express slow MyHC. These results suggest that although culture conditions allow for slow MyHC expression in myoblasts, such expression seems to be repressed by extrinsic factors in vivo.

Additional experiments utilizing retroviruses as heritable markers of cell fate in vivo further solidified these findings. When retroviral vectors encoding the reporter gene *lacZ* were injected directly into muscles of postnatal rats, clusters of multiply labeled fibers arising from progeny of single satellite cells were observed (23). The basal lamina, a connective sheath surrounding each muscle fiber, did not appear to prevent migration of labeled myoblasts into multiple fibers. Moreover, rat myoblast clones were shown to contribute progeny to both slow and fast muscle fiber types in their vicinity in vivo (24). These results demonstrate that mammalian myoblasts fuse randomly with all fiber types encountered and adopt the pattern of myogenic gene expression characteristic of the host muscle fiber.

Transplantation studies further developed the notion of employing myoblasts for gene delivery, using allografts of minced muscle tissue (35) or pieces of intact muscle (36), and also by injection of muscle precursor cells (37–40). In these studies, isoforms of the enzyme glucose-6-phosphate isomerase (GPI) were employed as markers to differentiate contributions of donor and host myoblasts to myofibers. The detection of hybrid fibers expressing isoforms containing subunits derived from donor and host provided evidence that grafts of muscle precursor cells could alter the genetic makeup of, and contribute muscle proteins to, mature myofibers.

These initial experiments were of importance in establishing that myoblasts can fuse with all muscle fiber types in their vicinity, becoming fully integrated into mature muscle tissue that has access to the circulation and is innervated. In addition, muscle precursor cells of one genotype that are injected into muscle tissue of another genotype fuse to form hybrid muscle fibers, where they are capable of expressing donor genes. These findings paved the way for later studies examining applications of myoblast transplantation for the correction of various diseases.

B. Methodology: Purification, Growth, and Transduction of Primary Myoblasts

The ease of isolating myoblasts from both mouse and human muscle and purifying, growing, and transducing them in vitro is a major advantage of using myoblasts rather than other cell types for gene transfer. Primary myoblasts can be isolated from any mouse strain—including strains carrying genetic mutations or transgenic strains (41,42)—providing a broad array of genotypes either for study in tissue culture or for transplantation. Moreover, because myoblasts may be isolated from a specific donor for implantation into a syngeneic host, problems of immunoincompatibility are obviated. Although established myoblast cell lines, such as the C2 myogenic cell line, may also be used for implantation, these cells can proliferate and form tumors when implanted into mice (43). In contrast, despite their impressive capacity to proliferate in culture, primary muscle cells do not form tumors upon injection into mouse muscle (43) and in the case of human myoblasts exhibit Hayflick-like senescence but not transformation (44).

Myoblasts can be isolated from muscle tissues from individuals of all ages, although both the yield and number of doublings tend to be higher if obtained from younger donors. Primary cultures are derived from postnatal muscle using mechanical or enzymatic dissociation methods (43,45) and readily obtained from human biopsy or autopsy tissue (46). Since such cultures are composed of a mixture of cell types, the population of myoblasts must be further purified. For primary cultures isolated from mice, this is accomplished using cell culture conditions that favor myoblast growth at the expense of other cell types, such that a pure population of myoblasts can be obtained within 2 weeks of normal growth (25,43). Human myoblasts can be purified by sorting in a fluorescence activated cell sorter (FACS) employing fluorescent antibodies specific to the muscle surface antigen H31, or NCAM (45). The cells that are isolated are capable of self-renewal and can undergo at least 40 cell doublings without differentiating (45). This implies that a kilogram of cells for transplantation use may be derived from a 5 mm^3 biopsy. Mouse (47) and rat (48) primary cells have also been isolated by FACS using antibodies to $\alpha 7$ integrin. Thus, a large population of rodent or human myoblasts may be easily obtained, purified, and expanded in cell culture.

Recombinant genes can be stably introduced into isolated and purified myoblasts using a number of methods, including lipofection, calcium-mediated transfection, or (more readily) by retroviral infection. Using conditions optimized for retroviral infection of myoblasts at high efficiency, 99% of primary myoblasts in culture are easily transduced without use of a selectable marker (49). This enables the creation of pure populations of primary myoblasts expressing a gene of interest, free of contamination by most nonexpressing cells. Myoblasts do not lose their ability to mature and differentiate by the process of being genetically altered.

III. APPLICATIONS OF MYOBLAST-MEDIATED EX VIVO GENE DELIVERY

Primary mouse myoblasts stably express recombinant genes following transduction. Myoblasts retrovirally transduced with the bacterial *lacZ* gene and injected into mouse skeletal muscle fuse with muscle fibers and express high levels of β-galactosidase (Fig. 3). The β-galactosidase expression can be observed in hybrid myofibers for at least 6 months (43). Other studies have shown that stable levels of recombinant proteins are produced for at least 10 months (50). Myoblasts that have been genetically engineered to express a recombinant gene may thus be used for stable delivery of that gene into the body (Fig. 4).

Although not widely viewed as a secretory tissue, skeletal muscle is highly vascularized and recombinant proteins secreted from myoblasts readily gain access to circulation. Initial studies using C2C12 myoblasts genetically altered to express human growth hormone (hGH) first demonstrated this to be the case (51,52). hGH was chosen as the gene of interest because it has a very short half-life in mouse serum (4 minutes) (53), providing a stringent test for sustained production and secretion into the circulation over time. After injection of genetically engineered myoblasts into mouse muscle, stable physiological levels of hGH could be detected for at least 3 months (Fig. 5). These results showed that myoblasts, by fusing with preexisting multinucleated myofibers, can serve as vehicles for systemic delivery of recombinant proteins. Thus, skeletal muscle may be used as a factory for production of a range of secreted gene products for treatment of nonmuscle-related

(a) (b)

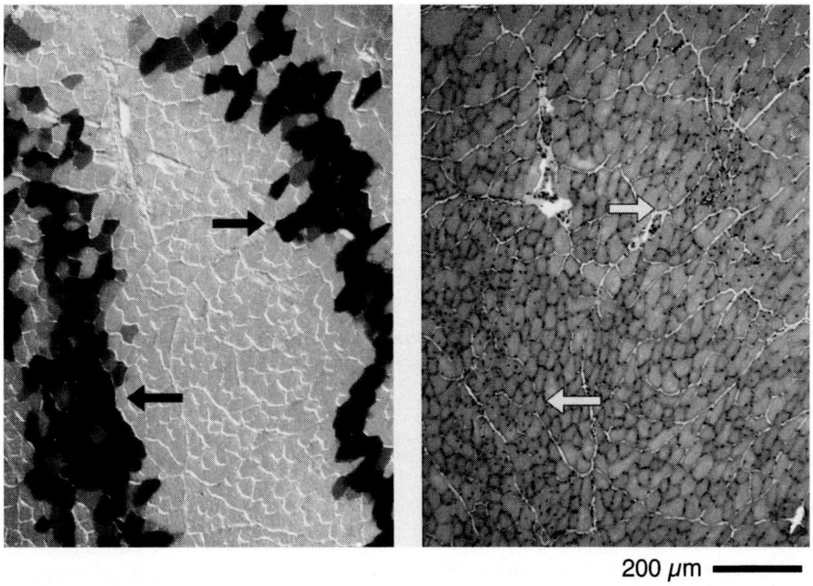

Figure 3 Incorporation of β-galactosidase–expressing myoblasts into skeletal muscle. Primary mouse myoblasts transduced with the reporter gene lacZ, encoding the bacterial β-galactosidase enzyme, were injected into mouse leg skeletal muscle, where they formed hybrid myofibers with host muscle. Injected muscles were isolated and frozen, and cryostat sections were prepared for histological analysis. (a) Hybrid myofibers producing β-galactosidase at the implantation sites can be seen as dark fibers after staining with the enzyme's substrate X-gal. (b) An adjacent section was stained with hematoxylin/eosin to show tissue architecture and demonstrates that the hybrid fibers are of normal diameter and morphology and are an integral part of the muscle tissue. The centrally located nuclei that can be observed are indicative of myofibers that have undergone regeneration and represent a normal response to a needle injection. The arrows denote corresponding regions in the two sections.

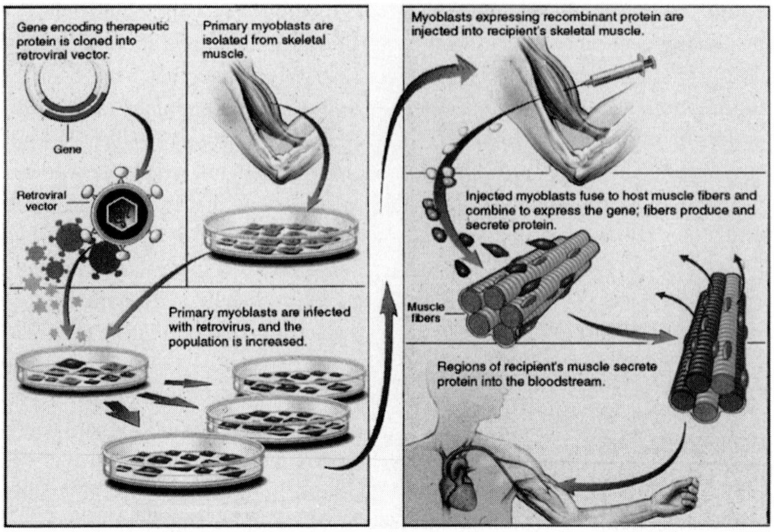

Figure 4 Muscle-mediated gene therapy. Muscle-mediated gene therapy by implantation of genetically engineered myoblasts allows for delivery of diverse therapeutic proteins, either directly to muscle or (as shown) to the systemic circulation. (Adapted with permission from The New England Journal of Medicine, 1995, vol. 333, p. 1555. Copyright ©1995 Massachusetts Medical Society. All rights reserved.)

disorders. Because muscle is capable of carrying out post-translational modifications normally performed by other tissues (such as gamma carboxylation essential for production of functional coagulation factors in the liver), such recombinant nonmuscle proteins are biologically active even when produced by muscle (54–57). Applications of myoblast-mediated gene delivery to treat diseases affecting both muscle and other tissues will be discussed in the following section.

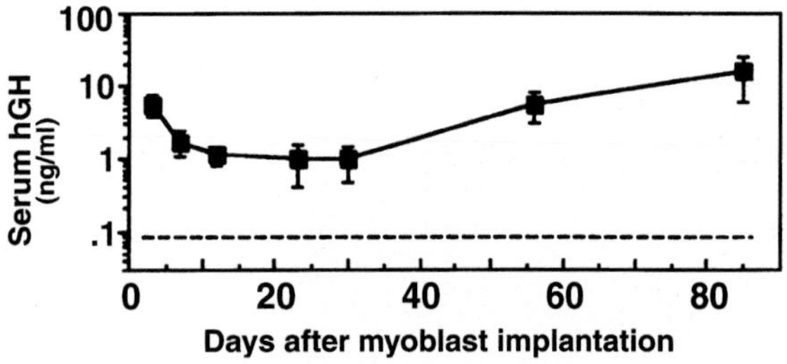

Figure 5 Systemic delivery of human growth hormone. A population of C2C12 myoblasts retrovirally transduced with hGH were implanted into hind limbs of 24 syngeneic mice, and serum hGH levels were monitored by radioimmunoassay of tail blood. Greater than 90% of the implanted cells expressed and secreted hGH as determined by clonal analysis in culture. Each point represents the mean ± SD for 4–24 mice; the dashed line shows the mean ± SD for serum samples taken from 5 uninjected control mice. Expression of hGH by implanted myoblasts persisted for at least 85 days in vivo. (Reprinted with permission from Science, 1991, 254(5037):1509–12. Copyright ©1991 American Association for the Advancement of Science.)

IV. DISEASE TARGETS FOR MYOBLAST-MEDIATED GENE TRANSFER

A. Muscular Dystrophies

The concept of applying myoblast transplantation to the treatment of disease was a natural outcome of the many studies establishing myoblasts as potent vehicles for delivering donor genes into host muscle. The first approaches centered on the use of allografts of normal precursor cells to insert donor nuclei, containing a normal genome, into genetically abnormal muscle. While not technically gene therapy (since donor myoblasts were not genetically engineered in any way), such "cell therapy" experiments were important in establishing the utility of myoblast-mediated gene delivery for the treatment of disease and are the only studies involving myoblast transplantation that have translated into human clinical trials to date. The first disorder to which this therapeutic approach was applied was Duchenne muscular dystrophy (DMD), the most common of heritable human muscular dystrophies. DMD affects 1 in 3000 males and causes progressive muscle weakness beginning in childhood; patients with severe forms rarely survive past early adulthood. DMD is caused by mutations in the gene *dystrophin* (58), a large gene encoding a structural protein involved in anchoring skeletal myofibers to the extracellular matrix. By implanting myoblasts that contained normal copies of the *dystrophin* gene into dystrophin-deficient muscle, researchers hoped to rescue the genetic defect in humans as previously achieved in mdx mice, the mouse model of disease (40). In mdx mice, the implanted myoblasts were able to render host myofibers dystrophin-positive while counteracting the characteristic cycle of fiber degeneration and regeneration characteristic of mdx muscle (40,59).

Clinical trials in which donor myoblasts taken from normal human muscle were introduced into DMD patients were initiated at multiple institutions (60–66). All of these studies demonstrated that myoblast implantation into humans has no adverse effects. However, all but one group reported the disappointing finding that only a very small percentage of host myofibers resulted in dystrophin expression. At the protein level, these results could have been due to reversion or occasional expression by mutant host fibers of a truncated dystrophin detectable by antibodies. One group, however, provided definitive evidence that donor dystrophin transcripts were being synthesized by PCR (61). Experiments combining fluorescent in situ hybridization (FISH) together with immunohistochemistry were recently conducted to examine the fate of individual myoblasts after implantation into muscles of DMD patients (67,68). This combination of techniques allowed the localization of both the dystrophin protein and the donor nuclei themselves, permitting more quantitative assessment of the efficiency of myoblast transfer. Findings from these studies showed that a large proportion of donor myoblasts successfully integrated into host myofibers in almost every subject; donor nuclei were interspersed with and aligned with host nuclei. Furthermore, these experiments demonstrated that increased dystrophin expression observed in recipient muscle was contributed by the donor nuclei and was not due to spontaneous reversion of the mutated *dystrophin* gene since the antibodies used were specific to the product for the deleted gene regions in the recipient. Moreover, the dystrophin produced by single nuclei spanned regions including 20–30 nuclei. Why only a subset of transduced myofibers expressed dystrophin is still not understood. One hypothesis is that variables related to the DMD disease state itself, such as increased fibrosis with patient age, impaired myoblast access. An alternative hypothesis is that nuclei were not transcriptionally active in regions of fibers undergoing degeneration.

For treatment of muscular dystrophies by gene therapy, a large proportion of muscle fibers must be transduced in order to produce a beneficial outcome. Furthermore, myoblasts must be implanted into all muscles, some of which are difficult to access, such as the diaphragm and heart. Failure of these latter muscles is the cause of death in patients with DMD. These represent major challenges to myoblast-mediated gene delivery in treating inherited myopathies and suggest that a cell-based method may not be practical. Histochemical staining and enzymatic activity assays of muscle transplanted with β-galactosidase–expressing myoblasts show that the total number of labeled fibers and the total β-galactosidase activity is maximal at the implantation site and decreases in parallel with increasing distance from the site (69). Although myoblasts were thought to be able to migrate from the circulation to damaged muscle (70), this is certainly not a frequent event. Thus, in order to target a high percentage of myofibers in multiple muscles of large organisms such as humans, delivery of viral vectors and naked DNA encoding either full-length or truncated dystrophin genes (71–73), or in the future the ubiquitous utrophin (74), may be most effective.

B. Lysosomal Storage Diseases and Serum Protein Deficiencies: Treatment by Secreted Circulating Recombinant Proteins

As described above, studies with hGH showed that myofibers efficiently secrete recombinant proteins that readily gain access to the circulation. Myoblast-mediated gene transfer has been further employed to express therapeutic proteins not normally made by muscle (50–52, 54–57,75–78). Here we describe in further detail progress made in studies in which genes encoding β-glucuronidase, clotting factor IX, and erythropoietin were transferred to muscle using myoblasts.

Lysosomal storage diseases are one subset of disorders that may be appropriate for muscle-mediated gene therapy (79). These recessive disorders are caused by detrimental build-up of lysosomal enzyme substrates within affected tissues due to a single missing or dysfunctional lysosomal enzyme. Because these enzymes are marked with a specific targeting signal (mannose 6-phosphate) (80), missing lysosomal enzymes manufactured by muscle and delivered to the serum can be internalized by distant tissues and appropriately transported to lysosomes via mannose 6-phosphate receptors. By implanting into muscle genetically engineered primary myoblasts encoding β-glucuronidase, a lysosomal enzyme, one group was able to demonstrate in vivo expression of the recombinant protein in adult β-glucuronidase–deficient mice (76). Production and secretion of the missing lysosomal enzyme by muscle led to correction of phenotypic abnormalities in the liver and spleen of treated animals.

A second disorder well suited to myoblast-mediated gene therapy is hemophilia B. Hemophilia B is a blood clotting disease caused by a deficiency of a protein, clotting factor IX. Because conventional protein-replacement therapies face drawbacks including the necessity for frequently repeated treatments and the risk of contaminating bloodborne pathogens in plasma-derived factors, gene therapy may provide a safer and more convenient alternative (81). Studies in which C2C12 myoblasts were transduced with a gene encoding human factor IX and implanted into immunocompetent mice led to a peak expression of recombinant protein (1 μg/mL) at day 12 and subsequent decline back to basal levels thereafter (54). The drop in human factor IX expression was shown to be due to production of specific antibodies targeted against the protein in wild-type mice. Other experiments (55–57) demonstrated that primary myoblasts engineered to constitutively express factor IX led to stable, low-level production of the protein in immunodeficient nude or SCID mice for many months. A more recent study (50) achieved stable production of human factor IX at therapeutic levels in SCID mice, using a promoter with muscle creatine enhancers to drive high levels of muscle-specific expression, for at least 8 months. Of importance, recombinant factor IX manufactured in muscle undergoes the gamma carboxylation required for functional activity of the protein (54–57). This finding demonstrates that muscle cells have efficient mechanisms for posttranslational modifications normally carried out by other tissue types such as liver. Moreover, the problems with immunogenicity are likely to affect only a percentage of hemophiliacs, as not all are null mutations but have some, albeit reduced, level of factor IX (82). Until recently, only dog models were available, however, now a mouse model that lacks factor IX has been created by homologous recombination (83), which should facilitate future preclinical gene therapy studies.

A third class of disorders for which myoblast-mediated expression of recombinant proteins into the circulation may be beneficial is in the treatment of erythropoietin-responsive anemias. Recombinant erythropoietin (Epo) replacement therapy has been employed for successful treatment of anemia associated with end-stage renal disease (84) and is being tested as a therapy for a broad array of other anemias (85). Epo is a mammalian hormone that controls the production of erythrocytes, hemoglobin-carrying cells that deliver oxygen to tissues of the body (86). Anemic patients can currently be treated by repeated administration of recombinant Epo; such treatments, however, require frequent hospital visits by patients and are costly. Thus, Epo delivery by gene therapy could provide patients with long-term delivery of the protein, eliminating the need for multiple treatments. However, as with many gene therapies, regulated expression is desirable for Epo, since dosage must be tailored to the particular application and to the individual patient.

Studies of muscle-mediated delivery of Epo by gene therapy appear promising. Epo-secreting primary or C2 myoblasts have been introduced bilaterally into skeletal muscles of mice (76,77). Implantation of engineered cells led to an elevated hematocrit for 3 months, a direct measure of Epo production. At 3 months posttransplantation, implanted myoblasts were observed to have fused and fully differentiated into myofibers (77). Moreover, in an animal model of renal failure in which anemia is induced by nephrectomy of immunocompromised nude mice, injection into muscle of C2 myoblasts secreting human Epo led to reversal of the anemic phenotype (78). Levels of recombinant serum Epo measured by ELISA remained elevated for the 2 months during which the animals were assessed following myoblast implantation. These studies lend credibility to using myoblast-mediated expression of recombinant Epo as a viable treatment for anemias.

Thus, myoblast-mediated gene transfer appears to be well suited for expression of recombinant proteins to the circulation. Unlike applications aimed at treating inherited myopathies, not all fibers need to be transduced with the gene of interest in order to achieve a therapeutic effect. Indeed, such therapies can be highly localized to a particular region of a single muscle. For a variety of disorders where patients may benefit from delivery of a recombinant gene product to the blood stream, myoblast-mediated gene transfer to muscle tissue appears to be a promising treatment method. Stable, long-term expression of physiological levels can be achieved with therapeutic effects, and because there is no immune response, repeated administration of genetically engineered myoblasts is possible, unlike AAV or adenoviral gene delivery.

C. Vascular Insufficiencies and Cancer

During the past decade, a great deal has been learned about growth factors that induce angiogenesis, the sprouting of new blood vessels from preexisting vessels. There has been much interest in the use of angiogenic factors to stimulate new vessels to grow as a treatment for maladies including stroke, peripheral arterial disease, and myocardial infarction. As the genes that encode these proteins have been cloned, the concept of therapeutic angiogenesis has moved quickly into the realm of gene therapy, and clinical trials are already underway as low levels provide therapeutic effects. Factors produced by genetically engineered myoblasts are continuous, by contrast with injection of pure proteins, naked DNA, and viral vectors, and may be advantageous.

The angiogenic factor that has received the most attention to date is vascular endothelial growth factor (VEGF), a potent mitogen that was isolated by virtue of its ability to stimulate growth of endothelial cells and to increase permeability in vascular endothelium (hence its other designation—vascular permeability factor) (87–91). VEGF plays an important role in the induction of angiogenesis by tumors (92) and in the angiogenic response of normal tissue to decreased oxygen availability. VEGF is also known to serve as a critical signal during the initial embryonic development of the vasculature by a process known as vasculogenesis, or the de novo growth of blood vessels from precursor cells (93,94). In this case, VEGF induces endothelial cell migration via specific receptors. Therefore, VEGF is a crucial regulator of both modes of growth and development of the vasculature pre- and postnatally.

Because of the potential clinical benefits of stimulating new blood vessel growth, much effort in recent years has been invested in the delivery of VEGF to tissues that are insufficiently vascularized. Injection of VEGF protein has resulted in angiogenic sprouting of vessels in muscle that was partially deprived of blood and oxygen and therefore ischemic (95–97). However, presumably because of vascular permeabilizing and/or vasodilating properties, bolus injections of the protein have been reported to be deleterious, causing hypotension (98,99). As a result, recent investigations have assessed the feasibility of localized delivery of VEGF by gene transfer using plasmid DNA injection or adenoviral vectors. Both of these delivery methods lead to transient production of the recombinant protein and to angiogenic sprouting from preexisting vessels in matrigel in vitro (100,101), in adipose tissues in vivo (102), as well as in ischemic skeletal or cardiac muscle (103–106).

The effects of long-term stable production of VEGF were recently investigated using the myoblast-mediated gene transfer techniques described above (107). This resulted in many unexpected findings. Myoblasts were transduced with a retrovirus carrying a murine cDNA encoding the heparin-binding $VEGF_{164}$ and injected into the muscles of immunodeficient SCID mice. A physiological response to VEGF was observed in every mouse that received VEGF-producing cells. At day 11 postimplantation, mice appeared outwardly normal and no differences were observed between VEGF and control muscle upon dissection. However, histological analysis of frozen muscle sections revealed that the implantation sites of VEGF-expressing myoblasts, but not control myoblasts, were invariably associated with regions of infiltrating mononuclear cells, identified by fluorescent antibody staining to multiple markers as endothelial cells and macrophages. By day 44–47, 100% of legs injected with VEGF myoblasts contained large hemangiomas composed of vascular channels and pools of blood, whereas control legs appeared normal (Fig. 6). These studies demonstrate that myoblast-mediated VEGF gene delivery is extremely potent and provide evidence that this single growth factor can lead to a cascade of events resulting in the formation of complex tissues of multiple cell types. These results also show for the first time that exogenous VEGF expression at high levels or long duration can have deleterious effects, a factor of importance as clinical trials of VEGF gene delivery by plasmid DNA injection or adenoviral-mediated delivery are underway. Moreover, because myoblast implantation affords higher expression levels of longer duration than other gene-transfer techniques, a physiological response to VEGF was observed in nonischemic muscle for the first time. Thus, the dose and duration of VEGF expression appear critical in determining a range of effects.

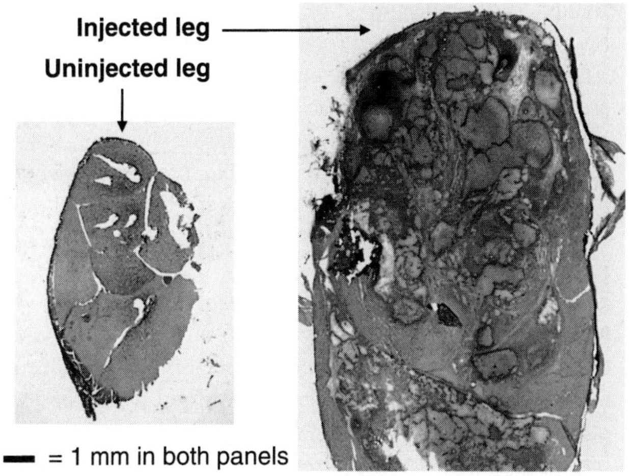

Figure 6 Formation of vascular structures in VEGF-myoblast-implanted legs. Myoblasts expressing the murine $VEGF_{164}$ gene were injected into mouse hind limb. Histological analysis of injected muscles were conducted at day 44–47 postimplantation using hematoxylin/eosin staining of cryostat sections. Uninjected control legs were normal both in size and in morphology (left panel), whereas legs injected with VEGF myoblasts (right panel) were greater than twice the diameter of control legs and consisted primarily of hemangioma and pools of blood. Both panels are shown at the same magnification. These results demonstrate the importance of regulating recombinant gene expression in gene therapy applications. (Adapted and reprinted from Ref. 107 with permission, copyright ©1998 Cell Press.)

These results point both to the potency of myoblast-mediated gene transfer and the necessity of regulation of recombinant gene expression for gene therapy applications. In the case of myoblast-mediated delivery of VEGF, too much of a good thing clearly can lead to adverse and unwanted effects. Gene therapy has mostly been plagued by insufficient levels of the protein of interest. However, these VEGF results illustrate that current methods of gene delivery can be limited by a lack of ability to control gene expression. Both the ability to increase expression levels if an insufficient amount of a recombinant protein is being produced and the option to intentionally reduce or cease expression are likely to be necessary for the health of the patient in many cases.

In addition to studies aimed at triggering the growth of new blood vessels, other experiments are currently geared towards preventing blood vessel development in special circumstances. Because tumor growth and metastasis require persistent new blood vessel growth (108,109), therapies targeted at blocking this growth could lead to an arrest of tumor development. One of the most promising avenues for preventing angiogenesis in tumors may lie in the utilization of recently discovered antiangiogenic agents.

Early in the twentieth century it was first noticed that primary tumors are able to suppress the growth of a second tumor inoculum (110). Resistance to secondary tumor challenge was shown to be inversely proportional to the size of the second tumor inoculum and directly proportional to the size of the primary tumor (111,112). Moreover, removal of certain tumors can lead to rapid growth of metastases (113). Isolation of fractions taken from serum and urine that were capable of inhibiting endothelial cell proliferation in vitro and metastatic tumor growth in vivo led to the discovery of two antiangiogenic proteins, angiostatin (114) and endostatin (115), proteolytic products of plasminogen and collagen XVIII, respectively. A recent study demonstrated that viral vectors encoding angiostatin cDNA could inhibit endothelial cell proliferation in vitro and glioblastoma growth in vivo (116). An interesting therapy for cancer could be to engineer myoblasts to express these proteins, such that their secretion may inhibit growth of tumors at distant sites. Reconfirmation that desired blood vessel synthesis at sites of injury, for example, is not impaired would be critical. Since angiostatin and endostatin are difficult to produce in adequate amounts in bacteria, gene therapy protocols will be invaluable for discerning their biological function and possible application as anticancer agents in vivo.

V. REGULATABLE RETROVIRAL VECTORS AND THE RETROTET-ART SYSTEM

Until recently, all vectors employed in gene therapy protocols have depended on constitutive promoters to drive expression of the transgene. As made abundantly clear in the recent study of the effects of myoblast-mediated delivery of VEGF on normal adult muscle (107), regulation of gene expression is extremely important for safe treatment of patients. Both delivery by plasmid transfection or adenoviral vectors, the two VEGF gene-transfer techniques currently being used in clinical trials, typically lead to transient gene expression that may be desirable in the case of angiogenic gene delivery. However, rather than count on inherent but uncontrollable limitations of the gene-delivery systems, it may prove better to use a system that delivers sustained and excessive levels but has been modified with regulatable control elements. This theoretically allows levels and timing of expression to be tailored to those that are deemed optimal on a case-by-case basis. An advantage of retrovirally transduced myoblast implantation is that it allows localized delivery of a recombinant gene at sustained levels; addition of inducible elements to retroviral vectors provides a mechanism for fine-tuning gene expression to the physiological levels required.

There are four characteristics that an ideal inducible system should possess. First, the regulatable system should demonstrate specificity—it should not require endogenous factors for activation or interfere with cellular regulatory pathways. Second, the system should be efficient, demonstrating induction to high levels of gene expression from starting low basal levels and the potential for repression back to uninduced levels. Third, it must be dose-dependent, responding to its inducer by modulating its expression in a sensitive and homogeneous manner. Last, none of its components should elicit a host immune response or be toxic. To date, there are four regulatable systems displaying some or most of these characteristics: the ecdysone, RU486, FK506/rapamycin, and tetracycline-inducible systems. The first three systems are derived from members of the nuclear receptor superfamily (for ecdysone and RU486) or immunosuppressant compounds (for FK506/rapamycin) (for review, see Refs. 117,118), and they may have potential effects on host genes in some cases. This section will focus on the attributes and recent advances of the tetracycline system, which has been extensively studied in our laboratory and has already been incorporated into myoblast implantation strategies.

The tetracycline-inducible system was originally developed by Bujard and coworkers (119,120) and has become one of the most widely used methods of regulating gene expression to date. All elements of the system are prokaryotic; thus, pleiotropic effects and endogenous ligands are avoided. In addition, because the inducer becomes an integral part of the transactivator directly responsible for turning on gene expression, there are no intermediate steps in the induction pathway. The tetracycline system thus allows for a more direct correlation between the amount of transcription factor capable of binding DNA and the concentra-

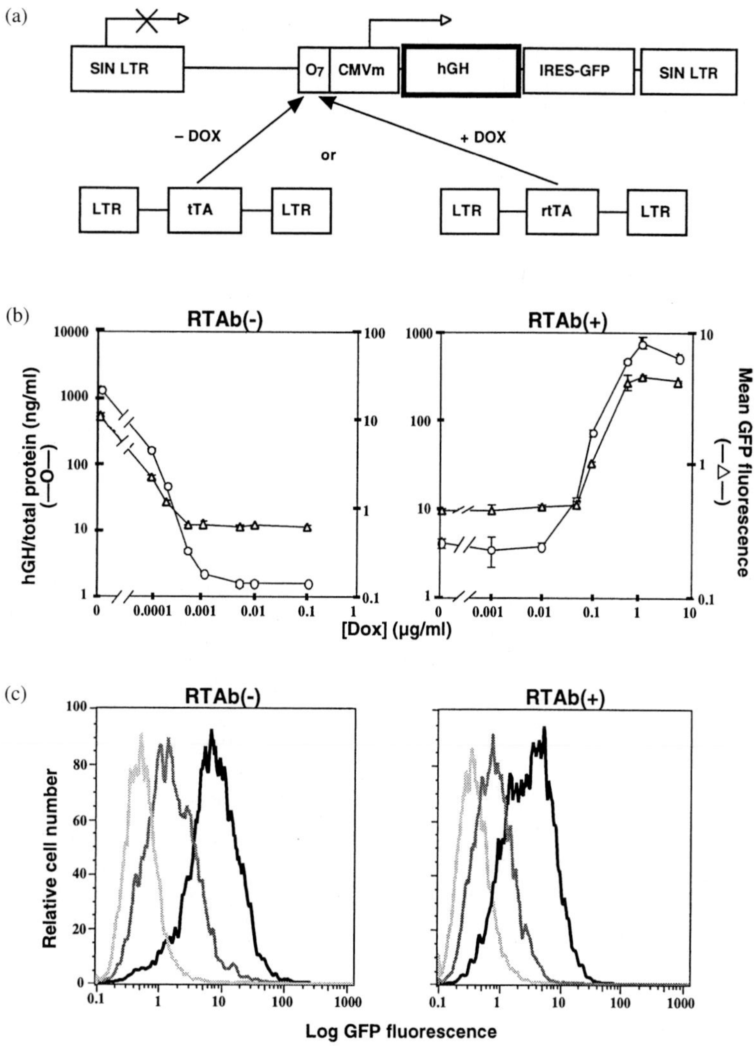

Figure 7 Tetracycline-inducible expression using tTA and rtTA. (a) Schematic of a binary retroviral system allowing tetracycline-inducible expression of both hGH and green fluorescent protein (GFP). The expression of both proteins is ensured by the use of an internal ribosomal entry site (IRES), allowing both genes to be encoded within the same mRNA transcript. The reporter virus contains a self-inactivating (SIN) retroviral backbone to avoid interference of the viral long terminal repeat (LTR) with the tet-responsive promoter (O_7-CMVm). The diagram represents the system after integration into the chromosome; hence, the SIN LTR exists in both the 5′ and 3′ positions. Tet-sensitive transactivators (either tTA or rtTA) are provided constitutively from a second retrovirus. (b) Dose response of the binary tet-inducible system shown in (a). RTAb(−) cells transduced with tet reporter virus and tTA virus, and RTAb(+) cells transduced with tet reporter virus and rtTA virus, were assessed for their dox dose response of hGH (○) expression and GFP (△) expression. Both systems exhibit concentration dependence over several orders of magnitude. (c) Histogram plots of GFP expression obtained from FACS analysis are shown in overlay at three selected doses [RTAb(−): 0.1 μg/mL (light gray), 0.001 μg/mL (dark gray), and 0 μg/mL (black); RTAb(+): 0 μg/mL (light gray), 0.1 μg/mL (dark gray), and 5 μg/mL (black)]. These plots show that with changing concentrations of dox, populations uniformly shift to intermediate and high levels of expression. (Adapted and republished from Ref. 124 with permission of the Proceedings of the National Academy of Sciences USA, 2101 Constitution Ave., NW, Washington, DC 20418. Reproduced by permission of the publisher via Copyright Clearance Center, Inc.)

tion of exogenous inducer [tetracycline (tet) or its synthetic analog doxycycline (dox)]. The pharmacokinetics of tet are well understood and, at the levels required for the inducible system, are well known to be safe for human use.

In its original and simplest form, the tet transactivator (tTA) is a hybrid factor comprising a bacterial tetracycline repressor (tetR) and the viral transactivator domain VP16 (119). When bound to tet, tTA is prevented from binding to tet operator sequences juxtaposed to a minimal promoter and gene expression is turned off. In the absence of tet, tTA is free to bind to the inducible promoter and gene expression is induced. A relatively recent modification of the system allows for induction of gene expression in the presence, not the absence, of tet (120). A second chimeric protein containing a mutated version of tetR was developed and designated as ''reverse'' tTA (rtTA); this transactivator binds to tet operator sequences in the presence of tet. Both tTA and rtTA have been demonstrated to efficiently regulate expression in tissue culture, fruit flies, and mice (121–124).

A major advance in broadening the utility of the tet system was the employment of retroviruses. Retroviral gene delivery is much more rapid and efficient than transfection using plasmids. Retroviral vectors also do not form concatemers and thus should not form a repressive chromatin environment sometimes associated with plasmids (125). Genes can be introduced into tens of thousands of myoblasts at high efficiency, generating polyclonal populations within a week (49) an advantage over the few stable clones routinely obtained. For these reasons, retroviruses are well suited for delivery of tet-inducible systems to primary cells isolated directly from tissue. Initial studies using tet-regulatable cassettes, however, met with a number of problems. In one case, the inclusion of an autoregulatory feedback loop necessitated high background levels of expression in order to ''jump-start'' the system (126). In other cases, overcomplexity of transcription and translation units produced low viral titers (127–131).

Bohl and colleagues (132) first overcame this problem by using simplified retroviral vectors in which the necessary elements were dispersed over more than one retroviral vector. In this study, one retrovirus encoded rtTA whereas the other contained an inducible Epo cassette. After multiple rounds of infection, primary myoblasts exhibited induction of about 200-fold in expression of the protein. When the engineered myoblasts were transplanted into mice, Epo expression could be repetitively turned on and off over a 5-month period by controlling levels of dox in drinking water. In an improvement of this approach, inclusion of a selectable marker such as GFP allows for purification by flow cytometry of regulatable populations of cells (124) (Fig. 7).

In the past year, two additional advancements of the tet system have increased its applicability for gene therapy purposes. The tetR transcriptional elements are modular; one may replace the VP16 transactivator domain of tTA, for instance, with the KRAB transrepressor domain to create a tet-regulated repressor of transcription (133). Expression of two tet modulators within the same cell, however, leads to formation of nonfunctional heterodimers because the modulators have identical dimerization domains (Fig. 8) (134). Based on sequence information and known crystal structures of tetR as well as mutational analysis (135–137), mutually distinct dimerization domains deriving from sepa-

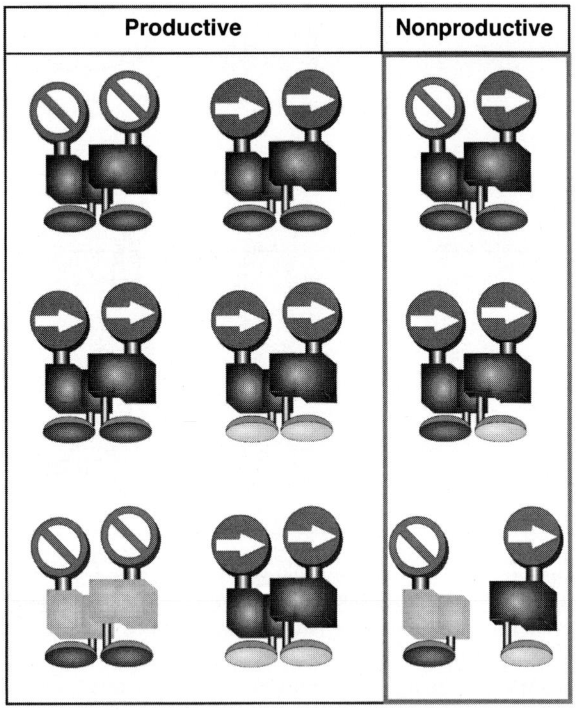

Figure 8 The need for tet modulators with distinct dimerization domains. Co-expression of tetR fusion proteins with different functional domains such as repressor domains (represented in the top row by the ''do-not-enter'' sign), and activator domains (represented by the ''go'' sign), or DNA-binding domains with distinct specificity (symbolized in the middle row by the light gray and dark gray ''feet''), leads to formation of both functional homodimers and nonfunctional heterodimers. Such nonfunctional heterodimers can be eliminated by engineering distinct dimerization domains into the tetR portion of the tet modulators (symbolized by the dark gray and light gray shaded midsections in the bottom row). (Republished from Ref. 134 with permission of the Proceedings of the National Academy of Sciences USA, 2101 Constitution Ave., NW, Washington, DC 20418. Reproduced by permission of the publisher via Copyright Clearance Center, Inc.)

rate classes of gram-negative bacteria have been identified (138,139). The ability to engineer tet modulators with specific dimerization domains allows tet activators and tet repressors to be expressed within the same cell without risk of forming a nonfunctional heterodimer. The development of such a tetracycline-inducible retroviral system, designated the RetroTet-ART (activators and repressors expressed together) system (138), allows for gene expression to be completely extinguished or induced in a fully dose-dependent manner—as a result, the dynamic range of gene expression has been greatly increased (up to 5 or 6 orders of magnitude) (Fig. 9). This improvement is a significant advantage in applications where basal expression from the inducible promoter must be extinct. The RetroTet-ART system was demonstrated to be able to reversibly silence expression of p16, a growth arrest protein (138).

In a second modification of the tet-inducible system, the DNA-binding domain of tetR was altered to interact with a modified tet operator sequence (139). The original and adapted binding sequences were engineered into tTA and rtTA proteins harboring distinct dimerization domains. By placing two separate genes under control of old and new tet operator sequences and expressing both of the modified tTA and rtTA proteins, Baron and colleagues were able to either repress expression of both genes or express either gene alone simply by changing the dox concentration (Fig. 10) (139). A means of turning on both genes at once has yet to be achieved. Thus, the activity of two different genes can be reversibly controlled in a mutually exclusive manner.

In summary, tet-regulatable retroviral systems are capable of being repressed and expressed in a fully inducible

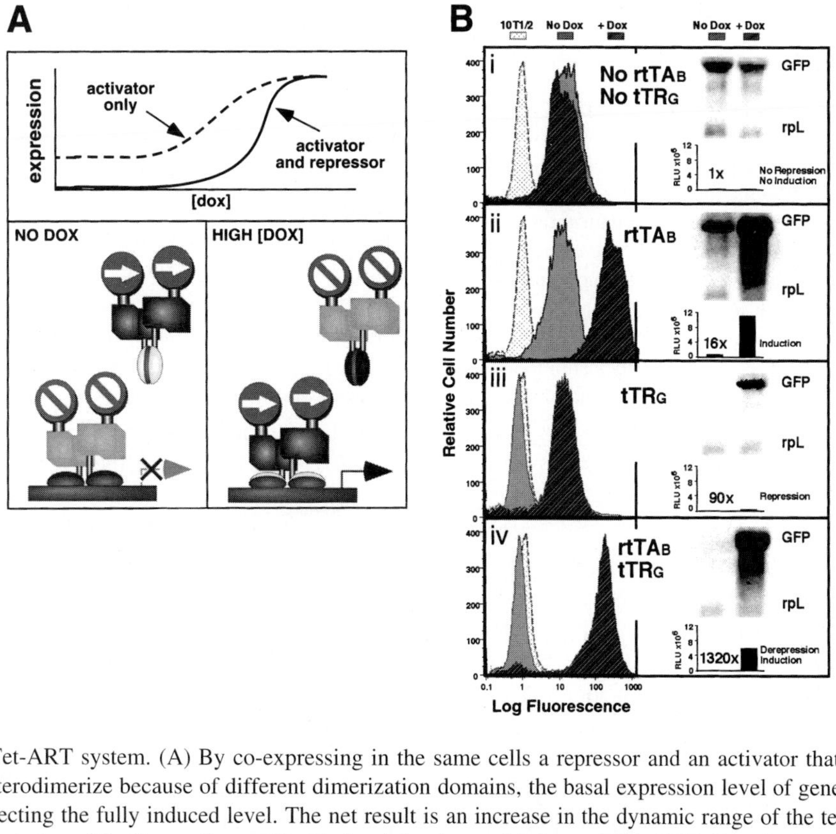

Figure 9 The RetroTet-ART system. (A) By co-expressing in the same cells a repressor and an activator that respond oppositely to dox and that do not heterodimerize because of different dimerization domains, the basal expression level of genes under tet control can be reduced without affecting the fully induced level. The net result is an increase in the dynamic range of the tet system. (Republished from Ref. 134 with permission of the Proceedings of the National Academy of Sciences USA, 2101 Constitution Ave., NW, Washington, DC 20418. Reproduced by permission of the publisher via Copyright Clearance Center, Inc.) (B) Proof of concept of the RetroTet-ART system is demonstrated by FACS (left) and northern blot (right) analysis. 10T1/2 fibroblasts were transduced with the GFP reporter retrovirus (i). Subsequently, cells were transduced with the transactivator retrovirus (ii), the transrepressor virus (iii), or with both transactivator and transrepressor virus (iv). With the addition of both transactivator and transrepressor, the dynamic range of gene expression is increased. Gene expression can be fully extinguished, and induced to maximal levels, as shown in (iv). (From Ref. 138 with permission.)

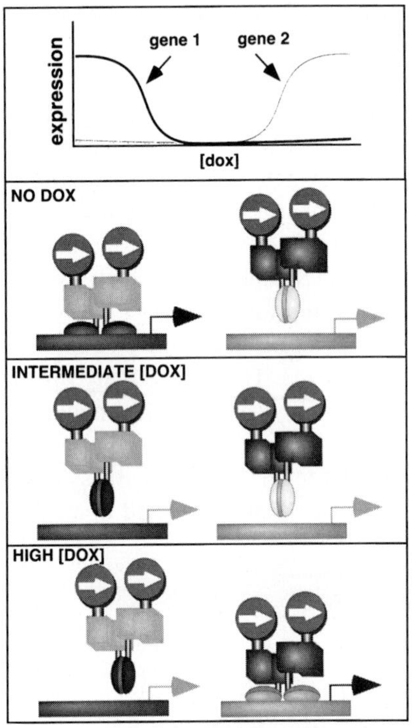

Figure 10 Tet-regulated expression of two separate genes. By co-expressing two tetR-based activators that contain DNA-binding domains with distinct specificity, respond oppositely to dox, and do not heterodimerize, two independent genes can be regulated by the same inducer. Because of the characteristic dose response of the wild-type and ''reverse'' tetR, the expression of each gene can be turned off at an intermediate concentration of dox and activated at markedly different dox concentrations. (Republished from Ref. 134 with permission of the Proceedings of the National Academy of Sciences USA, 2101 Constitution Ave., NW, Washington, DC 20418. Reproduced by permission of the publisher via Copyright Clearance Center, Inc.)

manner both in vitro and in vivo. Tet has been used for decades in humans and animals, and only at higher doses above those required for induction of transgenes have few if any deleterious effects been observed. In addition, when the rtTA protein was delivered to mice by ex vivo gene delivery using myoblasts, no immune response to foreign elements was observed (132). Retroviruses are efficient means of delivering tet-regulatable vectors to large numbers of primary cultures of cells, including myoblasts. Thus, there is much reason to believe that the tet-regulatable retroviral systems, in conjunction with myoblast-mediated gene delivery, may be well suited for gene therapy applications in humans in the future.

VI. FUTURE PROSPECTS FOR MYOBLAST-MEDIATED THERAPIES

A. Inherited Myopathies

As noted earlier, a problem in using the ex vivo delivery approach to treat inherited myopathies is that for such therapies to be effective, a large proportion of skeletal muscle must be targeted. Direct intramuscular implantation of myoblasts leads to fusion of the injected myoblasts to a majority of fibers in the region of the injection site; the number of fibers to which genes are delivered by this approach decreases with increasing distance from the site (69). Thus, in order for a sufficiently large percentage of fibers to be treated, many closely spaced injections would be necessitated. This requirement imposes a major limitation to the utility of myoblast-mediated gene transfer in treating human muscular dystrophies, which often affect cardiac and diaphragm muscles as well as skeletal muscles. Unless a myoblast population is isolated that can efficiently migrate to damaged or degenerated muscle, this approach seems too inefficient to be useful.

Recently, the observation by Ferrari and colleagues (140) that cells originating from bone marrow can become incorporated into regions of induced muscle degeneration has been met with much interest. This finding was significant because it elucidated the possibility that such bone marrow–derived cells can travel through the circulation and enter into skeletal muscle tissue (141). A possible solution to the problem of targeting skeletal muscles throughout the body may lie in introducing genetically engineered muscle precursor cells to the circulation, where they can reach muscles throughout the entire body. One study has examined the feasibility of intraarterial delivery of genetically labeled, immortalized L6 myoblasts to skeletal muscle (70). After infusion of these cells into the arterial circulation, a small number of labeled fibers were observed in skeletal leg muscle, showing that the circulation may be capable of delivering muscle precursor cells to differentiated myofibers, although some were also found in the lung. Alternatively, if muscle stem cells of the bone marrow could be isolated, genetically engineered ex vivo, and injected back into the patient, they could serve as a continual pool of circulating therapeutic effectors for the treatment of myopathies.

The existence of a muscle stem cell has been suggested from several pieces of evidence. Populations of cells that are capable of self-renewal and that give rise to differentiated cells have been identified both in the myogenic C2 cell line (142) and in clones of human myoblasts (143). In addition, a recent paper showed, using two genetic markers with different modes of inheritance to examine the fate of myoblasts transplanted into skeletal muscle, that only a discrete minority of transplanted myoblasts participate in regeneration of host muscle (144). This minority population of cells appears to divide slowly in vitro but proliferates rapidly in vivo upon transplantation into regenerating muscle (144). If methods for characterizing and isolating this muscle stem cell population could be devised, such cells could be genetically engineered ex vivo and then introduced to patients, either by infusion into the circulation or through introduction to the bone marrow.

B. Circulating Therapeutic Proteins

The utility of myoblast-mediated gene delivery has broadened to include disorders that benefit from long-term secretion of recombinant proteins into the circulation, including treatment of lysosomal storage deficiencies, hemophilia B, anemias, and possibly cancer. For application of myoblasts in delivering genes encoding recombinant secreted proteins, a hurdle limiting its utility in the therapeutic realm is the necessity of utilizing syngeneic cells in order to avoid immunological rejection of transplanted cells (145). Although myoblasts may be both isolated from and implanted back into the same individual, such procedures are both time consuming and costly. An alternative strategy would be to encapsulate myoblasts in an immuno-isolated environment prior to implantation. Using this approach, myoblasts are enclosed within a matrix, for example, an alginate matrix (although other materials may be used), that allows secreted proteins to leave the capsules. The recipient's immune cells are prevented from coming into contact with the myoblasts, obviating the need for a genetically identical donor. This technology has been shown to be effective in delivering myoblasts engineered to secrete

The Myoblast Song

© 1995 by Matt Springer
(to the tune of "When You Had Left Our Pirate Fold" ("A Paradox")
from Gilbert and Sullivan's *The Pirates of Penzance*)

So many of us work on cells and DNA and protein gels
and western blots and cloning genes and RT-PCR.
But out of all I've seen in lab—both in the present and the past,
there's none I like as much as the ingenious myoblast.
A myoblast, a myoblast, the most amazing myoblast;
that's in the present or the past, the most ingenious myoblast.

A myoblast, a myoblast, it's what we all should try a blast;
it's theirs or yours or his or hers or my-o-blast.

Their myogenic phenotype turns myoblasts into a pipe
that's long and multinucleate and later turns to meat.
You let them fuse, you let them bake—and then you've got a sirloin steak!
We'd all be vegetarian if not for myoblasts.
A myoblast, a myoblast, there's meat because there's myoblasts;
and so we'd starve (at least we'd fast) if it were not for myoblasts.

A myoblast, a myoblast, it hasn't got a chloroplast
because you never see in plants a my-o-blast.

They grow and die and die and grow and when they grow they grow so slow,
but oh do I just love them so, primary myoblasts.
You grow them in a culture dish—and then you hope and then you wish,
and wonder why the cells all die, those evil myoblasts.
The myoblasts, the myoblasts, those little evil myoblasts,
that's in the present or the past, they die because they're myoblasts.

A myoblast, a myoblast, without them we would be harassed;
oh what a useful object is a my-o-blast.

I'd love to stay and chat awhile, to run away is not my style;
unfortunately I must go and babysit my cells.
The cells will look like they're alright—and then they'll all die overnight.
I haven't got a life because I'm growing myoblasts!
Those myoblasts, those myoblasts, frustrating little myoblasts.
I have no life; I am aghast, because I'm growing myoblasts.

A myoblast, a myoblast, I promise this will be the last
time that I sing to you about a my-o-blast!

mouse growth hormone (26) and human factor IX (27) intraperitoneally. Encapsulated myoblasts were shown to be retrievable as long as 213 days postimplantation. These cells were found to be fully viable and capable of secreting recombinant proteins ex vivo at undiminished rates even at this late time point (27). More recently, encapsulated primary myoblasts were used to deliver VEGF to mice subcutaneously and intraperitoneally, causing an angiogenic response (28). This type of technology provides a promising method of attaining nonautologous gene therapy in which universal donor cells can be created simply by encapsulation in a benign, immunoprotective environment.

VII. SUMMARY

The types of disorders considered as potential targets for gene therapy has changed with the development of the field. Initially, most studies centered on developing therapies for single gene defect disorders; however, these present the greatest challenges. Thus, increasingly more attention is being paid to complex diseases involving more than one gene, such as cardiovascular disease and cancer, as these appear more tractable. In addition, although efforts attempting to correct genes that are defective are under development, currently methods for complementing their defects through recombinant expression of related genes are more readily achieved. As the strategies for gene therapy develop in complexity, the methods available for treatment of disorders must also increase in their level of sophistication. Because of its many advantages, myoblast-mediated gene delivery may be a method well suited for addressing these needs for certain types of diseases. Myoblasts can be multiply transduced ex vivo with a variety of retroviral cassettes, each containing separate genes. The availability of improved tet-inducible retroviral vectors allows for fine control of recombinant gene expression levels. The two systems together—ex vivo gene transfer using myoblasts and regulatable retroviral vectors for transducing myoblasts—contribute a powerful toolbox with which to develop gene therapies for a number of human diseases. Should myogenic stem cells prove to be readily isolated, cultivated, and able to migrate to muscle tissue, a large percentage of muscle could be targeted with relative ease, allowing for broad application in the treatment of both inherited myopathies and nonmuscle-related disorders.

REFERENCES

1. Blaese RM, Culver KW, Miller AD, et al. T lymphocyte-directed gene therapy for ADA-SCID: initial trial results after 4 years. Science 1995; 270:475–480.
2. van Deutekom JC, Hoffman EP, Huard J. Muscle maturation: implications for gene therapy. Mol Med Today 1998; 4:214–220.
3. Marshall DJ, Leiden JM. Recent advances in skeletal-muscle-based gene therapy. Curr Opin Genet Dev 1998; 8: 360–365.
4. Kafri T, Blomer U, Peterson DA, et al. Sustained expression of genes delivered directly into liver and muscle by lentiviral vectors. Nat Genet 1997; 17:314–317.
5. Kessler PD, Podsakoff GM, Chen X, et al. Gene delivery to skeletal muscle results in sustained expression and systemic delivery of a therapeutic protein. Proc Natl Acad Sci USA 1996; 93:14082–14087.
6. Xiao X, Li J, Samulski RJ. Efficient long-term gene transfer into muscle tissue of immunocompetent mice by adeno-associated virus vector. J Virol 1996; 70:8098–8108.
7. Snyder RO, Spratt SK, Lagarde C, et al. Efficient and stable adeno-associated virus-mediated transduction in the skeletal muscle of adult immunocompetent mice. Hum Gene Ther 1997; 8:1891–1900.
8. Fisher KJ, Jooss K, Alston J, et al. Recombinant adeno-associated virus for muscle directed gene therapy. Nat Med 1997; 3:306–312.
9. Clark KR, Sferra TJ, Johnson PR. Recombinant adeno-associated viral vectors mediate long-term transgene expression in muscle. Hum Gene Ther 1997; 8:659–669.
10. Wolff JA, Malone RW, Williams P, et al. Direct gene transfer into mouse muscle in vivo. Science 1990; 247: 1465–1468.
11. Wolff JA, Ludtke JJ, Acsadi G, et al. Long-term persistence of plasmid DNA and foreign gene expression in mouse muscle. Hum Mol Genet 1992; 1:363–369.
12. Lin H, Parmacek MS, Morle G, et al. Expression of recombinant genes in myocardium in vivo after direct injection of DNA. Circulation 1990; 82:2217–2221.
13. Kitsis RN, Buttrick PM, McNally EM, et al. Hormonal modulation of a gene injected into rat heart in vivo. Proc Natl Acad Sci USA 1991; 88:4138–4142.
14. Buttrick PM, Kass A, Kitsis RN, et al. Behavior of genes directly injected into the rat heart in vivo. Circ Res 1992; 70:193–198.
15. Ulmer JB, Donnelly JJ, Parker SE, et al. Heterologous protection against influenza by injection of DNA encoding a viral protein. Science 1993; 259:1745–1749.
16. Manickan E, Rouse RJ, Yu Z, et al. Genetic immunization against herpes simplex virus. Protection is mediated by CD4+ T lymphocytes. J Immunol 1995; 155:259–265.
17. Wang B, Ugen KE, Srikantan V, et al. Gene inoculation generates immune responses against human immunodeficiency virus type 1. Proc Natl Acad Sci USA 1993; 90: 4156–4160.
18. Davis HL, Michel ML, Whalen RG. DNA-based immunization induces continuous secretion of hepatitis B surface antigen and high levels of circulating antibody. Hum Mol Genet 1993; 2:1847–1851.
19. Hartikka J, Sawdey M, Cornefert-Jensen F, et al. An improved plasmid DNA expression vector for direct injection into skeletal muscle. Hum Gene Ther 1996; 7:1205–1217.

20. Aihara H, Miyazaki J. Gene transfer into muscle by electroporation in vivo. Nat Biotechnol 1998; 16:867–870.
21. Mir LM, Bureau MF, Rangara R, et al. Long-term, high level in vivo gene expression after electric pulse-mediated gene transfer into skeletal muscle. CR Acad Sci III 1998; 321:893–899.
22. Blau HM, Springer ML. Muscle-mediated gene therapy. N Engl J Med 1995; 333:1554–1556.
23. Hughes SM, Blau HM. Migration of myoblasts across basal lamina during skeletal muscle development. Nature 1990; 345:350–353.
24. Hughes SM, Blau HM. Muscle fiber pattern is independent of cell lineage in postnatal rodent development. Cell 1992; 68:659–671.
25. Springer ML, Rando T, Blau HM. Gene delivery to muscle. In: Boyle AL, ed. Current Protocols in Human Genetics. New York: John Wiley Sons, 1997:Unit 13.4.
26. al-Hendy A, Hortelano G, Tannenbaum GS, et al. Correction of the growth defect in dwarf mice with nonautologous microencapsulated myoblasts—an alternate approach to somatic gene therapy. Hum Gene Ther 1995; 6:165–175.
27. Hortelano G, al-Hendy A, Ofosu FA, et al. Delivery of human factor IX in mice by encapsulated recombinant myoblasts: a novel approach towards allogeneic gene therapy of hemophilia B. Blood 1996; 87:5095–6103.
28. Springer ML, Hortelano G, Bouley D, Wong J, Kraft PE, Blau HM. Systemic delivery of VEGF from implanted encapsulated myoblasts. Submitted.
29. Mauro A. Satellite cell of skeletal muscle fibers. J Biophys Biochem Cytol 1961; 9:493–495.
30. Campion DR. The muscle satellite cell: a review. Int Rev Cytol 1984; 87:225–251.
31. Barany M. ATPase activity of myosin correlated with speed of muscle shortening. J Gen Physiol 1967; 50(suppl):197–218.
32. Schmalbruch H. Handbook of Microscopic Anatomy. Vol. 2. New York: Springer-Verlag, 1985.
33. Hughes SM, Cho M, Karsch-Mizrachi I, et al. Three slow myosin heavy chains sequentially expressed in developing mammalian skeletal muscle. Dev Biol 1993; 158:183–199.
34. Cho M, Webster SG, Blau HM. Evidence for myoblast-extrinsic regulation of slow myosin heavy chain expression during muscle fiber formation in embryonic development. J Cell Biol 1993; 121:795–810.
35. Partridge TA, Grounds M, Sloper JC. Evidence of fusion between host and donor myoblasts in skeletal muscle grafts. Nature 1978; 273:306–308.
36. Watt DJ, Morgan JE, Clifford MA, et al. The movement of muscle precursor cells between adjacent regenerating muscles in the mouse. Anat Embryol 1987; 175:527–536.
37. Watt DJ, Lambert K, Morgan JE, et al. Incorporation of donor muscle precursor cells into an area of muscle regeneration in the host mouse. J Neurol Sci 1982; 57:319–331.
38. Watt DJ, Morgan JE, Partridge TA. Use of mononuclear precursor cells to insert allogeneic genes into growing mouse muscles. Muscle Nerve 1984; 7:741–750.
39. Morgan JE, Watt DJ, Sloper JC, et al. Partial correction of an inherited biochemical defect of skeletal muscle by grafts of normal muscle precursor cells. J Neurol Sci 1988; 86:137–147.
40. Partridge TA, Morgan JE, Coulton GR, et al. Conversion of mdx myofibres from dystrophin-negative to-positive by injection of normal myoblasts. Nature 1989; 337:176–179.
41. Charlton CA, Mohler WA, Radice GL, et al. Fusion competence of myoblasts rendered genetically null for N-cadherin in culture. J Cell Biol 1997; 138:331–336.
42. Yang JT, Rando TA, Mohler WA, et al. Genetic analysis of alpha 4 integrin functions in the development of mouse skeletal muscle. J Cell Biol 1996; 135:829–835.
43. Rando TA, Blau HM. Primary mouse myoblast purification, characterization, and transplantation for cell-mediated gene therapy. J Cell Biol 1994; 125:1275–1287.
44. Webster C, Blau HM. Accelerated age-related decline in replicative life-span of Duchenne muscular dystrophy myoblasts: implications for cell and gene therapy. Somat Cell Mol Genet 1990; 16:557–565.
45. Webster C, Pavlath GK, Parks DR, et al. Isolation of human myoblasts with the fluorescence-activated cell sorter. Exp Cell Res 1988; 174:252–265.
46. Blau HM, Webster C. Isolation and characterization of human muscle cells. Proc Natl Acad Sci USA 1981; 78: 5623–5627.
47. Blanco-Bose WE, Yoo C, Kramer R, et al. Purification of mouse primary myoblasts by sorting for α7B1 integrin expression. In preparation.
48. Kaufman SJ, Foster RF. Replicating myoblasts express a muscle-specific phenotype. Proc Natl Acad Sci USA 1988; 85:9606–9610.
49. Springer ML, Blau HM. High-efficiency retroviral infection of primary myoblasts. Somat Cell Mol Genet 1997; 23:203–209.
50. Wang JM, Zheng H, Blaivas M, et al. Persistent systemic production of human factor IX in mice by skeletal myoblast-mediated gene transfer: feasibility of repeat application to obtain therapeutic levels. Blood 1997; 90: 1075–1082.
51. Barr E, Leiden JM. Systemic delivery of recombinant proteins by genetically modified myoblasts. Science 1991; 254:1507–1509.
52. Dhawan J, Pan LC, Pavlath GK, et al. Systemic delivery of human growth hormone by injection of genetically engineered myoblasts. Science 1991; 254:1509–1512.
53. Peeters S, Friesen HG. A growth hormone binding factor in the serum of pregnant mice. Endocrinology 1977; 101: 1164–1183.
54. Yao SN, Kurachi K. Expression of human factor IX in mice after injection of genetically modified myoblasts. Proc Natl Acad Sci USA 1992; 89:3357–3361.
55. Yao SN, Smith KJ, Kurachi K. Primary myoblast-mediated gene transfer: persistent expression of human factor IX in mice. Gene Ther 1994; 1:99–107.
56. Dai Y, Roman M, Naviaux RK, et al. Gene therapy via primary myoblasts: long-term expression of factor IX pro-

tein following transplantation in vivo. Proc Natl Acad Sci USA 1992; 89:10892–10895.
57. Roman M, Axelrod JH, Dai Y, et al. Circulating human or canine factor IX from retrovirally transduced primary myoblasts and established myoblast cell lines grafted into murine skeletal muscle. Somat Cell Mol Genet 1992; 18: 247–258.
58. Hoffman EP, Brown RH, Jr., Kunkel LM. Dystrophin: the protein product of the Duchenne muscular dystrophy locus. Cell 1987; 51:919–928.
59. Morgan JE, Hoffman EP, Partridge TA. Normal myogenic cells from newborn mice restore normal histology to degenerating muscles of the mdx mouse. J Cell Biol 1990; 111:2437–2449.
60. Law PK, Bertorini TE, Goodwin TG, et al. Dystrophin production induced by myoblast transfer therapy in Duchenne muscular dystrophy. Lancet 1990; 336:114–115.
61. Gussoni E, Pavlath GK, Lanctot AM, et al. Normal dystrophin transcripts detected in Duchenne muscular dystrophy patients after myoblast transplantation. Nature 1992; 356:435–438.
62. Huard J, Bouchard JP, Roy R, et al. Human myoblast transplantation: preliminary results of 4 cases. Muscle Nerve 1992; 15:550–560.
63. Karpati G, Ajdukovic D, Arnold D, et al. Myoblast transfer in Duchenne muscular dystrophy. Ann Neurol 1993; 34: 8–17.
64. Mendell JR, Kissel JT, Amato AA, et al. Myoblast transfer in the treatment of Duchenne's muscular dystrophy. N Engl J Med 1995; 333:832–838.
65. Morandi L, Bernasconi P, Gebbia M, et al. Lack of mRNA and dystrophin expression in DMD patients three months after myoblast transfer. Neuromuscul Disord 1995; 5: 291–295.
66. Miller RG, Sharma KR, Pavlath GK, et al. Myoblast implantation in Duchenne muscular dystrophy: the San Francisco study. Muscle Nerve 1997; 20:469–478.
67. Gussoni E, Wang Y, Fraefel C, et al. A method to codetect introduced genes and their products in gene therapy protocols. Nat Biotechnol 1996; 14:1012–1016.
68. Gussoni E, Blau HM, Kunkel LM. The fate of individual myoblasts after transplantation into muscles of DMD patients. Nat Med 1997; 3:970–977.
69. Rando TA, Pavlath GK, Blau HM. The fate of myoblasts following transplantation into mature muscle. Exp Cell Res 1995; 220:383–389.
70. Neumeyer AM, DiGregorio DM, Brown RH, Jr. Arterial delivery of myoblasts to skeletal muscle. Neurology 1992; 42:2258–2262.
71. Ragot T, Vincent N, Chafey P, et al. Efficient adenovirus-mediated transfer of a human minidystrophin gene to skeletal muscle of mdx mice. Nature 1993; 361:647–650.
72. Kochanek S, Clemens PR, Mitani K, et al. A new adenoviral vector: Replacement of all viral coding sequences with 28 kb of DNA independently expressing both full-length dystrophin and beta-galactosidase. Proc Natl Acad Sci USA 1996; 93:5731–5736.
73. Kumar-Singh R, Chamberlain JS. Encapsidated adenovirus minichromosomes allow delivery and expression of a 14 kb dystrophin cDNA to muscle cells. Hum Mol Genet 1996; 5:913–921.
74. Tinsley J, Deconinck N, Fisher R, et al. Expression of full-length utrophin prevents muscular dystrophy in mdx mice. Nat Med 1998; 4:1441–1444.
75. Dhawan J, Rando TA, Elson SE, et al. Myoblast-mediated expression of colony stimulating factor-1 (CSF-1) in the cytokine-deficient op/op mouse. Somat Cell Mol Genet 1996; 22:363–381.
76. Naffakh N, Pinset C, Montarras D, et al. Long-term secretion of therapeutic proteins from genetically modified skeletal muscles. Hum Gene Ther 1996; 7:11–21.
77. Hamamori Y, Samal B, Tian J, et al. Persistent erythropoiesis by myoblast transfer of erythropoietin cDNA. Hum Gene Ther 1994; 5:1349–1356.
78. Hamamori Y, Samal B, Tian J, et al. Myoblast transfer of human erythropoietin gene in a mouse model of renal failure. J Clin Invest 1995; 95:1808–1813.
79. Svensson EC, Tripathy SK, Leiden JM. Muscle-based gene therapy: realistic possibilities for the future. Mol Med Today 1996; 2:166–172.
80. Pfeffer S. Targeting of proteins to the lysosome. Curr Topics Microbiol Immunol 1991; 170:43–63.
81. Chuah MK, Collen D, VandenDriessche T. Gene therapy for hemophilia: hopes and hurdles. Crit Rev Oncol Hematol 1998; 28:153–171.
82. Hedner U, Davie EW. Introduction to homeostasis and the vitamin K-dependent coagulation factors. In: Scriver C, Beaudet AL, Sly WS, Valle D, eds. The Metabolic Basis of Inherited Disease. Vol. 2. New York: McGraw-Hill, 1989:2107–2134.
83. Wang L, Zoppe M, Hackeng TM, et al. A factor IX-deficient mouse model for hemophilia B gene therapy. Proc Natl Acad Sci USA 1997; 94:11563–11566.
84. Evans RW. Recombinant human erythropoietin and the quality of life of end-stage renal disease patients: a comparative analysis. Am J Kidney Dis 1991; 18:62–70.
85. Naffakh N, Danos O. Gene transfer for erythropoiesis enhancement. Mol Med Today 1996; 2:343–348.
86. Koury MJ, Bondurant MC. The molecular mechanism of erythropoietin action. Eur J Biochem 1992; 210:649–663.
87. Senger DR, Galli SJ, Dvorak AM, et al. Tumor cells secrete a vascular permeability factor that promotes accumulation of ascites fluid. Science 1983; 219:983–985.
88. Leung DW, Cachianes G, Kuang WJ, et al. Vascular endothelial growth factor is a secreted angiogenic mitogen. Science 1989; 246:1306–1309.
89. Plouet J, Schilling J, Gospodarowicz D. Isolation and characterization of a newly identified endothelial cell mitogen produced by AtT-20 cells. Embo J 1989; 8:3801–3806.
90. Ferrara N, Henzel WJ. Pituitary follicular cells secrete a novel heparin-binding growth factor specific for vascular endothelial cells. Byophys Res Commun 1989; 161: 851–855.

91. Conn G, Soderman DD, Schaeffer MT, et al. Purification of a glycoprotein vascular endothelial cell mitogen from a rat glioma-derived cell line. Proc Natl Acad Sci USA 1990; 87:1323–1327.
92. Hanahan D, Folkman J. Patterns and emerging mechanisms of the angiogenic switch during tumorigenesis. Cell 1996; 86:353–364.
93. Pardanaud L, Yassine F, Dieterlen-Lievre F. Relationship between vasculogenesis, angiogenesis and haemopoiesis during avian ontogeny. Development 1989; 105:473–485.
94. Risau W, Flamme I. Vasculogenesis. Annu Rev Cell Dev Biol 1995; 11:73–91.
95. Takeshita S, Pu LQ, Stein LA, et al. Intramuscular administration of vascular endothelial growth factor induces dose-dependent collateral artery augmentation in a rabbit model of chronic limb ischemia. Circulation 1994; 90: II228–234.
96. Takeshita S, Zheng LP, Brogi E, et al. Therapeutic angiogenesis. A single intraarterial bolus of vascular endothelial growth factor augments revascularization in a rabbit ischemic hind limb model. J Clin Invest 1994; 93:662–670.
97. Bauters C, Asahara T, Zheng LP, et al. Site-specific therapeutic angiogenesis after systemic administration of vascular endothelial growth factor. J Vasc Surg 1995; 21: 314–324.
98. Hariawala MD, Horowitz JR, Esakof D, et al. VEGF improves myocardial blood flow but produces EDRF-mediated hypotension in porcine hearts. J Surg Res 1996; 63: 77–82.
99. Horowitz JR, Rivard A, van der Zee R, et al. Vascular endothelial growth factor/vascular permeability factor produces nitric oxide-dependent hypotension. Evidence for a maintenance role in quiescent adult endothelium. Arterioscler Thromb Vasc Biol 1997; 17:2793–800.
100. Mesri EA, Federoff HJ, Brownlee M. Expression of vascular endothelial growth factor from a defective herpes simplex virus type 1 amplicon vector induces angiogenesis in mice. Circ Res 1995; 76:161–167.
101. Muhlhauser J, Merrill MJ, Pili R, et al. VEGF165 expressed by a replication-deficient recombinant adenovirus vector induces angiogenesis in vivo. Circ Res 1995; 77: 1077–1086.
102. Magovern CJ, Mack CA, Zhang J, et al. Regional angiogenesis induced in nonischemic tissue by an adenoviral vector expressing vascular endothelial growth factor. Hum Gene Ther 1997; 8:215–227.
103. Isner JM, Pieczek A, Schainfeld R, et al. Clinical evidence of angiogenesis after arterial gene transfer of phVEGF165 in patient with ischaemic limb. Lancet 1996; 348:370–374.
104. Takeshita S, Weir L, Chen D, et al. Therapeutic angiogenesis following arterial gene transfer of vascular endothelial growth factor in a rabbit model of hindlimb ischemia. Biochem Biophys Res Commun 1996; 227:628–635.
105. Tsurumi Y, Takeshita S, Chen D, et al. Direct intramuscular gene transfer of naked DNA encoding vascular endothelial growth factor augments collateral development and tissue perfusion. Circulation 1996; 94:3281–3290.
106. Mack CA, Patel SR, Schwarz EA, et al. Biologic bypass with the use of adenovirus-mediated gene transfer of the complementary deoxyribonucleic acid for vascular endothelial growth factor 121 improves myocardial perfusion and function in the ischemic porcine heart. J Thorac Cardiovasc Surg 1998; 115:168–176.
107. Springer ML, Chen AS, Kraft PE, et al. VEGF gene delivery to muscle: potential role for vasculogenesis in adults. Mol Cell 1998; 2:549–558.
108. Gimbrone MA, Jr., Leapman SB, Cotran RS, et al. Tumor dormancy in vivo by prevention of neovascularization. J Exp Med 1972; 136:261–276.
109. Brem S, Brem H, Folkman J, et al. Prolonged tumor dormancy by prevention of neovascularization in the vitreous. Cancer Res 1976; 36:2807–2812.
110. Ehrlich P, Apolant H. Beobachtungen über maligne Mausetumoren. Berl Klin Wochenschr 1905; 42:871–874.
111. Gorelik E. Concomitant tumor immunity and the resistance to a second tumor challenge. Adv Cancer Res 1983; 39: 71–120.
112. Ruggiero RA, Bustuoabad OD, Bonfil RD, et al. ''Concomitant immunity'' in murine tumours of non-detectable immunogenicity. Br J Cancer 1985; 51:37–48.
113. Gershon RK, Carter RL, Kondo K. Immunologic defenses against metastases: impairment by excision of an allotransplanted lymphoma. Science 1968; 159:646–648.
114. O'Reilly MS, Holmgren L, Shing Y, et al. Angiostatin: a novel angiogenesis inhibitor that mediates the suppression of metastases by a Lewis lung carcinoma. Cell 1994; 79: 315–328.
115. O'Reilly MS, Boehm T, Shing Y, et al. Endostatin: an endogenous inhibitor of angiogenesis and tumor growth. Cell 1997; 88:277–285.
116. Tanaka T, Cao Y, Folkman J, et al. Viral vector-targeted antiangiogenic gene therapy utilizing an angiostatin complementary DNA. Cancer Res 1998; 58:3362–3369.
117. Rossi FM, Blau HM. Recent advances in inducible gene expression systems. Curr Opin Biotechnol 1998; 9: 451–456.
118. Harvey DM, Caskey CT. Inducible control of gene expression: prospects for gene therapy. Curr Opin Chem Biol 1998; 2:512–518.
119. Gossen M, Bujard H. Tight control of gene expression in mammalian cells by tetracycline-responsive promoters. Proc Natl Acad Sci USA 1992; 89:5547–5551.
120. Gossen M, Freundlieb S, Bender G, et al. Transcriptional activation by tetracyclines in mammalian cells. Science 1995; 268:1766–1769.
121. Mayford M, Bach ME, Huang YY, et al. Control of memory formation through regulated expression of a CaMKII transgene. Science 1996; 274:1678–1683.
122. Kistner A, Gossen M, Zimmermann F, et al. Doxycycline-mediated quantitative and tissue-specific control of gene expression in transgenic mice. Proc Natl Acad Sci USA 1996; 93:10933–10938.
123. Bello B, Resendez-Perez D, Gehring WJ. Spatial and temporal targeting of gene expression in Drosophila by means

of a tetracycline-dependent transactivator system. Development 1998; 125:2193–2202.
124. Kringstein AM, Rossi FM, Hofmann A, et al. Graded transcriptional response to different concentrations of a single transactivator. Proc Natl Acad Sci USA 1998; 95: 13670–13675.
125. Garrick D, Fiering S, Martin DI, et al. Repeat-induced gene silencing in mammals. Nat Genet 1998; 18:56–59.
126. Hofmann A, Nolan GP, Blau HM. Rapid retroviral delivery of tetracycline-inducible genes in a single autoregulatory cassette. Proc Natl Acad Sci USA 1996; 93: 5185–5190.
127. Hwang JJ, Scuric Z, Anderson WF. Novel retroviral vector transferring a suicide gene and a selectable marker gene with enhanced gene expression by using a tetracycline-responsive expression system. J Virol 1996; 70: 8138–8141.
128. Lindemann D, Patriquin E, Feng S, et al. Versatile retrovirus vector systems for regulated gene expression in vitro and in vivo. Mol Med 1997; 3:466–476.
129. Paulus W, Baur I, Boyce FM, et al. Self-contained, tetracycline-regulated retroviral vector system for gene delivery to mammalian cells. J Virol 1996; 70:62–67.
130. Hoshimaru M, Ray J, Sah DW, et al. Differentiation of the immortalized adult neuronal progenitor cell line HC2S2 into neurons by regulatable suppression of the v-myc oncogene. Proc Natl Acad Sci USA 1996; 93: 1518–1523.
131. Sah DW, Ray J, Gage FH. Bipotent progenitor cell lines from the human CNS. Nat Biotechnol 1997; 15:574–580.
132. Bohl D, Naffakh N, Heard JM. Long-term control of erythropoietin secretion by doxycycline in mice transplanted with engineered primary myoblasts. Nat Med 1997; 3: 299–305.
133. Deuschle U, Meyer WK, Thiesen HJ. Tetracycline-reversible silencing of eukaryotic promoters. Mol Cell Biol 1995; 15:1907–1914.
134. Blau HM, Rossi FM. Tet B or not tet B: advances in tetracycline-inducible gene expression. Proc Natl Acad Sci USA 1999; 96:797–799.
135. Hillen W, Berens C. Mechanisms underlying expression of Tn10 encoded tetracycline resistance. Annu Rev Microbiol 1994; 48:345–369.
136. Kisker C, Hinrichs W, Tovar K, et al. The complex formed between Tet repressor and tetracycline-Mg2+ reveals mechanism of antibiotic resistance. J Mol Biol 1995; 247: 260–280.
137. Schnappinger D, Schubert P, Pfleiderer K, et al. Determinants of protein-protein recognition by four helix bundles: changing the dimerization specificity of Tet repressor. Embo J 1998; 17:535–543.
138. Rossi FM, Guicherit OM, Spicher A, et al. Tetracycline-regulatable factors with distinct dimerization domains allow reversible growth inhibition by p16. Nat Genet 1998; 20:389–393.
139. Baron U, Schnappinger D, Helbl V, et al. Generation of conditional mutants in higher eukaryotes by switching between the expression of two genes. Proc Natl Acad Sci USA 1999; 96:1013–1018.
140. Ferrari G, Cusella-De Angelis G, Coletta M, et al. Muscle regeneration by bone marrow-derived myogenic progenitors. Science 1998; 279:1528–1530.
141. Partridge T. The ‘Fantastic Voyage’ of muscle progenitor cells. Nat Med 1998; 4:554–555.
142. Yoshida N, Yoshida S, Koishi K, et al. Cell heterogeneity upon myogenic differentiation: down-regulation of MyoD and Myf-5 generates ‘reserve cells’. J Cell Sci 1998; 111: 769–779.
143. Baroffio A, Hamann M, Bernheim L, et al. Identification of self-renewing myoblasts in the progeny of single human muscle satellite cells. Differentiation 1996; 60:47–57.
144. Beauchamp JR, Morgan JE, Pagel CN, et al. Dynamics of myoblast transplantation reveal a discrete minority of precursors with stem cell-like properties as the myogenic source. J Cell Biol 1999; 144:1113–1122.
145. Chang PL. Microencapsulation—an alternative approach to gene therapy. Transfus Sci 1996; 17:35–43.

5

Design and Use of Herpes Simplex Viral Vectors for Gene Therapy

Darren Wolfe, William F. Goins, David J. Fink, and Joseph C. Glorioso, III
University of Pittsburgh School of Medicine, Pittsburgh, Pennsylvania

I. INTRODUCTION

A. General Overview of Issues Related to Vector Design

The exploitation of genetic sequences as novel pharmaceutical agents has launched a new generation of molecular-based treatments of human disease referred to as gene therapy. In contrast to drugs, which act by modifying existing gene product activity, gene therapy aims to target the cause of the disease by altering the genetic makeup of the cell in order to correct the disease phenotype. Successful gene therapy requires the identification of therapeutic genes that will correct a genetic defect or ameliorate a disease process and the design and construction of suitable vehicles for delivery and expression of these genes in vivo. While identification of genes with therapeutic potential is rapidly proceeding, the engineering of effective gene-transfer vectors remains the central impediment in making gene therapy a practical reality. Nevertheless, considerable progress has been made in vector design, and clinical trials for the treatment of a number of diseases are underway. Success in these initial gene therapy endeavors will no doubt provide incentive for research into additional gene therapy applications, holding promise for creating a new age of molecular medicine in which genomics and functional genetics dovetail with genetic diagnostics and gene therapy.

While remarkable progress has been made toward the development of gene vector technologies, substantial hurdles remain. These include the development of strategies for vector targeting, modifications to increase transgene stability, the regulation of gene expression, and the circumvention of undesirable immune responses. The delivery of transgenes into target cells can be accomplished by either viral or nonviral vectors, with viral strategies remaining the most prevalent in human clinical trials. Virus-mediated gene delivery requires efficient methods for vector construction, vector production, and target cell infection. In this review, the relative merits and potential applications of herpes simplex virus type 1 (HSV-1) vectors will be discussed. In the context of vector development, the natural history of HSV infection in the host will be reviewed, highlighting unique features of the virus biology. Remaining potential pitfalls as well as approaches to their solution will also be discussed.

B. Potential Advantages of HSV Vectors

Although each viral gene-transfer vector possesses distinct attributes, successful gene therapy will require construction of gene-transfer vectors that are tailored to specific applications. The human herpesviruses represent promising candidate vectors for several types of gene therapy applications that include neuropathological disorders, cancer, pain control, autoimmune syndromes, and metabolic diseases.

Herpesviruses are large DNA viruses, with the potential to accommodate multiple transgene cassettes, that have evolved mechanisms that allow life-long persistence in a nonintegrated latent state without causing disease in an immunocompetent host. Among the herpesviruses, HSV-1 is an attractive vehicle for gene transfer to the nervous system since natural infection of humans results in a usually benign, life-long persistence of viral genomes in neurons. This latent state is characterized by the absence of lytic viral protein expression, and the presence of these latent genomes does not alter nerve cell function or survival. The HSV-1 genome contains a unique, neuron-specific promoter complex that remains active during latency, the latency active promoter (LAP). This promoter can be adapted to express therapeutic proteins without compromising the latent state or stimulating immune rejection of transduced cells. The establishment of latency does not appear to require the expression of viral lytic functions. Essential genes that are required for expression of the viral lytic functions can therefore be deleted to create completely replication-defective vectors that nonetheless effectively establish a latent state but cannot cause disease or reactivate from latency. Experimental HSV infection is not limited to neurons; the virus is capable of infecting most mammalian cell types and does not require cell division for infection and gene expression. Accordingly, HSV may be generally useful for gene transfer to a variety of nonneuronal tissues, particularly where short-term transgene expression is required to achieve a therapeutic effect.

Considerable technical progress has been made in developing HSV-1 into a practical gene-transfer vector. The obstacles requiring satisfactory resolution in order to realize the full potential of these vectors include (a) the elimination of vector toxicity, (b) the development of efficient methods for vector construction and high titer vector production, (c) the design of promoter cassettes that provide for adequate level and duration of transgene expression, and (d) targeting of transgene expression to specific cell populations through the use of tissue-specific promoters or by altering the virus host range through modifying receptor utilization for attachment and entry. In this chapter we will concentrate on the design, production, and utilization of replication-deficient genomic HSV vectors.

II. VECTOR DESIGN STRATEGIES

A. Biology of the Viral Lytic Cycle

HSV-1 is a double-stranded DNA virus whose capsid is surrounded by a dense layer of proteins, the tegument, contained within a lipid bilayer envelope (Fig. 1a). Glycoproteins embedded in the viral envelope mediate infection of the host cell, which takes place in two identifiable stages: (a) attachment to the cell surface and (b) fusion with the cell membrane, resulting in virus penetration. The envelope of HSV-1 contains at least 10 glycoproteins (gB, gC, gD, gE, gG, gH, gI, gJ, gL, and gM) and 4 nonglycosylated integral membrane proteins (products of the UL20, UL34, UL45, and UL49.5 genes). Of the 10 glycoproteins, gB, gD, gH, and gL are essential for viral infection (1–4) while gC, gE, gG, gI, gJ, and gM are dispensable for infection in vitro (5–7).

Attachment of the viral particle is mediated by several glycoproteins (5,6,8). The sequential attachment steps in infection result in fusion of the viral envelope with the cell surface membrane and entry of the viral capsid into the cell cytoplasm. Even though the molecular events of penetration are not entirely understood, it is clear that multiple viral glycoproteins are required (e.g., gB, gD, and gH/gL) (2,4,9–11). In addition, following new virion assembly, viral glycoproteins are also involved in a less well-defined process of egress and release of mature particles from the infected cell membrane. Viral particles are also capable of spreading from cell to cell across cell junctions, a process requiring the functional activities of several glycoproteins that are not required for initial infection (e.g., gI/gE) (12,13).

The genome structure of HSV can be divided into viral genes that are essential or accessory for replication in cell culture (Fig. 1b). The accessory functions may be deleted without significantly hampering virus growth in culture, however, removal of essential genes necessitates the use of complementing cell lines that express the essential products in order to propagate these viral recombinants. In human infections, HSV binds to and enters epidermal cells following direct contact with an infected individual that is shedding virus or has an active lesion. Following virus attachment, the viral capsid penetrates the surface membranes of epithelial cells of the skin or mucosa and is transported to the nuclear membrane where viral DNA is injected through a nuclear pore (Fig. 2a). Once inside the nucleus, the viral DNA is circularized and transported to nuclear domain 10 (ND10) structures (14,15), where the immediate early (IE) genes are expressed as part of the sequential cascade of lytic gene synthesis (16) (Fig. 2b). Transcription of the five IE genes (ICP0, ICP4, ICP22, ICP27, and ICP47) does not require de novo viral protein synthesis. Expression of the IE genes is controlled by promoters that contain one or more copies of an enhancer element responsive to the viral tegument protein VP16 (also called Vmw 65 or αTIF), a transactivator that is transported into the nucleus along with viral DNA (17–19). The IE genes ICP4 and ICP27 encode products that are required for expression of the early (E) and late (L) genes (20–23), the former (E) gene class specifying primarily enzyme functions required for viral DNA synthesis and the latter (L) comprising primarily virion structural components. ICP4 regulates viral promoter function (21), while ICP27 affects the processing and transport of viral RNA (24,25). The IE gene products ICP0 and ICP22 contribute to viral gene transcription but are not essential to virus replication

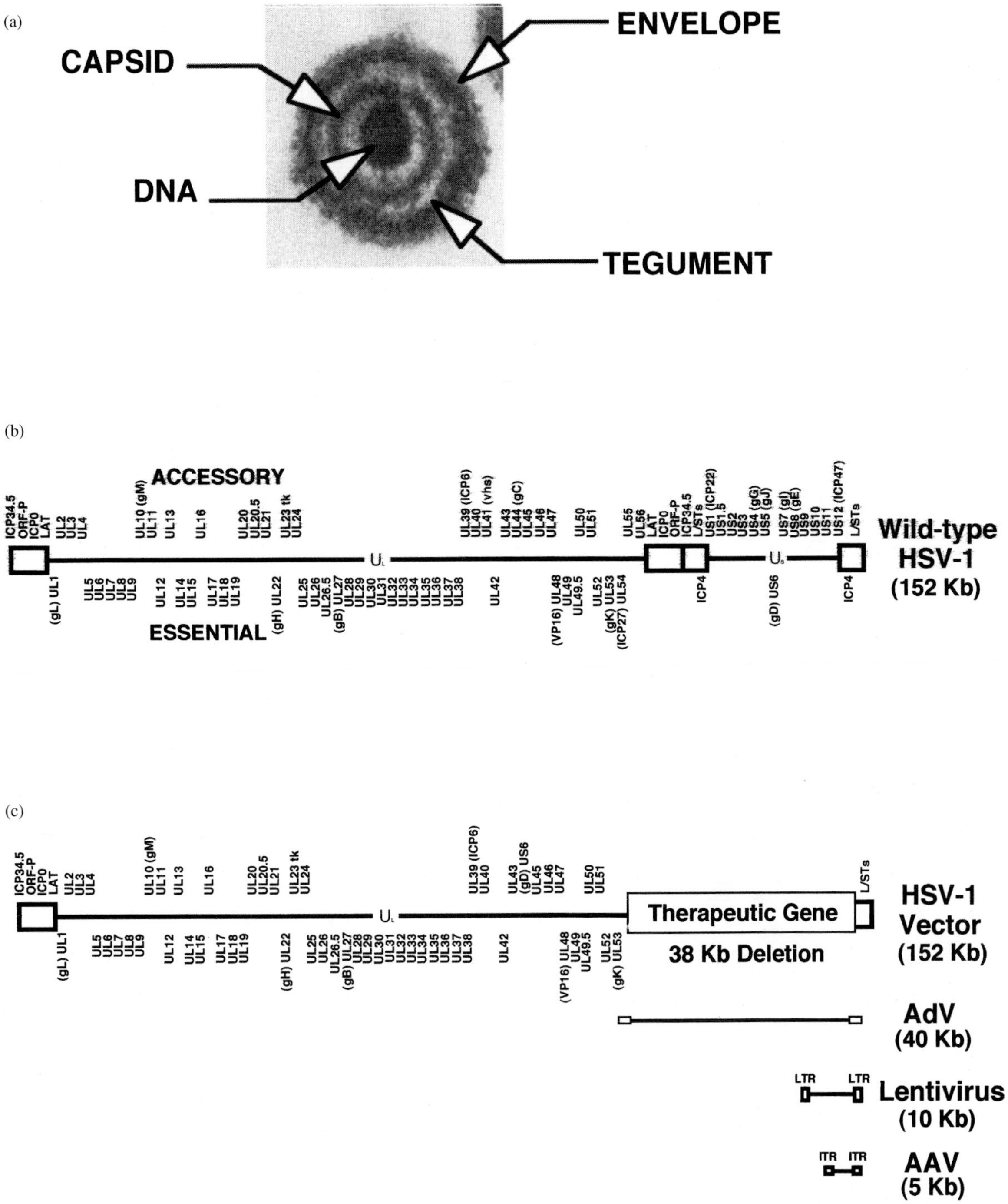

Figure 1 HSV-1 virion structure and genome organization. (a) Electron micrograph of the HSV particle showing the capsid, tegument, and glycoprotein-containing lipid envelope. (b) Schematic representation of the HSV genome showing the unique long (U_L) and unique short (U_S) segments, each bounded by inverted repeat (IR) elements. The location of the essential genes required for viral replication in vitro and the nonessential or accessory genes, which may be deleted without affecting replication in vitro, are indicated. The five IE genes, various glycoprotein genes, LAT, and other important loci are shown. (c) Comparison of viral vector payload capacities. Schematic diagram shows various viral vector genomes currently in use for gene transfer and gene therapy studies, including the overall size of the entire vector genome. The HSV-1 vector, which contains a 38 Kb deletion of sequences comprising the joint region and the entire unique short (U_S) segment of the viral genome ($ICP4^-$, $ICP22^-$, $ICP27^-$), can accommodate foreign transgene sequences that are larger than lentivirus or AAV vectors and equivalent in size to the complete adenoviral (AdV) genome.

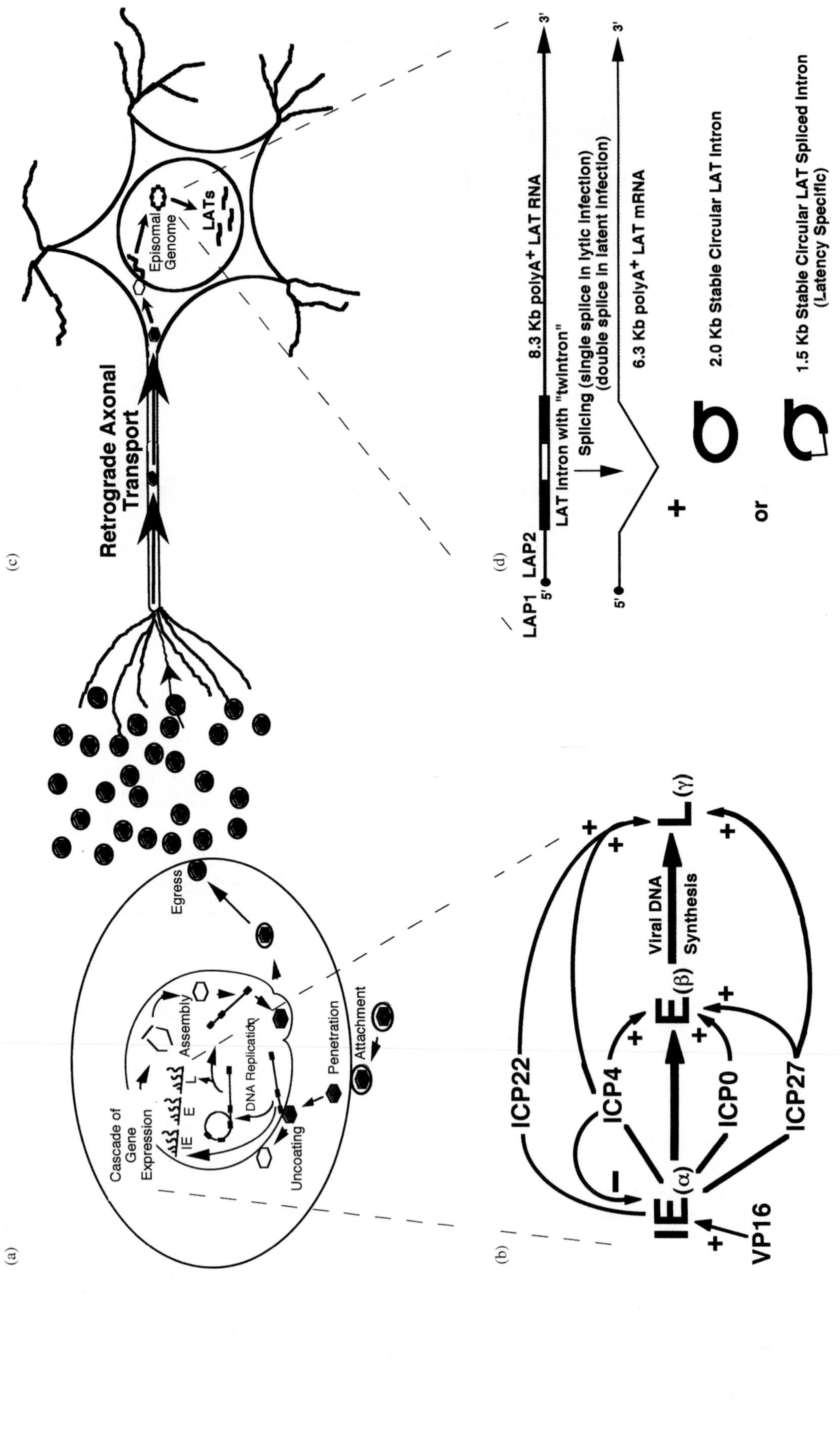
(a)
Cascade of Gene Expression
IE E L
Assembly
DNA Replication
Uncoating
Penetration
Attachment
Egress
(b)
IE(α)
E(β)
L(γ)
VP16
ICP22
ICP4
ICP0
ICP27
Viral DNA Synthesis
(c)
Retrograde Axonal Transport
Episomal Genome
LATs
(d)
LAP1 LAP2
5'
3'
8.3 Kb polyA+ LAT RNA
LAT intron with "twintron"
Splicing (single splice in lytic infection)
(double splice in latent infection)
6.3 Kb polyA+ LAT mRNA
2.0 Kb Stable Circular LAT Intron
or
1.5 Kb Stable Circular LAT Spliced Intron
(Latency Specific)

in cultured cells (26–29). ICP0 is a promiscuous transactivator that exerts its effect prior to the transcription initiation event; it is not a DNA-binding protein (30). ICP22 has been found to regulate the level of ICP0 expression (31). ICP47 does not affect transcription but rather has been reported to interfere with a transporter function (TAP) that is responsible for loading MHC class I molecules with antigenic peptides (32–35). Expression of late genes is dependent on both viral DNA synthesis and IE gene functions (21,23,36,37). Following translation of the late gene products, which become viral structural components of the capsid, tegument, and envelope, genome-length copies of viral DNA are packaged into the newly assembled capsids. Tegument proteins accumulate around the capsid and the immature particle buds through the inner nuclear membrane where the viral glycoproteins are localized. Double-membrane enveloped virus containing virus-encoded glycoproteins modified by the Golgi apparatus enzymes fuse with the cell membrane, forming a mature, extracellular virus particle with a single membrane bilayer (38). The infectious particles can infect neighboring cells by cell-to-cell transmission or can be released for infection of distal cells. With the exception of sensory neurons, cell lysis accompanies productive viral infection.

B. Complementation of Essential Genes and Elimination of Cytotoxicity

Since HSV genes are expressed in a sequential cascade during lytic infection (16), removal of the single essential IE gene ICP4 severely inhibits the expression of later E and L genes (21), resulting in a defective vector incapable of producing virus particles. In addition, the IE gene products, with the exception of ICP47, are individually toxic to most cell types when expressed at high levels by transfection (39). The elimination of multiple IE genes reduces the cytotoxicity of HSV-based vectors for cell lines and primary neuronal cell cultures (40–44) (Fig. 3). Cytotoxicity of a genomic HSV vector deleted for ICP4, ICP22, and ICP27 in cultured Vero cells is reduced compared to a virus only deficient for ICP4 (44). Such mutants are also less toxic to primary neurons (41) or undifferentiated cells such as bone marrow stem cells (J. C. Glorioso, unpublished observation). Mutants deleted for ICP0, ICP4, and ICP27 and defective for ICP22 expression in noncomplementing cells are essentially nontoxic, even when infected at very high multiplicities (45); in this regard they are similar to UV-irradiated particles that do not express viral functions (46). We created a mutant background for gene therapy applications that require short-term, high-level expression by constructing an HSV-1 vector deleted for multiple viral functions including the IE genes ICP4, ICP22, ICP27, and ICP47. We chose to remove the ICP47 gene in this vector to avoid interference with antigen presentation in applications intended for induction of specific immunity, but we did not delete the ICP0 gene because this gene product improves transgene expression and permits efficient construction of recombinant vectors (47,48). In this mutant background we eliminated the virion host shut-off function (vhs) encoded by UL41, because this virus tegument component indiscriminately interferes with translation of mRNA in infected cells (49–51). A similar vector background has been used to express transgenes for up to 21 days in cultured primary neurons without causing neuronal cell death (41). For applications involving infection of bone marrow stem cells or cancer cells in vivo, the transient arrest of cell division offered by ICP0 and subsequent recovery of

Figure 2 HSV-1 life cycle in the host. (a) Lytic infection. Primary lytic infection of epithelial or mucosal cells results from the attachment and penetration of HSV particles to host cells, a complex process involving many HSV surface glycoproteins. Following transport of the capsid to the nuclear membrane and injection of linear dsDNA into the nucleus, the genome circularizes and begins to express the lytic HSV gene functions in a highly regulated sequential cascade, yielding the expression of proteins involved in viral DNA synthesis and virion structural components. Following assembly of newly synthesized particles within the nucleus, virion maturation results in the egress of these virions from the infected cell. (b) Schematic diagram of the sequential cascade of lytic gene expression. The five IE or α genes are expressed immediately upon infection through transactivation by the VP16 tegument protein. The ICP4, ICP27, and ICP0 IE gene functions are responsible for the activation of the early or β genes that are primarily involved in viral DNA synthesis. In addition, ICP4 acts to shut off expression of the IE genes. Following viral DNA replication, ICP4, ICP22, and ICP27 participate in the activation of true viral late or γ genes, which mainly encode virion structural components. (c) Latent infection. When virion particles encounter and bind to axonal termini that innervate the site of primary infection, viral capsids are transported in a retrograde manner to the nerve cell body. At this point the circular viral genome can persist as an episomal molecule in a latent state within the neuron wherein viral lytic gene expression is silenced and a series of latency-associated transcripts (LATs) are produced. (d) Gene expression during latency. The major 2.0 Kb latency-associated transcript (LAT) arises from the large 8.3 Kb polyA$^+$ through a splicing event that yields an unstable 6.3 Kb LAT and a circular LAT lariat of 2.0 Kb. The location of the latency active promoter (LAP) regions LAP1 and LAP2 relative to the LATs is depicted.

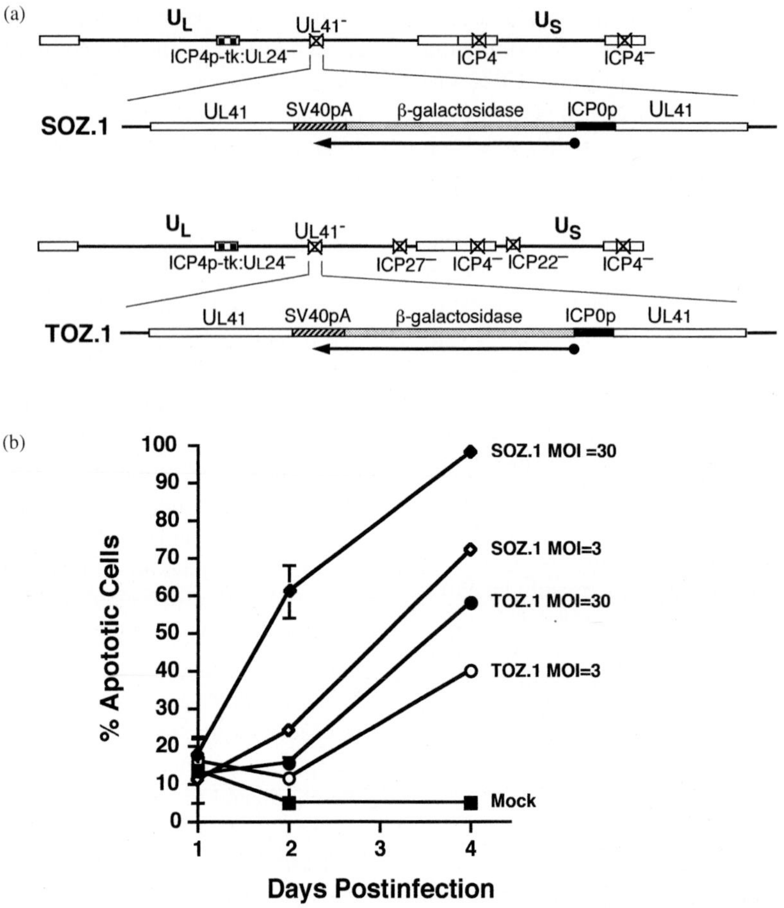

Figure 3 Reduced toxicity following infection of primary dorsal root ganglia neurons. (a) Schematic representation of the first-generation SOZ.1 (ICP4⁻, UL41⁻:ICP0p-lacZ: UL24⁻:ICP4p-tk) and the third generation TOZ.1 (ICP4⁻, ICP22⁻, ICP27⁻, UL41⁻: ICPOp-lacZ, UL24⁻:ICP4p-tk) replication defective vectors displaying the lacZ transgene inserted into the UL41 locus under the control of the ICP0 promoter using the SV40 polyadenylation signal. (b) The number of primary dorsal root ganglion (DRG) neurons undergoing apoptosis was determined at various times following infection with either SOZ.1 or TOZ.1 Even at an MO1 of 30, TOZ.1 was less toxic than the first-generation vector (SOZ.1) at the lower MOI (3.0).

cell growth at high multiplicity of infection should prove advantageous, because transducted cells will produce high levels of transgene product prior to induction of differentiation or cell death, respectively.

C. Vector Transgene Capacity

The treatment of monogenic diseases requires only limited vector capacity, but complex applications may require the delivery of large or multiple independent genetic sequences. A comparison of the genome structure and capacity of several current vector systems is shown in Figure 1c. The size of the HSV-1 genome (152 Kb) is an attractive feature for transfer of large amounts of exogenous genetic sequences. Approximately half of the HSV-1 coding sequences are nonessential for virus replication in cell culture and therefore may be deleted to increase transgene capacity without blocking viral replication (Fig. 1b). The latency region of the virus genome represents approximately 8 Kb of sequence that can be removed and the joint region of the virus is composed of 15 Kb of redundant sequence that can be eliminated without compromising virus replication (52). In one set of experiments we removed an 11 Kb section of the U_S region of the genome (J.C. Glorioso and S. Laquerre, unpublished) containing gD, the only essential gene in this region, which can be propagated on a cell line that expresses gD in trans (4). Approximately 44 Kb of HSV sequence can potentially be removed and vectors propagated in cells engineered to complement just three viral functions (ICP4, ICP27, and gD). Transgene expression cassettes can also be inserted into deleted essential gene loci to avoid transfer of foreign sequences to wild-type virus by recombination that could potentially occur between the vector and wild-type genomes in vivo. We have observed that some nonessential genes (e.g., IE genes ICP0 and ICP22) are toxic to some cell types, yet the products of these genes are required for high titer vector production. The toxicity of these products makes it difficult to produce a complementing cell line carrying these genes. However, it is possible to engineer the promoters for these genes in a manner to make their function dependent upon viral IE genes present only in complementing cells (44). By the judicious selection of viral gene deletions and promoter alterations, high titer vectors can be produced with minimal complementation.

We have developed a panel of novel HSV-1 vectors with a background suitable for expression of multiple transgenes using a rapid gene-insertion procedure (53). To take advantage of the reduced cytotoxicity resulting from the deletion of ICP4, ICP22, and ICP27 genes (41,43), we designed a single vector in which nine viral genes were deleted, removing a total of 11.6 Kb of viral DNA that was replaced with multiple transgenes under control of different promoters. These HSV multigene vectors were constructed with either four or five independent transgenes at distinct loci (47) with all the transgenes simultaneously expressed for up to 7 days. These multigene vectors demonstrate the potential for using HSV-1 vectors for the expression of complex sets of transgenes that have coordinated or complementary functions.

D. Amplicons as an Alternative Vector System

Often referred to as ''defective'' HSV-1 vectors, amplicons are plasmids engineered to contain both an HSV origin of replication and packaging signals and a bacterial origin of replication (54). Amplicons are propagated in bacteria and then co-transfected with a defective HSV ''helper'' virus to create a mixed population of HSV particles containing either the defective HSV helper genome or concatemers of the plasmid packaged within an HSV capsid. In concept, the production of virion-packaged amplicons utilizes transient complementation of the entire HSV genome to provide replication machinery and viral structural components. A comparison of replication-defective genomic HSV vectors and helper virus–free amplicons are shown in Figure 4. Amplicons have been used to express reporter genes

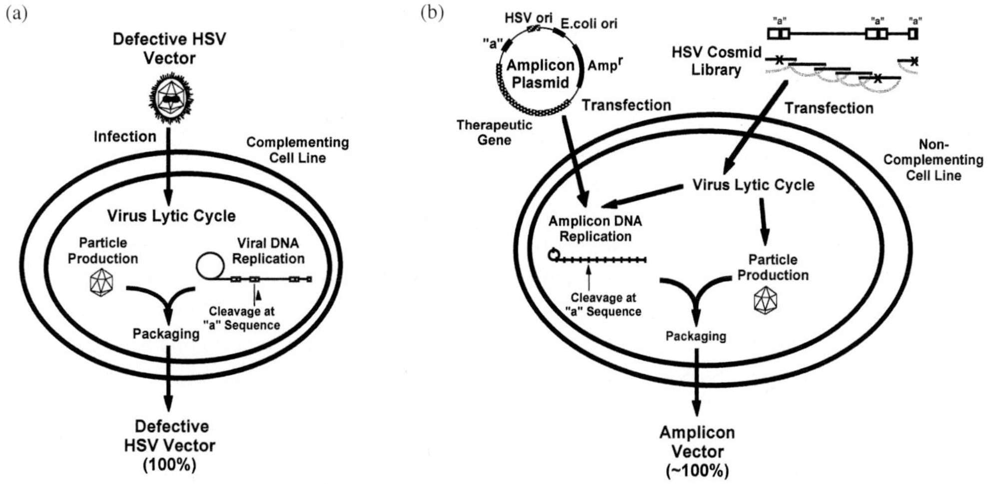

Figure 4 Strategies for HSV-1 vector design. (a) The production of defective full-length genomic HSV vectors is carried out in cell lines engineered to provide the deleted essential genes in *trans.* These vectors can be produced in high titers, are capable of long-term persistence in neurons in vivo, can accommodate large or multiple transgenes, and are incapable of replicating in neurons or other cells because of the missing essential genes. (b) Helper virus–free amplicons can be readily propagated in bacteria using the bacterial origin of replication (*E. coli* ori) and then transfected into a noncomplementing cell line along with five cosmids that encompass the entire HSV genome. Unlike the standard amplicon system in which the final preparation consists either of a mixture of amplicon concatemers and defective HSV particles, only amplicon concatemers get packaged into new virus particles since the overlapping cosmids lack the HSV packaging sequence (''a'' sequence). The helper-free amplicon preparations suffer from low titer yields, decreased stability of the amplicon DNA, and decreased transgene payload.

(55–61) or biologically active peptides (55,62–70) transiently in tissue culture systems.

In vivo, prolonged expression of both a *lacZ* reporter gene (59,71–75) and of the TH gene (71) following amplicon injection into brain have been reported. However, the production of amplicons requires repeated passaging of the amplicon/helper virus preparation, which results in the emergence of recombinant wild-type virus, which, although estimated to occur at the low frequency of 10^{-5} (71,72), results in the death of 10% of infected animals in experiments in vivo (71). The production of true helper virus–free amplicon preparations using multiple restriction fragments of the helper virus genome, which lack packaging signals, has recently been reported (76). However, the maximal yield obtained with that method has remained low ($<10^7$ pfu/mL), and expression in vivo has not been fully tested (76). The presence of cytotoxic helper virus and the generation of replication-competent contaminants represents technical hurdles to the effective production and use of amplicons in patients. Helper-free amplicons will likely require the development of new helper systems to make their use practical enough for human applications.

III. VECTOR TARGETING

One method to achieve cell-specific expression of the therapeutic gene is targeting vector recognition and infection of cells to unique receptors present on the target cell. Exploration of this approach has been limited thus far, but several recent reports have shown convincing targeting of adenovirus (77–79) or retrovirus (80–83). Targeted viral infection requires (a) the identification of cell-specific surface receptor(s) to which viral binding/entry can be directed and (b) the modification of viral glycoproteins to recognize novel receptors while eliminating the binding of these viral ligands to native receptors, a process that ideally should be accomplished without compromising infectivity. These steps can be combined if it is possible to replace the natural receptor-binding domain of viral glycoproteins responsible for infection with binding domains specific for alternate receptors.

The complexity of the glycoproteins in the viral membrane and the fact that multiple glycoproteins are required for the sequential steps of virus attachment and entry have made redirecting HSV infection difficult. Although HSV attachment is a multistage event, initial virus attachment is cooperatively mediated by numerous glycoproteins (5,6,8). Binding of viral particles to cell surface heparan sulfate (HS) and other glycosaminoglycans (GAGs) (10,84–90) is mediated by exposed domains of glycoproteins C (91–94) and B (86,92). Initial virus binding to cell surface HS enhances but is not essential for subsequent gD-mediated binding to specific viral receptors. Several distinct herpesvirus entry mediators (HVEM or HveA) have been identified by screening a cDNA expression library in HSV refractory CHO cells. The first HSV receptor was determined to be a member of the TNFα/NGF receptor family (95). Recently, a number of other entry mediators have been identified, including HveB (poliovirus receptor–related protein 2 [Prr2]) (96) and HveC (97), a member of the immunoglobulin superfamily that has no structural relation to HveA. Finding multiple, unrelated receptors capable of mediating HSV infection via gD suggests that several distinct receptor-binding domains exist within gD. Because HS binding enhances gD binding to a specific receptor, it is possible that targeted infection might be accomplished by manipulation of the specificity of gD while leaving the HS-binding activity of gC and gB intact.

Following the sequential binding of the virus to HS and HVEM, the virus envelope and the cell membrane fuse, resulting in entry of the capsid containing the viral genome. A role for gD in virus penetration is supported by the finding that recombinant virus deleted for gD is capable of binding to cells but unable to penetrate (9,11). In addition, infection can be neutralized by anti-gD antibodies that do not block cell adhesion (9,11). Mutants deleted for gH/gL or gB are also blocked in virus penetration but are not defective in attachment (1,2,98). The ability of gD to bind to a range of cellular receptors suggests that the partial or complete substitution of gD with other sequences capable of mediating viral entry may provide a means of HSV vector targeting. Mutation of, or antibody binding to, N-terminal amino acids of gD eliminates HveA binding while leaving HveC binding and the penetration function intact, but the reverse has yet to be accomplished (99). Future studies will determine whether the insertion of a novel binding ligand into the gD N-terminus will substitute for gD binding to HveA and HveC and restore the role of gD in penetration.

In initial studies to manipulate the cell-attachment properties of HSV, we focused on the elimination of HS binding by removal of these binding domains from the virus envelope leaving intact the secondary binding step mediated by gD. The subsequent replacement of the HS-binding ligands with avid specific receptor-binding sequences might achieve at least partial targeting. A double-mutant virus, KgBpK$^-$gC, in which the coding sequence for the nonessential gC gene was removed from the viral genome in combination with site-specific deletion of the HS-binding domain of the gB (92) (Fig. 5b), was derived from wild-type KOS strain. This mutant demonstrated an 80% reduction in binding to Vero cells compared to wild-type virus (Fig. 5d). By replacing the HS-binding domain of gC with the coding sequence of erythropoietin (EPO) in the back-

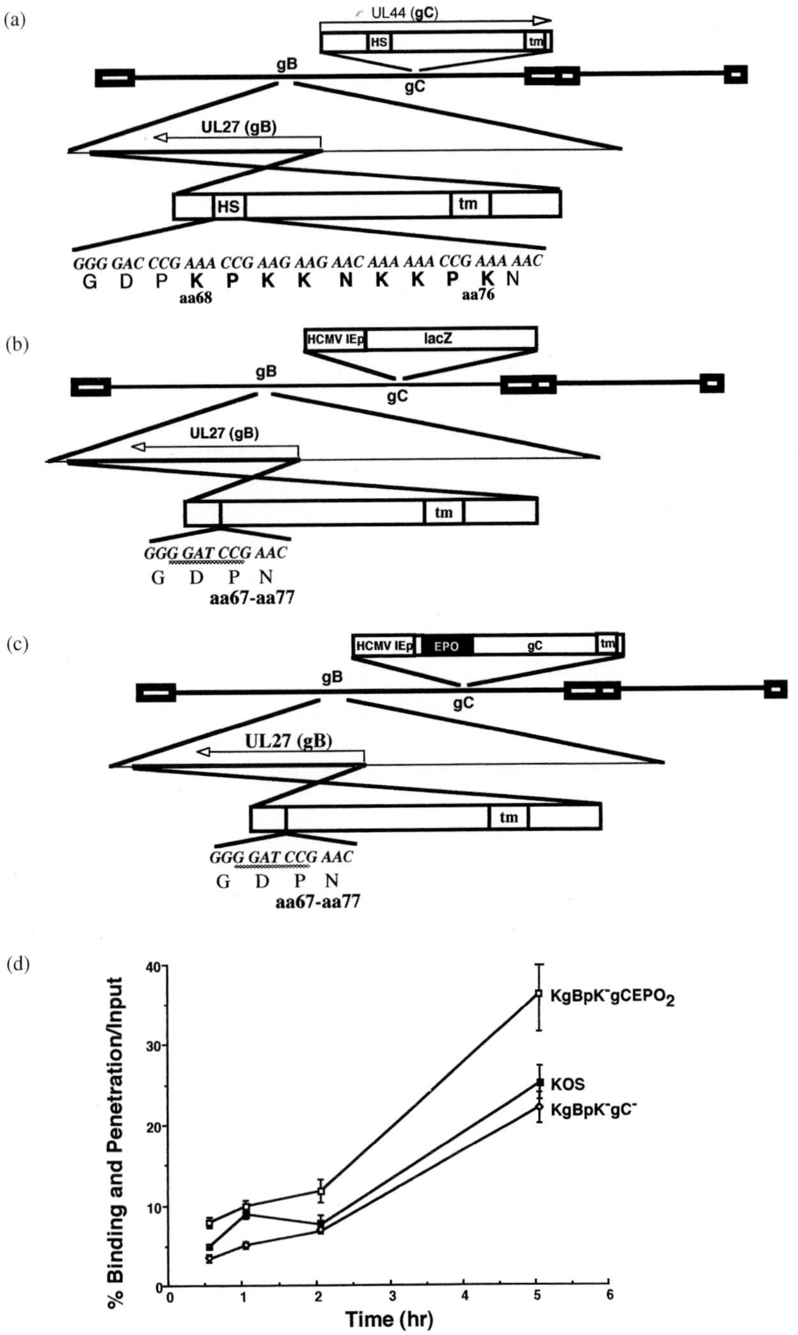

Figure 5 Targeted binding of HSV-1 particles expressing gC:EPO fusion molecules to EPO receptor (EPO-R)–bearing cells. (a) Diagram of the KOS wild-type HSV-1 genome depicting the location of the two HSV glycoproteins (gB and gC) involved in heperan sulfate binding. The heperan sulfate–binding domain of gB consisting of a series of polylysine (pK) residues is shown in greater detail. (b) The KgBpK$^-$gC$^-$ recombinant virus deleted for binding to heperan sulfate was constructed by deleting the polylysine region from the essential gB gene and deletion of the nonessential gC gene by insertion of an HCMV IEp-lacZ expression cassette into the gC locus. (c) The gC:EPO$_2$ recombinant (KgBpK$^-$gCEPO$_2$) was constructed by introducing EPO into the gC gene, replacing aa#1–162 in the KgBpK$^-$gC$^-$ recombinant virus, which could readily be purified by X-gal staining. (d) The percentage of radiolabeled wild-type HSV-1 (KOS), the recombinant deleted for heperan sulfate binding (KgBpK$^-$gC$^-$), and the EPO-expressing (KgBpK$^-$gCEPO$_2$) viruses that bound to K566 cells bearing the EPO-R was determined and is expressed compared to input virus. These data demonstrate that the KgBpK$^-$gCEPO$_2$ recombinant virus binds to the EPO-R, and this binding conferred increased infectivity of the KgBpK$^-$gCEPO$_2$ virus for cells bearing the EPO-R (K562).

ground of the $KgBpK^-gC^-$ mutant virus (Fig. 5c), we demonstrated that the gC:EPO fusion protein was incorporated into the budding virion and that recombinant virus was specifically retained on a soluble EPO-receptor column (100). The gC:EPO virus demonstrated a twofold increase in infection of K562 cells (Fig. 5d) (J. C. Glorioso and S. Laquerre, unpublished), which express the EPO receptor. The EPO-expressing particle also stimulated the proliferation of FD-EPO cells (100), an EPO-dependent cell line, indicative of virus binding. However, virus attachment was followed by delivery of the viral particle to endosomes resulting in virus degradation, thus preventing the normal pathway of entry resulting in productive infection. These studies stress the requirement for appropriate receptor interactions to ensure virus entry by the normal route of virus penetration. Experiments are in progress to modify the binding specificity of gD in the background of a virus mutant defective for IE genes but not HS-binding activity.

IV. VECTOR TRANSGENE EXPRESSION

A. Lytic Gene Promoters

We have explored the activity of many viral and cellular promoters in the background of replication-defective viral vectors (47,101–109). These lytic gene promoters display transient activity in both neuronal and nonneuronal cells. Thus, viral IE promoters are effective for applications that require only transient transgene expression. The human cytomegalovirus (HCMV) IE gene promoter produced vigorous transgene expression for up to 21 days postinfection in vivo (R. Ramakrishnan, unpublished) and in neuronal cell cultures in the background of a vector deleted for ICP4, ICP27, and ICP22 (41). Studies in rabbits have demonstrated transgene expression under control of the HCMV promoter for at least one year following infection of rabbit joints (D. P. Wolfe, W. F. Goins and J. C. Glorioso, unpublished). Other promoters, such as SV40 and various retroviral LTRs, are also transiently active (104,110) following infection of brain. Cellular promoters such as the muscle-specific MCK enhancer support muscle-specific expression in myotubes in culture (G. Akkaraju, unpublished). Several reports have described long-term transgene expression from similar promoters in neurons (111–114), but expression declined significantly after the first week and may represent activity of aborted reactivation events. However, many therapeutic applications will require prolonged transgene expression from latent genomes. For this purpose, we and others have studied the native latency gene promoters in considerable detail.

B. Biology of Latency and the Latency Active Promoter

Following infection of epithelial cells of skin or mucous membrane, viral particles come into contact with sensory neuron axon terminals in which the particle is transported along microtubules to the nerve cell body where the viral DNA enters the nucleus (115,116) (Fig. 2c). Although the virus can express lytic functions in sensory neurons (117–119), lytic gene expression is curtailed through a set of largely undefined molecular events and the virus enters a latent state. Latency is typified by expression of a series of latency-associated transcripts (LATs) from the repeat regions flanking the long unique segment (U_L) of the viral genome partially antisense to and overlapping the 3′ end of ICPO mRNA (120–122) (Fig. 2d). Two co-linear, nonpolyadenylated (poly A^-) LAT RNA species of 2.0 and 1.5 Kb (123,124), which accumulate in the nuclei of latently infected neurons (125), are stable nonlinear intron lariats derived from a large, unstable 8.3 Kb polyadenylated primary transcript (126–130). The virus can remain latent for the life of the individual, although sporadically viral genomes may reactivate in response to a variety of stimuli including immune suppression, UV light, fever, and stress (116,131).

The promoter/regulatory region that controls LAT expression is of interest to gene therapy applications since that promoter remains active during latency when all other viral promoters are silenced. LAT expression is differentially directed by two latency-active promoters, LAP1 (132–135) and LAP2 (135–137). LAP1, predominantly responsible for LAT expression during latency (132,135), is located 5′ proximal to the unstable 8.3 Kb LAT. LAP2, primarily responsible for LAT expression during lytic infection but also capable of driving low-level expression of LAT in the absence of LAP1 during latency (135), is located immediately upstream of the 2.0 Kb LAT intron (135–137). Deletion of both LAP1 and LAP2 completely eliminates expression of detectable levels of LAT during latency in animals (135), demonstrating that both promoters contribute to LAT expression during latency in neurons in vivo. The continuous expression of the LAT region of the HSV genome during neuronal latency suggests that it should be possible to exploit the LAT promoter to express therapeutic genes from latent viral genomes in neurons. Both LAP1 and LAP2 have been employed to achieve long-term transgene expression from the HSV vector genome during latency. For example, a LAP1-β-globin recombinant produced transgene expression in murine peripheral neurons during latency (132), but the level of product decreased over time (138). Other examples include recombinants with LAP1 driving expression of β-glucuronidase (139), NGF (138), β-galactosidase (113,136, 138,140), or murine α-interferon (104) that either displayed a similar expression pattern or were not active in latently infected animals (104,113,138). These data suggest that LAP1 may lack the *cis* elements required for long-term transgene expression in the context of the HSV viral genome. However, long-term transgene expression was achieved when LAP1 was juxtaposed to the Moloney murine leukemia virus (MoMLV) promoter (113), unlike recombinants employing either LAP1 or the LTR alone, suggesting that the elements responsible for extended expression lie elsewhere within the LAT promoter/regulatory region. These *cis*-acting elements may be complemented by elements within the MoMLV promoter, thus allowing transgene expression to continue during latency. When LAP2 was added to the LAP1-reporter cassette in the ectopic site within the genome, long-term expression was restored although the transcription start site was not determined (140). The LAP1/LAP2 complex was capable of driving long-term transgene expression when a lacZ reporter gene cassette was introduced into the LAT intron in the native LAT locus (141) (X. Chen and J. C. Glorioso, unpublished) (Fig. 3) or when a LAP2-lacZ expression cassette was present in an ectopic locus within the viral genome (137). We have also shown that a LAP2-NGF cassette present either in the tk or Us3 loci of the vector expressed this gene product in latently infected rodent neurons both in culture and in vivo (102). Although expression of β-galactosidase from the LAP-lacZ vectors could be detected in neurons of the mouse PNS for up to 300 days (137) (X. Chen and J. C. Glorioso, unpublished), prolonged expression in the CNS was at very low levels detectable only by RT-PCR techniques (X. Chen and J. C. Glorioso, unpublished). In an effort to increase expression from LAP2 in the brain, we have constructed recombinants in which the GFP reporter gene was fused to the internal ribosome entry site (IRES) of encephalomyocarditis virus and placed within the LAT intron downstream of LAP2 in the native LAT locus; a similar recombinant previously yielded high levels of transgene expression in the PNS (142). Our recombinant produced long-term expression in trigeminal and dorsal root ganglion neurons in culture (D. P. Wolfe, W. F. Goins, and J. C. Glorioso, unpublished), but expression in CNS was difficult to detect. Recently, we have determined that both the HCMV IE gene promoter and LAP2 are capable of long-term nerve growth factor expression in rabbits following intraarticular injection with a replication-defective HSV vector (D. P. Wolfe and J. C. Glorioso, unpublished). These unanticipated findings will be important for designing treatment regimens where continuous therapeutic protein production will be required to achieve a therapeutic outcome.

C. Drug-Regulated Promoters

For many applications it may be desirable to regulate expression of a therapeutic transgene in vivo, either to limit toxic effects from high level expression or to more closely resemble physiological expression profiles. We created a viral vector with regulatable transgene expression by using an autoregulatory loop that consisted of a promoter with five tandem copies of the 17-bp Gal4 DNA recognition element that could be transactivated by vector-encoded chimeric Ga14/VP16 protein (Fig. 6a), based on the ability of the chimeric protein to transactivate promoters containing this site (143–145) despite the repressive presence of nucleosomes (146,147). The constitutive Ga14/VP16 transactivator was able to induce transgene expression from a Ga14-sensitive minimal promoter in the background of the virus (106). Regulation was achieved by replacing the constitutive transactivator with a chimeric molecule consisting of the hormone-binding domain of the mutated progesterone receptor fused to the transactivation domain of VP16 and DNA-binding domain of Gal4 (148,149). In the presence of the progesterone analog RU486, the inactive chimeric transactivator assumes a conformation, allowing it to bind to and transactivate the Gal4 recognition site–containing promoter driving transgene expression. Compared to control (Fig. 6b), the completion of the autoregulatory loop following administration of RU486 (Fig. 6c) resulted in substantial enhancement of expression of the transgene in the CNS (106) (Fig. 6d). Following infection of the rat hippocampus with the regulatable virus, levels of viral vector–derived transgene expression is stimulated by administration of the inducing agent RU486 (150).

V. APPLICATIONS

A. Neurodegenerative Disease

The ability of HSV-1 to establish a latent state in neurons for the life of the host suggests that HSV vector–mediated gene transfer may be best suited for treatment of conditions broadly classed as neurodegenerative diseases. HSV-derived vectors have the potential to treat diseases in which the continued expression of a therapeutic gene would prevent the loss of neurons induced to undergo apoptosis. In experimental animal models, delivery of the trophic factor NGF has been shown to block the loss of cholinergic phenotype of septal cholinergic neurons following axotomy (151), and glial-derived neurotrophic factor (GDNF) has been shown to prevent the death of nigral dopaminergic

(a)

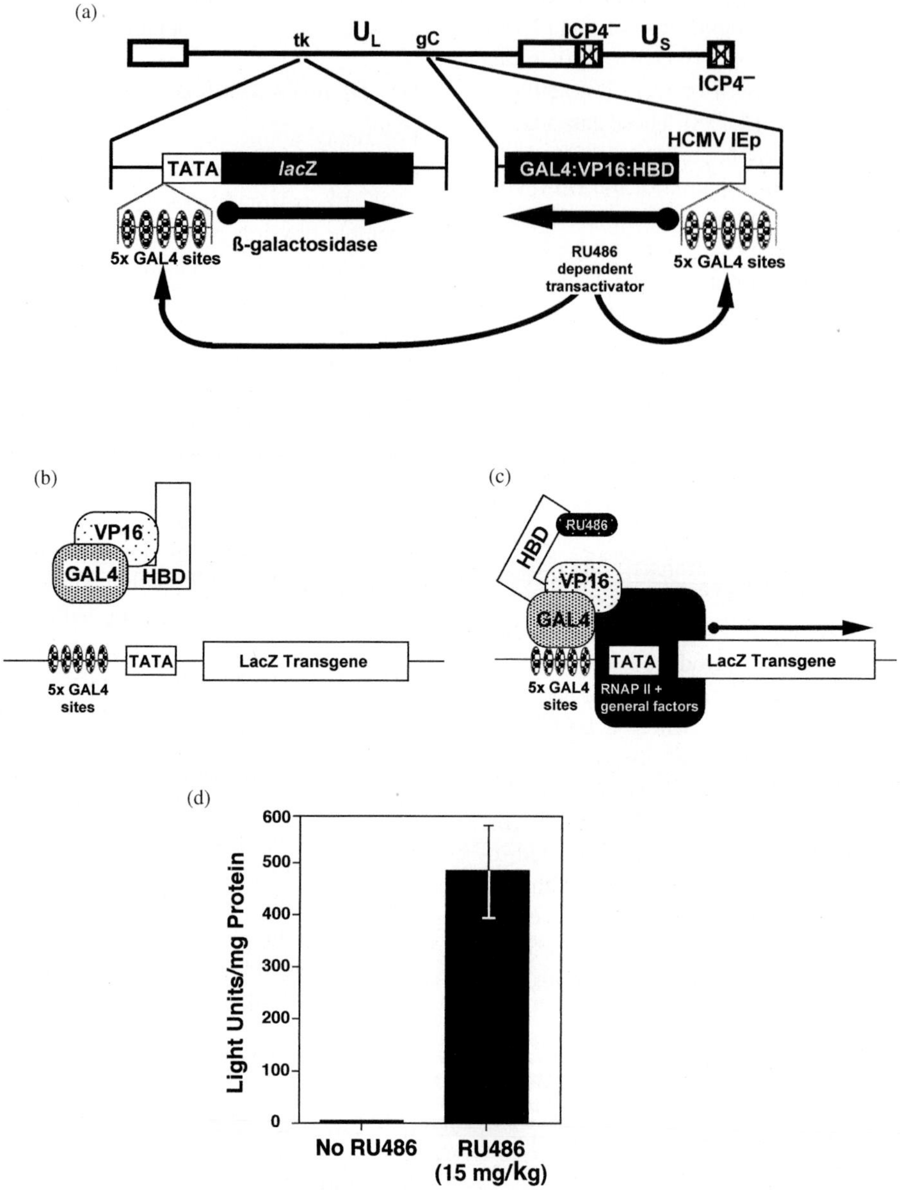

Figure 6 In vivo regulated transgene activation from HSV vectors by drug-inducible recombinant transactivator (RTA). (a) The GLVP RTA vector contains the inducible chimeric transactivator GAL4:VP16:HBD, composed of the yeast GAL4 DNA-binding domain fused to the HSV VP16 transactivation domain fused in frame to a mutant form of the progesterone receptor hormone-binding domain, which can be activated by RU486. In addition, the vector contains a promoter-reporter cassette ($GAL4_5$TATA-lacZ) that is responsive to activation by the transactivator (RTA). (b) In the absence of the drug, the GAL4:VP16:HBD recombinant transactivator cannot bind to the GAL4 sites in the minimal TATA box promoter, resulting in no expression of the β-galactosidase transgene. (c) Following administration of RU486, the tripartite transactivator undergoes a conformational change that allows the RTA to bind to the GAL4 binding sites to yield β-galactosidase expression. (d) Quantitation of β-galactosidase transgene expression in the presence of RU486 displays activation of the transgene promoter by the inducible transactivator following injection of the vector into rat CNS.

neurons induced by 6-hydroxydopamine (6-OHDA) or 1-methyl-4-phenyl-1,2,3,6-tetrahydropyridine (MPTP) (152–154). In the peripheral nervous system (PNS), administration of the ciliary neurotrophic factor (CNTF) or GDNF has been shown to prevent axotomy-induced death of motor neurons and the chronic neurodegenerative characteristic of the Wobbler mouse (155–157). In the central nervous system (CNS) the blood-brain and brain-CSF barriers limit delivery of such factors as traditional drugs to specific brain regions. Utilizing stereotactic injection of an HSV-based expression vector directly to the site of disease could allow local expression of transgenes that may overcome these limitations. For the PNS, cytokine-like side effects limited the dose of CNTF that could be administered in therapeutic trials for the treatment of amyotrophic lateral sclerosis or the use of NGF to treat diabetic neuropathy, and no beneficial effect was shown in humans despite impressive results in animal models (158,159). Local delivery of HSV-based NGF or CNTF expression vectors or the systemic release of these products may overcome the unwanted side effects associated with high doses of the neurotrophins that possess limited biological half-life following direct administration of the proteins.

In order to study the neuroprotective effects of neurotrophic factors in vitro and in vivo, we engineered a series of vectors that express β-NGF from either the human HCMV IE promoter or the HSV latency promoter LAP2 (Fig. 7a). The vectors driving NGF expression from the latency promoter produced long-term β-NGF expression in mouse trigeminal ganglia (TG) and were able to ameliorate the toxic effects of hydrogen peroxide neurotoxicity in primary DRGs in culture (102) (Fig. 7b). We have employed similar vectors expressing Bcl-2 (Fig. 8a) to protect cortical neurons in culture and in vivo in a drug-induced model of Parkinson's disease (109) (Fig. 8b). We are currently examining the ability of these vectors to ameliorate the PNS neurodegeneration seen in taxol-induced, cisplatinum-induced, and diabetic neuropathies, where LAP-driven therapeutic gene expression should be effective. We are also analyzing our LAP2 promoter system for use in other applications where transgene expression during latency could be effective. These include the production of

(a)

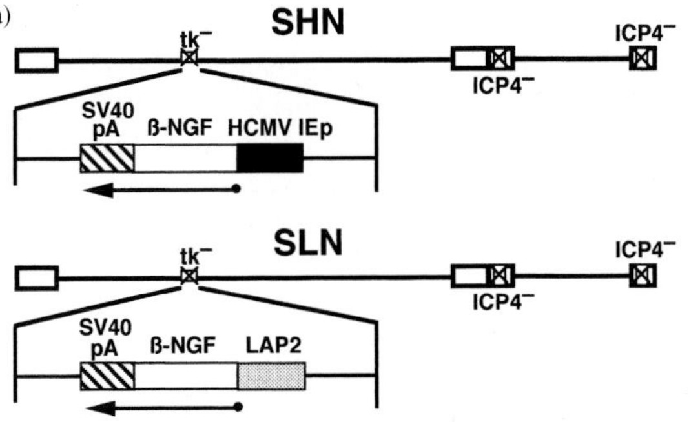

(b)

	3 days		14 days	
	Cell Viability	Protective Enzymes Induced*	Cell Viability	Protective Enzymes Induced*
SLN	−	−	+	+
SHN	+	+	−	−
Control	−	−	−	−
NGF Protein	+	+	+	+

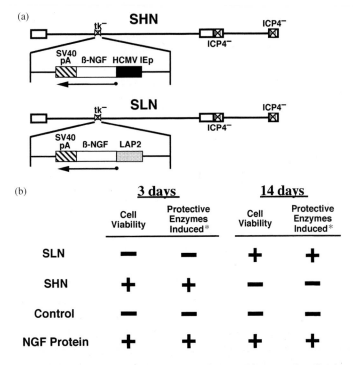

Figure 7 Neuroprotective effects of HSV vector-mediated NGF expression. (a) Diagram of replication-defective HSV-1 β-NGF gene-transfer vectors containing either the strong HCMV IE promoter (SHN) or the HSV LAP2 promoter (SLN) driving expression of the murine β-NGF cDNA inserted into the thymidine kinase (tk) gene locus of a recombinant deleted for both copies of ICP4. (b) NGF driven from the HCMV IE promoter (SHN) at 3 days or LAP2 (SLN) at 14 days postinfection was able to protect primary dorsal root ganglia (DRG) neurons from peroxide-induced cell death and stimulate the synthesis of antioxidant enzymes such as catalase and SOD unlike a control vector does not express the transgene. *Catalase anal superoxide dismutase.

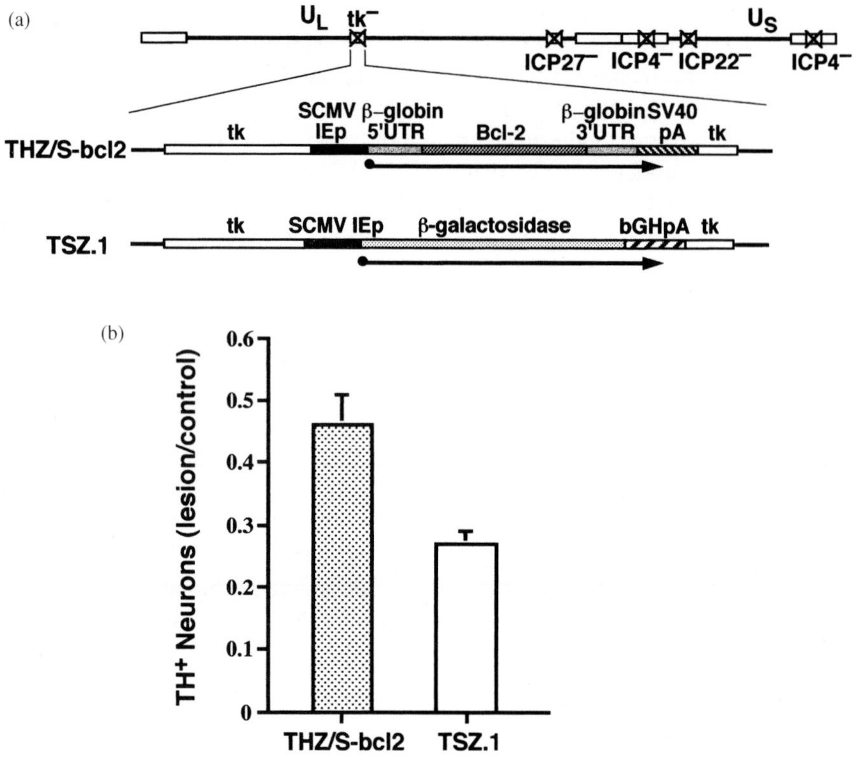

Figure 8 Neuroprotective effects of HSV vector-mediated Bcl-2 expression. (a) Diagram of replication-defective HSV-1 Bcl-2 expression vector (THZ/S-bcl2) containing the strong SCMV IE promoter juxtaposed to the Bcl-2 cDNA in a expression cassette utilizing the β-globin 5′ and 3′ untranslated regions (UTR) inserted into the thymidine kinase (tk) gene locus of a recombinant deleted for both copies of ICP4, as well as ICP27 and ICP22. The control vector (TSZ.1) contains an SCMV IEp-lacZ expression cassette inserted into the tk locus of the same vector backbone. (b) THZ/S-bcl2 vector-mediated Bcl-2 expression in the substantia nigra of 6-hydroxy dopamine (6-OHDA) lesions resulted in a significantly greater number of tyrosine hydroxylase positive (TH^+) neurons that survived toxic insult compared to injection of the control virus (TSZ.1).

factors, such as enkephalin, that regulate the function of local nonneuronal tissues and the transmission of pain signals to the brain (108).

B. Muscular Dystrophy

Muscle is recognized as an excellent target for gene delivery for vaccines, production of soluble products, and treatment of neuromuscular disease. Recently, we have explored the use of HSV vectors for gene transfer to muscle with the eventual aim of using this viral vector to deliver genes for treatment of muscular dystrophy including the Duchenne type, one of the most prevalent heritable human diseases. Duchenne muscular dystrophy (DMD) is a devastating muscle-wasting syndrome caused by a lack of dystrophin expression at the sarcolemma of muscle fibers (160–162). This protein appears to function in the maintenance of muscle membrane integrity. Dystrophin is one of the largest known human genes, and mutations arise at high frequency, making it one of the most common genetic diseases, affecting 1 in 2000 males. There is no treatment, and affected children usually die in their late teens of heart or respiratory failure.

Two different approaches have been considered for the treatment of DMD: myoblast transplantation and gene therapy. Myoblast transplantation (MT) consists of implantation of normal myobast precursors (satellite cells) into diseased muscle to create a reservoir of myoblasts capable of fusing to damaged myofibers and expressing the deficient dystrophin gene product (163–165). MT in both animals and human trials has not been successful primarily due to transplantation rejection and difficulty associated with effective delivery. Gene therapy also suffers limitations of gene delivery requiring a systemic approach involving intravenous inoculation of vector, since approximately 40% of the body's lean weight can be attributed to muscle.

A number of vectors have been tried for gene delivery to muscle including naked DNA, retroviruses, and adenoviruses. Naked DNA proved to be inefficient although stable gene delivery was possible (166,167), and retroviruses have not been found to efficiently infect differentiated muscle fibers (168,169). In addition, the dystrophin cDNA is 14 Kb in size, and thus standard adenoviral (AV) vectors are unable to accommodate the full-length coding sequence. Recently, completely "gutted" AV vectors have been reported that can accommodate the dystrophin gene (170–172), however, these vectors are contaminated with helper virus, which results in immune rejection of the vector-delivered transgene. Moreover, AV vectors infect mature muscle fibers poorly (and myoblasts preferentially) (173–176), the mature fibers having a low density of the AV receptor. Unfortunately, the number of myoblasts capable of fusing with damaged fibers decrease during disease progression, requiring gene delivery to muscle fibers. Adenovirus is also highly immunogenic, perhaps because of the high doses of vector required for infection of muscle, which will make repeat dosing difficult. Indeed, repeat dosing of AV has not been generally possible due to the production of neutralizing antibodies after first administration of vector (177).

Manipulation of HSV vectors may resolve some of these difficulties. HSV can easily accommodate the full-length dystrophin cDNA plus tissue specific regulatory sequences (258) and infects muscle with much greater efficiency (178), requiring only 1% as much infectious virus as adenovirus to achieve the same level of transduction of myoblasts and myotubes (178), and HSV infects both types of muscle cells equally both in vitro and in vivo (178). However, like AdV, HSV infects mature muscle poorly. HSV is significantly impeded by the muscle basal lamina, which acts as a physical barrier to infection (179). The use of multiply deleted vectors described above in vivo improves transgene delivery and expression including dystrophin, although expression is lost within 2 weeks (258). Recent experiments have shown that bone marrow stem cells (CD34+) are capable of differentiating into multiple cell lineages, including the various blood cells, endothelial cells lining newly formed blood vessels, and given the appropriate stimuli (e.g., morphogins for muscle or bone) these cells are pluripotent and can differentiate into myoblasts, cartilage, and bone (180–182). These recent experiments, coupled with our findings that highly defective HSV vectors infect bone marrow stem cells very efficiently without causing cell death and are able to express a transgene long term (>8 weeks) in circulating blood, suggests the possibility that dystrophin can be introduced into CD34+ cells from DMD patients along with a gene (e.g., myoD) that induces differentiation into myoblasts with subsequent incorporation into degenerating muscle tissue. This approach would provide a systemic treatment obviating the need for excessive multiple injection of all muscle tissue and circumventing the problem of inflammatory responses to the vector and the basal lamina barrier. Experiments to test this promising new possibility are ongoing.

C. Cancer

Cancer gene therapy may offer a treatment modality to patients who have exhausted all other treatment regimens. There are a number of considerations in applying gene therapy to cancer, which include the selection of the appropriate therapeutic gene(s), the specific effect or mechanism, target tissue, and method of gene delivery. The overriding problem is that cancer is generally a systemic disease, and thus even if gene transfer is effective in destroying a tumor locally, metastases will promote continued disease.

Strategies to treat cancer by gene therapy can be considered in two categories: (a) tumor cell destruction by expression of transgenes whose products induce cell death or sensitize the cells to chemo- (183) or radiation therapy (184) and (b) tumor vaccination through expression of transgenes whose products recruit, activate, or co-stimulate immunity or provide tumor antigens. Because these strategies are complementary, it has also been suggested that they can be used in combination. Examples include the use of pro-drug–activating genes (185), cytokines (186), MHC products such as costimulatory molecules (187–189), allotypic class I or class II molecules (187–190), and tumor antigens (191,192), which together may assist in the recruitment and activation of nonspecific inflammatory responses (193) or the induction of tumor-specific immunity.

Suicide gene therapy for the treatment of cancer in experimental animals and in Phase I human clinical protocols (183,194–198) has met with limited success. Transfer of the HSV gene thymidine kinase (tk) into tumor cells results in tumor cell death when combined with the antiviral drug ganciclovir (GCV). tk has been shown to convert the prodrug into a toxic nucleotide analog that, upon incorporation into nascent DNA, results in the interruption of DNA replication by chain termination. A uniquely powerful characteristic of the tk-GCV approach is that only a small fraction of the tumor cells need to be transduced with the suicide gene to result in significant antitumor activity—an activity known as the "bystander effect" (194,195,198–200). It has been demonstrated that cell-to-cell transfer of activated GCV via gap junctions between transduced tumor cells and untransduced neighboring cells is a major mechanism of the bystander effect (201–204). We have tested the ability of tk-overexpressing HSV vectors to act as a treatment for established tumors in rodent glioma models and observed significant increases in survival time (205). However, suicide gene therapy has a realistic chance as a cure only if it can be augmented by the actions of alternate gene therapy methodologies (202,206–209).

There is also a considerable amount of recent interest in using cytokine genes, costimulatory molecules, tumor antigens, and recruitment molecules to enhance the immune response to the tumor. Antitumor immunity should prove effective in treatment of metastatic cancer. The development of antitumor immunity could circumvent the need for replication-competent vectors since tumor-specific cytotoxic T lymphocytes constantly move through the brain parenchyma searching for target cells. A growing body of literature suggests that local expression of cytokines can enhance CTL activation at least in animal model systems and these bear testing in human brain cancer. HSV offers the potential for combinational gene therapy in this regard since multiple immunomodulatory genes can be recombined into the virus and comparatively tested (47).

HSV may be well suited for treatment of gliolastoma and other primary brain tumors or tumors that arise as metastases from other non-CNS tissues. Gliomas, for example, often produce large masses in the brain with the tumor invading the normal surrounding brain tissue making the complete surgical resection of these tumors impossible. The intact blood-brain barrier makes infiltrating tumor cells inaccessible by systemic delivery. Moreover, the architecture of newly synthesized blood vessels within the tumor is irregular and blood flow uneven, suggesting that distribution of antitumor agents would be difficult.

In an attempt to enhance the cell killing seen in suicide gene therapy, we have taken two approaches. In the first, we created a replication defective HSV-1–based vector, which expresses the human TNF-α gene product in conjunction with the HSV-tk gene (TH:TNF) (105) (Fig. 9a). TNF-α has been demonstrated to possess an array of antitumor activities, including potent cytotoxicity exerted directly on tumor cells (210), enhancement of the expression of HLA antigens (211), and ICAM-1 (212) on tumor cell surfaces, enhancement of interleukin-2 receptors on lymphocytes (213), and promotion of the activation of such effector cells as natural killer (NK) cells, lymphokine-activated killer (LAK) cells, and cytotoxic T lymphocytes (CTL) (214–216). However, despite this promising antitumor profile, the clinical use of TNF-α has been constrained by the toxicity of systemic TNF-α delivery (217,218). The possibility that local production of TNF-α at the site of tumor growth may allow for effective use of this cytokine as an antitumor agent provided the impetus for constructing and testing TNF-α–expressing, replication-deficient vectors. The results of both cell culture and in vivo experiments with our TNF vector showed that the effectiveness of combination immune stimulation with TNF-α and suicide gene therapy with HSV-tk was significantly enhanced (105) (Fig. 9b). Continuing with this approach, we introduced the connexin 43 gene into a HSV-tk expression vector to increase transfer of the modified prodrug to neighboring cells. The expression of connexin was found to increase the GCV-mediated bystander effect in tumor cells in which connexin was poorly expressed both in vitro and in vivo (P. Marconi, M. Tamura, and J. C. Glorioso, unpublished). Experiments are in progress to combine these three genes in one vector in order to further augment GCV-activated killing of tumor cells focusing on animal models of brain cancers.

As an alternative to the replication-defective vectors, HSV vectors compromised for their ability to replicate in normal nondividing neurons while retaining their ability to replicate in the tumor cells are now being tested in patients (219,220). The use of conditional replication-competent viruses could in theory allow for spread in tumor tissue without damaging normal brain, thus increasing the effectiveness. Such mutants include those lacking the viral thymidine kinase (221–224), the ribonucleotide reductase (225,226), a protein kinase (227), or a gene (γ34.5) required for growth specifically in neurons (228–230). Deleting these genes in combination creates viruses that are highly compromised for their ability to replicate in and kill neuronal cells yet retain the ability to replicate in and kill tumor cells. However, such highly compromised viruses grow poorly in tumor cells, and although multiple deletions increase safety, efficacy is compromised. If direct killing of tumor cells were coupled with gene expression that can activate anticancer pro-drugs in situ, perhaps the effectiveness of these anticancer vectors would be enhanced. There are also safety concerns in using conditionally replication-competent vectors related to toxicity for endothelial cells, normal glial cells, and microglia with the potential of the virus gaining access to the meningial fluid where the virus can cause meningitis and destruction of appendymal cells lining the ventricles of the brain. These potential problems may be greatly reduced if the vector contains ligands that will target it to tumor cells or at least block infection of neuronal cells. Specific cell lysis may also be possible if an essential viral gene such as ICP4 were transcriptionally regulated by a glial-specific promoter, further ensuring that the virus would replicate only in tumor tissue.

D. Arthritis

Arthritis is a long-term, painful disease associated with lower life expectancy, dramatically impairing the quality

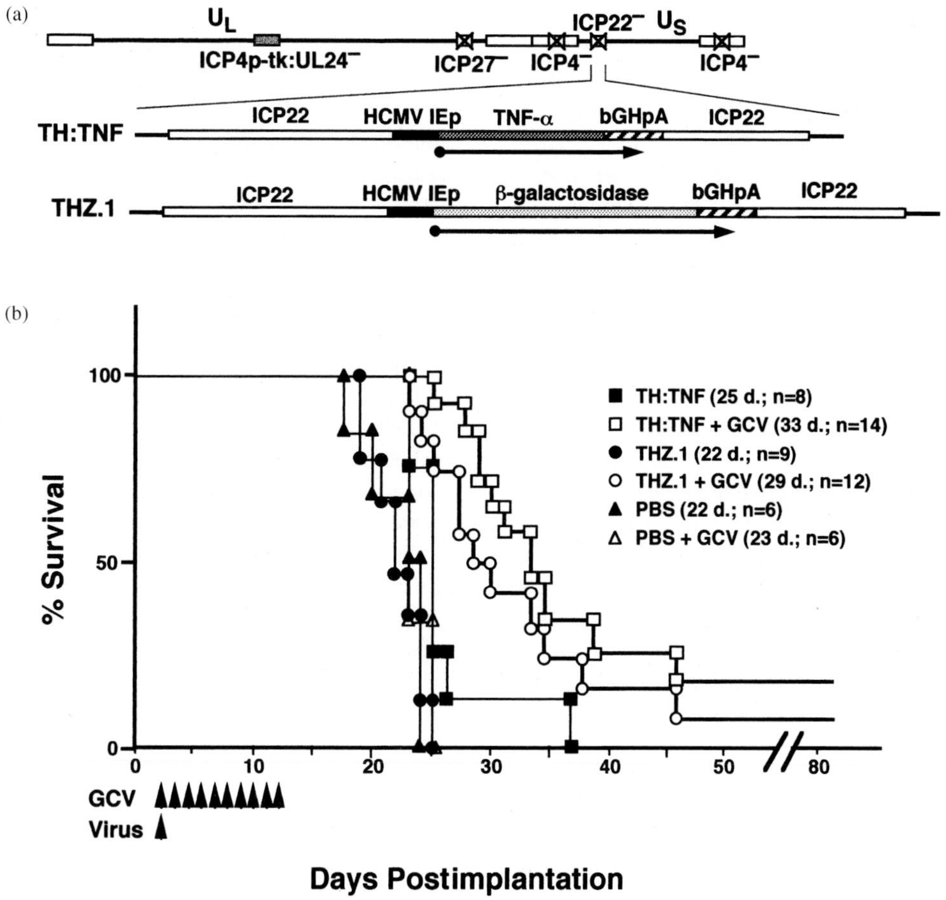

Figure 9 Treatment of TNF-α–resistant tumors (U87-MG) with the TH:TNF vector. (a) Schematic representation of the TH:TNF ($ICP4^-$, $ICP22^-$:HCMV IEp-TNF-α, $ICP27^-$, $UL24^-$:ICP4p-tk) and THZ.1 ($ICP4^-$, $ICP22^-$:HCMV IEp-lacZ, $ICP27^-$, $UL24^-$:ICP4p-tk) vectors displaying the transgenes (TNF-α cDNA and lacZ) inserted into the ICP22 locus under the control of the HCMV promoter using the bovine growth hormone (bGH) polyadenylation region. (b) Kaplan-Meier survival plot of athymic nude mice with intracerebral U87-MG tumors treated by a single viral injection and daily GCV administration for 10 days. The key includes the number of animals per treatment (n) and median survival times.

of life for disease sufferers, and it is the leading cause of morbidity in the elderly (231,232). The most common forms of the disease are osteoarthritis (OA), afflicting over 50% of individuals aged 65 years or greater, and rheumatoid arthritis (RA), which afflicts 1–2% of individuals worldwide.

All forms of arthritis share two common intraarticular pathologies, synovial inflammation and degeneration of articular cartilage, which may occur separately or together (233). In OA, for example, the major pathology is loss of articular cartilage, with inflammation usually being low or absent. In lupus erythematosus, joints become inflamed without cartilage erosion. In RA, inflammation and cartilage loss occur together, leading to the loss of joint function and pain. Comprehensive treatment of arthritis will require both anti-inflammatory and chondroprotective effects, perhaps with regimes that simultaneously provide both approaches. A number of drugs are moderately successful as anti-inflammatory agents yet provide incomplete treatment for many arthritis sufferers (234). However, there are currently no effective treatments for cartilage loss, often resulting in the loss of joint function and degeneration of the bone. In these cases, joint replacement surgery becomes the only realistic therapeutic avenue. The effectiveness of antiarthritic therapy will not improve dramatically by continuing along traditional lines of drug therapy. Recent advances in understanding the cellular and molecular pathophysiology of arthritis now permit the design of rational therapies for treating this group of diseases. In particular, it has now become clear that, irrespective of the etiology of the disease, much of the intraarticular pathology of arthritis is driven by cytokines though their action may be secondary to other disturbances (235).

Interleukin-1 (IL-1) and TNF-α are elevated in synovial fluids from arthritic joints (236,237) and have emerged as key mediators of arthritic pathology (238). These cytokines are chondrodestructive as well as inflammatory and damage cartilage by accelerating chondrocyte-mediated breakdown of the matrix and inhibit repair synthesis (239–241). Inflammation of the joint mediated by these cytokines occurs by a multifaceted mechanism including the upregulation of endothelial adhesion molecules, the induction of chemotactic cytokines such as IL-8, the degranulation of polymorphonuclear leukocytes, and the induction of other, downstream mediators such as IL-6, nitric oxide, and prostaglandins (242,243). Antagonists of these two cytokines have been found to be an effective treatment in a variety of animal models of RA and OA (244–246). Recent human clinical trials of anti-TNF-α antibodies have shown dramatic short-term efficacy in RA (247), and results from a trial of soluble IL-1 receptor antagonist type I (IL-1Ra) have been published (248). Partial success in these trials permits considerable optimism that antagonists of IL-1 and TNF-α, used singly or together, will produce superior results in treating arthritis. While attempts to block these two mediators by small, orally active drugs have met with some success, new methods of gene transfer may prove invaluable in delivering therapeutic proteins directly to the diseased tissue.

We have developed HSV vectors to deliver the IL-1 and TNF-α antagonists, IL-1Ra and sTNF-αR, to cells lining the joint in a rabbit model of arthritis (249–257). HSV-based vectors are able to efficiently infect rabbit synovial cells in vivo after intraarticular injection and produce high levels of transgene with modest doses of virus (10^7 pfu). HSV has the additional advantage that multiple transgenes, including cytokine inhibitors, can be produced from a single vector. Production of antiarthritic transgenes encoding secreted proteins from the synovial lining of arthritic joints also has several advantages. As seen with many clinical trials, systemic delivery of drugs often produce unwanted side effects. Following HSV-mediated delivery directly to the diseased joint, the highest concentration of the gene product accumulates within the joint space, thus maximizing the effectiveness of the transgene while minimizing systemic side effects.

We administered HSV vectors carrying lacZ, IL-1sR, or TNF-αsR to arthritic rabbit knee and measured the glycosaminoglycan (GAG) content of the fluids, an index of cartilage breakdown and the onset of arthritis. The GAG influx was unaffected by the presence of the lacZ gene delivered by a control HSV vector but was reduced by either the sIL-1R or TNFαsR at both 3 and 7 days postinfection (259). Visual inspection of treated knees suggested that these transgenes reduced swelling and were indistinguishable from normal. These results suggest that HSV may be a useful vector for gene therapy of arthritis. However, transgene expression was limited to 7 days as measured by the presence of β-gal–positive synovial cells or the presence of soluble IL-receptor in synovial fluid. Based on studies with vectors expressing NGF following intraarticular injection of a highly defective vector, we tested for release TNF-αsR after similar inoculation of a vector capable of expressing both NGF and TNF-αsR (D. P. Wolfe, W. F. Goins, and J. C. Glorioso, unpublished). NGF was found in the joint space, however, TNF-αsR was not released either in vivo or in vitro from differentiated PC-12 cells in culture, suggesting that a targeting sequence may be required for release of cytokine inhibitors from neurons. Experiments are in progress to test this approach. If successful, it may be possible to treat inflammation of joints using peripheral neurons as a depot for targeting these anti-inflammatory molecules to joints from a site in the body where long-term expression will be possible without the vector itself inducing an inflammatory response.

E. Pain Management

Another application for HSV-based gene therapy is the treatment of chronic pain. There exists a vast unmet need for effective treatments for chronic pain. The local production of endorphins may be an attractive alternative to drug therapy in the treatment of chronic pain since they are naturally occurring peptides that are effective in blocking pain transmission at the level of the spinal cord but do not result in dependency or alter brain function as observed with morphine. We have demonstrated that HSV vectors containing the pro-proenkephalin cDNA can be used to express enkephalin in DRG neurons innervating the rat foot. Capsaicin-stimulated local neurons are less sensitive to painful radiant heat than animals injected with a control lacZ vector or unstimulated (108). This effect can be reversed by intrathecal injection of an endorphin antagonist, naloxone, indicating that the loss of heat pain sensitivity is due to an effect of vector-produced endorphin locally. Moreover, we observed that endorphins were not released unless the neuron was sensitized by capsaicin, raising the interesting possibility that despite continuous expression of enkephalin by the vector, endorphins are retained in synaptic vesicles in the neurons until the pain stimulator is applied. This important finding suggests that pain management in this way will be an exciting approach not requiring regulated transgene product formation because product release itself is regulated in response to pain.

VI. SUMMARY AND FUTURE DIRECTIONS

This overview of HSV biology and gene transfer has focused on the use of highly defective HSV genomic vectors that are blocked very early in the virus lytic cycle. These vectors express few viral functions and are highly reduced in vector toxicity, even for primary neurons in culture, which are readily killed by less defective HSV vectors. Moreover, these vector backgrounds are suitable for expression of multiple transgenes or single large genes (e.g., dystrophin) in applications where expression of single or multiple gene products are required to achieve a therapeutic outcome (e.g., tumor-cell killing and vaccination). Expression of these transgenes can be coordinated, or even sequentially using strategies similar to those employed by the virus to regulate its own genes. Expression can also be controlled by drug-sensitive transactivators, which may prove to be important for regulating the timing and duration of transgene expression. HSV vectors may be most suited for expression of genes in the nervous system where the virus has evolved to remain life-long in a latent state. The highly defective viruses deleted for multiple IE genes are able to efficiently establish resistance in neurons and serve as a platform for long-term gene expression using the latency active LAP2 promoter system. These mutants cannot reactivate from latency and cannot spread to other nerves or tissues following infection of cells. Delivery of these vectors requires direct inoculation of tissue to achieve direct contact with neurons. Ideally, HSV vectors would be most effective if infection could be targeted to specific cell types using enveloped particles defective for their normal receptor recognition ligands but modified to contain novel attachment and entry functions. This area of research is still very early in development, and it remains to be determined to what extent this will be feasible. Finally, it should be emphasized that current viral delivery systems may each become reduced to highly defective transfer vectors retaining only those elements required for vector DNA maintenance and transgene expression. Fortunately, the natural biology of many persistent viruses, including HSV-1, indicates that long-term vector maintenance will be possible, and we continue to learn from the highly evolved biology of persistent and latent viruses in order to mimic their strategies for gene transfer and therapy.

REFERENCES

1. Cai W, Gu B, Person S. Role of glycoprotein B of herpes simplex virus type 1 in viral entry and cell fusion. J Virol 1988; 62:2596–2604.
2. Desai P, Schaffer P, Minson A. Excretion of non-infectious virus particles lacking glycoprotein H by a temperature-sensitive mutant of herpes-simplex virus type 1: evidence that gH is essential for virion infectivity. J Gen Virol 1988; 69:1147–1156.
3. Hutchinson L, Goldsmith K, Snoddy D, Ghosh H, Graham FL, Johnson DC. Identification and characterization of a novel herpes simplex virus glycoprotein, gK, involved in cell fusion. J Virol 1992; 66:5603–5609.
4. Ligas M, Johnson D. A herpes simplex virus mutant in which glycoprotein D sequences are replaced by β-galactosidase sequences binds to but is unable to penetrate into cells. J Virol 1988; 62:1486–1494.
5. Spear P. Membrane fusion induced by herpes simplex virus. In: Bentz J, ed. Viral Fusion Mechanisms. Boca Raton, FL: CRC Press, 1993:201–232.
6. Spear PG. Entry of alphaherpesviruses into cells. Sem Virol 1993; 4:167–180.
7. Steven AC, Spear PG. Herpesvirus capsid assembly and envelopment. In: Chiu W, Burnett R, Garcea R, eds. Structural Biology of Viruses. New York: Oxford University Press, 1997; 512–533.
8. Mettenleiter TC. Initiation and spread of α-herpesvirus infections. Trends Microbiol 1994; 2:2–3.
9. Fuller AO, Spear PG. Specificities of monoclonal and polyclonal antibodies that inhibit adsorption of herpes simplex virus to cells and lack of inhibition by potent neutralizing antibodies. J Virol 1985; 55:475–482.
10. Fuller AO, Lee WC. Herpes simplex virus type 1 entry through a cascade of virus-cell interactions requires different roles of gD and gH in penetration. J Virol 1992; 66: 5002–5012.
11. Highlander SL, Sutherland SL, Gage PJ, Johnson DC, Levine M, Glorioso JC. Neutralizing monoclonal antibodies specific for herpes simplex virus glycoprotein D inhibit virus penetration. J Virol 1987; 61:3356–3364.
12. Dingwell K, Brunetti C, Hendricks R, et al. Herpes simplex virus glycoproteins E and I facilitate cell-to-cell spread in vivo and across junctions of cultured cells. J Virol 1994; 68:834–845.
13. Dingwell KS, Doering LC, Johnson DC. Glycoproteins E and I facilitate neuron-to-neuron spread of herpes simplex virus. J Virol 1995; 69:7087–7098.
14. Maul G, Everett R. The nuclear location of PML, a cellular member of the C3HC4 zinc-binding domain protein family, is rearranged during herpes simplex virus infection by the C3HC4 viral protein ICP0. J Gen Virol 1994: 1223–1233.
15. Mullen M-A, Gerstberger S, Ciufo DM, Mosca JD, Hayward GS. Evaluation of colocalization interactions between the IE110, IE175, and IE63 transactivator proteins of herpes simplex virus within subcellular punctate structures. J Virol 1995; 69:476–491.
16. Honess R, Roizman B. Regulation of herpes simplex virus macromolecular synthesis. I. Cascade regulation of the synthesis of three groups of viral proteins. J Virol 1974; 14:8–19.

17. Mackem S, Roizman B. Differentiation between alpha promoter and regulatory regions of herpes simplex virus type 1: the functional domains and sequence of a movable alpha regulator. Proc Natl Acad Sci USA 1982; 79:4917–4921.
18. Campbell MEM, Palfeyman JW, Preston CM. Identification of herpes simplex virus DNA sequences which encode a trans-acting polypeptide responsible for stimulation of immediate early transcription. J Mol Biol 1984; 180:1–19.
19. Preston C, Frame M, Campbell M. A complex formed between cell components and an HSV structural polypeptide binds to a viral immediate early gene regulatory DNA sequence. Cell 1988; 52:425–434.
20. Dixon RAF, Schaffer PA. Fine-structure mapping and functional analysis of temperature-sensitive mutants in the gene encoding the herpes simplex virus type 1 immediate early protein VP175. J Virol 1980; 36:189–203.
21. DeLuca NA, Schaffer PA. Activation of immediate-early, early, and late promoters by temperature-sensitive and wild-type forms of herpes simplex virus type 1 protein ICP4. Mol Cell Biol 1985; 5:1997–2008.
22. Sacks W, Greene C, Aschman D, Schaffer P. Herpes simplex virus type 1 ICP27 is essential regulatory protein. J Virol 1985; 55:796–805.
23. McCarthy AM, McMahan L, Schaffer PA. Herpes simplex virus type 1 ICP27 deletion mutants exhibit altered patterns of transcription and are DNA deficient. J Virol 1989; 63: 18–27.
24. Sandri-Goldin R, Hibbard M. The herpes simplex virus type 1 regulatory protein ICP27 coimmunoprecipitates with anti-sm antiserum, and the C terminus appears to be required for this interaction. J Virol 1996; 70:108–118.
25. Sandri-Goldin RM. Interactions between a herpes simplex virus regulatory protein and cellular mRNA processing pathways. Methods 1998; 16:95–104.
26. Prod'hon C, Machuca I, Berthomme H, Epstein A, Jacquemont B. Characterization of regulatory functions of the HSV-1 immediate-early protein ICP22. Virology 1996; 226:393–402.
27. Rice S, Long M, Lam V, Spencer C. RNA polymerase II is aberrantly phosphorylated and localized to viral replication compartments following herpes simplex virus infection. J Virol 1994; 68:988–1001.
28. Sacks WR, Schaffer PA. Deletion mutants in the gene encoding the herpes simplex virus type 1 immediate-early protein ICP0 exhibit impaired growth in cell culture. J Virol 1987; 61:829–839.
29. Stow N, Stow E. Isolation and characterization of a herpes simplex virus type 1 mutant containing a deletion within the gene encoding the immediate early polypeptide Vmw 110. J Gen Virol 1986; 67:2571–2585.
30. Everett RD. Transactivation of transcription by herpes simplex virus products: reqquirements for two herpes simplex virus type 1 immediate early polypeptides for maximum activity. EMBO J 1984; 3:3135–3141.
31. Carter K, Roizman B. The promoter and transcriptional unit of a novel herpes simplex virus 1 alpha gene are contained in, and encode a protein in frame with, the open reading frame of the alpha22 gene. J Virol 1996; 70: 172–178.
32. Fruh K, Ahn K, Djaballah H, et al. A viral inhibitor of peptide transporters for antigen presentation. Nature 1995; 375:415–418.
33. Hill A, Jugovic P, York I, et al. Herpes simplex virus turns off the TAP to evade host immunity. Nature 1995; 375: 411–415.
34. Hill A, Ploegh H. Getting the inside out: the transporter associated with antigen processing (TAP) and the presentation of viral antigen. Proc Natl Acad Sci USA 1995; 92: 341–343.
35. York I, Roop C, Andrews D, Riddell S, Graham F, Johnson D. A cytosolic herpes simplex virus protein inhibits antigen presentation to CD8+ T lymphocytes. Cell 1994; 77: 525–535.
36. Holland LE, Anderson KP, Shipman C, Wagner EK. Viral DNA synthesis is required for efficient expression of specific herpes simplex virus type 1 mRNA. Virology 1980; 101:10–24.
37. Mavromara-Nazos P, Roizman B. Activation of herpes simplex virus 1 $\gamma 2$ genes by viral DNA replication. Virology 1987; 161:593–598.
38. Roizman G, Batterson W. Herpesviruses and their replication. In: Fields BN, ed. Virology. New York: Raven Press, 1985:497–526.
39. Johnson PA, Miyanohara A, Levine F, Cahill T, Friedmann T. Cytotoxicity of a replication-defective mutant herpes simplex virus type 1. J Virol 1992; 66:2952–2965.
40. Johnson P, Wang M, Friedmann T. Improved cell survival by the reduction of immediate-early gene expression in replication-defective mutants of herpes simplex virus type 1 but not by mutation of the viron host shutoff function. J Virol 1994; 68:6347–6362.
41. Krisky DM, Wolfe D, Goins WF, et al. Deletion of multiple immediate early genes from herpes simplex virus reduces cytotoxicity and permits long-term gene expression in neurons. Gene Ther 1998; 5:1593–1603.
42. Marconi P, Krisky D, Oligino T, et al. Replication-defective HSV vectors for gene transfer in vivo. Proc Natl Acad Sci USA 1996; 93:11319–11320.
43. Samaniego L, Webb A, DeLuca N. Functional interaction between herpes simplex virus immediate-early proteins during infection: gene expression as a consequence of ICP27 and different domains of ICP4. J Virol 1995; 69: 5705–5715.
44. Wu N, Watkins SC, Schaffer PA, DeLuca NA. Prolonged gene expression and cell survival after infection by a herpes simplex virus mutant defective in the immediate-early genes encoding ICP4, ICP27, and ICP22. J Virol 1996; 70:6358–6368.
45. Samaniego LA, Neiderhiser L, DeLuca NA. Persistence and expression of the herpes simplex virus genome in the absence of immediate-early proteins. J Virol 1998; 72: 3307–3320.

46. Leiden J, Frenkel N, Rapp F. Identification of the herpes simplex virus DNA sequences present in six herpes simplex virus thymidine kinase-transformed mouse cell lines. J Virol 1980; 33:272–285.
47. Krisky DM, Marconi PC, Oligino TJ, et al. Development of herpes simplex virus replication defective multigene vectors for combination gene therapy applications. Gene Ther 1998; 5:1517–1530.
48. Samaniego L, Wu N, DeLuca NA. The herpes simplex virus immediate-early protein ICP0 affects transcription from the viral genome and infected-cell survival in the absence of ICP4 and ICP27. J Virol 1997; 71:4614–4625.
49. Kwong AD, Kruper JA, Frenkel N. Herpes simplex virus virion host shutoff function. J Virol 1988; 62:912–921.
50. Oroskar A, Read G. Control of mRNA stability by the virion host shutoff function of herpes simplex virus. J Virol 1989; 63:1897–1906.
51. Read GS, Frenkel N. Herpes simplex virus mutants defective in the virion-associated shutoff of host polypeptide synthesis and exhibiting abnormal synthesis of α (immediate early) viral polypeptides. J Virol 1983; 46:498–512.
52. Jenkins FJ, Casadaban MJ, Roizman B. Application of the mini-Mu-phage for target-sequence-specific insertional mutagenesis of the herpes simplex virus genome. Proc Natl Acad Sci USA 1985; 82:4773–4777.
53. Krisky DM, Marconi PC, Oligino T, Rouse RJD, Fink DJ, Glorioso JC. Rapid method for construction of recombinant HSV gene transfer vectors. Gene Ther 1997; 4: 1120–1125.
54. Spaete R, Frenkel N. The herpes simplex virus amplicon: a new eucaryotic defective-virus cloning amplifying vector. Cell 1982; 30:295–304.
55. Casaccia-Bonnefil P, Benedikz E, Shen H, et al. Localized gene transfer into organotypic hippocampal slice cultures and acute hippocampal slices. J Neurosci Methods 1993; 50:341–351.
56. Freese A, Geller A. Infection of cultured striatal neurons with a defective HSV-1 vector: implications for gene therapy. Nucleic Acids Res 1991; 19:7219–7223.
57. Geller A, Breakefield X. A defective HSV-1 vector expresses *Escherichia coli* β-galactosidase in cultured peripheral neurons. Science 1988; 241:1667–1669.
58. Geller A, Freese A. Infection of cultured central nervous system neurons with a defective herpes simplex virus 1 vector results in stable expression of Escherichia coli β-galactosidase. Proc Natl Acad Sci USA 1990; 87: 1149–1153.
59. Ho DY, McLaughlin JR, Sapolsky RM. Inducible gene expression from defective herpes simplex virus vectors using the tetracycline-responsive promoter system. Brain Res Mol Brain Res 1996; 41:200–209.
60. Pechan PA, Fotaki M, Thompson RL, et al. A novel 'piggyback' packaging system for herpes simplex virus amplicon vectors. Hum Gene Ther 1996; 7:2003–2013.
61. Shering AF, Bain D, Stewart K, et al. Cell type-specific expression in brain cell cultures from a short human cytomegalovirus major immediate early promoter depends on whether it is inserted into herpesvirus or adenovirus vectors. J Gen Virol 1997; 78:445–459.
62. Battleman D, Geller A, Chao M. HSV-1 vector-mediated gene transfer of the human nerve growth factor receptor p75hNGFR defines high-affinity NGF binding. J Neurosci 1993; 13:941–951.
63. Bergold PJ, Casaccia-Bonnefil P, Zeng XL, Federoff HJ. Transsynaptic neuronal loss induced in hippocampal slice cultures by a herpes simplex virus vector expressing the GluR6 subunit of the kainate receptor. Proc Natl Acad Sci USA 1993; 90:6165–6169.
64. Geller A, During M, Haycock J, Freese A, Neve R. Long-term increases in neurotransmitter release from neuronal cells expressing a constitutively active adenylate cyclase from a herpes simplex virus type 1 vector. Proc Natl Acad Sci USA 1993; 90:7603–7607.
65. Geschwind M, Kessler J, Geller A, Federoff H. Transfer of the nerve growth factor gene into cell lines and cultured neurons using a defective herpes simplex virus vector transfer to the NGF gene into cells by a HSV-1 vector. Brain Res 1994; 24:327–335.
66. Ho D, Mocarski E, Sapolsky R. Altering central nervous system physiology with a defective herpes simplex virus vector expressing the glucose transporter gene. Proc Natl Acad Sci USA 1993; 90:3655–3659.
67. Jia WW, Wang Y, Qiang D, Tufaro F, Remington R, Cynader M. A bcl-2 expressing viral vector protects cortical neurons from excitotoxicity even when administered several hours after the toxic insult. Brain Res Mol Brain Res 1996; 42:350–353.
68. Lawrence MS, Ho DY, Dash R, Sapolsky RM. Herpes simplex virus vectors overexpressing the glucose transporter gene protect against seizure-induced neuron loss. Proc Natl Acad Sci USA 1995; 92:7247–7251.
69. Miyatake S, Iyer A, Martuza RL, Rabkin SD. Transcriptional targeting of herpes simplex virus for cell-specific replication. J Virol 1997; 71:5124–5132.
70. Miyatake S, Martuza RL, Rabkin SD. Defective herpes simplex virus vectors expressing thymidine kinase for the treatment of malignant glioma. Cancer Gene Ther 1997; 4:222–228.
71. During M, Naegele J, O'Malley K, Geller A. Long-term behavioral recovery in parkinsonian rats by an HSV vector expressing tyrosine hydroxylase. Science 1994; 266: 1399–1403.
72. Geller A, Keyomarsi K, Bryan J, Pardee A. An efficient deletion mutant packaging system for defective herpes simplex virus vectors: potential applications to human gene therapy and neuronal physiology. Proc Natl Acad Sci USA 1990; 87:8950–8954.
73. Geller AI, Yu L, Wang Y, Fraefel C. Helper virus-free herpes simplex virus-1 plasmid vectors for gene therapy of Parkinson's disease and other neurological disorders. Exp Neurol 1997; 144:98–102.
74. Jin B, Belloni M, Conti B, et al. Prolonged in vivo gene expression driven by a tyrosine hydroxylase promoter in

a defective herpes simplex virus amplicon vector. Hum Gene Ther 1996; 7:2015–2024.

75. New KC, Rabkin SD. Co-expression of two gene products in the CNS using double-cassette defective herpes simplex virus vectors. Brain Res Mol Brain Res 1996; 37:317–323.
76. Fraefel C, Song S, Lim F, et al. Helper virus-free transfer of herpes simplex virus type 1 plasmid vectors into neural cells. J Virol 1996; 70:7190–7197.
77. Rogers BE, Douglas JT, Ahlem C, Buchsbaum DJ, Frincke J, Curiel DT. Use of a novel cross-linking method to modify adenovirus tropism. Gene Ther 1997; 4:1387–1392.
78. Wickham TJ, Tzeng E, Shears II LL, et al. Increased in vitro and in vivo gene transfer by adenovirus vectors containing chimeric fiber proteins. J Virol 1997; 71: 8221–8229.
79. Wickham TJ, Haskard D, Segal D, Kovesdi I. Targeting endothelium for gene therapy via receptors up-regulated during angiogenesis and inflammation. Cancer Immunol Immunother 1997; 45:149–151.
80. Kasahara N, Dozy M, Kan YW. Tissue-specific targeting of retroviral vectors through ligand-receptor interactions. Science 1994; 255:1373–1376.
81. Marin M, Noel D, Valsesia-Wittman S, et al. Targeted infection of human cells via major histocompatibility complex class I molecules by moloney murine leukemia virus-derived viruses displaying single-chain antibody fragment-envelope fusion proteins. J Virol 1996; 70:2957–2962.
82. Russell SJ, Hawkins RE, Winter G. Retroviral vectors displaying functional antibody fragments. Nucleic Acids Res 1993; 21:1081–1085.
83. Somia NV, Zoppe M, Verma IM. Generation of targeted retroviral vectors by using single-chain variable fragment: an approach to in vivo gene delivery. Proc Natl Acad Sci USA 1995; 92:7570–7574.
84. Banfield BW, Leduc Y, Esford L, Schubert K, Tufaro F. Sequential isolation of proteoglycan synthesis mutants by using herpes simplex virus as a selective agent: evidence for a proteoglycan-independent virus entry pathway. J Virol 1995; 69:3290–3298.
85. Gruenheid S, Gatzke L, Meadows H, Tufaro F. Herpes simplex virus infection and propagation in a mouse L cell mutant lacking heparan sulfate proteoglycans. J Virol 1993; 67:93–100.
86. Herold B, Visalli R, Susmarski N, Brandt C, Spear P. Glycoprotein C-independent binding of herpes simplex virus to cells requires cell surface heparan sulfate and glycoprotein B. J Gen Virol 1994; 75:1211–1222.
87. Shih M, Wudunn D, Montgomery R, Esko J, Spear P. Cell surface receptors for herpes simplex virus are heparan sulfate proteoglycans. J Cell Biol 1992; 116:1273–1281.
88. Spear PG, Shieh MT, Herold BC, WuDunn D, Koshy TI. Heparan sulfate glycosaminoglycans as primary cell surface receptors for herpes simplex virus. Adv Exp Med Biol 1992; 313:341–353.
89. Williams RK, Straus SE. Specificity and affinity of binding of herpes simplex virus type 2 glycoprotein B to glycosaminoglycans. J Virol 1997; 71:1375–1380.
90. Wudunn D, Spear P. Initial interaction of herpes simplex virus with cells is binding to heparan sulfate. J Virol 1989; 63:52–58.
91. Herold BC, Gerber SI, Polonsky T, Belval BJ, Shaklee PN, Holme K. Identification of structural features of heparin required for inhibition of herpes simplex virus type 1 binding. Virology 1995; 206:1108–1116.
92. Laquerre S, Argnani R, Anderson DB, Zucchini S, Manservigi R, Glorioso JC. Heparan sulfate proteoglycan binding by herpes simplex virus type 1 glycoproteins B and C which differ in their contribution to virus attachment, penetration, and cell-to-cell spread. J Virol 1998; 72: 6119–6130.
93. Tal-Singer R, Peng C, Ponce de Leon M, et al. Interaction of herpes simplex virus glycoprotein gC with mammalian cell surface molecules. J Virol 1995; 69:4471–4483.
94. Trybala E, Berghtrom T, Svennerholm B, Jeansson S, Glorioso JC, Olufsson S. Localization of the functional site in herpes simplex virus type 1 glycoproteins C involved in binding to cell surface heparan sulfate. J Gen Virol 1994; 75:743–752.
95. Montgomery RI, Warner MS, Lum BJ, Spear PG. Herpes simplex virus 1 entry into cells mediated by a novel member of the TNF/NGF receptor family. Cell 1996; 87: 427–436.
96. Warner MS, Geraghty RJ, Martinez WM, et al. A cell surface protein with herpesvirus entry activity (HveB) confers susceptibility to infection by mutants of herpes simplex virus type 1, herpes simplex virus type 2, and pseudorabies virus. Virology 1998; 246:179–189.
97. Geraghty RJ, Krummenacher C, Cohen GH, Eisenberg RJ, Spear PG. Entry of alphaherpesviruses mediated by poliovirus receptor-related protein 1 and poliovirus receptor. Science 1998; 280:1618–1620.
98. Hutchinson L, Browne H, Wargent V, et al. A novel herpes simplex virus glycoprotein, gL, forms a complex with glycoprotein H (gH) and affects normal folding and surface expression of gH. J Virol 1992; 66:2240–2250.
99. Nicola AV, Ponce de Leon M, Xu R, et al. Monoclonal antibodies to distinct sites on herpes simplex virus (HSV) glycoprotein D block HSV binding to HVEM. J Virol 1998; 72:3595–3601.
100. Laquerre S, Anderson DB, Stolze DB, Glorioso JC. Recombinant herpes simplex virus type 1 engineered for targeted binding to erythropoietin receptor bearing cells. J Virol 1998; 72:9683–9697.
101. Fink DJ, Ramakrishnan R, Marconi P, Goins WF, Holland TC, Glorioso JC. Advances in the development of herpes simplex virus-based gene transfer vectors for the nervous system. Clin Neurosci 1996; 3:1–8.
102. Goins WF, Lee KA, Cavalcoli JD, et al. Herpes simplex virus type 1 vector-mediated expression of nerve growth factor protects dorsal root ganglia neurons from peroxide toxicity. J Virol 1999; 73:519–532.
103. Marconi P, Simonato M, Zucchini S, et al. Replication-defective herpes simplex virus vectors for neurotrophic

factor gene transfer in vitro and in vivo. Gene Ther 1999; 6:904–912.
104. Mester JC, Pitha P, Glorioso JC. Anti-viral activity of herpes simplex virus vectors expressing alpha-interferon. Gene Ther 1995; 3:187–196.
105. Moriuchi S, Oligino T, Krisky D, et al. Enhanced tumor-cell killing in the presence of ganciclovir by HSV-1 vector-directed co-expression of human TNF-α and HSV thymidine kinase. Cancer Res 1998; 58:5731–5737.
106. Oligino T, Poliani PL, Marconi P, et al. In vivo transgene activation from an HSV-based gene vector by GAL4: VP16. Gene Ther 1996; 3:892–899.
107. Rasty S, Goins WF, Glorioso JC. Site-specific integration of multigenic shuttle plasmids into the herpes simplex virus type 1 (HSV-1) genome using a cell-free Cre-*lox* recombination system. In: Adolph K, ed. Methods in Molecular Genetics. San Diego: Academic Press, 1995: 114–130.
108. Wilson SP, Yeomans DC, Bender MA, Lu Y, Goins WF, Glorioso JC. Antihyperalgesic effects of infection with a preproenkephalin-encoding herpes virus. Proc Natl Acad Sci USA 1999; 96:3211–3216.
109. Yamada M, Oligino T, Mata M, Goss JR, Glorioso JC, Fink DJ. HSV vector-mediated expression of Bcl-2 prevents 6-hydroxydopamine induced degeneration of neurons in the substantia nigra in vivo. Proc Natl Acad Sci USA 1999; 96:4078–4083.
110. Rasty S, Thatikunta P, Gordon J, Khalili K, Amini S, Glorioso J. Human immunodeficiency virus tat gene transfer to the murine central nervous system using a replication-defective herpes simplex virus vector stimulates transforming growth factor beta 1 gene expression. Proc Natl Acad Sci USA 1996; 93:6073–6078.
111. Bloom DC, Jarman RG. Generation and use of recombinant reporter viruses for study of herpes simplex virus infections in vivo. Methods 1998; 16:117–125.
112. Carpenter DE, Stevens JG. Long-term expression of a foreign gene from a unique position in the latent herpes simplex virus genome. Hum Gene Ther 1996; 7:1447–1454.
113. Lokensgard JR, Bloom DC, Dobson AT, Feldman LT. Long-term promoter activity during herpes simplex virus latency. J Virol 1994; 68:7148–7158.
114. Preston CM, Mabbs R, Nicholl MJ. Construction and characterization of herpes simplex virus type 1 mutants with conditional defects in immediate early gene expression. Virology 1997; 229:228–239.
115. Cook ML, Stevens JG. Pathogenesis of herpetic neuritis and ganglionitis in mice: evidence of intra-axonal transport of infection. Infect Immun 1973; 7:272–288.
116. Stevens JG. Human herpesviruses: a consideration of the latent state. Microbiol Rev 1989; 53:318–332.
117. Rodahl E, Stevens J. Differential accumulation of herpes simplex virus type 1 latency-associated transcripts in sensory and autonomic ganglia. Virology 1992; 189:385–388.
118. Speck PG, Simmons A. Divergent molecular pathways of productive and latent infection with a virulent strain of herpes simplex virus type 1. J Virol 1991; 65:4004–4005.
119. Speck P, Simmons A. Synchronous appearance of antigen-positive and latently infected neurons in spinal ganglia of mice infected with a virulent strain or herpes simplex virus. J Gen Virol 1992; 73:1281–1285.
120. Croen KD, Ostrove JM, Dragovic LJ, Smialek JE, Straus SE. Latent herpes simplex virus in human trigeminal ganlia. Detection of an immediate early gene ''anti-sense'' transcript by in situ hybridization. N Engl J Med 1987; 317:1427–1432.
121. Deatly AM, Spivack JG, Lavi E, Fraser NW. RNA from an immediate early region of the HSV-1 genome is present in the trigeminal ganglia of latently infected mice. Proc Natl Acad Sci USA 1987; 84:3204–3208.
122. Stevens JG, Wagner EK, Devi-Rao GB, Cook ML, Feldman LT. RNA complementary to a herpesviruses α gene mRNA is prominent in latently infected neurons. Science 1987; 255:1056–1059.
123. Deatly AM, Spivack JG, Lavi E, O'Boyle D, Fraser NW. Latent herpes simplex virus type 1 transcripts in peripheral and central nervous systems tissues of mice map to similar regions of the viral genome. J Virol 1988; 62:749–756.
124. Wagner EK, Flanagan WM, Devi-Rao GB, et al. The herpes simplex virus latency-associated transcript is spliced during the latent phase of infection. J Virol 1988; 62:4577–4585.
125. Devi-Rao GB, Goddart SA, Hecht LM, Rochford R, Rice MK, Wagner EK. Relationship between polyadenylated and nonpolyadenylated HSV type 1 latency-associated transcripts. J Gen Virol 1991; 65:2179–2190.
126. Alvira MR, Cohen JB, Goins WF, Glorioso JC. Genetic studies exposing the splicing events involved in HSV-1 latency associated transcript (LAT) production during lytic and latent infection. J Virol 1999; 73:3866–3876.
127. Farrell MJ, Dobson AT, Feldman LT. Herpes simplex virus latency-associated transcript is a stable intron. Proc Natl Acad Sci USA 1991; 88:790–794.
128. Krummenacher C, Zabolotny J, Fraser N. Selection of a nonconsensus branch point is influenced by an RNA stem-loop structure and is important to confer stability to the herpes simplex virus 2-kilobase latency-associated transcript. J Virol 1997; 71:5849–5860.
129. Rodahl E, Haarr L. Analysis of the 2-kilobase latency-associated transcript expressed in PC12 cells productively infected with herpes simplex virus type 1: evidence for a stable, nonlinear structure. J Virol 1997; 71:1703–1707.
130. Zabolotny J, Krummenacher C, Fraser NW. The herpes simplex virus type 1 2.0-kilobase latency-associated transcript is a stable intron which branches at a guanosine. J Virol 1997; 71:4199–4208.
131. Blondeau JM, Aoki FY, Glavin GB. Stress-induced reactivation of latent herpes simplex virus infection in rat lumbar dorsal root ganglia. J Psychosom Res 1993; 37:843–849.
132. Dobson AT, Sederati F, Devi-Rao G, et al. Identification of the latency-associated transcript promoter by expression of rabbit β-globin mRNA in mouse sensory nerve ganglia latently infected with a recombinant herpes simplex virus. J Virol 1989; 63:3844–3851.

133. Zwaagstra J, Ghiasi H, Nesburn AB, Wechsler SL. In vitro promoter activity associated with the latency-associated transcript gene of herpes simplex virus type 1. J Gen Virol 1989; 70:2163–2169.
134. Batchelor AH, O'Hare PO. Regulation and cell-type-specific activity of a promoter located upstream of the latency-associated transcript of herpes simplex virus type 1. J Virol 1990; 64:3269–3279.
135. Chen X, Schmidt MC, Goins WF, Glorioso JC. Two herpes simplex virus type-1 latency active promoters differ in their contribution to latency-associated transcript expression during lytic and latent infection. J Virol 1995; 69: 7899–7908.
136. Nicosia M, Deshmane SL, Zabolotny JM, Valyi-Nagy T, Fraser NW. Herpes simplex virus type 1 latency-associated transcript (LAT) promoter deletion mutants can express a 2-kilobase transcript mapping to the LAT region. J Virol 1993; 67:7276–7283.
137. Goins WF, Sternberg LR, Croen KD, et al. A novel latency-active promoter is contained within the herpes simplex virus type 1 U_L flanking repeats. J Virol 1994; 68: 2239–2252.
138. Margolis TP, Bloom DC, Dobson AT, Feldman LT, Stevens JG. Decreased reporter gene expression during latent infection with HSV LAT promoter constructs. Virology 1993; 197:585–592.
139. Wolfe JH, Deshmane SL, Fraser NW. Herpesvirus vector gene transfer and expression of β-glucuronidase in the central nervous system of MPS VII mice. Nat Genet 1992; 1: 379–384.
140. Lokensgard JR, Feldman LT, Berthomme H. The latency-associated promoter of herpes simplex virus type 1 requires a region downstream of the transcription start site for long-term expression during latency. J Virol 1997; 71: 6714–6719.
141. Ho DY, Mocarski ES. Herpes simplex virus latent RNA (LAT) is not required for latent infection in the mouse. Proc Natl Acad Sci USA 1989; 86:7596–7600.
142. Lachmann RH, Efstathiou S. Utilization of the herpes simplex virus type 1 latency-associated regulatory region to drive stable reporter gene expression in the nervous system. J Virol 1997; 71:3197–3207.
143. Carey M, Leatherwood J, Ptashne M. A potent GAL4 derivative activates transcription at a distance in vitro. Science 1990; 247:710–712.
144. Chasman DI, Leatherwood M, Carey M, Ptashne M, Kornberg RD. Activation of yeast polymerase II transcription by herpesvirus VP16 and GAL4 derivative in vitro. Mol Cell Biol 1989; 9:4746–4749.
145. Sadowski I, Ma J, Triezenberg S, Ptashne M. GAL4/VP16 is an unusually potent transcriptional activator. Nature 1988; 335:563–564.
146. Axelrod JD, Reagan MS, Majors J. GAL4 disrupts a repressing nucleosome during activation of GAL 1 transcription in vivo. Genes Devel 1993; 7:857–869.
147. Xu L, Schaffner W, Rungger D. Transcription activation by recombinant GAL4/VP16 in the *Xenopus* oocyte. Nucl Acids Res 1993; 21:2775.
148. Vegeto E, Allan GF, Schrader WT, Tsai M-J, McDonnell DP, O'Malley BW. The mechanism of RU486 antagonism is dependent on the conformation of the carboxy-terminal tail of the human progesterone receptor. Cell 1992; 69: 703–713.
149. Wang Y, Jr BOM, Tsai S, O'Malley B. A novel regulatory system for gene transfer. Proc Natl Acad Sci USA 1994; 91:8180–8184.
150. Oligino T, Poliani PL, Wang Y, Tsai SY, O'Malley BW, Glorioso JC. Drug inducible transgene expression in brain using a herpes simplex virus vector. Gene Ther 1998; 5: 491–496.
151. Lucidi-Phillipi CA, Clary DO, Reichardt LF, Gage FH. TrkA activation is sufficient to rescue axotomized cholinergic neurons. Neuron 1996; 16:653–663.
152. Beck K, Valverde J, Alexi T, et al. Mesencephalic dopaminergic neurons protected by GDNF from axotomy-induced degeneration in the adult brain. Nature 1995; 373: 339–341.
153. Hoffer B, Hoffman A, Bowenkamp K, et al. GDNF reverses toxin-induced injury to midbrain dopaminergic neurons in vivo. Neurosci Lett 1995; 182:107–111.
154. Kearns C, Gash D. GDNF protects nigral dopamine neurons against 6-hydroxydopamine in vivo. Brain Res 1995; 672:104–111.
155. Sagot Y, Aebischer P, Kato AC, Schmalbruch H, Baetge E, Tan SA. Polymer encapsulated cell lines genetically engineered to release ciliary neurotrophic factor can slow down progressive motor neuronopathy in the mouse. Eur J Neurosci 1995; 7:1313–1322.
156. Lindsay RM. Therapeutic potential of the neurotrophins and neurotrophin-CNF combinations in peripheral neuropathies and motor neuron diseases. Ciba Found Symp 1996; 196:39–48.
157. Ishiyama T, Mitsumoto H, Pioro EP, Klinkosz B. Genetic transfer of the wobbler gene to a C57BL/6J × NZB hybrid stock: natural history of the motor neuron disease and response to CNTF and BDNF cotreatment. Exp Neurol 1997; 148:247–255.
158. Cedarbaum JM, Stambler N. Performance of the Amyotrophic Lateral Sclerosis Functional Rating Scale (ALSFRS) in multicenter clinical trials. J Neurol Sci 1997; 152: S1–S9.
159. McGuire D, Ross MA, Petajan JH, Parry GJ, Miller R. A brief quality-of-life measure for ALS clinical trials based on a subset of items from the sickness impact profile. The Syntex-Synergen ALS/CNTF Study Group. J Neurol Sci 1997; 152:S18–S22.
160. Hoffman E, Brown R, Kunkel L. Dystrophin: the protein product of the Duchenne muscular dystrophy locus. Cell 1987; 51:919–928.
161. Arahata K, Ishiura S, Ishiguro T, et al. Immunostaining of skeletal and cardiac muscle surface membrane with antibody against Ducheme muscular dystrophy peptide. Nature 1988; 333:861–863.
162. Zubryzcka-Gaarn E, Bulman D, Karpati G, al. e. The Duchenne muscular dystrophy gene is localized in the sacro-

lemma of human skeletal muscle. Nature 1988; 333: 466–469.
163. Huard J, Acsadi G, Jani A, Massie B, Karpati G. Gene transfer into skeletal muscles by isogenic myoblasts. Hum Gene Ther 1994; 5:949–958.
164. Karpati G, Acsadi G. The principles of gene therapy in Duchenne muscular dystrophy. Clin Invest Med 1994; 17: 531–541.
165. Morgan J, Pagel C, Sherrat T, Partridge T. Long-term persistence and migration of myogenic cells injected into pre-irradiated muscles of mdx mice. J Neurol Sci 1993; 115: 191–200.
166. Acsadi G, Dickson G, Love D, et al. Human dystrophin expression in mdx mice after intramuscular injection of DNA constructs. Nature 1991; 352:815–818.
167. Danko I, Fritz J, Latendresse J, Herweijer H, Schultz E, Wolff J. Dystrophin expression improves myofiber survival in mdx muscles following intramuscular plasmid DNA injection. Hum Mol Genet 1993; 2:2055–2061.
168. Dunckley MG, Love DR, Davies KE, Walsh FS, Morris GE, Dickson G. Retroviral-mediated transfer of a dystrophin minigene into mdx mouse myoblasts in vitro. FEBS Lett 1992; 296:128–134.
169. Salvatori G, Ferrari G, Messogiorno A, et al. Retroviral vector-mediated gene transfer into human primary myogenic cells leads to expression in muscle fibers in vivo. Hum Gene Ther 1993; 4:713–723.
170. Floyd SS, Clemens PR, Ontell MR, et al. Ex vivo gene transfer using adenovirus-mediated full-length dystrophin delivery to dystrophic muscle. Gene Ther 1998; 5:19–30.
171. Haecker SE, Stedman HH, Balice-Gordon RJ, et al. In vivo expression of full-length human dystrophin from adenoviral vectors deleted of all viral genes. Hum Gene Ther 1996; 7:1907–1914.
172. Kochanek S, Clemens PR, Mitani K, Chen H-H, Chan S, Caskey CT. A new adenoviral vector: replacement of all viral coding sequences with 28 kb of DNA independently expressing both full-length dystrophin and β-galactosidase. Proc Natl Acad Sci USA 1996; 93:5731–5736.
173. Acsadi G, Jani A, Massie B, et al. A differential efficiency of adenovirus-mediated in vivo gene transfer into skeletal muscle cells of different maturity. Hum Mol Genet 1994; 3:579–584.
174. Quantin B, Perricaudet L, Tajbakhsh S, Mandel J-L. Adenovirus as an expression vector in muscle cells in vivo. Proc Natl Acad Sci USA 1992; 89:2581–2584.
175. Ragot T, Vincent N, Chafey P, et al. Efficient adneovirus-mediated transfer of a human minidystrophin gene to skeletal muscle of mdx mice. Nature 1993; 321:647–650.
176. Vincent N, Ragot T, Gilgenkrantz H, et al. Long-term correction of mouse dystrophic degeneration by adenovirus-mediated transfer of a minidystrophin gene. Nat Genet 1993; 5:130–134.
177. Yang Y, Nunes F, Berencis K, Gonczol E, Engelhardt J, Wilson J. Inactivation of E2a in recombinant adenoviruses improves the prospect for gene therapy in cystic fibrosis. Nat Genet 1994; 7:362–369.
178. Huard J, Goins WF, Glorioso JC. Herpes simplex virus type 1 vector mediated gene transfer to muscle. Gene Ther 1995; 2:385–393.
179. Huard J, Feero W, Watkins S, Hoffman E, Rosenblatt D, Glorioso J. The basal lamina is a physical barrier to herpes simplex virus-mediated gene delivery to mature muscle fibers. J Virol 1996; 70:8117–8123.
180. Gardner JP, Rosenzweig M, Marks DF, et al. T-lymphopoietic capacity of cord blood-derived CD34+ progenitor cells. Exp Hematol 1998; 26:991–999.
181. Li J, Sensebe L, Herver P, Charbord P. Nontransformed colony-derived stromal cell lines from normal human marrows. III. The maintenance of hematopoiesis from CD34+ cell populations. Exp Hematol 1997; 25:582–591.
182. Venditti A, Buccisano F, DelPoeta G, et al. Multiparametric analysis for the enumeration of CD34+ cells from bone marrow and stimulated peripheral blood. Bioorganic Med Chem Lett 1998; 1:67–70.
183. Moolten FL. Tumor chemosensitivity conferred by inserted herpes thymidine kinase genes: paradigm for a prospective cancer control strategy. Cancer Res 1986; 46: 5276–5281.
184. Hanna NN, Mauceri HJ, Wayne JD, Hallahan DE, Kufe DW, Weichselbaum RR. Virally directed cytosine deaminase/5-fluorocytosine gene therapy enhances radiation response in human cancer xenografts. Cancer Res 1997; 57:4205–4209.
185. Freeman SM, Whartenby KA, Freeman JL, Abboud CN, Marrogi AJ. In situ use of suicide genes for cancer therapy. Sem Oncol 1996; 23:31–45.
186. Finke S, Trojaneck B, Moller P, et al. Increase of cytotoxic sensitivity of primary human melanoma cells transfected with the interleukin-7 gene to autologous and allogeneic immunologic effector cells. Cancer Gene Ther 1997; 4: 260–268.
187. Chen L, Ashe S, Brady W, et al. Costimulation of antitumor immunity by the B7 counterreceptor for the T lymphocyte molecules CD28 and CTLA-4. Cell 1992; 71: 1093–1102.
188. Katsanis E, Xu Z, Bausero MA, et al. B7-1 expression decreases tumorigenicity and induces partial systemic immunity to murine neuroblastoma deficient in major histocompatibility complex and costimulatory molecules. Cancer Gene Ther 1995; 2:39–46.
189. Galea-Lauri J, Farzaneh F, Gaken J. Novel costimulators in the immunue gene therapy of cancer. Cancer Gene Ther 1996; 3:202–214.
190. Schmidt W, Steinlein P, Buschle M, et al. Transloading of tumor cells with foreign major histocompatibility complex class I peptide ligand: a novel general strategy for the generation of potent cancer vaccines. Proc Natl Acad Sci USA 1996; 93:9759–9763.
191. Henderson RA, Finn OJ. Human tumor antigens are ready to fly. Adv Immunol 1996; 62:217–256.
192. Pecher G, Finn OJ. Induction of cellular immunity in chimpanzees to human tumor-associated antigen mucin by vac-

cination with MUC-1 cDNA-transfected Epstein-Barr virus-immortalized autologous B cells. Proc Natl Acad Sci USA 1996; 93:1699–1704.

193. Herrlinger U, Kramm CM, Johnston KM, et al. Vaccination for experimental gliomas using GM-CSF-transduced glioma cells. Cancer Gene Ther 1997; 4:345–352.

194. Ram Z, Culver KW, Walbridge S, Blaese RM, Oldfield EH. In situ retroviral-mediated gene transfer for the treatment of brain tumors in rats. Cancer Res 1986; 46: 5276–5281.

195. Ezzeddine ZD, Martuza RL, Platika D, et al. Selective killing of glioma cells in culture and in vivo by retrovirus transfer of the herpes simplex virus thymidine kinase gene. New Biol 1991; 3:608–614.

196. Culver K, Ram Z, Walbridge S, Ishii H, Oldfield E, Blaese R. In vivo gene transfer with retroviral vector-producer cells for treatment of experimental brain tumors. Science 1992; 256:1550–1552.

197. Barba D, Hardin J, Ray J, Gage FH. Thymidine kinase-mediated killing of rat brain tumors. J Neurosurg 1993; 79:729–735.

198. Caruso M, Panis Y, Gagandeep S, Houssin D, Salzmann JL, Klatzmann D. Regression of established macroscopic liver metastases after in situ transduction of a suicide gene. Proc Natl Acad Sci USA 1993; 90:7024–7028.

199. Short MP, Choi BC, Lee JK, Malick A, Breakefield XO, Martuza RL. Gene delivery to glioma cells in rat brain by grafting of a retrovirus packaging cell line. J Neurosci Res 1990; 27:427–439.

200. Burger P, Scheithauer B. Tumors of the central nervous system. Atlas of Tumor Pathology. Vol. Third Series, Fascicle 10. Washington, DC: Armed Forces Institute of Pathology, 1994:59.

201. Bi WL, Parysek LM, Warnick R, Stambrook PJ. In vitro evidence that metabolic cooperation is responsible for the bystander effect observed with HCV Tk retroviral gene therapy. Hum Gene Ther 1993; 4:725–731.

202. Freeman SM, Abboud CN, Whartenby KA, et al. The ''bystander effect'': tumor regression when a fraction of the tumor mass is genetically modified. Cancer Res 1993; 53: 5274–5283.

203. Kato K, Yoshida J, Mizuno M, Sugita K, Emi N. Retroviral transfer of herpes simplex thymidine kinase into glioma cells targeting of gancyclovir cytotoxic effect. Neurol Med Chir (Tokyo) 1994; 34:339–344.

204. Wu JK, Cano WG, Meylaerts SA, Qi P, Vrionis F, Cherington V. Bystander tumoricidal effect in the treatment of experimental brain tumors. Neurosurgery 1994; 35: 1094–1102.

205. Oligino T, Krisky D, Marconi P, Fink DJ, Glorioso JC. Herpes simplex gene therapy vectors for the treatment of cancer. In: Kornblith PL, Walker MD, eds. Advances in Neuro-Oncology II. Armonk, NY: Futura Publishing Company, Inc., 1997:517–539.

206. Boviatsis EJ, Park JS, Sena-Esteves M, et al. Long-term survival of rats harboring brain neoplasms treated with ganciclovir and a herpes simplex virus vector that retains an intact thymidine kinase gene. Cancer Res 1994; 15: 5745–5751.

207. Barba D, Hardin J, Sadelain M, Gage FH. Development of antitumor immunity for following thymidine kinase-mediated killing of experimental brain tumors. Proc Natl Acad Sci USA 1994; 91:4348–4352.

208. Chen SH, Shine HD, Goodman JC, Grossman RG, Woo SL. Gene therapy for brain tumors: regression of experimental gliomas by adenovirus-mediated gene transfer in vivo. Proc Natl Acad Sci USA 1994; 91:3054–3057.

209. Perez-Cruet M, Trask TW, Chen SH, et al. Adenovirus-mediated gene therapy of experimental gliomas. J Neurosci Res 1994; 39:506–511.

210. Han SK, Brody SL, Crystal RG. Suppression of in vivo tumorigenicity of human lung cancer cells by retrovirus-mediated transfer of the human tumor necrosis factor-alpha cDNA. Am J Respir Cell Mol Biol 1994; 11:270–278.

211. Cao G, Kuriyama S, Du P, et al. Complete regression of established murine hepatocellular carcinoma by in vivo tumor necrosis factor α gene transfer. Gastroenterology 1997; 11:270–278.

212. Watanabe Y, Kuribayashi K, Miyatake S, et al. Exogenous expression of mouse interferon cDNA in mouse neuroblastoma C1300 cells results in reduced tumorigenicity by augmented anti-tumor immunity. Proc Natl Acad Sci USA 1989; 86:9456–9460.

213. Pfizenmaier K, Pfizenmaier K, Scheurich P, Schluter C, Kronke M. Tumor necrosis factor enhances HLA-A, B, C and HLA-DR gene expression in human tumor cells. J Immunol 1987; 138:975–980.

214. Ostensen ME, Thiele DL, Lipsky PE. Enhancement of human natural killer cell function by the combined effects of tumor necrosis factor alpha or interleukin-1 and interferon-alpha or interleukin-2. J. Biol Res Mod 1987; 8: 53–61.

215. Plaetinck G, Declercq W, Tavernier J, Jabholz M, Fiers W. Recombinant tumor necrosis factor can induce interleukin 2 receptor expression and cytolytic activity in a rat x mouse T cell hybrid. Eur J Immunol 1987; 17:1835–1838.

216. Rothlein R, Czajkowski M, O'Neill MM, Marlin SD, Merluzzi VJ. Induction of intercellular adhesion molecule 1 on primary and continuous cell lines by pro-inflammatory cytokines. Regulation by pharmacologic agents and neutralizing antibodies. J Immunol 1988; 141:1665–1669.

217. Ranges GE, Figari IS, Espevik T, Palladino Jr. MA. Inhibition of cytotoxic T cell development by transforming growth factor beta and reversal by recombinant tumor necrosis factor alpha. J Exp Med 1987; 166:991–998.

218. Owen-Schaub LB, Gutterman JU, Grimm EA. Synergy of tumor necrosis factor and interleukin 2 in the activation of human cytotoxic lymphocytes: effect of tumor necrosis factor alpha and interleukin 2 in the generation of human lymphokine-activated killer cell cytotoxicity. Cancer Res 1988; 48:788–792.

219. Brown SM, Rampling R, Cruikshank G, et al. A phase 1

dose escalation trial of intratumoural injection with ICP34.5 -ve HSV1 into recurrent malignant glioma (abstr). 23rd International Herpesvirus Workshop, York, United Kingdom, 1998.
220. Markert JM, Medlock M, Martuza R, Rabkin S, Hunter W. Initial report of phase I trial of genetically-engineered HSV-1 in patients with malignant glioma (abstr). 23rd International Herpesvirus Workshop, York, United Kingdom, 1998.
221. Boviatsis E, Chase M, Wei M, et al. Gene transfer into experimental brain tumors mediated by adenovirus, herpes simplex virus, and retrovirus vectors. Hum Gene Ther 1994; 5:183–191.
222. Kosz-Vnenchak M, Coen D, Knipe D. Restricted expression of herpes simplex virus lytic genes during establishment of latent infection by thymidine kinase-negative mutant viruses. J Virol 1990; 64:5396–5402.
223. Markert J, Malick A, Coen D, Martuza R. Reduction of elimination of encephalitis in experimental glioma therapy model with attenuated herpes simplex mutants that retain susceptibility to acyclovir. Neurosurgery 1993; 32: 597–603.
224. Martuza R, Malick A, Markert J, Ruffner K, Coen D. Experimental therapy of human glioma by means of a genetically engineered virus mutant. Science 1991; 252: 854–856.
225. Mineta T, Rabkin S, Martuza R. Treatment of malignant gliomas using ganciclovir-hypersensitive, ribonucleotide reductase-deficient herpes simplex viral mutant. Cancer Res 1994; 54:3963–3966.
226. Yamada Y, Kimura H, Morishima T, Daikoku T, Maeno K, Nishiyama K. The pathogenicity of ribonucleotide reductase-null mutants of herpes simplex virus type 1 in mice. J Infect Dis 1991; 164:109–1097.
227. Fink DJ, Sternberg LR, Weber PC, Mata M, Goins WF, Glorioso JC. In vivo expression of β-galactosidase in hippocampal neurons by HSV-mediated gene transfer. Hum Gene Ther 1992; 3:11–19.
228. Chambers R, Gillespie GY, Soroceanu L, et al. Comparison of genetically engineered herpes simplex viruses for the treatment of brain tumors in a scid mouse model of human malignant glioma. Proc Natl Acad Sci USA 1995; 92:1411–1415.
229. MacLean A, ul-Fareed M, Robertson L, Harland J, Brown S. Herpes simplex virus type 1 deletion variants 1714 and 1716 pinpoint neurovirulence-related sequences in Glasgow strain 17+ between immediate early gene 1 and the 'a' sequence. J Gen Virol. 1991; 72:631–639.
230. Whitley R, Kern E, Chatterjee S, Chou J, Roizman B. Replication establishment of latency, and induced reactivation of herpes simplex virus γ_1 34.5 deletion mutants in rodent models. J Clin Invest 1993; 91:2837–2843.
231. Praemer A, Furner S, Rice D. Musculoskeletal Conditions in the United States. Park Ridge, IL: American Academy of Orthopaedic Surgeons, 1992.
232. Yelin E. Arthritis. The cumulative impact of a common chronic condition. Arthritis Rheum 1992; 35:489–497.
233. Harris E. Rheumatoid arthritis. Patholophysiology and implications for therapy. N Engl J Med 1990; 322: 1277–1289.
234. Pinals R. Pharmacologic treatment of osteoarthritis. Clin Ther 1992; 14:336–346.
235. Henderson B. Therapeutic modulation of cytokines. Ann Rheum Dis 1996; 59:519–523.
236. Hopkins S, Humphreys M, Jayson M. Cytokines in synovial fluid. I. The presence of biologically active and immunoreactive IL-1. Clin Exp Immunol 1988; 72:422–427.
237. Westacott C, Whicher J, Barnes I, Thompson D, Swan A, Dieppe P. Synovial fluid concentration of five different cytokines in rheumatic diseases. Ann Rheum Dis 1990; 49:676–681.
238. Arend WP, Dayer JM. Inhibitor of the production of interleukin-1 and tumor necrosis factor α in rheumatoid arthritis. Arthritis Rheum 1995; 38:151–160.
239. Tyler J. Articular cartilage cultured catabolin (pig interleukin 1) synthesizes a decreased number of normal proteoglycan molecules. Biochem J 1985; 227:869–878.
240. Pettipher E, Higgs G, Henderson B. Interleukin-1 induces leukocyte infiltration and cartilage proteoglycan degradation in the synovial joint. Proc Natl Acad Sci USA 1986; 83:8749–8753.
241. Saklatvala J. Tumor necrosis factor α stimulates resorption and inhibits synthesis of proteoglycans in cartilage. Nature 1986; 322:547–548.
242. Dinarello C. The interleukin-1 family: 10 years of discovery. FASEB J 1995; 8:1314–1319.
243. Piquet P, Grau G, Vassalli P. Tumor necrosis factor (TNF) and immunopathology. Immunol Res 1991; 10: 122–129.
244. Schwab J, Anderle S, Brown R, Dalldorf F, Thompson R. Pro- and anti-inflammatory roles of interleukin-1 in recurrence of bacterial cell wall-induced arthritis in rats. Infect Immun 1991; 59:4436–4442.
245. van den Berg WB, Joosten LAB, Helsen M, Van de Loo FAJ. Amelioration of established murine collagen-induced arthritis with anti-IL-1 treatment. Clin Exp Immunol 1994; 95:237–243.
246. Wooley P, Dutcher J, Widmer M, Gillis S. Influence of a recombinant human soluble tumor necrosis factor Fc fusion protein on type II collagen-induced arthritis in mice. J Immunol 1993; 151:6602–6607.
247. Elliott M, Maini R, Feldman M, et al. Treatment of rheumatoid arthritis with chimeric monoclonal antibodies to tumor necrosis factors α. Arthritis Rheum 1993; 36: 1681–1690.
248. Drevlow B, Lovis R, Haag M, et al. Recombinant human interleukin-1 receptor type 1 in the treatment of patients with active arthritis. Arthritis Rheum 1996; 39:257–265.
249. Bandara G, Robbins PD, Georgescu HI, Mueller GM, Gloroios JC, Evans CH. Gene transfer to synoviocytes: prospects for gene treatment of arthritis. DNA Cell Biol 1992; 11:227–231.

250. Evans CH, Robbins PD. Prospects for treating arthritis by gene therapy. J Rheumatol 1994; 21:779–782.
251. Evans CH, Robbins PD. Gene therapy for arthritis. In: Wolff J, ed. Gene Therapeutics: Methods and Applications of Direct Gene Transfer. Boston: Birkhauser Press, 1994: 320–343.
252. Evans CH, Robbins PD. Gene therapy as a treatment of rheumatoid arthritis. Exp Opin Invest Drugs 1995; 4: 843–852.
253. Evans CH, Robbins PD. Possible orthopaedic applications of gene therapy. J Bone Joint Surg Am 1995; 77: 1103–1114.
254. Evans CH, Robbins PD. Progress toward the treatment of arthritis by gene therapy. Ann Med 1995; 27:543–546.
255. Evans CH, Robbins PD, Ghivizzani SC, et al. Clinical trial to assess the safety, feasibility, and efficacy of transferring a potentially anti-arthritic cytokine gene to human joints with rheumatoid arthritis. Hum Gene Ther 1996; 7:1261–1280.
256. Evans CH, Ghivizzani SC, Robbins PD. Blocking cytokines with genes. J Leukocyte Biol 1998; 64:55–61.
257. Glorioso JC, Robbins PD, Krisky D, et al. Progress in the development of herpes simplex virus gene vectors for treatment of rheumatoid arthritis. Drug Delivery Rev 1997; 27:41–57.
258. Akkaraju GR, Huard J, Hoffman EP, et al. Herpes simplex virus vector-mediated dystrophin gene transfer and expression in MDX mouse skeletal muscle. J Gene Med 1999; 1:280–289.
259. Oligino T, Ghivizzani SC, Wolfe D, et al. Intra-articular delivery of a herpes simplex virus IL-1Ra gene vector reduces inflammation in a rabbit model of arthritis. Gene Ther 1999; 6:1713–1720.

6

Alphavirus-Based Vectors for Vaccine and Gene Therapy Applications

Thomas W. Dubensky, Jr. and John M. Polo
Chiron Corporation, Emeryville, California

Douglas J. Jolly
Chiron Corporation, San Diego, California

I. INTRODUCTION

Alphavirus vectors are a group of relatively new gene-transfer systems that have shown great promise for preventative and therapeutic vaccines for both infectious disease and cancer. These vectors also are being applied toward gene therapy applications where only transient expression of the transgene is appropriate, for example, in growth factor–delivery applications. In addition, alphavirus vectors have been exploited in a variety of other ways, including (1) as diagnostic tools for pathogenic viruses, (2) for production of recombinant proteins, and (3) for basic gene expression studies.

Alphavirus vectors, as well as other vectors derived from positive-stranded RNA viruses such as picornaviruses (poliovirus) and flaviviruses (yellow fever virus, Kunjin virus), constitute a new class of vectors known as replicons. Replicon vectors retain the genes from the parent virus encoding the replicase and thus can direct their self-amplification in the transduced cell, resulting in high levels of transgene expression. In addition to high transgene expression levels, several other properties of alphavirus replicon vectors make them ideal candidates for vaccine and particular gene therapy applications. These features include a broad host range (both within a host and across species) and the ability to infect nondividing cells. The alphavirus replicons are termed "suicide vectors" because the RNA-based amplification and expression is always transient, with no potential for permanent transduction of the host cell. This transient nature of alphavirus replicons may in fact provide an important safety advantage for these vectors, avoiding risks of immune tolerance related to persistent antigen expression in vaccine applications or transformation from prolonged expression of growth factors in gene therapy applications.

Alphaviral vectors are relatively simple. Typically, only four out of the seven virus genes are delivered with the transgene, and they provide all necessary enzymatic functions required for expression. As discussed in detail below, a variety of vector formats have been developed from the alphavirus replicon. The first format is a recombinant vector particle, which consists of the replicon packaged into a virion "coat," thus retaining the transduction efficiency and broad tropism of infectious virus. Targeting of such alphavirus replicon particles has been demonstrated recently, which may be especially useful for cancer applications, particularly ablation approaches intended for the diseased cell. The second format is a layered plasmid DNA vector, in which the replicon is launched when introduced into the target cell. This vector format combines the advantages of "naked" plasmid DNA vectors with those of the alphavirus replicon. Significantly, both vector formats have been shown to be highly efficacious in animal models of human infectious disease, stimulating robust humoral, cellular, and mucosal immune responses specific for the replicon-encoded antigen.

A primary limitation for commercial application of viral-based gene transfer vectors is the development of manufacturing methods that are efficient and result in a high yield. RNA polymerase II–mediated expression of alphaviral RNA genes not only allows the use of the plasmid DNA replicon vector format, but also makes large-scale efficient production of the vector particles possible through the generation of stable packaging cell lines. Each of the alphavirus vector formats is therefore amenable to large-scale production and enhanced commercial feasibility.

II. ALPHAVIRUSES

A. Natural History, Genus Members, and Epidemiology

Alphaviruses comprise a large group of genetically, structurally, and serologically related arthropod-borne viruses of the Togaviridae family (reviewed in Refs. 1–3). These viruses are distributed worldwide, although no individual alphavirus has such a broad distribution. Alphaviruses persist in nature through an alternating replication cycle between mosquito and vertebrate hosts, with birds, rodents, horses, and primates being among the defined natural vertebrate hosts. Humans are not considered a major host, but rather the recipient of an accidental infection. Therefore, alphaviruses are characterized by a wide host range, with a large number of different animal and insect species capable of being infected experimentally or naturally.

Within the *Alphavirus* genus, viruses have been classified antigenically and by their relative clinical features in humans. Antigenic classification segregates the alphaviruses into three major complexes: the western equine encephalitis virus (WEE) complex, the Venezuelan equine encephalitis virus (VEE) complex, and the Semliki Forest virus (SFV) complex. Four other viruses, eastern equine encephalitis (EEE), Barmah Forest, Middelburg, and Ndumu, receive individual classification.

Disease manifestations of the different alphaviruses range from entirely asymptomatic to lethal, with the majority being either subclinical or resulting in acute, temporarily incapacitating febrile illness. Based on their relative clinical features, the viruses may be grouped according to those associated primarily with central nervous system involvement and those associated primarily with fever, rash, and polyarthritis. Included in the former group are the VEE, EEE, and some members of the WEE complexes. Infection with this group can result in permanent sequelae, including death. The latter group includes the SF complex and the prototype alphavirus, Sindbis virus (SIN). Although epidemics have been reported, infection by viruses of this group is generally self-limiting, without permanent sequelae.

Among the alphaviruses, three species are being developed into vectors for possible human application: SIN, SFV, and VEE. The reasons for selecting these viruses are both historical and based on particular phenotypes of each alphavirus species, which are expected to translate into desired features of its derived vector.

B. Molecular Biology and Replication

The molecular biology and replication strategy of alphaviruses has been well characterized using Sindbis virus and Semliki Forest virus as models (reviewed in Ref. 3). Alphaviruses are enveloped icosahedral viruses that contain an RNA genome. The virions are comprised of a genome-containing icosahedral nucleocapsid surrounded by a host-derived lipid envelope from which two envelope glycoproteins, E1 and E2, protrude as heterodimers. The glycoprotein heterodimers, in turn, associate as trimers, forming the virion ''spikes.'' Both the nucleocapsid and surrounding envelope glycoproteins exhibit a highly ordered $T = 4$ symmetry, as determined by cryoelectron microscopy at 28 Å resolution (4). It is these envelope glycoproteins, and in particular glycoprotein E2, that determine the receptor-specific host range of viral infection.

The approximately 12 kb RNA genome of alphaviruses is single-stranded, capped, polyadenylated, and of positive polarity. Introduction of the genome RNA into the cytoplasm of susceptible host cells by natural or artificial means is sufficient to initiate a productive viral infection. It is this property that allowed for highly refined molecular characterization of the virus and eventual vector development (discussed below) by the assembly of a full-length Sindbis virus cDNA clone from which ''infectious'' viral RNA could be transcribed in vitro using a bacteriophage RNA polymerase (5). Genome modifications at the cDNA level are easily recovered and examined in vivo by transcription of RNA and direct introduction into suitable cells.

After virus adsorption, penetration, and genome RNA uncoating, the cytoplasmic replication process is initiated by direct translation of four nonstructural replicase proteins (nsP1-nsP4) from the 5′ two thirds of the viral genome (Fig. 1). The four nsPs are translated as a polyprotein and processed postranslationally into mature monomeric units by a protease activity present in nsP2. Both the nonstructural polyproteins and their derived monomeric units participate in the RNA replication process, which involves nsP binding and initiation at highly conserved sequence elements (CSEs) present in the 5′ and 3′ ends as well as at the highly active internal subgenomic promoter. The positive strand genome serves as template for synthesis of a full-length complementary negative strand RNA. The negative strand, in turn, serves as template for the synthesis of additional positive strand genome RNA for packaging plus an abundant subgenomic mRNA.

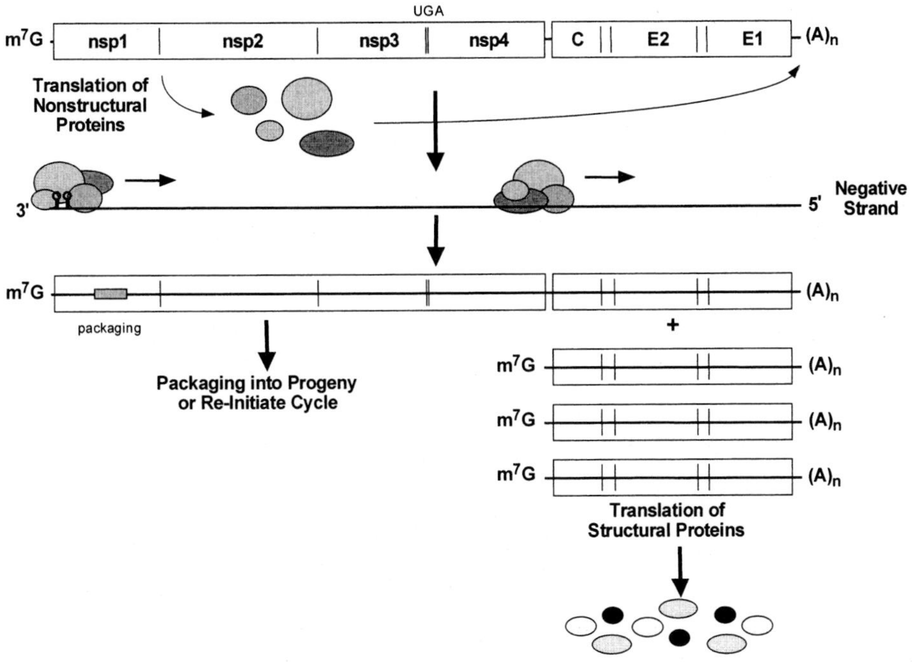

Figure 1 Schematic illustration of the alphavirus genome organization and replication strategy. The approximately 11.7 kb genome of alphaviruses is single stranded and of positive polarity. The RNA consists of two regions that contain the nonstructural replicase (nsp1–4) genes and the structural (C, E2, E1) genes. Nonstructural protein-mediated replication occurs entirely in the cytoplasm of the infected cell and proceeds through a genome-length negative strand RNA intermediate. Transcription of an abundant subgenomic mRNA encoding the structural proteins is directed by an internal ''junction region'' promoter. (Courtesy of J. Polo, Chiron Corporation.)

Alphavirus structural proteins necessary for virion formation are translated from an abundantly transcribed subgenomic RNA, which corresponds to the 3′ one third of the genome. Translation produces a single polyprotein that is processed posttranslationally into the individual proteins capsid (C), glycoproteins E2 and E1, plus the corresponding leader/signal sequences (E3, 6k) for glycoprotein insertion into the endoplasmic reticulum. The structural gene polyprotein is processed by a combination of viral (capsid autoprotease) and cellular proteases (e.g., signal peptidase). Alphavirus structural proteins are produced at very high levels due to the abundance of transcribed subgenomic mRNA as well as a translational enhancer element present within the mRNA 5′ ends (6–8).

III. DEVELOPMENT OF ALPHAVIRUS VECTORS

Unlike the other viral systems described in this book, development of expression vectors from alphaviruses was limited initially by an inability to manipulate the RNA genomes of these viruses. This obstacle was overcome by the pioneering work of Rice et al. (5), who demonstrated that functional genome RNA could be transcribed in vitro from a full-length cDNA clone of SIN. Transfection of genome RNA directly into the cytoplasm of cultured cells mimicked natural virus infection and resulted in productive SIN replication. The critical success factor in these experiments was correct juxtapositioning of a bacteriophage SP6 RNA promoter adjacent to SIN genomic cDNA, such that transcription initiation occurred within three nucleotides of the authentic viral 5′-end. Subsequently, full-length cDNA clones, from which infectious RNA could be transcribed in vitro, were constructed for other alphaviruses, including SFV (9), Ross River virus (RRV) (10), and VEE (11). As described below, the focus on alphaviruses as a platform for gene expression has grown tremendously in recent years. A variety of alphavirus-based expression systems now have been developed, with the ultimate goal of in vivo gene delivery.

A. Replicons and Vector Particles

The first and most common strategy used for engineering of alphaviruses into expression vectors is that of a propagation-incompetent RNA replicon. Using the full-length SIN

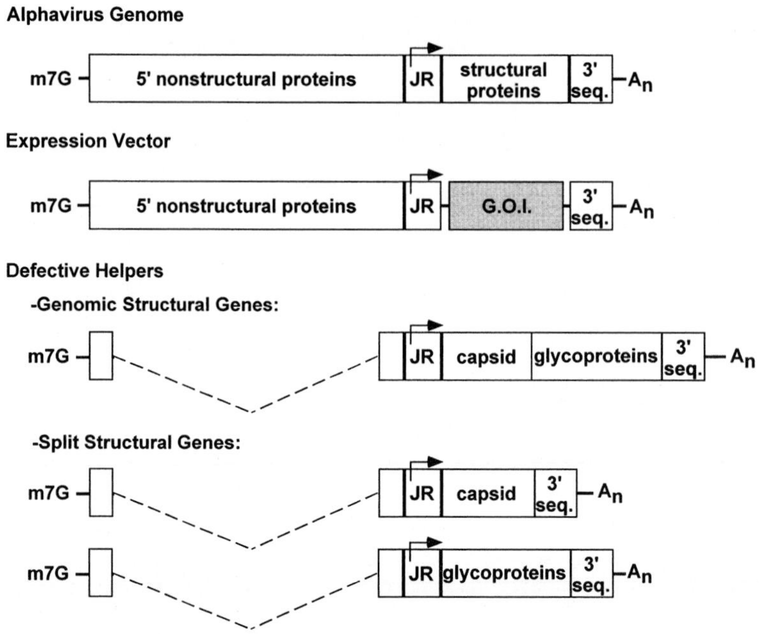

Figure 2 Schematic illustration of alphavirus genomic and vector RNA configurations. Alphavirus vector ''replicons'' contain a heterologous gene of interest substituted in place of the virus structural protein genes, resulting in a nonpropagating suicide vector. Packaging of RNA replicons into vector particles is performed by co-transfection with one or more defective helper RNAs encoding the structural genes, but lacking the RNA packaging signal. (Courtesy of J. Polo, Chiron Corporation.)

cDNA clone, the first such vector was constructed by replacing the entire structural polyprotein gene region with a heterologous gene while maintaining transcriptional control via the highly active subgenomic RNA promoter (12) (Fig. 2). As such, these vectors retained the entire complement of replicase genes (nsP1–4) and the 5′- and 3′-end *cis* sequences needed for replication. Following transcription in vitro, vector replicon RNA was transfected into cultured cells, resulting in expression levels of heterologous protein approaching 10^8 molecules per cell. Because SIN replicons do not synthesize the structural proteins necessary for packaging into particles, expression is limited to only those cells initially transfected. Replicons analogous to the SIN system have also been developed for SFV and VEE (13,14).

One mechanism used by alphaviruses to maximize structural protein expression is a translation enhancer element that is located near the 5′ end of subgenomic RNA, downstream of the capsid AUG initiation codon (6–8). Thus, the enhancer element typically is not maintained in replicon vectors to avoid unwanted expression of virus structural proteins. However, heterologous gene expression from replicons was found to be 10- to 20-fold lower compared to expression of virus structural protein genes. Two approaches have been used to recover an optimum level of foreign gene expression. In the first approach, capsid gene sequences that included the translation enhancer and autoprotease domains but lacked the RNA-binding domain were reintroduced into SIN and SFV vector constructs immediately upstream and fused with the heterologous gene (6–8). Posttranslational cleavage of the capsid portion provided high levels of intact heterologous protein. In the second approach, translation enhancement was obtained by inserting immediately upstream of the heterologous gene a sequence from the untranslated region of β-globin (15).

Regardless of heterologous gene expression levels, the utility of transfecting vector replicon RNA into cells, especially in vivo, is limited by poor transfection efficiency and lability of RNA. Therefore, methods were developed to encapsidate the replicon RNA into mature virion particles that structurally resemble virus and allow for delivery by a normal receptor-mediated pathway. Initially, alphavirus replicons were packaged using wild-type helper virus to co-infect cells that had been transfected with RNA (12). However, as these preparations contained significant levels of wild-type helper virus, a noninfectious packaging helper that could be transcribed in vitro and co-transfected into cells, together with replicon RNA, was developed (13,16)

(Fig. 2). This noninfectious helper was termed a ''defective helper'' (DH), due to extensive deletion of the virus nonstructural protein genes and the RNA packaging signal (17). However, by retaining the 5′- and 3′-end *cis* replication sequences, as well as the structural polyprotein open reading frame under the control of the native subgenomic promoter, amplification of the DH RNA can by programmed in *trans* by the vector-supplied replicase. The titer of packaged vector particles achieved using this co-transfection system approximates that of wild-type virus.

Although co-transfection of replicon and defective helper RNA was an efficient method for producing alphavirus vector particle preparations, substantial levels of replication-competent virus (RCV) contaminated vector preparations. Both RNA recombination (18) and RNA co-packaging (19) have been demonstrated following co-transfection of alphavirus RNAs. Indeed, the defective helper co-transfection method used for vector packaging was not immune from these events (13,16), with RCV being consistently detected. Thus, an emphasis was placed on the development of strategies to eliminate the generation of contaminating RCV.

A first strategy to eliminate RCV was developed with the SFV vector system and incorporated a specific mutation into the cleavage site of glycoprotein precursor pE2 that rendered the protein insensitive to processing by normal cellular proteases (20). The lack of pE2 processing resulted in the formation of pE2-containing vector particles that were unable to infect cells. Treatment of vector particle preparations with chymotrypsin properly cleaved pE2 and ''activated'' the vector preparations. Although not specifically designed to prevent RNA recombination or co-packaging, the pE2 cleavage mutation provided a mechanism to eliminate the spread of such recombinants formed during vector packaging. More recent data indicate that such cleavage defects may be overcome by second site suppressor mutations in the protein, allowing for functional vector particles that still maintain unprocessed pE2 (21–23). Thus, a need for additional approaches remained.

A second strategy addressing the RCV issue and now standard for alphavirus vectors is based on separation of the structural polyprotein into separate defective helper cassettes for the capsid protein gene and the envelope glycoprotein genes (Fig. 2). This vector packaging approach requires the co-transfection of three in vitro transcribed RNAs (a vector and two defective helpers) into cells but is still highly efficient when performed by electroporation. Triple RNA transfection has been used successfully for SIN (24,25), VEE (14), and SFV (26) vector systems to produce high-titer vector particles, while reducing the level of contaminating RCV below the limit of detection by plaque assay or undiluted serial passage. The separation of capsid and envelope glycoprotein genes into distinct cassettes brings into consideration the capsid translational enhancer element discussed previously in the context of vector replicons. Unlike the capsid protein defective helper that maintains its native element, the glycoprotein defective helpers would no longer have such an element available. Therefore, SIN and SFV glycoprotein helpers have been designed to retain the capsid protein gene translational enhancer and protease domains, much like the replicons described above (25,26). In an alternative approach, variations of the SIN defective helpers were assembled in capsid-E2 and capsid-E1 configurations and shown to package co-transfected vector RNA (27). It is certainly possible that a final alphavirus vector product for human application may include some combination of the above safety strategies.

B. Double Subgenomic Promoter Replicating Virus Vectors

In contrast to the replicon vectors described above, double subgenomic (ds) virus vectors have been constructed specifically to be not only replication competent but propagation competent as well. Using a full-length Sindbis virus cDNA clone, Hahn et al. (28) inserted an additional subgenomic promoter into the viral 3′-end noncoding region, immediately downstream from the structural protein genes. Heterologous sequences encoding the desired gene product are placed under the transcriptional control of this second subgenomic promoter. Similar to the replicon vector, dsSIN vector plasmids require linearization and in vitro transcription for subsequent RNA transfection into cultured cells. Introduction of dsSIN vector RNA transcripts into cells directly initiates productive viral replication and the generation of high-titer recombinant viral vector preparations. Cytoplasmic replication of the dsSIN vector gives rise to two subgenomic mRNAs, one from each promoter. Expression of the virus structural proteins occurs from the native subgenomic promoter, while expression of the heterologous gene results from the duplicated promoter via a distinct subgenomic mRNA species.

Because the dsSIN vectors are self-propagating, there exists no theoretical need for large-scale transient packaging approaches for vector production. Rather, the recombinant virus vector that is produced initially will spread throughout the culture, further increasing the yield. Unfortunately, the overall utility of the dsSIN virus vector configuration has been limited by the appearance of deletion mutants during multiple cell culture passages. These deletions typically occur within heterologous gene sequences, especially those greater than 1–2 kb in length, and overtake the nondeleted recombinant virus vector population within a few passages. The occurrence of deletions was reduced somewhat in a subsequent generation of dsSIN vectors, when the duplicated subgenomic promoter was placed upstream of the native subgenomic promoter and virus structural protein genes (29). However, for both dsSIN vector configurations, the most effective means to prevent spontaneous deletions is to use vector stocks produced directly from the initial RNA transfection.

The dsSIN vectors, as well as analogous vectors derived from VEE (30), have shown significant potency as vaccine vehicles in a number of animal models (29–32). The dsSIN vectors also are being used in a particularly interesting approach toward preventing the natural spread of mosquito-transmitted viruses. SIN vector expression of specific RNA sequences from dengue and California serogroup viruses was highly effective for intracellular immunization of mosquitoes by inhibiting virus infection (33,34).

C. DNA-Based Expression of Alphaviruses

The positive-stranded nature of alphavirus genome RNA and availability of cDNA constructs from which infectious RNA may be transcribed in vitro and subsequently tested in cells has facilitated the development of these viruses as expression vectors. However, the procedure for producing transcripts in vitro is not efficient and may be extremely difficult to manufacture in a large-scale setting. Furthermore, the fidelity of bacteriophage polymerases is up to 100-fold lower than RNA polymerase II (pol II). Of particular interest, this poor fidelity of bacteriophage polymerases has been exploited for selection of positive-stranded RNA viruses with phenotypes that differ from their wild-type counterpart (35). While RNA transfection using the electroporation process has been optimized to work at near 100% efficiency in bench scale procedures, this process is not easily amenable to scale-up. Combined with the fact that RNA is relatively labile, these limitations provided the motivation to develop efficient means for pol II–based expression of alphavirus genomes.

It was first demonstrated that alphavirus infection could be launched directly within a transfected cell from genomic-length cDNA copies positioned precisely within a pol II expression cassette (36–38). Alphavirus vector components also were expressed directly from transfected plasmids and included both the replicon and defective helper RNAs. In addition, co-transfection of the DNA constructs was used successfully to produce vector replicon particles (38). The ability to transfect alphavirus plasmid DNA vector constructs directly into cultured cells and animals has enhanced the utility of these vectors and facilitated their overall development. In addition, pol II–based expression of alphaviruses has made the systems much easier to use by eliminating several in vitro manipulation steps.

Plasmid DNA replicons hold significant promise as vectors for nucleic acid–based immunization. In general, DNA-based vaccines have provided optimism for the medical community that safe and effective vaccines for multiple infectious diseases and cancer are on the horizon. Unfortunately, while DNA vaccines have shown tremendous efficacy in many preclinical animal models (reviewed in Ref. 39), their efficacy in primates and humans has been less promising. Results from initial phase I human clinical trials have been somewhat disappointing, with either poor or no immune responses elicited to DNA encoded antigens (40–42). One attraction of alphavirus vectors is that the self-amplifying nature of replicons may provide high antigen expression levels in the immunized animal. Since a threshold level of antigen is required for induction of an immune response, it is expected that replicon-based expression will enhance both the consistency and magnitude of the antigen-specific response. This approach combines the simplicity of plasmid vectors with alphavirus replicons to increase the potency of DNA vaccines. Alphavirus plasmid replicons are layered DNA vectors which, when inoculated directly into animal muscle, transcribe the self-amplifying RNA vector replicon from a pol II–based expression cassette. As described in a later section, alphavirus DNA replicons have been shown to be more efficacious than conventional CMV promoter/intron-based plasmid expression vectors in preclinical mouse models.

Plasmid replicon vectors have been derived from all three alphaviruses under commercial development for human application, including SIN, SFV (43), and VEE (44). The plasmids all have been constructed in a similar manner and consist of the replicon cDNA precisely inserted within a pol II expression cassette. The alphavirus plasmid replicons are quite unlike conventional plasmid expression vectors, in which transcription of mRNA encoding a heterologous gene is driven directly from the pol II promoter. As shown schematically in Figure 3, the poll II promoter of alphavirus plasmid vectors transcribes only the replicon vector, which in turn directs expression of the heterologous gene from an RNA-dependent RNA polymerase. Thus, the primary difference between these vector configurations is the mechanism of mRNA transcription and the abundance of transcripts. In the case of the alphavirus plasmids, heterologous genes are expressed as an alphavirus subgenomic mRNA transcribed directly from the 26S promoter. This promoter is active only in the cytoplasm as the negative-stranded RNA complement of the replicon.

Similar to cDNA clones for in vitro transcription from bacteriophage promoters, plasmid DNA-based alphavirus vectors typically require the precise juxtaposition of an

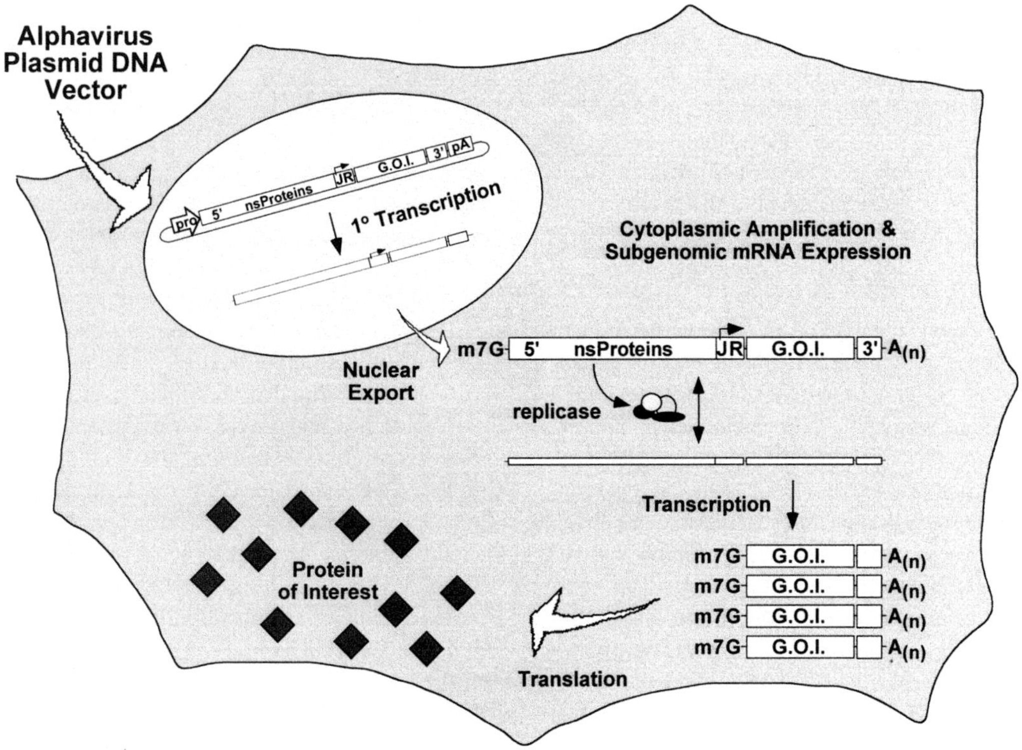

Figure 3 Schematic illustration of the ''layered amplification'' expression strategy for plasmid DNA-based alphavirus vectors. Contained within an RNA polymerase II cassette is the cDNA sequence of an alphavirus vector replicon and linked heterologous gene to be expressed. Following primary transcription and vector transport into the cytoplasm, RNA amplification and high level expression is catalyzed by the vector-encoded replicase proteins. (Courtesy of J. Polo, Chiron Corporation.)

RNA polymerase II promoter with the viral 5′ end in order to obtain biological activity (36,38). However, SFV plasmid DNA replicons recently were described with the expected transcription initiation site at least 50 bps upstream from the authentic viral 5′ end. These DNA vectors appeared to function in transfected cells at a level similar to constructs in which transcription initiation occurred at the authentic alphaviral 5′ end (45). Reasons for the discrepancy between these results, plus other reports demonstrating a requirement for authenticity of in vitro transcribed replicon 5′ ends for function, are unknown. Although several pol II promoters have been used, most constructions currently being evaluated in preclinical animal models contain the CMV immediate early promoter. Theoretically, the level of heterologous protein expression should not be affected by relative promoter strength, because amplification of the RNA replicon is exponential. However, in contrast to this prediction, the highest expression levels appear to be seen using the CMV promoter to launch transcription of the replicon (38).

Several mechanisms may contribute to the observed promoter dependence of alphavirus plasmid replicon efficiency. Not surprisingly, because alphavirus RNA did not evolve in the nucleus, the replicon appears to be transported inefficiently from that compartment to the cytoplasm. Nuclear export seems to be improved in plasmid constructs that incorporate an intron or a transport element, as demonstrated by an increase in the percentage of cells expressing functional replicon in transfection experiments (46). On the other hand, there is no evidence that real or cryptic splicing occurs in the replicon from alphavirus plasmid vector transfected cells. Aberrantly spliced RNAs have not been observed in BHK cells transfected with a plasmid expressing full-length Sindbis virus, as detected by Northern blot analysis (38). The much larger size of alphavirus plasmid replicons, as compared to conventional plasmid expression vectors, may limit their transfection efficiency, either at the cell or nuclear membranes. Data related to this issue are conflicting, as one study found plasmids containing full-length Sindbis virus cDNA transfected equally well as their threefold smaller plasmid DNA expression vector counterparts (38), while another study found that transfection efficiency of linear DNA smaller than 500 bps was size dependent (47). In all likelihood, a strong promoter may overcome many inhibitory mechanisms and simply increase the chance of at least one functional replicon RNA molecule being transported to the cytoplasm of the transfected cell. One replicon is sufficient to direct amplification and expression of the encoded heterologous gene.

Unlike observations for the 5′ end, there are fewer constraints at the 3′ end of alphavirus plasmid replicons affecting vector activity. Strict requirements have been seen for a polyadenylate tract, typically 25–40 nucleotides in length, immediately following the 3′ alphavirus nontranslated region. Additional nonviral nucleotides beyond the polyadenylate tract do not seem to prevent activity (46), and multiple plasmids have been constructed with different elements after the polyadenylate tract. Plasmid replicons that incorporate an HDV ribozyme for cleavage immediately after the polyadenylate tract expressed higher levels of reporter protein in BHK cells (38). These data suggest that structures mimicking the 3′ end of wild-type virus are most efficient.

While the initial work on pol II–based expression of alphaviruses has focused on the development of DNA-based replicons, the utility of pol II expression has been expanded significantly to include defective helpers and packaging cell lines. Not only can replicon particles now be produced by co-transfecting cells with plasmid DNAs, rather than in vitro transcribed RNAs, but packaging cell lines (described below) also can be used to avoid co-transfection altogether. RNA polymerase II–based expression of alphavirus genomes has facilitated a rapid development of these vectors and, importantly, has resulted in formats that are amenable to large-scale manufacture.

D. Replicon Packaging Cell Lines

Traditional RNA co-transfection methods for the packaging of alphavirus vector replicons into particles were described above. These methods are suitable for the relatively small-scale production needs of basic gene expression and preclinical animal studies. It is also likely that materials produced in this manner may be useful for initial clinical studies in humans. However, the eventual commercial utility of alphavirus vectors for vaccine and other applications will require a scalable and consistent means of vector manufacture. Lessons learned from the retroviral vector field suggest that these hurdles might be overcome by the development of stable vector packaging cell lines. Unfortunately, strategies that directly mimic those of the retroviral vector systems are not viable due to the lytic nature of alphavirus replication, the toxicity associated with high-level structural protein expression, and the inevitable shut-off of transcription from RNA polymerase II promoters.

To address these issues, alphavirus vector packaging cell lines (PCL) optimally would be constructed to express very high levels of the structural proteins under the control of an inducible promoter that is not impacted by effects on host macromolecular synthesis. Indeed, such an alphavirus PCL system recently was generated by our group and has successfully captured each of these properties (48) (Fig. 4). The alphavirus PCL employed a strategy whereby one or more stably integrated RNA polymerase II cassettes produced transcripts containing the Sindbis virus structural protein genes under the control of their native subgenomic RNA promoter. As such, basal levels of expression were undetectable by Western blot prior to the induction event, which was mediated entirely by nonstructural replicase proteins supplied in *trans* by the input alphavirus replicon to be packaged. The transcripts also contained 5′- and 3′-end replication signals necessary for RNA amplification by the vector-supplied replicase, thus providing a mechanism to mimic high-level virus replication and expression. The vector-inducible PCL system is somewhat analogous to an alphavirus reporter cell line, where infection of the reporter cells induces expression of luciferase by a replicase-mediated event (49).

Alphavirus-based PCL described by Polo et al. (48) include a variety of structural protein expression cassette modifications that provided increasingly higher levels of packaging activity. Early versions of the PCL utilized a single structural protein cassette and were designed primarily to show proof-of-concept but did not address the generation of contaminating RCV. By separating the structural genes into distinct cassettes for the capsid protein and envelope glycoproteins, second-generation PCL no longer were plagued by the problems of RCV in vector particle preparations.

The availability of split structural gene alphavirus PCL provides a variety of options for packaging vectors. The PCL may be transfected directly with replicon RNA or alternatively with plasmid replicon DNA (48) to avoid prior in vitro transcription and fidelity issues associated with using bacteriophage RNA polymerases (35). In addition, PCL also may be used to amplify a previously generated seed stock of packaged vector particles (48). The latter approach of vector particle amplification appears to hold the most promise for large-scale commercial manufacture of alphavirus vector preparations. By using sequentially larger PCL cultures, it should be possible to propagate and

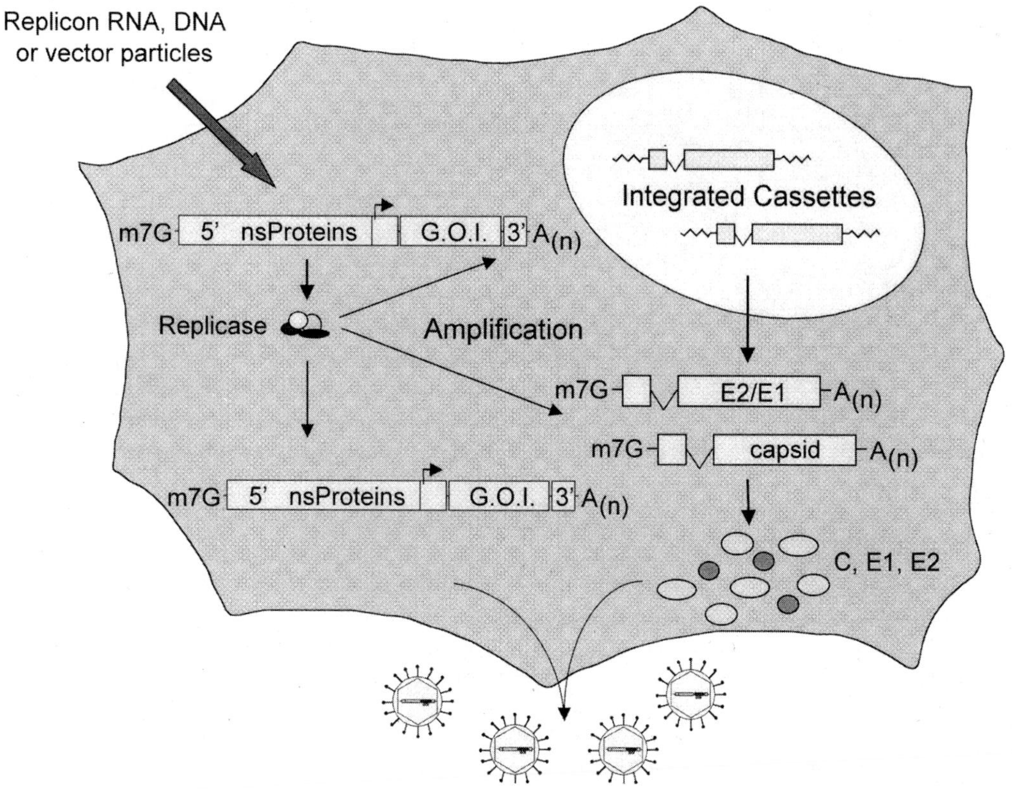

Figure 4 Schematic illustration of an alphavirus packaging cell line (PCL). Structural protein expression cassettes are stably integrated into the genome of PCL, resulting in the constitutive transcription of packaging RNAs. Upon introduction of vector replicon into the PCL by a variety of means, the vector-encoded nonstructural proteins induce expression of the structural proteins leading to high-level packaging of vector particles. (Courtesy of J. Polo, Chiron Corporation.)

expand vector particles much like virus is grown in cultured cells. Preliminary data shown in Figure 5 indicate the feasibility of this method to produce high-titer ($>10^8$ IU/mL) replicon particle preparations free from contaminating RCV.

An eventual goal for the alphavirus field also might include the development of vector-producer cell lines (VPCL). VPCL typically would comprise the packaging cell line components described above, with the addition of a stably incorporated cassette for transcription of the vector replicon itself. Similar to packaging cell lines, a VPCL system also must address the lytic nature of alphavirus infection. Three potential approaches include the use of inducible promoters, noncytopathic replicons, and parental cell lines, such as mosquito cells, in which alphaviruses are not lytic. A system based entirely on inducible promoters may prove most challenging, because transcription of a single functional vector replicon would be sufficient to initiate RNA replication and the subsequent cascade of events culminating in structural protein and vector particle production.

E. Noncytopathic Vectors

Alphavirus infection of mammalian cells is lytic, resulting from virus-mediated downregulation of host cell macromolecular synthesis (reviewed in Ref. 3). In addition, alphaviruses have been shown to induce apoptosis in several types of cells (50,51). While structural protein expression plays a significant role in these events, particularly an accelerated onset of cytopathic effects, infection by alphavirus-derived vectors lacking the structural protein genes also culminates in host cell shut-off, albeit over a delayed time frame (52). For particular gene-delivery applications, such as vaccination, cancer therapeutics, and growth factor expression, high-level production for a relatively short duration should be suitable or even advantageous. However, for other gene delivery or recombinant protein production applications, a

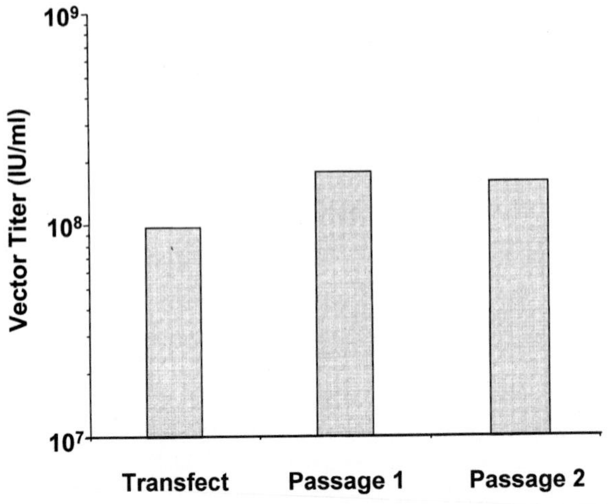

Figure 5 Serial propagation of alphavirus vector particles using a packaging cell line (PCL). To demonstrate feasibility of large-scale vector production by sequential particle amplification, split structural gene PCL were transfected initially with SIN-βgal vector RNA. Vector particle–containing supernatants were harvested and a small aliquot of supernatant was used to "seed" a naïve culture of PCL for additional vector production (Passage 1). The passage 1 supernatant, in turn, was used to seed another naïve culture of PCL (Passage 2). Vector particle titers for each sample were determined on BHK cells, and the samples were shown to be free from replication-competent virus by plaque assay. (Courtesy of J. Polo, Chiron Corporation.)

substantial benefit may be obtained from increasing the duration of expression. Furthermore, minimizing the vector effect on host cell function for any application is also likely to be desirable. Therefore, noncytopathic versions of alphavirus vectors are being developed.

The feasibility of generating noncytopathic vectors is supported by the natural biology of these viruses, whereby infection of mosquitoes and cultured mosquito cells results in persistent infection, with little evidence of cytopathology (53). In addition, it has been shown that propagation of Sindbis virus in BHK cell cultures enriched for the presence of defective interfering (DI) virus particles resulted in a persistent infection (54). From these persistently infected BHK cells, a clonal variant of Sindbis virus was plaque purified and found to exhibit the noncytopathic phenotype independently, in the absence of DI particles.

Recently, the noncytopathic Sindbis virus variant has been revisited. Mapping studies substituted cDNA fragments from the variant into a full-length Sindbis virus clone and identified the causal mutation within nonstructural protein gene 2 (55). By localizing the mutation, substitution of the mutant nsP2 gene into SIN replicons was then possible as a means to generate noncytopathic vectors.

In an alternative approach, noncytopathic SIN vector replicons were selected for directly by expressing a drug resistance marker as the heterologous gene (35,56). Following introduction of SIN replicons expressing puromycin acetyltransferase (PAC) into BHK cells, drug selection was applied. Although the vast majority of cells succumbed to vector replication and/or drug toxicity, a small number of resistant foci survived. Resistance of these cells to puromycin was the result of PAC expression from mutant replicons that were no longer cytopathic but retained the ability to replicate in a persistent manner.

A panel of noncytopathic SIN and SFV variants also has been generated in BHK cells using the neomycin phosphotransferase selectable marker (27). Interestingly, the causal mutation in one SIN variant from these studies was mapped to the same nsP2 residue 726 as described by Dryga et al. (55) and Frolov et al. (56). However, the other SIN and SFV variants from this new panel were not restricted to mutations in the carboxy terminus of nsP2. Rather, changes in other domains of the nsP2 protein, such as the amino terminus, also were shown to result in a noncytopathic phenotype.

The noncytopathic phenotype of alphavirus variants isolated in BHK cells appears to be limited to a select group of cell lines (27,56), and in vivo characterization is not yet available. This observed restriction may be attributable to different levels of interferon response among cell types or it may indicate variation in specific host factors that impact the level of viral replication. Nevertheless, similar strategies for selection may provide a powerful approach to obtain additional vector variants in cell types that are more relevant to commercial application.

F. Vector Particles with Modified Tropism

Not only is targeted gene transfer by viral-based vectors an important safety advantage, but for certain applications the ability to preferentially transduce a particular organ or cell type is essential for efficacy. In the case of cancer gene therapy, some tumors can be accessed directly, while systemic malignancies cannot. Thus, for such therapy to be effective, the viral vector must be able to seek out the diseased cells in a background of normal cells. The broad host range and ability of alphavirus vectors to infect both dividing and nondividing cells limits their utility for systemic ablative approaches to cancer gene therapy without prior modification of the wild-type tropism. A central feature of all arboviruses, which include the alphaviruses, is an ability to efficiently infect both insect and vertebrate hosts. To exhibit such broad host range, arboviruses must use a receptor that is highly conserved across multiple species. Preferential targeting by Sindbis virus vectors has focused on modification of the viral envelope glycoprotein E2, which binds to the well-conserved and high-affinity laminin receptor (57). Although the E2/E1 glycoprotein heterodimer serves as a functional unit, E2 alone appears to mediate receptor binding and contains most of the viral neutralization epitopes, while E1 mediates endosomal fusion. Development of alphavirus vectors that can preferentially target malignant cells overexpressing specific cell surface proteins in vivo may provide an effective gene therapy treatment for cancer.

The seminal work suggesting that alphavirus vector particles may be targeted identified specific regions within the E2 glycoprotein of Sindbis virus that could be substituted with epitopes from a heterologous virus (58). In this study, infectious Sindbis virus chimeras were generated that contained a neutralization epitope from Rift Valley fever virus (RVFV) within the E2 glycoprotein. Mice immunized with the chimeric virus were protected against lethal RVFV challenge. These results indicated that the chimeric SIN particles could recognize and bind the T-cell receptor for the RVFV epitope and that incorporation of a receptor-specific ligand into permissive regions of envelope glycoprotein E2 could redirect the tropism of alphaviruses. In a subsequent investigation, it was shown that the normal host range of SIN could be abrogated by incorporation of a short sequence within E2 (59).

Targeting of SIN replicon particles has been accomplished by insertion of the IgG F_c binding domain of *Staphylococcus aureus* protein A (PA) or receptor-specific ligands into the E2 glycoprotein region defined by Dubuisson and Rice (59,60). Targeting of PA-substituted chimeric SIN particles to a desired cell type was accomplished by decorating the particles with a monoclonal antibody directed towards a cell-specific receptor. This method now has been used to target a number of human cancer cell lines that normally are refractory to infection by wild-type SIN envelopes, including epidermal, epithelial, glioblastoma, and lymphoma cells, as well as cells expressing human CD4 (60–62). For commercial application, those monoclonal antibodies that were demonstrated to retarget SIN particles likely would need to be ''humanized'' in order to permit readministration. In a second method, chimeric SIN particles were generated by the insertion of a 4.5 kb sequence corresponding to the α- and β-chorionic gonadotropin (CG) genes directly into an E2 defective helper packaging construct (62). The SIN replicon particles produced using this configuration were able to infect cell lines expressing the CG/leuteinizing hormone receptors. However, the vector particle titers produced using this approach were quite low, most likely due to the large size of α-/β-CG, and indicated limitations in the extent of perturbation to the alphavirus particle with cell-specific ligands. Chimeric alphavirus particles in which relatively small ligands are tolerated may offer an advantage compared to the monoclonal antibody–decorated particles, due to expected lower costs of manufacturing and a less complex final product.

Alphavirus vectors with modified tropism may be required for particular applications where the targeting of a particular diseased cell or tissue type is critical for efficacy, for example, in cancer. The pharmacokinetics of retargeted Sindbis replicon particles in vivo remains as yet unknown. However, it has been shown that SIN particles modified by either method have a dramatically reduced capability of infecting BHK cells (59,60), the normal cell host used for virus propagation in culture. This result is promising, as it suggests that retargeted alphavirus particles may be highly selective in vivo for infecting a desired host cell. In addition, retargeted alphavirus vectors may be particularly well suited for cancer gene therapy, as cells transduced with these vectors ultimately will undergo apoptosis (50,51,63–65). The overall ablative effect of these vectors in vivo may likely be enhanced even further by pro-drug strategies that provide a bystander effect, as shown by sensitization of human tumor cell lines to killing by ganciclovir when transduced with retargeted Sindbis virus particles encoding herpes simplex virus thymidine kinase (61).

Finally, when considering the targeting of alphavirus vectors or any virus-based vector, it should be remembered that viruses have multistep lifecycles, and thus phenotypic changes in tropism may also result from mutation of the nonstructural replicase genes as well as noncoding *cis* sequence elements. The approaches that have been used to target Sindbis virus–based particles may be applicable for targeting other viral-based gene therapy vectors. If successful, this strategy conceivably could become a new paradigm for the treatment of cancer.

IV. APPLICATIONS OF ALPHAVIRUS REPLICONS

A. Vaccines

The high level of heterologous gene expression obtained with alphavirus replicons has stimulated considerable interest in these vectors for vaccine applications. Both plasmid DNA–and particle-based vectors derived from the alphaviruses SIN, SFV, and VEE are currently being developed as vaccine agents. Initial studies with these vectors focused exclusively on particle-based replicons; while more recent work also has evaluated the efficacy of plasmid DNA-based alphavirus replicons. Each vector format likely will have its own distinct advantages and potential limitations.

One consideration for both systems is the level of gene expression. It is not known whether the very high levels of vector expression in cultured cells will be reproduced entirely in vivo, where interferon or other innate immune responses are present. The level of antigen expression is a critical issue for vaccine efficacy and relates directly to the immunization dose required for a broad and robust immune response. This, in turn, impacts both vector-specific immune responses in the vaccinated individual and commercial feasibility of a given delivery system.

As viral infection inherently is more efficient than DNA transfection in vivo, the vector particle format is expected to be more efficient than the DNA-based replicons for vaccine applications. Gene expression in a vector particle–infected cell occurs exclusively in the cytoplasm, avoiding problems related to transport of plasmid DNA to the nucleus and RNA back to the cytoplasm. However, the DNA-based alphavirus vectors may also provide a safety advantage compared to their viral particle counterpart, due to the elimination of issues related to replication-competent virus.

1. Efficacy of Immunization in Small Animal and Primate Models

Multiple publications have demonstrated the comparatively robust potency of using the alphavirus particle and DNA formats for induction of antigen-specific immune responses in mice. A summary of recent investigations is provided in Table 1 (14,32,48,66–74). Vaccination of mice with as few as 100 vector particles resulted in the stimulation of influenza (flu) HA-specific antibody (75). In general, immunization of diverse strains of mice with SIN, SFV, or VEE replicon particles, at doses of 10^4–10^7 IU, has produced humoral and cellular responses at levels sufficient to protect against lethal challenge with the corresponding infectious agent from which the antigen was obtained. Such resistance to lethal challenge in vaccinated mice has been shown with flu (14) and herpes simplex virus (48) and in guinea pigs vaccinated against the particularly virulent filovirus, Marburg (MBGV) (74). Significantly, mice immunized with VEE replicon particles encoding HIV MA/CA antigen developed a relatively robust mucosal response at a distal location, as shown by detection of anti-MA/CA IgA-specific antibody in vaginal washes (32). In contrast, flu HA-specific IgA antibody was detected in the respiratory tract of SFV replicon immunized mice only when given intranasally (72).

In those studies where it has been examined, immunization with alphavirus vector particles has resulted in a sustained immune response against the vector-encoded antigen (30). An additional important observation was that immunization with vector encoding a first antigen did not interfere with the level of protection induced during a sequential immunization with vector encoding a second, distinct antigen. These data suggest minimal immune responses to the replicon- or particle-specific proteins or, alternatively, that sufficient replicon-driven antigen expression and presentation occurs prior to any vector-specific immune response.

Table 1 Recent Immunization Studies with Alphavirus Vectors

Parent alphavirus	Vector format	Antigen	Animal model	Challenge	Ref.
Sindbis	Virus[a]	Influenza NP	Mice	Yes	66
Sindbis	Virus	Malaria CS	Mice	Yes	66
Sindbis	Particles	HSV-1 gB	Mice	No	48
Sindbis	DNA	HSV-1 gB	Mice	Yes	67
Semliki Forest	Particles	SIV gp160	Primates	Yes	68
Semliki Forest	Particles	HIV gp160	Primates	Yes	69
Semliki Forest	Particles	Louping ill prME/NS1	Mice	Yes	70
Semliki Forest	Particles	Murray Valley PrM/E	Mice	No	71
Semliki Forest	Particles	Influenza HA/NP	Mice	Yes	73
Semliki Forest	DNA	Influenza HA/NP	Mice	Yes	72
VEE	Particles	HIV MA/CA	Mice	No	32
VEE	Particles	Influenza HA	Mice	Yes	14
VEE	Particles	Lassa N	Mice	Yes	14
VEE	Particles	Marburg NP/GP	Primates	Yes	74

[a] Expression of epitope in the context of infectious virus, using a second subgenomic promoter.

The successful induction of antigen-specific immune responses in smaller animals has led to recent investigations in primates. Results of initial primate studies have been promising as well and to date have included reports with both SFV and VEE replicons. The MBGV investigation also included immunization of cynomolgus monkeys (74). Animals given three vaccinations of VEE replicon encoding GP presented no signs of illness after challenge with a high dose of MBGV. VEE replicons were particularly efficacious at inducing anti-MBGV antibody, as postchallenge ELISA titers in vaccinated guinea pigs and monkeys were absent or modest, respectively. No viremia was detected in vaccinated monkeys following challenge.

In both SIV and SHIV primate challenge models of HIV infection, immunization studies also have shown some promise, although not to the extent of the MBGV investigation. Monkeys were vaccinated with SFV or VEE replicon particles expressing either env or MA/CA from HIV or SIV and subsequently challenged with the corresponding virus, SIV or SHIV (67,68). Pig-tailed macaques were protected against challenge with a virulent strain of SIV after immunization with SFV replicon particles given by a combination of intramuscular and intravenous routes (67). The general observation in these initial studies was induction of both humoral and cellular antigen-specific immune responses, but at a level that only reduced the viral load compared to unvaccinated controls (68). However, as HIV load is predictive of time of progression to AIDS in infected individuals, these results are indeed encouraging.

Plasmid DNA-based alphavirus replicons have been shown to be quite efficacious in vaccinated mice as compared to conventional plasmid DNA expression vectors. In two separate investigations (43,67) mice were protected against lethal challenge doses of influenza or HSV when immunized with significantly lower levels of DNA-based replicon compared to conventional CMV promoter-based expression plasmids. For each of these studies, the immune correlates of protection against lethal virus challenge were both humoral and cellular. In the flu study, SFV-based DNA was 1000-fold more efficacious at inducing an antibody response. The CD4+ immune response in the alphavirus plasmid immunized mice was mainly of the T_H1 type, as demonstrated by a high IgG2a/IgG1 ratio (43). Using a SIN-based DNA plasmid, CTL precursors were induced by replicon-expressed HSV glycoprotein B also at 1000-fold lower levels of DNA compared to animals immunized with conventional plasmid (67). More recently, we have extended this first dosing investigation by comparing Sindbis replicon (pSIN) and conventional (pCI) plasmid DNA vectors expressing HIV gp160 across a range of intramuscular doses for their ability to induce humoral and cellular immune responses in Balb/C mice (27). The results of these studies were similar to our earlier observations with the HSV model system; alphavirus replicon plasmid was much more effective at inducing HIV gp160-specific CTL precursors, compared to the conventional DNA plasmid. The results are summarized in Table 2, along with the HSV data reported previously (67).

Although chromosomal integration may be a safety concern for conventional plasmid DNA vectors, this may not be an issue for alphavirus plasmid replicons. Expression of the nonstructural proteins and vector RNA self-amplification eventually results in apoptosis for cells transfected with the alphavirus plasmid replicon (43,46). Thus, it would appear that the "suicidal" alphavirus plasmid vectors have an attractive safety advantage compared to conventional plasmids, because cells transduced with the former vector will not persist.

2. Relative Efficacy Between Alphavirus Vectors

While SIN-, SFV-, and VEE-based vectors have individually been shown to be efficacious in animal models, the relative potency of these vectors is unknown. Of particular interest, VEE has been shown to target lymphocytes (30), which could enhance potency of this system through direct antigen presentation in transduced cells and/or from efficient cross-priming by phagocytosis of replicon-infected cells undergoing apoptosis by neighboring antigen-presenting cells. Replicon particles derived from particular strains of Sindbis virus have also been shown recently to infect immature human dendritic cells (27). Whether this property extends to an enhanced efficacy in vivo for induction of antigen-specific immune responses is unknown. For practical, if not commercial, reasons, it will likely be important to compare these (and possibly other) alphaviruses directly with each other to determine relative efficacy. Decisions as to which alphavirus vector to develop clinically will be related in part to safety, potency, and ability to manufacture.

3. Mechanisms of Replicon-Induced Immune Response

As noted previously, the ability of some alphavirus replicon particles to target antigen-presenting cells may be important for the relative potency of this vector system. Additionally, high levels of double-stranded RNA (dsRNA) are produced during the course of replicon amplification and may enhance the immune response through a variety of mechanisms, including increased class I self-antigen presentation and/or direct activation of dendritic cells (76). Other ways in which replicon-mediated immunization may affect vaccine potency include adjuvant effects by the vec-

Table 2 Immune Threshold Doses Comparing SIN Replicon and Conventional Plasmid DNA Immunization in Mice

HSV model	Immunogen		
Parameter	pSIN-HSV gB	pCI-HSV gB	Fold difference
Protection	0.1 μg	3.0 μg	30
Bulk CTL	0.01 μg	10 μg	1000
CTL precursors (at 10 μg)	1 in 30,000	1 in 86,000	3
CTL precursors (at 1 μg)	1 in 43,186	≥ 2,000,000	NA
Ab induction	0.01 μg	1.0 μg	100
HIV model	**Immunogen**		
Parameter	**pSIN-HIV gp160**	**pCI-HIV gp160**	**Fold difference**
Bulk CTL	0.03 μg	3.0 μg	100
CTL precursors (at 0.3 μg)	1 in 25,000	1 in 1,051,853	42
Ab induction	0.03 μg	0.1 μg	3

tor replicase or the induction of apoptosis in replicon-containing cells and subsequent cross-priming of antigen presenting cells. These mechanisms, combined with antigen expression level, likely contribute in varying degrees to the extent and breadth of the immune response.

B. Gene Therapy

Although most investigations to date using alphavirus vectors in vivo have been vaccine related, more recent publications have explored their use for cancer as well as neurological and cardiovascular diseases. Cancer is a natural disease target for alphavirus vectors, and ablative therapies were discussed in the targeting section. The alphavirus vectors would be presumed to be efficacious for both preventative and therapeutic vaccines for cancers where tumor-specific antigens have been identified. In a recent study, in vitro transcribed SFV replicon encoding a model antigen was shown to protect immunized mice from challenge with tumor expressing the model antigen, and therapeutic immunization prolonged the survival of mice bearing an established tumor (77). It is expected that induction of interferons and increased expression of class I antigens should enhance directly the tumor-specific immune response as a result of alphavirus vector transduction or by expression of particular cytokines encoded by the replicon. However, while initial experiments have demonstrated expression in cultured tumor cells of IL-12 by an SFV vector (78) or IL-2 by a SIN vector (27), there have been no reports related to the in vivo expression of these or any other cytokines. Nevertheless, cancer is an attractive target for alphavirus vectors, and such applications are certain to be explored further.

It is well known that alphaviruses are neurotropic, with virus crossing the blood-brain barrier following high levels of viremia. The extent of alphavirus virulence in animals is determined both by the virus and strain, as well as the age of the injected animal (3,79,80). Wild-type VEE is distinctly more neurovirulent than either SIN or SFV, and injected adult mice succumb to infection following intracranial or subcutaneous administration of infectious virus. Consequently, only SIN and SFV vectors have been utilized for in vitro and in vivo neuronal gene transfer investigations. Two recent studies have shown that SIN and SFV vectors preferentially infect neurons with greater than 90% efficiency in rat hippocampal slice cultures (81,82). Significantly, the onset of cytopathogenicity was delayed in these cultures compared to other cultured cell types, for example, BHK or 293 cells, as the neurons appeared to be morphologically normal and viable for up to at least 5 days postinfection. Vectors have been constructed that will allow co-expression of GFP along with a selected gene, facilitating physiological analysis in transduced neurons. Reporter gene expression in vivo has been described in the nucleus caudata/putamen and nucleus accumbens septi of mice receiving a steriotactic injection with SIN-lac Z replicon particles (83–85). Whether alphavirus vectors will be useful for various neurological applications will require a better understanding of replicon-induced cytopathogenicity and/or apoptosis in neurons, as well as the level of inflammation. If the outcome of these further investigations is favorable, SIN and SFV vectors could prove to be useful for a number of neurodegenerative diseases. In particular, high-level transient expression of neurotrophic factors, such as NT-3 (neurotrophin 3), GDNF (glial-derived neurotrophic factor), BDNF (brain-derived neurotrophic factor), and

NGF (nerve growth factor), may be therapeutic for these diseases.

Finally, it is expected that alphavirus vectors may be quite useful for a variety of cardiovascular and wound-healing applications where a finite period of robust expression of the transgene is desirable. SIN and SFV vectors function efficiently in muscle, and high reporter gene expression levels were observed in cultured human and rat aortic smooth muscle cells and cardiac myocytes, as well as in smooth muscle cells, but not endothelial cells, in vivo (27,86). Based on success in animal models of ischemic disease, first-generation adenovirus E1 gene-deleted vectors expressing pro-angiogenic growth factors are being tested in phase I clinical trials by direct cardiac injection in patients with coronary artery disease (87–89). Alphavirus replicon particles also may have utility for ischemic diseases, with the attractive feature that, as a result of cytoplasmic expression, these vectors are highly unlikely to result in a host cell permanently transduced with a growth factor. However, as both the adenovirus and alphavirus vectors induce apoptosis, it remains to be determined whether death of transduced cardiac cells will negate any therapeutic benefit. Other possible growth factor applications for alphavirus vectors include diabetic ulcers, severe fractures and osteoporosis, and osteoarthritis. The availability of high-titer preparations of alphavirus replicon particles that are free from detectable replication competent virus is likely to encourage exploration of these applications and many others applications in the near future.

V. ADDITIONAL APPLICATIONS OF ALPHAVIRUS VECTORS

A. Inducible Alphavirus Vector Systems for Expression of Recombinant Proteins

The various approaches developed to induce expression of foreign genes or alphaviral structural proteins from alphavirus vector and defective helper RNAs also have been used to produce recombinant proteins and vector particles for other virus systems and to make diagnostic cell lines for adventitious viruses. For these applications, the gene(s) of interest are substituted for the structural protein genes in either the replicon or the DH constructions. Similar to methods used for producing alphavirus replicon particles, DHs encoding heterologous genes may be introduced into cells either by transfection of in vitro transcribed RNA or from a stably integrated expression cassette. The potential for inducibly regulating very high levels of protein production by programming the amplification of DH RNAs in *trans* with vector-encoded replicase has led to a rapid development of these hybrid alphavirus-based systems.

Alphavirus-based vectors are an attractive system for the production of recombinant proteins due to their rapid and high-level expression (12). The level of protein produced from a VEE replicon in BHK cells was reported to be 20% of the total cell protein (14). Both in vitro transcribed RNA as well as DNA-based SFV vectors have been used to produce recombinant proteins (45,83). The broad host range of alphaviruses allows for protein production in a variety of cell lines by infecting at high multiplicity with a vector particle stock. Reported yields of recombinant protein produced by these methods have been 20–30 pg/cell (45). One concern for this system may be fidelity of the alphavirus replicase, which could result in a product with lower specific activity and/or unanticipated antigenicity in humans. This issue can be addressed by generating cell lines stably transformed with a DH construct encoding the protein of interest. Induction of the DH is accomplished by infection of the cell line with a replicon particle. Because RNA polymerase II has a higher fidelity than the alphavirus replicase, it would be expected that recombinant proteins produced by this method may be less susceptible to mutation.

B. Inducible Alphavirus Vector Systems for Production of Other Virus-Based Vectors

Retrovirus vectors based on Moloney murine leukemia virus (MLV) have been tested in more patients and in more gene therapy clinical trials than any other vector system (90). Integration of the MLV vector into the host chromosome allows for long-term expression of the foreign gene. While retrovirus vectors have been used extensively, they have been difficult to produce at high titer from stable producer cell lines. Using hybrid SFV vectors, two methods have been developed for alphavirus-mediated production of MLV vectors. One attraction of these systems is that cytoplasmic transcription of MLV vector RNA circumvents the editing of particular genetic elements, for example, introns, from the vector, as would typically occur following nuclear transcription.

In the first approach, BHK cells were electroporated with three in vitro transcribed SFV replicon RNAs encoding MLV *env, gag-pol,* or the MLV vector with 5′ and 3′LTRs (91,92). The replicon RNAs independently programmed their own amplification and expression of retroviral vector elements. Construction of an SFV replicon encoding a functional MLV vector was difficult, since the 5′ end of alphavirus subgenomic mRNA necessarily contains a 38 bp sequence from the 26S promoter. To produce MLV vector RNA that could be reverse transcribed into

DNA and integrate into the host chromosome, this 38 bp sequence (SF) was repeated near the 3′ end of the subgenomic RNA, between the U3 and R regions. The SFV replicon encoding the MLV vector contained the following ordered genetic elements: SF-R-U5-Ψ-promoter/foreign gene-U3-SF-R. Thus, each proviral LTR transcribed in cells by this method had the following structure: U3-SF-R-U5. Electroporation of BHK cells with the three in vitro transcribed hybrid SFV/MLV RNAs produced titers of approximately 1×10^6 cfu/mL.

In the second approach, MLV vector packaging cells (PCL) derived from murine or human cell lines were electroporated with a single in vitro transcribed replicon RNA encoding an MLV vector (93,94). The MLV vector RNA was packaged in *trans* by retroviral structural proteins expressed constitutively by the PCL. However, as alphavirus replicons inhibit host cell protein synthesis, the retroviral vector titers of approximately 1×10^5 cfu/mL produced by this method were lower than the former method. An approach that has not yet been reported would be to insert all of the retroviral genetic elements into individual DH expression cassettes and then to derive stable cell lines containing these constructions. Synthesis of the retrovirus vector–specific RNAs and proteins then would be induced by introduction of a replicon, similar to the generation of alphavirus vector particles from stable packaging cell lines (48). Alphavirus hybrid vectors ultimately may not be the best method for production of retrovirus vector particles, because stable MLV vector producer cell lines now can be generated that produce vector particle titers of 5×10^8 cfu/mL over several days in a GMP manufacturing setting (90). However, these approaches may be useful to produce other virus-based gene-transfer vectors, where current methods are problematic.

C. Inducible Alphavirus Vector Systems for Diagnostic Applications

A particularly promising application of alphavirus vectors is the generation of diagnostic cell lines. Several cell lines have been developed for the detection of adventitious viruses in clinical samples or the determination of titers for alphavirus replicon particle preparations. All of the diagnostic cell lines share a similar property of 26S promoter induction by the alphavirus replicase, resulting in expression of a reporter protein, which is easily quantitated and compared to a reference standard. Diagnostic cell lines for alphavirus replicon particles contain a stably integrated expression cassette of the same basic configuration as a defective helper (49). Infection with replicon particles results in the induction of this cassette and synthesis of large amounts of β-galactosidase reporter from the subgenomic message. Using a variation of this theme with a bit more complexity, additional cell lines were made in which induction of integrated alphavirus vectors encoding β-galactosidase was used to detect herpesviruses (95). In one application, Vero cells contained the cDNA of a SIN/LacZ replicon with expression regulated by the herpes simplex virus type 1 (HSV-1)–infected cell protein 8 promoter (UL29 gene). Induction of the SIN replicon and expression of β-galactosidase occurred in response to infection of the diagnostic cell line with HSV-1. A second Vero cell line contained, in addition to the SIN/LacZ replicon cDNA, a DH cassette encoding the SIN structural proteins. This cell line produced SIN/LacZ replicon particles in response to infection with HSV-1 and was more sensitive for HSV detection because the SIN/LacZ particles could in turn spread throughout the culture. A similar diagnostic assay for human cytomegalovirus (HCMV) also was produced in mink lung cells that contained the SIN/LacZ replicon cDNA under the control of the HCMV early gene UL45 promoter (95). An important observation with these diagnostic cell lines is that SIN replicon RNA was not produced, even at a basal level, in the absence of induction by the relevant herpesvirus. Replicon production at any level would subsequently self-amplify and induce apoptosis. Therefore, cell lines in which basal expression occurred would not be stable.

The ability to use alphavirus expression systems to efficiently produce recombinant proteins, other virus-based vector particles, and diagnostic cell lines for herpesviruses has significantly advanced the overall utility of these vectors beyond vaccine and gene therapy applications. The replicon particle titering cell lines should facilitate the commercialization of alphavirus vectors, while the diagnostic cell lines will be useful for any virus that is difficult to detect, when controlling genetic elements are understood and can be used to develop new assays. An important feature of these cell lines is that alphavirus-programmed expression is very rapid, with high levels of β-galactosidase being detected within 12–24 hours, timing which is critical for many clinical diagnoses.

VI. ISSUES RELATED TO COMMERCIALIZATION OF ALPHAVIRUS VECTORS

Manufacturing of gene therapy vectors is a central issue in the development and successful commercialization of the technology in general, and has been the rationale for the efforts described in this chapter to develop methods for producing alphavirus vectors that are amenable to large-scale manufacture. No products have been licensed for sale in the United States or elsewhere at this time that can be described conventionally as a gene therapy product, but several precedents exist (e.g., live viral vaccines, recombinant protein products). The expectations of the U.S. Food and Drug Administration (FDA) have been clearly set out in several relevant ''Points to Consider'' and ''Guidelines'' documents (see FDA web site at http://www.fda.gov/cber/).

Practically speaking, it is possible to perform preclinical animal experiments and even small early phase human clinical trials with material made in small batches using technology that has not been developed into large-scale production methods. However, these animal and clinical experiments may be difficult to interpret or even misleading, because the properties of the vector system in terms of safety, efficacy, and potency can change if the method of manufacture has been substantially modified. Therefore, although product scale-up and progress towards a process employing clinical Good Manufacturing Principles (cGMP) will be an ongoing activity as clinical trials proceed, it is important to start with a process from which efficient large-scale production can be accomplished. Scale-up procedures for the alphavirus replicon packaging cell lines described in this chapter are now being tested. The following discussion represents expectations of this replicon particle production format and other related issues.

A. Batch Culture System

Extensive experience exists for optimizing and scaling up vector production with murine retroviral vectors and using these preparations in clinical trials (96). Many of the issues for production of alphavirus replicon particles are similar, but initial materials likely will be made by batch mode rather than continuous production.

The alphavirus replicon PCL carry integrated expression cassettes encoding the structural protein genes such that synthesis is induced after introduction of replicon into the cells. The replicon programs amplification of both itself and the structural protein gene cassettes, resulting in the production of alphavirus vector particles. In turn, these particles expand throughout a large growing culture of PCL as a pseudo-infection, leading to cell death and a large burst of replicon particle production. This strategy is necessary because of the toxicity of both the structural proteins and the replicase genes encoded by the replicon. As described in the replicon packaging cell lines section, vector particle seed stocks may be produced by transfecting the PCL with a plasmid DNA alphavirus replicon. The seed stock then can be amplified by subsequent sequential passaging in fresh PCL cultures. Similar considerations exist with other virus-based gene-transfer systems, such as vectors derived from adenovirus, (97), adeno-associated virus (98), and herpesvirus (99). In this way, the alphavirus replicon production system strongly resembles the production of viral vaccines, such as for poliovirus or varicella zoster virus (100,101). Vector is then harvested from the culture over a few days, clarified, purified, and concentrated using techniques similar to those of other gene therapy vectors (102).

It will be necessary to bank and test master and working banks of the packaging cell line and create a master and working stock of the relevant vector. An incidental advantage over the retroviral vector system is that, like adenoviral vectors, the same bank of packaging cell line can be used with multiple replicons encoding distinct genes of interest.

B. Scale

It is not yet clear at what scale this process will need to be performed either for early phase I trials or for large-scale pivotal trials, as the indications and doses necessary have not been finally determined. A few assumptions can illustrate how important this issue is. Doses for immunotherapy applications are expected to be within the range of 1×10^6 to 1×10^{10} infectious units (IU) per patient. Assuming that the current PCL will yield about 1×10^8 IU/mL of culture harvested and that the yield after purification is 25%, then the volume of culture for 100 doses is from 40 mL to 40 L. The high-end number is quite feasible and in line with scales of production for recombinant proteins (103). However, this is true only for a process that is compatible with such scale. For example, it seems unlikely that techniques involving transient transfection or ultra-centrifugation could be used in such a situation.

C. Testing

The testing required on banks and clinical material should be designed to provide assurance that the vector can be produced with predictable safety and potency. Safety issues can be broken down into those that are associated with most biological materials (e.g., sterility, free from contamination with mycoplasma and other human pathogens etc.) and specific issues associated with the vector or its production. An important vector-specific issue is preventing contamination of replicon particle preparations with replication-competent virus (RCV, see below) but also includes issues such as the potential use of BHK cells as the parent line for packaging cells. If this were the case, it would be the first time, to our knowledge, that the BHK cell line has been used to make clinical material. BHK cells are capable of making intracisternal A type particles (104), so it is likely that there would be a need to test for their presence in final preparations. It should be noted that CHO cells are used to make a number of recombinant protein products, and they also make intracisternal type A particles (105). The potency issues will be addressed with some combination of vector particle quantitation assay plus a test for expression of the gene encoded by the replicon. The particle quantitation assay may be plaque formation on the PCL but may eventually use RT-PCR or indicator cell lines that express a reporter protein in response to particle infection.

D. Replication-Competent Alphavirus

One agent that has received considerable time and effort to reduce to undetectable levels is replication-competent virus. One of the attractions of working with laboratory attenuated strains of Sindbis virus is their relatively benign clinical profile (1–3). Nonetheless, it is never desirable to administer replicating infectious viruses to patients if this is not the active agent. However, because testing destroys a sample, it is only possible to state that the probability of a patient receiving such an agent is below a defined level.

Given these circumstances, it is necessary to design, standardize, and eventually validate tests with a defined sensitivity measured by spiking preparations with low levels of replication-competent virus (106). At present the most direct assay is to add the vector sample to fresh monolayer of BHK cells. Any RCV present is expected to amplify in the BHK cells and be detected by the observance of cytopathic effects in the entire culture. However, the issues of interference by high-titer vector and the actual sensitivity remain to be carefully calibrated. This can be addressed to some extent by serial undiluted passaging of culture fluids on fresh BHK cell monolayers. As noted above, the doses for human use remain undefined, but clearly the larger the quantity of vector, the more likely that a rare event will occur and be detected. Whether such an event can be tolerated will depend on the perceived risk: benefit ratio and the actual feasibility of further decreasing its probability.

E. Clinical Applications and a Development Strategy for the Vector System

As noted above, the clinical applications where alphavirus replicons are expected to be useful are antigen-specific immunotherapy, including vaccines and cancer, as well as gene therapy applications that include wound healing and cardiac ischemia. It is expected that the risk: benefit ratio will determine the extent to which preclinical safety studies in animals will be necessary. In practical terms this means that the choice of a dire or life-threatening indication such as cancer or HIV infection as initial targets may allow earlier entry into the clinic and the creation of a clinical track record linked to the agent, its method of production, and subsequent testing. Provided there is no strong evidence of treatment-related toxicity, it should then be easier to move to non–life-threatening diseases and vaccine applications, using a comparable production process.

VII. CONCLUSIONS

It was little more than a decade ago that the genomes of alphaviruses could first be functionally manipulated, with the construction of a full-length ''infectious'' cDNA clone of Sindbis virus. This work opened the door to rapid construction of novel alphavirus-based vectors and subsequent testing in cultured cells and animals. Alphavirus replicon vector formats and methods for their commercial scale manufacture have been developed to the point where testing in human clinical trials is in the foreseeable future. The first applications likely to be tested in the clinic are preventative and therapeutic vaccines for infectious disease. Hopefully the promising results observed to date in animal models with both the plasmid- and particle-based alphavirus replicon vectors will translate to efficacy in humans.

Beyond in vivo vaccine and gene therapy applications, alphavirus-based vectors continue to be a useful tool in the laboratory for basic gene expression studies. Particularly interesting is the recent work with hippocampal slice cultures, where neurons are preferentially transduced over glial cells. Several diagnostic cell lines have now been developed for the detection of herpesviruses in which SIN replicons expressing a reporter protein are induced by the test virus. These cell lines may serve as a model for the development of assays for several adventitious viruses that currently lack sensitive and rapid detection methods. Finally, alphavirus vectors may prove to be useful for the production of many diverse gene transfer vectors described in this book, for which efficient methods are currently not available. It is likely that the rapidly increasing publicity surrounding alphavirus vectors will lead to many more creative applications.

REFERENCES

1. Schlesinger S, Schlesinger MJ. Togaviridae: The viruses and their replication. In: Fields BN, ed. Virology. 3rd ed. Philadelphia: Lippincott, 1996:825–842.
2. Johnston RE, Peters CJ. Alphaviruses. In: Fields BN, ed. Virology. 3rd ed. Philadelphia: Lippincott, 1996:843–898.
3. Strauss JH, Strauss CG. The alphaviruses: gene expression, replication, and evolution. Microbiol Rev 1994; 58: 491–562.

4. Paredes AM, Brown DT, Rothnagel R, Chiu W, Schoepp RJ, Johnston RE, Venkataram Prasad BV. Three-dimensional structure of a membrane-containing virus. PNAS 1993; 90:9095–9099.
5. Rice CM, Levis R, Strauss JH, Huang HV. Production of infectious RNA transcripts from Sindbis Virus cDNA clones: mapping of lethal mutations, rescue of a temperature-sensitive marker, and in vitro mutagenesis to generate defined mutants. J Virol 1987; 61:3809–3819.
6. Frolov I, Schlesinger S. Translation of Sindbis Virus mRNA: effects of sequences downstream of the initiating codon. J Virol 1994; 68:8111–8117.
7. Frolov I, Schlesinger S. Translation of Sindbis virus mRNA: analysis of sequences downstream of the initiating AUG codon that enhance translation. J Virol 1996; 70: 1182–1190.
8. Sjöberg EM, Suomalainen M, Garoff H. A significantly improved Semliki Forest virus expression system based on translation enhancer segments from the viral capsid gene. Bio/Technology 1994; 12:1127–1131.
9. Liljestrom P, Lusa S, Huylebroeck D, Garoff H. In vitro mutagenesis of a full-length cDNA clone of Semliki Forest virus: the small 6,000-molecular-weight membrane protein modulates virus release. J Virol 1991; 65:4107–4113.
10. Kuhn RJ, Niesters HGM, Hong Z, Strauss JH. Infectious RNA transcripts from Ross River virus cDNA clones and the construction and characterization of defined chimeras with Sindbis virus. Virology 1991; 182:430–441.
11. Davis NL, Willis LV, Smith JF, Johnston RE. In vitro synthesis of infectious Venezuelan equine encephalitis virus RNA from a cDNA clone: analysis of a viable deletion mutant. Virology 1989; 171:189–204.
12. Xiong C, Levis R, Shen P, Schlesinger S, Rice CM, Huang HV. Sindbis virus: an efficient, broad host range vector for gene expression in animal cells. Science 1989; 243: 1188–1191.
13. Liljeström P, Garoff H. A new generation of animal cell expression vectors based on the Semliki Forest virus replicon. Biotechnology 1991; 9:1356–1361.
14. Pushko P, Parker M, Ludwig GV, Davis NL, Johnston RE, Smith JG. Replicon-helper systems form attenuated Venezuelan equine encephalitis virus: expression of heterologous genes in vitro and immunization against heterologous pathogens in vivo. Virology 1997; 239:389–401.
15. Strong TV, Hampton TH, Louro I, Bilboa G, Conry RM, Curiel DT. Incorporation of β-globin untranslated regions into a Sindbis virus vector for augmentation of heterologous mRNA expression. Gene Therapy 1997; 4:624–627.
16. Bredenbeek PJ, Frolov I, Rice CM, Schlesinger S. Sindbis virus expression vectors: packaging of RNA replicons by using defective helper RNAs. J Virol 1993; 67:6439–6446.
17. Levis R, Weiss BG, Tsiang M, Huang H, Schlesinger S. Deletion mapping of Sindbis virus DI RNAs derived from cDNAs defines the sequences essential for replication and packaging. Cel 1986; 44:137–145.
18. Weiss BG, Schlesinger S. Recombination between Sindbis virus RNAs. J Virol 1991; 65(8):4017–4025.
19. Geigenmüller-Gnirke U, Weiss B, Wright R, Schlesinger S. Complementation between Sindbis viral RNAs produces infectious particles with a bipartite genome. Proc Natl Acad Sci USA 1991; 88(4):3253–3257.
20. Berglund P, Sjöberg M, Garoff H, Atkins GJ, Sheahan BJ, Liljeström P. Semliki Forest virus expression system: production of conditionally infectious recombinant particles. Bio/Technology 1992; 11:916–920.
21. Davis NL, Brown KW, Greenwald GF, Zajac AJ, Zacny VL, Smith JF, Johnston RF. Attenuated mutants of Venezuelan equine encephalitis virus containing lethal mutations in the PE2 cleavage signal combined with a second-site suppressor mutation in E1. Virology 1995; 212: 102–110.
22. Heidner HW, McKnight KL, Davis NL, Johnston RE. Lethality of PE2 incorporation into SIN virus can be suppressed by second-site mutations in E2 and E2. J Virol 1994; 68:2683–2692.
23. Tubulekas I, Liljestrom P. Suppressors of cleavage-site mutations in the p62 envelope protein of Semliki Forest virus reveal dynamics in spike structure and function. J Virol 1997; 72:2825–2831.
24. Frolov I, Hoffman TA, Pragai BM, Dryga SA, Huang HV, Schlesinger S, Rice CM. Alphavirus-based expression vectors: strategies and applications. PNAS 1996; 93: 11371–11377.
25. Frolov I, Frolova E, Schlesinger S. Sindbis virus replicons and Sindbis virus: assembly of chimeras and of particles deficient in virus RNA. J Virol 1997; 71:2819–2829.
26. Smerdou C, Liljestrom P. Two-helper RNA system for production of recombinant Semliki Forest virus particles. J Virol 1999; 73:1092–1098.
27. Polo JM, Belli BA, Driver DA, Sherrill S, Perri S, Gardner J, Hariharan MJ, Banks TA, Dubensky, Jr. TW. Unpublished observations.
28. Hahn CS, Hahn YS, Braciale TJ, Rice CM. Infectious Sindbis virus transient expression vectors for studying antigen processing and presentation. Proc Natl Acad Sci USA 1992; 89:2679–2683.
29. Pugachev KV, Mason PW, Shope RE, Frey TK. Double-subgenomic Sindbis virus recombinants expressing immunogenic proteins of Japanese encephalits virus induce significant protection in mice against lethal JEV infection. 1995; 212:587–594.
30. Davis NL, Brown KW, Johnston RE. A viral vaccine vector that expresses foreign genes in lymph nodes and protects against muscosal challenge. J Virol 1996; 70: 3781–3787.
31. Charles PC, Brown KW, Davis NL, Hart MK, Johnston RE. Mucosal immunity induced by parenteral immunization with a live attenuated Venezuelan equine encephalitis virus vaccine candidate. Virology 1997; 228:153–160.
32. Caley IJ, Betts MR, Iribeck DM, Davis N, Swanstrom R, Frelinger JA, Johnston RE. Humoral, mucosal, and cellular

immunity in response to a human immunodeficiency virus type 1 immunogen expressed by a Venezuelan equine encephalitis virus vaccine vector. J Virol 1997; 71: 3031–3038.
33. Olson KE, Higgs S, Gaines PJ, Powers AM, Davis BS, Kamrud KI, Carlson JO, Blair CD, Beaty BJ. Genetically engineered resistance to dengue-2 virus transmission in mosquitoes. Science 1996; 272:884–886.
34. Powers AM, Olson KE, Higgs S, Carlson JO, Beaty BJ. Intracellular immunization of mosquito cells to LaCrosse virus using a recombinant Sindbis virus vector. Virus Res 1994; 32:57–67.
35. Agapov EV, Frolov I, Lindenbach BD, Pragai BM, Schlesinger S, Rice CM. Noncytopathic Sindbis virus RNA vectors for heterologous gene expression. Proc Natl Acad Sci USA 1998; 95:12989–12994.
36. Driver DA, Latham EM, Polo JM, Belli BA, Banks TA, Chada S, Brumm D, Chang SMW, Mento SJ, Jolly DJ, Dubensky TW. Layered amplification of gene expression with a DNA gene delivery system. Ann NY Acad Sci 1995; 772:261–264.
37. Herweijer H, Latendresse JS, Williams P, Zhang G, Danko I, Schlesinger S, Wolff JA. A plasmid-based self-amplifying Sindbis virus vector. Hum Gene Ther 1995; 6: 1161–1167.
38. Dubensky Jr. TW, Driver DA, Polo JM, Belli BA, Latham EM, Ibanez CE, Chada S, Brumm D, Banks TA, Mento SJ, Jolly DJ, Chang SMW, Sindbis virus DNA-based expression vectors: utility for in vitro and in vivo gene transfer. J Virol 1996; 70:508–519.
39. Donnelly JJ, Ulmer JB, Liu MA. DNA vaccines. Life Sci 1997; 60(3):163–172.
40. Calarota S, Bratt G, Nordlund S, Hinkula J, Leandersson AC, Sandstrom E, Wahren B. Cellular cytoxic response induce by DNA vaccination in HIV-1-infected patients. Lancet 1998; 351:1320–1325.
41. MacGregor RR, Boyer JD, Ugen KE, Lacy KE, Gluckman SJ, Bagarazzi ML, Chattergoon MA, Baine Y, Higgins TJ, Ciccarelli RB, Coney LR, Ginsberg RS, Weiner DB. First human trial of a DNA-based vaccine for treatment of human immunodeficiency virus type 1 infection: safety and host response. J Infect Dis 1998; 178:92–100.
42. Wang R, Doolan DL, Le TP, Hedstrom RO, Coonan KM, Charoenvit Y, Jones TR, Hobart P, Margalith M, Ng J, Weiss WR, de Sedegah M, Taisne C, Norman JA, Hoffman SL. Induction of antigen-specific cytotoxic T lymphocytes in humans by a malaria DNA vaccine. Science 1998; 282: 476–480.
43. Berglund P, Smerdou C, Fleeton MN, Tubulekas I, Liljestrom P. Enhancing immune responses using suicidal DNA vaccines. Nat Biotechnol 1998; 16:562–565.
44. Smith JF, Crise B. Personal communication.
45. DiCiommo DP, Bremner R. Rapid, high level protein production using DNA-based Semliki Forest virus vectors. J Biol. Chem 1998; 273:18060–18066.
46. Driver DA, Polo JM, Belli BA, Banks TA, Hariharan M, Dubensky, Jr., TW. Plasmid DNA-based alphavirus expression vectors for nucleic acid immunization. Drugs 1998; 1:678–685.
47. Wolff J. American Society for Gene Therapy meeting, Washington, DC, May 1999.
48. Polo JM, Belli BA, Driver DA, Frolov I, Sherrill S, Hariharan MJ, Townsend K, Perri S, Mento SJ, Jolly DJ, Chang SMW, Schlesinger S, Dubensky TW. Stable alphavirus packaging cells lines for Sindbis virus-and Semliki Forest virus-derived vectors. PNAS 1999; 96:4598–4603.
49. Olivo PD, Frolov I, Schlesinger S. A cell line that expresses a reporter gene in response to infection by Sindbis Virus: a prototype for detection of positive strand RNA viruses. Virology 1994; 198:381–384.
50. Levine B, Goldman JE, Jiang HH, Griffin DE, Hardwick JM. Bcl-2 protects mice against fatal alphavirus encephalitis. Proc Natl Acad Sci 1996; 93:4810–4815.
51. Griffin DE, Hardwick JM. Regulators of apoptosis on the road to persistent alphavirus infection. Annu Rev Microbiol 1997; 51:565–592.
52. Frolov I, Schlesinger S. Comparison of the effects of Sindbis virus and Sindbis virus replicons on host cell protein synthesis and cytopathogenicity in BHK cells. J Virol 1994; 68:1721–1727.
53. Stollar V. Togaviruses in cultured arthropod cells. In: Schlesinger RW, ed. The Togaviruses—Biology, Structure, Replication. New York: Academic Press, Inc., 1980: 584–621.
54. Weiss B, Rosenthal R, Schlesinger S. Establishment and maintenance of persistent infection by Sindbis virus in BHK cells. J Virol 1980; 33:463–474.
55. Dryga SA, Dryga OA, Schlesinger S. Identification of mutations in a Sindbis virus variant able to establish persistent infection in BHK cells: the importance of mutation in the nsP2. gene. J Virol 1997; 228:74–83.
56. Frolov I, Agapov E, Hoffman Jr. TA, Pragai BM, Lippa M, Schlesinger S, Rice CM. Selection of RNA replicons capable of persistent noncytopathic replication in mammalian cells. J Virol 1999; 73:3854–3865.
57. Wang K-S, Kuhn RJ, Strauss EG, Ou S, Strauss JH. High-affinity laminin receptor is a receptor for Sindbis virus in mammallan cells. J Virol 1992; 66:4992–5001.
58. London SD, Schmaljohn AL, Dalrymple JM, Rice CM. Infectious enveloped RNA virus antigenic chimeras. Proc Natl Acad Sci USA 1992; 89:207–211.
59. Dubuisson J, Rice CM. Sindbis virus attachment: isolation and characterization of mutants with impaired binding to vertebrate cells. J Virol 1993; 67:3363–3374.
60. Ohno K, Sawai K, Iijima Y, Levin B, Meruelo D. Cell-specific targeting of Sindbis virus vectors displaying IgG-binding domains of protein A. Nature Biotech 1997; 15: 763–767.
61. Iijima Y, Ohno K, Ikeda H, Sawai K, Levin B, Meruelo D. Cell-specific targeting of a thymidine kinase/ganciclovir gene therapy system using a recombinant Sindbis virus vector. Int J Cancer 1999; 80:110–118.
62. Sawai K, Meruelo D. Cell-specific transfection of choriocarcinoma cells by using Sindbis virus hCG expressing

chimeric vector. Biochem Biophys Res Comm 1998; 248: 315–323.
63. Glasgow GM, McGee MM, Tarbatt CJ, Mooney DA, Sheahan BJ, Atkins GJ. The Semliki Forest virus vector induces p53-independent apoptosis. J Gen Virol 1998; 79: 2405–2410.
64. Levine B, Huang Q, Isaacs JT, Reed JC, Griffin DE, Hardwick JM. Conversion of lytic to persistent alphavirus infection by the bcl-2 cellular oncogene. Nature 1993; 361: 739–742.
65. Lewis J, Wesselingh SL, Griffin DE, Hardwick JM. Alphavirus-induced apoptosis in mouse brains correlates with neurovirulence. J Virol 1996; 70:1828–1835.
66. Tsuji M, Bergmann CC, Takita-Sonoda Y, Murata K-I, Rodrigues EG, Nussenzweig RS, Zavala F. Recombinant Sindbis viruses expressing a cytotoxic T-lymphocyte epitope of a malaria parasite or of influenza virus elicit protection against the corresponding pathogen in mice. J Virol 1998; 72:6907–6910.
67. Hariharan MJ, Driver DA, Townsend K, Brumm D, Polo JM, Belli BA, Catton DJ, Hsu D, Mittlestaedt D, McCormack JE, Karavodin L, Dubensky Jr. TW, Chang SMW, Banks TA. DNA immunization against herpes simplex virus: enhanced efficacy using a Sindbis virus-based vector. J Virol 1998; 72:950–958.
68. Mossman SP, Bex F, Berglund P, Arthos J, O'Neil SP, Riley D, Maul DH, Bruck C, Momin P, Burny A, Fultz PN, Mullis JI, Liljestrom P, Hoover EA. Protection against lethal simian immunodeficiency virus SIVsmmPBj14 disease by a recombinant Semliki Forest virus gp160 vaccine and by a gp120 subunit vaccine. J Virol 1996; 70: 1953–1960.
69. Berglund P, Quesada-Rolander M, Putkonen P, Biberfeld G, Thorstensson R, Liljestrom P. Outcome of immunization of cynomolgus monkeys with recombinant Semliki Forest virus encoding human immunodeficiency virus type 1 envelope protein and challenge with a high dose of SHIV-4 virus. AIDS Res Hum Retro 1997; 13:1487–1495.
70. Fleeton MN, Sheahan BJ, Gould EA, Atkins GJ, Liljestrom P. Recombinant Semliki Forest virus particles encoding the prME or NS1 proteins of louping ill virus protect mice from lethal challenge. J Gen Virol 1999; 80:1189–1198.
71. Colombage G, Hall R, Pavy M, Lobigs M. DNA-based and alphavirus-vectored immunisation with PrM and E proteins elicits long-lived and protective immunity against the flavivirus, murray valley encephalitis virus. Virology 1998; 250:151–163.
72. Malone JG, Bergland PJ, Liljestrom P, Rhodes GH, Malone RW. Mucosal immune responses associated with polynucleotide vaccination. Behring Inst Mitt 1997; 98: 63–72.
73. Berglund P, Fleeton MN, Smerdou C, Liljestrom P. Immunization with recombinant Semliki Forest virus induces protection against influenza challenge in mice. Vaccine 1998; 17:497–507.
74. Hevey M, Negley D, Pushko P, Smith J, Schmaljohn A. Marburg virus vaccines based upon alphavirus replicons protect guinea pigs and nonhuman primates. Virology 1998; 251:28–37.
75. Zhou X, Berglund P, Zhao H, Liljeström P, Jondal M. Generation of cytotoxic and humoral immune responses by nonreplicative recombinant Semliki Forest virus. PNAS 1995; 92:3009–3013.
76. Cella M, Salio M, Sakakibara Y, Langen H, Julkunen I, Lanzavecchia A. Maturation, activation, and protection of dendritic cells induced by double-stranded RNA. J Exp Med 1999; 189:821–829.
77. Ying H, Zaks TZ, Wang R-F, Irvine KR, Kammula US, Marincola FM, Leitner WW, Restifo NP. Cancer therapy using a self-replicating RNA vaccine. Nat Med 1999; 5: 823–827.
78. Zhang J, Asselin-Paturel C, Bex F, Bernard J, Chehimi J, Willems F, Caignard A, Berglund P, Liljestrom P, Burny A, Chouaib S. Cloning of human IL-12 p40 and p35 DNA into the Semliki Forest virus vector: expression of IL-12 in human tumor cells. Gene Ther 1997; 4:367–374.
79. Grieder FB, Davis NL, Aronson JF, Charles PC, Sellon DC, Suzuki K, Johnston RE. Specific restrictions in the progression of Venezuelan equine encephalitis virus induced disease resulting from single amino acid changes in the glycoproteins. Virology 1995; 206:994–1006.
80. Griffin D. Molecular pathogenesis of Sindbis virus encephalitis in experimental animals. Adv Virus Res 1989; 36:255–271.
81. Enrengruber MU, Lundstrom K, Schweitzer C, Heuss C, Schlesinger S, Gahwiler BH. Recombinant Semliki Forest virus and Sindbis virus efficiently infect neurons in hippocampal slice cultures. PNAS 1999; 96:7041–7046.
82. Maletic-Savatic M, Malinow R, Svoboda K. Rapid dendritic morphogenesis in CA1 hipppocampal dendrites induced by synaptic activity. Science 1999; 283:1923–1926.
83. Lundstrom K. Alphaviruses as tools in neurobiology and gene therapy. J Recept Sig Transduc Res 1999; 19: 673–686.
84. Altman-Hamamdzic S, Groseclose C, Ma J-X, Hamamdzic D, Vrindavanam NS, Middaugh LD, Parratto NP, Sallee FR. Expression of β-galactosidase in mouse brain: utilization of a novel nonreplicative Sindbis virus vector as a neuronal gene delivery system. Gene Ther 1997; 4: 815–822.
85. Gwag BJ, Kim EY, Ryu BR, Won SJ, Ko HW, Oh YJ, Cho YG, Ha SJ, Sung YC. A neuron-specific gene transfer by a recombinant defective Sindbis virus. Mol Brain Res 1998; 63:53–61.
86. Roks AJM, Pinto YM, Paul M, Pries F, Stula M, Eschenhagen T, Orzechowski HD, Gschwendt S, Wilschut J, van Gilst WH. Vectors based on Semliki Forest virus for rapid and efficient gene transfer into non-endothelial cardiovascular cells: comparison to adenovirus. Cardio Res 1997; 35:498–504.
87. Lee JS, Feldman AM. Gene therapy for therapeutic myocardial angiogenesis: a promising synthesis of two emerging technologies. Nat Med 1998; 4:732–742.

88. Rosengart TK, Patel SR, Crystal RG. Therapeutic angiogenesis: protein and gene therapy delivery strategies. J Cardio Risk 1999; 6:29–40.
89. Safi Jr. J, Gloe TR, Riccioni T, Kovesdi I, Capogrossi MC. Gene therapy with angiogenic factors: a new potential approach to the treatment of ischemic diseases. J Mol Cell Cardiol 1997; 29:2311–2325.
90. DePolo NJ, Harkleroad CE, Bodner M, Watt AT, Anderson CG, Greengard JS, Murthy KK, Dubensky Jr. TW, Jolly DJ. The resistance of retroviral vectors produced from human cells to serum inactivation in vivo and in vitro is primate species dependent. J Virol 1999; 73:6708–6714.
91. Li KJ, Garoff H. Production of infectious recombinant Moloney murine leukemia virus particles in BHK cells using Semliki Forest virus-derived RNA expression vectors. PNAS 1996; 93:11658–11663.
92. Li KJ, Garoff H. Packaging of intron-containing genes into retrovirus vectors by alphavirus vectors. PNAS 1998; 95: 3650–3654.
93. Wahlfors JJ, Xanthopoulos KG, Morgan RA. Semliki Forest virus-mediated production of retroviral vector RNA in retroviral packaging cells. Human Gene Ther 1997; 8: 2031–2041.
94. Wahlfors JJ, Morgan RA. Production of minigene-containing retroviral vectors using an alphavirus-retrovirus hybrid vector system. Human Gene Ther 1999; 10:1197–1206.
95. Ivanova L, Schlesinger S, Olivo PD. Regulated expression of a Sindbis virus replicon by herpesvirus promoters. J Virol 1999; 73:1998–2005.
96. Fong TC, Sauter SL, Ibanez CE, Sheridan PL, Jolly DJ. The use and development of retroviral vectors to deliver cytokine genes for cancer therapy. Crit Rev Drug Carrier Systems 2000; in press.
97. Hitt M, Bett AJ, Addison CL, Prevec L, Graham FL. In: Adolph KW, ed. Methods in Molecular Genetics. San Diego: Academic, 1995:13–30.
98. Samulski RJ, Sally M, Muzyczka N. Adeno-associated Viral Vectors. Cold Spring Harbor, NY: Cold Spring Harbor Laboratory Press, 1999:131.
99. Laquerre C, Goins WF, Moriuchi S, Oligino TJ, Krisky DM, Marconi P, Soares MK, Cohen JB, Glorioso JC. Gene-Transfer Tool: Herpes Simplex Virus Vectors. Cold Spring Harbor, NY: Cold Spring Harbor Laboratory Press, 1999:173–208.
100. Montagnon B, Vincent-Falquet JC, Fanget B. Thousand litre scale microcarrier culture of vero cells for killed polio virus vaccine. Promising results. Fifth General Meeting of ESACT, Copenhagen, Denmark, 1982. Dev Biol Standard 1984; 55:37–42.
101. Gershon AA, LaRussa P, Steinberg S, Silverstein S. Varicella vaccine. The American experience. J Infect Dis 1992; 166:S63–S68.
102. Kotani H, Newton PB III, Zhang S, Chiang YL, Otto E, Weaver L, Blaese RM, Anderson WF, McGarrity GJ. Improved methods of retroviral vector transduction and production for gene therapy. Hum Gene Ther 1994; 5: 19–28.
103. Prior CP, Doyle KR, Duffy A, Hope JA, Moellering DJ, Prior M, Scott RW, Tolbert WR. The recovery of highly purified biopharmaceuticals from perfusion cell culture bioreactors. J Parenteral Sci Tech 1989; 43:15–23.
104. Reuss FU. Expression of intracisternal A-particle-related retroviral element-encoded envelope proteins detected in cell lines. J Virol 1992; 66:1915–1923.
105. Anderson KP, Low ML, Lie YS, Keller G, Dinowitz M. Endogenous origin of defective retroviruslike particles from a recombinant Chinese hamster ovary cell line. Virology 1991; 181:305–311.
106. Sajjadi N. Development of retroviral-based gene therapy products: a quality control perspective. Qual Assur J 1997; 2:113.

7

Gene Delivery with Polyethylenimine

S. M. Zou and Jean-Paul Behr
Laboratoire de Chimie Génétique, CNRS–URA 1386, Illkirch, France

D. Goula and Barbara Demeneix
Laboratoire de Physiologie Générale et Comparée, CNRS–UMR 8572, Muséum National d'Historie Naturelle, Paris, France

I. INTRODUCTION

In order for gene therapy to become a realistic prospect, gene transfer must be vastly improved. Indeed, getting the pro-drug DNA into the cell and into the nucleus remains a major bottleneck, and currently available gene transfer techniques are failing to provide sufficient expression of the desired protein products. Even recombinant viral methods still show limited performances in clinical situations, and nonviral methods are considered to be of still lower efficiency.

For DNA to be of therapeutic use, its transfer into the cell must be followed by a cascade of events beginning in the nucleus and culminating in the synthesis of a large number of effector protein molecules. Vector systems must thus deliver the exogenous DNA to the nucleus. This requires cell targeting, efficient cell membrane rupture mechanisms, and nuclear transport. Membrane rupture can occur either directly at the cell surface or after endocytosis.

In this chapter we consider how the properties of polyethylenimine (PEI), a cationic polymer, can be exploited to optimize each of these steps. Although most gene therapy approaches will involve gene transfer in vivo, results from in vitro work are pertinent to the discussion for two main reasons. First, results obtained on cultured cells can provide insights into transfer mechanisms, and second, they are directly applicable to cell-based therapies that are based on ex vivo gene delivery. Taken together, the results discussed here show PEI to be one of the best synthetic vectors currently available for in vitro gene transfer. Moreover, PEI is proving to be an extremely versatile and effective carrier for in vivo delivery, especially for delivering genes into the mammalian brain and lung.

Before reviewing the use of PEI in in vitro and in vivo settings, we will deal with some of the theories behind its mode of action at the levels of DNA compaction, interaction with the cell membrane, and cell entry. To this end our discussion will encompass the properties of polycationic lipids, because it was work on these compounds that produced the logic for testing the gene-transfer capacity of PEI.

First, complex formation between DNA and cationic lipids or polymers is a process that is still largely empirical and uncontrolled. Basically, the anionic plasmid and cationic vector will collapse into particles. It is important to note that with polycationic (as distinct from monocationic) molecules, like charges borne on the molecule will repel each other, thus extending the molecule and optimizing counterion collapse on interaction with the polyanionic DNA. Such properties will also affect interaction with the cell membrane, because high charge density will favor interactions with the cell surface (unfortunately also with the extracellular matrix and with the complement system). Indeed, provided the net charge of the complex formation is cationic (with an excess ratio of cationic charges to nucleic acid phosphates), cooperative ionic interaction will again enable the complexes to bind to polyanionic glycosaminoglycans of the cell membrane (1,2). In vitro studies with both cationic lipids and cationic polymers have shown that electrostatic interactions between the negatively charged cell membranes and the positively charged DNA/vector complexes are enhanced by increasing the overall charge of the complexes, which in turn is achieved by increasing the ratio of vector to DNA (3,4). Moreover, electron microscopy has been used to follow these interactions in vitro, and such studies show that on adherent cells, interactions of positively charged complexes with the cell membrane will lead to endocytosis (1).

As to the process of membrane rupture, again, if an extended polycation (such as spermine) is used as headgroup for a lipid, it will have a favorable effect because its overall molecular shape will be a wedge, which upon packing with DNA leads to nonbilayer phases capable of perturbing cellular membranes. Another membrane-rupturing property of polyamines could come from the buffering potential of amine functions remaining nonprotonated at physiological pH. This hypothesis is supported by the observation that transfection with lipopolyamines cannot be improved either by the addition of fusogenic peptides (5) or with chloroquine (6). Moreover, the potentiometric protonation states of the amines show that at physiological pH only three of the four nitrogens in the spermine head are cationic. The pKa of the last amine is 5.5 (7), halfway between the extracellular and intralysosomal pH values. This feature contrasts with the headgroups of monovalent-cationic lipids, which contain a constitutively charged ammonium that cannot provide any buffering capacity in endosomes. The buffering hypothesis is again bolstered by results obtained with cationic polymers such as polyamidoamine (8) and polyethylenimine (9). These macromolecules bear a large number of amine groups, and again, as for the lipopolyamines, not all of these amines are protonated at physiological pH. In fact, in PEI, one in every third atom is an amino nitrogen that can be protonated, making PEI the cationic polymer having the highest charge density potential. Moreover, the overall protonation level of PEI increases from 20 to 45% between pH 7 and 5 (10) (Fig. 1A).

Thus, certain polycationic vectors can provide a substrate for a protonation process, which will result in a distribution of decreasing pK as it goes on and on, further resulting in a buffering capacity below neutral pH. This will not only tend to inhibit the action of the lysosomal nucleases

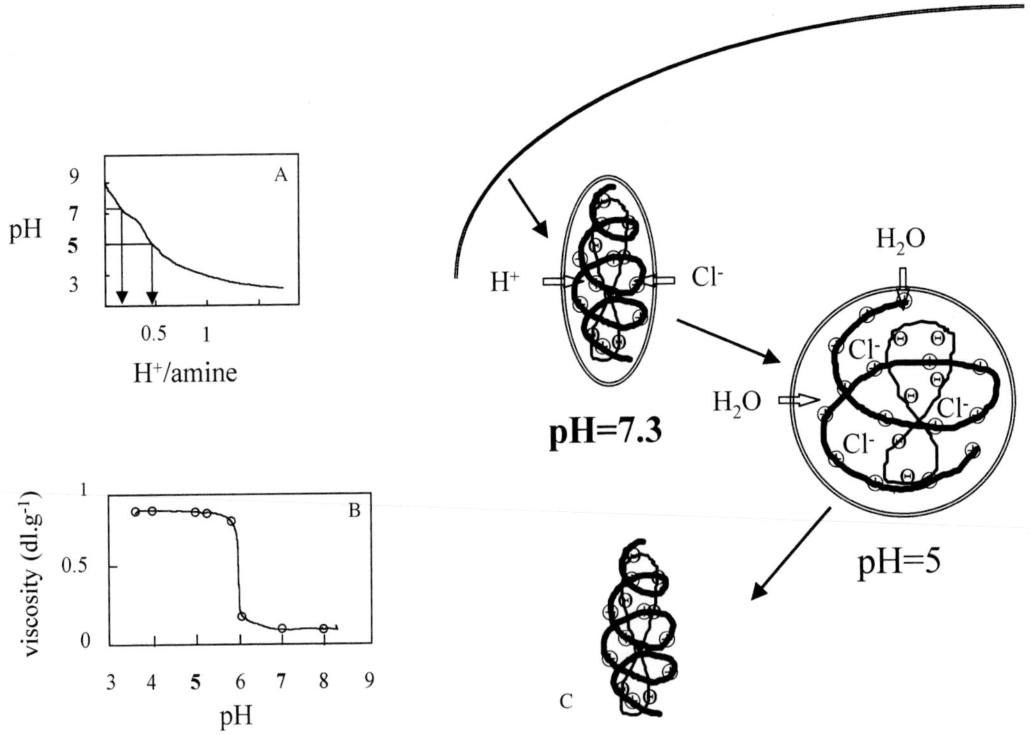

Figure 1 The proton sponge hypothesis: (A) Titration curve showing overall protonation level of PEI versus pH; (B) viscosity of a PEI solution versus pH; (C) extensive H^+ and Cl^- entry into the PEI-containing vacuole leads to polymer expansion and osmotic swelling.

(that have an acid optimal pH), but will also alter the osmolarity of the vesicle. Indeed, the accumulation of protons brought in by the endosomal ATPase is coupled to an influx of chloride anions (11). In the presence of a protonatable polycation such as PEI there will be a large increase in the ionic concentration within the endosome, resulting in a swelling of the polymer by internal charge repulsion and concomitant osmotic swelling of the endosome due to water entry. The sudden swelling of PEI at pH 6 is demonstrated by its 20-fold increase in viscosity (Fig. 1B). With both of these phenomena occurring simultaneously, endosomal membrane stability is sorely impaired. A diagram of the hypothetical sequence of events leading from DNA condensation to endosome lysis and intracellular release of the DNA is provided in Fig. 1C.

The steps following cell entry and endosome release are intracellular trafficking and nuclear membrane crossing, dissociation of complexes occurring either in the cytoplasm or the nucleus. Little is known about how these steps occur, but we do know that they are inefficient. A good analytical approach for dissecting these components is to follow the expression of complexes injected directly into the cytoplasm or nucleus of cells in culture (12). Indeed, complexing DNA with PEI enhances transgene expression fourfold when complexes are injected directly into the cytoplasm of COS-7 cells (Fig. 2a). This increased efficiency is apparently due to nucleic acid compaction by PEI, rather than charge ratio of the complexes, as it is already maximal at an amine to phosphate ratio of 2 (Fig. 2b) where DNA is fully condensed. The work of Pollard and coworkers (12) also shows that breakdown of the nuclear envelope, as occurs in cell division, is not necessary for penetration of DNA-PEI complexes into the nucleus. This is in agreement with previously published data on transfection of postmitotic cells such as differentiated neurons (4,13). The next stage in gene transfer is dissociation of the complexes. Microinjection experiments showed that, in contrast to cationic lipids, PEI does not prevent gene expression when complexes are injected into the nucleus (12). Plasmid release, presumably by exchange with cellular DNA, must be rapid because expression kinetics are similar with naked or PEI-complexed DNA.

We will now consider the gene-transfer performances of different forms of the cationic polymer PEI in ex vivo and in vivo settings. We will mainly make reference to two medium molecular weight forms of PEI, the branched 25 kDa polymer (Aldrich) and the fully linear 22 kDa polymer (Euromedex, France).

II. EX VIVO GENE DELIVERY

A frequent problem when transfecting cells in culture is the presence of serum, which generally lowers efficiency or increases the variability of many gene-transfer vectors. This same factor can of course hinder their in vivo use. To overcome this limitation, one can proceed by sequential addition of a cationic vector to the DNA. Complexes produced in such a manner provide higher transfection efficiencies in the presence of serum (14).

When a cationic vector is used at an excess ratio of cationic charges to nucleic acid phosphates, the resulting

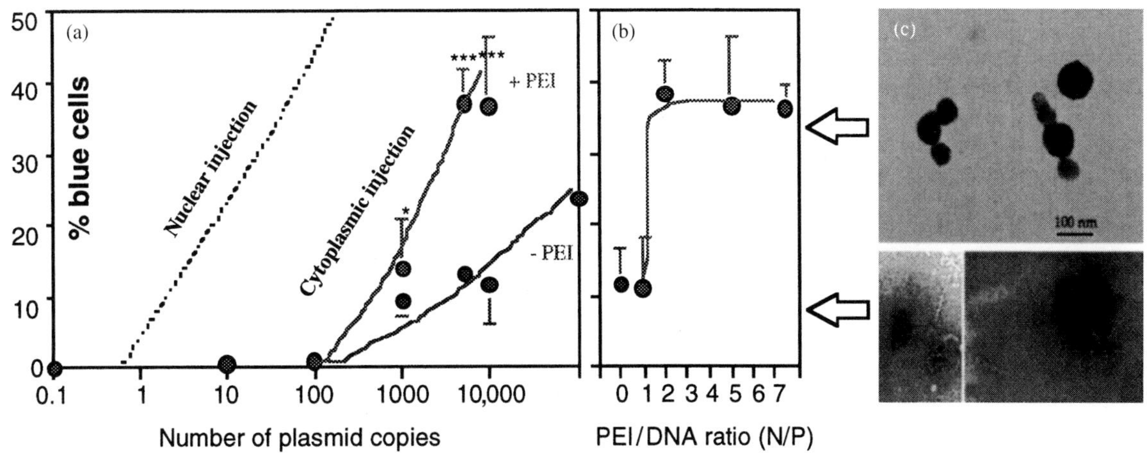

Figure 2 Intracellular microinjection of pCMV-gal DNA into COS-7 cells. (a) Comparison of transfection efficiencies following nuclear or cytoplasmic (±PEI) injection. (b) Effect of PEI/DNA ratio on transgene expression after cytoplasmic injection. (c) Electron microscopy photograph of PEI/DNA complexes at low and high N/P ratio.

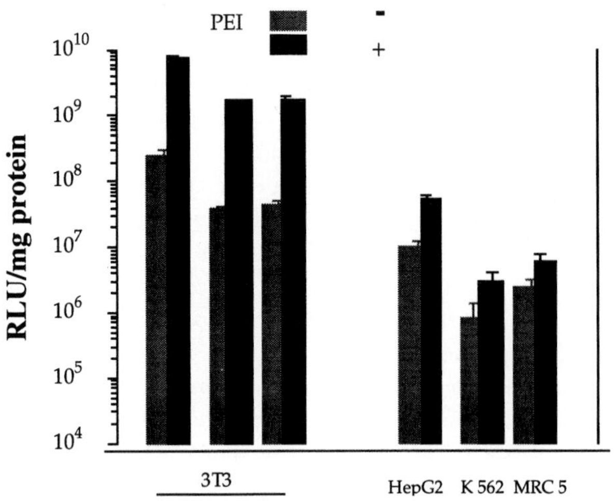

Figure 3 PEI-mediated transfection of various cell types is increased by gentle centrifugation (+) of the complexes onto the cells in culture.

particles fix to the cell surface. Transfection efficiency increases concomitantly with charge ratio until toxicity results. This coarse optimization can, however, be much more finely tuned. One approach considers that the transfection efficiency of small vector-DNA complexes may be limited by Brownian motion, as recently described for retroviruses (15). To counter this, we used centrifugation (5 min at 280 *g*) of cells covered by the transfection mixture and found that it increased PEI transfection efficiencies up to 50-fold (Fig. 3) (14).

III. IN VIVO DELIVERY

A. Principles: Using Polycationic Vectors In Vivo

As when working with polycationic lipids, different amine: phosphate ratios are required for optimal transfection efficiencies with PEI in vitro and in vivo (9). In both the newborn and adult central nervous systems, complexes with amine: phosphate ratios of 6 provide the best transfection efficiencies, whereas ratios of 9 amines per DNA phosphate were found to be optimal in vitro (13; D. Goula et al., unpublished observations). Theoretically, ratios of 6 should produce almost neutral complexes because only one in five of the protonatable amines carried by the PEI are in fact protonated at pH 7. However, preliminary data show that complexes bear net positive charges above amine: phosphate (N:P) ratios of 3:1 (16). This is the consequence of an increased basicity of some of the PEI amine functions when complexed with DNA.

B. Formulation Affects Size and Performance of Complexes

The solution in which the complexes are prepared is a major factor affecting both the net charge borne by the complex, its size, and hence its transfection efficiency. Indeed, we have compared the sizes and transfection efficiencies of complexes prepared with 22 kDa linear PEI in two different iso-osmotic solutions: 5% glucose and 150 mM NaCl (17). When plasmid DNA was formulated with 22 kDa PEI in 5% glucose, it produced a homogeneous population of complexes with mean diameters ranging from 30 to 100 nm according to the amount of PEI used (Fig. 4). In contrast, formulation in physiological saline produced complexes an order of magnitude greater (≥ 1 μm). Increasing the N:P ratio from 2 to 6 or 10 decreased the size of particles formulated in glucose. More than 60% of the particles had diameters of 50–60 nm, and this size was reproducible over a wide range of DNA concentrations (10–500 μg/mL). However, a similar increase in N:P ratio had no effect on particles formulated in NaCl (Fig. 4B and C).

Carrying out electron microscopy on particles formed in either NaCl or glucose confirmed these findings. Particles formed in NaCl were clumped and of highly irregular shape (Fig. 4d), whereas complexes produced in glucose were discrete spheres or toroids (Fig. 4E). Again, size measurement showed particles formulated in glucose to have a mean size (diameter or length) of 37 $\pm$ 26 nm (n = 83) with very few particles in oligomeric structures.

IV. DELIVERY TO THE CENTRAL NERVOUS SYSTEM

A. Intrathecal Delivery

One of the most promising aspects of PEI-based gene transfer comes from results obtained in vivo. Indeed, the main limitation of current nonviral gene-transfer methods is their relatively low efficiencies in vivo, cationic lipids often requiring dilution with neutral lipids to achieve delivery. No such molecular adjustments with neutral compounds are required with PEI. In both the adult and the newborn mouse brain, PEI-DNA complexes provide levels of transfection equal to those found in vitro for the same amount of DNA applied to primary neuronal cultures (up to 10^6 RLU, approximately 3.5 ng luciferase, per μg DNA injected). The best levels of expression in both models are obtained with polymers having a medium MW, either 25 kDa branched

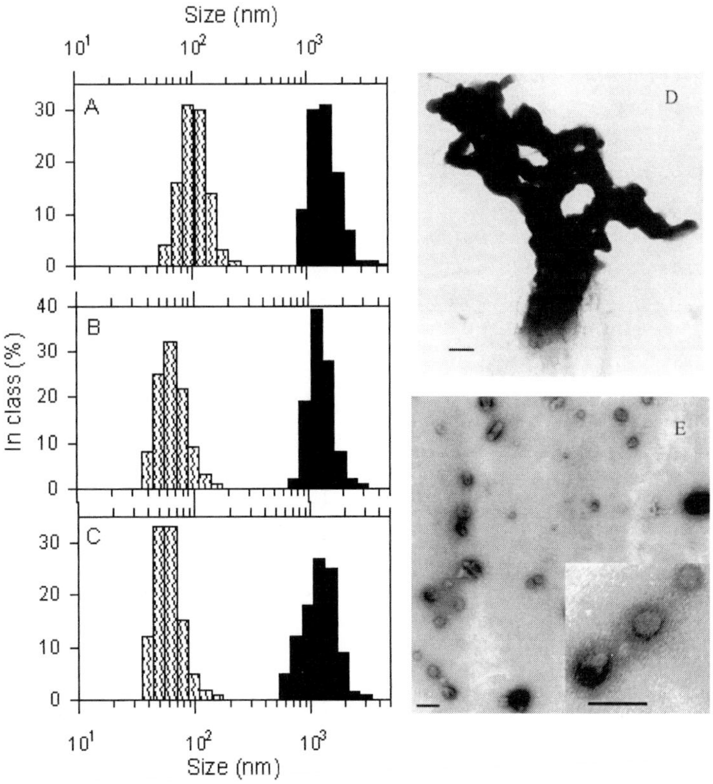

Figure 4 PEI-DNA complexes have different sizes according to the solutions used for formulation. (A–C) Complexes were prepared by separate dilution of PEI (N/P = 2, 6, and 10 for A, B, and C, respectively) and DNA (20 μg) into 500 μL of NaCl 0.15 M (plain bars) or 5% glucose (hatched bars), followed by mixing of the two solutions (glucose/DNA to glucose/PEI or NaCl/DNA to NaCl/PEI). After 10–20 min, particle size was determined by quasi-elastic light scattering (QUELS) on a Zetamasters 3 (Malvern Instruments, Orsay, France). (D, E) Electron micrographs of PEI 22kDa-DNA complexes prepared in NaCl 0.15 M (D, N/P = 2) or in 5% (w/w) glucose (E, N/P = 5); bars represent 100 nm.

(13) or 22 kDa linear (D Goula et al., unpublished results). In the adult brain we have used double immunostaining with antibodies against cell-specific markers and transgene products to show that both neurons and glia can be transduced by PEI transfection in vivo (13,18). Moreover, toxicity is low, no mortality being observed in injected animals and no necrosis at the site of injection. Also of interest is that when transfecting neuronal cells in culture, no interference with membrane excitability is seen (19).

B. Intraventricular Injection

Injection of DNA-PEI 22 kDa complexes formulated in glucose into the brain ventricles of adult mice showed the complexes to be highly diffusible in the cerebrospinal fluid, diffusing from a single site of injection throughout the entire brain ventricular spaces (18). These complexes are of low mean size (<100 nm). There is another report in the literature on size of complexes formed with 22 kDa PEI. Dunlap and coworkers (20) examined DNA-lipospermine or DNA-PEI complexes by scanning force microscopy imaged in low-salt (15 mM NaCl) conditions. These authors found, as did Tang and Szoka (21) using branched 25 kDa PEI, that the complexes were small (<100 nm in both cases), but they did not test their transfection performance in vivo or in physiological fluids. We also have found that complexes formed with 25 kDa PEI are of small size in NaCl, and moreover for this polymer we find no size difference whether formulated in NaCl or glucose. However, there must be an intrinsic difference in complexes formed with branched or linear PEI, and indeed when tested in vivo we find more efficient and reproducible results with the 22 kDa polymer. Moreover, not only are the particles formed with the linear 22 kDa polymer in 5% glucose stable and highly diffusible, but they are also efficient for gene transfer. This is shown by the fact that not only were positive cells found throughout the brain, but more importantly, between 10 and 20 cells expressing the transgene were generally found in *each* brain section.

V. INTRAVENOUS DELIVERY

In the light of the findings that complexes formulated in glucose provided efficient gene expression in the CNS (13,18), we chose to examine the effects of injecting complexes formulated with 22 kDa PEI in 5% glucose directly into the blood system and to examine transgene expression in a variety of organs. Complexes were delivered into adult mice through the tail vein. Two marker genes were used, β-galactosidase and luciferase. High levels of luciferase expression (10^7 RLU or 35 ng luciferase/mg protein) were found in the lung when DNA was complexed with PEI at a ratio of 4 nitrogen equivalents per DNA phosphate. This level of expression is 4 orders of magnitude greater than control levels. Our controls were animals injected with an equivalent amount of naked DNA, whereas the only other report to show a similar 4 orders of magnitude increase was that of Y. Liu and coworkers (22), who used uninjected animals as controls. Using the same basis of comparison—uninjected animals—PEI vectorization provides levels of transgene expression 5 orders of magnitude greater than background. This result is bolstered by the β-galactosidase expression data, obtained with two different constructs, having cytoplasmic and nuclear localization directed proteins. In both cases the lung was seen to strongly express the transgene with no histological abnormality (17).

Tail vein injection resulted in lower levels of transfection in the heart, spleen, liver, and kidney. Expression was dose and time dependent in all tissues examined (Fig. 5) (17). In the lung, β-galactosidase staining showed transgene expression in clusters of 10 or more pulmonary cells including the alveolar endothelium, squamous and great alveolar epithelial cells (type I and II pneumocytes), and septal cells. These findings indicate that the complexes pass the capillary barrier in the lung.

One of the problems of injection of DNA-PEI complexes into the blood stream is that even slightly positively charged complexes will attract circulating proteins such as albumin. They may also, to variable extents, activate the complement system (23). To assess the effect of interaction with serum components on transfection efficiency, we preincubated DNA-PEI complexes with mouse serum for 10 minutes prior to injection of the suspension into the tail vein. We found (Fig. 6) that this preincubation completely changed the profile of expression in the target tissues, with lungs and liver now expressing equivalent amounts of luciferase protein ($\sim 5.10^5$ RLU/mg protein). This contrasts with that seen when complexes are injected without prior incubation in serum, where lung expression is more that 2 orders of magnitude greater than that seen in the liver at the same time point (Fig. 5). The decreased levels of expression in the lungs may be due to the fact that preincubation with serum changes the size or the charge of the complexes and thus their interaction with different cell types. These possibilities are currently being investigated.

VI. FUTURE DIRECTIONS

A. Targeting

One of the main goals of gene-therapy researchers will be to obtain not only efficient gene transfer, but also transfer that is targeted to specific tissues. Targeting can be achieved either by use of cell-specific promoters or by addition of cell-specific ligands, receptors, or antibodies. Targeting by addition of cell-specific molecules to the vector could have two major advantages; first, it will reduce undesirable toxic effects in tissues that do not require treatment, and second, ideally should increase efficiency if most of the transgenes reach their target rather than be dispersed in irrelevant destinations. PEI has already proven to be a good starting point for the production of such modified vectors. Several cases have been reported. Zanta and coworkers (24) showed that a 5% substitution of PEI amine functions with galactose gave selective transfection of hepatocytes in the presence of 10% serum. A number of experimental paradigms showed this transfection to be dependent on asialoglycoprotein receptor–mediated endocytosis: removal of the targeting galactose residues or their replacement by glucose suppressed transfection, as did addition of excess asialofetuin to the culture medium. The second example is that from the group of E. Wagner (6). These authors coupled a variety of cell-binding ligands to PEI and showed selective transfection of neuroblastoma, melanoma, and leukemia cell lines. In this series of experiments and those reported by Zanta et al., the importance of the ligand-receptor interaction was demonstrated by the fact that transfection was observed at low PEI cation: DNA anion ratios, where ligand-free PEI is inefficient. Finally, integrin-mediated transfection of epithelial cells could be obtained with a RGD-peptide–containing PEI (25).

As yet only one report (26) has appeared on the behavior of these modified PEIs in in vivo situations. It is conceivable that if they bear low net charges, they may behave like "stealth" liposomes and avoid rapid elimination in the reticuloendothelial system.

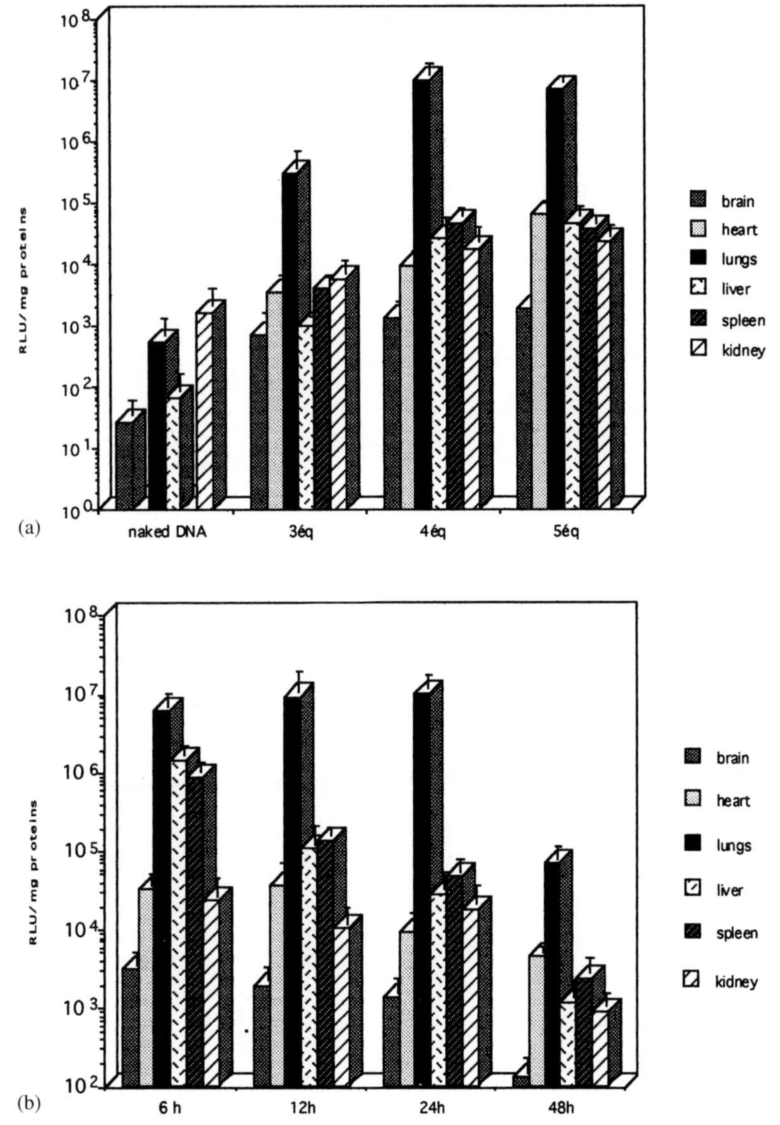

Figure 5 Optimization of PEI-DNA formulation for intravenous gene delivery. (a) Transgene expression is a function of PEI nitrogen-to-DNA phosphate (N/P) ratio. Mice were injected through the tail vein with 125 μg CMV-luciferase complexed with increasing amounts of 22 kDa PEI in 500 μL of 5% glucose. Animals were sacrified 24 hours later, tissues removed, and homogenized. Luciferase assays were carried out as described in Ref. 13. Protein content was measured using a Bradford assay. Means $\pm$ SEM are given; $n \geq 4$ in all cases. (b) Transgene expression as a function of time postinjection. Mice were injected through the tail vein with 125 μg of CMV-luciferase complexed with 22 kDa PEI at a N/P ratio of 4 in 500 μL of 5% glucose. Animals were sacrified the times indicated. Other details as in (a).

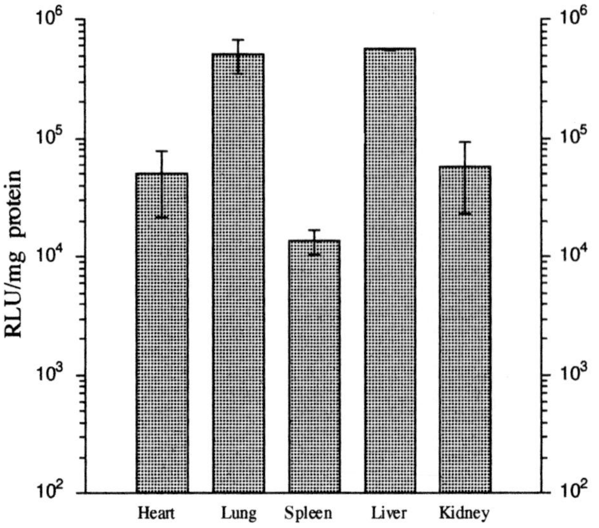

Figure 6 The effect of serum on gene transfer following i.v. injection in mice. Prior to injection, 50 μg of pCMV-luc plasmid were complexed with 22 kDa PEI at N/P = 10 in 400 μL, of 5% glucose supplemented with 100 μL of fresh murine serum. After homogenization the complexes were injected intravenously. Twenty-four hours later, luciferase activity was assayed (data is given as mean value SD, n = 4).

B. Sustained Expression

Another central problem remaining to be addressed is that of duration of expression. Indeed, as for adenoviral vectors that, like plasmid DNA, do rely on integration in the genome but have an episomal location in the nucleus, transgene expression following PEI-based gene transfer is not long-lasting. In the brain of adult mice we found measurable luciferase expressions up to 2 weeks posttransfection, and this was not improved by using a ''housekeeping'' promoter such as β-actin (13). Moreover, in the lungs, as with other synthetic vector systems, expression is ephemeral, reaching a peak at 24 hours and declining rapidly thereafter (17). In other systems the levels and duration of gene expression have been shown to be greatly affected by different plasmid constructs and the features that govern gene expression and protein production, such as promoters, polyadenylation sequences, and signal peptides (27). How these different factors affect in vivo expression in different tissues requires detailed investigation.

VII. CONCLUSION

PEI is clearly a most promising vector for gene delivery in a number of ex vivo and in vivo settings. The work presented here shows that correct formulation allows for control of DNA condensation and size of the resulting complexes. These factors will in turn affect not only interaction with the cell membrane and release from the endosome, but also intracellular trafficking and possibly nuclear entry, dissociation of complexes, and gene expression. Analyzing and improving each of these steps will help to lead to the ultimate goal of high, sustained, regulatable gene expression in targeted tissues.

ACKNOWLEDGMENTS

We acknowledge with gratitude our coworkers Bassima Abdallah, Corrine Benoist, and Isabelle Seugnet (MNHN, Paris). This work has been supported by the Centre National de la Recherche Scientifique, the Association Française de Lutte contre la Mucoviscidose, the Association Francaise contre les Myopathies, la Ligue contre le Cancer, and the Association pour la Recherche contre le Cancer.

REFERENCES

1. Labat-Moleur F, Steffan AM, Brisson CC, Perron H, Feugeas O, Furstenberger P, Oberling F, Brambilla E, Behr JP. Gene Ther 1996; 3:1010–1017.
2. Mislick KA, Baldeschwieler JD. Proc Natl Acad Sci USA 1996; 93:12349–12354.
3. Behr J, Demeneix B, Loeffler J, Perez-Mutul J. Proc Natl Acad Sci USA 1989; 86:6982–6986.
4. Boussif O, Lezoualc'h F, Zanta MA, Mergny M, Scherman D, Demeneix B, Behr J-P. Proc Natl Acad Sci USA 1995; 92:7297–7303.
5. Remy JS, Kichler A, Mordinov V, Schuber F, Behr JP. Proc Natl Acad Sci USA 1995; 92:1744–1748.
6. Kircheis R, Kichler A, Wallner G, Kursa M, Ogris M, Felzmann T, Buchberger M, Wagner E. Gene Ther 1997; 4: 409–418.
7. Behr JP. Bioconj Chem 1994; 5:382–389.
8. Haensler J, Szoka FC. Bioconj Chem 1993; 4:32–39.
9. Behr JP, Demeneix BA. Curr Res Mol Ther 1998; 1:5–12.
10. Suh J, Paik H-J, Hwang BK. Bioorg Chem 1994; 22: 318–327.
11. Nelson N. Trends Pharmacol Sci 1991; 12:71–75.
12. Pollard H, Remy J, Loussouarn G, Demolombe S, Behr J, Escande D. J Biol Chem 1998; 273:7507–7511.
13. Abdallah B, Hassan A, Benoist C, Goula D, Behr JP. Demeneix BA. Hum Gene Ther 1996; 7:1947–1954.
14. Boussif O, Zanta MA, Behr JP. Gene Ther 1996; 3: 1074–1080.
15. Chuck AS, Clarke MF, Palsson BO. Hum Gene Ther 1996; 7:1527–1534.
16. Erbacher P, Zou S, Steffan AM, Remy JS. Pharm Res 1998a; 15:1332–1339.

17. Goula D, Benoist C, Mantero S, Merlo G, Levi G, Demeneix B. Gene Ther 1998; 5:1291–1295.
18. Goula D, Remy J, Erbacher P, Wasowicz M, Levi G, Abdallah B, Demeneix B. Gene Ther 1998; 5:712–717.
19. Lambert RC, Maulet Y, Dupont JL, Mykita S, Craig P, Volsen S, Feltz A. Mol Cell Neurosci 1996; 7:239–246.
20. Dunlap DD, Maggi A, Soria MR, Monaco L. Nucleic Acids Res 1997; 25:3095–3101.
21. Tang MX, Szoka FC. Gene Ther 1997; 4:823–832.
22. Liu Y, Mounkes LC, Liggitt HD, Brown CS, Solodin I, Heath TD, Debs RJ. Nat Biotechnol 1997; 15:167–173.
23. Plank C, Mechtler K, Szoka, Jr. FC, Wagner E. Hum Gene Ther 1996; 7:1437–1446.
24. Zanta MA, Boussif O, Adib A, Behr JP. Bioconj Chem 1997; 8:839–844.
25. Erbacher P, Remy JS, Behr JP. Gene Ther. 1999; 6: 138–145.
26. Kren BT, Bandyopadhyay P, Steer CJ. Nat Med 1998; 4: 285–290.
27. Hartikka J, Sawdey M, Cornefert-Jensen F, Margalith M, Barnhart K, Nolasco M, Vahlsing HL, Meek J, Marquet M, Hobart P, Norman J. Hum Gene Ther 1996; 7:1205–1217.

8

Receptor-Mediated Gene Transfer

Kurosh Ameri
The University of Sheffield, Sheffield, England

Ernst Wagner
Boehringer Ingelheim Austria, Vienna, Austria

I. INTRODUCTION

Crucial requirements in gene therapy are a successful delivery of the therapeutic gene into the right target cells and a controlled expression in the transfected cell at the appropriate levels and over the required period. The current gene-delivery systems are not optimal in these aspects. Recently increased attention has been given to nonviral delivery vehicles such as naked plasmid DNA, cationic liposome-DNA complexes (lipoplexes), polymer/DNA-based systems (polyplexes) delivery, and combinations thereof (1–4). These delivery systems are attractive because of their simplicity (they can be generated from a few defined components) and the flexibility in synthesis and assembly of the gene-transfer particle. If desired, they can be designed to be protein-free/nonimmunogenic and can be very flexible regarding the size of DNA to be transported. However, the efficiency in gene delivery does not meet the requirements for most therapeutic applications.

Several mechanisms have evolved during biological evolution that enable the transport of molecules into cells. Natural mechanisms enabling material transport or exchange ranges from simple diffusion, active transport, phagocytosis, and receptor-mediated endocytosis to viral infection, bacterial conjugation, and natural transformation mechanisms (uptake of DNA) seen in some microorganisms. These natural pathways can be used in a new, artificial setting as a transfer route to deliver genes into cells. This chapter describes the nonviral delivery systems that take advantage of the receptor-mediated import to target and transfer genes into specific cells. Special attention will be given to the many barriers that need to be overcome for gene transfer to be efficient. Factors such as DNA condensation, particle size of the DNA complex, route of administration, stability of the transferred gene in vivo, physical barriers that need to be overcome in order to reach target sites, and other in vivo confrontations will be discussed. The current concepts on binding of DNA complexes to the cell surface receptor and internalization and intracellular trafficking will be reviewed, as well as strategies for enhanced intracellular vesicular release or nuclear targeting.

II. CONCEPT OF RECEPTOR-MEDIATED GENE TRANSFER

Gene-transfer vehicles must fulfill at least two major delivery tasks: to deliver the therapeutic gene from the site of administration into the appropriate tissue on the surface of the target cell, and to facilitate the transfer of the gene into the nucleus of this cell. Incorporation of receptor ligands has been considered to support both tasks, i.e., targeting and enhanced cellular internalization of the transferred (therapeutic) gene. Receptor-mediated delivery of molecules is a cellular process by which various ligands bind to specific cell surface receptors, resulting in subsequent internalization and trafficking of receptor/ligand within the cell, as reviewed in Ref. 5. Cell targeting is a result of the specific binding of a ligand to its cell surface receptor, and in most cases, due to this interaction, internalization is enhanced.

Specific cell binding and enhanced uptake can be mediated by one ligand but could be regarded as two separate processes, since some ligands might target and bind a specific cell surface receptor but not necessarily result in enhanced internalization, whereas other ligands have no cell-type specificity but efficiently mediate uptake. The vitality of these two points is very clear when working in vitro as well as in vivo. In vitro, targeting the gene of interest to specific cells is not a problem as such, since the delivered gene is in direct contact with the target cells only and hence need not seek out specific cells. However, it is necessary to enhance cellular uptake of the transferred gene. This can be achieved by utilizing ligands as intracellular delivery–enhancing elements. For in vivo administration of therapeutic gene, both cell targeting and enhanced cellular uptake of the complex carrying the DNA are crucial for successful gene therapy.

A. Receptor Ligands for Targeting Specific Cells

One major requirement for gene delivery is the specific cell targeting of the therapeutic gene. To promote specific interactions between the complex carrying the DNA and cells, a specific ligand able to recognize a specific receptor at the surface of target cell may be coupled to the carrier. Ligands, internalized via receptor-mediated delivery mechanisms, represent a wide variety of macromolecules with varying physiological activities, including nutrient provision (e.g., LDL, transferrin), modified molecules from the circulation (e.g., ASGP, plasminogen activator-inhibitor complexes), growth factors and hormones (e.g., insulin, VEGF, EGF), and some lysosomal enzymes. Some of these ligands may be coupled to DNA complexes, targeting them to specific cells. Ligands can be proteins such as transferrin or asialoglycoproteins and small natural or synthetic molecules such as folic acid, peptides, or sugar derivatives. Examples of ligands that have been used as conjugates with certain polycationic carriers for targeted gene transfer are shown in Table 1.

Table 1 Ligands Used in Receptor-Mediated Gene Transfer

Ligands	Refs.
α_2-Macroglobulin	11,12
Anti-CD 3	13,14
Anti-CD 5	15
Anti-CD 117	16
Anti-EGF	17
Anti-HER2	18
Anti-IgG	19,20
Anti-secretory component Fab	21–23
Anti-Tn	24
Anti-thrombomodulin	25
Antibody ChCE7	26
Asialoglycoproteins	27–36
EGF	37
Fibroblast growth factor (FGF2)	38
Folate	39–41
Glycosylated synthetic ligands	42–55
IgG (FcR ligand)	19,56
Insulin	57,58
Invasin	59
Lectins	60–62
Malarial circumsporozoite protein	63
RGD-motif (integrin binding)	64
Steel factor (CD117 ligand)	65
Surfactant proteins A and B	66,67
Transferrin	68–77

A general aspect to be considered in the selection of a ligand to be coupled to the carrier is that some ligands are very specific in targeting certain cells or tissues in the body (e.g., asialoglycoproteins/hepatocytes), others are not (e.g., transferrin (Tf)/iron supply to many cell types). Some ligands are internalized very efficiently (e.g., Tf, anti-CD3 antibody bound to the T-cell receptor–associated surface molecule CD3), whereas still others may be internalized either very slowly or not at all. Thus, the choice of ligand for efficient gene transfer is fundamental. One may also take advantage of the ligand binding and internalization enhancement as two separate processes, utilizing two different ligands: one for targeting and the other for internalization. Hypothetically, two different ligands could also be used, where one ligand serves a cell-binding function only, with the other ligand enhancing the cellular internalization process. The target cell must contain the cognate receptors, enabling the ligands to work in concert. Efficient internalization will only take place with cell types containing both receptor types, enabling the two ligands to work in concert. In this regard, the cell biology of specific cell types may also play an important role for efficient targeting. For example, cellular targeting ligand coupled to the DNA complex can be used as an element to target only the corresponding cell, whereas internalization can be achieved via phagocytosis. Any cell containing the corresponding receptor will be targeted, but internalization will only take place at cell types with competent phagocytic apparatus. Thus, other factors also play a role, such as the size of the carrier-DNA complex, which will be discussed in Section III.

B. Enhanced Intracellular Uptake by Receptor-Mediated Mechanisms

The concept of receptor-mediated gene transfer is notable for its natural delivery mechanism of infectious and cytotoxic agents such as viruses, microorganisms and toxins, and macromolecules such as cell nutrients, growth factors, and hormones into cells via cellular internalization processes such as receptor-mediated endocytosis, potocytosis, and phagocytosis (5,6). There are basically two mechanisms of endocytosis: clathrin-dependent receptor-mediated endocytosis (coated pit endocytosis) (7) and clathrin-independent endocytosis (8). Clathrin-dependent receptor-mediated endocytosis involves the binding of a ligand to a specific cell surface receptor, resulting in the clustering of the ligand-receptor complexes in clathrin-coated pits, invagination into the cell, budding off of the coated pits from the cell surface membrane to form intracellular coated vesicles, and maturation (uncoating, fusion of vesicles) into endosomes. Within these endosomes, ligands and receptors are sent to their appropriate (intra)cellular destinations (e.g., lysosome, Golgi apparatus, nucleus, or cell surface membrane) (Fig. 1).

The clathrin-independent mechanisms resulting in uncoated pits include phagocytosis, pinocytosis, and potocytosis. Phagocytosis is a mechanism of internalizing large particles and microorganisms (>0.5 μm). This mode of internalization is initiated by receptors on the phagocyte recognizing the particle either directly or indirectly via opsonization of the particle. Internalization is primarily mediated via pseudopod action rather than pits (invaginations) on the cell surface. The engulfed particle, initially situated in the early phagosome, is eventually destroyed along the endocytosed pathway. Thus, cell capability to recognize particles via receptors and to form pseudopods seem to be a major characteristic mediating phagocytic internalization. Other forms of internalization that do not utilize clathrin do, however, seem to rely on pits (invaginations) on the cell surface. Such internalization systems include macropinocytosis, pinocytosis, potocytosis, and transcytosis. Potocytosis and transcytosis may utilise caveolae as routes for internalization (6,9,10).

The specific pathways explained above can be used to enhance the delivery of foreign genes into cells (see Table 1). Many receptors contain motifs in their cytoplasmic domains that act as recognition sequences for initiating the process of enhanced intracellular uptake of macromolecules. With ligand interaction, the rate of receptor internalization is increased. Whether the intracellular pathways of the internalized molecule and biochemical consequences are the same for different forms of endocytosis and ligands remains unclear (38,58,78,79).

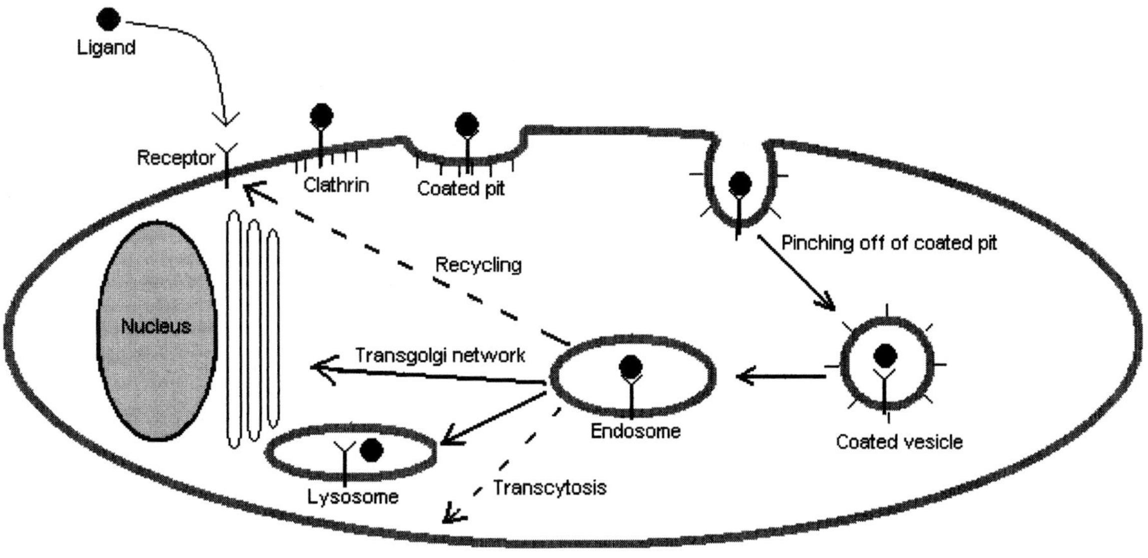

Figure 1 Receptor-mediated endocytosis.

III. EXTRACELLULAR BARRIERS FOR GENE DELIVERY

The development of gene-delivery vehicles is confronted with two major hindrances: the transferred genetic material must overcome the extracellular barriers in order to reach the target cells, and once it reaches and contacts the target cells, it must then traverse several target cell membranes and subcellular compartments to achieve nuclear localization, whereby heterologous gene expression can take place.

A schematic diagram of the potential intracellular and extracellular fate of a gene-transfer vector is shown in Figure 2. Strategies must be developed to design DNA complexes capable of surviving blood and other biological fluids and able to escape extracellular physical barriers and reaching the target cells. The specific strategies must take into account the physicochemical characteristics of the DNA complexes, such as size, shape, and flexibility of the complex, overall charge, charge density, and nonelectrostatic interactions at the surface of the complex. Besides these physical properties, it may also be possible to utilize active endogenous cellular transport mechanisms, such as transcytosis (80,81).

In vitro gene-delivery and ex vivo gene-therapy approaches are predominantly concerned with gene-delivery barriers presented by the cell itself. In vivo gene therapy must also be concerned with extracellular barriers. Here the route of administration of the therapeutic gene also plays a major role (82,83). In systemic administration, where the vector is introduced into the body intravenously, the harsh blood circulation pathway and environment and the various cells and organs encountered by the vector before reaching the target cells are major obstacles determining the fate of the transferred DNA (see, e.g., Ref. 84). On the other hand, local administration methods such as direct injection of the vectors into the target region are not confronted with the circulation problem but nevertheless still encounter barriers such as extracellular matrix or inflammatory and immune responses.

A. Physical Restrictions of Transfection Particles

Size seems to be a general critical factor for drug targeting (85). Because of size restriction, (several) hundred nm large particles cannot penetrate endothelial and epithelial barriers (86) or extravasate from the vascular to the interstitial space. Particle size is also an important factor when considering organ clearance and intraorgan distribution. For example, particles that are too large to pass through the vascular endothelium to the liver parenchyma are engulfed and degraded by liver Kupffer cells, phagocytic cells residing next to the vascular epithelial cells.

DNA is a negatively charged, flexible molecule, both of which characteristics hinder the DNA from being transported efficiently into and across cells, which in this case represent the physical barriers. To overcome these physical drawbacks, the DNA molecule needs to be compacted and

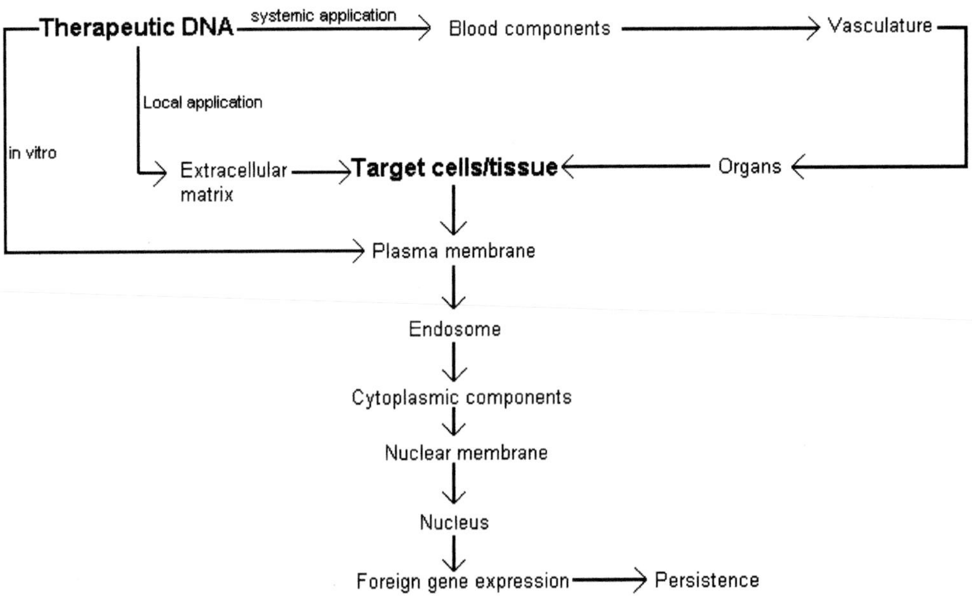

Figure 2 Extracellular and intracellular pathways for gene delivery (in vivo—systemic or local application; in vitro—cultured cells).

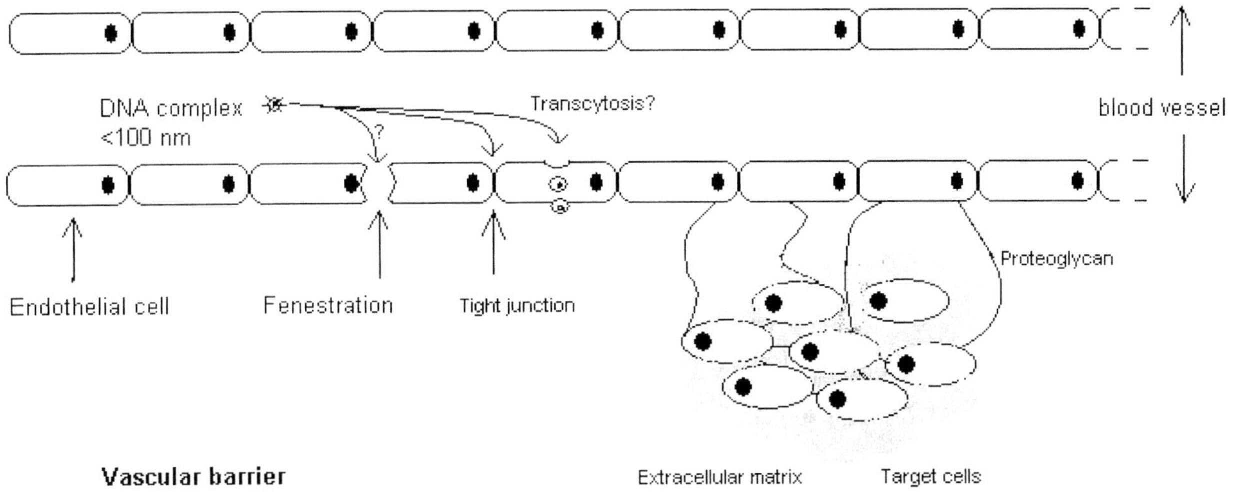

Figure 3 Vascular barrier for gene delivery.

the negative charges minimized for efficient gene transfer. These requirements can be achieved by taking advantage of molecules capable of binding and condensing DNA (87). The structure of condensed DNA complexes has been analyzed in several reports (e.g., Refs. 71,88–90). DNA polycation complexes have been characterized by electron microscopy (shape, size), laser light scattering (size), electrophoretic mobility (reflects charge and size of complexes), zeta potential measurements (charge), circular dichroism (conformation of DNA), and centrifugation techniques (molecular weight and condensation). The results give some insight into how to generate DNA complexes sufficiently small to traverse the endothelial layer, possibly through fenestrations or vesicular transport systems such as transcytosis (Fig. 3). In addition, the compact DNA complexes are more stable against enzymatic or mechanical degradation, which may take place during DNA transport processes to the target cells/tissue.

However, preparation of effective DNA complex molecules for in vivo delivery of DNA remains a major hurdle. The extent of DNA condensation depends on a number of variables, including the ratio of positively charged DNA-binding element (''cationic carrier'') to negatively charged DNA, the size and modification of the DNA-binding element, size, sequence, and state of the DNA, and also the procedure of complex formation (16,91), strongly influencing the in vitro and in vivo gene-transfer efficiency. The net charge of the DNA-cationic carrier complex affects its solubility. Complexes with an excess of either DNA or positively charged carrier are stabilized in solution by the negative or positive charges. At molar charge ratios (positive charges of carrier to negative charges of DNA phosphates; see Ref. 1) close to 1 (i.e., electroneutrality), hydrophobic domains of DNA-binding elements such as polylysine are considered responsible for low solubility in water. This may lead to aggregation and precipitation of complexes.

Methods of formulation still have to be improved for generating homogenous and stable complexes capable of overcoming physical barriers. DNA-polylysine conjugate complexes have been prepared in several ways. Wu and Wu (27) mixed the compounds at high salt concentration, where electrostatic binding is strongly reduced. Slow reduction of the salt concentration by dialysis into physiological buffer results in a thermodynamically controlled complex formation. Charge ratios of polylysine-DNA smaller than 1 and enhanced hydrophilicity due to the conjugated asialoglycoprotein presumably are essential for the solubility of the complex.

Wagner et al. (71) described a different approach using transferrin-polylysine DNA complexes. Flash mixing of dilute compounds in physiological phosphate-free buffer results in formation of kinetically controlled complexes. Charge ratios of polylysine-DNA from smaller than 1:2 to larger than 2:1 have been applied. At ratios of electroneutrality or higher, donut-like and rod-like particles of 80–120 nm diameter are formed. Complexes containing transferrin-conjugated polylysine have increased solubility compared to the use of unmodified polylysine.

Interestingly, donuts of similar sizes are formed independent of whether small or large (up to 48 kbp) DNA is used in the complex formation. Using a standard expression plasmid of approximately 5 kbp, several DNA molecules are incorporated into one particle. In an attempt to generate unimolecular DNA complexes, Perales and colleagues (22,46) added polylysine conjugates slowly, in several small portions, to a vortexing solution of DNA in approximately 0.5–0.9 M sodium chloride until a charge ratio of polylysine-DNA of approximately 0.7 is reached. The slow addition of polylysine has been reported to generate monomeric DNA complexes, with sizes of approximately 15–30 nm. These complexes aggregate immediately; aggregation is reversed by subsequent addition of salt. The promising findings have been reported to be applicable for in vivo gene-transfer applications (22,46).

Recent reports on the size of DNA complexes with polyethylenimine (PEI) or transferrin-polyethylenimine describe the strong influence of parameters such as DNA concentration and charge ratio as well as ionic strength of solution or serum content of culture medium. Mixing DNA-PEI complexes at N:P (PEI nitrogen:DNA phosphate) molar ratios below 6 in 150 mM saline results in rapid aggregation; aggregation can be avoided by complex formation at low ionic strength (25 mM aqueous buffer), generating particles with an average diameter of approximately 40–50 nm (92).

B. Undesired Interactions with Plasma, Degradative Enzymes, Matrix, and Nontarget Tissue

DNA complexes, when administered in vivo, are surrounded by a variety of compounds present in blood plasma. Salts, lipids, carbohydrates, proteins, or enzymes contribute to changes in the physicochemical properties of the DNA complex. Some of these factors (''opsonins'') may coat the DNA complex, causing aggregation, dissociation, or degradation of the DNA complex. This may influence the composition of the complex as well as the bioavailability. Thus, the DNA complexes, even when reaching the target cells/tissue, may no longer exhibit the physical properties necessary for efficient transfer into cells.

Previous studies have demonstrated the inactivation of polylysine-based DNA complexes by blood components (93). One of the factors was identified as the complement system (94). More recently, the interaction of DNA-PEI complexes with plasma was analyzed on the biochemical level. Upon incubation of the DNA complexes with human plasma, specific proteins (IgM, fibrinogen, fibronectin, and complement C3) bind to the complexes (see also Section V.B). By coating the DNA-PEI complexes with polyethylene glycol (PEG) through covalent coupling to PEI, plasma protein binding was found to be strongly reduced.

Another problem encountered in the blood stream are degradative enzymes. There are nucleases in the blood stream that degrade extracellular DNA (such as generated by degradation of invading microorganisms or dead host cells). Cationic DNA-binding elements may provide some protection (32).

Other undesired interactions include ones with the extracellular matrix and nontarget cells/tissue. There is a complex network of proteins and proteoglycans, termed extracellular matrix, that fill the intercellular space (95, 96). The matrix helps bind the cells in tissues together and also provides a lattice through which cells can move.

Once the DNA complex has traveled across the vascular barrier into the interstitial space, it must avoid interactions with the extracellular matrix in order to reach and bind the target cells/tissue. Extracellular matrices in animals are composed of different combinations of collagens, proteoglycans, hyaluronic acid, fibronectin, and other glycoproteins. These components could serve as specific barriers by binding the DNA complexes. For example, hyaluronic acid binds cations very effectively. With this in mind, DNA condensed by polycations, resulting in a net positive charge, could also interact with the extracellular matrix, binding, dissociating, or aggregating the DNA complex. Thus, proper formulations when preparing the DNA complexes will be necessary to avoid such interactions. Optimizing the DNA complexes bearing an overall low charge ratio close to neutrality would be one way to avoid such interactions (97). Unfortunately, a net positive charge has been found desirable for interaction with the cellular plasma membrane and entry into the target cell, while such a positive charge might favor entrapment of the DNA complexes by negatively charged extracellular matrix components.

Interaction with nontarget cells/tissue is another difficult-to-overcome hurdle. In Section II the cellular internalization mechanisms using receptor specific ligands were presented as a solution. Ligands may target cells very efficiently, but it must be kept in mind that they do not inhibit nonspecific interactions with nontarget cells, which could result in cellular binding and internalization via any additional process. The nonspecific interactions with nontarget cells may be due to factors such as particle size, charge, and in vivo protein coating of the DNA complexes. For example, interaction with unwanted cells may take place due to an excess positive charge of the complex. It has been shown in cell culture that minor changes in the DNA: polylysine conjugate ratio, resulting in a positively charged DNA complex, may convert a ligand-specific transfer into a completely unspecific process (16). Ideally, the DNA complex should be masked in a fashion that only allows ligand receptor interactions with the target cell and no other interactions with nontarget cells.

C. Inflammatory and Immunological Responses

As a result of introducing foreign molecules into the body, individual immune cells are stimulated to produce antibodies, a process termed humoral immunity. In addition to this humoral response, specific T cells may also be activated (cellular immunity). These two processes constitute the specific immune response. There is, however, also a nonspecific immune response, including phagocytosis, inflammation, and other nonspecific host-resistance mechanisms, such as the complement system (98,99). These nonspecific mechanisms develop immediately against virtually any foreign molecule, even those the host has never encountered. Thus, the nonspecific immune response is a major extracellular barrier for the DNA complex, which in this case is the foreign molecule. The ultimate goal is to formulate and construct polyplexes in a manner that avoids eliciting any immune response.

Inflammatory response is a major problem for any gene delivery system (100), since it may take place independently of the route of administration and result in a greater access of phagocytes to the foreign molecules, for example, due to an increased capillary permeability caused by retraction of the endothelial cells. During an inflammatory response, leukocytes, particularly neutrophil polymorphs and to a lesser extent macrophages, migrate out of the capillaries into the surrounding tissue. At the site of inflammation the phagocytes recognize the foreign molecules via receptors on their surface, which allow them to attach nonspecifically and phagocytose foreign molecules. Attachment is greatly enhanced and specified upon opsonization of foreign molecules, such as by the C3b component of complement. Both neutrophils and macrophages have receptors that specifically bind to C3b, allowing them to recognize their target.

A variety of macromolecules, such as proteins, lipoproteins, some nucleic acids, and many polysaccharides, can act as immunogens under appropriate conditions. Positively charged DNA complexes have the ability to activate the complement system (94). A number of synthetic cationic molecules frequently used in gene delivery and their complexes with DNA have recently been examined for their complement-activating properties. Complement activation by polylysine is strongly dependent on chain length and on the charge ratio. Longer chains and greater surface charge density are strong activators of the complement system. The positive charges on the DNA complex are accessible to the complement protein C3b. Opsonization of such particles by C3b leads to the initiation of a cascade of events presumably resulting in the clearance of DNA complexes by the retinoculoendothelial system. Coating of the positive charges of the DNA complexes with other macromolecules may inhibit interactions with components of complement, hence decreasing complement activation and clearance of the complexes from the blood circulation (101). It has already been demonstrated that modification of the surface of liposomes reduces interaction with blood components (102–104) and stabilizes DNA-liposome complexes (105). Coating of polycation-DNA complexes by PEG also reduces interaction of DNA complexes with blood components (94; M. Ogris and E. Wagner, unpublished data).

IV. INTRACELLULAR PATHWAYS AND BARRIERS

In order to achieve foreign therapeutic gene expression within the target cell nucleus, the DNA must be internalized by receptor-mediated endocytosis, followed by release from the endosomal entrapment. Transported to the nucleus, the DNA must be released from the carrier molecules, leading to foreign gene expression, with appropriate persistence.
To tackle the intracellular barriers, a DNA complex needs to:

Have the ability to bind specific cell surface receptors for endocytosis
Have the appropriate size for target cell internalization
Escape from the endosome to avoid enzymatic degradation
Survive the cytoplasmic environment
Be targeted towards the nucleus with subsequent nuclear entry
Be disassembled so it can be recognized by the cell's transcription machinery and be expressed under control and only in the desired target tissue popolation

The above requirements can be achieved by taking advantage of several elements to be incorporated into the DNA complex (Fig. 4): DNA binding, condensing and protective elements, cell-targeting elements (ligands), endosomal-releasing agents, and possibly nuclear localization signals. Thus, DNA-binding elements and ligands help to overcome both extracellular and intracellular barriers.

A. Receptor-Mediated Internalization

To transfer DNA safely and efficiently into the cell, it is necessary to overcome the repulsive forces that exist between negatively charged DNA and target cell plasma membrane, to recognize target cell receptors, and to determine the size of the DNA complex to permit the specific internalization process to proceed. Carrier elements capable of binding DNA are utilized to condense the DNA into

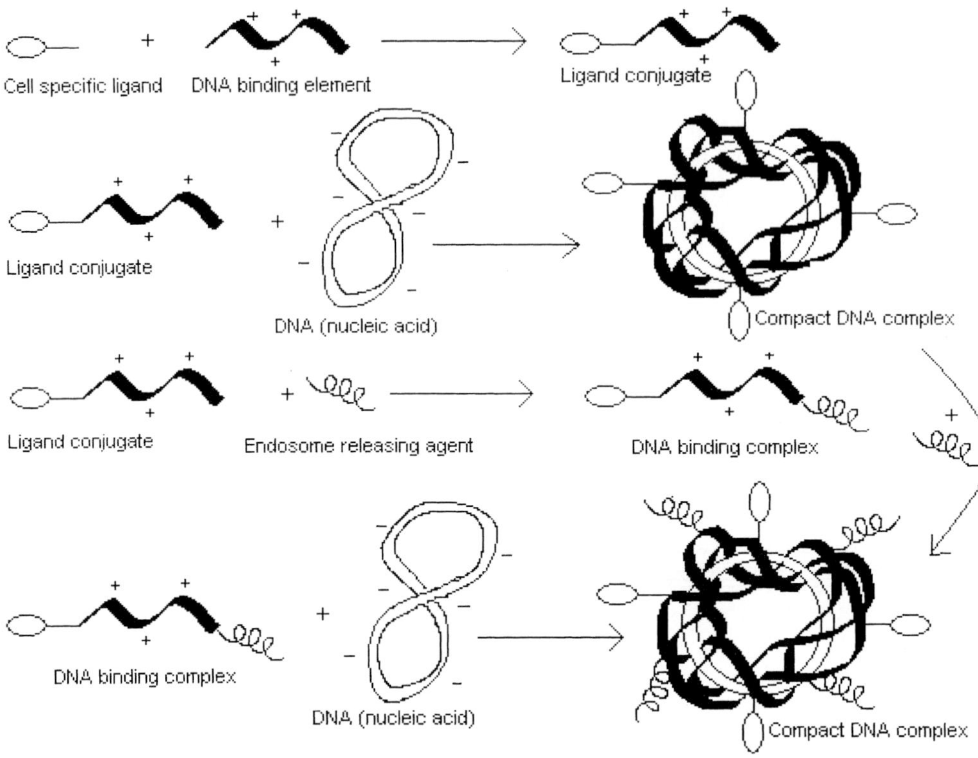

Figure 4 Assembly of DNA complexes.

a size preferred by the target cell for being internalized. These DNA-binding elements also neutralize the negative charges of the DNA, hence omitting repulsive forces to exist between the DNA and the cell plasma membrane. In addition, this condensation may also serve a protective function (see Section III). Cell-targeting ligands (see Section II and Table 1) can be coupled to the DNA-binding elements, forming a conjugate capable of interacting with and condensing the DNA, targeting it to a specific cell.

1. Polycationic Nucleic Acid Binding and Condensing Carriers

DNA-binding carrier elements should achieve interaction with the genetic material in a reversible, noncovalent, nondamaging manner. Several carriers, such as cationic lipids, lipopolyamines, polycations (cationic polymers) like polylysine or polyethylenimine, or histones, have been used for binding and condensing DNA into sizes that can be taken up by cells (106–110). For the majority of the cases, polylysine has served as the DNA-binding element, condensing the DNA into toroid-shaped complexes of 80–100 nm (71). A series of other DNA-binding compounds have also been used in DNA complexes: polycations such as polyarginine (111) protamine (71), or HMG1 (112) as well as intercalative agents (compounds) like bisacridine (43) or ethidium dimers (72). Use of intercalators in transfections in the absence of polycations has been largely unsuccessful; essential requirements like condensing of the DNA and interactions with phospholipids may be missing. Thus, DNA condensation is vital for efficient transfer into cells; not just any molecule that binds DNA results in an appropriate condensation. The cationic portion of the DNA complex can enhance binding to the cell (in addition to ligand-mediated receptor binding), and may also facilitate and mediate the transfer of the DNA to the cytoplasm, either by fusion with the cell surface or vesicular membranes or by disruption of the vesicular membranes (see Section IV B).

2. Ligand Conjugates

Achieving nonspecific cellular internalization via a net positive charge of the DNA complex could result in cytotoxic side effects, such as disruption of cell membranes. In addition, interaction can take place with any cell and other anionic molecules such as the components of the extracellular matrix, especially when the therapeutic gene is administered in vivo. Coupling ligands to the DNA-binding carrier partially solves this problem by enabling the complex to target the DNA to specific cells, binding them strongly by ligand-receptor interactions instead of simple nonspecific charge interaction and thus minimizing interactions with unwanted cells.

The DNA-binding element should be bound to the ligand without its DNA binding, condensing, and protective characteristics being affected and without effecting the cell-targeting property of the ligand. Such as molecular conjugate containing both DNA-binding and cell-targeting properties can combine with DNA, forming the conjugated-DNA complex. This complex should contain the DNA in a highly condensed state, with the ligands positioned to be free to interact with the target cell receptors.

Conjugates are commonly synthesized by covalently coupling the ligand to the DNA-binding element. More than 15 years ago, reports were published describing the concept of exploiting natural endocytosis pathways of ligands for the delivery of DNA macromolecules. A method was published for the covalent coupling of DNA to protein ligands, such as alpha2-macroglobulin, formulating the concept of receptor-mediated endocytosis (11). Alternative approaches use compositions containing DNA associated with the ligand in noncovalent mode, using the ligand linked to liposomes (113). This concept was expanded with approaches such as modifying proteins (transferrin and asialoglycoprotein) with positively charged *N*-acylurea groups that enable electrostatic binding to DNA to generate DNA-binding ligands for receptor-mediated gene transfer (114). A chemically more defined approach involves conjugates of asialoorosomucoid and the polycation poly(L)-lysine (27). Complexes of these DNA-binding conjugates with DNA plasmids encoding CAT marker genes or therapeutically relevant genes were shown to result in gene expression both in vitro in cultured HepG2 hepatoma cells and in vivo in the liver of rats or rabbits (27–34) (see also Section V). This was the beginning of the "receptor-mediated gene transfer" era, where ligand-polycation conjugates were complexed with DNA to condense, target, and transfer the gene into specific cells. Since then, many successful attempts have been made to synthesize ligand conjugates, for example, conjugation of transferrin, folic acid, anti-CD3 antibody, to the DNA-binding elements polylysine, protamines, histones, intercalators, and complexing them with DNA for achieving targeted gene transfer (see Table 1).

Taking transferrin as an example, conjugate synthesis (Fig. 5) involves the modification of transferrin and DNA-binding elements (polycations) with bifunctional reagents such as succinimidyl3-(2-pyridyldithio)propionate (Fig. 5a) (27,68). In the first steps, the activated (succinimidyl) esters can separately react with some amino groups of transferrin and the polycation. Subsequent steps result in disufide bonds (reducible) between the polycation and transferrin. Alternatively, a bifunctional reagent containing a maleimido group has been used (75), resulting in a (non-reducible) thioether linkage. Such an approach is not necessarily specific because the actual site of ligation between transferrin and the polycation is unknown. Conjugate synthesis can also be achieved in a more specific manner, e.g., via ligation through the transferrin carbohydrate moiety (Fig. 5b) (72). Transferrin contains two carbohydrate chains that are attached by *N*-glycosylation to Asn-413 and Asn-611. The glycan chains have a biantennary structure, composed of a mannotriosidodi-*N*-acetylchitobyose core bearing two *N*-acetylneuraminyl-*N*-acetyllactosamine units. The glycosylation on the transferrin has no known influence on receptor binding or any other biological function (apart from the clearance of asialotransferrin from the plasma). Thus, this site of the transferrin carbohydrate moieties is a good choice for attachment of polylysine and other nucleic acid–binding elements, without disturbing the cell receptor–targeting characteristics of transferrin. In order to couple the transferrin to the amino groups of polylysine, the transferrin carbohydrate groups must be activated. The terminal point of the transferrin carbohydrate chains consists of sialic acids. The two terminal exocyclic carbon atoms of the sialic acids can be selectively removed by periodate oxidation, resulting in the formation of aldehyde groups at the end of the carbohydrate chains.

The concept has been applied to other targeting ligands (Table 1). Ideally, the chosen ligand must be recognized by specific cell surface receptors, bound with high affinity and internalized. Most research in this field has been performed by targeting the liver-specific asialoglycoprotein receptor and the ubiquitous transferrin receptor. Other possibilities, such as using antibodies to target specific cells, have been investigated successfully. Anti-CD3 antibody coupled to carrier-DNA complex has been shown to be very efficient in targeting T cells by binding the CD3 T-cell receptor complex (13). Malignant B cells have also been successfully targeted by aids of antiidiotype antibodies (20). Others have achieved selective targeting of cells by using the ligand folic acid to target cells that target the folic acid receptor (39–41). It has been demonstrated that the growth factor receptors HER-2 (18), EGF-R (17,37), and FGF2-R (38), also highly overexpressed in many human tumors, serve as good targets. Transferring genes into macrophages by mannose/fucose, or galactose-specific membrane lectin is another example demonstrating that the receptor characteristics of cells can be exploited to target the cell via an appropriate ligand (42–55).

Recently the DNA-delivery activity of the cationic polymer polyethylenimine (PEI) has been combined with the concept of receptor-mediated gene delivery by incorporating cell-binding ligands (transferrin, antiCD3 antibody,

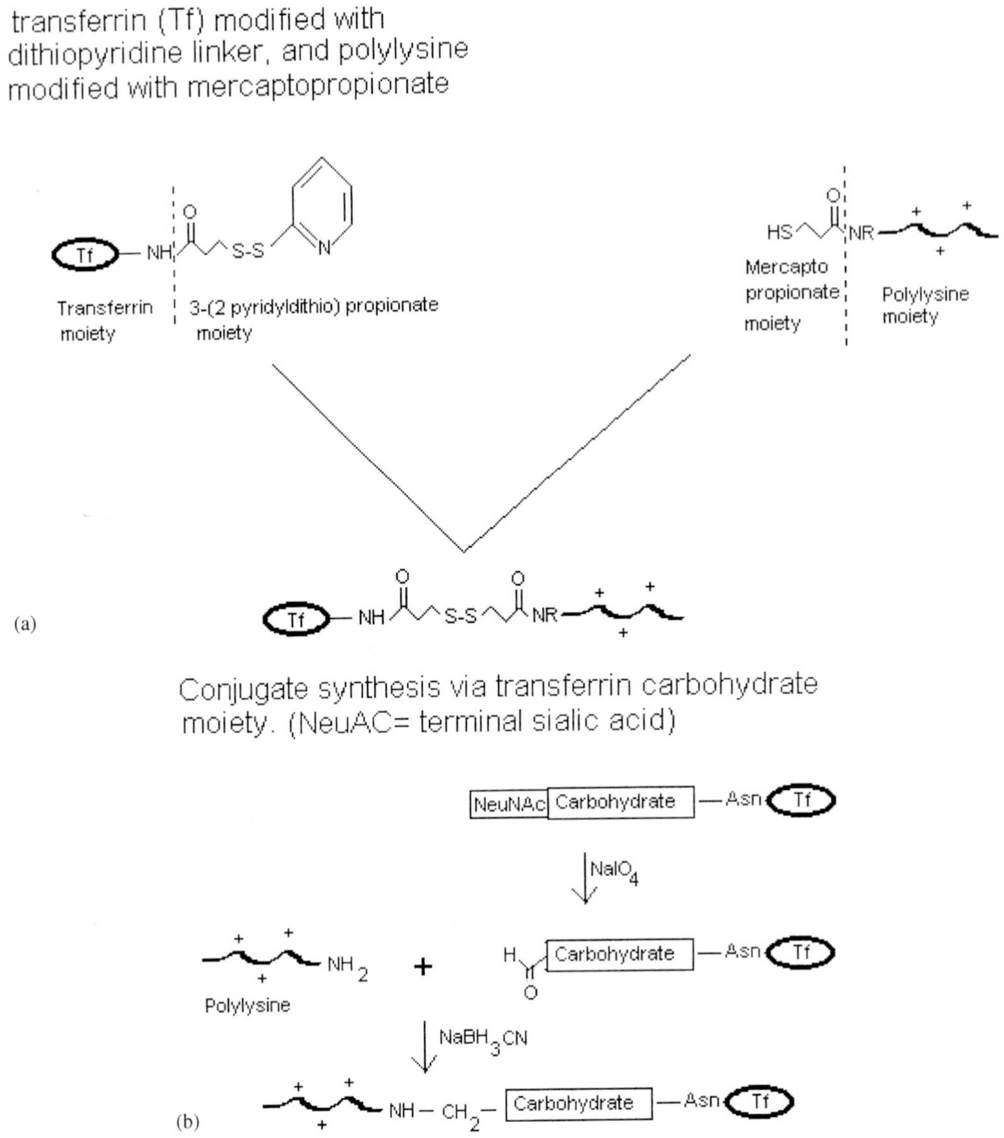

Figure 5 Synthesis of ligand-polycation conjugates (a) by a heterobifunctional linker reagent, SPDP, and (b) by ligation through a carbohydrate moiety.

lactose) by covalent linkage to PEI. Incorporation of cell-binding ligand results in an up to 1000-fold increased transfection efficiency (55,77). This activity was obtained with electroneutral particles but depends on ligand-receptor interaction, resulting in enhanced cellular internalization. It is important to note that coupling of the ligand did not disturb the DNA-condensing and transfer capability of PEI, which is a required aspect in formation of a DNA-conjugate complex.

In conclusion, enhancing cellular internalization by incorporating ligands to the carrier not only enhances cellular internalization, but also avoids problems such as cytotoxicity of positively charged complexes and undesired interactions with other cells and molecules, which would otherwise arise due to the need of a net positive charge of the DNA complex required for efficient (non–ligand-mediated) transfection.

B. Endosomal Escape

Another barrier that greatly impairs the efficiency of gene transfer the entrapment and degradation of the DNA com-

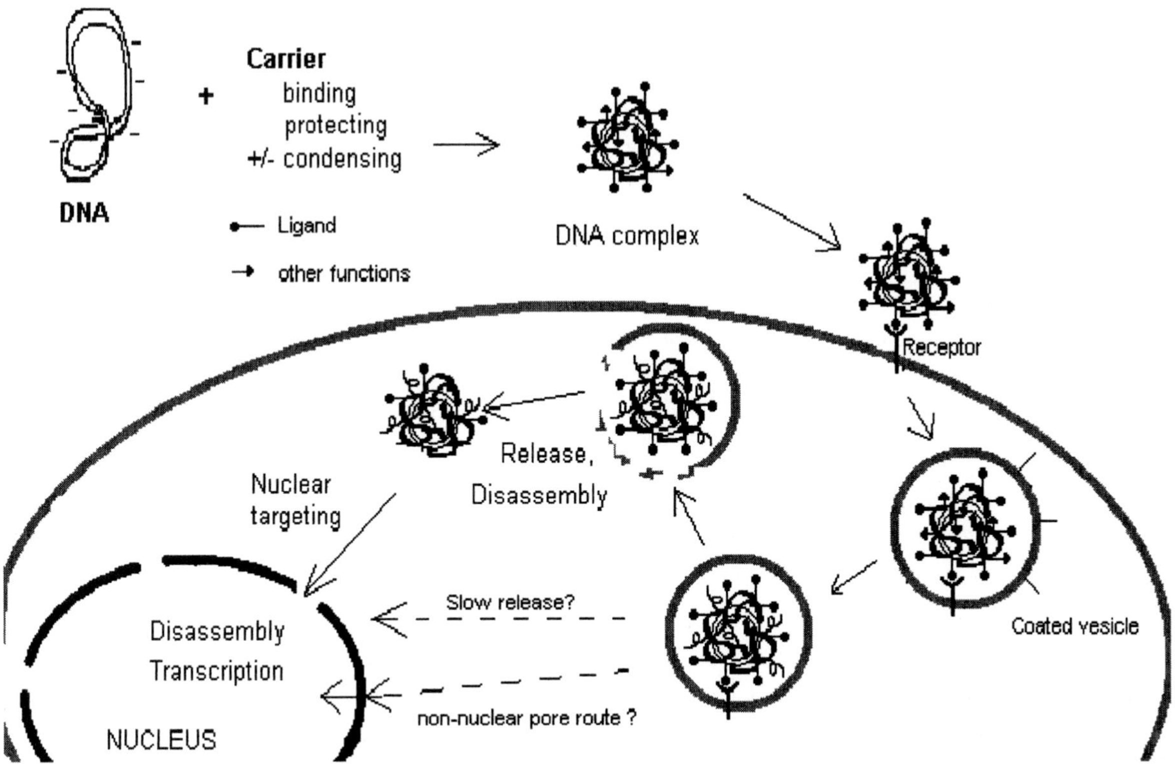

Figure 6 Intracellular release of DNA complexes.

plex within intracellular vesicles after budding off of the coated pits from the plasma membrane (Fig. 6). Entrapment and degradation can be regarded as two separate barriers, since overcoming vesicular degradation only would result in the accumulation of the transferred gene in the vesicles, limiting further transport into the nucleus. Thus, after cellular internalization, the transferred gene needs to overcome certain parameters, such as enzymatic degradation during vesicular fusion into lysosomes, and once this is done, it needs to then be released from the vesicles in order to reach the nucleus.

Several strategies have been developed to ensure the protection/release of DNA complexes from intracellular vesicles. The strategies involve incorporation or linkage of vesicular destructive elements to the DNA complexes, which perturb the integrity of vesicle membranes, allowing the luminal contents to spill into the cytoplasm in a non-damaged manner. The fundamental aspect here is to perturb the vesicular membrane without damaging the DNA complex and other cellular membranes. Thus, the endosome-releasing elements must either become active within the membranous vesicle or possess the ability to distinguish between vesicular membrane and the cell membrane.

1. Enhancement of Gene Transfer by Endosomal Releasing Agents

Application of endosome (vesicular)-releasing agents to the transfection process has shown to augment gene transfer. Lysosomotropic agents, glycerol, virus particles, membrane active peptides, and proteins possess properties that can reorganize vesicle membranes in a fashion promoting vesicular release of the DNA complex.

a. Lysosomotropic Agents. Lysosomotropic agents are weak base amines that can inhibit lysosomal function specifically (115–116). Examples of such agents are ammonium chloride and the weakly basic alkylamines such as methylamine, propylamine, chloroquine, procaine, and spermidine. These agents are termed lysosomotropic because they accumulate in the endosomes/lysosomes. This accumulation is partly due to the initially low lysosomal pH and partly because of continuous pumping of protons into the endosome/lysosome.

In several cell lines, such as erythroid cell line K562, gene expression is strongly enhanced by adding chloroquine to the transfection medium. This enhancement is primarily due to the prevention of intravesicular (lysosomal) degradation, followed by vesicular membrane disruption triggered by osmotic effects (see below). Chloroquine is also the most commonly used lysosomotropic agent in gene-transfer experiments (69). It is believed that chloroquine accumulates in the endosomal/lysosomal compartment, acting osmotically, vacuolarizing, and eventually disrupting the vesicle. In this case, the transferred gene is protected and released from intracellular vesicles. Bafilomycin or monensin, two other agents that also prevent endosomal/lysosomal acidification but do not accumulate, do not enhance transfection. The effectiveness of chloroquine in enhancing gene transfer is also dependent on cell type, which ensures vesicular accumulation of the lysosomotropic agent. For example, K562 cells, in comparison to other living cells (117), have a defect in their vesicular pump system determining the accumulation of chloroquine in endocytic vesicles (118). The use of chloroquine is limited due to cytotoxic properties.

b. Glycerol. Glycerol is a trihydric sugar alcohol and is the alcoholic component of fats. Several reports describe the interaction of glycerol with cellular membranes (119,120). Incubation of DNA-polylysine complexes in the presence of glycerol has resulted in a substantially enhanced transfection efficiency in primary fibroblasts and some cell lines. Regarding this, glycerol probably acts in intracellular vesicles after DNA complex internalization, rather than at the cellular membrane. The presence of glycerol alone is not sufficient for efficient gene transfer. For glycerol to have its maximum effect, other factors such as DNA complex net positive charge and type of DNA-binding carrier play a major role. Thus, a combined action of glycerol and polylysine on vesicular membrane seems to be responsible for enhancing gene transfer (120). It should, however, be noted that many cell types do not show the strong enhancement by glycerol.

c. Virus Particles. Adenovirus particles are capable of inducing endosomal lysis during the process of adenoviral infection. Upon acidification of the endosome, the capsid proteins (e.g., the penton proteins) undergo conformational changes to an active form capable of disrupting the endosomal membrane causing release of the contents into the cytoplasm. This observation potentiated the exploration of utilizing adenovirus (viruses that enter cells via receptor-mediated endocytosis) as means of overcoming vesicular entrapment during gene transfer (Fig. 7). Adenovirus has been successfully incorporated in DNA complexes, enhancing transfection efficiency 100- to 1000-fold (35,36,60,74,121–128). Incorporation may be achieved by adding adenovirus freely, where endomolysis action is in *trans,* or by directly linking the virus to the DNA complex. Various methods of linkage have been applied as an alternative method for ensuring cointernalization of the adenovirus, which is not always the case when the virus is added in *trans.* Most of these methods have been investigated with DNA complexes with polylysine as the DNA-binding element. There are several methods of covalently coupling polylysine to the exterior of the adenovirus. Approaches

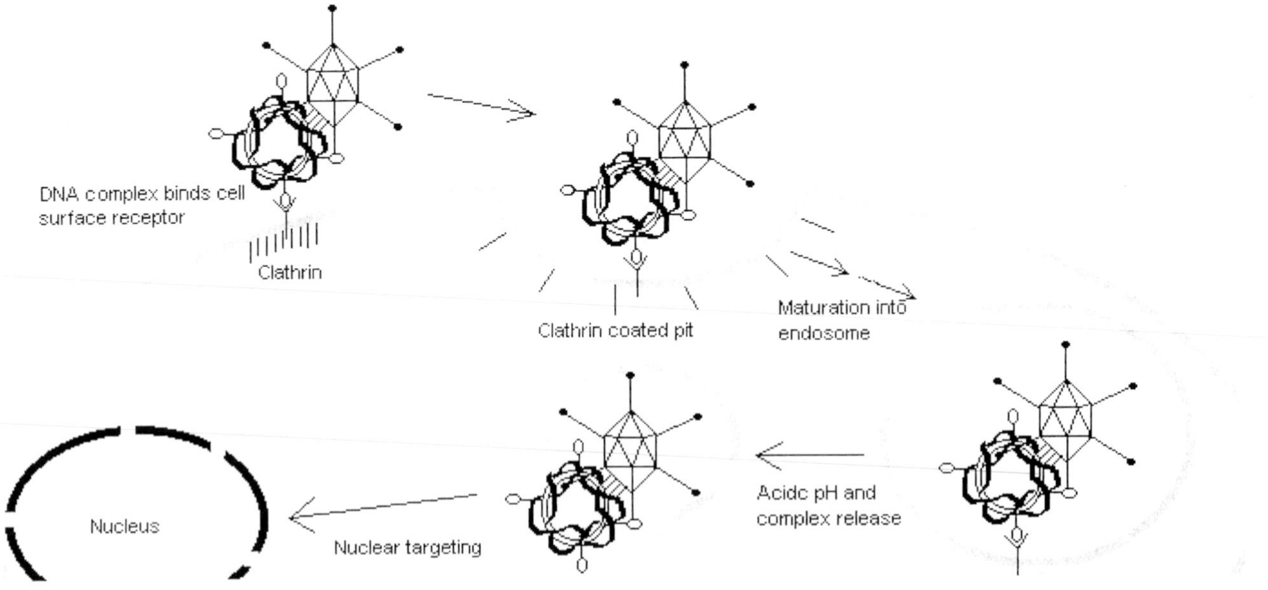

Figure 7 Adenovirus-enhanced receptor-mediated gene transfer.

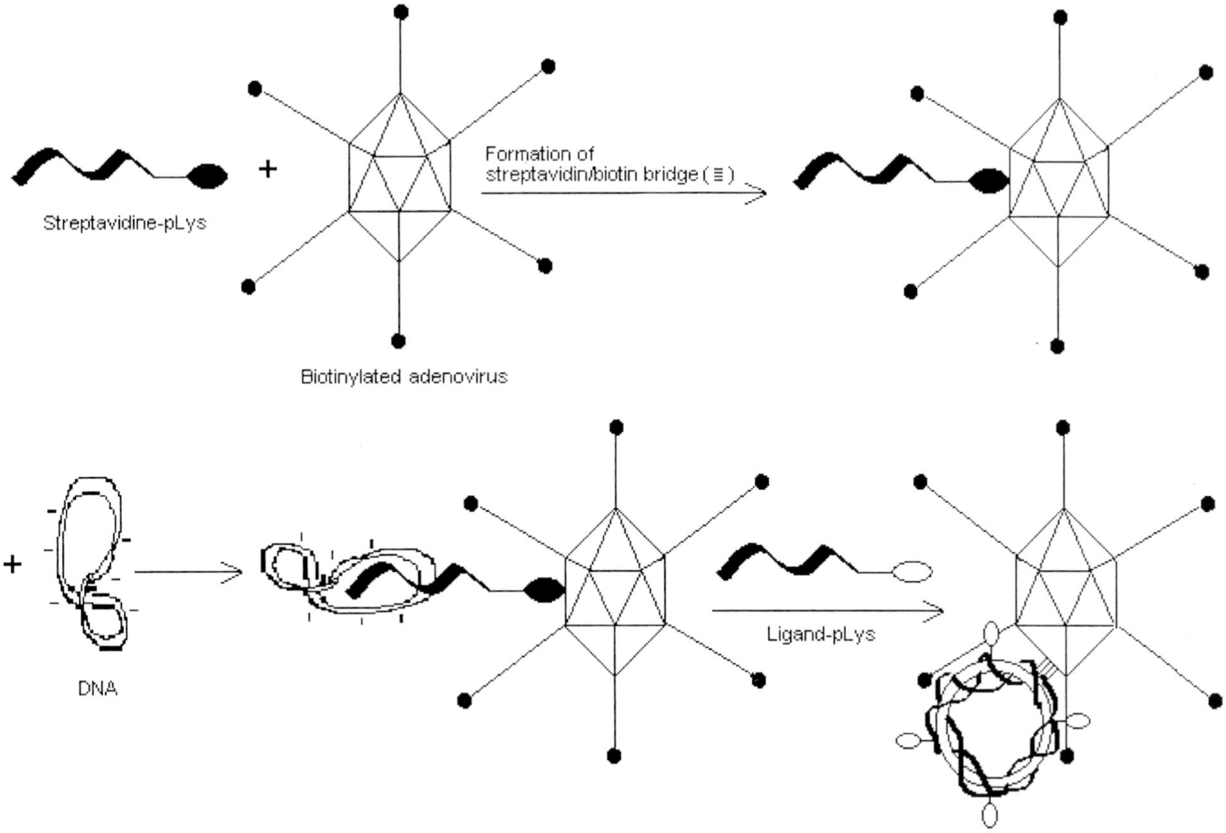

Figure 8 Assembly of adenovirus-enhanced transfection complexes. pLys, Polylysine.

including an enzymatic transglutaminase method, or chemical coupling methods, have been applied successfully. Alternative approaches are those involving noncovalent coupling methods, such as an immunological linkage strategy, with an anticapsid monoclonal antibody effecting the linkage between the adenovirus and polylysine DNA-binding moiety (antibody bridge), ionic interactions, or biotin-streptavidin bridge (Fig. 8), which are more convenient to use than covalent linkages, since covalent linkages suffer from precipitation and storage problems. To achieve a streptavidin-biotin linkage, the adenovirus needs to become biotinylated (via a reaction with biotin) and the DNA-binding element (e.g., polylysine) streptavidinylated. In order to achieve streptavidinylation, streptavidin is coupled to the DNA-binding element (polylysine) by a linker. After addition of biotinylated adenovirus to streptavidinylated DNA-binding element, adenovirus-polylysine conjugates are formed. Addition of these conjugates to DNA allows complex formation. Depending on the methodology, this complex can result in a fraction neutralization of the DNA negative charges. A calculated amount of ligand-polylysine conjugate can be added to the DNA complex to neutralize the remainder of the DNA. Such complexes consisting of DNA, adenovirus-polylysine, and ligand-polylysine are refered to as ''ternary complexes.''

Only the membrane-destabilizing function of the adenovirus capsid is required, thus the viral genome can be inactivated with methoxypsoralen plus irradiation, retaining endosome disruption properties (122,125). One problem with the inclusion of adenovirus is that the transferred gene may also enter cells via the adenovirus receptor, thus compromising ligand-specific gene transfer. Strategies to inhibit uptake via adenovirus receptor include coupling of polylysine to periodate oxidized adenovirus. This treatment modifies the adenovirus fiber, which is necessary for virus attachment. An alternative approach is to target an antibody against the adenovirus fiber. Ablating binding to adenovirus receptor does not interfere with subsequent endosomolyic activity. In addition to human adenovirus, CELO (chicken adenoviral strain) has also been successfully linked to DNA complexes, enhancing receptor-mediated gene transfer, although not as efficiently as adenovirus

(60). However, a major drawback in using viruses is their inflammatory response of cells to virus entry per se as well as their immunogenicity.

Since many other viruses also enter cells via the endocytic pathways, they may be utilized as gene-transfer enhancers, provided that they display an endosmolytic function. The use of human rhinoviruses (picornaviruses), which are RNA viruses, has been described and investigated for releasing vesicular entrapped DNA complexes into the cytoplasm (129). One major drawback of using rhinoviruses is the toxicity to human cells due to host protein synthesis machinery shut-off. One way to circumvent the viral-induced drawbacks is to use only the endosomolytic portion of the virus or synthetic derivatives thereof.

d. Membrane-Disruptive Proteins and Peptides. For many biological processes such as entry of viruses and bacterial toxins into cells to be exercised, cellular membrane barriers need to be bypassed, which is usually achieved by membrane reorganization processes. The membrane reorganization process is the result of specific actions of certain membrane-disruptive elements (peptides and proteins). In most cases, the membrane active elements are peptide domains with amphipathic sequences. Under appropriate conditions the amphipathic sequences can interact with lipid membranes, perturbing them. This characteristic can be specifically used to influence gene transfer; membrane-active peptides can be derived from viral peptide sequences such as the N-terminus of influenza virus hemagglutinin subunit HA-2 or the N-terminus of rhinovirus VP-1, or they may be designed sythetically from the derived peptides by molecular modeling, for example, GALA, KALA, EGLA, or JTS1 (129–133).

Viruses that enter the cell via the receptor-mediated endocytosis pathway have evolved specific mechanisms that ensure the release of their genome from the intracellular vesicles into the cytoplasm. The mechanisms leading to vesicular release are associated with viral proteins that specifically perturb membranes in either a disruptive or a fusogenic manner. The membrane-disruptive peptides are tools of membrane-free viruses (such as adenovirus), whereas the membrane-fusion peptides belong to enveloped viruses (such as influenza virus). These fusogenic or endosomolytic protein domains are activated in a pH-dependent manner, and this characteristic can be utilized to enhance gene transfer (129–133), in a manner similar to whole virus particles, as mentioned above. The virus-derived peptides can be incorporated into polylysine-DNA complexes either by covalently linking to polylysine or via biotinylation of the elements, which allows binding to streptavidinylated polylysine. Simple noncovalent ionic interactions between positively charged polylysine-DNA complex and the negatively charged residues of the membrane-destabilizing element is another possibility to achieve linkage. The linkage procedures should be also applicable to other DNA-binding elements. The membrane-destabilizing peptides have been shown to enhance receptor-mediated gene transfer up to 1000-fold in cell cultures.

Other larger viral proteins have also been investigated for enhancing transfection by endosomal release. Adenovirus penton proteins have been attached to DNA via a synthetic oligolysine-extended penton-binding adapter peptide. This complex transfers the DNA into the cell via adenovirus receptor and results in intracellular release (134).

One of the characteristics involved in virulence activity of microorganisms is the formation of substances (toxins, enzymes, and other proteins) that cause damage to the host (135–137). Some of the virulence factors act specifically on cell membranes. This action can be direct, for example, the action of streptolysin O, resulting in cell lysis, or indirect, specifically acting on intracellular vesicular membranes, resulting in the release of entrapped virulence factors, having entered the cell via an endocytic pathway. Various bacterial lysing proteins (cytolysins) and other toxins have been utilized as devices to enhance gene transfer. For example, streptolysin O and staphylococcal alpha toxin have been used as intracellular delivery reagents. Perfringolysin O has also been used to enhance delivery of DNA into cultured cells (138). For this purpose, the biotinylated protein was bound to DNA-polylysine complexes by a streptavidin bridge. Another well-studied exotoxin capable of enhancing gene transfer is the diphteria toxin. A recombinant transmembrane domain of this toxin has been coupled to polylysine with subsequent incorporation into DNA-asialoorosomucoid polylysine complexes (139).

e. Slow Release from Vesicular Reservoirs. Partial hepatectomy or microtubular disruption by colchicine treatment has been shown to prolong gene expression after intravenous injection of DNA-asialoorosomucoid polylysine complexes (33,34). This prolonged expression is due to the continous existence and survival of plasmid DNA in cells of treated cells. This survival is due to protection of the DNA complex from the lysosomal or cytoplasmic environment as a result of DNA complex persistence in the endosomal compartment, and the prolonged gene expression is due to a constant slow supply of plasmid DNA to the nucleus. The slow release is not a direct endosomolytic action. How the DNA complex reaches the nucleus in this case remains unclear.

2. Endosomal Escape Mediated by Cationic Carrier

In contrast to DNA-binding elements such as polylysine, there are other elements that possess specific properties enabling them to combine DNA-binding and condensing activity with membrane-perturbing capacity, thus not requiring the presence of endomolytic agents for enhancing transfection. The membrane-perturbing activity of such DNA-binding elements may be associated with their ionic state or conformational flexibility, resulting in membrane-specific interactions.

PEI, lipopolyamines, and polyamidoamine polymers (dendrimers) are efficient transfection agents per se (106–108). Most of these agents possess buffering capacity below physiological pH. This buffering capacity is due to residues of these agents not being protonated at physiological pH, making them efficient ''proton sponges.'' Upon acidification in the intracellular vesicle, the further protonation of the polymers triggers chloride influx, resulting in osmotic swelling (endosome swelling) and thus destabilization (rupture) of the intracellular vesicle membrane, resulting in the escape of the DNA complex, and hence gene-transfer enhancement in the sense that DNA is free to travel to the nucleus.

Incorporation of cell-binding ligands (such as Tf, lactose, or anti-CD3 antibody) into DNA-PEI complexes results in an up to 1000-fold increase in transfection efficiency through the mechanism of receptor-mediated endocytosis (55,77) demonstrating the vitality of ligands for eventual enhanced gene transfer and expression. Expression level is not dependent on endosomolytic agents such as chloroquine. However, Tf-PEI–mediated gene transfer can be augmented up to 10-fold by the addition of an endosome-destabilizing influenza peptide.

There are also designed cationic peptide carriers that can bind nucleic acids and permeabilize lipid bilayers at the same time. One example is the cationic amphiphilic peptide KALA, mentioned above (133).

C. Nuclear Entry

1. Mitotic and Postmitotic Cells

In growing cells, DNA may passively enter the nucleus during mitosis when the nuclear membrane is broken down (140). However, many cells and cell types are nondividing with the nuclear membrane staying intact, thus, the transferred gene needs to enter the nucleus differently than in dividing cells. In this case, nuclear entry and trafficking may represent a major inter-intracellular barrier for successful in vivo gene transfer. Thus, understanding the mechanisms of nuclear entry is vital and will be a large step towards designing gene-delivery systems that are more efficient in transferring the DNA into the cell nucleus.

2. Nuclear Import Mechanisms

The transport of DNA from the cytoplasm into the nucleus is essential for gene expression, but the factors important in this process remain poorly understood. In the majority of cell types, transport of DNA into the cell nucleus is inefficient. For example, less than 1% of NIH 3T3 fibroblasts have been shown to express β-galactosidase after cytoplasmic injection of reporter gene. In contrast, β-galactosidase has been efficiently expressed when injected into the cytoplasm of primary rat muscle cells. How DNA complexes find their way to the nucleus remains unclear. Per se, the DNA complex import into the nucleus may not be directed, although import of DNA into the nucleus may be sequence specific as has been demonstrated by intact protein-free SV40 DNA (141).

When DNA is injected into the muscle cell far from the nuclei, expression decreases. This may be the result of cytoplasmic sequestration, preventing nuclear accumulation of DNA. The movement of DNA towards the nucleus may be inhibited by its binding to cytoplasmic elements and/or by entrapment within the cytoskeletal mesh (142). Compact DNA structures may overcome such entrapments.

Expression of transferred DNA has been inhibited by WGA, suggesting that DNA may enter the nucleus by the WGA-sensitive process common to large karyophilic proteins and RNA (142) [WGA blocks the nuclear pore complex (NPC) machinery because of the presence of *N*-acetylglucosamine residues on nucleoporins]. However, recently it has been shown that nuclear localization of DNA does not require the addition of cytoplasmic protein factors necessary for protein import (143). Nevertheless, DNA entry appears to be regulated by NPC. The NPC accomodates both passive diffusion and active transport. Molecules less than 20 nm in diameter passively diffuse through NPC into and out of the nucleus. Larger macromolecules require active transport for nuclear entry. The exact mechanism by which exogenous DNA passes through the NPC has not yet been determined, although it may be similar to the transport of proteins larger than 15 kDa actively into the nucleus.

Certain viruses such as hepatitis B virus also utilize the active nuclear import mechanism. Viral core particles containing synthesized DNA bind to the nuclear pore complex; the viral polymerase, which is covalently linked to the viral DNA, acts as NLS. Core particles (35 nm) exceed the maximal diameter of the nuclear pores, thus requiring disassembly before the viral genome is internalized.

Regarding nuclear protein import, several major processes need to be distinguished: (1) the steps leading to the import process—signals guiding the protein transport to the nuclear membrane, including cytoplasmic recognition of the import protein by transport factors, and nuclear pore targeting, (2) the actual molecular mechanism of translocation of the protein from the cytoplasmic side of NPC to the nuclear side of NPC into the nucleus, the nuclear pores being the site of translocation, (3) release of the import protein into the nucleus, and (4) recycling of transport factors.

Several distinct nuclear import signals guide the import of proteins into the nucleus. These signals are part of the primary sequence of the protein destined to be targeted into the nucleus. The best characterized ones are the SV4O LTA type NLS (nuclear localization signal) and M9 (an import signal of hnRNP AI protein) import signals.

It has been suggested that shuttling of import receptors may be a major process in nuclear transport of proteins. In this hypothesis, the import receptor binds the protein in the cytoplasm. The molecule is then carried through the NPC into the nucleus, where it is released from the transport receptor. The receptor returns to the cytoplasm, ready for transporting the next molecule into the nucleus. In this model, the binding of the transport receptor to the molecule may be regulated by the different environments of the nucleus and cytoplasm.

Four major factors (transport factors) are required for the NLS-dependent protein import: importins alpha and beta (karyopherin alpha and beta), GTPase Ran/TC4, and NTF2 (nuclear transport factor 2, p10). These factors interact for successful transport of proteins into the nucleus. Proteins (with NLS signal) with sizes up to 25 nm interact in the cytoplasm with soluble NLS receptor (importins alpha and beta). The karyopherin beta 1 (importin beta) mediates docking to nucleoporins, the components of the nuclear pore, located at the cytoplasmic and nucleoplasmic faces of the nuclear pore complex (NPC). Nucleopore cytoplasmic filaments may also be involved in the nuclear targeting process. GTPase Ran and p10 (NTF2) are required to translocate the docked NLS peptide into the nucleus. The influenza virus nucleoprotein particle is one example of a molecule taken up by this pathway.

The M9 domain of hnRNP A1 contains 38 amino acid residues (M9 import signal), sufficient for import purposes into the nucleus. It bears no sequence similarity to classical NLS. Nuclear import of ribonucleoprotein A1 is mediated by another distinct import pathway, by binding to karyopherin beta 2 (transportin—an import receptor of the M9 pathway). It also requires Ran.

It is very likely that, in addition to NLS and M9-dependent import, more pathways into the nucleus exist. This may be an advantage in the sense of regulating import of distinct classes of molecules separately. Several reviews have appeared on nuclear protein import (144,145).

The efficient transport of DNA complex into the nucleus is an active process that probably requires a nuclear localization signal. Several NLS have been identified in proteins with a nuclear fate, the sequences being very basic, with >50% of their amino acids being lysine residues, e.g., Phe-Lys-Lys-Lys-Arg-Lys-Val, directing the nuclear import of SV-40 large T antigen, or the NLS (Lys-Lys-Lys-Tyr-Lys-Leu-Lys) within HIV-1 matrix protein. Substitution of one of the lysine residues results in total failure of nuclear import. Thus, it is possible that DNA-binding elements rich in lysine (e.g., polylysine) may play a role in the nuclear import of DNA complexes. Injection of DNA-polylysine mixtures into the cytoplasm of mouse ES cells has led to transgenic animals with about 50% efficiency (compared to intranuclear injection of naked DNA). In contrast, injection of naked DNA into the cytoplasm does not lead to transgenesis. However, polylysine serves as a protective agent, thus it is unlikely that polylysine acts as a nuclear targeting signal. To make the DNA import process more efficient, it may be necessary to direct the transport to the nucleus by incorporating nuclear localization signals into the DNA complex. This is strongly supported by recent findings (146) that incorporation of a single SV40 LTA NLS into a DNA plasmid molecule can dramatically enhance transfection efficiency.

To sum it up, it would be desirable to engineer DNA complexes with specific nuclear targeting and translocating elements enabling the DNA complex to be (1) recognized in the cytoplasm by nuclear import receptors (by interacting with transport motifs either directly on the DNA sequence or on a protein from the DNA complex), (2) targeted to the nuclear pore complex, (3) translocated efficiently through the nuclear pore, and (4) released at the nucleoplasmic face of the nuclear pore complex into the appropriate nuclear compartment for subsequent disassembly and expression.

3. Complex Disassembly, Release of DNA

The cell nucleus is crowded, containing large amounts of DNA, RNA, and protein. In addition, nuclear processes such as replication, transcription, translation, and DNA repair processes are constantly active in specific compartments, resulting in a nuclear jam (147,148). Within all the mass of cellular DNA, RNA, and proteins and the nuclear processes, the DNA complex needs to become—either disassembled or reorganized in a suitable fashion—exposed, enabling the nuclear expression machinery to recognize and express it.

D. Persistence of Gene Expression

Four main factors endanger the persistence of transferred DNA within the nucleus: (1) degradation by intranuclear nucleases, (2) DNA loss, mainly during cell division, although DNA may also be rapidly lost even when cells are not dividing, (3) loss of transfected cell because of apoptotic, inflammatory, or immune response, and (4) silencing of the introduced gene by transcriptional shut-off.

Protection of DNA may be achieved via the proper ratio of DNA to DNA binding carrier (e.g., polylysine). Saturating the binding capacity of the DNA backbone with the DNA-binding moiety may avoid the access of DNA to nucleases and increase the stability of the DNA in the nucleus (nuclear retention), resulting in prolonged expression.

DNA loss other than degradative loss can be prevented by including specific sequences to the transferred DNA that ensure either integration of the DNA into host chromosome or extrachromosomal replication of the transferred DNA with equal segregation to daughter cells. These persistence-ensuring sequences can be derived from certain viruses or from chromosomes.

Retroviruses and adeno-associated virus (AVV) stably insert their genome into the host genome. The integration mechanisms have been characterized (retrovirus: LTR sequences, integrase protein; AAV: ITR sequences, rep protein) and may be exploited by incorporation of the corresponding nucleic acid and protein elements into a virus-like particle (DNA complex). During its lysogenic cycle AAV integrates into a specific site, denoted AAVS1, on human chromosome 19 (149). This property has been utilized to achieve site-specific integration of plasmid DNA in 293 cells. When the AAV-encoded recombinase rep is supplied in *cis* or *trans,* plasmids containing the AAV ITRs are integrated at AAVS1. In this way DNA can be directed to a specific region of a human chromosome and thus may avoid the problem of random insertional mutations created by integrative vectors such as retroviral vectors.

Other viruses such as herpesvirus (e.g., Epstein-Barr virus) can persist in infected cells without integrating their genome into the host. This persistence is partially due to the replicative property of viral DNA via *cis*-acting origin of replication, which is activated by the *trans*-acting gene product of the viral EBNA-1, and additional nuclear retention mechanisms. The viral persistence mechanisms can be utilized in designing extrachromosomal replicating DNA constructs (episomal vectors) by integrating the appropriate sequence elements, recognizable in mammalian cells, into the DNA construct to be transferred (e.g., EBV Ori P, EBNA-1). DNA constructs containing these sequences have the ability to replicate once per cell cycle with nuclear retention without interfering with the host chromosomes. An alternative to using viral origin of replication human genomic sequences may be used to mediate DNA construct replication (150).

Other origins of replication characterized include those of bovine papilloma virus or SV40 (151). However, these replication origins also require viral proteins for activation, which may have oncogenic or toxic properties. The viral-replication origins are species specific and may also replicate more than once per cell cycle, resulting in mutations in the transferred gene.

The next challenge is the generation of artificial chromosomes for maintenance of large genomic sequences. The basic DNA sequence requirements for human chromosome function are thought to be similar to those identified in yeast, which include a centromere, telomeres, and origins of replication. These elements have been used to construct YACs (152), and their transfer has been demonstrated by spheroblast fusion. Researchers are now trying to construct human artificial chromosomes (HACs) (153). It is important to define the minimal sequence requirements for functional human chromosomal elements.

HACs may serve as valuable DNA constructs containing the requirements for achieving gene expression persistence. An opening door towards this goal is the recent generation of mitotically and cytogenetically stable artificial chromosome derived from transfecting human HT 1080 cells with alpha satellite plus telomere DNA and genomic carrier DNA, forming de novo microchromosomes with functioning centromeres (154). The only sequence that has been shown to form de novo centromeres after transfection is alphoid DNA with telomere DNA and genomic carrier DNA. However, centromeric function of human chromosome is not always associated with alphoid repeats. There are other nonalphoid genomic regions characterized by neo-centromeric activity (sometimes, a centromere can appear at a new position in a chromosome by a process called centromere activation). Transfection experiments with DNA present at the neo-centromere should demonstrate whether this DNA can also form centromeres de novo.

With advancement, HACs could be used to introduce therapeutic genes into cells. To utilize HACs for human gene therapy, efficient methods for delivery will be required. A receptor-mediated gene-transfer system is a very promising choice capable of targeting and transferring any large DNA construct into cells. Bacterial artificial chromosomes have already been delivered into mammalian cells using psoralen-inactivated adenovirus-PEI carrier (126).

Persistence of the transferred gene is required but not necessarily sufficient. It does not necessarily mean that gene expression is going to be efficient and long-lasting. A failure of gene therapy in clinical trials may not always be due to gene delivery, but rather to novel confrontations at the expression level. Specific expression cassettes determine the efficiency of expression after the gene has been transferred and maintained in the nucleus. The major elements of the expression cassette are those that ensure strong, controllable (switchable), and cell-specific (tissue-restricted) expression of the therapeutic gene. Studies using viral promoters (e.g., CMV promoter/enhancer) have observed a transcriptional shut-off (''silencing'') of the introduced expression cassettes. This can be avoided by the use of natural, cell-specific promoter/enhancer sequences. These are also attractive due to the opportunity for transcriptional targeting as a further filter for specificity (155). Some examples of this include steroid-inducible promoters, tumor-specific promoters, muscle-specific promoters, hypoxia-responsive elements, hepatitis B virus–derived promoters for liver-specific expression, and multidrug-resistant gene promoter (156). Here lies the attractiveness of nonviral receptor-mediated gene transfer—any gene construct, regardless of the size may be transferred.

V. PRACTICAL APPLICATION

A. Receptor-Mediated Gene Delivery In Vitro (Ex Vivo)

One approach for performing somatic gene therapy is the ex vivo strategy. In this approach gene transfer is performed in cell culture (in vitro) and the resulting transfected cell is transplanted into the organism. Application of receptor-mediated gene transfer to transfect endothelial cells (124,157), fibroblasts, B cells, vessels, and primary tumor cells has potentiated several ex vivo approaches. For example, clotting factor VIII, which is deficient in hemophilia A, can be produced by transfected primary fibroblasts at levels more than 10-fold higher than those generated by retroviral vectors, enabling factor VIII–expressing fibroblast implants for in situ expression of this protein (158).

The highly efficient delivery in vitro has resulted in the development of other ex vivo approaches. For example, treatment for malignant melanoma has been designed by application of gene-modified cancer cell vaccines. DNA complexes are used to deliver immunostimulator genes (such as interleukin-2) into melanoma cells in vitro. After irradiation (to block tumor cell growth), the transfected cells are applied in vivo to trigger an antitumor immune response. This treatment has been translated into a medical protocol and is being evaluated in clinical trials (159,160).

B. Receptor-Mediated Gene Delivery In Vivo

The first encouraging results for in vivo gene transfer were obtained by targeting, by intravenous injection, the liver asialoglycoprotein receptor using asialoorosomucoid covalently linked to poly(L)lysine carrying the CAT marker gene (29–31,33,34). DNA expression proved to be liver specific. Other organs such as kidney, spleen, and lungs did not produce detectable quantities of CAT activity. Gene-expression persistence was improved by applying partial hepatectomy, a procedure for stimulation of hepatic regeneration and DNA synthesis, beginning 12 hours after surgery, resulting in CAT activity up to 11 weeks postsurgery.

Related approaches have been utilized to target the liver with different sized DNA complexes. Small (about 12 nm) galactosylated DNA-polylysine complexes encoding human factor IX have been shown to target the hepatic asialoglycoprotein receptor, with up to 140 days of detectable protein in serum of transfected rats (46). This result was achieved without partial hepatectomy. In a related approach, the polymeric immunoglobulin receptor has been targeted by 25 nm DNA complexes bearing antigen-binding fragment of an antibody enabling gene transfer to rat pneumocytes following intravenous administration (22,23). It appears that the procedure for preparing DNA complexes (see Section III) may at least partially determine the success of in vivo gene-transfer approaches by influencing extracellular barriers.

These promising results suggest that receptor-mediated gene transfer can be utilized for in vivo systemic gene transfer into cancer cells to target tumor-specific receptors or receptors that are differentially expressed on tumors (161). Physical parameters of the transfection complex can strongly influence such an approach. Local injection of DNA complexes directly into subcutaneously growing tumors produced significant reporter gene expression, with DNA-transferrin PEI complexes or adenovirus-linked DNA-transferrin polylysine complexes being 10- to 100-fold more efficient than naked DNA (162). Intravenous application of transferrin PEI-DNA complexes through the tail vein into tumor-bearing mice resulted in gene expression in the tail and lung; there was no expression in the tumor, but serious toxicity (162,163). By first coating the DNA complexes with polyethyleneglycol (PEG) through covalent coupling to PEI, complexes are stabilized in size and do not bind plasma proteins (163). These PEGylated PEI complexes or optimized adenovirus-linked DNA complexes, when injected intravenously into mice, were far less toxic; gene expression was almost exclusively found at the application site (in the tail) and the tumor (162,163). Although these first results are encouraging, further optimization of in vivo gene-delivery systems is required for the development of useful therapies for human patients.

REFERENCES

1. Felgner PL, Barenholz Y, Behr JP, Cheng SH, Cullis P, Huang L, Jessee JA, Seymour L, Szoka F, Thierry AR, Wagner E, Wu G. Nomenclature for synthetic gene delivery systems. Hum Gene Ther 1997; 8:511–512.
2. Cotten M, Wagner E. Non-viral approaches to gene therapy. Current Op Biotech 1993; 4:705–710.
3. Ledley F. Non-viral gene therapy. Current Op Biotech 1994; 5:626–636.

65. Schwarzenberger P, Spence SE, Gooya JM, Michiel D, Curiel DT, Ruscetti FW, Keller JR. Targeted gene transfer to human hematopoietic progenitor cell lines through the c-kit receptor. Blood 1996; 87:472–478.
66. Baatz JE, Bruno MD, Ciraolo PJ, Glasser SW, Stripp BR, Smyth KL, Korfhagen TR. Utilization of modified surfactant-associated protein B for delivery of DNA to airway cells in culture. Proc Natl Acad Sci USA 1994; 91: 2547–2551.
67. Ross GF, Morris RE, Ciraolo G, Huelsman K, Bruno M, Whitsett JA, Baatz JE, Korfhagen TR. Surfactant protein A-polylysine conjugates for delivery of DNA to airway cells in culture. Hum Gene Ther 1995; 6:31–40.
68. Wagner E, Zenke M, Cotten M, Beug H, Birnstiel ML. Transferrin-polycation conjugates as carriers for DNA uptake into cells. Proc Natl Acad Sci USA 1990; 87: 3410–3414.
69. Cotten M, Laengle-Rouault F, Kirlappos H, Wagner E, Mechtler K, Zenke M, Beug H, Birnstiel ML. Transferrin-polycation-mediated introduction of DNA into human leukemic cells: stimulation by agents that affect the survival of transfected DNA or modulate transferrin receptor levels. Proc Natl Acad Sci USA 1990; 87:4033–4037.
70. Zenke M, Steinlein P, Wagner E, Cotten M, Beug H, Birnstiel ML. Receptor-mediated endocytosis of transferrin-polycation conjugates: an efficient way to introduce DNA into hemaptopoietic cells. Proc Natl Acad Sci USA 1990; 87:3655–3659.
71. Wagner E, Cotten M, Foisner R, Birnstiel ML. Transferrin-polycation-DNA complexes: the effect of polycatións on the structure of the complex and DNA delivery to cells. Proc Natl Acad Sci USA 1991; 88:4255–4259.
72. Wagner E, Cotten M, Mechtler K, Kirlappos H, Birnstiel ML. DNA-binding transferrin conjugates as functional gene-delivery agents: synthesis by linkage of polylysine or ethidium homodimer to the transferrin carbohydrate moiety. Bioconjugate Chem 1991; 2:226–231.
73. Cotten M, Wagner E, Birnstiel ML. Receptor-mediated transport of DNA into eukaryotic cells. Methods Enzymol 1993; 217:618–644.
74. Wagner E, Zatloukal K, Cotten M, Kirlappos H, Mechtler K, Curiel DT, Birnstiel ML. Coupling of adenovirus to transferrin-polylysine/DNA complexes greatly enhances receptor-mediated gene delivery and expression of transfected genes. Proc Natl Acad Sci USA 1992; 89: 6099–6103.
75. Taxman DJ, Lee ES, Wojchowski DM. Receptor-targeted transfection using stable maleimido-transferrin/thio-poly-L-lysine conjugates. Anal Biochem 1993; 213:97–103.
76. Cheng PW. Receptor ligand-facilitated gene transfer: Enhancement of liposome-mediated gene transfer and expression by transferrin. Hum Gene Ther 1996; 7:275–282.
77. Kircheis R, Kichler A, Wallner G, Kursa M, Ogris M, Felzmann T, Buchberger M, Wagner E. Coupling of cell-binding ligand to polyethylenimine for targeted gene delivery. Gene Ther 1997; 4:409–418.
78. Edwards RJ, Carpenter DS, Minchin RF. Uptake and intracellular trafficking of asialoglycoprotein-polylysine-DNA complexes in isolated hepatocytes. Gene Ther 1996; 3: 937–940.
79. Fra AM, Williamson E, Simons K, Parton RG. De novo formation of caveolae in lymphocytes by expression of VIP21-caveolin. Proc Natl Acad Sci USA 1995; 92: 8655–8659.
80. Middleton J, Neil S, Wintle J, Lewis JC, Moore H, Lam C, Auer M, Hub E, Rot A. Transcytosis and surface presentation of IL-8 by venular endothelial cells. Cell 1997; 91: 385–395.
81. Predescu D, Horvat R, Predescu S, Palade GE. Transcytosis in the continuous endothelium of the myocardial microvasculature is inhibited by N-ethylmaleimide. Proc Natl Acad Sci USA 1994; 91:3014–3018.
82. Nomura T, Nakajima S, Kawabata K, Yamashita F, Takakura Y, Hashida M. Intratumoral pharmacokinetics and in vivo gene expression of naked plasmid DNA and its cationic liposome complexes after direct gene transfer. Cancer Res 1997; 57:2681–2686.
83. Thierry AR, Rabinovich P, Peng B, Mahan LC, Bryant JL, Gallo RC. Characterisation of liposome-mediated gene delivery: expression, stability and pharmacokinetics of plasmid DNA. Gene Ther 1997; 4:226–237.
84. Bijsterbosch MK, Manoharan M, Rump ET, De Vrueh RLA, Van Aeghel R, Tivel KL, Biessen EAL, Bennett FC, Dan Cook P, Van Berkel TJC. In vivo fate of phosphorothioate antisense oligodeoxynucleotides: predominant uptake by scavenger receptors on endothelial liver cells. Nucleic Acids Res 1997; 25:3290–3296.
85. Davis SS. Biomedical applications of nanotechnology—implications for drug targeting and gene therapy. Trends Biotechnol 1997; 15:217–224.
86. Lampugnani MG, Dejana E. Interendothelial junctions: structure, signalling and functional roles. Current Opinion Cell Biol 1997; 9:674–682.
87. Kabanov AV, Kabanov VA. DNA complexes with polycations for the delivery of genetic material into cells. Bioconjugate Chem 1995; 6:7–20.
88. Dunlap DD, Maggi A, Soria MR, Monaco L. Nanoscopic structure of DNA condensed for gene delivery. Nucleic Acids Res 1997; 25:3095–3101.
89. Labat-Moleur F, Steffan AM, Brisson C, Perron H, Feugeas O, Furstenberger P, Oberling F, Brambilla E, Behr JP. An electron microscopy study into the mechanism of gene transfer with lipopolyamines. Gene Ther 1996; 3: 1010–1017.
90. Wolfert MA, Seymour LW. Atomic force microscopic analysis of the influence of the molecular weight of poly(L)lysine on the size of polyelectrolyte complexes formed with DNA. Gene Ther 1996; 3:269–273.
91. Kichler A, Zauner W, Morrison C, Wagner E. Ligand-polylysine mediated gene transfer. In: Artificial Self-Assembling Systems for Gene Delivery. Felgner, P.L. (ed.), ACS, Washington DC. 1996, pp. 120–128.

92. Ogris M, Steinlein P, Kursa M, Mechtler K, Kircheis R, Wagner E. The size of DNA/transferrin-PEI complexes is an important factor for gene expression in cultured cells. Gene Ther 1998; 5:1425–1433.
93. Wagner E, Curiel D, Cotten M. Delivery of drugs, proteins and genes into cells using transferrin as a ligand for receptor-mediated endocytosis. Adv Drug Del Rev 1994; 14: 113–136.
94. Plank C, Mechtler K, Szoka F, Wagner E. Activation of the complement system by synthetic DNA complexes: a potential barrier for intravenous gene delivery. Hum Gene Ther 1996; 7:1437–1446.
95. Ekblom P, Timpl R. Cell-to-cell contact and extracellular matrix. A multifaceted approach emerging. Current Opinion Cell Biol 1996; 8:599–601.
96. Iozzo RV, Murdoch AD. Proteoglycans of the extracellular environment: clues from the gene and protein side offer novel perspectives in molecular diversity and function. FASEB J 1996; 10:598–624.
97. Schwartz B, Benoist C, Abdallah B, Scherman D, Behr JP, Demeneix BA. Lipospermine-based gene transfer into the newborn mouse brain is optimized by a low lipospermine/DNA charge ratio. Hum Gene Ther 1995; 6: 1515–1524.
98. Prodeus AP, Zhou X, Maurer M, Galli SJ, Carroll MC. Impaired mast cell-dependent natural immunity in complement C3-deficient mice. Nature 1997; 390:172–175.
99. Wolbink GJ, Brouwer MC, Buysmann S, Ten Berge IJM, Hack EC. CRP-mediated activation of complement in vivo. J Immunol 1996; 157:473–479.
100. Rodman DM, San H, Simari R, Stephan D, Tanner F, Yang Z, Nabel GJ, Nabel EG. In vivo gene delivery to the pulmonary circulation in rats: transgene distribution and vascular inflammatory response. Am J Respir Cell Mol Biol 1997; 16:640–649.
101. Wiertz EJ, Mukherjee S, Ploegh HL. Viruses use stealth technology to escape from the host immune system. Mol Med Today 1997; 3:116–123.
102. Deol P, Khuller GK. Lung specific stealth liposomes: stability, biodistribution and toxicity of liposomal antitubercular drugs in mice. Biochim Biophys Acta 1997; 1334: 161–172.
103. Du H, Chandaroy P, Hui SW. Grafted poly-(ethylene glycol) on lipid surfaces inhibits protein adsorption and cell adhesion. Biochim Biophys Acta 1997; 1326:236–248.
104. Goren D, Horowitz AT, Zalipsky S, Woodle MC, Yarden Y, Gabizon A. Targeting of stealth liposomes to erb-2 (Her/2) receptor: in vitro and in vivo studies. Br J Cancer 1996; 74:1749–1756.
105. Hong K, Zheng W, Baker A, Paphadjopoulos D. Stabalization of cationic liposome-plasmid DNA complexes by polyamines and poly(ethylene glycol)-phospholipid conjugates for efficient in vivo gene delivery. FEBS Lett 1997; 400:233–237.
106. Haensler J, Szoka FC. Polyamidoamine cascade polymers mediate efficient transfection of cells in culture. Bioconjugate Chem 1993; 4:372–379.
107. Boussif O, Lezoualc'h F, Zanta MA, Mergny M, Scherman D, Demeneix B, Behr JP. A novel, versatile vector for gene and oligonucleotide transfer into cells in culture and in vivo: polyethylenimine. Proc Natl Acad Sci USA 1995; 92:7297–7301.
108. Tang MX, Szoka FC. The influence of polymer structure on the interactions of cationic polymers with DNA and morphology of the resulting complexes. Gene Ther 1997; 4:823–832.
109. Fritz JD, Herweijer H, Zhang G, Wolff JA. Gene transfer into mammalian cells using histone-condensed plasmid DNA. Hum Gene Ther 1996; 7:1395–1404.
110. Blessing T, Remy JS, Behr JP. Molecular collapse of plasmid DNA into stable virus-like particles. Proc Natl Acad Sci USA 1998; 95:1427–1431.
111. Emi N, Kidoaki S, Yoshikawa K, Saito H. Gene transfer mediated by polyarginine requires a formation of big carrier-complex of DNA aggregate. Biochem Biophys Res Comm 1997; 231:421–424.
112. Mistry AR, Falciola L, Monaco L, Taliabue R, Acerbis G, Knight A, Harbottle RP, Soria M, Bianchi ME, Coutelle C, Hart SL. Recombinant HMG1 protein produced in pichia pastoris: a nonviral gene delivery agent. Bio Techniques 1997; 22:718–729.
113. Stavridis JC, Deliconstantinos G, Psallidopoulos MC, Armenakas NA, Hadjiminas DJ, Hadjiminas J. Construction of transferrin-coated liposomes for in vivo transport of exogeneous DNA to bone marrow erythroblasts in rabbits. Exp Cell Res 1986; 164:568–572.
114. Huckett B, Gordhan H, Hawtrey R, Moodley N, Ariatti M, Hawtrey A. Binding of DNA to albumin and transferrin modified by treatment with water soluble carbodiimides. Biochem Pharmacol 1986; 35:1249–1257.
115. Seglen PO. Inhibitors of lysosomal function. Methods Enzymol 1983; 96:737–764.
116. Pless DD, Wellner RB. In vitro fusion of endocytic vesicles: effects of reagents that alter endosomal pH. J Cell Biochem 1996; 62:27–39.
117. Cain CC, Sipe DM, Murphy RF. Regulation of endocytic pH by the NA+, K+ ATPase in living cells. Proc Natl Acad Sci USA 1989; 86:544–548.
118. Sipe DM, Jesurum A, Murphy RF. Absence of NA+, K+ ATPase regulation of endosomal acidification in K562 erythroleukemia cells. J Biol Chem 1991; 266: 34690–3474.
119. Li S., Thacker J. High-efficiency stable DNA transfection using cationic detergent and glycerol. Biochem Biophys Res Comm 1997; 231:531–534.
120. Zauner W, Kichler A, Mechtler K, Schmidt W, Wagner E. Glycerol and polylysine synergize in their ability to rupture vesicular membranes and increase transferrin-polylysine mediated gene transfer. Exp Cell Res 1997; 232:137–145.
121. Curiel DT, Agarwal S, Wagner E, Cotten M. Adenovirus enhancement of transferrin-polylysine-mediated gene delivery. Proc Natl Acad Sci USA 1991; 88:8850–8854.

122. Cotten M, Wagner E, Zatloukal K, et al. High-efficiency receptor-mediated delivery of small and large (48kb) gene constructs using the endosome disruption activity of defective or chemically inactivated adenovirus particles. Proc Natl Acad Sci USA 1992; 89:6094–6098.
123. Curiel DT, Wagner E, Cotten M, Birnstiel ML, Agarwal S, Li CM, Loechel S, Hu PC. High-efficiency gene transfer mediated by adenovirus coupled to DNA-polylysine complexes. Hum Gene Ther 1992; 3:147–154.
124. Kupfer JM, Ruan XM, Liu G, Matloff J, Forrester J, Chaux A. High-efficiency gene transfer to autologous rabbit jugular vein grafts using adenovirus-transferrin/polylysine-DNA complexes. Hum Gene Ther 1994; 5:1437–1443.
125. Cotten M, Saltik M, Kursa M, Wagner E, Maass G, Birnstiel ML. Psoralen treatment of adenovirus particles eliminates virus replication and transcription while maintaining the endosomolytic activity of the virus capsid. Virology 1994; 205:254–261.
126. Baker A, Cotten M. Delivery of bacterial artificial chromosomes into mammalian cells with psoralen-inactivated adenovirus carrier. Nucleic Acid Res 1997; 25:1950–1956.
127. Baker A, Saltik M, Lehrmann H, Killisch I, Mautner V, Lamm G, Christofori G, Cotten M. Polyethylenimine (PEI) is a simple, inexpensive and effective reagent for condensing and linking plasmid DNA to adenovirus for gene delivery. Gene Ther 1997; 4:773–782.
128. Fasbender A, Zabner J, Chillon M, Moninger Th.O, Puga AP, Davidson BL, Welsh MJ. Complexes of adenovirus with polycationic polymers and cationic lipids increase the efficiency of gene transfer in vitro and in vivo. J Biol Chem 1997; 272:6479–6489.
129. Zauner W, Blaas D, Küchler E, Wagner E. Rhinovirus mediated endosomal release of transfection complexes. J Virol 1995; 69:1085–1092.
130. Plank C, Oberhauser B, Mechtler K, Koch C, Wagner E. The influence of endosome-disruptive peptides on gene transfer using synthetic virus-like gene transfer systems. J Biol Chem 1994; 269:12918–12924.
131. Gottschalk S, Sparrow JT, Hauer J, Mims MP, Leland FE, Woo SLC, Smith LC. A novel DNA-peptide complex for efficient gene transfer and expression in mammalian cells. Gene Ther 1996; 3:448–457.
132. Kichler A, Mechtler K, Behr JP, Wagner E. The influence of membrane-active peptides and helper lipids on lipospermine/DNA complex mediated gene transfer. Bioconjugate Chem 1997; 8:213–221.
133. Wyman TB, Nicol F, Zelphati O, Scaria PV, Plank C, Szoka FC. Design, synthesis and characterization of a cationic peptide that binds to nucleic acids and permeabilizes bilayers. Biochemistry 1997; 36:3008–3017.
134. Fender P, Ruigrock RWH, Gout E, Buffet S, Chroboczek J. Adenovirus dodecahedron, a new vector for human gene transfer. Nature Biotechnol 1997; 15:52–56.
135. Hakansson S, Schesser K, Persson C, Galyov EE, Rosqvist R, Homble F, Wolf-Watz H. The YopB protein of Yersinia pseudotuberculosis is essential for the translocation of Yop effector proteins across the target cell plasma membrane and displays a contact-dependent membrane disrupting activity. EMBO J 1996; 15:5812–5823.
136. Plotkowski MC, Meirelles MN. Concomitant endosome-phagosome fusion and lysis of endosomal membranes account for *Pseudomonas aeruginosa* survival in human endothelial cells. J Submicrosc Cytol Pathol 1997; 29: 229–237.
137. Satin B, Norais N, Telford J, Rappuolli R, Murgia M, Montrcucco C, Papini E. Effect of helicobacter pylori vacuolating toxin on maturation and extracellular release of procathepsin D and on epidermal growth factor degradation. J Biol Chem 1997; 272:25022–25028.
138. Gottschalk S, Tweten RK, Smith LC, Woo SLC. Efficient gene delivery and expression in mammalian cells using DNA coupled with perfringolysin O. Gene Ther 1995; 2: 498–503.
139. Fisher KJ, Wilson JM. The transmembrane domain of diphtheria toxin improves molecular conjugate gene transfer. J Biochem 1997; 321:49–58.
140. Wilke M, Fortunati E, Broek M, Hoogeveen AT, Scholte BJ. Efficacy of a peptide-based gene delivery system depends on mitotic activity. Gene Ther 1996; 3:1133–1142.
141. Dean DA. Import of DNA is sequence specific. Exp Cell Res 1997; 230:293–302.
142. Dowty ME, Williams P, Zhang G, Hagstrom JE, Wolff JA. Plasmid DNA entry into postmitotic nuclei of primary rat myotubes. Proc Natl Acad Sci USA 1995; 92: 4572–4576.
143. Hagstrom J, Ludtke J, Bassik M, Sebestyen M, Adams S, Wolff J. Nuclear import of DNA in digitonin-permeabilized cells. J Cell Sci 1997; 110:2323–2331.
144. Görlich D, Mattaj IW. Nucleocytoplasmic transport. Science 1996; 271:1513–1518.
145. Pennisi E. The nucleus's resolving door. Science 1998; 279:1129–1131.
146. Zanta MA, Belguise Valladier P, Behr JP. Gene delivery: a single nuclear localization signal peptide is sufficient to carry DNA to the cell nucleus. Proc Natl Acad Sci USA 1999; 96:91–96.
147. Laemmli UK, Tjian R. Nucleus and gene expression-a nuclear trafic jam: unraveling multicomponent machines and compartments. Current Opinion Cell Biol 1996; 8: 299–302.
148. Singer RH, Green MR. Compartmentalization of eukaryotic gene expression: causes and effects. Cell 1997; 91: 291–294.
149. Surosky RT, Urabe M, Godwin SG, McQuiston SA, Kurtzman GJ, Ozawas K, Natsoulis G. Adeno-associated virus Rep proteins target DNA sequence to a unique locus in the human genome. J Virol 1997; 71:7951–7959.
150. Calos MP. The potential of extrachromosomal replicating vectors for gene therapy. TIG 1996; 12:463–466.
151. Wohlgemuth JG, Kang SH, Bulboaca GH, Nawotka KA, Calos MP. Long-term gene expression from autonomosly replicating vectors in mammalian cells. Gene Ther 1996; 3:503–512.

152. Huxley C. Mammalian artificial chromosomes: a new tool for gene therapy. Gene Ther 1994; 1:7–12.
153. Rosenfeld MA. Human artificial chromosomes get real. Nature Genetics 1997; 15:333–335.
154. Harrington JJ, Bokkelen GV, Mays RW, Gustashaw K., Willard HF. Formation of de novo centromeres and construction of first-generation human artificial microchromosomes. Nature Genetics 1997; 15:345–355.
155. Miller N, Whelan J. Progress in transcriptionaly targeted and regulatable vectors for gene therapy. Hum Gene Ther 1997; 8:803–815.
156. Dillon N. Regulating gene expression in gene therapy. Trends Biotech 1993; 11:167–173.
157. Cheng Q, Cant CA, Moll T, Hofer-Warbinek R, Wagner E., Birnstiel ML, Bach FH, de Martin R. NF-kB Subunit-specific regulation of the IkB promoter. J Biol Chem 1994; 269:13551–13557.
158. Zatloukal K, Cotten M, Berger M, Schmidt W, Wagner E., Birnstiel ML. In vivo production of human factor VIII in mice after intrasplenic implantation of primary fibroblasts transfected by receptor-mediated, adenovirus-augmented gene delivery. Proc Natl Acad Sci USA 1994; 91: 5148–5152.
159. Zatloukal K, Schneeberger A, Berger M, Schmidt W, Kosik F, Kutil R, Cotten M., Wagner E, Buschle M, Maass G, Payer E, Stingl G, Birnstiel ML. Elicitation of a systemic and protective anti-melanoma immune response by an IL-2 based vaccine: assessment of critical parameters. J Immunol 1995; 154:3406–3419.
160. Schreiber S, Kämpgen E, Wagner E, et al. Immunotherapy of metastatic malignant melanoma by a vaccine consisting of autologous interleukin 2-transfected cancer cells: outcome of a phase I study. Hum Gene Ther 1999; 10: 983–993.
161. Nguyen DM, Wiehle SA, Roth JA, Cristiano RJ. Gene delivery into malignant cells in vivo by conjugated adenovirus/DNA complex. Cancer Gene Ther 1997; 4: 183–190.
162. Kircheis R, Schüller S., Brunner S, Ogris M, Heider KH, Zauner W, Wagner E. Polycation-based DNA complexes for tumor-targeted gene delivery in vivo. J Gene Med 1999; 1:111–120.
163. Ogris M, Brunner S, Schüller S, Kircheis R, Wagner E. PEGylated DNA/Transferrin-PEI complexes: reduced interaction with blood components, extended circulation in blood and potential for systemic gene delivery. Gene Ther 1999; 6:595–605.

9

Modification of Melanoma Cells via Ballistic Gene Delivery for Vaccination

Ulrich R. Hengge
University of Essen, Essen, Germany

Dirk Schadendorf
University of Mannheim, Mannheim, Germany

I. INTRODUCTION

Gene therapy is an emerging field for treating diseases using DNA as the remedy. It can be used to treat systemic diseases as well as various organ disorders. The goal of gene therapy is to treat a specific disease process with the protein product of the introduced gene. This protein can be used either locally or systemically (e.g., clotting factors and hormones) (1).

An essential component of the revolution in molecular biology has been the arrival of transfer methods by transfection or transduction. In principal, three different ways of introducing genetic material exist: (1) viral vectors, (2) calcium phosphate, DEAE-dextran, or liposomes, and (3) physical methods such as direct injection, electroporation, or the gene gun (2). Each of these methods has its own inherent strengths and weaknesses and is especially suitable for a particular application. In 1987, Sanford and coworkers invented a new addition to the armamentarium of gene-delivery vehicles called the ''biolistic method of gene transfer'' (3). Other terms include ''particle bombardment'' and ''gene gun.'' In principal, the technique implies that DNA is coated onto 1–5 μm heavy metal particles (usually gold or tungsten) that have been accelerated using helium to sufficient velocity to penetrate the target cells. Historically, the first cells to be penetrated were plant cells (3,4). The most notable application involved the production of the first transgenic crop (i.e., the transfection of maize) (5,6).

In order to design potential treatment strategies for gene therapy, it is relevant to discuss two general approaches: the in vivo and the ex vivo approaches of gene transfer (Fig. 1). In the in vivo approach the desired genes are introduced directly into the target organ, while in the ex vivo approach the target cells are cultured from biopsy specimens and the desired gene is inserted while these cells are being propagated in tissue culture. The genetically modified target cells are grown in culture and eventually grafted back onto the donor. Both the in vivo and the ex vivo approaches have their relative advantages and disadvantages, which reflect their potential applications. The biggest advantage of the in vivo approach is that it is simple and direct. In the case of skin, it takes advantage of its easy accessibility. The biggest disadvantage is that expression of the desired gene is usually transient because the gene is introduced locally and only into a limited number of target cells. Generally, stem cells have not been successfully targeted using in vivo approaches, with the potential exception of hematopoiesis and liposomal gene transfer (7,8). However, it should be noted that transient expression of the desired gene may be adequate for a variety of applications such as genetic vaccination.

A plethora of different techniques has been developed in gene therapy to enhance the uptake of DNA (containing the gene of interest) (2). Initially, chemical DNA transfection used calcium chloride and DEAE-dextran to transfer genetic material followed by the use of cationic lipids or

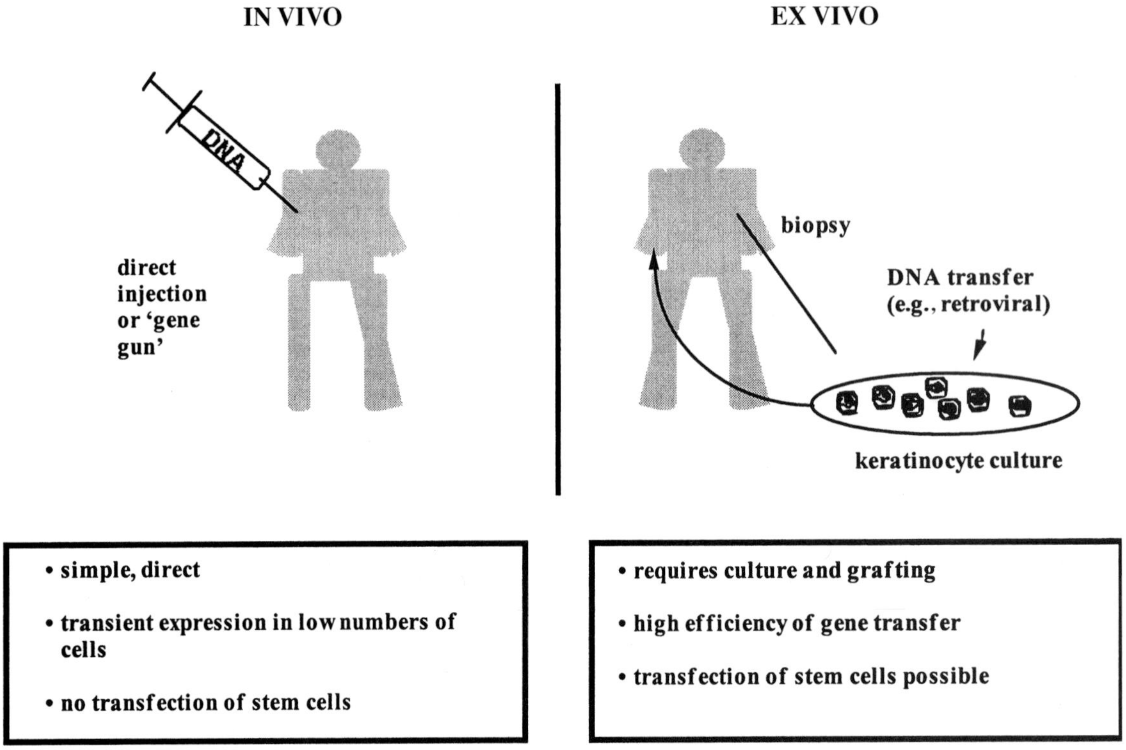

Figure 1 In vivo and ex vivo gene transfer—schematic outline.

liposomes. Because of the low transfection efficiency and the substantial in vivo toxicity of cationic lipids, other methods of gene transfer have increasingly been developed to insert DNA into cells. Viral gene transfer has exploited the capability of recombinant viruses such as retrovirus, adenovirus, or adeno-associated virus to infect cells and efficiently transport the genetic material containing the gene of interest into the cells. In addition, three physical techniques have been developed to introduce DNA into target tissues (2). These physical techniques are similar in that they can directly introduce DNA into the target organ such as skin. Consequently, these techniques will generally be used for in vivo approaches. While the particle bombardment technique will be extensively reviewed in this chapter, direct injection using a syringe and a small needle has been added as another alternative for gene transfer. Upon direct injection of DNA into skin or muscle, the DNA is taken up by the target cells and the desired genes are transiently expressed (9–12). In the case of injected muscle, the transgene can be detected for up to 1 year with some albeit low level of expression.

A variety of tissues has been successfully transfected using direct injection such as epidermis, muscle, thyroid, liver, lung, synovia, and melanoma (13–17). The exact mechanisms of how epithelial cells or muscle cells, the first tissue demonstrated to take up and express naked DNA, accomplish this is not yet clear, but there is evidence that a specialized transport process for small molecules, called potocytosis, may be involved (18,19). The existence of DNA-binding proteins on keratinocyte and muscle membranes is currently being investigated in the laboratory.

Feasibility studies have shown that plasmid DNA can also be expressed upon microinjection into the nucleus of mammalian cells (mouse fibroblast cell line LMTK) but not when injected into the cytoplasm (20). Furthermore, ultrasound has been demonstrated to allow gene transfer into mammalian cells in culture (21).

Alternative ways of introducing genetic material into the skin consist of various techniques to overcome the epidermal barrier that limits the delivery of plasmid DNA. Such methods comprise applying a pulsed electric field on topically applied plasmid DNA (22). A simpler way for gene transfer to the skin is constant puncturing using a device with oscillating fine needles (23). Topical application of plasmid DNA complexed to various cationic lipids has been demonstrated to allow gene transfer to the skin (24), although this approach has not worked for others. Topical application of plasmid DNA coding for the murine interleukin-10 gene to the scarified cornea has been shown to suppress an ongoing ocular inflammation caused by herpetic keratitis (25). The corneal route also proved effective in generating an immune response when expression plasmids coding for the herpes simplex glycoprotein B were applied (25).

The focus of this chapter is to review the basic elements of the gene gun and its operation. We will highlight its applications to transfect cultured cells, tissue explants, and living animals. Particular emphasis will be placed on genetic vaccination using plasmid DNA to induce humoral and cytotoxic T-cell responses. A large variety of tissues and cell types from multiple species have been successfully transfected using this technique.

II. HISTORY OF BALLISTIC GENE TRANSFER

The pioneering studies by Sanford et al. demonstrated that a gene could be expressed in intact plant cells after biolistic transfer (3,4). The original gene gun as invented by Sanford and coworkers involved the placement of DNA-coated microprojectiles in an aqueous slurry on a small plastic bullet. This bullet was placed into a 22-caliber barrel in front of a gun powder cartridge. Upon firing, the cartridge propelled a plastic bullet in the barrel until it was stopped by a solid plate. The plate had a central small hole that allowed the microprojectiles to continue their trajectory into the target tissue. Target organs or cells were placed in a chamber for bombardment. Subsequently, the gunpowder device has been replaced because it created too much tissue damage and the velocity of the projectiles was not readily adjustable. Therefore, the helium device was developed as a collaboration of the Sanford and Johnston group that used high-pressure helium restrained by a piercable kapton disks. Another kapton disk, called macroprojectile, is positioned approximately 1 cm in front of the restraining membranes. The DNA-coated microprojectiles are placed in a dry state in front of this macroprojectile (Fig. 2). Another centimeter in front of the macroprojectile, a stopping screen is securely placed. Right in front of this stopping screen a small orifice is put in contact with the tissue culture dish or the appropriate tissue. When the high-pressure helium gas is released by piercing the restraining membrane, a

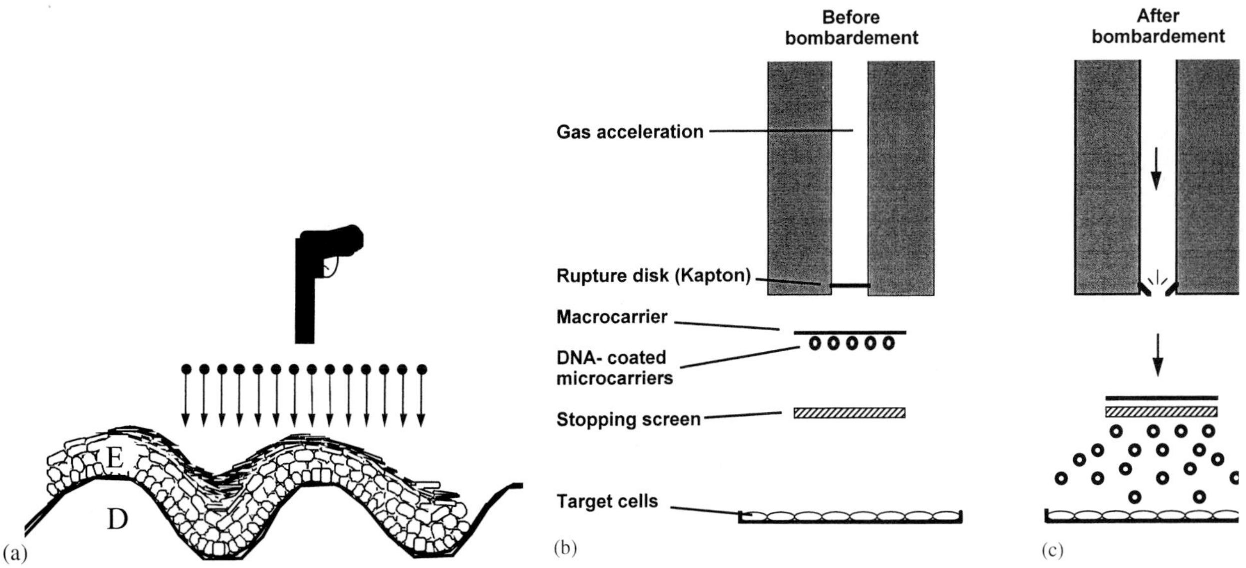

Figure 2 (a) Schematic of biolistic gene transfer. (b) Detailed view of the biolistic process (see text for details). (a) Colloidal gold particles are loaded with plasmid DNA encoding a cytokine and paramagnetic beads on the carrier disc. E = Epidermis; D = dermis. (b) Pressure via helium gas is applied onto a burst disc causing its rupture and an acceleration of the loaded carrier disc. (c) The particle-carrying disc is abruptly stopped at a stopping grid causing a sudden release of the paramagnetic gold particles, which will subsequently hit the cells maintained in the petri culture disk at the bottom of the apparatus. Gold particles coated with paramagnetic particles and the plasmid DNA encoding human recombinant IL-7 or IL-12 will hit the tumor cells and pass the nucleus packed with chromatin. Because of the charge of the nuclear chromatin, the passing gold particles will lose most of their coated paramagnetic beads and plasmid DNA. Subsequently, cells hit are easily recovered by magnetic separation and selected for live cells, if necessary, by attachment to culture dishes.

shock wave will be produced. This supersonic shock wave hits the macroprojectile, which is then launched against the stopping screen, allowing the microprojectiles to continue on into the target cells. An important technical feature is that the macroprojectiles seal off the chamber when they hit the stopping screen in order to protect the target tissue. All the single parts of the device are contained in a cylindrical chamber the size of a soft drink can. In the chamber, where the microprojectiles are released, a vacuum is maintained in order to avoid deceleration by the air. The device is attached to a gas line and a vacuum line, and an electric battery pack is used as power supply. This design is currently available from Biorad (PDS 1000/He; Hercules, CA). Its design involves a restraining membrane that ruptures at the desired gas pressure.

The distance the microprojectiles travel to the cells affects the transfection efficiency in several ways. First, especially for small particles, the velocity decreases with the travel distance. The velocity is an important variable with tissues explants, but not so with cultured cells. By placing the target cells closer to the stopping screen, the blast effect of the shock wave is increased. This effect is especially important for working with sensitive cell types. The area of bombardment increases with the distance from the stopping screen. On average, the bombarded area covers a 10 cm culture plate, when it is placed about 8 cm from the screen. The usual pressure of 25 mmHg (0.03 atm) is generally used to transfect most cultured cells. Second, studies on the plasmid delivery have determined that about 20 biologically active 6 kb plasmids can be carried on one single 0.5 μm microprojectile (26). Since commonly the microparticles are about 1–1.6 μm in size, considerably more copies of plasmid DNA can be loaded on one particle (27). However, the coating of individual particles is quite uneven. In general, tissues are bombarded with gold particles having a diameter range of 1–5 μm. Tungsten particles are 3.9 μm in size. Microprojectiles are coated with DNA as described by Klein et al. (4). Briefly, 25 μL of a gold or tungsten suspension are mixed with 25 μL of 2.5 M $CaCl_2$ and 5 μL of 1 M spermidine. After 10 minutes of incubation the microprojectiles are pelleted and the supernatant is removed. The pellet is washed once in 70% ethanol prior to resuspension in 100% ethanol. The DNA-coated particles are spread onto macrocarrier discs, and the ethanol is allowed to evaporate prior to loading the gun. Further refinement of the particle homogenicity will improve the DNA coating and will potentially lead to higher numbers of intact plasmid copies being delivered into the cells.

In the meantime, Agracetus (Madison, WI) has designed a similar device, called Accell (28,29), which uses a large electrical discharge to vaporize a water droplet to create the impelling shock wave. Other adopted versions have been constructed for application in very sensitive tissues such as soft plants or seedlings as a hand-held apparatus (HandGun or Blowpipe) (30) or air-driven (pneumatic or jet gun) devices (31,32).

III. APPLICATIONS IN OTHER FIELDS

Technologies for introducing foreign genes into cells are critical for both basic studies of gene function as well as for the production of transgenic organisms with commercial value. Particle bombardment was primarily devised to overcome barriers to genetic transformation of many plant species. Broad experience has been generated in the transfection of plants without removing cell walls and living animals using this technique. Also, in basic biology the gene gun technology has been useful to study the regulation of gene expression. This was made possible by analyzing the structure and function of *cis*- and *trans*-acting transcription factors. Therefore, one approach was to assess the activity of promoters, 3′ regions, and associated enhancer elements by using chimeric genes fused to a coding sequence of a marker gene that can be easily detected (33). In particular, particle bombardment has been helpful to study the promoter hypermethylation in barley endosperm (34) and in following the promoter activity during various developmental stages of tomatoes (35,36). Using particle bombardment the causal agent of plant diseases such as the strawberry mild yellow edge disease could be identified as a potexvirus (37).

A. Plants

A lot of knowledge has been derived from applying the gene gun to plants and microbes, which were among the early targets of ballistic gene transfer. First, for both plants and microbes, the gene gun has proven capable of transforming recalcitrant species. The most notable example has been the creation of transgenic maize (5,6,38,39), soybean (40), tobacco (41), and wheat (42). In plants (e.g., soybean) particle bombardment has achieved stable transfection that was transmitted to subsequent generations (40). In addition, transgenic rice has been made resistant against the yellow stem borer (*Scirpophaga incertulas*), a major cause of insect pest in rice, by introduction of the insecticidal crystal protein gene of *Bacillus thuringiensis* (43,44). Transgenic wheat has been generated that is resistant to a frequently used herbicide in horticulture by gene gun transfer of the appropriate resistance gene (phosphinothricin acetyltransferase) (42,45). The generation of such crops has important agronomic implications.

Moreover, the first organelle transfections (tobacco chloroplasts) were accomplished with the gene gun (46,47) as have the mitochondria of yeast, thus allowing the manipulation of organelle genomes in the same way as nuclear genomes (48). In this example, mutants that were unable to grow photosynthetically as a result of a defective atpB gene were restored by bombardment with plasmid DNA encoding the functional atpB gene. Prior to particle bombardment the study of the mitochondrial genome has been hampered by the double-membrane preventing the introduction of foreign genes.

Particle bombardment of microbes has received limited attention, probably because genetic material can be readily introduced into bacteria. However, the transformation of a number of biologically important microbes remains a significant barrier. Recent results indicate that *Magnoportha griseia,* a fungal pathogen of rice, has been successfully transformed using the gene gun. Mycelium of fungi such as *Erysiphe graminis,* an obligate plant pathogen, have also been successfully transformed using particle bombardment (49).

The biolistic transfer has also been useful in reverse genetics studying the interactions of the hard-to-clone potatovirus Y and plants such as tobacco (50). Similarly, particle bombardment has been found to be several orders of magnitude more efficient than mechanical inoculation in squash, cucumber, melon, and watermelon when the infectivity of cloned zucchini yellow mosaic potyvirus was studied (51). Moreover, the gene gun has been employed to inoculate RNA into various pollens of plants (e.g., lily, tulip, and freesia) in order to study the expression kinetics of RNA (52) and for the assessment of promoter activity during fruit ripening under various environmental conditions such as varying temperatures and light (53–55). In addition, the photoregulation of gene expression has been studied in particle-mediated gene transfer in various crop plants (35).

B. Animals

One newer application of particle bombardment technology is the direct insertion of genes into tissues and organs of living animals (56). In experiments using simple organisms such as the mating *Tetrahymena thermophila,* transformations have been achieved in the germline and in somatic cells (57).

Bombarding the epidermis of anesthetized mice resulted in the expression of the transgene for up to 14 days (58). The assessment of the promoter strength in various tissues has generally revealed the transient nature of expression upon particle-mediated gene transfer (59,60). The transient nature of expression is probably attributable to the fact that most microprojectiles come to rest in the first few layers of the epidermis. By the third day most of the remaining microprojectiles were found in the dermis, since most of the epidermal cells have sloughed as part of their normal turnover (58). To avoid gold particles, the biolistic transfer has been modified employing ice crystals or pressurized air as carriers for DNA (31,32,61,62). On histological sections the bombarded skin revealed very little damage or inflammation with few microscopic hematomas being present. Up to 20% of cells in the target field stained positive for the reporter gene. In general, less than 5% of the introduced genes were expressed in the dermis. In mice ears expression persisted for up to 10 days, declining rapidly from initially high levels. However, gold particles have been demonstrated to penetrate into the ear cartilage and further. Generally, the microprojectiles retained the DNA and DNA was not deposited significantly in the path of the particles. Similar results were obtained using fresh isolated ductal segments of rat and human mammary glands (28).

Other tissues such as muscle, liver, pancreas, cornea, and brain have also successfully been transfected using the gene gun (28,63–65). Some studies were performed to assess the prolongation of graft survival by localized immunosuppression upon expression of CTLA-4 immunoglobulin (64). In liver, the transgene activity per bombarded area was comparable to skin at one day after bombardment but declined rapidly after 5 days (28,58). When human growth hormone (hGH) was expressed from a fatty acid–binding protein promoter, hGH was detected for up to 3 days in blood (1.1 ng/mL) and for up to 23 days in liver tissue.

Recently, other species such as chicken and fish eggs and mouse, oyster, and drosophila embryos, which were usually transfeced inefficiently, have been targeted successfully utilizing the gene gun (66–69). Various cell lines of epithelial, endothelial, fibroblast, and lymphocyte origin have also been successfully transfected in culture (28,70). Stably transformed clones have been recovered from several cell lines following bombardment with a plasmid conferring resistance to the antibiotic G418 and subsequent selection. Remarkably, the viability upon particle bombardment remained high (85–95%) (33). These results suggest that particle bombardment can be used to transform cell lines that have proven difficult to transform.

These promising results have led to the speculation that this process of DNA transfer could be employed in the generation of antibodies and gene therapy. Immunization with plasmid DNA encoding microbial agents would represent an attractive application of particle bombardment technology. In this regard, DNA technology seems superior to conventional protein vaccination considering economical and logistic aspects (availability, stability, storage). Antigens produced in host tissues such as muscle and skin can elicit humoral and cellular immune responses including class I major histocompatibility (MHC)–restricted cytotoxic T lymphocytes (CTL), which are thought to be important in tumor and virus defense. The mechanisms of antigen processing and presentation to T lymphocytes are only partly understood. Class I MHC molecules present on the surface of antigen-producing myocytes or keratinocytes are probably sensitized with antigenic peptides derived from the antigen that can engage the T-cell receptor. Humoral immune responses may be explained following the secretion of antigen from transfected somatic cells or by the release of antigen from lytic cells (71,72). Exogenous proteins released by this fashion could be taken up and presented to CD4-positive T cells by antigen-presenting cells in the draining lymph nodes. The presentation of genetically produced antigens to CD8-positive CTL is less clear. Besides the scenario that transfected nonprofessional cells such as keratinocytes present the antigen directly, antigens could be taken up by antigen-presenting cells via phagocytosis and gain access to the MHC class I pathway leading to the induction of antigen-specific CTL-mediated immunity (73–75).

In addition to the therapeutic antigen, immunostimulatory cytokines such as GM-CSF, IL-1, or IL-12 in DNA form can be used as a vaccine cocktail (76–81). At least in some cases the co-expression of co-stimulatory molecules such as B7.1 has further enhanced the immune response (82). Alternatively, the immunization can be performed with the complete expression library of pathogenic organisms (83,84) leading to the expression of all proteins coded by the infectious agent's DNA independent of their immunogenicity.

Using particle bombardment, a polyclonal immune response against various pathogens such as Ebola virus (85), hepatitis B and C (86–89), herpes simplex (90,91), malaria (76,92), mycoplasma (83,93), papillomavirus (94), prions (95), rotavirus (96), and tuberculosis (97,98) has been reported. Two diseases with a major impact on socioeconomic health served as a model: influenza and HIV. Pioneering work has been performed by Johnston et al. and Liu et al., who demonstrated protection against heterologous strains of influenza (99–104). On the other hand, therapeutic and prophylactic vaccines against HIV have represented a great challenge for researchers. Several lines of progress have been made in mice (105–110) and nonhuman primates (111–113). Recombinant DNA vaccines against HIV are currently in clinical trials conducted by Weiner et al. (personal communication).

Various researchers have demonstrated the dependence of the immune response from the method and route of DNA administration. More specifically, saline injections of DNA vaccines into the skin have revealed a Th1-type antibody response, whereas gene gun immunizations produced a predominantly Th2-type immune response (i.e., IgG1) (110,114,115). In addition, the nature of the antigen also seemed to influence the type of immune response (115). The elicitation of a Th1-type immune response following the biolistic approach has been achieved by co-delivery of vectors expressing IL-2, IL-7, or IL-12 (110). Various other factors such as the time period between immunizations have been identified to augment the Th1-type immunity (110). Direct comparison of the epidermal versus the intramuscular route suggested a higher rate of seroconversion and higher antibody titers following epidermal immunization (29,116). The importance of antigen-presenting cells for the generation of an immune response has been clearly demonstrated in chimeric mice grafted with partially MHC-matched spleen cells (74,75) and in studies where direct transfection of dendritic cells with plasmid DNA has led to an effective immunization (73). This method of generating CTLs would alleviate the need for expanding and loading dendritic cells in culture prior to reinfusion into the host. Other adjuvants such as immunostimulatory CpG motifs may offer additional benefit (117,118). Furthermore, the presence of muscle cells following intramuscular injection of plasmid DNA has not been found necessary for effective immunizations (119). In contrast, the elicitation of antibody and CTL responses was dependent on the presence of the injected skin sites for at least 48 hours (119,120). Further studies have shown that injected skin that was transplanted to naive mice up to 24 hours postinjection could elicit a primary immune response (120). Variation of the delivery concept have included biodegradable microspheres showing an enhanced immunization potential compared to naked DNA (121). Successful immunization using plasmid DNA has also been shown in the female genital tract where vaginal mucosa expressed the introduced gene producing high levels of secretory IgA antibodies that were not consistently produced by other routes (122).

This section has summarized the evolutional steps of the particle bombardment technology and has attempted to present some of the experimental data that has been obtained in various cell and tissue systems. The overall importance of this relatively atraumatic technology lies in the ease of inducing an effective DNA vaccination. However, the preferential Th2 type of the immune reaction needs to be kept in mind when considering potential target diseases. Based on recent experiments where protective immunity has been achieved in various animal models, this new technology using particle bombardment can be considered a potentially useful strategy for prophylactic or therapeutic vaccination of human beings.

IV. BALLISTIC GENE TRANSFER IN CANCER TREATMENT

The era of gene therapy has become a clinical reality. Since the first therapeutic experiments in 1970 more than 250 additional clinical gene therapy trials were approved and more than 2000 patients were treated worldwide by the end of 1996 (123). Almost 25% of these studies had no therapeutic intent and were gene-marking trials. The majority (60%) of the trials were intended to treat cancer. The great majority of investigators used immunization strategies with cytokine gene–modified tumor cells. Since melanoma is supposedly one of the most immunogenic tumors, it was therefore a favorable target for gene-modified cancer vaccines (summarized in Table 1). Based on animal tumor models, a number of clinical protocols have been developed to treat cancer patients with cytokine gene–modified tumor cells.

As discussed above, there are several nonviral methods of gene transfer that seem to be less risky in general, particularly in terms of integration into the host genome or potential infectiousness when compared to viral vector systems. Transfer techniques in use are calcium phosphate precipitation, DEAE-dextrane transfection, electroporation, in vitro DNA microinjection, receptor-mediated DNA transfection, liposomal DNA complexes, direct DNA injection in vivo, and ballistic gene transfer (1,2,124). Most of these techniques have been known for years and are well established in small-scale approaches in the laboratory but are not useful for clinical application because of the low transfection efficiency or certain technical requirements that cannot be fulfilled in clinical trials.

A. Melanoma and Tumor Immunology

Melanoma is a malignant tumor of neuroectodermal origin with an increasing incidence and mortality. It needs to be detected and eliminated early, since melanoma is characterized by its high resistance to conventional therapies, including surgery and chemotherapy (125–127). On the other hand, melanoma is supposed to be one of the most immunogenic tumors, which is demonstrated by tumor-infiltrating lymphocytes (TIL) destroying melanoma cells (128–130). This may also be responsible for the occurrence of spontaneous partial or complete melanoma regression and for the concomitant destruction of melanocytes in benign lesions, leading to clinical phenomena such as halo nevi, uveitis, and vitiligo in melanoma patients.

Table 1 Clinical Trials Designed to Treat Melanoma Patients by Cytokine Gene Transfer

Gene	Cell target	Vector	Investigator	No. of patients
IL-2	Allogeneic tumor lines	RVV	Osanto/Schrier	35
IL-2	Allogeneic tumor lines	RVV	Parmiani/Cascinelli/Foa	6
IL-2/B7	Allogeneic tumor lines	RVV	Parmiani/Cascinelli/Foa	0
IL-4	Allogeneic tumor lines	RVV	Parmiani/Cascinelli/Foa	6
IL-2	Allogeneic tumor lines	RVV	Das Gupta	3
IL-2	Allogeneic tumor lines	RVV	Ecomonu	0
IL-2	Allogeneic tumor lines	RVV	Gänsbacher	12
IL-7	Allogeneic tumor lines	RVV	Ecomonu	4
IL-2	Fibroblasts + autologous tumor	Lipofection	Mertelsmann/Lindemann	14
IL-4	Fibroblasts + autologous tumor	RVV	Lotze	18
IL-12	Fibroblasts + autologous tumor	RVV	Lotze	14
IL-2	Autologous tumor	RVV	Gore/Collins	12
IL-2	Autologous tumor	RMT	Stingl/Bröcker/Mertelsmann	12
IL-7	Autologous tumor	Ballistic	Schadendorf	10
IL-12	Autologous tumor	Ballistic	Schadendorf	6
GM-CSF	Autologous tumor	RVV	Rankin	33
GM-CSF	Autologous tumor	RVV	Ellem	10
GM-CSF	Autologous tumor	RVV	Chang	3
GM-CSF	Autologous tumor	Ballistic	Mahvi	2
IFN-γ	Autologous tumor	RVV	Seigler	20

RVV: Retroviral vectors; RMT: receptor-mediated gene transfer; TF: transfection.
Source: Adapted from Ref. 123.

It is generally accepted that the spontaneous generation of cancer cells is a common event, and that the immune system assures a strict surveillance with the detection and elimination of these cells. In order to fight cancer, the idea to use the destructive power of immunological reactions is easily visualized in autoimmune diseases and by the rejection of allografts in transplantation medicine. A number of clinical observations in human malignant melanoma suggest a particularly vigorous immune response (128–131). In recent years, it has become increasingly clear that T lymphocytes may play a critical role in antitumor immune responses and surveillance (128,132). Furthermore, CD8+ T lymphocytes derived from melanoma lesions or the peripheral blood were shown to be able to mediate impressive tumor regressions in vivo (133,134). The availability and further characterization of such tumor-specific T-cell clones in recent years led to the identification of several melanoma-associated antigens (reviewed in Ref. 132). There are different approaches to utilize the host's immune system to fight the tumor including the augmentation of the immunogenicity of tumor cells by cytokine gene transfer (reviewed in Refs. 135–137).

B. Rationale for Cytokine Gene Transfer

In recent decades, the identification and cloning of cytokines provided an important set of tools for the manipulation of immunological responses. Systemic infusions of interleukin-2 (IL-2), originally named T-cell growth factor, into patients suffering from advanced melanoma were shown to achieve comparable clinical responses as conventional therapies. The effects, however, were associated with dramatic side events (138). Today, IL-2 and interferon-alpha (IFN α) are commonly used in combination with conventional chemotherapies (chemoimmunotherapy) in order to improve response rates and survival (127).

Since 1989, a different immunotherapy approach using cytokines in a more physiological (paracrine) mode has been tested in various animal tumor models. Starting from the pioneering work of Tepper and coworkers (139), who showed that tumor cells after transfection with the IL-4 gene were rejected, and work by Fearon and colleagues (140), who demonstrated that—following gene transfer—locally secreted IL-2 can bypass T-helper function in a poorly immunogenic murine tumor leading to the generation of a antitumor response including protection against subsequent challenge with parental tumor cells, numerous cytokines have been tested in such tumor-bearing animal models (reviewed in Refs. 136,137). Gene transfer of cytokine genes such as IL-2, IL-4, IL-7, IL-12, IFN-γ, TNF-α, and GM-CSF were shown to be able to induce a systemic antitumor immune memory demonstrated by a subsequent challenge with wild-type tumor cells at a distant site. This antitumor immunity required CD8+ T cells and in part CD4+ T cells (136,137). Possibly, CD8+ and CD4+ T lymphocytes were activated directly by transfected tumor cells or, more likely indirectly via antigen-presenting cells (APC) (71). Certain cytokines are active in some, but not in all animal tumor models (136,137). Recently, the combination of cytokine genes such as IL-7 and the co-stimulatory B7 molecule seemed to significantly enhance the antitumor effect (141). The goal of a cytokine gene transfer into tumor cells is the induction of local inflammation as a mode of action in inducing systemic antitumor immunity. As shown in Figure 3, the idea is that cytokine gene–transfected tumor cells cause a local influx of immunological effector cells such as natural killer (NK) cells, macrophages, and dendritic cells (DC) leading to a local inflammation at the site of vaccination (Fig. 3a). Subsequent destruction of the gene-altered tumor cells will occur (Fig. 3b) and proteins of the destroyed tumor cells will be taken up by antigen-presenting cells (APC). Intracellular antigen

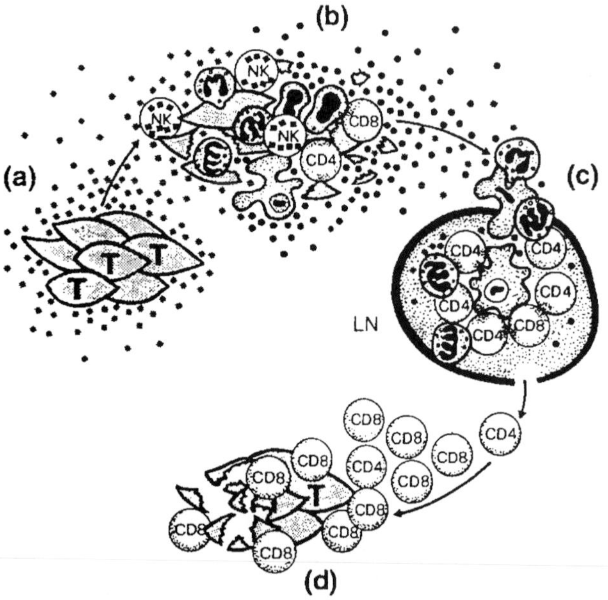

Figure 3 Rationale of cytokine gene transfer. Cytokine gene transfer into tumor cells causes a local secretion of cytokines (a) leading to an influx of immunological effector cells such as T-lymphocytes, NK-cells and dendritic cells (CD) and destruction of tumor cells and inflammation (b). Destroyed tumor cells are taken up by antigen-presenting cells (APC), which will migrate to the lymph node (LN) (c). After induction and expansion of tumor-specific T cells in the lymph node, tumor-reactive T cells of $CD4^+$ and $CD8^+$ phenotype will enter the circulation and destroy any (micro-)metastases detected at distant locations.

processing and presentation of relevant peptide epitopes in the context of MHC complexes after migration into the lymph node leads to the induction of T-cell responses (Fig. 3c). Subsequently, tumor antigen–specific T lymphocytes circulate through the organism destroying remaining (micro-)metastases.

In conclusion, experimental tumor models using gene-modified tumor cells demonstrated the antitumor effects of various cytokines and point to the need for CTL induction for long-lived tumor immunity. Although these results are encouraging because they show the feasibility of the approach, a long way remains before one can imagine treating patients in a tumor-specific manner leading to a *curative* T-cell response.

C. Cytokine Gene Transfer by Particle Bombardment

Naked DNA coated on gold microprojectiles that is directly propelled into in vivo target cells is an elegant method of gene transfer (Fig. 2). This ballistic transfer is also applicable for an in vitro gene transfer, allowing a subsequent selection of transfected from nontransfected cells. That can be achieved by selection over weeks for antibiotic resistance co-expressed with the gene of interest or by using the recently described ballisto-magnetic transfer system (142,143). This gene transfer technology, which combines ballistic transfer of biological molecules and magnetic cell sorting, was originally developed to study gene regulation at the chromatin level. It opens now the possibility to transfect large cell numbers for gene therapy protocols in a reasonable amount of time. Using this technique, more than 10^8 cells can be transfected each day, eliminating the need for viral vector systems. This system is convenient when a cancer vaccine must be prepared from autologous tumor cells in a short time frame. Colloidal gold particles were resuspended in a mixture of DNA and a suspension of colloidal supraparamagnetic particles and were coated onto carrier membranes (Fig. 2). The accelerating system for ballistic transfer is based on the biolistic PDS-100/He apparatus (1550 psi rupture disk, 500 mmHg of vacuum, Bio-Rad). The biolistic unit was modified by a pressure outlet manifold, a multiparticle carrier assembly, and an adjustable bearing to carry a 10 cm Petri dish. Ballistomagnetic transfer of biomolecules up to 10^8 cells seeded onto 10 cm Petri dishes is achieved by simultaneous delivery of particles from seven particle carrier membranes that are arranged in a way to cover the entire area of the Petri dish evenly (Fig. 2). Subsequent enrichment of transduced cells by magnetic selection using a high-gradient magnetic separation column without the need for an in vitro selection over months allows the fast, easy, and cost-effective vaccination of suitable patients. The column can be washed with PBS buffer, and finally the column is removed again from the separator and eluted with PBS (magnetic fraction). The collected fractions are further processed according to experimental conditions required for the subsequent assay. Examples of data obtained using the ballistomagnetic vector system to transfer both chains of the IL-12 gene are shown in Figure 4. The bioactivity of IL-12–containing supernatants of human melanoma cells transduced by particle bombardment was analyzed and confirmed with a bioassay analyzing the release of IFN-γ from PBL upon contact to cell culture supernatants (Fig. 5).

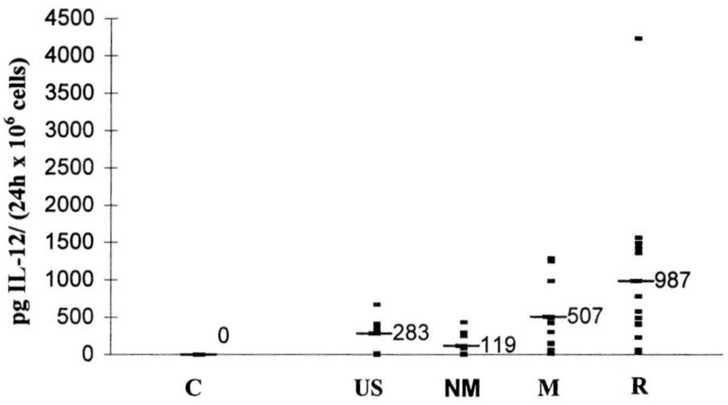

Figure 4 Cytokine release. Primary melanoma cell cultures from 15 metastases of patients were analyzed for the release of IL-12 from tumor cells after gene transfer. Gold particles coated with p35- and p40-encoding vector constructs were used for ballistic transfer. Cell fractions were magnetically separated and aliquots of all fractions were analyzed for IL-12 secretion after 24 hours by ELISA. Nontransfected cells (C) did not secrete any IL-12. The whole cell mixture after ballistic transfer without separation (US) released a mean of 283 pg IL-12 (24 h; 10^6 cells), which increased to 507 pg IL-12 (24 h; 10^6 cells) after magnetic separation (M) compared to 119 pg IL-12 (24 h; 10^6 cells) in the nonmagnetic cell fraction (NM). Irradiation (100 Gy) of the magnetic fraction (R) further increased IL-12 secretion to 987 pg IL-12 (24 h; 10^6 cells).

D. Results of IL-7 and IL-12 Gene Transfer in Melanoma Treatment

Clinical phase I studies were iniated aiming at the induction of T-cell–mediated cytotoxicity and tumor immunity by immunizing melanoma patients (142–144). Autologous melanoma cells were gene-modified by genetic manipulation in order to attract immunological competent cells to the tumor and to elicit a systemic antitumor immunity. Therefore, melanoma metastases from melanoma patients who have failed to respond to other therapies were surgically removed and melanoma cells were expanded in vitro

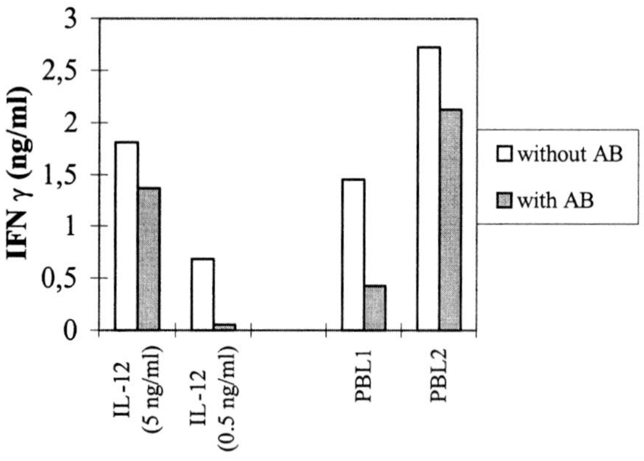

Figure 5 Bioactivity. In order to test the bioactivity of the IL-12 secreted, interferon-γ release from PBL obtained from two healthy donors was analyzed. Both PBL preparations secreted IFN-γ in a dose-dependent fashion after addition of recombinant IL-12 (left panel), which could be blocked by a goat antihuman IL-12 antiserum (2 μg/mL—gray columns). Even higher release of IFN-γ was observed upon addition of cell culture supernatant of IL-12–transfected melanoma cells (right panel). That effect could only partly be blocked by antihuman IL-12 antiserum, however, supernatants of nontransfected cells had no effect on IFN-γ secretion (not shown). Proliferation kinetics of five human melanoma cell lines were not affected upon addition of recombinant IL-12 (1 pg/mL to 1 μg/mL) up to 7 days (not shown).

(Fig. 6). Autologous melanoma cells were transfected either with both chains of the IL-12 gene (144) or with the IL-7 gene (144). Patients are vaccinated s.c. with 5×10^{-6} to 5×10^{-7} autologous cells at week 1, week 2, week 3, and week 6. In parallel, DTH reactivity and an extensive immunological monitoring including flow cytometry, NK and LAK activity as well as CTL analysis were performed. The cytokine gene-transfer protocol used a newly developed gene-transfer technology, which combines ballistic transfer of biological molecules and magnetic cell sorting (143).

Evaluation of the first 10 patients immunized with autologous, IL-7 gene–modified melanoma cells demonstrated the safety, the lack of toxicity, and the feasibility of such an approach. However, no major clinical response was achieved (144). Eight of 10 patients completed the initial three s.c. vaccinations with IL-7 gene–modified cells and were eligible for immunological evaluation. Nonspecific cytotoxicity (NK and LAK activity) increased upon vaccination in 4 of 8 and 7 of 8 patients, respectively. Furthermore, peripheral blood lymphocytes were found to contain an increased number of tumor-reactive T cells after immunization. The number of tumor-reactive as well as cytolytic Tcell lines was significantly higher after vaccination, as determined by a limited dilution analysis in 7 patients. Furthermore, in 3 of 6 patients, the frequency of cytolytic microcultures increased 2.6- to 28-fold. The magnitude of the T-cell reactivity was found to be highly associated with the patients' Karnofsky index and recall antigen skin reactivity before vaccination. Nevertheless, only one mixed clinical response was observed during the treatment period. In a subsequent study, 6 patients were immunized with autologous IL-12 gene–modified melanoma cells (144). Clinically, there was no major toxicity except for mild fever. All patients completed more than four vaccinations and were eligible for immunological evaluation. Postvaccination, the number of tumor-reactive proliferative as well as cytotoxic T cells was significantly increased in 2 patients (up to 15-fold). Two patients developed DTH reactivity against autologous melanoma cells, and one had

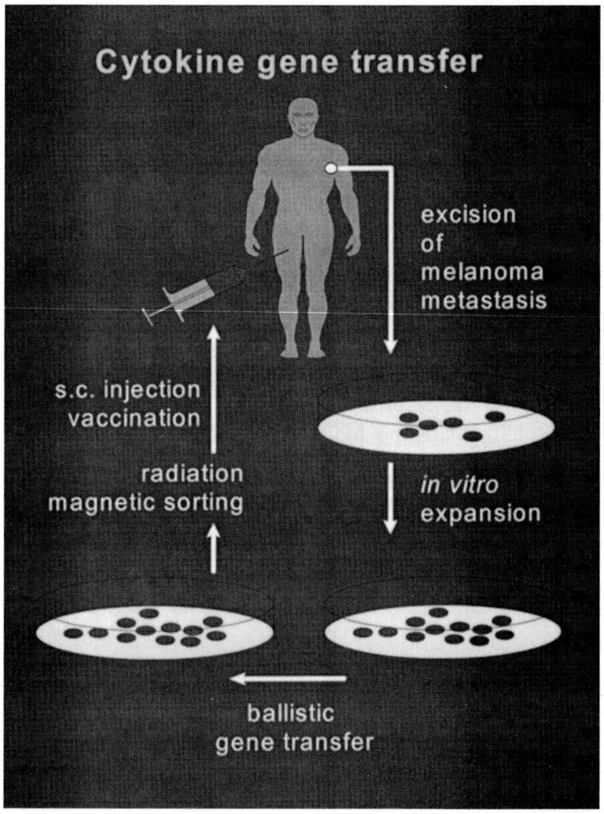

Figure 6 Outline of vaccination preparation used for immunization of patients with advanced melanoma. Surgical excision of melanoma metastases and subsequent expansion of tumor cells ex vivo, gene transfer using the magneto-ballistic transfer technique, and irradiation is followed by s.c. injection of genetically modified, cytokine-secreting, autologous melanoma cells at weekly intervals.

a minor clinical response. Biopsies taken from that patient's metastases revealed a heavy infiltration of CD4- and CD8-positive T lymphocytes. In conclusion, vaccination of patients with advanced melanoma using autologous, gene-modified melanoma cells induced immunological changes even in far advanced, terminally ill patients, which can be interpreted as an increased antitumor immune response (143,144).

V. CONCLUSION AND PERSPECTIVES

Tumor immunology has made great progress in recent years. Recent animal studies have indicated that a potent protective immune response can be generated in vivo using cytokine gene–modified tumor cells. Locally secreted cytokines such as IL-2, IL-4, IL-7, IL-12, or GM-CSF and others from genetically modified tumor cells were shown to mediate tumor rejection and long-lived antitumor immunity. Based on these successful animal studies, various clinical protocols for the treatment of human cancer, predominantly using cytokine gene modifications, were initiated in recent years.

In the next few years, the large number of ongoing clinical studies using gene therapeutic strategies will provide the necessary scientific basis to proceed on the new avenue of medicine. At present, it seems safe to conclude that gene therapeutic strategies involving cytokine gene–modified tumor cells can influence the immunological tumor-host relationship, however, in most cases the response seems not to be strong enough to completely eradicate the tumor in patients who are highly pretreated and far advanced with metastatic disease. Although gene therapy is still in its infancy, the potential of this new therapeutic opportunity is already evident. Because an enormous amount of work is currently being done on the development of suitable vector systems and genetic tools, it is only a matter of time until gene therapy will be a standard treatment option in medicine and cancer therapy. One should keep in mind that standard therapy modalities such as chemotherapy required decades before at least a few cancer entities could be cured. So far, chemotherapy has not achieved a major benefit for patients with advanced malignant melanoma.

ACKNOWLEDGMENTS

The work was supported by the DFG and would not have been possible without the contributions of Drs. B. Wittig, P. Möller, Y. Sun, B. Henz, K. Jurgovsky, and the excellent technical assistance of A. Sucker and T. Dorbic. The authors are grateful to Jonathan C. Vogel (NIH, Dermatology Branch), who was critically involved in establishing the direct injection method of naked plasmid DNA.

REFERENCES

1. Vogel JC. Keratinocyte gene therapy. Arch Dermatol 1993; 129:1478–1483.
2. Hengge UR. Gene therapy for blistering diseases. In: Sterry W, Pleyer U, eds. Oculodermal Diseases. Amsterdam: Aeolus Press, 1997:297–316.
3. Sanford JC, Klein TM, Wolf ED, Alen N. Delivery of substances into cells and tissues using a particle bombardment process. Particulate Sci Technol 1987; 5:27–37.
4. Klein TM, Wolf ED, Wu R, Sanford JC. High velocity microprojectiles for delivering nucleic acids into living cells. Nature 1987; 327:70–73.
5. Fromm ME, Morrish F, Armstrong C, Williams R, Thomas J, Klein TM. Inheritance and expression of chimeric genes in the progeny of transgenic maize plants. Biotechnology 1990; 8:833–839.
6. Gordon-Kamm WJ, Spencer TM, Magano ML, Adams TR, Daines RJ, Start WG, O'Brien JV, Chambers SA, Adams WR, Willets NG, Rice TB, Mackey CJ, Krueger RW, Kausch AP, Lemaux PG. Transformation of maize cells and regeneration of fertile plants. Plant Cell 1990; 2: 603–618.
7. Zhu N, Liggitt D, Liu Y, Debs R Systemic gene expression after intravenous DNA delivery into adult mice. Science 1993; 261:209–211.
8. Liu Y, Mounkes LC, Liggitt HD, Brown CS, Solodin I, Heath TD, Debs RJ. Factors influencing the efficiency of cationic liposome-mediated intravenous gene delivery. Nat Biotechnol 1997; 15:167–173.
9. Wolff JA, Malone RW, Williams P, Chong W, Ascadi G, Jani A, Felgner PL. Direct gene transfer into mouse muscle in vivo. Science 1990; 247:1465–1468.
10. Hengge UR, Chan EF, Foster RA, Walker PS, Vogel JC. Cytokine gene expression in epidermis with biological effects following injection of naked DNA. Nat Genetics 1995; 10:161–166.
11. Hengge UR, Walker PS, Vogel JC. Expression of naked DNA in pig, mouse and human skin. J Clin Invest 1996; 97:2911–2916.
12. Hengge UR, Williams M, M Goos, Vogel JV. Efficient expression of naked plasmid DNA in mucosal epithelium: prospective for the treatment of skin lesions. J Invest Dermatol 1998 Oct;111(4):605–608.
13. Sikes ML, O'Malley BW Jr., Finegold MJ, Ledley FD. In vivo gene transfer into rabbit thyroid follicular cells by direct DNA injection. Hum Gene Ther 1994; 5:837–844.
14. Hickman MA, Malone RW, Lehmann-Bruinsma K, Sih TR, Knoell D, Szoka FC, Walzem R, Carlson DM, Powell JS. Gene expression following direct injection of DNA into liver. Hum Gene Ther 1994; 5:1477–1488.
15. Yovandich J, O'Malley B, Sikes M, Ledley FD. Gene transfer to synovial cells by intraarticular administration of plasmid DNA. Hum Gene Ther 1995; 6:603–610.
16. Tsan MF, White JE, Shepard B. Lung-specific direct in vivo gene transfer with recombinant plasmid DNA. Am J Physiol 1995; 268:1052–1056.

17. Yang JP, Huang L. Direct gene transfer to mouse melanoma by intratumor injection of free DNA. Gene Ther 1996; 3:542–548.
18. Anderson RG, Kamen BA, Rothberg KG, Lacey SW. Potocytosis: sequestration and transport of small molecules by caveolae. Science 1992; 255:410–411.
19. Dowty ME, Williams P, Zhang G, Hagstrom JE, Wolff JA. Plasmid DNA entry into postmitotic nuclei of primary rat myotubes. Proc Natl Acad Sci USA 1995; 92: 4572–4576.
20. Capecci MR. High efficiency transformation by direct microinjection of DNA into cultured mammalian cells. Cell 1980; 22:479–488.
21. Kim HJ, Greenleaf JF, Kinnick RR, Bronk JT, Bolander ME. Ultrasound-mediated transfection of mammalian cells. Hum Gene Ther 1996; 7:1339–1346.
22. Zhang L, Li L, Hoffmann A, Hoffmann RM. Depth-targeted efficient gene delivery and expression in the skin by pulsed electric fields: an approach to gene therapy of skin aging and other diseases. Biochem Biophys Res Commun 1996; 220:633–636.
23. Ciernik IF, Krayenbühl BH, Carbone DP. Puncture-mediated gene transfer to the skin. Hum Gene Ther 1996; 7: 893–899.
24. Li L, Hoffmann RM. The feasibility of targeted selective gene therapy of the hair follicle. Nat Med 1995; 7: 705–706.
25. Daheshia M, Kuklin N, Kanangat S, Manickan E, Rouse BT. Suppression of ongoing ocular inflammatory disease by topical administration of plasmid DAN encoding IL-10. J Immunol 1997; 159:1945–1952.
26. Armaleo D, Ye GN, Klein TM, Shark KB, Sanford JC, Johnston SA. Biolistic nuclear transformation of saccharomyces cerevisiae and other fungi. Curr Genet 1990; 17: 97–103.
27. Yoshida Y, Kobayashi E, Endo H, Hamamoto T, Yamanaka T, Fujimura A, Kagawa Y. Introduction of DNA into rat liver with a hand-held gene gun: distribution of the expressed enzyme, [32P]DNA, and Ca2+ flux. Biochem Biophys Res Commun 1997; 234:695–700.
28. Yang NS, Burkholder J, Roberts B, Martinell B, McCabe D. In vivo and in vitro gene transfer to mammalian somatic cells by particle bombardment. Proc Natl Acad Sci USA 1990; 87:9568–9572.
29. Haynes JR, Fuller DH, Eisenbraun MD, Ford MJ, Pertmer TM. Accell particle-mediated immunization elicits humoral, cytotoxic, and protective immune responses. AIDS Res Hum Retroviruses 1994; 10:43S–45S.
30. Gal-On A, Meiri E, Elman C, Gray DJ, Gaba V. Simple hand-held devices for the efficient infection of plants with viral-encoding constructs by particle bombardment. J Virol Methods 1997; 64:103–110.
31. Oard JH, Paige DF, Simmonds JA, Gradziel TM. Transient gene expression in maize, rice and wheat cells using an air gun apparatus. Plant Pysiol 1990; 92:334–339.
32. Vahlsing HL, Yankauckas MA, Sawdey M, Gromkowski SH, Manthorpe M. Immunization with plasmid DNA using a pneumatic gun. J Immunol Methods 1994; 175:11–22.
33. Klein TM, Arentzen R, Lewis PA, Fitzpatrick-McElligott S. Transformation of microbes, plants and animals by particle bombardement. Biotechnology 1992; 10:286–291.
34. Sorensen MB, Muller M, Skeritt J, Simpson D. Hordein promoter methylation and transcriptional activity in wild-type and mutant barley endosperm. Mol Gen Genet 1996; 250:750–760.
35. Bruce WB, Christensen AH, Klein T, Fromm M, Quail PH. Photoregulation of a phytochrome gene promoter from oat transferred into rice by particle bombardment. Proc Natl Acad Sci USA 1989; 86:9692–9696.
36. Baum K, Groning B, Meier I. Improved ballistic transient transformation conditions for tomato fruit allow identification of organ-specific contributions of I-box and G-box to the RBCS2 promoter activity. Plant J 1997; 12:463–469.
37. Lamprecht S, Jelkmann W. Infectious cDNA clone used to identify strawberry mild yellow edge-associated potexvirus as causel agent of the disease. J Gen Virol 1997; 78: 2347–2353.
38. Murry LE, Elliott LG, Capitant SA, West JA, Hanson KK, Scarafia L, Johnston S, DeLuca-Flaherty C, Nichols S, Cunanan D. Transgenic corn plants expressing MDMV strain B coat protein are resistant to mixed infections of maize dwarf mosaic virus and maize chlorotic mottle virus. Biotechnology 1993; 11:1559–1564.
39. Register JC, Peterson DJ, Bell PJ, Bullock WP, Evans IJ, Frame B, Greenland AJ, Higgs NS, Jepson I, Jiao S, Lewnau CJ, Sillick JM, Wilson HM. Structure and function of selectable and non-selectable transgenes in maize after introduction by particle bombardment. Plant Mol Biol 1994; 25:951–961.
40. Christou P, McCabe DE, Swain WF. Stable transformation of soybean callus by DNA-coated gold particles. Plant Physiol 1988; 87:671–674.
41. Godon C, Caboche M, Daniel-Vedele F. Transient plant gene expression: a simple and reproducible method based on flowing particle gun. Biochimie 1993; 75:591–595.
42. Becker D, Brettschneider R, Lorz H. Fertile transgenic wheat from microprojectile bombardment of scutellar tissue. Plant J 1994; 5:299–307.
43. Christou P. Rice transformation: bombardment. Plant Mol Biol 1997; 35:197–203.
44. Nayak P, Basu S, Das S, Basu A, Ghosh S, Ramakrishnan NA, Ghish M, Sen SK. Transgenic elite indica rice plants expressing CryIAc delta-endotoxin of Bacillus thruingiensis are resistant against yellow stem borer (Scirpophaga incertulas). Proc Natl Acad Sci USA 1997; 94: 2111–2116.
45. Takumi S, Shimada T. Variation in transformation frequencies among six common wheat cultivars through particle bombardment of scutellar tissues. Genes Genet Syst 1997; 72:63–69.
46. Boynton JE, Gillham NW, Harris EH, Hosler JP, Johnson AM, Jones AR, Randolph-Anderson BL, Robertson D, Klein TM, Shark KB. Chloroplast transformation in Chlamydomonas with high velocity microprojectiles. Science 1988; 240:1534–1538.

47. Daniell H. Foreign gene expression in chloroplasts of higher plants mediated by tungsten particle bombardment. Methods Enzymol 1993; 217:536–556.
48. Johnston SA, Anziano PQ, Shark K, Sanford JC, Butow RA. Mitochondrial transformation in yeast by bombardment with microprojectiles. Science 1988; 240: 1538–1541.
49. Christiansen SK, Knudsen S, Giese H. Biolistic transformation of the obligate plant pathogenic fungus, Erysiphe graminis f.sp. hordei. Curr Genet 1995; 29:100–102.
50. Fakhfah H, Vilaine F, Makni M, Robaglia C. Cell-free and biolistic inoculation of an infectious cDNA of potato virus Y. J Gen Virol 1996; 77:519–523.
51. Gal-On A, Meiri E, Huet H, Hua WJ, Raccah B, Gaba V. Particle bombardment drastically increases the infectivity of cloned DNA of zucchini yellow mosaic potyvirus. J Gen Virol 1995; 76:3223–3227.
52. Tanaka T, Nishihara M, Seki M, Sakamoto A, Tanaka K, Irifune K, Morikawa H. Successful expression in pollen of various plant species of in vitro synthesized mRNA introduced by particle bombardment. Plant Mol Biol 1995; 28:337–341.
53. Wilmink A, van de Ven BC, Dons JJ. Activity of constitutive promoters in various species from the Liliaceae. Plant Mol Biol 1995; 28:949–955.
54. Molina A, Diaz I, Vasil IK, Carbonero P, Garcia-Olmedo. Two cold-inducible genes encoding lipid transfer protein LTP4 from barley show differential responses to bacterial pathogens. Mol Gen Genet 1996; 252:162–168.
55. van der Fits L, Memelink J. Comparison of the activities of CaMV 35S and FMV 34S promoter derivatives in Catharanthus roseus cells transiently and stably transformed by particle bombardment. Plant Mol Biol 1997; 33:943–946.
56. Heiser WC. Gene transfer into mammalian cells by particle bombardment. Anal Biochem 1994; 217:185–196.
57. Cassidy-Hanley D, Bowen J, Lee JH, VerPlank LA, Gaertig J, Gorovsky MA, Bruns PJ. Germline and somatic transformation of mating Tetrahymena thermophila by particle bombardment. Genetics 1997; 146:135–147.
58. Williams RS, Johnston SA, Riedy M, DeVit MJ, McElligott SG, Sanford JC. Introduction of foreign genes into tissues of living mice by DNA-coated microprojectiles. Proc Natl Acad Sci USA 1991; 88:2726–2730.
59. Cheng L, Ziegekhoffer PR, Yang NS. In vivo promoter activity and transgene expression in mammalian somatic tissues evaluated by using particle bombardment. Proc Natl Acad Sci USA 1993; 90:4455–4459.
60. Thompson TA, Gould MN, Burkholder JK, Yang NS. Transient promoter activity in primary rat mammary epithelial cells evaluated using particle bombardment gene transfer. In Vitro Cell Dev Biol 1993; 29A:165–170.
61. Furth PA, Shamay A, Hennighausen L. Gene transfer into mammalian cells by jet injection. Hybridoma 1995; 14: 149–152.
62. Seki M, Komeda Y, Iida A, Yamada Y, Morikawa H. Transient expression of β-glucuronidase in Arabidopsis thaliana leaves and roots and Brassica napus stems using a pneumatic particle gun. Plant Mol Biol 1991; 17:259–263.
63. Jiao S, Cheng L, Wolff JA, Yang NS. Particle bombardment-mediated gene transfer and expression in rat brain tissues. Biotechnology 1993; 11:497–502.
64. Gainer A, Korbut GS, Rajotte RV, Warnock GL, Elliott JF. Expression of CTLA-4-Ig by biolistically transfected mouse islets promotes islet allograft survival. Transplantation 1997; 63:1017–1021.
65. Tanelian DL, Barry MA, Johnston SA, Le T, Smith G. Controlled gene gun delivery and expression of DNA within the cornea. Biotechniques 1997; 23:484–488.
66. Zelenin AV, Alimov AA, Titomirov AV, Kazansky AV, Gorodetsky SI, Kolesnikov V. High-velocity mechanical DNA transfer of the chloramphenicolacetyl transferase gene into rodent liver, kidney and mammary gland cells in organ explants and in vivo. FEBS Lett 1991; 280:94–96.
67. Zelenin AV, Alimov AA, Zelenina IA, Semenova ML, Rodova MA, Chernov BK, Kolesnikov VA. Transfer of foreign DNA into the cells of developing mouse embryos by microprojectile bombardment. FEBS Lett 1993; 315: 29–32.
68. Cadoret JP, Boulo V, Gendreau S, Mialhe E. Promoters from drosophila heat shock protein and cytomegalovirus drive transient expression of luciferase introduced by particle bombardment into embryos of the oyster crassostrea gigas. J Biotechnol 1997; 56:183–189.
69. Muramatsu T, Mizutani Y, Ohmori Y, Okumura JI. Comparison of three nonviral transfection methods for foreign gene expression in early chicken embryos in ovo. Biochem Biophys Res Comm 1997; 230:376–380.
70. Burkholder JK, Decker J, Yang NS. Rapid transgene expression in lymphocyte and macrophage primary cultures after particle bombardment-mediated gene transfer. J Immunol Methods 1993; 165:149–156.
71. Pardoll DM, Beckerleg AM. Exposing the immunology of naked DNA. Immunity 1995; 3:165–169.
72. Mc Donnell WM, Askari FK. DNA vaccines. N Engl J Med 1996; 334:42–45.
73. Condon C, Watkins SC, Celluzzi CM, Thompson K, Falo LD. DNA-based immunization by in vivo transfection of dendritic cells. Nat Med 1996; 2:1122–1128.
74. Doe B, Selby M, Barnett S, Baenziger J, Walker CM. Induction of cytotoxic T lymphocytes by intramuscular immunization with plasmid DNA is facilitated by bone marrow-derived cells. Proc Natl Acad Sci USA 1996; 93: 8578–8583.
75. Iwasaki A, Torres CA, Ohashi PS, Robinson HL, Barber BH. The dominant role of bone marrow-derived cells in CTL induction following plasmid DNA immunization at different sites. J Immunol 1997; 159:11–14.
76. Doolan DL, Sedegah M, Hedstrom RC, Hobart P, Charoenvit Y, Hoffman SL. Circumventing genetic restriction of protection against malaria with multigene DNA immunization: CD8 + cell-, interferon gamma-, and nitric oxide-dependent immunity. J Exp Med 1996; 183:1739–1746.

77. Mahvi DM, Burkholder JK, Turner J, Culp J, Malter JS, Sondel PM, Yang NS. Particle-mediated gene transfer of granulocyte-macrophage colony-stimulating factor cDNA to tumor cells: implications for a clinically relevant tumor vaccine. Hum Gene Ther 1996; 7:1535–1543.
78. Rofolfo M, Zilocchi C, Melani C, Cappetti B, Arioli I, Parmiani G, Colombo MP. Immunotherapy of experimental metastases by vaccination with interleukin gene-transduced adenocarcinoma cells sharing tumor-associated antigens. J Immunol 1995; 157:5536–5542.
79. Geissler M, Gesien A, Tokushige K, Wands JR. Enhancement of cellular and humoral immune responses to hepatitis C virus core protein using DNA-based vaccines augmented with cytokine-expressing plasmids. J Immunol 1997; 158:1231–1237.
80. Rakhmilevich AL, Turner J, Ford MJ, McCabe B, Sun WH, Sondel PM, Grota K, Yang NS. Gene gun-mediated skin transfection with interleukin 12 gene results in regression of established primary and metastatic murine tumors. Proc Natl Acad Sci USA 1996; 93:6291–6296.
81. Sin JI, Sung JH, Suh YS, Lee AH, Chung JH, Sung YC. Protective immunity against heterologous challenge with encephalomyocarditis virus by VP1 DNA vaccination: effect of coinjection with a granulocyte-macrophage colony stimulating factor gene. Vaccine 1997; 15:1827–1833.
82. Conry RM, LoBuglio AF, Curiel DT. Phase Ia trial of a polynucleotide anti-tumor immunization to human carcinoembryonic antigen in patients with metastatic colorectal cancer. Hum Gene Ther 1996; 7:775–772.
83. Barry MA, Lai WC, Johnston SA. Protection against mycoplasma infection using expression-library immunization. Nature 1995; 377:632–635.
84. Ulmer JB, Liu MA. ELI's coming: expression library immunization and vaccine antigen discovery. Trends Microbiol 1996; 4:169–170.
85. Xu L, Sanchez A, Yang Z, Zaki SR, Nabel EG, Nichol ST, Nabel GJ. Immunization for Ebola virus infection. Nat Med 1998; 4:37–42.
86. Michel M. DNA-mediated immunization: prospects for hepatitis B vaccination. Res Virol 1995; 146:261–265.
87. Davis HL, McCluskie MJ, Gerin JL, Purcell RH. DNA vaccine for hepatitis B: evidence for immunogenicity in chimpanzees and comparison with other vaccines. Proc Natl Acad Sci USA 1996; 93:7213–7218.
88. Lagging LM, Meyer K, Hoft D, Houghton M, Belshe RB, Ray R. Immune response to plasmid DNA encoding hepatitis C virus core protein. J Virol 1995; 69:5859–5863.
89. Tokushige K, Wakita T, Pachuk C, Moradpour B, Weiner DB, Zurawski VR Jr., Wands JR. Expression and immune response to hepatitis C virus core DNA-based vaccine constructs. Hepatology 1996; 24:14–20.
90. Ghiasi H, Cai S, Slanina S, Nesburn AB, Wechsler SL. Vaccination of mice with herpes simplex virus type 1 glycoprotein D DNA produces low levels of protection against lethal HSV-1 challenge. Antiviral Res 1995; 28:147–157.
91. Manickan E, Rouse RJ, Yu Z, Wire WS, Rouse BT. Genetic immunization against herpes simplex virus. Protection is mediated by CD4+ lymphocytes. J Immunol 1995; 155:259–265.
92. Sedegah M, Hedstrom R, Hobart P, Hoffman SL. Protection against malaria by immunization with plasmid DNA encoding circumsporozoite protein. Proc Natl Acad Sci USA 1994; 91:9866–9670.
93. Lai WC, Bennett M, Johnston SA, Barry MA, Pakes SP. Protection against mycoplasma pulmonis infection by genetic vaccination. DNA Cell Biol 1995; 14:643–651.
94. Donnelly JJ, Martinez D, Jansen KU, Ellis RW, Montgomery DL, Liu MA. Protection against papillomavirus with a polynucleotide vaccine. J Infect Dis 1996; 173:314–320.
95. Krasemann S, Groschup M, Hunsmann G, Bodemer W. Induction of antibodies against human prion proteins (PrP) by DNA-mediated immunization of PrP0/0 mice. J Immunol Methods 1996; 199:109–118.
96. Choi AH, Knowlton DR, McNeal MM, Ward RL. Particle bombardment-mediated DNA vaccination with rotavirus VP6 induces high levels of serum rotavirus IgG but fails to protect mice against challenge. Virology 1997; 232: 129–138.
97. Huygen K, Content J, Denis O, Montgomery DL, Yawman AM, Deck RR, De Witt CM, Orme IM, Baldwin S, D'Souza C, Drowart A, Lozes E, Vandenbussche P, Van Vooren JP, Liu MA, Ulmer JB. Immunogenicity and protective efficacy of a tuberculosis DNA vaccine. Nat Med 1996; 2:893–898.
98. Tascon RE, Colston MJ, Ragno S, Stavropoulos E, Gregory D, Lowrie DB. Vaccination against tuberculosis by DNA injection. Nat Med 1996; 2:888–892.
99. Tang D, DeVit M, Johnston SA. Genetic immunization is a simple method for eliciting and immune response. Nature 1992; 356:152–154.
100. Fynan EF, Webster RG, Fuller DH, Haynes JR, Santoro JC. DNA Vaccines: protective immunizations by parenteral, mucosal, and gene-gun inoculations. Proc Natl Acad Sci USA 1993; 90:11478–11482.
101. Montgomery DL, Shiver JW, Leander KR, Perry HC, Friedman A, Martinez D, Ulmer JB, Donnelly JJ, Liu MA. Heterologous and homologous protection against Influenza A by DNA vaccination: optimization of DNA vectors. DNA Cell Biol 1993; 12:777–783.
102. Ulmer JB, Donnelly JJ, Parker SE, Rhodes GH, Felgner PL, Dwarki VJ, Gromkowski SH, Deck RR, DeWitt CM, Friedmann A, Hawe LA, Leander KR, Martinez D, Perry HC, Shiver JW, Montgomery DL, Liu MA. Heterologous protection against influenza by injection of DNA encoding a viral protein. Science 1993; 259:1745–1748.
103. Donnelly JJ, Friedman A, Ulmer JB, Liu MA. Further protection against antigenic drift of influenza virus in a ferret model by DNA vaccination. Vaccine 1997; 15: 865–868.
104. Robinson HL, Boyle CA, Feltquate DM, Morin MJ, Santoro JC, Webster RG. DNA immunization for influenza virus: studies using hemagglutinin- and nucleoprotein-expressing DNAs. J Infect Dis 1997; 176:S50–S55.

105. Wang B, Boyer J, Srikantan V, Coney L, Carrano R, Phan C, Merva M, Dang K, Agadjanan M, Gilbert L, Ugen KE, Williams WV, Weiner DB. DNA inoculation induces neutralizing immune responses against human immunodeficiency virus type 1 in mice and nonhuman primates. DNA Cell Biol 1993; 12:799–805.
106. Fuller DH, Haynes JR. A qualitative progression in HIV type 1 glycoprotein 120-specific cytotoxic cellular and humoral immune responses in mice receiving a DNA-based glycoprotein 120 vaccine. AIDS Res Hum Retroviruses 1994; 10:1433–1441.
107. Heydenburg-Fuller D, Haynes JR. A qualitative progression in HIV type 1 glycoprotein 120-specific cytotoxic cellular and humoral immunw responses in mice receiving a DNA-based glycoprotein 120 vaccine. AIDS Res Hum Retroviruses 1994; 11:1433–1441.
108. Wang B, Merva M, Dang K, Ugen KE, Boyer J, Williams WV, Weiner DB. DNA inoculation induces protective in vivo immune responses against cellular challenge with HIV-1 antigen-expressing cells. AIDS Res Hum Retroviruses 1994; 10:S35–41.
109. Barnett SW, Rajasekar S, Legg H, Doe B, Fuller DH, Haynes JR, Walker CM, Steimer KS. Vaccination with HIV-1 gp120 DNA induces immune responses that are boosted by a recombinant gp120 protein subunit. Vaccine 1997; 15:869–873.
110. Prayaga SK, Ford MJ, Haynes JR. Manipulation of HIV-1 gp120-specific immune responses elicited via gene gun-based DNA immunization. Vaccine 1997; 15:1349–1352.
111. Bagarazzi ML, Boyer JD, Javadian MA, Chattergoon MA, Shah AR, Cohen AD, Bennett MK, Ciccarelli RB, Ugen KE, Weiner DB. Systemic and mucosal immunity is elicited after both intramuscular and intravaginal delivery of human immunodeficiency virus type 1 DNA plasmid vaccines to pregnant chimpanzees. J Infect Dis 1999 Oct; 180(4):1351–1355.
112. Fuller DH, Corb MM, Barnett S, Steimer K, Hynes JR. Enhancement of immunodeficiency virus-specific immune responses in DNA-immunized rhesus macaques. Vaccine 1997a; 15:924–926.
113. Fuller DH, Simpson L, Cole KS, Clements JE, Panicali DL, Montelaro RC, Murphey-Corb M, Haynes JR. Gen gun-based nucleic acid immunization alone or in combination with recombinant vaccinia vectors suppresses virus burden in rhesus macaques challenged with a heterologous SIV. Immunol Cell Biol 1997; 75:389–396.
114. Feltquate D, Heaney S, Webster RG, Robinson HL. Different T helper cell types and antibody isotypes generated by saline and gene gun DNA immunization. J Immunol 1997; 158:2278–2284.
115. Cardoso AI, Sixt N, Vallier A, Fayolle J, Buckland R, Wild TF. Measles virus DNA vaccination: antibody isotype is determined by the method of immunization and by the nature of both the antigen and the coimmunized antigen. J Virol 1998; 72:2516–2518.
116. Nakano I, Maertens G, Major ME, Vivitski L, Dubuisson J, Fournillier A, deMartynoff G, Trepo C, Inchauspe G. Immunization with plasmid DNA encoding hepatitis C virus envelope E2 antigenic domains induces antibodies whose immune reactivity is linked to the injection mode. J Virol 1997; 71:7101–7109.
117. Krieg AM, Yi AK, Matson S, Waldschmidt YJ, Bishop GA, Teasdale R, Koretzky GA, Klinman DM. CpG motifs in bacteria trigger direct B-cell activation. Nature 1995; 374:546–549.
118. Lipford GB, Bauer M, Blank C, Reiter R, Wagner H, Heeg K. CpG-containing synthetic oligonucleotides promote B and cytotoxic T cell responses to protein antigen: a new class of vaccine adjuvants. Eur J Immunol 1997; 27: 2340–2344.
119. Torres CAT, Iwasaki A, Barber BH, Robinson HL. Differential dependence on target site tissue for gene gun and intramuscular DNA immunizations. J Immunol 1997; 158: 4529–4532.
120. Klinman DM, Sechler JMG, Conover J, Gu M, Rosenberg AS. Contribution of cells at the site of DNA vaccination to the generation of antigen-specific immunity and memory. J Immunol 1998; 160:2388–2392.
121. Hedley ML, Curley J, Urban R. Microspheres containing plasmid-encoded antigens elicit cytotoxic T-cell responses. J Virol 1998; 72:4931–4939.
122. Livingston JB, Lu S, Robinson H, Anderson DJ. Immunization of the female genital tract with a DNA-based vaccine. Infect Immun 1998; 66:322–329.
123. Marcel T, and Grausz JD. The TMC worldwide gene therapy enrollment report, end 1996. Hum Gene Ther 1997; 8:775–800.
124. Ledley FD. Nonviral gene therapy: the promise of genes as pharmaceutical products. Hum Gene Ther 1995; 6: 1129–1144.
125. Ahmann DL, Creagan ET, Hahn RG, Edmonson JH, Bisel HF, Schaid DJ. Complete responses and long-term survivals after systemic chemotherapy for patients with advanced malignant melanoma. Cancer 1989; 63:224–227.
126. Johnson TM, Smith JW, Nelson BR, and Chang A. Current therapy for cutaneous melanoma. J Am Acad Dermatol 1995; 32:689–707.
127. Garbe C. Chemotherapy and chemoimmunotherapy in disseminated malignant melanoma. Melanoma Res 1993; 3: 291–299.
128. Oettgen HF, Old LJ. The history of cancer immunotherapy. In: De Vita VT, Hellman S, Rosenberg SA, eds. Biologic Therapy of Cancer, Principles and Practice. Philadelphia: Lippincott, 1991:87–99.
129. Parkinson DR, Houghton AN, Hersey P, Borden EC. Biologic therapy for melanoma. In: Balch CM, Houghton AN, Milton GW, Sober AJ, Soong SJ, eds. Cutaneous Melanoma. Philadelphia: Lippincott, 1992:522–535.
130. Dagleish A. The case for therapeutic vaccines. Melanoma Res 1996; 6:5–10.
131. Mackensen A, Carcelain G, Viel S, Raynal MC, Michalaki H, Triebel F, Bosq J, Hercend T. Direct evidence to support the immunosurveillance concept in a human regressive melanoma. J Clin Invest 1994; 93:1391–1402.

132. Maeurer MJ, Storkus WJ, Kirkwood JM, Lotze MT. New treatment options for patients with melanoma: review of melanoma-derived T-cell epitope-based peptide vaccines. Melanoma Res 1996; 6:11–24.
133. Kawakami Y, Eliyahu S, Delgado CH, Robbins PF, Sakaguchi K, Appella E, Yannelli JR, Aderna GJ, Miki T, Rosenberg SA. Identification of a human melanoma antigen recognized by tumor-infiltrating lymphocytes associated with in vivo tumor rejection. Proc Natl Acad Sci USA 1994; 91:6458–6462.
134. Robbins PF, El-Gamil M, Kawakami Y, Rosenberg SA. Recognition of tyrosinase by tumor-infiltrating lymphocytes from a patient responding to immunotherapy. Cancer Res 1994; 54:3124–3126.
135. Möller P, Schadendorf D. Somatic gene therapy and its implication for the treatment of malignant melanoma. Arch Dermatol Res 1997; 289:71–77.
136. Vieweg J, and Gilboa E. Considerations for the use of cytokine-secreting tumor cell preparations for cancer treatment. Cancer Invest 1995; 13:193–201.
137. Schadendorf D. Cytokines, autologous cell immunostimulatory and gene therapy for cancer treatment. In: Bos JD, ed. Skin Immune System. 2d ed. Boca Raton, FL: CRC Press, 1997:657–669.
138. Rosenberg SA, Lotze MT, Muul LM, Leitman S, Chang AE, Ettinhhausen SE, Matory YLJM, Shilow E, Vetto JF. Observation on the systemic administration of autologous lymphokine-activated killer cells and recombinant interleukin-2 to patients with cancer. N Engl J Med 1985; 313:1485–1492.
139. Tepper RI, Pattengale PK, Leder P. Murine interleukin 4 displays potent anti-tumor activity in vivo. Cell 1989; 57: 503–512.
140. Fearon ER, Pardoll DM, Itaya T, Golumbek P, Livitsky HI, Simons JW, Karasuyama H, Vogelstein B, Frost P. Interleukin-2 production by tumor cells bypasses T helper function in the generation of an antitumor response. Cell 1990; 60:397–403.
141. Cayeux S, Beck C, Aicher A, Dörken B, Blankenstein T. Tumor cells cotransfected with interleukin-7 and B7.1 genes induce CD25 and CD28 on tumor-infiltrating T lymphocytes and are strong vaccines. Eur J Immunol 1995; 25:2325–2331.
142. Schadendorf D, Henz BM, Wittig B. Interleukin 7 trials for melanoma treatment. Mol Med Today 1996; 2:143–144.
143. Möller P, Sun YS, Dorbic T, Möller H, Makki A, Jurgovsky K, Schroff M, Henz BM, Wittig B, Schadendorf D. Vaccination with IL-7-gene modified autologous melanoma cells can enhances the anti-melanoma lytic activity in peripheral blood of advanced melanoma patients—a clinical phase I study. Br J Cancer 1998; 77:1907–1916.
144. Sun Y, Jurgovsky K, Möller P, Alijagic S, Dorbic T, Georgieva J, Wittig B, Schadendorf D. Vaccination with IL-12-gene modified autologous melanoma cells—preclinical results and a first clinical phase I study. Gene Ther 1998; 5:481–490.

10

Polymer-Encapsulated Cells for Gene Therapy

Dwaine F. Emerich
Alkermes, Inc., Cambridge, Massachusetts

Elizabeth Razee
CytoTherapeutics, Inc., Lincoln, Rhode Island

I. INTRODUCTION

A major goal of gene therapy research is the development of effective treatments for clinical disorders, including those with underlying central nervous system (CNS) dysfunction. Progressive CNS diseases are characterized by the progressive deterioration of both cognitive and motor function that lead to prolonged periods of increasing incapacity. Among the most problematic and prevalent neurological disorders are those associated with the loss of specific populations of brain neurons. Today, approximately 12 million people in the United States alone suffer from such neurological disorders (Table 1). Estimated costs in the United States of public expenditures and secondary medical expenses for treating patients with neurological disorders exceed $400 billion annually. Expenses directly attributed to the organic neurological disease account for only about 25% of that amount. Beyond monetary costs to the health care economy, however, the medical, societal, familial and personal costs cascading from these diseases defy calculation. Despite significant advances in technology and in our understanding of CNS disorders, effective treatments for progressive neurological disorders remain elusive.

Neural transplantation research, however, shows promise as an effective treatment for neurological diseases. Neural transplantation is rooted in the use of grafting tissue into damaged areas of the CNS to study the development and regenerative capacity of the brain. Extending from these roots was the appealing logic of replacing lost or damaged populations of neurons. Supporting this inherent appeal were the demonstrations that grafted tissue survives, integrates with the host brain, and promotes functional recovery in animal models of acute injury or neurodegenerative disorders (1–17). In addition, reconstructing damaged neuronal circuits, living tissue, and cell cultures may also be used as "vehicles" for delivering therapeutic molecules, including gene products, directly to the brain (18–25).

Despite their promise as means to treat or repair the CNS, the ability to identify appropriate tissue sources for use in human neural transplantation remains a major stumbling block to their widespread clinical evaluation. The use of human tissue, while it has enjoyed acceptance in the form of whole organ transplantation, is complicated by poor availability. However, societal, legal, and ethical issues encumber the use of neural tissue because it is most frequently derived from human fetuses. Gene-transfer technology, though, could enable the production of cells that express a novel genetic program that enables them to locally manufacture and secrete regulated quantities of specific molecules once implanted into the brain.

While cell lines have been used successfully in numerous experimental models, concern has remained that these immortalized, or dividing, cells may become neoplastic due to the transforming element incorporated into their genome. The use of xenogeneic genetically modified cells, which are encapsulated within immunoisolatory membranes to protect them from host rejection, may provide

Table 1 Annual Cost of Neurological Diseases

Disease	Prevalence (U.S.)	Annual cost (billion dollars)
Dementias	4,000,000–5,000,000	113.2
Head injury	1,000,000	48.3
Mental retardation	575,000	35.1
Spinal cord injury	175,000	22.6
Stroke	3,000,000	17.9
Other	~1,000,000	8.1
Multiple sclerosis	200,000–500,000	5.0
Cerebral palsy	600,000–750,000	1.2
Epilepsy	2,000,000	3.0
Total	10,000,000–14,000,000	254.4

an alternative method. In this chapter, we will track the use of immunoisolated cells from the initial cell biology and encapsulation process, through several preclinical research models and, ultimately, to human clinical trials (Fig. 1). Specifically, we will examine (1) some of the fundamental engineering aspects of cell encapsulation, (2) preclinical animal model data demonstrating the therapeutic potential of genetically modified, encapsulated cell therapy for Alzheimer's disease (AD) and Huntington's disease (HD), and (3) the current state of initial clinical trials examining the use of encapsulated xenogeneic implants.

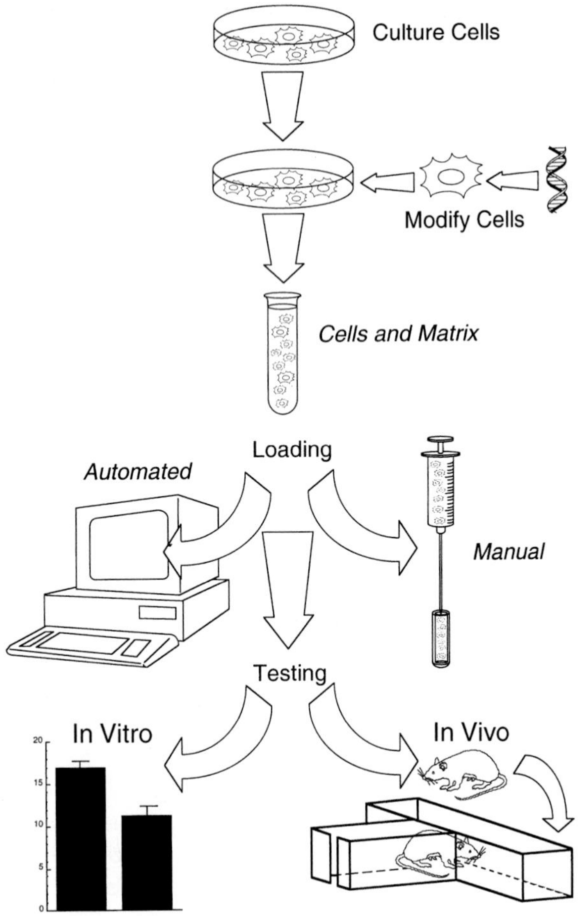

Figure 1 Flow diagram illustrating the steps involved in using genetically modified polymer-encapsulated cells for CNS implantation. Cells are cultured and modified in vitro prior to either manual or automated loading into hollow-fiber membranes. Following in vitro characterization the cells are transplanted into the desired region of the brain and in vivo tests are conducted to determine the potential efficacy produced by the products secreted from the encapsulated cells.

II. OVERCOMING THE OBSTACLE OF THE BLOOD-BRAIN BARRIER IN DELIVERING GENE PRODUCTS TO THE CNS

A significant impediment to the development of treatments for CNS diseases is the ability to deliver therapeutics directly to the brain. Relative to other body systems, the brain uses the blood-brain barrier (BBB) as a unique structural means of modulating both the local and global exchange of metabolic products (28). Systemic capillaries have endothelial cells that are fenestrated and contain clefts between cells, which permit the passage of large molecules. Systemic capillaries also actively transport materials from the circulation to local tissue by means of endocytosis and vesicular transport. Capillaries in the brain, however, function in a distinctly different manner and form a barrier that results from a continuous layer of endothelial cells that are bound together with tight junctions restricting transcellular and pericellular transport of bloodborne molecules. The BBB excludes the transport of molecules into the brain based on electric charge, lipid solubility, and molecular weight and protects the brain from fluctuations in large, lipid-insoluble substances and proteins. The only substances excepted from this are those essential to brain metabolism or the synthesis of brain proteins and neurotransmitters, some exogenous compounds that are structurally similar to endogenous molecules, and some inorganic ions that make use of specific transport systems to facilitate their entry into the brain.

By combining low passive permeability together with highly selective transport between the blood and the brain, the BBB provides an exquisite system to regulate the internal chemical environment of the CNS. The very features of this system that protect the brain create a barrier for both researchers and clinicians to introduce drugs to the brain as well as for investigators of gene therapy.

Since the impermeability of the BBB prevents the use of systemically administered enzyme- or protein-producing cells, or genetic vectors, other methods of bypassing the BBB have been the subject of intensive experimental and clinical investigation. Intraventricular infusions of molecules using pumps, chemical conjugation to specific carriers that are capable of crossing the BBB, and implantable polymers that slowly release the drug of choice are all being explored (see Table 2). Still other approaches have concentrated on direct genetic transfer of genetic material to cells in vivo using viral and chemical agents. These approaches are not covered here but are expertly reviewed in this volume. Ex vivo approaches, on the other hand, have relied on genetic transfer to cultured neuronal and nonneuronal cells that are subsequently implanted into the desired brain region. Polymer encapsulation of genetically modified cells is a technological hybrid that combines some of the advantages of in vivo gene therapy, implantable polymers, and direct cell grafting (Table 3).

III. THE CONCEPT OF IMMUNOISOLATION AND ENCAPSULATION OF CELLS

Single cells, as well as clusters of cells, can be enclosed within a selective, semipermeable membrane barrier to deliver specific therapeutic agents in the host. The membrane barrier surrounds the cells and is engineered with size-selective pores to permit oxygen and required nutrients to pass through to the cells, as well as to permit bioactive cell secretions to pass through to the host tissue. At the same time, the membrane restricts the passage of larger cytotoxic agents from the host immune defense system.

There are two main implications of membrane encapsulation. First, it reduces or eliminates the need for chronic immunosuppression of the host. Second, theoretically, it

Table 2 Advantages and Disadvantages of Non–Cell-Based Delivery Methods to the Central Nervous System

Method	Advantages	Disadvantages
Intraventricular infusion	Able to achieve high concentrations of molecule in CSF Widely used and accepted surgical approach; proven efficacy in infectious and inflammatory indications Permits repeated and variable dosing Long-term, chronic infusions possible but difficult Frequent refilling may be needed Delivery of proteins not restricted on the basis of size Delivery of DNA possible	Invasive surgical procedure with an inherant risk of complications Technology does not permit direct delivery to parenchyma Diffusion from CSF to tissue is limited Very low-level dosing difficult Risk of mechanical failure, blockage, etc. Compound must be stable at body temperature Risk of side effects from nonspecific delivery to the CSF
Implantable polymers	Suitable for placement into surgical cavities or injection into deep structures Demonstrated efficacy in neurooncology applications Delivery into both CSF and parenchyma possible Able to control the rate of release Delivery of proteins and DNA possible Delivery is not limited due to the size of the molecule Biodegradable polymers are available High concentrations of macromolecules may be delivered	Invasive surgical procedure Diffusion may be limited Difficult to control or change the rate of delivery Biocompatibility with brain tissue may be an issue depending on the type of polymer Surgery may be needed to discontinue delivery Long-term delivery difficult Compound must be stable at body temperature
Carrier drugs	Invasive surgery not needed Suitable for widespread delivery to the CNS Multiple carrier technologies available Able to deliver proteins, DNA, and nonpolypeptide moieties Sustained release possible but difficult Drugs can be delivered to specific CNS sites	Design of carrier systems complex Potential immunigenicity to the carrier molecule Frequent and repeated administration may be needed Nonspecific effects may result from a lack of localized delivery

Table 3 Advantages and Disadvantages of Transplantation of Unencapsulated, Micro- and Macroencapsulated Cells

Unencapsulated implants	Microencapsulation	Macroencapsulation
	Advantages	
Permits anatomical integration between the host and transplanted tissue	Permits use of allo- and xenografts without immunosuppression	Permits use of allo- and xenografts without immunosuppression
Good cell viability and neurochemical diffusion	Thin wall and spherical shape are optimal for cell viability and neurochemical diffusion	Good mechanical stability
		Good cell viability and neurochemical diffusion
		Retrievable
	Disadvantages	
May require immunosuppression	Mechanically and chemically fragile	Internal characteristics (i.e., diameter) may potentially limit neurochemical diffusion and cell viability
Tissue availability limited	Limited retrievability	Need for multiple implants may produce significant tissue displacement/damage
Limited retrievability		
Societal and ethical issues		

permits cells from a variety of sources to be used, including those from nonhuman sources. The ability to select from a wide range of cell sources potentially avoids the source constraints that have thus far limited the clinical application of generally successful investigative trials of unencapsulated cell transplantation. Indeed, cross-species immunoisolated cell therapy has been validated to varying degrees in small and large animal models of Parkinson's disease (19,27–33), HD (36–39), AD (22,40,41), and amyotrophic lateral sclerosis (ALS) (18,20,42).

Encapsulation is generally divided into two categories, micro and macro, each with some benefits and drawbacks (see Table 3). Microencapsulation involves surrounding cells with a thin, spherical, semi-permeable polymer film. The small size, thin wall, and spherical shape of microcapsules are structurally optimal for diffusion, cell viability, and release kinetics. Microcapsules are formed by ionic or hydrogen bonds between two weak polyelectrolytes with opposite charges. Microcapsules can be prepared by gelling droplets of a polyanion/cellular suspension (e.g., alginate) in a mixing divalent cationic bath, which immobilizes the cells in a negatively charged matrix, and then coating the immobilized cells with a thin film of a polycation, such as poly(L-lysine). The poly(L-lysine)–alginate bond creates a permselective membrane whose molecular weight cutoff is on the order of 30,000–70,000. Since poly(L-lysine) is not biocompatible, a second layer of alginate is generally added to the capsule surface (Figs. 2, 3). Polyelectrolyte-based techniques have the advantage of avoiding the use of organic solvents, and with proper permeability control, microcapsules represent a very effective configuration for

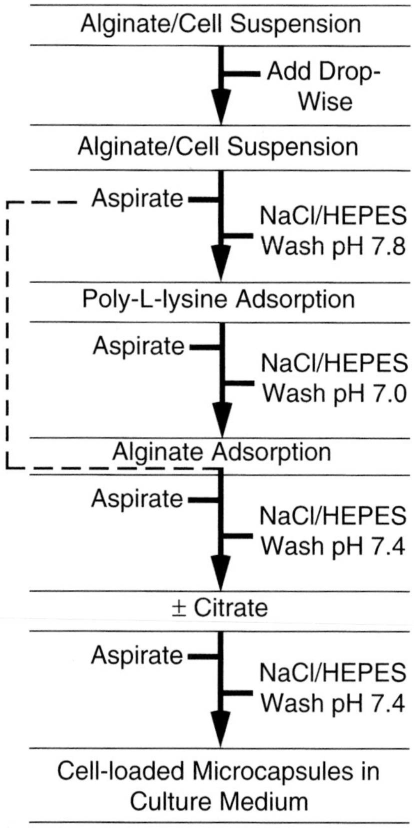

Figure 2 Flow diagram outlining the steps involved in the microencapsulation of cells. The poly(L-lysine) and alginate are sequentially adsorbed onto the alginate microspheres following immersion in a bath of H_2O.

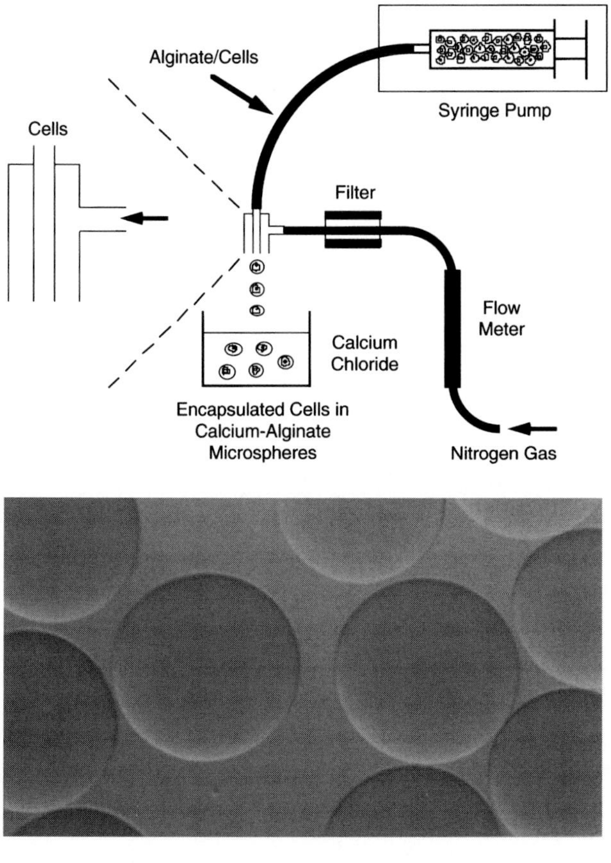

Figure 3 (Top) Schematic illustration of a syringe pump extrusion technique for encapsulating cells within alginate microcapsules. The alginate/cell suspension is extruded through the center of the annular spinneret while filtered nitrogen is passed through a surrounding outer tube. In this manner, droplets are sheared off the spinneret assembly and dropped into a container of $CaCL_2$. (Bottom) Light micrographs of microcapsules demonstrating the uniform size and shape obtained in a typical preparation.

cell viability and neurochemical diffusion. They are, however, mechanically and chemically fragile, as well as difficult to retrieve.

In contrast, macroencapsulation involves filling a hollow, usually cylindrical, permselective membrane with cells and then sealing the ends to form a capsule. Polymers used for macroencapsulation are stable, with a thicker wall than that found in microencapsulation. While thicker wall and larger implant diameters can enhance long-term implant stability, these features may also impair diffusion, compromise the viability of the tissue, and slow the release kinetics of desired factors. In theory, macrocapsules can also be retrieved from the recipient and replaced if necessary or desired.

Macroencapsulation is achieved by filling preformed thermoplastic fibers with a cell suspension. The hollow fiber is formed by pumping a solution of polymer in a water-miscible solvent through a nozzle concurrently with an aqueous solution. The polymer solution is pumped through an outer annular region of the nozzle, while the aqueous solution is pumped through a central bore. Upon contact with the water, the polymer precipitates and forms a cylindrical hollow fiber with a permselective inner membrane or ''skin.'' Further precipitation of the polymer occurs as the water moves through the polymer wall, forcing the organic solvent out and forming a trabecular wall structure. The hollow fiber is collected in a large aqueous water bath, where complete precipitation of the polymer and dissolution of the organic solvent occurs. The ends of the hollow fiber are then sealed to form a macrocapsules. This final step is not a trivial one, since reliably sealing the ends of capsules can be extremely difficult.

A second method of macroencapsulation, called coextrusion, avoids the sealing problem by entrapping cells within the lumen of a hollow fiber during the fabrication process. Pinching the fiber before complete precipitation of the polymer causes fusion of the walls, providing closure of the extremities while the cells are inside. The advantages of coextrusion over loading preformed capsules include (a) cells that are distributed more uniformly along the entire length of the fiber, (b) reduced shear stresses on the cells during the loading process, and (c) the potential for mass-production of capsules.

IV. CELLS AND EXTRACELLULAR MATRICES USED IN ENCAPSULATION

Cells used within hollow fiber membrane based devices fall into one of three basic types:

1. Primary postmitotic cells, such as porcine islets of Langerhans, bovine adrenal chromaffin cells, or porcine hepatocytes
2. Immortalized (or dividing) cells such as PC12 (derived from a rat pheochromacytoma) or fibroblasts
3. Cell lines that have been engineered to secrete a bioactive substance such as fibroblast cells, which secrete specific neurotrophic factors

In vivo, extracellular matrices (ECMs) provide control of cell function through the regulation of morphology, proliferation, differentiation, migration, and metastasis (43–46). Within a capsule, ECMs were originally employed to prevent aggregation of cells (immobilization) and central necrosis. Since then, ECMs have been found to be beneficial to the viability and function of cells that prefer immobilization and anchorage-dependent cell lines requiring a scaffolding. Currently employed matrices are derived from naturally occurring polysaccharides (sodium alginate, chitin, chitosan, or hyaluronic acid) or biologically derived materials (Matrigel, Vitrogen, Types I and IV collagen) (47,48). Relevant to the present chapter, collagen acts as a matrix for fibroblasts that have been genetically engineered to secrete trophic factors such as nerve growth factor (NGF) (36), ciliary neurotrophic factor (CNTF) (37), glial derived neurotrophic factor (GDNF) (49), and neurotrophin 4/5 (NT4/5) (39). All in all, successful cell encapsulation involves the choice of the cell to be encapsulated, the type of intracapsular matrix used, and the ability to control multiple membrane properties such as geometry, morphology and transport (Fig. 4).

V. PREPARATION OF MEMBRANES USED FOR CNS TRANSPLANTATION

The majority of thermoplastic ultrafiltration (UF) and microfiltration (MF) membranes used to encapsulate cells are manufactured from homogeneous polymer solutions by

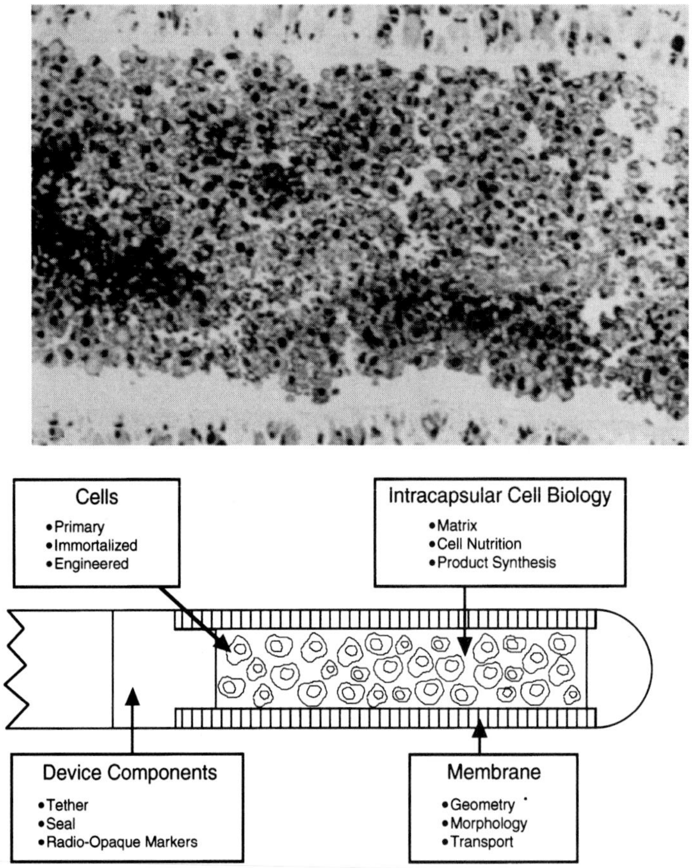

Figure 4 (Top) An example of encapsulated fibroblasts retrieved from monkey lateral ventricle illustrating many of the components listed above. Cells were modified to produce NGF and were encapsulated using Vitrogen as an extracellular matrix. Under these conditions, numerous hematoxylin and eosin-stained cells were visible and evenly distributed within the full length of the capsule one month following transplantation. These cells displayed a healthy morphology and numerous mitotic figures were observed. (Bottom) Diagram illustrating the different components of a macrocapsule contributing to successful implantation and cell viability. The manufacturing process involves several different aspects, each with its own complexities. The initial choice of cell types includes primary, immortalized, or engineered. Intracapsular cell biology issues following encapsulation include a consideration of the need to use a compatible extracellular matrix and other considerations specific to that cell type because they impact cell nutrition and product synthesis. A series of other device-related issues include membrane geometry, morphology, and transport of molecules into and out of the device. Finally, the device must be sealed and, depending on the site of implantation, could require a tether for subsequent retrieval or the inclusion radio-opaque markers for imaging purposes.

phase inversion. Ultrafiltration membranes have pore sizes ranging from 5 nm to 0.1 μm, while microfiltration (or microporous) membranes have pores ranging from 0.1 μm to 3 μm. Phase inversion is a versatile technique that allows for the formation of membranes with a wide variety of nominal molecular weight cutoffs, permeabilities, and morphologies. The morphology and membrane properties depend on the thermodynamic parameters and kinetics of the fabrication process. In this process, the polymer is first dissolved in an appropriate solvent. The solution is then cast as a flat sheet or extruded as a hollow fiber. As part of the casting or extrusion procedure, the polymer solution is precipitated by a phase transition, which can be brought about by changing the temperature or solution composition. This process involves the transfer of a single-phase liquid polymer solution into a two-phase system consisting of a polymer-rich phase that forms the membrane structure and a second liquid polymer-poor phase that forms the membrane pores. Any polymer that will form a homogeneous solution that under certain temperatures and compositions will separate into two phases can be used. Thermodynamic and kinetic parameters, such as the chemical potential of the components and the free energy of mixing of the components, determine the manner in which the phase separation takes place (50).

In cases where membrane strength limits the overall device strength, the membrane must be manufactured with certain considerations in mind, and the membrane dimensions, composition, and structure may have to be altered. Choosing a material that is inherently stronger (i.e., more ordered) or higher in molecular weight with which to cast the membrane should increase the overall mechanical properties. UF or MF membranes can be fabricated with macrovoids within the wall or as an open-cell foam where the microvoids are interconnected. By incorporating techniques that increase this isoreticulated structure within the membrane wall, the tensile strength can be increased at the same general membrane porosity, thus maintaining the same overall diffusive transport. The strength can also be improved by increasing the cross-sectional area of the membrane by thickening the walls. Decreasing the overall membrane porosity also increases the overall membrane strength. Examples of macrovoid containing structures are shown in Figure 5.

The outer morphology of the membranes can be altered during fabrication or by a posttreatment to improve the host tissue reaction. Using various phase inversion techniques, the outer surface of the membrane can range from a rejecting skin to a structure that is large enough to allow cells to enter into the wall itself (approximately 10 μm diameter). The combination of proper membrane transport and outer morphologies may also be achieved using composite membranes (51).

VI. MEMBRANE TRANSPORT CHARACTERIZATION

Membrane transport is typically characterized by the capability to retain marker molecules in convective sieving experiments. Here the rejection coefficient, R, is defined as:

$$R - 1 = \frac{C_f}{C_r} \tag{1}$$

where C_f and C_r are the concentrations of a marker in the filtrate and retentate, respectively.

Although standard convective measurements give an approximate idea of what size molecules can pass through a membrane, they are insufficient to predict the rate or selectivity in diffusion-based devices. Since immunoisolation systems are primarily diffusion based (52–54), it is essential to determine the diffusive transport properties of the membrane in order to understand the intracapsular environment of encapsulated cells, optimize the passage of essential metabolic species and molecules of interest, and assess the degree of immune exposure.

A. General Theory

In the absence of electrochemical or buoyant effects, the one-dimensional flux, N (g/cm^2 s), of a dissolved solute, i, may be represented by the following equation:

$$Ni = (-D\, \partial C/\partial x)_i + (1 - \sigma_i)\, \bar{\omega}_i \tag{2}$$

where D is the diffusion coefficient (cm^2/s), C is the concentration (g/cm^3), x is the distance (cm), σ is the Stavermen reflection coefficient (dimensionless), and v is the mass velocity per surface area (g/cm^2 s). The concentration- and pressure-dependent terms above represent the diffusive and convective components of solute transport. Equation (2) can usually only be integrated for special cases where the interdependence of convection and diffusion is known or where the two components can be assumed to be independent and additive. However, in cases of no transmembrane convection (velocity, $v_i = 0$), applicable for many immunoisolation devices, the second term drops out, and Eq. (2) becomes Fick's first law, which can be integrated assuming a homogeneous membrane and a solute concentration–independent diffusion coefficient (55), yielding:

$$N_i = [k_t\,(C_l - C_b)]_i = (k_t\,\Delta C)_i \tag{3}$$

where ΔC is the bulk solution concentration difference between the fiber lumen (1) and the bath (b) (g/cm^3), and

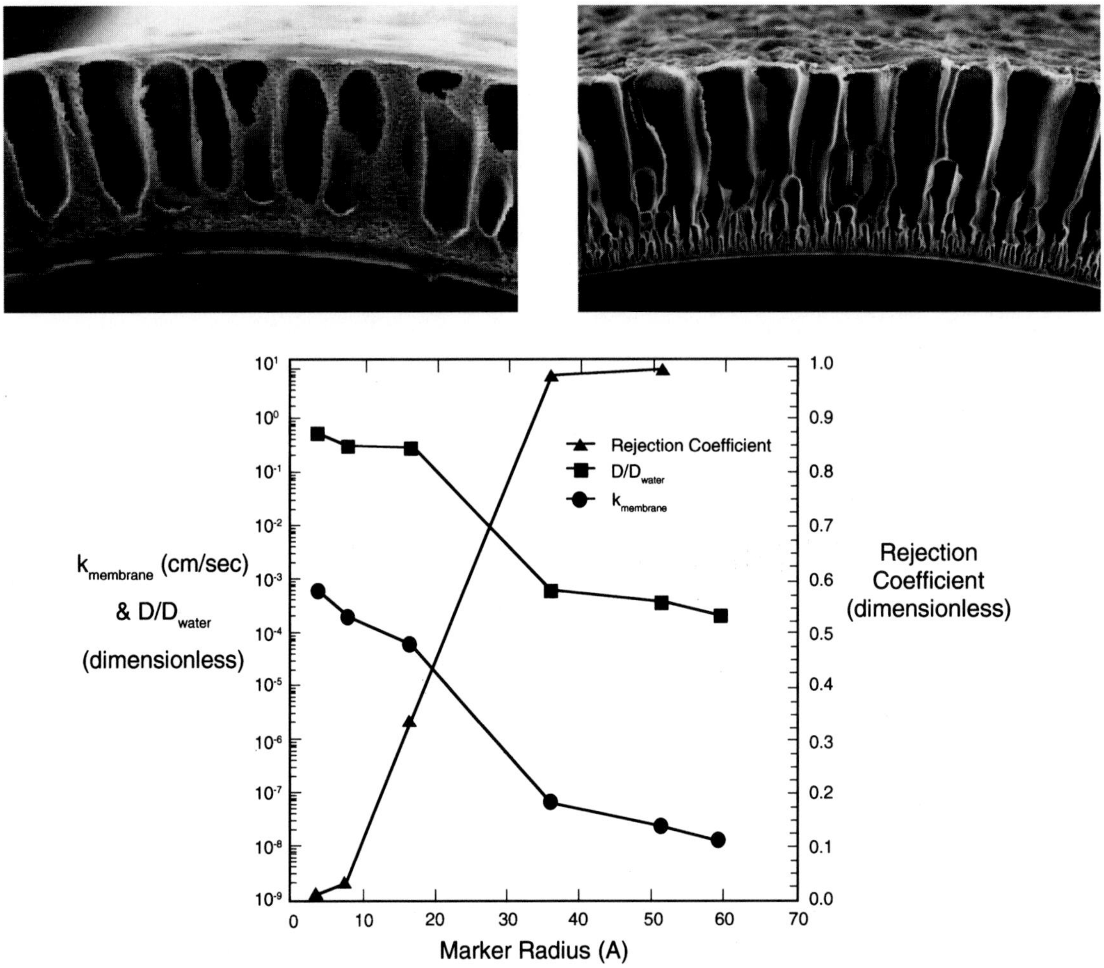

Figure 5 (Top) Scanning electron micrographs of typical macrovoid-containing membranes used in cell encapsulation studies. (Bottom) Convective rejection coefficient, membrane mass transfer coefficient, and relative membrane diffusivity relative to water versus molecular size for glucose and proteins.

k_t is the overall mass transfer coefficient (cm/s). Although nonlinearities in the concentration profile caused by chemical charge, or other interactions of the solute with the membrane material may make the internal concentration impossible to predict, they can usually be taken into account by using overall ''lumped-parameter'' mass transport coefficients. Ideally, solute concentration is uniform in the liquid region on either side of the membrane and decreases linearly across the membrane. In practice, such profiles are approximated only when the membrane resistance is large compared to the unstirred liquid resistances. However, even with aggressive stirring, the transport of small, rapidly diffusing solutes can lead to gradients within the media, which, if neglected, may cause large errors in calculated membrane mass transfer coefficients. The contribution of the unstirred liquid regions, often referred to as boundary layers, may be accounted for by defining the reciprocal overall mass transfer coefficient as an inverse sum of the coefficients for each region:

$$\frac{1}{k_t} = \frac{1}{k_b} + \frac{1}{k_m} + \frac{1}{k_l} \tag{4}$$

where the subscripts b, m, and l refer to the outside bath, membrane, and fiber lumen, respectively.

B. Small Solutes

To minimize the effect of boundary layers, the membrane diffusivity of rapidly diffusing small solutes can be measured using a flowing-type system in which solute diffuses from a recirculating bath fluid through the membrane wall and is carried away by buffer that is slowly pumped through the fiber lumen at a known flow rate. The mixing cup concentration of solute i, $(C_{mc})_i$, which is equal to the flux divided by the average velocity, is measured in the collected lumen fluid. Using Eq. (3) and assuming the buffer entering the fiber lumen is solute-free, the overall device-averaged mass transfer coefficient can be expressed in terms of the following easily measured variables:

$$(k_t)_i = \frac{(C_{mc})_i\ Q_f}{(A\ \Delta C_i)} \qquad (5)$$

where A is the log mean membrane surface area calculated for an annulus $(2\pi(r_2 - r_1)z/(\ln(r_2/r_1)$, r_2 and r_1 are the outer and inner radii, respectively, z is the length, and Q_f is the volumetric flowrate through the fiber lumen in μL/min.

1. Membrane $(k_m)_i$

The transport resistance of the membrane is a complicated function of bulk diffusivity, D, membrane thickness, tortuosity, equilibrium partition coefficient (which in turn is a function of porosity, pore size distribution, and membrane/solute interactions), and reduced pore diffusivity. In most practical situations, $(k_m)_i$ is impossible to calculate from fundamental principles and is instead calculated from measurements of overall mass transport. Effectively, $(k_m)_i$ can be viewed as the proportionality constant that relates the measured flux, N_i, to the concentration difference of solute "i" across the membrane if the solution concentration at the membrane/solution interface is known.

2. Bath Side Boundary $(k_b)_i$ and Fiber Lumen $(k_l)_i$ Boundary Lavers

These effects can be separately calculated using a Sherwood number analysis to yield the following equation:

$$\frac{(k_m)_i = 1}{\{(A/Q_f \ln [C_b/(C_b - C_{mc}] - (1/k_l + 1/k_b)\}_i} \qquad (6)$$

where Q_f is the volumetric flowrate through the fiber lumen in μL/min and C_b and C_{mc} are the bath side and mixing cup concentrations, respectively.

C. Large Solutes

Large solutes are practically defined as solutes with a molecular weight or size equal to or greater than the nominal molecular weight cutoff of the membrane (defined as the molecular weight at 90% rejection in a convective measurement). These solutes are sterically excluded from all but the largest pores, creating a membrane transport resistance at least an order of magnitude greater than the surrounding bath and lumen resistances. In encapsulation studies, k_l and k_b often account for less than 10% of the membrane resistance, and their contribution to the overall resistance is assumed to be insignificant. Accordingly, the elaborate calculations introduced for the smaller solutes to compensate for the boundary layer contributions are not necessary. The large solutes used in diffusion studies are typically both proteins (bovine serum albumin, immunoglobulin G, and apoferritin) and fluorescein-tagged dextrans (10–2000 K). Because long measurement times are necessary to attain detectable quantities of these large solutes, the membrane mass transfer coefficient, $(k_m)_i$, is usually measured in the static system, wherein a marker solution was loaded inside the fiber and allowed to diffuse through the membrane into the surrounding bath which was initially filled with solute-free buffer. In these cases, stirring is not required to reduce boundary layers because diffusion through the membrane is the rate-limiting step in transport. Equating the flux N_i from Eq. (3) with the flux across the membrane, the following is obtained:

$$N_i = \frac{V_b(dC_b/dt)}{A = \{k_t\Delta C\}_i} \qquad (7)$$

A mass balance equates the amount of solute leaving the fiber to the amount entering the bath, and integrating yields:

$$\ln\left[\frac{(C_l - C_b)_{n+1}}{(C_l - C_b')_n}\right] = -(k_m)_i At_n\left[\frac{1}{V_l} + \frac{1}{V_b}\right] \qquad (8)$$

where

$$(C_b)'_n = (C_b)_n\,(1 - V_r/V_b) \qquad (9)$$

$$(C_l)_{n+1} = (C_l)_n + (V_b/V_l)\,\{(C_b)'_n - (C_b)_{n+1})\} \qquad (10)$$

and t_n is time of sampling of the nth sample, $(C_l)_n$ and $(C_b)_n$ are the lumen and bath concentrations of the nth sample, respectively, and V_r is the replacement volume. Figure 5 shows the diffusive characterization, including the membrane mass transfer coefficient, relative membrane diffusivity (D_m/D_{H20}), and the convective sieving curve, of a membrane manufactured and characterized using these principles.

VII. USE OF ENCAPSULATED NGF-PRODUCING CELLS IN ANIMAL MODELS OF ALZHEIMER'S DISEASE

A. Background

Alzheimer's disease affects approximately 5% of the population over the age of 65 worldwide and is the most prevalent form of adult onset dementia. With the aging population, the incidence of AD is expected to triple over the next 75 years. The most prominent feature of AD is a progressive deterioration of cognitive and mnemonic ability, which has been suggested to be at least partially related to the degeneration of basal forebrain cholinergic neurons. At present, treatments are ineffective for slowing or preventing the loss of cholinergic neurons or the associated memory deficits. Several converging lines of evidence indicate that NGF has potent target-derived trophic and tropic effects upon cholinergic basal forebrain neurons:

1. The highest levels of NGF protein and mRNA are found in the target regions of basal forebrain cholinergic neurons (56,57).
2. Radiolabeled NGF is taken up by cholinergic terminals and specifically transported in a retrograde fashion to cholinergic basal forebrain perikarya (58,59).
3. Target-derived NGF binds to both low (p75) and high (*trk A*)-affinity NGF receptors, which in the adult rat, nonhuman primate, and human brains are found within cholinergic neurons of the basal forebrain (60–66).
4. NGF administration in rodents and nonhuman primates prevents the loss of basal forebrain cholinergic neurons following axotomy (24,67–73).
5. Both the memory deficits and basal forebrain atrophy displayed by aged rats can be reversed by intraventricular NGF infusions (74).

Together, these data indicate that the use of NGF may represent a useful treatment strategy for AD and/or other diseases characterized by basal forebrain-mediated cholinergic deficits. Accordingly, small preliminary clinical trials employing intraventricular mouse NGF for the treatment of AD have been conducted (75).

B. Anatomical Effects of NGF in Rodent and Primate Alzheimer's Disease Models

Although no model faithfully recapitulates the complex etiology and time-dependent loss of cholinergic neurons seen in AD patients, model systems have been developed to answer the very specific question: Can NGF prevent the death of damaged cholinergic neurons following acute trauma? The initial studies described here determined whether encapsulated baby hamster kidney (BHK) cells that had been modified to produce high and stable levels of human NGF could prevent the loss of cholinergic neurons following aspiration of the fimbria/formix (76) (Fig. 6). In this model, the cholinergic neurons within the medial septum atrophy and die in a manner that is reversible with concurrent administration of NGF. Rats received lesions of the fimbria/fornix following by intraventricular implants of BHK-NGF or BHK-control (nontransfected) cells. Control-implanted animals had an extensive loss of ChAT-positive cholinergic neurons ipsilateral to the lesion that was prevented by BHK-NGF capsule implants. Quantitation of ChAT-positive neurons for the two groups revealed that with the BHK-control capsules, only 14% of the neurons remained viable on the lesioned side compared to the nonlesioned side, whereas with the BHK-NGF capsules, 88% of the cholinergic neurons were rescued. Similar results were obtained in nonhuman primates (40), an essential prerequisite to human clinical trials. In these studies, cynomolgus primates received transections of the fornix followed by placement of encapsulated BHK-NGF or BHK-control cells into the lateral ventricle (Fig. 7). In the control animals, a significant reduction in the number of cholinergic neurons was observed in the medial septum and vertical limb of the diagonal band of Broca. Again, this loss of cholinergic neurons was prevented by implants of NGF-secreting cells. It also appeared that cholinergic neurons within the medial septum of NGF-treated animals were larger, more intensely labeled, and elaborated more extensive proximal dendrites than those displayed by BHK control animals (Fig. 8).

In addition to the effects on cell viability, BHK-NGF implants induced a robust sprouting of cholinergic fibers proximal to the implant site (Fig. 9). All monkeys receiving BHK-NGF implants displayed dense collections of NGF receptor-immunoreactive fibers throughout the entire dorso-ventral extent of the lateral septum. This effect was unilateral because the contralateral side displayed only a few cholinergic fibers in a manner similar to that seen in control-implanted monkeys. The cholinergic nature of this sprouting was confirmed by an identical pattern of fibers, which were both ChAT-immunoreactive and AChE-positive. These fibers ramified against the ependymal lining of the lateral ventricle adjacent to the transplant site and were particularly prominent within the dorsolateral quadrant of the septum corresponding to the normal course of the fornix. These results have been replicated in a group of aged nonhuman primates (41) (Figs 7, 9).

C. Behavioral Effects of NGF in Aged Rodents

One of the cardinal behavioral symptoms of AD is a progressive loss of cognitive ability. Just as no animal model faithfully mimics the complex etiology and pathophysiology of AD, comparable behavioral abnormalities are difficult to reproduce in animal models. However, the aged rodent does show a progressive degeneration of basal forebrain cholinergic neurons together with marked cognitive impairments, which are in part reversible by administering

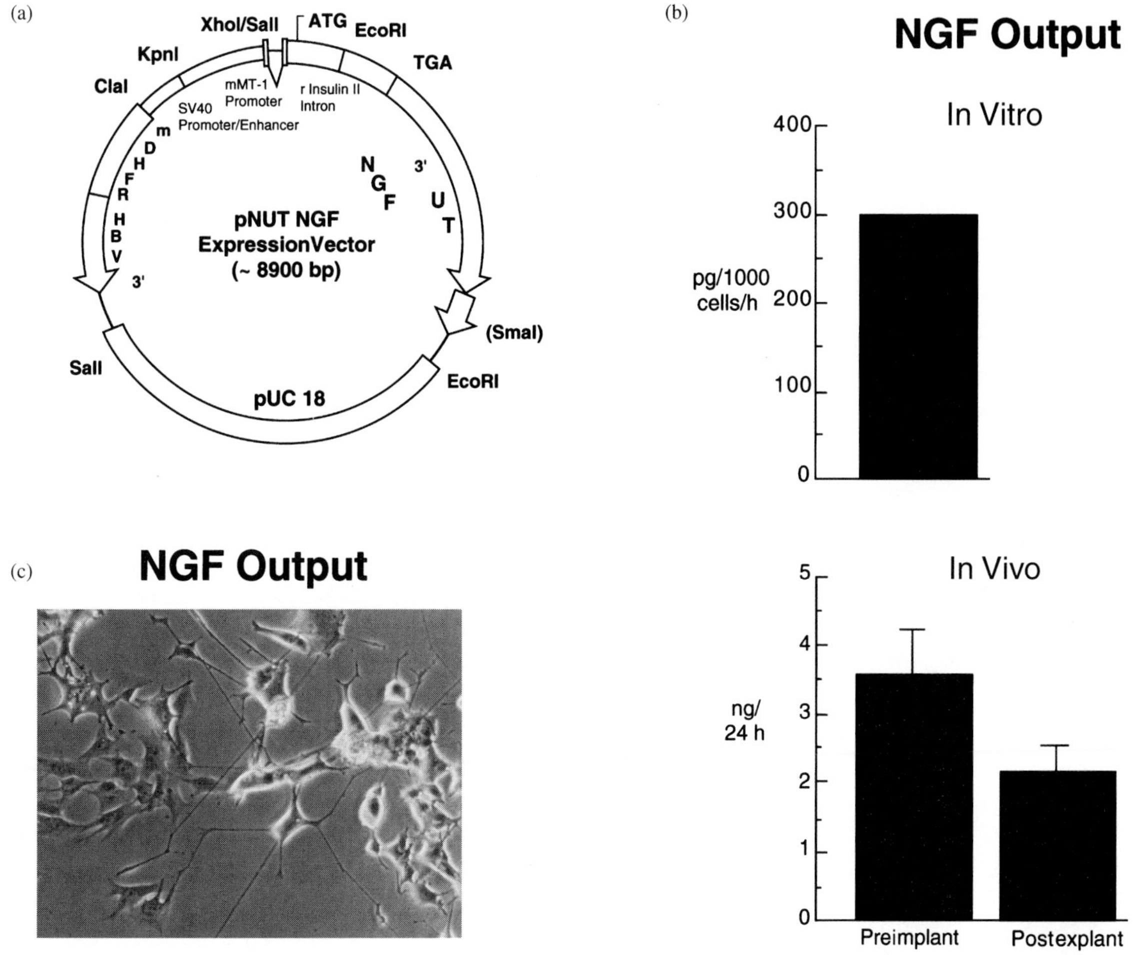

Figure 6 (a) Expression vector containing the human NGF gene. (b) NGF levels, as determined by ELISA, in unencapsulated (top) and encapsulated (bottom) BHK cells. The in vivo levels were determined from capsules that were retrieved from rodent striatum 3 months following implantation. (c) The biological activity of the NGF from encapsulated BHK cells is shown in phase contrast photomicrographs of PC12 cells treated with conditioned medium from BHK-NGF cell-loaded devices. Note that virtually all PC12A cells exhibit extensive neurite processes. Original magnification = 25 μm. (See Refs. 22, 40 for details.)

NGF. Lindner et al. (77) trained 3-, 18- and 24-month-old rats on a spatial learning task in a Morris water maze (Fig. 10). Cognitive function as measured in this task declined with age. Evidence of age-related atrophy of cholinergic neurons was observed in the striatum, medial septum, nucleus basalis, and vertical limb of the diagonal band. More importantly, these anatomical changes were most severe in those animals with the greatest cognitive impairments, suggesting a link between the two pathological processes. Following training, animals received bilateral intraventricular implants of encapsulated BHK-NGF or BHK-control cells. The 18- and 24-month-old animals receiving BHK-NGF cells showed a significant improvement in cognitive function. No improvements or deleterious effects were observed in the young, nonimpaired animals. Anatomically, the NGF released from the encapsulated cells increased the size of the atrophied basal forebrain and striatal cholinergic neurons to the size of the neurons in the young healthy rats. Furthermore, there was no evidence that the BHK-NGF cells produced changes in mortality, body weights, somatosensory thresholds, potential hyperalgesia, or activity levels, suggesting that the levels of NGF produced were not toxic or harmful to the aged rats.

It is likely that any cell-based gene therapy for a chronic disease like AD would require long-term delivery of the therapeutic gene product. However, the long-term effects

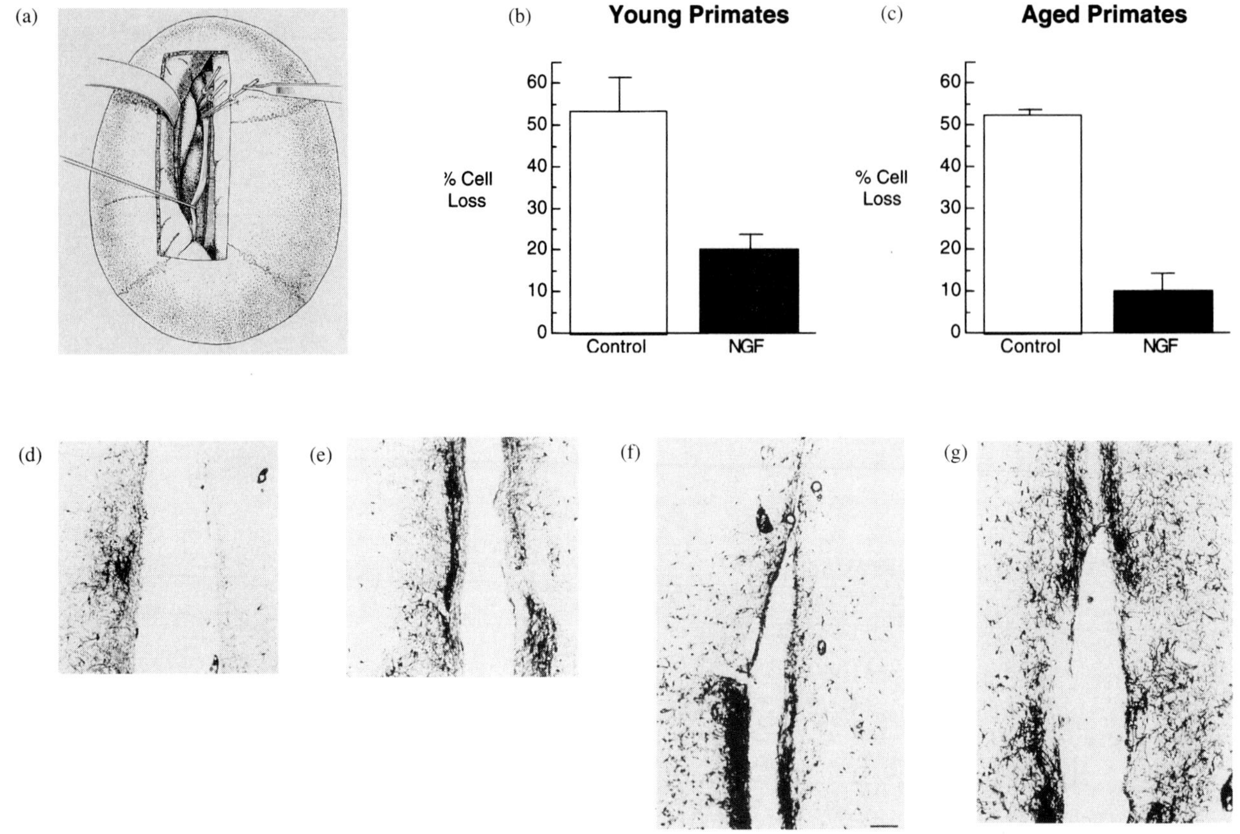

Figure 7 (a) Drawing of dorsal aspect of primate brain illustrating transection of the fornix and placement of polymer capsules containing NGF-producing BHK cells. Following a craniotomy, the cerebral hemisphere is retracted and the formix is unilaterally transected. The polymer capsules are then placed within the lateral ventricle located between the caudate (left) and septal nucleus (right). The upper portion of the capsules consists of a silastic tether that is clipped to permit closure of the dura. Quantification of p75 NGF receptor-immunoreactive neurons within the medial septum following fornix transections in young (b) and aged (c) monkeys. These figures show the percent loss of cholinergic neurons ipsilateral to the lesion and demonstrate that the loss of cholinergic neurons was significantly attenuated by implantation of BHK-NGF cells in both young and aged monkeys. The bottom figures are photomicrographs through the septal diagonal band complex of young (d and e) and aged (f and g) monkeys stained for the p75 NGF receptor from fornix transected cynomolgus monkeys receiving polymer-encapsulated implants of either a BHK-control transplant (d and f) or a BHK-NGF transplant (e and g). Note the extensive loss of p75 NGF receptor-immunoreactive neurons ipsilateral to the lesion (right) in the control-implanted monkeys. In contrast, numerous NGF receptor-positive neurons were observed in fornix transected monkeys receiving the BHK-NGF implant. Scale bar in F = 100 μm for d–g.

of NGF or any other neurotrophic factor are largely unknown. Polymer-encapsulated cells have been reported to survive and continue to secrete NGF for 13.5 months in rodents (78). No deleterious effects from NGF were detectable on body weight, mortality rate, motor/ambulatory function, or cognitive function as assessed with the Morris water maze and delayed matching to position in healthy young adult rats. In addition, there was no evidence that NGF from these encapsulated cells produced hyperalgesia, although tests of somatosensory thresholds did reveal effects related to the NGF delivery. These same animals exhibited a marked hypertrophy of cholinergic neurons within the striatum and nucleus basalis as well as a robust sprouting of cholinergic fibers within the frontal cortex and lateral septum proximal to the implant site. Together these results indicate that (1) encapsulated NGF-secreting cells prevent the loss of cholinergic neurons and induce sprouting of cholinergic fibers following axotomy in rodents and nonhuman primates, (2) NGF-secreting cells induce hypertrophy of cholinergic neurons and promote cognitive recovery in aged animals, (3) encapsulated BHK cells survive for prolonged periods of time while continuing to secrete biologically active NGF within the CNS, (4) the long-term delivery of NGF appears to be safe and without any signifi-

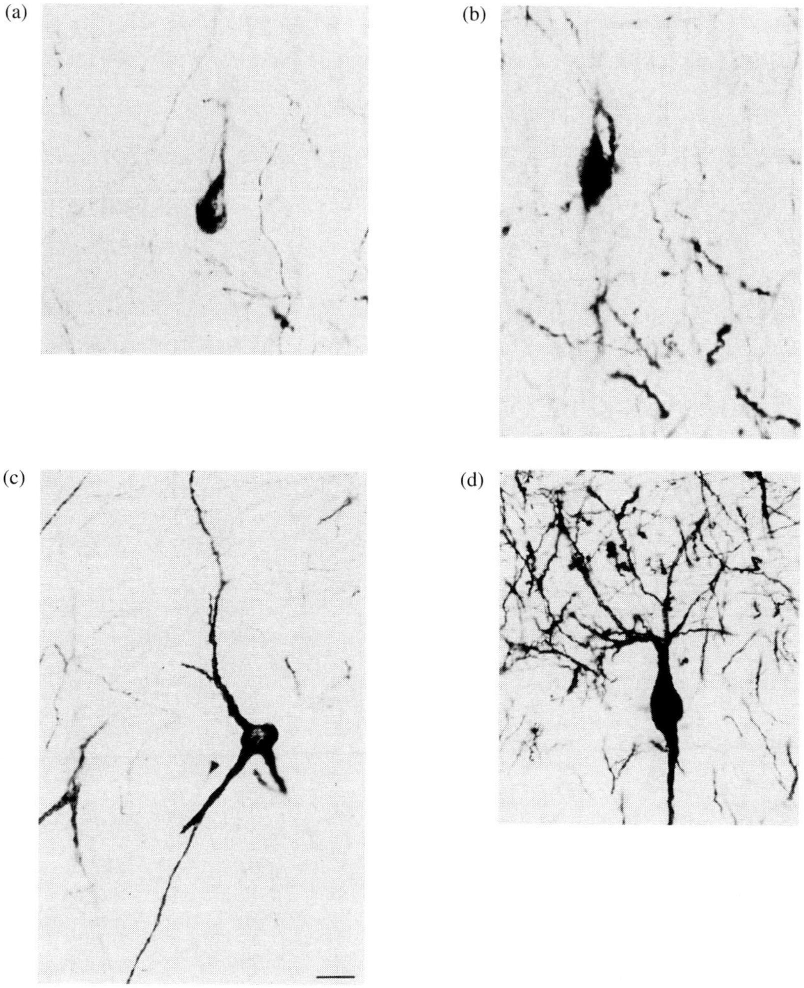

Figure 8 High-power photomicrographs illustrating the morphology of p75 NGF receptor-immunoreactive neurons within the medial septum of young monkeys receiving BHK-control (a and b) or BHK-NGF (c and d) implants. All neurons were located within the medial septum ipsilateral to the lesion/implants. Note the enlarged perikarya and extensive neuritic arbor displayed by monkeys receiving the BHK-NGF implants. In particular, the neuron in panel d displays an atypical "chandelier-like" morphology. In contrast, many neurons within the medial septum ipsilateral to the lesion/BHK-control implants appeared atrophic with a stunted neuritic branching pattern. Scale bar in c represents 50 μm for all panels.

cant deleterious behavioral effects, and (5) the anatomical changes associated with long-term NGF delivery are limited to the area immediately adjacent to the implanted device and not in more distant regions of the CNS.

VIII. USE OF POLYMER-ENCAPSULATED CELLS TO DELIVER NEUROTROPHIC FACTORS IN ANIMAL MODELS OF HUNTINGTON'S DISEASE

A. Background

Huntington's disease is an inherited, progressive neurological disorder characterized by a severe degeneration of basal ganglia neurons, particularly the intrinsic neurons of the striatum. Accompanying these pathological changes is a progressive dementia coupled with uncontrollable movements and abnormal postures. From the time of onset an intractable course of mental deterioration and progressive motor abnormalities begins, with death usually occurring within 15–17 years. Overall, the prevalence rate of HD in the United States is approximately 50 per 1,000,000 (79). At present there is no treatment that effectively addresses the behavioral symptoms or slows the inexorable neural degeneration in HD. Intrastriatal injections of excitotoxins such as quinolinic acid (QA) have been suggested to accurately model HD. Excitotoxic lesions of the striatum pro-

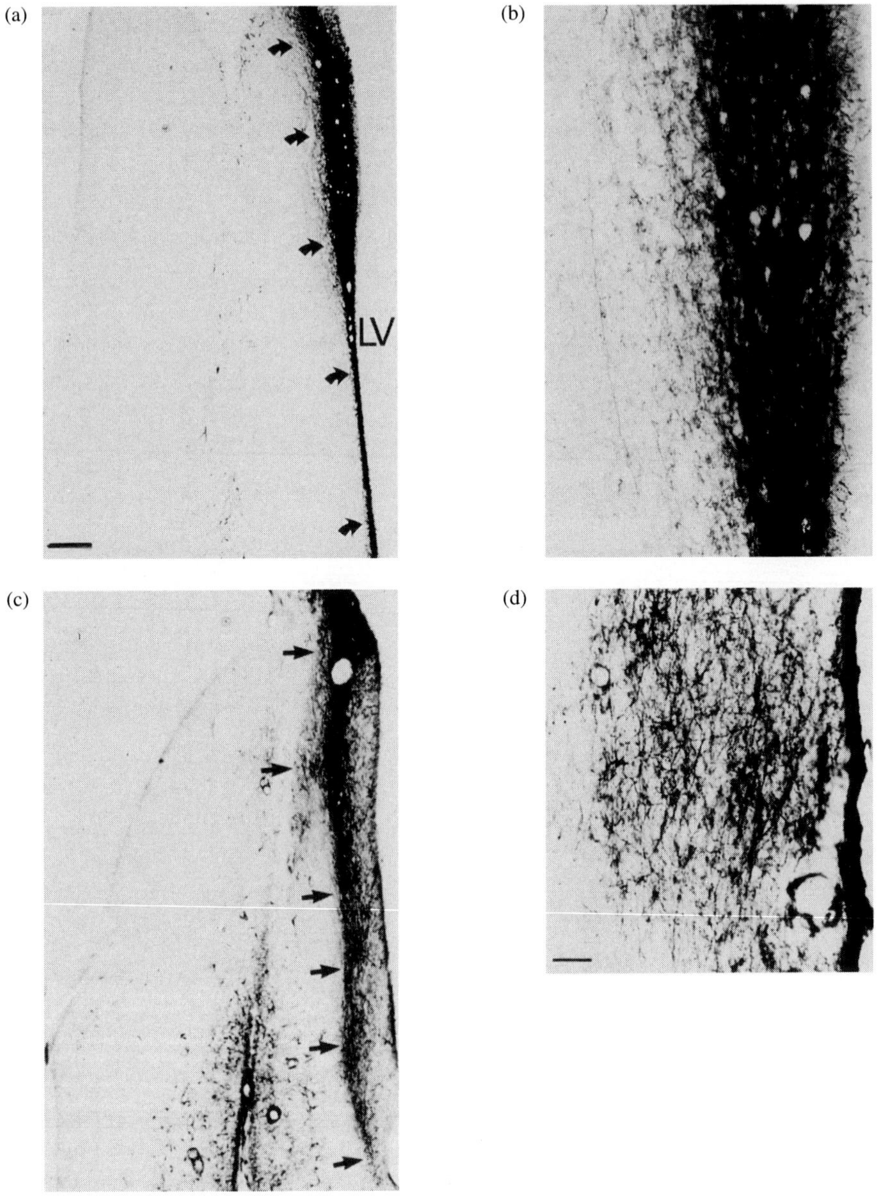

Figure 9 Sprouting of cholinergic fibers in young (a and b) and aged (c and d) NGF-treated monkeys. Low (a and c)-power photomicrographs of NGF receptor-immunostained sections illustrating a dense plexus of cholinergic fibers on the side of NGF treatment along the dorsoventral extent of the septum (arrows). This plexus was most extensive in the dorsal quadrant. High-power photomicrographs (b and d) illustrating the morphology of the NGF receptor-immunoreactive fibers, which coalesce as a dense bundle adjacent to the ventricle. LV = lateral ventricle. Scale bar in a A = 1000 μm for a and c, scale bar in d = 50 μm for b and d.

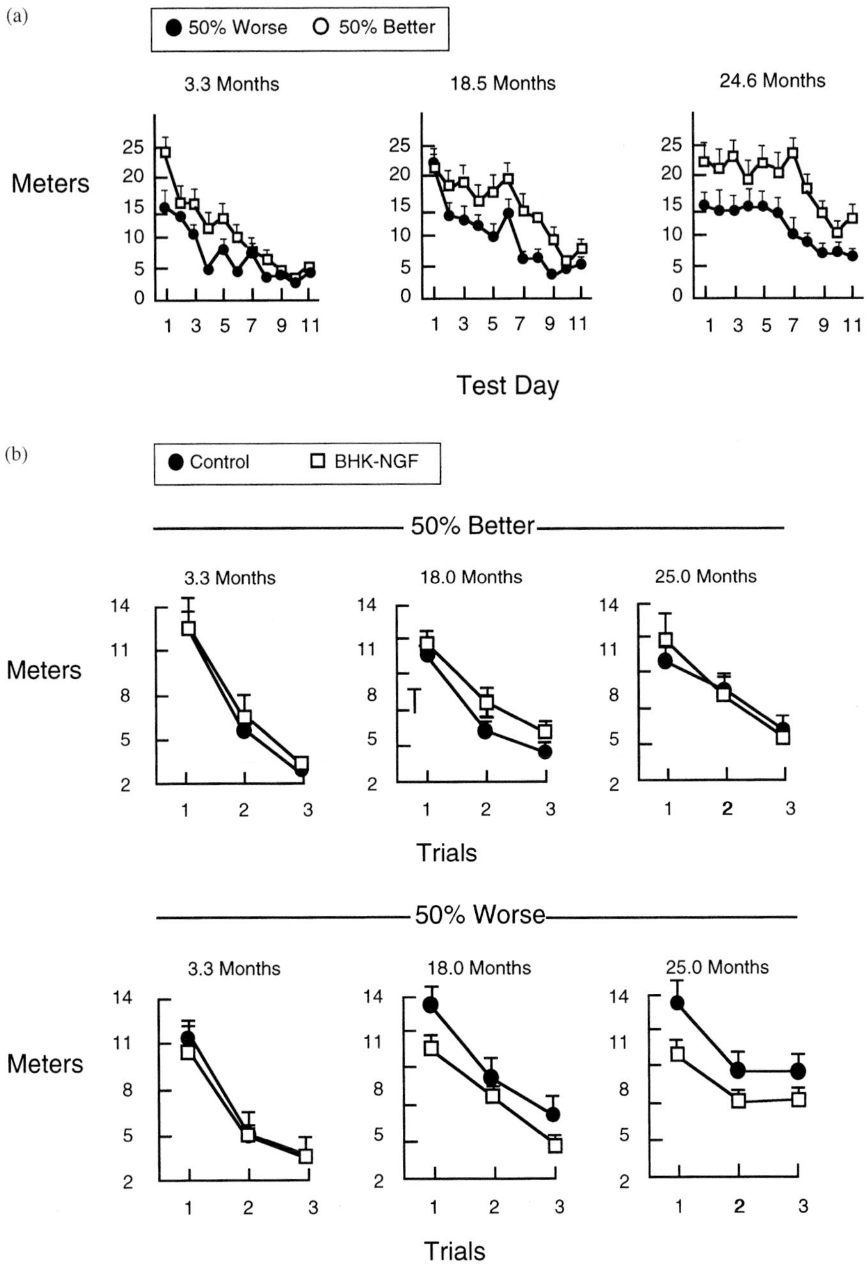

Figure 10 Cognitive function in young, middle-aged, and aged rats following implantation of encapsulated NGF-producing cells into the lateral ventricles. (a) Prior to implantation, animals were divided into the 50% worse and 50% better performers in a water maze task. (b) Following implantation, NGF was found to improve performance in the middle-aged and aged animals. Moreover, the improvements in cognitive performance were greatest in those animals that demonstrated the worst initial performance. (See Ref. 77 for details.)

duce a profile of neurochemical and pathological alterations, which bear a considerable homology to that observed in the striatum of HD patients upon postmortem examination (80–82). Behaviorally, excitotoxin-lesioned animals exhibit an abnormal profile of spontaneous locomotor activity as well as an exaggerated response to pharmacological challenges, which are reminiscent of those seen in HD patients (83,84). In addition, these animals are impaired on a variety of learning and memory tasks and have regulatory deficits which are symptomatic in HD patients (79,85,89).

It appears that intrastriatal injections of QA have become a useful model of HD and can serve to evaluate novel therapeutic strategies aimed at preventing, attenuating, or reversing neuroanatomical and behavioral changes associated with HD. The use of trophic factors in a neural protection strategy may be particularly relevant for the treatment of HD. Unlike other neurodegenerative diseases, genetic screening can identify virtually all individuals at risk who will ultimately suffer from HD. This provides a unique opportunity to design treatment strategies that can intervene prior to the onset of striatal degeneration. Thus, instead of replacing neuronal systems that have already undergone extensive neuronal death, trophic factor strategies could be designed to support host systems destined to die at later time in the patient's life.

B. Effects of NGF and CNTF in Rodent and Primate Models of Huntington's Disease

Infusions of trophic factors such as NGF or implants of cells genetically modified to secrete NGF have proven effective in preventing the neuropathological sequelae resulting from intrastriatal injections of excitotoxins including QA (86–88). Emerich and colleagues examined the ability of encapsulated CNTF-secreting cells to effect central striatal neurons in a series of defined animal models of HD (Fig. 11). In these experiments, rats received implants of BHK-NGF or BHK-CNTF cells into the lateral ventricles (36,37). One week later, the same animals received unilateral injections of QA (225 nmol) or the saline vehicle into the ipsilateral striatum. An analysis of Nissl-stained sections demonstrated that the size of the lesion was signifi-

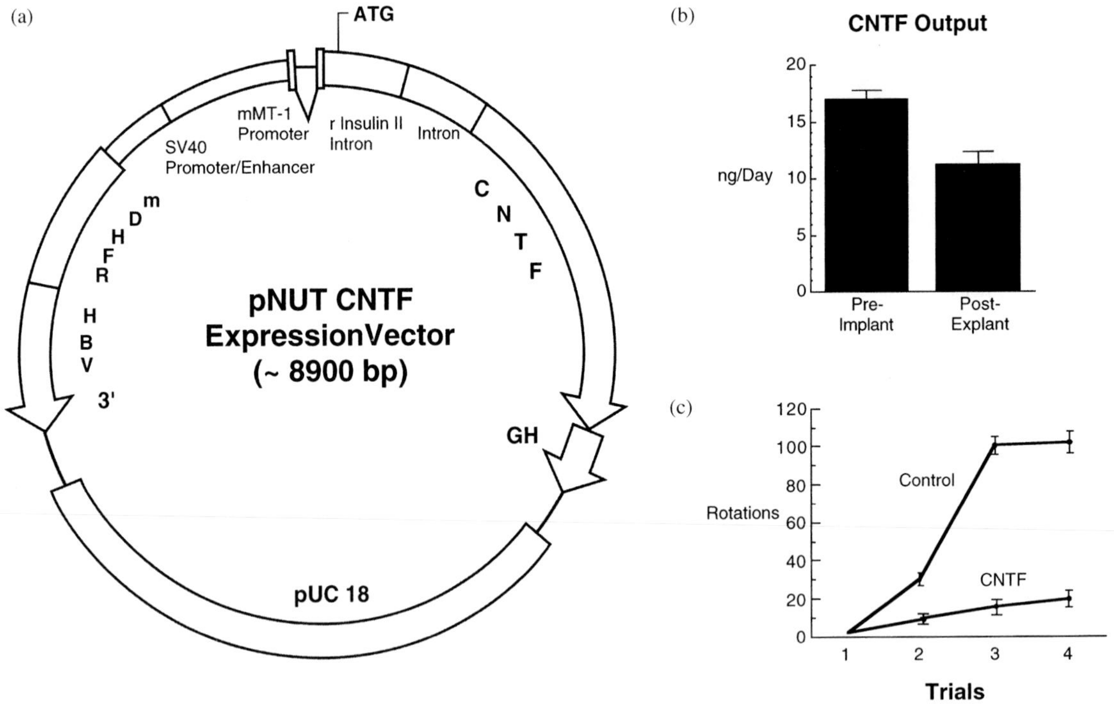

Figure 11 (a) Expression vector containing the human CNTF gene. (b) CNTF levels, as determined by ELISA, in encapsulated BHK cells immediately prior to implantation (left) and immediately following retrieval from rodent lateral ventricle 70 days following implantation. (c) Implants of encapsulated CNTF-producing cells reduce apomorphine-induced (1.0 mg/kg) rotations in rats after unilateral striatal injections of quinolinic acid. This figure shows the mean ± SEM number of rotations in a 30-minute test period. (See Ref. 37 for details.)

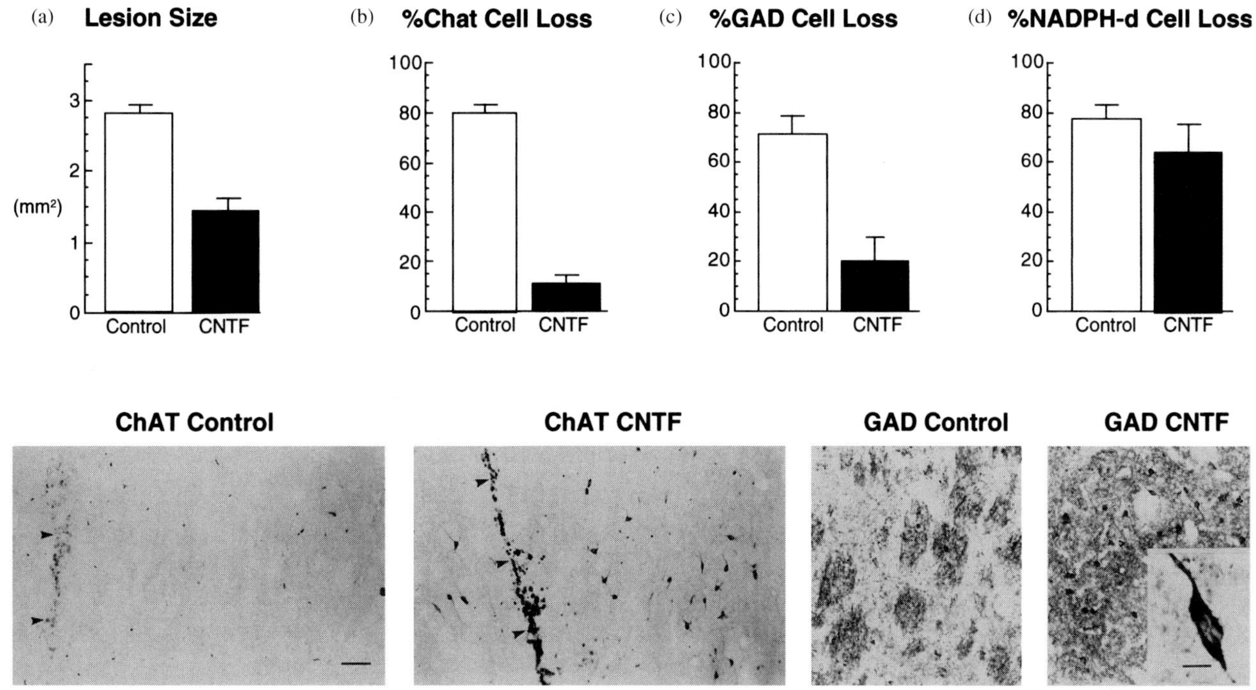

Figure 12 Lesion volume and neuronal cell counts in quinolinic acid-lesioned rats. Control-implanted animals displayed a marked lesion volume (a; determined by Nissl staining) and a significant loss of multiple types of striatal cell types including cholinergic (b), GABAergic (c) and diaphorase-positive neurons (d). The cholinergic and GABAergic neuronal losses were largely prevented in animals receiving CNTF implants, while the loss of diaphorase-positive neurons was not affected. In each case, data are presented as a percent loss of neurons on the lesioned/implanted side compared to intact contralateral side. Representative photomicrographs for cholinergic and GABAergic cells are shown for both control and CNTF-implanted animals. Note the appearance of numerous healthy-appearing cholinergic and GABAergic neurons in the CNTF-treated animals. Scale bar in ChAT control = 500 μm for ChAT control/CNTF, and scale bar in insert = 100 μm for GAD control/CNTF and 17 μm for insert.

cantly reduced in those animals receiving NGF and CNTF cells compared with those animals receiving control implants. Moreover, both NGF and CNTF cells attenuated the extent of host neural damage produced by QA as assessed by a sparing of specific populations of striatal cells, including cholinergic, diaphorase-positive, and GABAergic neurons (Fig. 12). Neurochemical analyses has confirmed the protection of multiple striatal cell populations using this strategy (89). These results clearly suggested that implantation of polymer-encapsulated trophic factor–releasing cells can protect neurons from excitotoxin damage. Importantly, behavioral studies offer additional and compelling evidence of the extent of neuronal protection that can be produced in animal models of HD (89). Trophic factor–secreting cells have provided extensive behavioral protection as measured by tests that assess both gross and subtle movement abnormalities. Moreover, these same animals show improved performance on learning and memory tasks, indicating that the anatomical protection afforded by trophic factors in this model is paralleled by a robust and relevant behavioral protection.

The ability of cellularly delivered trophic factors to preserve neurons within the striatum in a rodent model of HD led to similar studies in nonhuman primates, a step that is crucial to the initiation of clinical trials. A paradigm similar to the one employed in the rodent studies was used in nonhuman primates (38). Polymer capsules containing BHK cells, which were genetically modified to secrete CNTF, were grafted into the striatum of rhesus monkeys. Capsules were placed into the putamen and into the caudate nucleus. One week later a QA injection was placed into the putamen and caudate proximal to the capsule implants. As seen in the rodent studies, GABAergic and cholinergic neurons destined to degenerate were spared in CNTF-grafted animals. Although all animals had significant lesions, there was 3 fold and 7 fold increase in GABAergic neurons in the caudate and putamen, respectively, in CNTF-grafted animals relative to controls. Similarly, there was a 2.5-fold

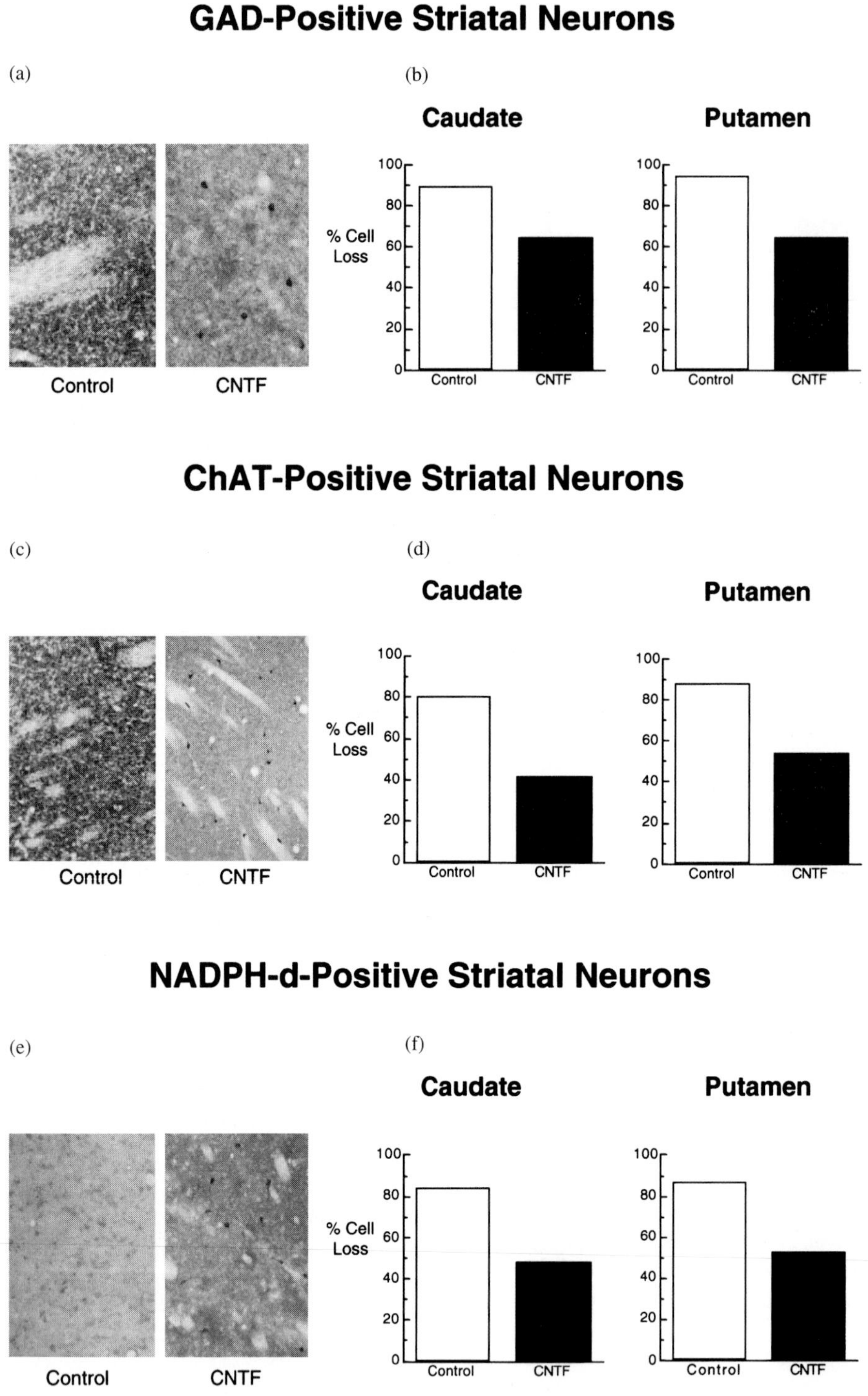

Figure 13 Neuronal cell counts in quinolinic acid–lesioned monkeys. Control-implanted animals displayed a significant loss of multiple types of striatal neurons including GABAergic (a and b), cholinergic (c and d), and diaphorase-positive neurons (e and f). Although neuronal loss was still present in animals receiving CNTF implants, it was significantly attenuated in both the caudate and putamen. In each case, data are presented as a percent of neurons on the lesioned/implanted side compared to the intact contralateral side. Representative photomicrographs for all three cell types are shown for both control and CNTF-implanted animals (a = GABAergic, c = cholinergic, and e = diaphorase-positive neurons).

and 4-fold increase in cholinergic neurons in the caudate and putamen, respectively, in CNTF-grafted animals (Fig. 13).

The ability to preserve GABAergic neurons in animals models of HD is an important, although not entirely sufficient, step in the development of a useful therapeutic. If the perikarya are preserved without sustaining their innervation, then the experimental therapeutic strategy under investigation is not likely to yield significant value. The striatum is a central station in series of loop circuits, which receive inputs from all of the neocortex, projecting to a number of subcortical sites, and then return information flow to the cerebral cortex. One critical part of this circuitry is the GABA-ergic projections to the globus pallidus and substantia nigra pars reticulata, the parts of the direct and indirect basal ganglia loop circuits. One approach to examining the integrity of this circuit is to use an antibody that recognizes GABA-ergic terminals (DARPP-32) to determine if the preservation of GABA-ergic somata within the striatum also results in the preservation of the axons of these neurons to critical extrastriatal sites. Using quantitative morphological assessment of DARPP-32 optical density, it has been shown that monkeys receiving QA lesions have significant reductions in DARPP-32 immunoreactivity within the globus pallidus and substantia nigra. The lesion-induced decrease in GABAergic innervation for both of these regions was prevented in CNTF-grafted monkeys, demonstrating that this treatment strategy protected GABAergic neurons destined to die following excitotoxic lesion as well as sustained the normal projection systems from this critical population of neurons (38) (Fig. 14, 15).

The intrinsic striatal cytoarchitecture can be preserved in monkeys by CNTF grafts, and once exposed to these grafts, these cells apparently maintain their projections. But

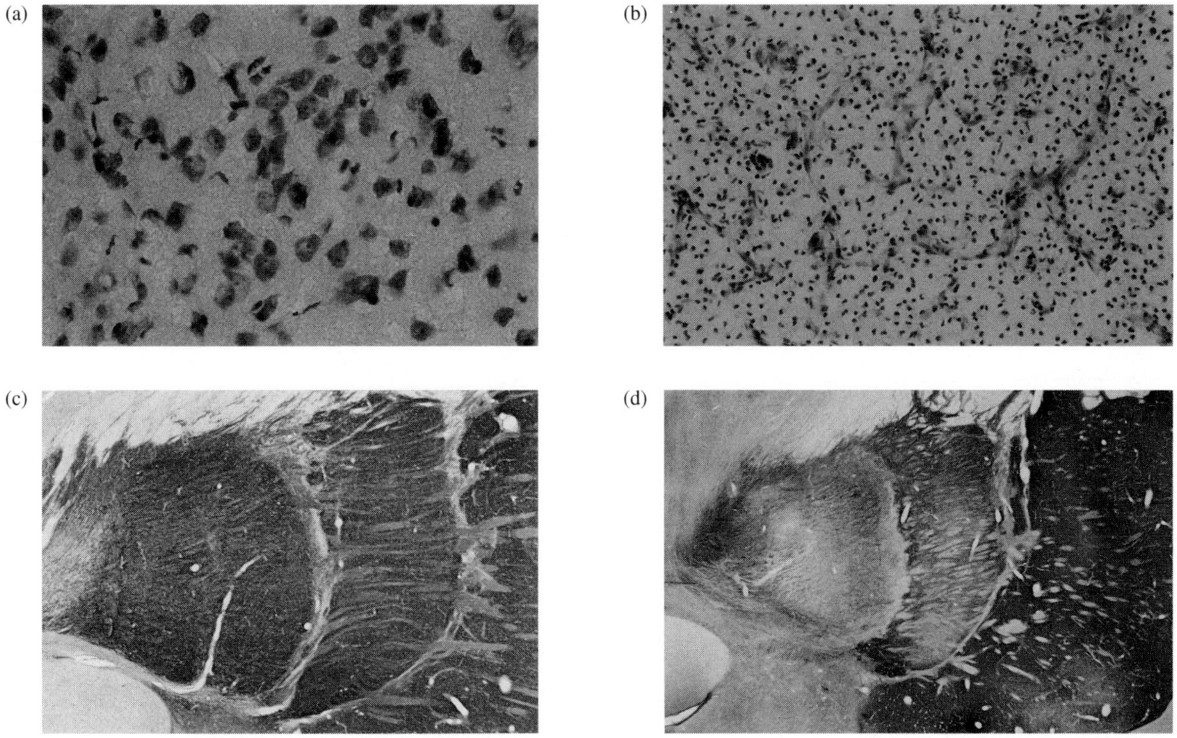

Figure 14 Photomicrographs of Nissl-stained sections through the striatum of monkeys that received quinolinic acid injections into the striatum followed by implants of encapsulated CNTF-secreting (a) or control (b) BHK cells. A paucity of healthy neurons is observed in the striatum of control-implanted monkeys, which is in stark contrast to the numerous healthy-appearing neurons seen in the same region of the CNTF-implanted monkeys. Together with the sparing of striatal neurons is a preservation of the GABAergic projection from the striatum to the globus pallidus. DARPP-32 immunocytochemistry revealed an intense, normal-appearing immunoreactivity within both the external and internal segments of the globus pallidus of CNTF-treated animals (c). In contrast, DARPP-32 immunoreactivity is reduced in control-implanted animals as a consequence of the QA lesion (d). The quantitative results from the DARPP-32 immunocytochemistry are presented in Figure 15, further highlighting the fact that this projection is sustained in these animals following CNTF treatment.

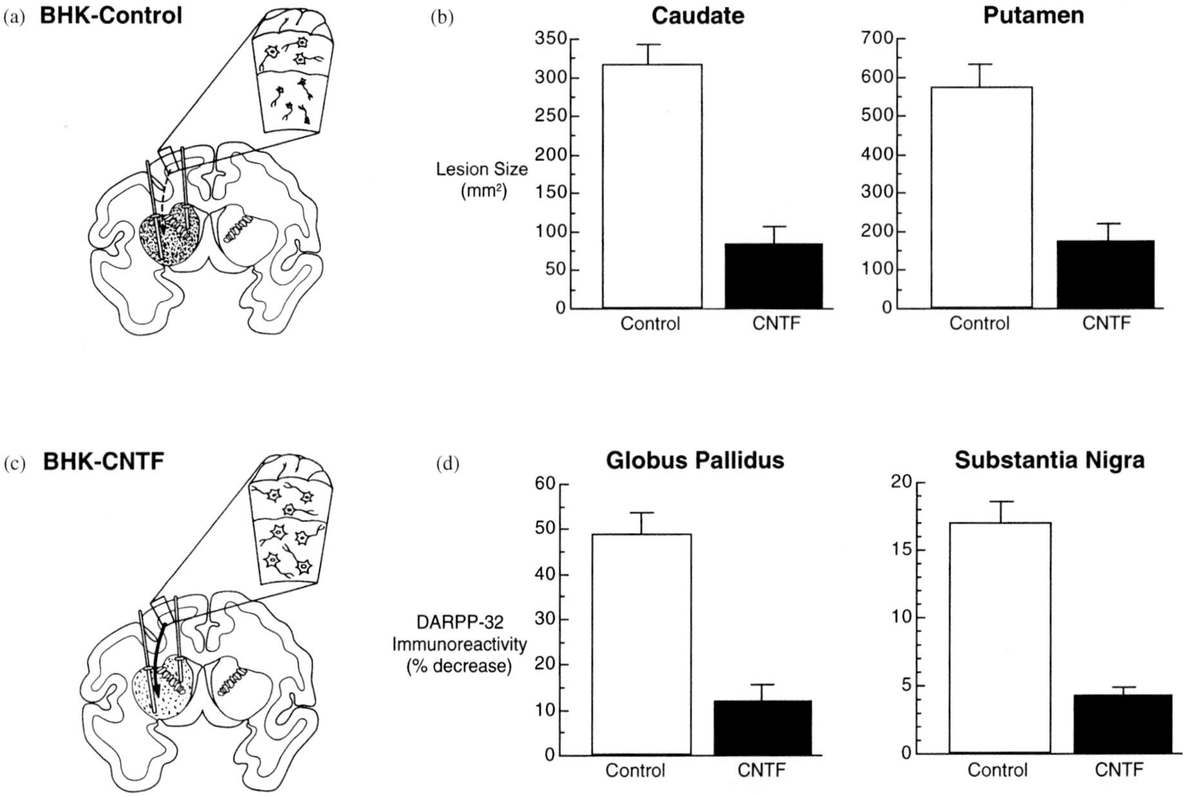

Figure 15 Quantitation of lesion size and DARPP-32 immunoreactivity in quinolinic acid-lesioned monkeys. (a and c) Schematics illustrating placement of capsules in the caudate and putamen of monkeys. CNTF treatment prevented the loss striatal neurons and decreased the volume of striatal damage (b) in both the caudate and putamen. The atrophy of cortical neurons innervating the striatum was also prevented [note dashed line in (a) and solid line in (c)] as is the projection from the striatum to the globus pallidus and the substantia nigra. The percent decrease of DARPP-32 immunoreactivity was significantly attenuated by prior CNTF treatment (d).

are afferents to the striatum, specifically from the cerebral cortex, also influenced by these grafts? This may be particularly important if some of the more devastating nonmotor symptoms seen in HD result from cortical changes secondary to striatal degeneration. Since layer V neurons from motor cortex send a dense projection to the postcommissural putamen, a region severely impacted by the QA lesion, the effects of QA lesions and CNTF implants on the number and size of cortical neurons in this region were examined. Although the QA lesion did not affect the number of neurons in this cortical area, layer V neurons were significantly reduced in cross-sectional area on the side ipsilateral to the lesion in control-grafted monkeys. This atrophy of cortical neurons was virtually completely reversed by CNTF grafts (38) (Fig. 16).

While the sparing of striatal neurons and maintenance of intrinsic circuitry is impressive, the magnitude of the effect is less than that seen in rodents. In primates, robust protection is limited to the area of the capsules. However, the area of the lesion remains extensive, and it is likely that diffusion of CNTF from the capsule may not be sufficient to protect more distant striatal regions undergoing degeneration. This concept is supported by a recent experiment that examined the effects of intraventricular grafts of encapsulated CNTF grafts in the nonhuman primate model of HD (90). In contrast to when the capsules were placed directly within brain parenchyma, intraventricular placements failed to engender neuroprotection for any striatal cell types, again suggesting that diffusion is a key factor in the efficacy of this experimental therapeutic strategy. If human trials are to yield clinically relevant positive effects, the means of CNTF delivery utilized in these studies needs to be improved. Whether this entails grafting more capsules, enhancing the CNTF delivery from the cells by changing the vector system or cell type employed, or changing the characteristics of the polymer membrane remains to be determined.

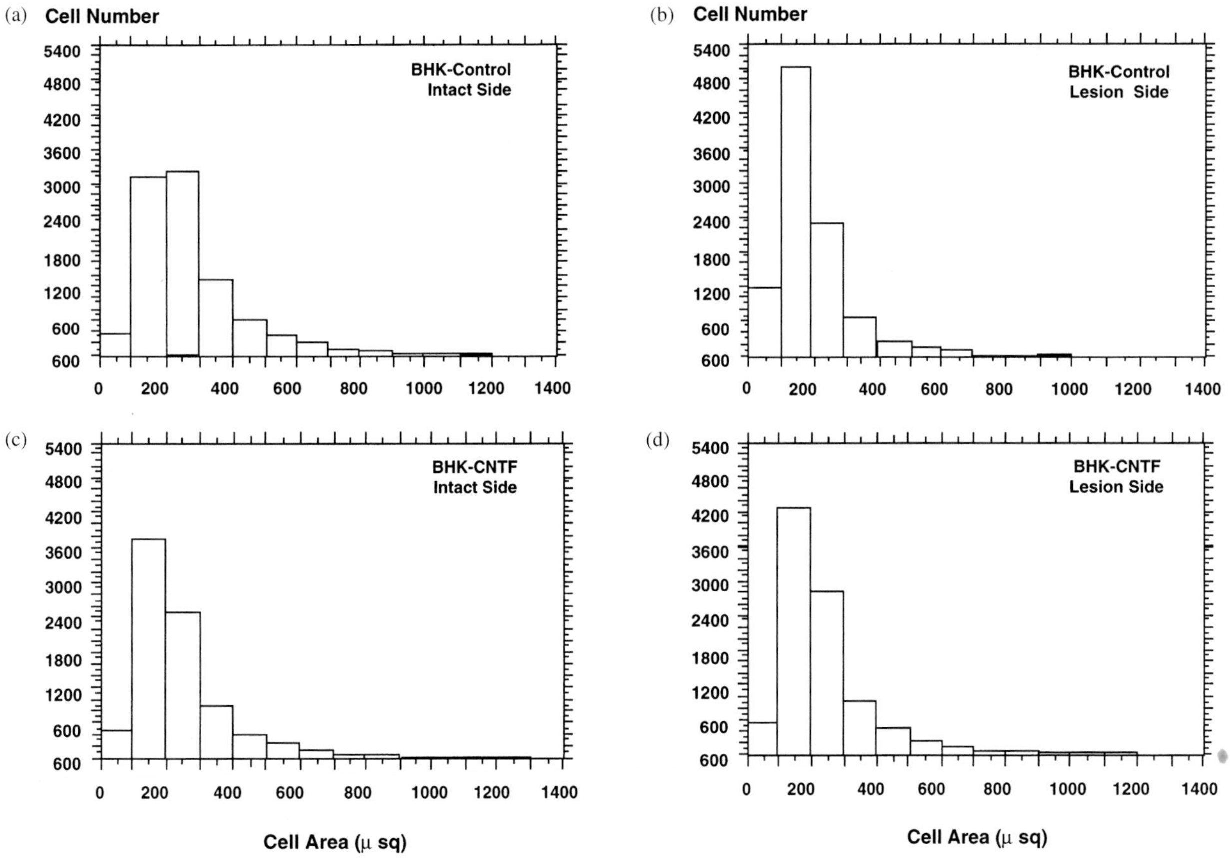

Figure 16 The cell size distribution of layer V neurons in the motor cortex of monkeys that received intrastriatal injections of quinolinic acid followed by implants of encapsulated BHK-control (a and b) or BHK-CNTF (c and d) cells. This figure demonstrates that CNTF-producing grafts prevented the atrophy of cortical neurons that innervate the striatum. Note that in the BHK control animals, there is an increase in the number of neurons in the 0–100 and 100–20 μm range and a decrease in the number of neurons in the 300–400 and 400–500 μm range ipsilateral to the lesion. This shift in cell size was not seen in those animals receiving BHK-CNTF grafts.

IX. AN INITIAL CLINICAL EXPERIENCE WITH ENCAPSULATION-BASED GENE THERAPY

Neuromuscular disorders such as ALS are marked by a progressive degeneration of spinal motor neurons. The challenge for research scientists and clinicians remains to understand the etiology of this fatal disease in order to develop an effective treatment. Different families of neurotrophic factors demonstrate therapeutic potential in vitro and in animal models of motor neuron disease (42,91–98). The cytokine CNTF has neuroprotective effects for motor neurons in wobbler mice (95) and homozygote pmn (progressive motorneuropathy) mice (42,96). The delivery of CNTF to motor neurons by peripheral administration proved difficult due to severe systemic side effects, short half-life of CNTF, and the inability of CNTF to cross the blood-brain barrier (99–101).

Continuous intrathecal delivery of CNTF proximal to the nerve roots in the spinal cord is a practical alternative that could result in fewer side effects and better efficacy of CNTF in ALS patients. After safety, toxicology, and preclinical evaluation, a clinical trial to establish safety has been performed in ALS patients using polymer-encapsulated BHK cells genetically modified to secrete CNTF (20). A total of six ALS patients with early stage disease indicated by a forced vital capacity (FVC) greater than 75% with no other major illness or treated with any investigational drugs for ALS were included. These patients were baseline tested for Tufts Quantitative Neuromuscular Evaluation (TQNE), the Norris scale, blood levels of acute reactive proteins, and CNTF levels in the serum and cerebrospinal fluid (CSF). BHK cells were encapsulated into 5-cm-long by 0.6-mm-diameter hollow membranes and implanted into the lumbar intrathecal space. The device included a silicone tether, which was sutured to the lumbo-

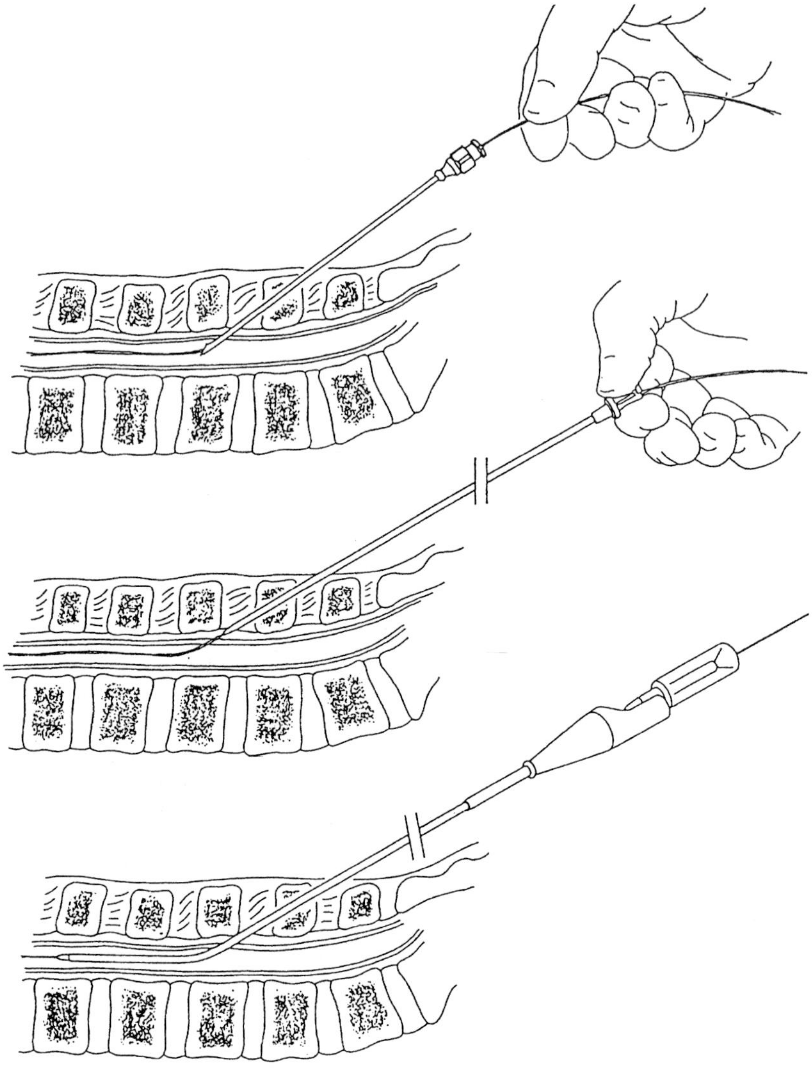

Figure 17 Under local anesthesia, a device containing CNTF-producing cells is implanted into the lumbar subarachnoid space via a small incision over the lumbar spine. A 19 gauge Tuohy needle is inserted into the subarachnoid space. A flexible-tip wire is inserted, the needle withdrawn, and a dilator passed through. A smaller cannula is then inserted over the wire and the cell-containing device is guided through the subarachnoid cannula. The silicone tether is secured to the lumbar fascia and the skin sutured closed over the entire device.

dorsal fascia, and the skin was closed over the device (Fig. 17).

CNTF concentration in the CSF was not detectable prior to implantation but was found in all six patients at 3–4 months postimplantation. All six explanted devices had viable cells and CNTF secretion of approximately 0.2–0.9 μg/day. No CNTF was detected in the serum. To establish a baseline, patients were evaluated monthly for their Norris scores commencing 4 months prior to the trial to establish a baseline. There was no significant improvement in the patients Norris scores during this study, and two of the patients exhibited a mild to dry cough.

X. SUMMARY AND CONCLUSIONS

Considerable evidence indicates that neural transplantation ameliorates the behavioral deficits seen in a number of animal models of neurodegenerative diseases. Recent studies in humans support these preclinical studies and clearly indicate that transplantation of fetal neural tissue shows promise for the treatment of human CNS diseases. Despite its promise in animals and humans, the use of human fetal tissue is complicated by a complex of societal and ethical considerations as well as by the ability to obtain adequate amounts of quality-controlled donor tissue. These considerations have led investigators to search for alternative means of using cell transplantation to deliver therapeutic compounds to the CNS. In this chapter we have described some of our preclinical and initial clinical experience and results with encapsulated cells as one possible means of correcting the behavioral and anatomical consequences of CNS diseases.

There are several promising results of and theoretical advantages to using encapsulated cells/tissue. The permselective membranes of the polymeric capsules allow bidirectional access of nutrients in for maintaining cell viability and biologically active, potentially therapeutic molecules out into the host brain. The membrane also prevents elements of the immune system from destroying the cells, allowing transplantation of cells from adult donors of the same species, or even other species, thereby greatly enhancing the availability of tissue sources for transplantation into patients. Animal studies have demonstrated that encapsulated cells survive, continue to release biologically active molecules, and promote functional recovery following implantation into rodent and primate models of CNS diseases. Polymer-encapsulated cell implants have the advantage of being retrievable should the transplant produce undesired effects or should the cells need to be replaced. Implants may also be designed to allow repeated and minimally invasive removal and replacement of cells over time.

Despite the promise of encapsulated cell implants, a number of concerns surround their use in the treatment of human neurodegenerative diseases. In some cases, the extent of diffusion from the implants appears to limit the therapeutic effectiveness of the encapsulated cells. If so, multiple implants could be needed, thus increasing the risk of significant tissue displacement and/or damage. While the ability to retrieve implants is advantageous, the need to externalize the implant to the skull could pose a route for infection of the host neural tissue. Should a capsule rupture during implantation or retrieval, a deleterious host immunological response could be induced. In fact, recent clinical trials for the treatment of chronic pain revealed a number of device breaks upon removal from the lumbar intrathecal space. Though the host immune system should reject any released cells following capsule damage, the potential for tumorous growth remains a significant concern. Alterations in the ability of the host immune system to reject cells following damage to implants could also change upon long-term residence of the cells within the host. Regulation of dosage may also prove challenging when delivered via encapsulated cells. Varying the numbers of cells within an implant, or even the use of multiple implants, may theoretically accomplish this, but it remains untested and highly speculative.

In conclusion, it appears that the implantation of encapsulated cells may provide an effective means of alleviating the symptoms of numerous human conditions/diseases. One particularly attractive avenue of research continues to be the application of trophic factors to minimize or halt the progression of neural degeneration or promote regeneration of damaged central nerves. However, caution must be applied when considering any novel therapy for treating brain disorders, and the wide-scale use of polymer neural implants should be considered only after rigourous scientific experimentation in animal models and their demonstrated efficacy and safety in human clinical trials.

REFERENCES

1. Bakay RA, Fiandaca MS, Barrow DL, Schiff A, Collins DC. Preliminary report on the use of fetal tissue transplantation to correct MPTP-induced Parkinson-like syndrome in primates. Appl Neurophysiol 1985; 48:358–361.
2. Bakay RA, Barrow DL, Fiandaca MS, Iuvone PM, Schiff A, Collins DC. Biochemical and behavioral correction of MPTP Parkinson-like syndrome by fetal cell transplantation. Ann NY Acad Sci 1987; 495:623–640.
3. Bankiewicz KS, Plunkett RJ, Jacobowitz DM, Porrino L, diPorzio U, London WT, Kopin IJ, Oldfield, EH. The effect of fetal mesencephalon implants on primate MPTP-induced parkinsonism. Histochemical and behavioral studies. J Neurosurg 1990; 72:231–244.
4. Bjorklund A, Dunnett SB, Stenevi U, Lewis ME, Iversen SD. Reinnervation of the denervated striatum by substantia nigra transplants: functional consequences as revealed by pharmacological and sensorimotor testing. Brain Res 1980; 199:307–333.
5. Bjorklund A, Stenevi U, Dunnett SB, Gage FH. Cross-species neural grafting in a rat model of Parkinson's disease. Nature 1982; 298:652–654.
6. Bjorklund A, Stenevi U. Intracerebral neural implants: neuronal replacement and reconstruction of damaged circuitries. Ann Rev Neurosci 1984; 7:279–308.
7. Bjorklund A, Stenevi U. Reformation of the severed septohippocampal cholinergic pathway in the adult rat by transplanted septal neurons. Cell Tiss Res 1977; 185: 289–302.
8. Bjorklund A, Gage FH, Stenevi U, Dunnett SB. Intracerebral grafting of neuronal cell suspensions VI. Survival and growth of intrahippocampal implants of septal cell suspensions. Acta Physiol Scand 1983; (suppl):49–58.
9. Bjorklund A, Gage FH, Schmidt RH, Stenevi U, Dunnett, SB. Intracerebral grafting of neuronal cellsuspensions VII. Recovery of choline acetyltransferase activity and acetylcholine synthesis in the denervated hippocampus reinner-

vated by septal suspension implants. Acta Physiol Scand 1983; (suppl):59–66.
10. Bjorklund A, Campbell K, Sirinathsinghji DJ, Fricker RA, Dunnett SB. Functional capacity of striatal transplants in the rat Huntington model. In: Dunnett SB, Bjorklund A, eds. Functional Neural Transplantation. New York: Raven Press, 1984; 157–195.
11. Brundin P, Strecker RE, Widner H, Clarke DJ, Nilsson OG, Astedt B, Lindvall O, Bjorklund A. Human fetal dopamine neurons grafted in a rat model of Parkinson's disease: immunological aspects, spontaneous and drug-induced behavior, and dopamine release. Exp Brain Res 1988; 70: 192–208.
12. Emerich DF, Black BA, Kesslak JP, Cotman CW, Walsh TJ. Transplantation of fetal cholinergic neurons into the hippocampus attenuates the cognitive and neurochemical deficits induced by AF64A. Brain Res Bull 1992; 28: 219–226.
13. Freed WJ, Morihisa JM, Spoor E, Hoffer BJ, Olson L, Seiger A, Wyatt RJ. Transplanted adrenal chromaffin cells in rat brain reduce lesion-induced rotational behavior. Nature 1981; 292:351–352.
14. Perlow MJ, Freed WJ, Seiger A, Olson L, Wyatt RJ. Brain grafts reduce motor abnormalities produced by destruction of nigrostriatal dopamine system. Science 1979; 204: 643–647.
15. Sanberg PR, Henault MA, Deckel AW. Locomotor hyperactivity: effects of multiple striatal transplants in an animal model of Huntington's disease. Pharmacol Biochem Behav 1986; 25:297–300.
16. Sanberg PR, Calderon SF, Garver DL, Norman AB. Brain tissue transplants in an animal model of Huntington's disease. Psychopharm Bull 1987; 23:476–482.
17. Segal M, Greenberger V, Pearl E. Septal transplants ameliorate spatial deficits and restore cholinergic function in rats with a damaged septo-hippocampal connection. Brain Res 1989; 500:139–148.
18. Aebischer P, Pochon NA-M, Heyd B, Déglon N, Joseph J-M, Zurn AD, Baetge EE, Hammang JP, Goddard M, Lysaght M, Kaplan F, Kato AC, Schleup M, Hirt L, Regli F, Porchet F, De Tribolet N. Gene therapy for amyotrophic lateral sclerosis (ALS) using a polymer encapsulated xenogenic cell line engineered to secrete hCNTF. Hum Gene Ther 1996; 7:851–860.
19. Aebischer P, Tresco PA, Winn SR, Greene LA, Jaeger CB. Long-term cross-species brain transplantation of a polymer encapsulated dopamine-secreting cell line. Exp Neurol 1991; 111:269–275.
20. Aebischer P, Schleup M, Déglon N, Joseph J-M, Hirt L, Heyd B, Goddard M, Hammang JP, Zurn AD, Kato AC, Regli F, Baetge EE. Intrathecal delivery of CNTF using encapsulated genetically modified xenogeneic cells in amyotrophic lateral sclerosis patients. Nature Med 1996; 2:696–699.
21. Breakefield XO. Combining CNS transplantation and gene transfer. Neurobiol Aging 1989; 10:647–648.
22. Kordower JH, Chen E-Y, Mufson EJ, Winn SR, Emerich DF. Intrastriatal implants of polymer-encapsulated cells genetically modified to secrete human nerve growth factor: trophic effects upon cholinergic and noncholinergic neurons. Neuroscience 1996; 72:63–77.
23. Frim DM, Schumacher JM, Short MP, Breakefield XO, Isacson O. Local response to intracerebral grafts of NGF-secreting fibroblasts:Induction of a peroxidative enzyme. Neurosci Abstr 1992; 18:1100.
24. Kawaja MD, Rosenberg MB, Yoshida K, Gage FH. Somatic gene transfer of nerve growth factor promotes the survival of axotomized septal neurons and the regeneration of their axons in adult rats. J Neurosci 1992; 12: 2849–2864.
25. Maysinger D, Piccardo P, Goiny M, Cuello AC. Grafting of genetically modified cells: effects of acetylcholine release in vivo. Neurochem Int 1992; 21:543–548.
26. Rowland LP, Fink ME, Rubin L. Cerebrospinal fluid: blood brain barrier, brain edema, and hydrocephalus. In: Kandel ER, Schwartz JH, Jessell TM, eds. Principles of Neural Science. Norwalk, CT: Appleton and Lange, 1991: 1050–1060.
27. Aebischer P, Wahlberg L, Tresco PA, Winn SR. Macroencapsulation of dopamine-secreting cells by coextrusion with an organic polymer solution. Biomaterials 1991; 12: 50–56.
28. Aebischer P, Goddard M, Signore P, Timpson R. Functional recovery in hemiparkinsonian primates transplanted with polymer encapsulated PC12 cells, Exp Neurol 1994; 126:1–12.
29. Kordower JH, Liu Y-T, Winn SR, Emerich DF. Encapsulated PC12 cell transplants into hemiparkinsonian monkeys: a behavioral, neuroanatomical and neurochemical analysis. Cell Transplant 1995; 4:155–171.
30. Tresco PA, Winn SR, Jaeger CB, Greene LA, Aebischer P. Polymer-encapsulated PC12 cells: longterm survival and associated reduction in lesioned-induced rotational behavior. Cell Trans 1992; 1:255–264.
31. Winn SR, Zielinski B, Tresco PA, Signore AP, Jaeger CB, Greene LA, Aebischer P. Behavioral recovery following intrastriatal implantation of microencapsulated PC12 cells. Exp Neurol 191; 113:322–329.
32. Winn SR, Wahlberg L, Tresco PA, Aebischer P. An encapsulated dopamine-releasing polymer alleviates experimental parkinsonism in rats. Exp Neurol 1989; 105:244–250.
33. Emerich DF, Frydel B, McDermott P, Krueger P, Lavoie M, Sanberg PR, Winn SR. Polymer-encapsulated PC12 cells promote recovery of motor function in aged rats. Exp Neurol 1993; 122:37–47.
34. Subramanian T, Emerich DF, Bakay RAE, Hoffman JM, Goodman MM, Shoup TM, Miller GW, Levey AI, Hubert GW, Batchelor S, Winn SR, Saydoff JA, Watts RL. Polymer-encapsulated PC12 cells demonstrate high affinity uptake of dopamine in vitro and 18F-dopa uptake and metabolism after intracerebral implantation in nonhuman primates. Cell Transpl 1997; 6:469–477.

35. Lindner MD; Emerich, DF Therapeutic potential of a polymer-encapsulated L-DOPA and dopamine-producing cell line in rodent and primate models of Parkinson's disease. Cell Transplant. 1998; 7:165–174.
36. Emerich DF, Hammang JP, Baetge EE, Winn SR. Implantation of polymer-encapsulated human nerve growth factor-secreting fibroblasts attenuates the behavioral and neuropathological consequences of quinolinic acid injections into rodent striatum. Exp Neurol 1994; 130:141–150.
37. Emerich DF, Lindner MD, Winn SR, Chen E-Y, Frydel BR, Kordower JH. Implants of encapsulated human CNTF-producing fibroblasts prevent behavioral deficits and striatal degeneration in a rodent model of Huntington's disease. J Neurosci 1996; 16:5168–5181.
38. Emerich DF, Winn SR, Hantraye PM, Peschanski M, Chen E-Y, Chu Y, McDermott P, Baetge EE, Kordower JH. Protective effects of encapsulated cells producing neurotrophic factor CNTF in a monkey model of Huntington's disease. Nature 1997, 386:395–399.
39. Emerich DF, Bruhn S, Chu Y, Kordower JH. Cellular delivery of CNTF but not NT4/5 prevents degeneration of striatal neurons in a rodent model of Huntington's disease. Cell Transpl 1998, 7:213–225.
40. Emerich DF, Winn SR, Harper J, Hammang JP, Baetge EE, Kordower JH. Implants of polymer-encapsulated human NGF-secreting cells in the nonhuman primate:rescue and sprouting of degenerating cholinergic basal forebrain neurons. J Comp Neurol 1994; 349:148–164.
41. Kordower JH, Winn SR, Liu Y-T, Mufson EJ, Sladek JR Jr., Baetge EE, Hammang JP, Emerich DF. The aged monkey basal forebrain:rescue and sprouting of axotomized basal forebrain neurons after grafts of encapsulated cells secreting human nerve growth factor. Proc Natl Acad Sci 1994; 91:10898–10902.
42. Sagot Y, Tan SA, Baetge EE, Schmalbruch H, Kato AC, Aebischer P. Polymer encapsulated cell lines genetically engineered to release ciliary neurotrophic factor can slow down progressive motor neuronopathy in the mouse. Eur J Neurosci 1995; 7:1313–1320.
43. Dunn JCY, Tompkins RG, Yarmush ML. Long-term in vitro function of adult hepatocytes in a collagen sandwich configuration. Biotechnol Prog 1991; 7:237–245.
44. Mooney DJ, Hansen L, Vacanti JP, Langer R, Farmer S, Ingber D. Switching from differentiation to growth in hepatocytes - control by extracellular-matrix. J Cell Physiol 1992; 151:497–505.
45. Rotem A, Toner M, Tompkins RG, Yarmush ML. Oxygen-uptake rates in cultured hepatocytes. Biotechnol Bioeng 1992; 40:1286–1291.
46. Uyama S, Kaufmann PM, Takeda T, Vacanti JP. Delivery of whole liver equivalent hepatocyte mass using polymer devices and hepatotrophic stimulation. Transplantation 1995; 55:932–935.
47. Emerich DF, Frydel B, Flanagan TR, Palmatier M, Winn SR, Christenson L. Transplantation of polymer encapsulated PC12 cells: use of chitosan as an immobilization matrix. Cell Trans 1993; 2:241–249.
48. Lacy PE, Hegre OH, Gerasimidi-Vazeou A, Gentile FT, Dionne KE. Maintenance of normoglycemia in diabetic mice by subcutaneous xenografts of encapsulated islets. Science 1991; 254:1782–1784.
49. Emerich DF, Winn SR, Lindner MD. Alleviation of behavioral deficits in aged rodents following implantation of encapsulated GDNF-producing fibroblasts. Brain Res 1996; 736:99–110.
50. Strathmann H. Production of microporous media by phase inversion processes. In: Lloyd DR, ed. Material Science of Synthetic Membranes. Washington, DC: American Chemical Society, 1985:165–196.
51. Brauker JH, Carrbrendel VE, Martinson LA, Crudele J, Johnston WD, Johnson WC. Neovascularization of synthetic membranes directed by membrane microarchitecture. J Biomed Mater Res 1995; 29:1517–1524.
52. Martinson L, Pauley R, Boggs D, Brauker JH, Sternberg SM, Johnson RC. Protection of xenografts with immunoisolation membranes. Cell Transpl 1993; 3:249.
53. Langer R, Vacanti JP. Tissue Engineering. Science 1993; 260:920–925.
54. Christenson L, Dionne KE, Lysaght MJ. Biomedical applications of immobilized cells. In: Goosen MFA, ed. Fundamentals of Animal Cell Encapsulation and Immobilization. Boca Raton, FL: CRC Press, 1993:7–41.
55. Lysaght MJ, Baurmeister U. Dialysis. In: Kirk-Othmer Encyclopedia of Chemical Technology. 4th ed. New York: John Wiley & Sons, 1993:59–74.
56. Korsching S, Auberger G, Heuman R, Scott J, Thoenen H. Levels of nerve growth factor and its mRNA in the central nervous system of the rat correlate with cholinergic innervation. EMBO J 1985; 4:1389–1393.
57. Sheldon DL, Reichardt LF. Studies on the expression of beta NGF gene in the central nervous system: level and regional distribution of NGF mRNA suggest that NGF functions as a trophic factor for several neuronal populations. Proc Natl Acad Sci USA 1986; 83:2714–2718.
58. Schwab ME, Otten U, Agid Y, Thoenen H. Nerve growth factor (NGF) in the rat CNS: absence of specific retrograde transport and tyrosine hydroxylase induction in locus coeruleus and substantia nigra. Brain Res 1979; 168:473–483.
59. Seiler M, Schwab ME. Specific retrograde transport of nerve growth factor (NGF) from cortex to nucleus basalis in the rat. Brain Res 1984; 300:33–39.
60. Hefti F, Hartikka J, Salviaterra P, Weiner WJ, Mash DC. Localization of nerve growth factor receptors on cholinergic neurons of the human basal forebrain. Neurosci Lett 1986; 69:275–281.
61. Kordower JH, Bartus RT, Bothwell M, Schatteman G, Gash DM. Nerve growth factor receptor immunoreactivity in the nonhuman primate (Cebus apella): Distribution, morphology, and colocalization with cholinergic enzymes. J Comp Neurol 1988; 277:465–486.
62. Kordower JH, Gash DM, Bothwell M, Hersh L, Mufson EJ. Nerve growth factor receptor and choline acetyltransferase remain colocalized in the nucleus basalis (Ch4) of Alzheimer's patients. Neurobiol Aging 1989; 10:287–294.

63. Batchelor PE, Armstrong DM, Blaker SN, Gage FH. Nerve growth factor receptor and choline acetyltransferase colocalization in neurons within the rat forebrain: response to fimbria-fornix transection. J Comp Neurol 1989; 284: 187–204.
64. Koh S, Oyler GA, Higgins GA. Localization of nerve growth factor receptor messenger RNA and protein in the adult rat brain. Exp Neurol 1989; 106:209–221.
65. Mufson EJ, Bothwell M, Hersh LB, Kordower JH. Nerve growth factor receptor immunoreactive profiles in the normal aged human basal forebrain: colocalization with cholinergic neurons. J Comp Neurol 1989; 285:196–217.
66. Steininger TL, Wainer BH, Klein, Barbacid M, Palfrey HC. High affinity nerve growth factor receptor (trk) immunoreactivity is localized in cholinergic neurons of the basal forebrain and striatum in the adult rat. Brain Res 1993; 612:330–335.
67. Hefti F. Nerve growth factor promotes survival of septal cholinergic neurons after fimbrial transections. J Neurosci 1986; 2155–2162.
68. Koliatsos VE, Clatterbuck RE, Nauta HJW, Knusel B, Burton LE, Hefti F, Mobley WC, Price DL. Human nerve growth factor prevents degeneration of basal forebrain cholinergic neurons in primates. Ann Neurol 1991; 30: 831–840.
69. Breakefield XO. Combining CNS transplantation and gene transfer. Neurobiol Aging 1989; 10:647–648.
70. Koliatsos VE, Applegate MD, Knusel B, Junard EO, Burton LE, Mobley WC, Hefti F, Price DL. Recombinant human nerve growth factor prevents retrograde degeneration of axotomized basal forebrain cholinergic neurons in the rat. Exp Neurol 1991; 112:161–173.
71. Montero CN, Hefti F. Rescue of lesioned septal cholinergic neurons by nerve growth factor: specificity and requirement for chronic treatment. J Neurosci 1988; 8: 2986–2999.
72. Tuszynski MH, U HS, Amaral DG, Gage FH. Nerve growth factor infusion in the primate brain reduces lesion-induced cholinergic neuronal degeneration. J Neurosci 1990; 10:3604–3614.
73. Tuszynski MH, U HS, Yoshida K, Gage FH. Recombinant human nerve factor infusions prevent cholinergic neuronal degeneration in the adult primate brain. Ann Neurol 1991; 30:625–636.
74. Fischer W, Wictorin K, Bjorklund A, Williams LR, Varon S, Gage FH. Amelioration of cholinergic neuron atrophy and spatial memory impairment in aged rats by nerve growth factor. Nature 1987; 329:65–67.
75. Olson L, Nordberg A, von Holst H, Backman L, Ebendal T, Alafuzoff I, Amberla K, Hartvig P, Herlitz A, Lilja A, Lundqvist H, Langstrom B, Meyerson B, Persson A, Vlitanen M, Winblad B, Seiger A. Nerve growth factor affects 11C-nicotine binding, blood flow, EEG, and verbal episodic memory in an Alzheimer patient (case report). J Neuronal Transmission (P-D. Sect.) 1992; 4:79–495.
76. Winn SR, Hammang JP, Emerich DF, Lee, A, Palmiter RD, Baetge EE. Polymer-encapsulated cells genetically modified to secrete human nerve growth factor promote the survival of axotomized septal cholinergic neurons. Proc Natl Acad Sci USA 1994; 91:2324–2328.
77. Lindner MD, Kearns CE, Winn SR, Frydel BR, Emerich DF. Effects of intraventricular encapsulated hNGF-secreting fibroblasts in aged rats. Cell Transp 1996; 5:205–223.
78. Winn SR, Lindner MD, Haggett G, Francis JM, Emerich DF. Polymer-encapsulated genetically-modified cells continue to secrete human nerve growth factor for over one year in rat ventricles behavioral and anatomical consequences. Exp Neurol 1996; 140:126–138.
79. Emerich DF, Sanberg PR. Animal Models in Huntington's disease. In: Boulton AA, Baker GB, Butterworth RF, eds. Neuromethods. Vol. 17. Animal Models of Neurological Disease. Totowa, NJ: Humana Press, 1992:65–134.
80. Beal MF, Kowall NW, Ellison DW, Mazurek MF, Swartz KJ, Martin JB. Replication of the neurochemical characteristics Huntington's disease by quinolinic acid. Nature 1986; 321:168–171.
81. Beal MF, Mazurek MF, Ellison DW, Swartz KJ, McGarvey U, Bird ED, Martin JB. Somatostatin and neuropeptide Y concentrations in pathologically graded cases of Huntington's disease. Ann Neurol 1988; 23:562–569.
82. Beal MF, Kowall NW, Swartz KJ, Ferranti RJ, Martin JB. Differential sparing of somatostatin-neuropeptide Y and cholinergic neurons following striatal excitotoxin lesions. Synapse 1989; 3:38–47.
83. Emerich DF, Zubricki EM, Shipley MT, Norman AB, Sanberg PR. Female rats are more sensitive to the locomotor alterations following quinolinic acid-induced striatal lesions: effects of striatal transplants. Exp Neurol 1991; 111:369–378.
84. Sanberg PR, Calderon SF, Giordano M, Tew JM, Norman AB. The quinolinic acid model of Huntington's disease: locomotor abnormalities. Exp Neurol 1989; 105:45–53.
85. Block F, Kunkel M, Schwarz M. Quinolinic acid lesion of the striatum induces impairment in spatial learning and motor performance in rats. Neurosci Lett 1993; 149: 126–128.
86. Frim DM, Uhler TA, Short MP, Exedine ZD, Klagsbrun M, Breakefield XO, Isacson O. Effects of biologically delivered NGF, BDNF, and bFGF on striatal excitotoxic lesions. Neuroreport 1993; 4:367–370.
87. Frim DM, Simpson J, Uhler TA, Short MP, Bossi SR, Breakefield XO, Isacson O. Striatal degeneration induced by mitochondrial blockade is prevented by biologically delivered NGF. J Neurosci Res 1993; 35:452–458.
88. Schumacher JM, Shor MP, Hyman BT, Breakefield XO, Isacson O. Intracerebral implantation of nerve growth factor-producing fibroblasts protects striatum against neurotoxic levels of excitatory amino acids. Neuroscience 1991; 45:561–70.
89. Emerich DF, Cain CK, Greco C, Saydoff JA, Hu ZY, Liu H, Lindner MD. Cellular delivery of human CNTF prevents motor and cognitive dysfunction in a rodent model of Huntington's disease. Cell Transplant 1997; 6:249–266.

90. Kordower JH, Chen E-Y, Chu Y-P, McDermott P, Baetge EE, Emerich DF. Intrastriatal but not intraventricular grafts of encapsulated CNTF-producing cells protects against striatal degeneration in a nonhuman primate model of Huntington's disease. Society for Neuroscience Abstracts, New Orleans, 1997.
91. Henderson CE. GDNF: a potent survival factor of motoneurons present in peripheral nerve and muscle. Science 1994; 266:1062–1064.
92. Hughes RA, Sendtner M, Thoenen H. Members of several gene families influence survival of rat motoneurons in vitro and in vivo. J Neurosci Res 1993; 36:663–671.
93. Kato AC, Lindsay RM. Overlapping and additive effects of neurotrophins and CNTF on cultured human spinal cord neurons. Exp Neurol 1994; 130:196–201.
94. Lewis ME, Neff NT, Contreras PC, Stong DB, Oppenheim RW, Grebow PE, Vaught JL. Insulin-like growth factor-I: potential for treatment of motor neuronal disorders. Exp Neurol 1993; 124:73–88.
95. Mitsumoto H, Ikeda K, Klinkosz B, Cedarbaum JM, Wong V, Lindsay RM. Arrest of motor neuron disease in wobbler mice cotreated with CNTF and BDNF. Science 1994; 265: 1107–1110.
96. Sendtner M, Schmalbruch H, Stöckli KA, Carroll P, Kreutzberg GW, Thoenen H. Ciliary neurotrophic factor prevents degeneration of motor neurons in mouse mutant progressive motor neuronopathy. Nature 1992; 358:502–504.
97. Sendtner M, Holtmann B, Kolbeck R, Thoenen H, Barde YA. Brain-derived neurotrophic factor prevents the death of motor neurons in newborn rats after nerve section. Nature 1992; 360:757–759.
98. Wong V, Arriaga R, Ip NY, Lindsay RM. The neurotrophins BDNF, NT-3 and NT-4/5, but not NGF, up-regulate the cholinergic phenotype of developing motor neurons. Eur J Neurosci 1993; 5:466–474.
99. The ALS CNTF Treatment Study (ACTS) Phase I-II Study Group. The pharmacokinetics of subcutaneously administered recombinant human ciliary neurotrophic factor (rhCNTF) in patients with amytrophic lateral sclerosis: relationship to parameters of the acute phase response. Clin Neuropharmacol 1995; 18:500–514.
100. The ALS CNTF Treatment Study (ACTS) Phase I-II Study Group. A phase I study of recombinant human ciliary neurotrophic factor (rHCNTF) in patients with amyotrophic lateral sclerosis. Clin Neuropharmacol 1995; 18:515–532.
101. Dittrich F, Thoenen H, Sendtner M. Ciliary neurotrophic factor: pharmacokinetics and acute-phase response in rat. Ann Neurol 1994; 35:151–163.

11

Molecular Interactions in Lipids, DNA, and DNA-Lipid Complexes

Rudolf Podgornik
University of Ljubljana, Ljubljana, Slovenia, and National Institute of Child Health and Human Development, National Institutes of Health, Bethesda, Maryland

Helmut H. Strey
University of Massachusetts, Amherst, Massachussetts

V. A. Parsegian
National Institute of Child Health and Human Development, National Institutes of Health, Bethesda, Maryland

I. INTRODUCTION

Designed by nature for information, valued by molecular biologists for manipulation, DNA is also a favorite of physical chemists and physicists (1). Its mechanical properties (2), its interactions with other molecules (3), and its modes of packing (4) present tractable but challenging problems, whose answers have in vivo and in vitro consequences. In the context of DNA transfection and gene therapy (5), what has been learned about molecular mechanics, interaction, and packing might teach us how to package DNA for more effective gene transfer. Among these modes of in vitro packaging are association with proteins, treatment with natural or synthetic cationic ''condensing agents,'' and combination with synthetic positively charged lipids (6).

In vivo, DNA is tightly held, not at all like the dilute solution form often studied in vitro (Fig. 1). This tight assembly necessarily incurs huge energetic costs of confinement, costs that create a tension under which DNA is expected to ravel or to unravel its message. Through direct measurement of forces between DNA molecules (7) and direct observation of its modes of packing (8), we might see not only how to use concomitant energies to design better DNA-transfer systems but also to reason better about the sequences of events by which DNA is read in cells.

What binds these structures? To first approximation, for large, flexible biological macromolecules, the relevant interactions resemble those found in among colloidal particles (9), where the size of the molecule (such as DNA molecules, lipid membranes, actin bundles) distinguishes it from simpler, smaller species (such as small solutes or salt ions). On the colloidal scale of tens of nm (10^{-9} m) only the interactions between macromolecules are evaluated explicitly, while the small molecular species only ''dress'' the large molecules and drive the interactions between them.

The electrical charge patterns of multivalent ions such as Mn^{+2}, Co^{3+}, or spermine^{+4}, cation binding to negative DNA, create attractive electrostatic and/or solvation forces that move DNA double helices to finite separations despite the steric knock of DNA thermal motion (10). Solvation patterns about the cation-dressed structures create solvation forces e.g., DNA-DNA repulsion because of water clinging to the surface and attraction from the release of solvent (11). Positively charged histones will spool DNA into carefully distributed skeins, themselves arrayed for systematic unraveling and reading (12). Viral capsids will encase DNA, stuffed against its own DNA-DNA electrostatic and solvation repulsion, to keep it under pressure for release upon infection (13). In artificial preparations the

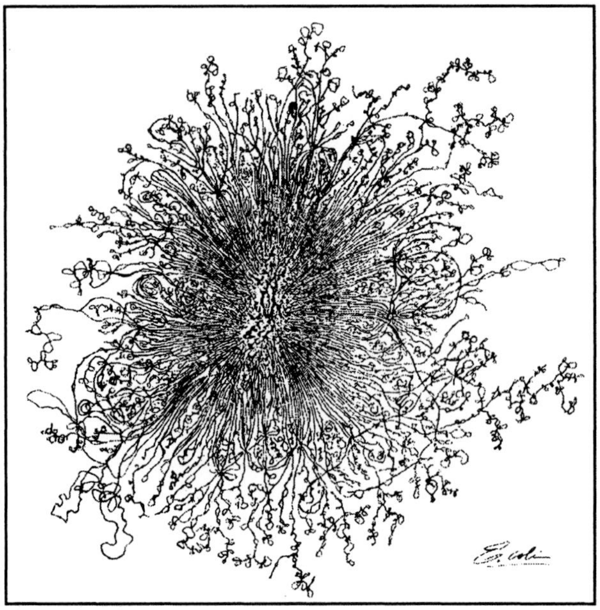

Escherichia coli DNA after osmotic shock

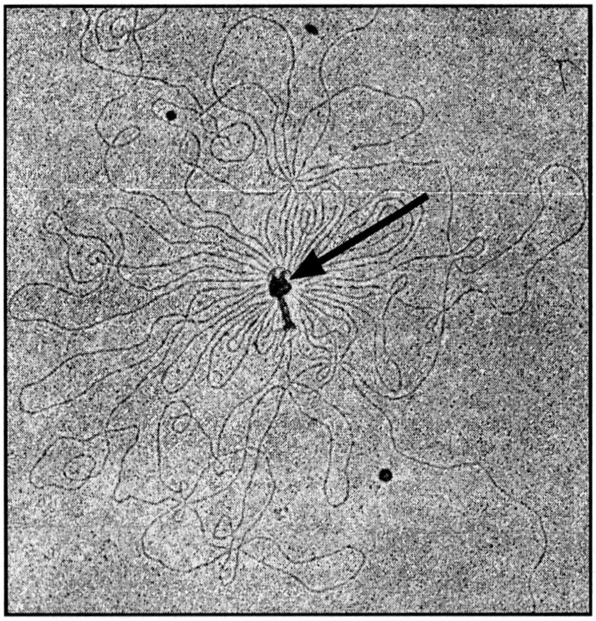

Bacteriophage T2 DNA after osmotic shock

Figure 1 In vivo DNA is highly compacted. The figure shows *Escherichia coli* DNA and T2 bacteriophage DNA after an osmotic shock that has allowed them to expand from their in vivo configurations. (*E. coli* picture courtesy of Ruth Kavenoff, Designergenes Inc., Los Angeles, CA. T2 picture from Ref. 108. Courtesy of Elsevier Publishing Company, Oxford, England.)

glue of positively charged and neutral lipids can lump negative DNA into ordered structures that can move through lipids and through water solutions (14).

Changes in the suspending medium can modulate intermolecular forces. One example is the change in van der Waals charge fluctuation forces (see below) between lipid bilayers when small sugars modifying the dielectric dispersion properties of water are added to the solution (15). More dramatic, the addition of salt to water can substantially reduce electrostatic interactions between charged molecules such as DNA or other charged macromolecules bathed by an aqueous solution (16). These changes can modify the behavior of macromolecules quantitatively or induce qualitatively new features into their repertoire, among these most notably precipitation of DNA by addition of organic polycations to the solution (10).

Similar observations can be made about a small molecule essential to practically every aspect of interaction between macromolecules. Through the dielectric constant it enters electrostatic interactions, through pH it enters charging equilibria, and through its fundamental molecular geometry it enters the hydrogen bond network topology around simple solutes. This is, of course, the water molecule (17). In what follows we will limit ourselves to only three basic properties of macromolecules—charge, polarity (solubility), and conformational flexibility—that appear to govern the plethora of forces encountered in biology. It is no surprise that the highly ordered biological structures, such as the quasi-crystalline spooling of DNA in viral heads or the multilamellar stacking of lipid membranes in visual receptor cells, can in fact be explained through the properties of a very small number of fundamental forces acting between macromolecules (Fig. 2). Detailed experimental as well as theoretical investigations have identified hydration, electrostatic, van der Waals or dispersion, and conformational fluctuation forces as the most fundamental interactions governing the fate of biological macromolecules. Our intent here is to sketch the measurements of these operative forces and to dwell on concepts that rationalize them. It is from these concepts, with their insight into what controls organizing forces, that we expect people to learn to manipulate and to package DNA in more rewarding ways.

II. MOLECULAR FORCES

A. The Origin of Molecular Forces

We divide these forces into two broad categories. First, there are interactions that are connected with fields emanating from sources within or on the macromolecules them-

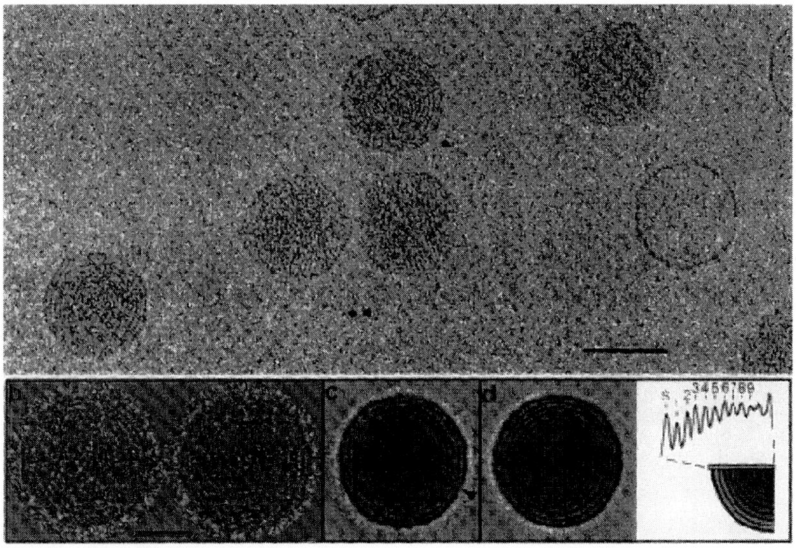

Cryo-micrographs and computer-processed images of T7 heads.
Bar = 50 nm.

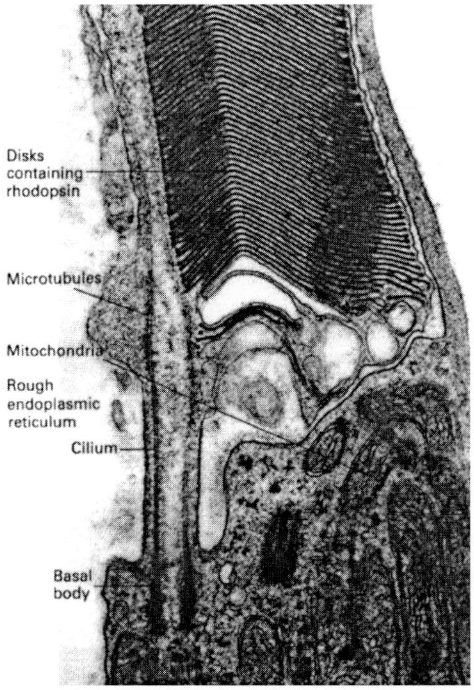

Electron micrograph of a part of human rod cell.

Figure 2 Highly ordered assemblies, ubiquitous among biological structures, can be explained through the properties of a very small number of fundamental forces acting between macromolecules. Cryomicrographs and computer-processed images of T7 phage heads showing ordered DNA spooling within the heads (from Ref. 13). Electron micrograph of a part of a human eye rod cell. (From Ref. 109. Courtesy of Cell Press, Cambridge, MA and Harcourt Brace & Co., Orlando, FL.)

selves (16). Among these are the electrostatic fields pointing from the fixed charge distributions on macromolecules into the surrounding space; there are also the fields of connectivity of hydrogen bond networks extending from the macromolecular surfaces into the bulk solution that are seen in hydration interactions. Second are the forces due to fluctuations that originate either in thermal Brownian motion or microscopic quantum jitter (15). These interactions include the van der Waals or dispersion forces that originate from thermal as well as quantum mechanical fluctuations of electromagnetic fields in the space between and within the interacting molecules, conformation-fluctuation forces from thermal gyrations by the macromolecule when thermal agitation pushes against the elastic energy resistance of the molecule, and confinement imposed by neighboring macromolecules (16). Attraction as well as repulsion can result from either category.

B. Hydration Force

The hydration force is connected with a very simple observation that it takes increasing amounts of work to remove water from between electrically neutral lipids in multilamellar arrays or from between ordered arrays of polymers at large polymer concentrations (18). Direct measurements of this work strongly suggest that it increases exponentially with the diminishing separation between colloid surfaces, with a certain decay length that depends as much on the bulk properties of the solvent as on the detailed characteristics of the interacting surfaces.

Hydration forces can be understood in different terms with no consensus yet on mechanism (11). Marčelja and coworkers (19) first proposed the idea that colloid surfaces perturb the vicinal water and that the exponential decay of the hydration force is due to the weakening of the perturbation of the solvent as a function of the distance between the interacting surfaces. They introduced an order parameter, P, as a function of the spatial coordinates between the surfaces, P(r), that would capture the local condition or local ordering of solvent molecules between the surfaces. The detailed physical nature of this order parameter is left unspecified, but since the theory builds on general principles of symmetry and perturbation expansions, molecular details are not needed. All one needs to know about P is that within the bulk water P = 0 and close to a macromolecular surface P remains nonzero. As a mnemonic device, one can envision P as an arrow associated with each water molecule. In the bulk the arrows point in all directions with equal probability. Close to a bounding macromolecular surface, they point preferentially towards or away from the surface (Fig. 3).

If we envisage solvent molecules between two perturbing surfaces we can decompose the total free energy into its energy and entropy parts. Energetically it would be most favorable for the surface-induced order to persist away from the surfaces, but that would create conflict between the apposing surfaces (see Fig. 3). Entropy fights any type of ordering and wants to eliminate all orderly configurations between the two surfaces, creating a homogeneous state of molecular disorder characterized by P = 0. Energy and entropy compromise to create a nonuniform profile of the order parameter between the surfaces; surface-induced order propagates but progressively decreases away from the surfaces.

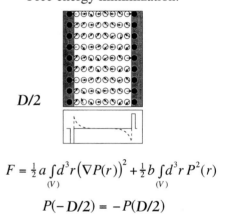

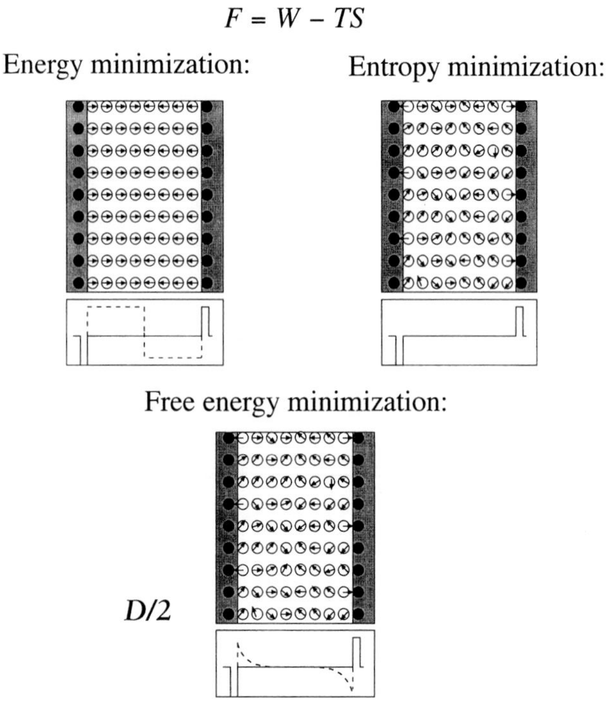

$$F = \tfrac{1}{2} a \int_{(V)} d^3r \left(\nabla P(r)\right)^2 + \tfrac{1}{2} b \int_{(V)} d^3r\, P^2(r)$$

$$P(-D/2) = -P(D/2)$$

Figure 3 The theory of hydration force. Marčelja and Radić (19) introduced an order parameter P that would capture the local condition, or local ordering, of solvent molecules between the surfaces. We represent it as a vector on each water molecule that is trapped between the two opposing surfaces. The detailed physical nature of this order parameter is left unspecified, but because the theory builds on general principles of symmetry and perturbation expansion, molecular details are not needed. Energy minimization leads to ordering of P at the two surfaces, whereas entropy favors completely disordered configurations. Free energy minimization leads to a nonmonotonic order parameter profile. For formalism, see main text.

Formalizing this qualitative discussion, we can decompose the total free energy due to the order parameter variations as

$$F = \frac{1}{2}a \int_{(v)} dV\, (\nabla P)^2 + \frac{1}{2}b \int_{(v)} dV\, P^2$$

where the first term stems from the entropic cost to create inhomogeneous order parameter distributions, div $P(r) \neq 0$, while the second one originates in the energy, preferring configurations with no net order parameter, i.e., $P(r) = 0$.

Minimizing this free energy *ansatz* with respect to all order parameter profiles and taking into account that for two equal surfaces their order parameters should describe ordering that points in opposite directions, one has to assume first of all that the vectorial order parameter has only one component that depends only on the transverse coordinate, $P(r) = P(z)$, as well as that $P(z = D/2) = -P(z = -D/2)$. Clearly the total separation between the surface is D. Solving now this mathematically well-defined problem, we end up with the following form of the free energy

$$F(D) = \frac{1}{2}\frac{P(D/2)^2}{a} \sinh^{-2}(D/2\lambda_H)$$

which decays approximately exponentially with D, with a decay length of $\lambda_H = (a/b)$. Measured decay lengths are usually within the range of 0.5–3 Å. Osmotic pressure between two apposed lipid surfaces has been measured extensively for different lipids (20). From these experiments one can deduce the ratio of P^2 (D/2) to (a λ_H), which for a great variety of lipids and lipid mixtures can be found within an interval of 10^{12}–10^{10} dynes/cm^2. From this simple theory, the hydration force should decay with a universal decay length, depending only on the bulk properties of the solvent, i.e., the constants a and b.

In order to generalize this simplification, Kornyshev and Leikin (21) formulated a variant of the hydration force theory to take into account explicitly also the nature of surface ordering. They derive a modified decay length that clearly shows how the surface order couples with the hydration force decay length. Without going too deeply into this theory, we note that if the interacting surfaces have two-dimensional ordering patterns characterized by a wave vector $Q = 2\pi/\lambda$, where λ is their characteristic scale, then the hydration force decay length should be

$$\lambda_{KL} = \frac{1}{2\sqrt{Q^2 + \lambda_H^{-2}}}$$

Given the experimentally determined variety of forces between phospholipids (20), it is indeed quite possible that even in the simplest cases the measured decay distances are not those of the water solvent itself.

The other important facet of this theory is that it predicts that in certain circumstances the hydration forces can become attractive (11). This is particularly important in the case of interacting DNA molecules, where this hydration attraction connected with condensing agents can hold DNAs into an ordered array even though the van der Waals forces themselves would be unable to accomplish that (22). This attraction is always an outcome of nonhomogeneous surface ordering and arises in situations where apposing surfaces have complementary checkerboard-like order (11). Unfortunately, in this situation many mechanisms can contribute to attractions; it is difficult to argue for one strongest contribution.

C. Electrostatic Forces

Electrostatic forces between charged colloid bodies are among the key components of the force equilibria in (bio)-colloid systems (23). At larger separations they are the only forces that can counteract van der Waals attractions and thus stabilize colloid assembly. The crucial role of the electrostatic interactions in (bio)colloid systems is well documented and explored following the seminal realization of Bernal and Fankuchen (24) that electrostatic interaction is the stabilizing force in TMV arrays.

Although the salient features of electrostatic interactions of fixed charges in a sea of mobile countercharges and salt ions are intuitively straightforward to understand, they are difficult to evaluate. These difficulties are clearly displayed by the early ambiguities in the sign of electrostatic interactions between two equally charged bodies that was first claimed to be attractive (Levine), then repulsive (Verwey-Overbeek), and finally realized to be usually repulsive except if the counterions or the salt ions are of higher valency (25).

Here we introduce the electrostatic interaction on an intuitive footing (Fig. 4). Assume we have two equally charged bodies with counterions in between. Clearly the minimum of electrostatic energy W (28) for the electrostatic field configuration E(r) is as follows (in MKS units):

$$W = \frac{1}{2}\epsilon\epsilon_0 \int E^2(r)dV$$

where the integration extends over all the volume with a nonzero electrostatic field, which would correspond to adsorption of counterions to the charges leading to their complete neutralization. However, at finite temperatures it is not the electrostatic energy but rather the free energy, $F = W - TS$, containing the entropy of the counterion distribution that should be minimized (26). The entropy of the mobile particles with the local density $\rho_i(r)$ (we assume there are more than one species of mobile particles, e.g., counterions and salt ions, tracked through the index, i) is taken as an ideal gas entropy (26),

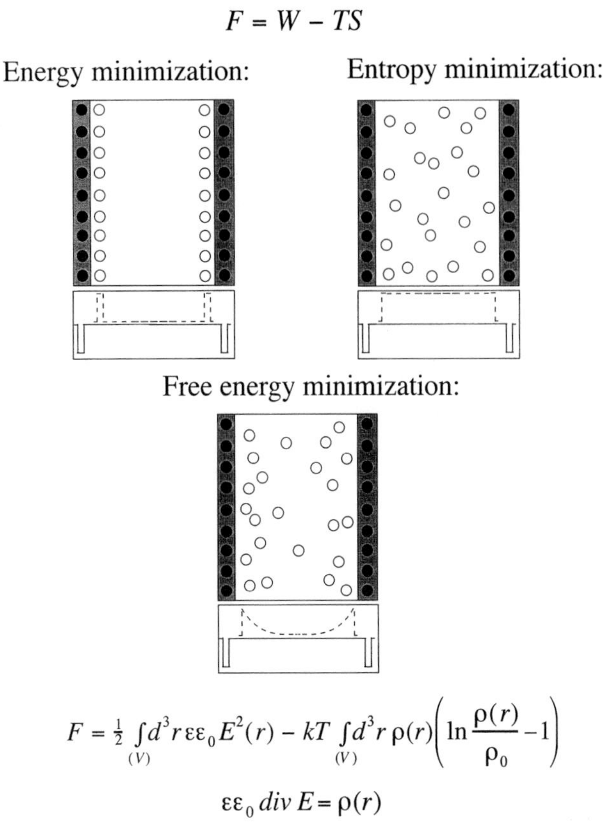

Figure 4 A pictorial exposition of the main ideas behind the Poisson-Boltzmann theory of electrostatic interactions between (bio)colloids. Electrostatic energy by itself would favor adsorption of counterions (white circles) to the oppositely charged surfaces (black circles). Entropy, to the contrary, favors a completely disordered configuration, a uniform distribution of counterions between the surfaces. The free energy works a compromise between the two principles leading to a nonmonotonic profile of the counterion density (25). As the two surfaces are brought close, the overlapping counterion distributions create repulsive forces between them.

$$S = k \int \sum_i \left(\rho_i(r) \ln\frac{\rho_i(r)}{\rho_{i0}} - (\rho_i(r) - \rho_{i0})\right) dV$$

where ρ_{i0} is the density of the mobile charges in a reservoir connected to the system under investigation. Entropy by itself would clearly lead to a uniform distribution of counterions between the charged bodies, $\rho_i(r) = \rho_{i0}$, while together with the electrostatic energy it obviously leads to a nonmonotonic profile of the mobile charge distribution between the surfaces, minimizing the total free energy of the mobile ions.

The above discussion, though being far from rigorous, contains all the important theoretical underpinnings known as the Poisson-Boltzmann theory (27). In order to arrive at the central equation corresponding to the core of this theory, one simply has to formally minimize the free energy, F = W − TS, together with the basic electrostatic equation (28) (Poisson equation) connecting the sources of the electrostatic field with the charge densities of different ionic species,

$$\epsilon\epsilon_0\, \mathrm{div}\mathrm{E}(r) = \sum_i e_i \rho_i(r)$$

where e_i is the charge on the mobile charged species i. The standard procedure now is to minimize the free energy, take into account the Poisson equation, and what follows is the well-known Poisson-Boltzmann equation, the solution of which gives the nonuniform profile of the mobile charges between the surfaces with fixed charges. This equation can be solved explicitly for some particularly simple geometries (27). For two charged planar surfaces the solution gives a screened electrostatic potential that decays exponentially away from the walls. It is thus smallest in the middle of the region between the surfaces and largest at the surfaces. The characteristic length of this decay, the Debye length,

$$\lambda_D = \sqrt{\frac{\epsilon\epsilon_0 kT}{\sum_i e_i^2 \rho_{i0}}}$$

away from the surfaces is independent of the surface charge. For uni-uni valent salts, the Debye screening length is numerically close to 3 Å/$\sqrt{I}$, where I is the ionic strength of the salt in moles per liter. The exponential decay of the electrostatic field away from the charged surfaces with a characteristic length independent (to the lowest order) of the surface charge is one of the most important results of the Poisson-Boltzmann theory.

Obviously as the surfaces come closer together, their decaying electrostatic potentials begin to interpenetrate (25). The consequence of this interpenetration is a repulsive force between the surfaces that again decays exponentially with the intersurface separation and a characteristic length again equal to the Debye length. For two planar surfaces at a separation, D, bearing sufficiently small charges, characterized by the surface charge density, σ, so that the ensuing electrostatic potential is never larger than kT/e, one can derive (27) for the interaction free energy per unit surface area, F(D), the expression

$$F(D) = \frac{\sigma^2 \lambda_D}{\epsilon\epsilon_0}(\coth(D/\lambda_D) - 1)$$

The typical magnitude of the electrostatic interaction in different systems of course depends on the magnitude of the surface charge. It would not be unusual in lipids to have surface charge densities in the range of one unit charge per 50–100 Å^2 (29).

The same type of analysis would also apply to two charged cylindrical bodies, e.g., two molecules of DNA, interacting across an electrolyte solution. What one evaluates in this case is the interaction free energy per unit length of the cylinders (30), g(R), that can be obtained in the form

$$g(R) = \frac{\mu^2}{2\pi\epsilon\epsilon_0} K_0(R/\lambda_D)$$

where $K_0(x)$ is the modified cylindrical Bessel function that has an asymptotic form of $K_0(x) \sim (1/\sqrt{x}) \exp(-x)$. It is actually possible to get an explicit form (30) of the interaction energy between two cylinders even if they are skewed by an angle, θ, between them. In this case the relevant quantity is the interaction free energy itself (if θ is nonzero, then the interaction energy does not scale with the length of the molecules) that can be obtained in a closed form as

$$F(R, \theta) = \frac{\mu^2\lambda_D}{2\pi\epsilon\epsilon_0}\sqrt{\frac{2\pi R}{\lambda_D}}\frac{e^{-R/\lambda_D}}{\sin\theta}$$

The predictions for the forces between charged colloid bodies have been reasonably well borne out for electrolyte solutions of uni-uni valent salts (31). In that case there is near quantitative agreement between theory and experiment. However, for higher valency salts the Poisson-Boltzmann theory not only gives the wrong numerical values for the strength of the electrostatic interactions, but also misses their sign. In higher-valency salts the correlations among mobile charges between charged colloid bodies due to thermal fluctuations in their mean concentration lead effectively to attractive interactions (32), that are in many respect similar to van der Waals forces.

D. van der Waals Forces

van der Waals charge fluctuation forces are special in the sense that they are a consequence of thermodynamic as well as quantum mechanical fluctuations of the electromagnetic fields (15). They exist even if the average charge, dipole moment or higher multipole moments, on the colloid bodies are zero. This is in stark contrast to electrostatic forces that require a net charge or a net polarization to drive the interaction. This also signifies that the van der Waals forces are much more general and ubiquitous than any other force between colloid bodies (9).

There are many different approaches to van der Waals forces (33). For interacting molecules, one can distinguish different contributions to the van der Waals force, stemming from thermally averaged dipole-dipole potentials (the Keesom interaction), dipole–induced dipole interactions (the Debye interaction), and induced dipole–induced dipole interactions (the London interaction) (34). They are all attractive, and their respective interaction energy decays as the sixth power of the separation between the interacting molecules. The magnitude of the interaction energy depends on the electromagnetic adsorption (dispersion) spectrum of interacting bodies, thus also the term dispersion forces.

For large colloidal bodies composed of many molecules, the calculation of the total van der Waals interaction is no trivial matter (15), even if we know the interactions between individual molecules composing the bodies. Hamaker assumed that one can simply add the interactions between composing molecules in a pairwise manner. It turned out that this was a very crude and simplistic approach to van der Waals forces in colloidal systems, as it does not take into account the highly nonlinear nature of the van der Waals interactions in condensed media. Molecules in a condensed body interact among themselves, thus changing their properties, which turn modify the van der Waals forces between them.

Lifshitz, following work of Casimir (9,15), realized how to circumvent this difficulty and formulated the theory of van der Waals forces in a way that already includes all these nonlinearities. The main assumption of this theory is that the presence of dielectric discontinuities as in colloid surfaces modifies the spectrum of electromagnetic field modes between these surfaces (Fig. 5). As the separation between colloid bodies varies, so do the eigenmode frequencies of the electromagnetic field between and within the colloid bodies. It is possible to deduce the change in the free energy of the electromagnetic modes due to the changes in the separation between colloid bodies coupled to their dispersion spectral characteristics (35).

From the work of Lifshitz it is now clear that if one associates the fluctuation free energy difference, F, with the change of the free energy of field harmonic oscillators at a particular eigenmode frequency, ω, as a function of the separation between the interacting bodies, D, and temperature, T,

$$F = kT\ln\left(2\sinh\frac{\hbar\omega(D)}{kT}\right) - kT\ln\left(2\sinh\frac{\hbar\omega(\infty)}{kT}\right)$$

this change is nothing but the van der Waals interaction energy. With this equivalence in mind, it is quite straightforward to calculate the van der Waals interaction free energy between two planar surfaces at a separation, D, and temperature, T; the dielectric constant between the two sur-

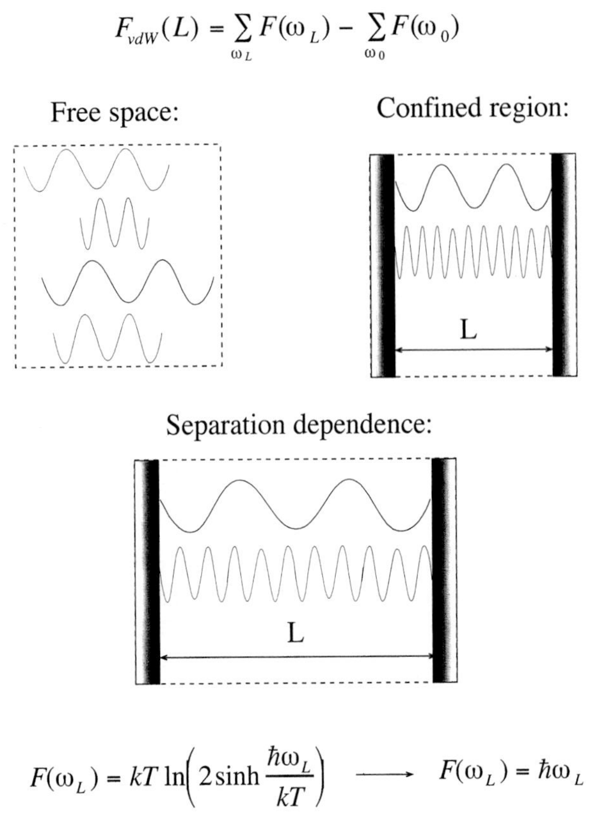

Figure 5 A pictorial introduction to the theory of Lifshitz–van der Waals forces between colloid bodies. Empty space is alive with electromagnetic (EM) field modes that are excited by thermal as well as quantum mechanical fluctuations. Their frequency is unconstrained and follows the black body radiation law. Between dielectric bodies only those EM modes survive that can fit in a confined geometry. As the width of the space between the bodies changes, so do the allowed EM mode frequencies. Every mode can be treated as a separate harmonic oscillator, each contributing to the free energy of the system. Since this free energy depends on the frequency of the mode, which in turn depends on the separation between the bodies, the total free energy of the EM modes depends on the separation between the bodies. This is the Lifshitz–van der Waals force (15).

faces is ϵ, and within the surfaces ϵ' must be known as a function of the frequency of the electromagnetic field (35). This is a consequence that in general the dielectric media comprising the surfaces as well as the space between them are dispersive, meaning that their dielectric functions depend on frequency of the electromagnetic field, i.e., $\epsilon = \epsilon(\omega)$. With this in mind one can derive the interaction free energy per unit surface area of the interacting surfaces in the form

$$F(D) = \frac{A}{12\pi D^2}$$

where the s.c. Hamaker coefficient, A, has been introduced as shorthand for

$$A = \frac{3kT}{4}\left(\frac{\epsilon(0) - \epsilon'(0)}{\epsilon(0) + \epsilon'(0)}\right)^2 + \frac{3\hbar}{4\pi}\int_0^\infty d\zeta \left(\frac{\epsilon(i\zeta) - \epsilon'(i\zeta)}{\epsilon(i\zeta) + \epsilon'(i\zeta)}\right)^2 .$$

The first term in the Hamaker constant is due to thermodynamic fluctuations, such as Brownian rotations of the dipoles of the molecules composing the media or the averaged dipole–induced dipole forces and depends on the static ($\omega = 0$) dielectric response of the interacting media, while the second term is purely quantum mechanical in nature (15). The imaginary argument of the dielectric constants is not that odd since $\epsilon(i\zeta)$ is an even function of ζ, which makes $\epsilon(i\zeta)$ also a purely real quantity (35).

In order to evaluate the magnitude of the van der Waals forces, one thus has to know the dielectric dispersion, $\epsilon(\omega)$, of all the media involved. This is no simple task and can be accomplished only for very few materials (34). Experiments seem to be a much more straightforward way to proceed. The values for the Hamaker constants of different materials interacting across water are between 0.3 and 2.0 $\times$ 10^{-20} J. Specifically for lipids, the Hamaker constants are quite close to theoretical expectations except for the phosphatidylethanolamines, which show much larger attractive interactions probably due to headgroup alignment (31). Evidence from direct measurements of attractive contact energies as well as direct force measurements suggest that van der Waals forces are more than adequate to provide attraction between bilayers for them to form multilamellar systems (36).

For cylinders the same type of argument applies, except that due to the geometry the calculations are a bit more tedious (37). Here the relevant quantity is not the free energy per unit area but the interaction free energy per unit length of the two cylinders of radius a, g(R), considered to be parallel at a separation R. The calculation (38) leads to the following form:

$$g(R) = \frac{3\ kT}{8\ \pi}(\pi a^2)\left(\Delta_\perp^2 + \frac{1}{4}\Delta_\perp\,\Gamma + \Gamma^2\frac{3}{2^7}\right)\frac{1}{R^5}$$

where

$$\Delta_\parallel = \frac{\epsilon_\parallel - \epsilon_m}{\epsilon_m}\quad \Delta_\perp = \frac{\epsilon_\perp - \epsilon_m}{\epsilon_\perp + \epsilon_m}$$

with $\epsilon_\parallel$ the parallel and $\epsilon_\perp$-the perpendicular components of the dielectric constant of the dielectric material of the cylinders, while ϵ_m is the dielectric constant of the bathing medium. The above equation contains only the part of the van der Waals force corresponding to thermodynamic fluctuations. The corresponding quantum mechanical contribution is, however, easy to write down in complete analogy with the planar case.

If the two interacting cylinders are skewed at an angle θ, then the interaction free energy $G(R, \theta)$, this time not per length, is obtained (38) in the form

$$G(R, \theta) = -\frac{3\ kT}{8\ \pi}(\pi\ a^2)^2 \left(\Delta_\perp^2 + \frac{1}{4}\Delta_\perp\ \Gamma + \Gamma^2\ \frac{2\cos^2\theta + 1}{2^7}\right)\frac{1}{R^4 \sin\theta}$$

The same correspondence between the thermodynamic and quantum mechanical parts of the interactions as for two parallel cylinders applies also to this case. Clearly the van der Waals force between two cylinders has a profound angular dependence that in general creates torque between the two interacting molecules.

Taking the numerical values of the dielectric constants for two interacting DNA molecules, one can calculate that the van der Waals forces are quite small, typically one to two orders of magnitude smaller than the electrostatic repulsions between them, and in general cannot hold the DNAs together in an ordered array. Other forces leading to condensation phenomena in DNA (10) clearly have to be added to the total force balance in order to get a stable array. There is as yet still no consensus on the exact nature of these additional attractions. It seems that they are due to the fluctuations of counterion atmosphere close to the molecules.

E. The DLVO Model

The popular Derjaguin-Landau-Verwey-Overbeek (DLVO) (9,25) model assumes that electrostatic double layer and van der Waals interactions govern colloid stability. Applied with a piety not anticipated by its founders, this model actually does work rather well in surprisingly many cases. Direct osmotic stress measurements of forces between lipid bilayers show that at separations less than ~10 Å there are qualitative deviations from DLVO thinking (39). For μm-sized objects and for macromolecules at greater separations, electrostatic double-layer forces and sometimes van der Waals forces tell us what we need to know about interactions governing movement and packing.

F. Geometric Effects

Forces between macromolecular surfaces are most easily analyzed in plane-parallel geometry. Because most of the interacting colloid surfaces are not planar, one has either to evaluate molecular interactions for each particular geometry or to devise a way to connect the forces between planar surfaces with forces between surfaces of a more general shape. The Derjaguin approximation (9) assumes that interactions between curved bodies can be decomposed into interactions between small plane-parallel sections of the curved bodies (Fig. 6). The total interaction between curved bodies would be thus equal to a sum where each term corresponds to a partial interaction between quasi plane-parallel sections of the two bodies. This idea can be given a completely rigorous form and leads to a connection between the interaction free energy per unit area of two interacting planar surfaces, F(D), and the force acting between two spheres at minimal separation D, f(D), one with the mean radius of curvature R_1 and the other

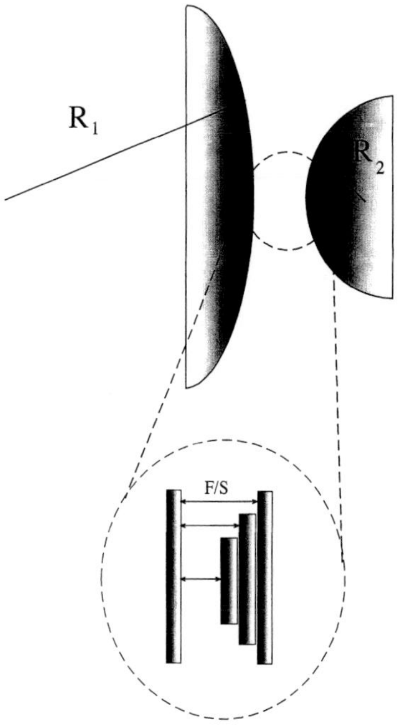

$$f(D) \cong 2\pi\left(\frac{R_1 R_2}{R_1 + R_2}\right)\frac{F(D)}{S}$$

Figure 6 The Derjaguin approximation. To formulate forces between oppositely curved bodies (e.g., cylinders, spheres) is very difficult. But it is often possible to use an approximate procedure. Two curved bodies (two spheres of unequal radii in this case) are approximated by a succession of planar sections, interactions between which can be calculated relatively easily. The total interaction between curved bodies is obtained through a summation over these planar sections.

one with R_2. The formal equivalence can be written as follows:

$$f(D) = 2\pi \frac{R_1R_2}{R_1 + R_2} F(D)$$

A similar equation can also be obtained for two cylinders in the form

$$f(D) = 2\pi \sqrt{R_1R_2}\, F(D)$$

These approximate relations clearly make the problem of calculating interactions between bodies of general shape tractable. The only caveat here is that the radii of curvature should be much larger than the proximal separation between the two interacting bodies, effectively limiting the Derjaguin approximation to sufficiently small separations.

Using the Derjaguin formula or evaluating the interaction energy explicitly for those geometries for which this indeed is not an insurmountable task, one can now obtain a whole zoo of DLVO expressions for different interaction geometries (Fig. 7). The salient features of all these expressions are that the total interaction free energy always has a primary minimum, which can only be eliminated by strong short-range hydration forces, and a secondary minimum due to the compensation of screened electrostatic repulsion and van der Waals–Lifshitz attraction. The position of the secondary minimum depends as much on the parameters of the forces (Hamaker constant, fixed charges, and ionic strength) as well as on the interaction geometry. One can state generally that the range of interaction between the bodies of different shapes is inversely proportional to their radii of curvature.

Thus the longest-range forces are observed between planar bodies, and the shortest between small (point-like) bodies. What we have not indicated in Figure 7 is that the interaction energy between two cylindrical bodies, skewed at a general angle θ and not just for parallel or crossed configurations, can be obtained in an explicit form. It follows simply from these results that the configuration of two interacting rods with minimal interaction energy is the one corresponding to $\theta = \pi/2$, i.e., corresponding to crossed rods.

G. Fluctuation Forces

The term ''fluctuation forces'' is a bit misleading in this context because clearly van der Waals forces already are fluctuation forces. What we have in mind is thus a generalization of the van der Waals forces to situations where the fluctuating quantities are not electromagnetic fields but other quantities subject to thermal fluctuations. No general observation as to the sign of these interactions can be made; they can be either repulsive or attractive and are as a rule

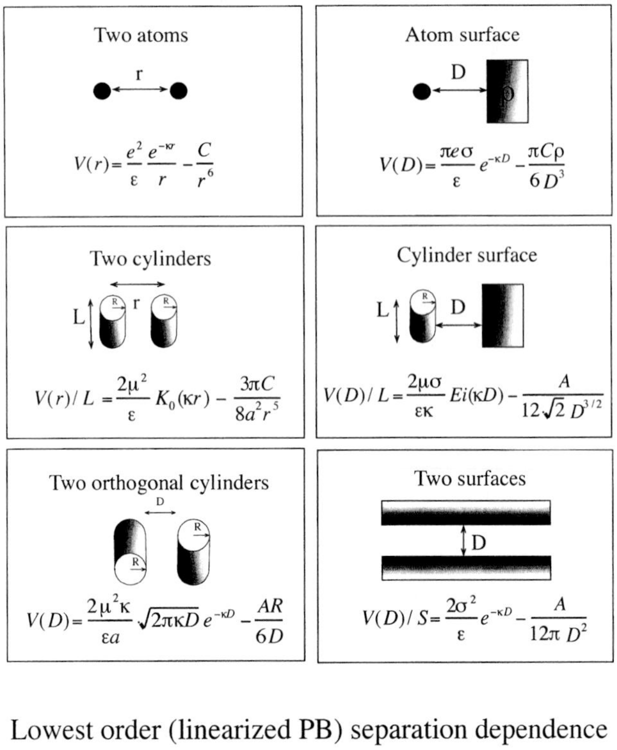

Figure 7 A menagerie of DLVO interaction expressions for different geometries most commonly encountered in biological milieu: two small particles, a particle and a wall, two parallel cylinders, a cylinder close to a wall, two skewed cylinders, and two walls. The DLVO interaction free energy is always composed of a repulsive electrostatic part (calculated from a linearized Poisson-Boltzmann theory) and an attractive van der Waals part. μ = Charge per unit length of a cylinder; σ = charge per unit surface area of a wall; C = a geometry-dependent constant, ϵ = the dielectric constant, κ = the inverse Debye length, and ρ = the density of the wall material.

of thumb comparable in magnitude to the van der Waals forces.

The most important and ubiquitous force in this category is the undulation or Helfrich force (40). It has a very simple origin and operates among any type of deformable bodies as long as their curvature moduli are small enough (comparable to thermal energies). It was shown to be important for multilamellar lipid arrays (41) as well as in hexagonal polyelectrolyte arrays (42) (Fig. 8).

The mechanism is simple. The shape of deformable bodies fluctuates because of thermal agitation (Brownian motion) (26). If the bodies are close to each other the conformational fluctuations of one will be constrained by the fluctuations of its neighbors. Thermal motion makes the

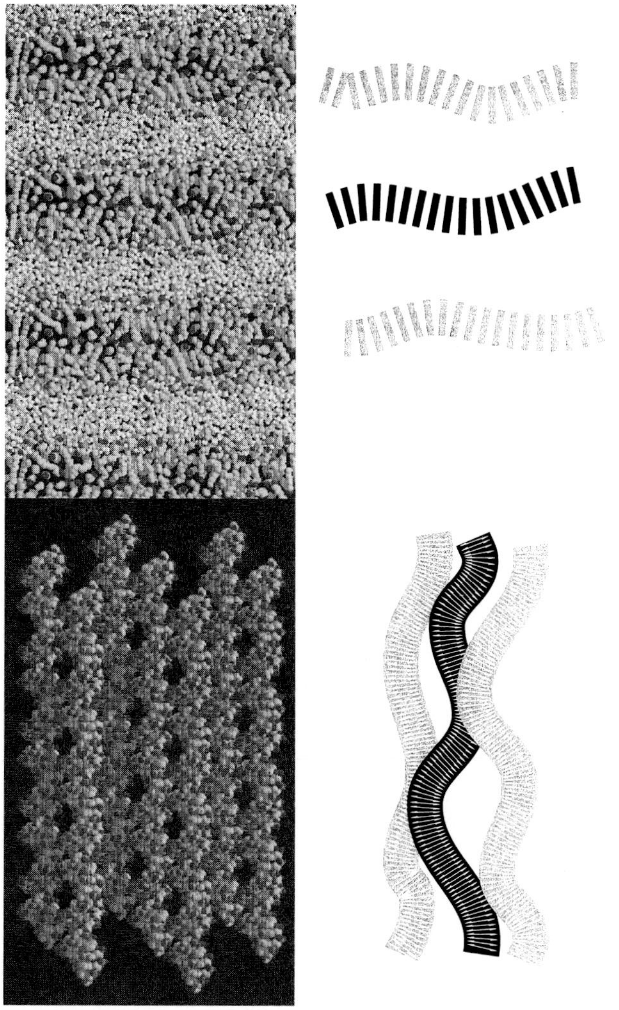

Figure 8 Thermally excited conformational fluctuations in a multilamellar membrane array or in a tightly packed polyelectrolyte chain array lead to collisions between membranes or polyelectrolyte chains. These collisions contribute an additional repulsive contribution to the total osmotic pressure in the array, a repulsion that depends on the average spacing between the fluctuating objects: $\langle D(x,y) \rangle$ for membranes and $\langle R(x,y) \rangle$ for polyelectrolyte chains. (The coordinates (x,y) point in the plane perpendicular to the average normal of the membrane, or perpendicular to the average direction of the polyelectrolyte chains.)

bodies bump into each other, which creates spikes of repulsive force between them. The average of this force is smooth and decays continuously with the mean separation between the bodies.

One can estimate this steric interaction for multilamellar lipid systems and for condensed arrays of cylindrical polymers. The only quantity entering this calculation is the elastic energy, F_{el}, of a single bilayer, which can be written in the form

$$F_{el} = \frac{1}{2} K_c \int dS \left(\frac{1}{R_1} + \frac{1}{R_2} \right)^2$$

where K_c is the elastic modulus, usually between 10 and 50 kT (43) for different lipid membranes, dS is the element of surface area, and R_1 and R_2 are the two main curvatures of the membrane. If the instantaneous deviation of the membrane from its overall planar shape in the (x,y) plane is now introduced as u(x,y), the presence of neighboring membranes introduces a constrain on the fluctuations of u(x,y) that one can write as

$$\langle u(x, y)^2 \rangle = \text{const. } D^2$$

where D is the average separation between the membranes in a multilamellar stack. The free energy associated with this constraint can now be derived as (40).

$$F \propto \frac{(kT)^2}{K_c D^2}$$

It has obviously the same dependence on D as the van der Waals force. This is, however, not a general feature of undulation interactions as the next example clearly shows. Also, we only indicated the general proportionality of the interaction energy. Calculation of the prefactors can be difficult (44), especially because the elastic bodies usually do not interact with idealized hard repulsions but rather through soft potentials that have both attractive as well as repulsive regimes.

The same line of thought can now be applied to flexible polymers in a condensed array (42). This system is a one-dimensional analog of the multilamellar membrane system. For polymers the elastic energy can be written as

$$F_{el} = \frac{1}{2} K_c \int_s ds \left(\frac{1}{R} \right)^2$$

where again K_c is the elastic modulus, usually expressed through a persistence length $L_p = K_c/(kT)$, and ds is the element of the contour length along the polymer and R its local radius of curvature. Using the same constraint for the average fluctuations of the polymer away from the straight axis, one derives for the free energy change due to this constraint the relationship

$$F \propto \frac{kT}{L_p^{1/3} D^{2/3}}$$

Clearly the D dependence for this geometry is very much different from the one for van der Waals force, which would be D^{-5}. There is thus no general connection between the van der Waals force and the undulation fluctuation force. Here again one has to indicate that if the interaction potential between fluctuating bodies is described by a soft potential, with no discernible hard core, the fluctuation interaction can have a profoundly different dependence on the mean separation (42).

Apart from the undulation fluctuation force, there are other fluctuation forces. The most important among them appears to be the monopolar charge fluctuation force (45), recently investigated in the context of DNA condensation. It arises from transient charge fluctuations along the DNA molecule due to constant statistical redistributions of the counterion atmosphere.

Although the theory of charge fluctuation forces is quite intricate and mathematically demanding (46), a simple argument will show the essential physics of it. Assume we have two point charges, e_1 and e_2, at a separation, R, interacting through screened coulomb potential with a screening length again equal to the Debye length, λ_D, obtained by solving the linearized Poisson-Boltzmann equation. Together with the self-energies of the two charges, the total energy of the system can be written in the form

$$W(R) = \frac{e_1^2}{4\pi\epsilon\epsilon_0\lambda_D} + \frac{e^2}{4\pi\epsilon\epsilon_0\lambda_D} + \frac{e_1e_2}{4\pi\epsilon\epsilon_0 R}$$

If the two charges are not fixed, but are allowed to fluctuate, i.e., to explore all statistically available configurations, the partition function for the system, $\Xi(R)$, can be obtained from

$$\Xi(R) = \iint de_1\, de_2\, e^{-\beta W(R)}$$

where the integrals run over all values of the two fluctuating charges. Evaluating these two integrals by extending the range of integration to $(+\infty, -\infty)$, which introduces only a small error in the final result, we obtain to the lowest order in the separation between the two charges the result

$$F(R) = -kT\ln\Xi(R) = -kT\ln\left(1 + \left(\frac{\lambda_D}{R}\right)^2 e^{-2\kappa R}\right) \cong -kT\left(\frac{\lambda_D}{R}\right)^2 e^{-2kR}$$

This simplified derivation already shows one of the salient features of the interaction potential for monopolar charge fluctuation forces, namely it is screened with half the Debye screening length. If there is no screening, however, the monopolar charge fluctuation force becomes the strongest and longest ranged among all the fluctuation forces. It is, however, much less general than the related van der Waals force, and at present it is still not clear what the detailed conditions should be for its appearance, the main difficulty being the question whether charge fluctuations in the counterion atmosphere are constrained or not.

H. Lessons

Molecular forces apparently convey a variety that is surprising considering the fact that they are all to some extent or another just a variant of electrostatic interactions. Quantum and thermal fluctuations apparently modify the underlying electrostatics, leading to qualitatively novel and unexpected features. The zoo of forces obtained in this way is what one has to deal with and understand when trying to make them work for us.

III. DNA MESOPHASES

A. Polyelectrolyte Properties of DNA

We can define several levels of DNA organization similarly to Ref. 1. Its structure is the sequence of base pairs. Its secondary structure is the famous double helix that can exist in several conformations. In solution, the B-helical structure dominates (47). The bases are perpendicular to the axis of the molecule and are 0.34 nm apart, and 10 of them make one turn of the helix. These parameters can vary for DNA in solution, where up to 10.6 base pairs can make a whole turn of the double helix (48). In the A structure the bases are tilted with respect to the direction of the helix, and this arrangement yields an internal hole, wider diameter, and closer packing (Fig. 9). Other conformations, such as the left-handed Z form, are rare. In solution, DNA's tertiary structure includes the many bent and twisted conformations in three dimensions.

DNA lengths can reach macroscopic dimensions. For instance, the human genome is coded in approximately 3 billion base pairs with a collective linear stretch on the order of a meter. Obviously, this molecule must undergo extensive compaction in order to fit in the cell nucleus. In natural environments DNA is packaged by basic proteins, which form chromatin structures to keep DNA organized. In the test tube, DNA can be packaged into very tight and dense structures as well, primarily by various ''condensing'' agents. Their addition typically induces a random coil-to-globule transition. At large concentrations, DNA molecules, like lipids, form ordered liquid crystalline phases (10).

In vitro, at concentrations above a critical value (49), polyelectrolyte DNA self-organizes in highly ordered mesophases. In this respect it is lyotropic. But contrary to the case of lipid mesophases, where the shape of constituent molecules plays a determining role, the organization of DNA in condensed phases is primarily a consequence of

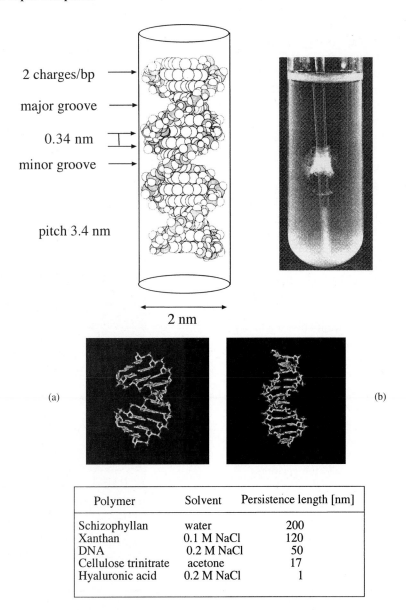

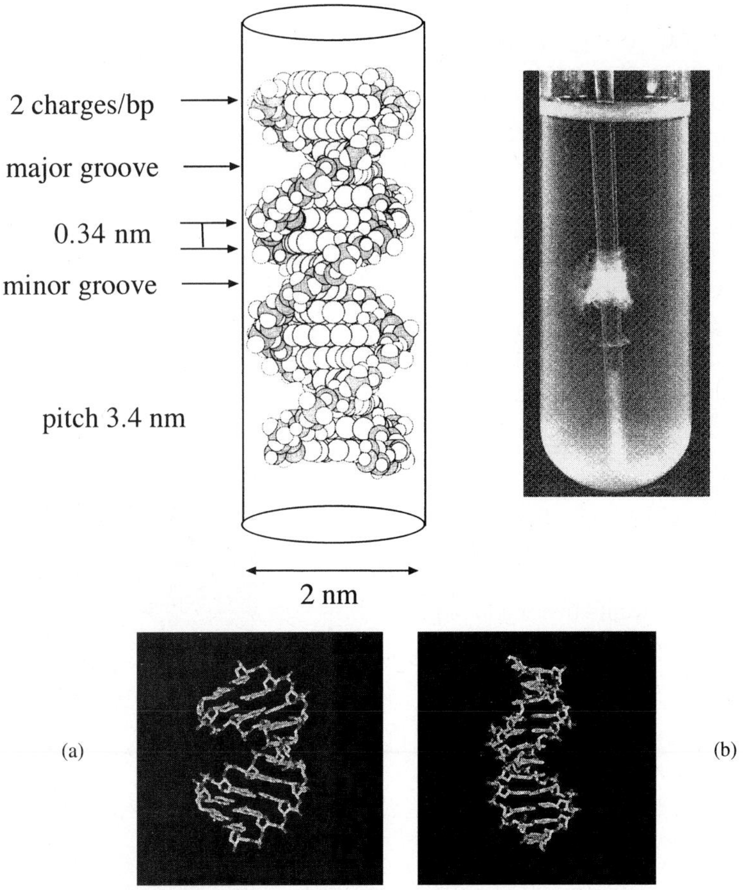

Polymer	Solvent	Persistence length [nm]
Schizophyllan	water	200
Xanthan	0.1 M NaCl	120
DNA	0.2 M NaCl	50
Cellulose trinitrate	acetone	17
Hyaluronic acid	0.2 M NaCl	1

Figure 9 Structural parameters of a DNA molecule. The two relevant configurations of the DNA backbone: (a) A-DNA, common at small hydrations or high DNA densities, and (b) B-DNA, common in solution at large hydrations and lower DNA densities. The test tube holds ethanol precipitated DNA in solution. Its milky color is due to the light scattering by thermal conformational fluctuations in the hexatic phase (see main text). Table indicates typical persistence lengths for different (bio)polymer chains.

its relatively large stiffness (8). The orientational ordering of DNA at high concentrations is promoted mostly by the interplay between entropically favored disorder or misalignment and the consequent price in terms of the high interaction energy. The mechanism of orientational ordering is thus the same as in standard short nematogens (50), the main difference being due to the large length of polymeric chains. The discussion that follows will concentrate on very long—on the order of 1000 persistence lengths—DNA molecules.

B. Flexibility of DNA Molecules in Solution

In isotropic solutions, DNA can be in one of several forms. For linear DNA, individual molecules are effectively straight over the span of a persistence length (defined as the exponential decay length for the loss of angular correlation between two positions along the molecule), while for longer lengths they form a worm-like random coil. The persistence length of DNA is about 500 (1). The persistence length has been determined by measuring the diffusion coefficient of different-length DNA molecules using dynamic light scattering and by enzymatic cyclization reactions (51). It depends only weakly on the base-pair sequence and ionic strength.

DNA can also be circular, as in the case of a plasmid. The closed form of a plasmid introduces an additional topological constraint on the conformation that is given by the linking number Lk (2). The linking number gives the number of helical turns along a circular DNA molecule. Because plasmid DNA is closed, Lk has to be an integer number. By convention, Lk of a closed right-handed DNA helix is positive. The most frequent DNA conformation for plasmids in cells is negatively supercoiled. This means that for such plasmids Lk is less than it would be for a torsionally relaxed DNA circle—negatively supercoiled DNA is underwound. This is a general phenomenon with important biological consequences. It seems that free energy of negative supercoiling catalyzes processes that depend on DNA untwisting, such as DNA replication and transcription, which rely on DNA (52). While the sequence of bases in exons determine the nature of proteins synthesized, it is possible that such structural features dictate the temporal and spatial evolution of DNA-encoded information.

C. Liquid Crystals

The fact that DNA is intrinsically stiff makes it form liquid crystals at high concentration (8). Known for about 100 years, the simplest liquid crystals are formed by rod-like molecules. Solutions of rods exhibit a transition from an isotropic phase with no preferential orientation to a nematic phase, a fluid in which the axes of all molecules point on average in one direction (Fig. 10). The unit vector in which the molecules point is called the nematic director, n. Nematic order is orientational order (50), in contrast to positional order that distinguishes between fluid and crystalline phases. Polymers with intrinsic stiffness can also form liquid crystals. This is because a long polymer with persistence length L_p acts much like a solution of individual rods that are all one persistence length long—polymer nematics (53).

If the molecules that comprise the liquid crystal are chiral, have a natural twist such as double-helical DNA, then their orientational order tends to twist. This twist originates from the interaction between two molecules that are both of the same handedness. This chiral interaction is illustrated

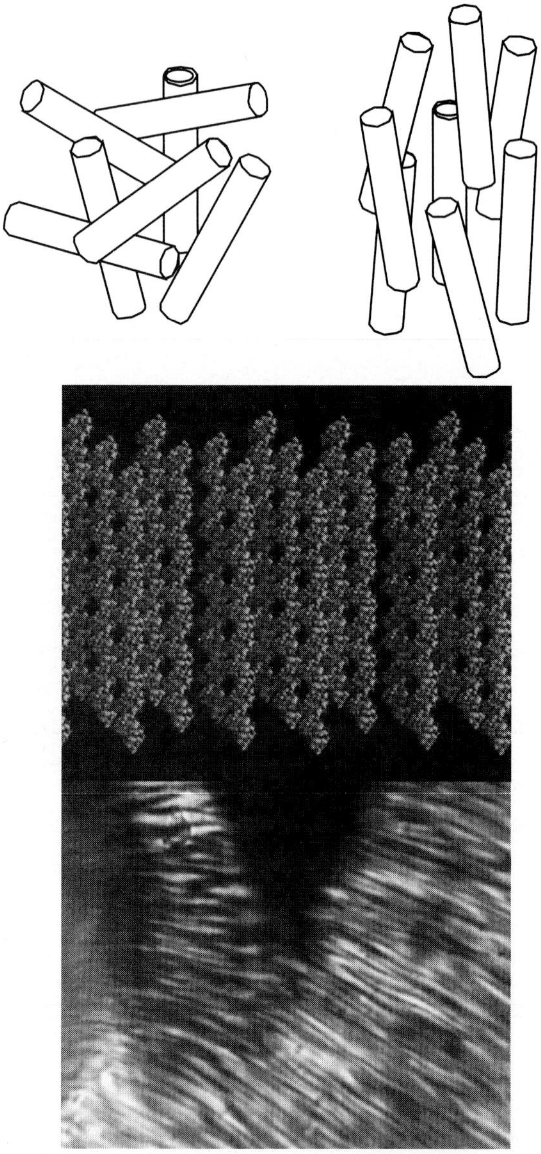

Figure 10 Nematic order in nondilute DNA solutions. The nematic state (50) is characterized by the average direction of the DNA molecules, here represented schematically by short cylinders. Locally DNAs are hexagonally packed with an average spacing that depends on applied osmotic pressure. Under crossed polarizers (bottom), the DNA nematic phase creates a characteristic striated texture. For long DNA molecules, the striations appear disordered.

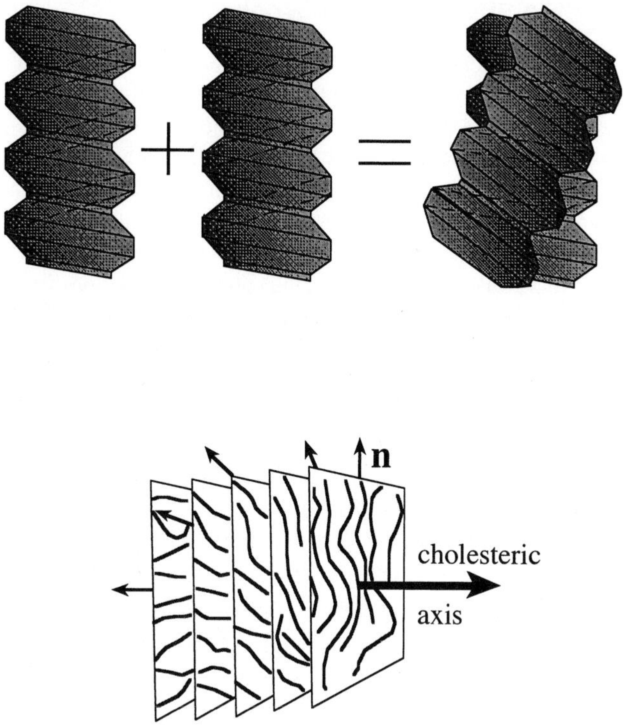

Figure 11 Chiral interaction for two helical or screw-like molecules. For steric reasons two helices pack best when slightly tilted with respect to each other. Instead of a nematic phase, chiral molecules form a cholesteric phase (50). The cholesteric phase is a twisted nematic phase in which the nematic director twists continuously around a cholesteric axis.

in Figure 11 for two helical or screw-like molecules. For steric reasons two helices pack best when tilted with respect to each other. Instead of a nematic phase, chiral molecules form a cholesteric phase (50). The cholesteric phase is a twisted nematic phase in which the nematic director twists continuously around the so-called cholesteric axis, as shown in Figure 11. Using the same arguments as for plain polymers, chiral polymers will form polymer cholesterics.

Both cholesteric and hexagonal liquid crystalline DNA phases were identified in the 1960s. This discovery was especially exciting because both phases were also found in biological systems. The hexagonal liquid crystalline phase can be seen in bacterial phages and the cholesteric phase seen in cell nuclei of dinoflagellates (8).

D. Measurements of Forces Between DNA Molecules

Liquid crystalline order lets us measure intermolecular forces directly. With the osmotic stress method, DNA liquid crystals are equilibrated against neutral polymer (such as PEG or PVP) solutions of known osmotic pressure, pH, temperature, and ionic composition (54). Equilibration of DNA under osmotic stress of external polymer solution is effectively the same as exerting mechanical pressure on the DNA subphase with a piston (Fig. 12). In this respect the osmotic stress technique is formally very much similar

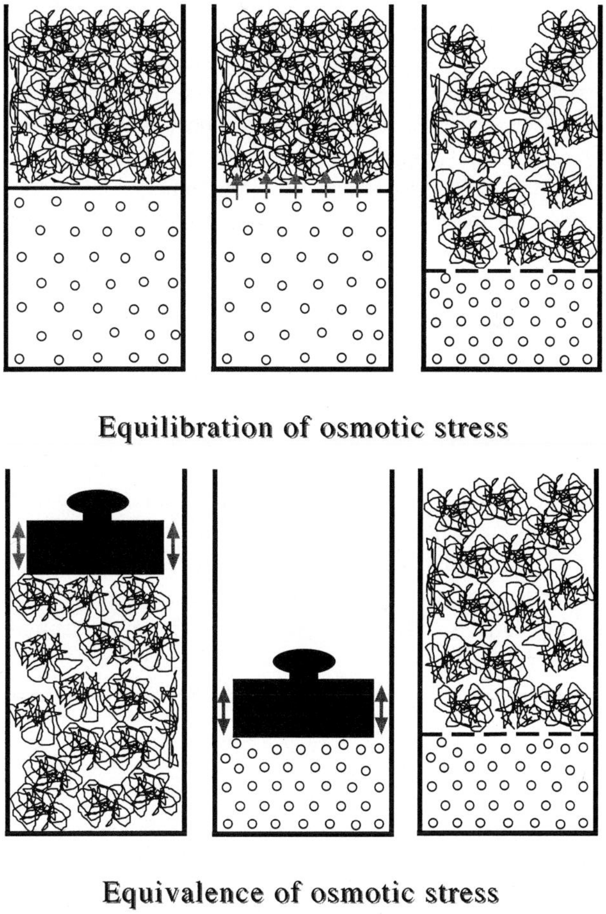

Figure 12 The osmotic stress method (18). DNA liquid crystals are equilibrated against solutions of a neutral polymer (such as PEG or PVP, depicted as disordered coils). These solutions are of known osmotic pressure, pH, temperature, and ionic composition (54). Equilibration of DNA under the osmotic stress of external polymer solution is effectively the same as exerting mechanical pressure on the DNA subphase with a piston that passes water and small solutes but not DNA. After equilibration under this known stress, DNA separation is measured either by x-ray scattering, if the DNA subphase is sufficiently ordered, or by densitometry (55). DNA density and osmotic stress thus determined immediately provide an equation of state (osmotic pressure as a function of the density of the DNA subphase) to be codified in analytic form over an entire phase diagram.

to the Boyle experiment, where one compresses a gas with mechanical pistons and measures the ensuing pressure. After equilibration under this known stress, DNA separation is measured either by x-ray scattering, if the DNA subphase is sufficiently ordered, or by straightforward densitometry (55). Known DNA density and osmotic stress immediately provide an equation of state (osmotic pressure as a function of the density of the DNA subphase) to be codified in analytic form for the entire phase diagram. Then, with the local packing symmetry derived from x-ray scattering (7,54), and sometimes to correct for DNA motion (42), it is possible to extract the bare interaxial forces between molecules, which can be compared with theoretical predictions as developed in Chapter 2. In vivo observation of DNA liquid crystals (56) shows that the amount of stress needed for compaction and liquid crystalline ordering is the same as for DNA in vitro.

E. Interactions Between DNA Molecules

Performed on DNA in univalent salt solutions, direct force measurements reveal two types of purely repulsive interactions between DNA double helices (4):

1. At interaxial separations less than ~3 nm (surface separation ~1 nm) an exponentially varying "hydration" repulsion is thought to originate from partially ordered water near the DNA surface.
2. At surface separations greater than 1 nm, measured interactions reveal electrostatic double-layer repulsion presumably from negative phosphates along the DNA backbone.

Measurements give no evidence for a significant DNA-DNA attraction expected on theoretical grounds (57). Though charge fluctuation forces must certainly occur, they appear to be negligible at least for liquid crystal formation in monovalent ion solutions. At these larger separations, the double-layer repulsion often couples with configurational fluctuations to create exponentially decaying forces, whose decay length is significantly larger than the expected Debye screening length (42).

Bare short-range molecular interactions between DNA molecules appear to be insensitive to the amount of added salt. This has been taken as evidence that they are not electrostatic in origin. The term "hydration force" associates these forces with perturbations of the water structure around DNA surface (54). Alternatively, short-range repulsion has been viewed as a consequence of the electrostatic force specific to high DNA density and counterion concentration (58).

F. High-Density DNA Mesophases

Ordering of DNA can be induced by two alternative mechanisms. First, attractive interactions between different DNA segments can be enhanced by adding multivalent counterions thought to promote either counterion-correlation forces (59) or electrostatic (60) and hydration attraction (22). In these cases DNA aggregates spontaneously. Alternatively, one can add neutral crowding polymers to the bathing solution that phase separate from DNA and exert osmotic stress on the DNA subphase (61). In this case the segment repulsions in DNA are simply counteracted by the large externally applied osmotic pressure. DNA is forced in this case to condense under externally imposed constraints. This latter case is formally (but only formally) analogous to a Boyle gas pressure experiment but with osmotic pressure playing the role of ordinary pressure, the main difference being that ordinary pressure is set mechanically, while osmotic pressure has to be set through the chemical potential of water, which is in turn controlled by the amount of neutral crowding polymers (such as PEG, PVP, or dextran) in the bathing solution (55).

At very high DNA densities, where the osmotic pressure exceeds 160 atm, DNA can exist only in a (poly)crystalline state (62). Nearest neighbors in such an array are all oriented in parallel and show correlated (nucleotide) base stacking between neighboring duplexes (Fig. 13). This means that there is a long-range correlation in the positions of the backbone phosphates between different DNA molecules in the crystal. The local symmetry of the lattice is monoclinic. Because of the high osmotic pressure, DNA is actually forced to be in an A conformation characterized by a somewhat larger outer diameter as well as a somewhat smaller pitch than in the canonical B conformation (see Fig. 9), which persists at smaller densities. If the osmotic pressure of such a crystal is increased above 400 atm, the helix begins to crack and the sample loses structural homogeneity (62).

Lowering the osmotic pressure does not have a pronounced effect on the DNA crystal until it is down to ~160 atm. Then the crystal as a whole simultaneously expands while individual DNA molecules undergo an A-B conformational transition (see Fig. 13) (62). This phase transformation is thus first order and, besides being a conformational transition for single DNAs is connected with the melting of the base stacking as well as positional order of the helices in the lattice. The ensuing low-density mesophase, where DNA is in the B conformation, is therefore characterized by short-range base-stacking order, short-range two dimensional (2D) positional order, and long-range bond orientational order (Fig. 14) (63). This order is connected with the spatial direction of the nearest neigh-

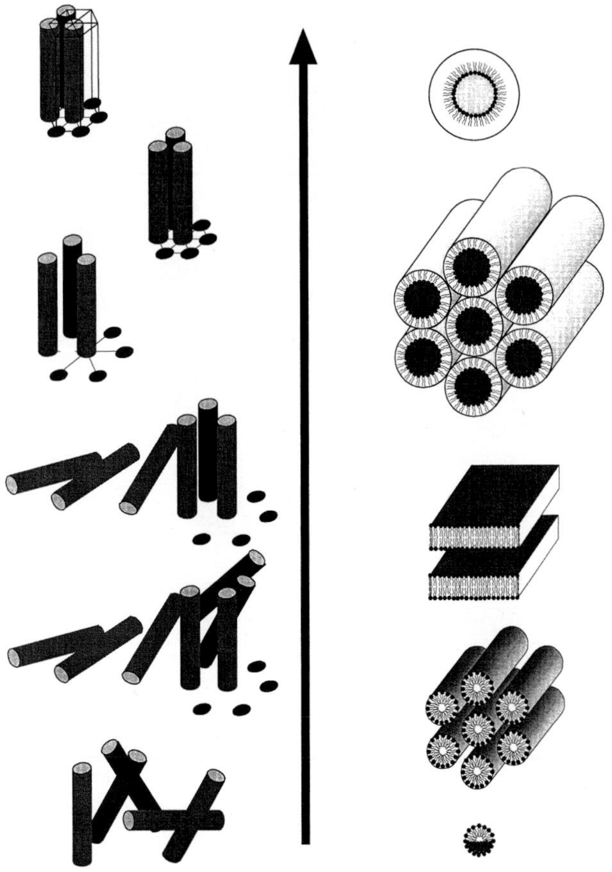

Figure 13 Schematic phase diagrams for DNA (left) and lipids (right). In both cases the arrow indicates increasing density in both cases. DNA starts (bottom) as a completely disordered solution. It progresses through a sequence of ''blue'' phases characterized by cholesteric pitch in two perpendicular directions (68), then to a cholesteric phase with pitch in only one direction. At still larger densities this second cholesteric phase is succeeded by a hexatic phase characterized by short-range liquid-like positional order and long-range crystal-like bond orientational or hexatic order (indicated by lines). At highest densities there is a crystalline phase, characterized by long-range positional order of the molecules and long-range base-stacking order in the direction of the long axes of the molecules. Between the hexatic and the crystalline forms, there might exist a hexagonal columnar liquid-crystalline phase that is similar to a crystal, but with base-stacking order only on short scales.

This lipid phase diagram (77) is a composite of results obtained for different lipids. It starts from a micellar solution and progresses through a phase of lipid tubes to a multilamellar phase of lipid bilayers. This is followed by an inverted hexagonal columnar phase of water cylinders and possibly goes to an inverted micellar phase. Most lipids show only a subset of these possibilities. Boundaries between the phases shown here might contain exotic cubic phases not included in this picture.

bors (64). It is for this reason that the phase has been termed a ''line hexatic'' phase. Hexatics usually occur only in 2D systems. They have crystalline bond orientational order but liquid-like positional order. There might be a hexatic-hexagonal columnar transition somewhere along the hexatic line, but direct experimental proof is lacking. The difference between the two phases is that the hexagonal columnar phase has also a crystalline positional order, a real 2D crystal (see Fig. 13) (65). It is the long-range bond orientational order that gives the line hexatic phase some crystalline character (66). The DNA duplexes are still packed in parallel, while the local symmetry perpendicular to the long axes of the molecules is changed to hexagonal. The directions of the nearest neighbors persist through macroscopic dimensions (on the order of mm), while their positions tend to become disordered after several (typically 5–10) lattice spacings. This mesophase has a characteristic x-ray scattering fingerprint (see Fig. 14). If the x-ray beam is directed parallel to the long axis of the molecules, it will show a hexagonally symmetrical diffraction pattern of broad liquid-like peaks (67).

Typical lattice spacings in the line hexatic phase are between 20 and 35 Å (i.e., between 600 and 300 mg/mL of DNA) (63). The free energy in this mesophase is mostly a consequence of the large hydration forces stemming from removal of water from the phosphates of the DNA backbone. Typically independent of the ionic strength of the bathing solution, these hydration forces (54) depend exponentially on the interhelical separation and decay with a decay length of about 3 Å (11) at these large densities.

When the osmotic pressure is lowered to about 10 atm (corresponding to interaxial spacing of about 35 Å, or DNA density of about 300 mg/mL), the characteristic hexagonal x-ray diffraction fingerprint of the line hexatic mesophase disappears continuously. This disappearance suggests the presence of a continuous, second-order transition into a low-density cholesteric (63). It is characterized by short-range (or effectively no) base-stacking order, short-range positional order, short-range bond orientational order, but long-range cholesteric order, manifested in a continuing rotation of the long axis of the molecules in a preferred direction. In this sense the cholesteric DNA mesophase would retain the symmetry of a one dimensional (1D) crystal. X-ray diffraction pattern of the DNA in the cholesteric phase is isotropic and has the form of a ring. Crossed polarizers, however, reveal the existence of long-range cholesteric order just as in the case of short chiral molecules. The texture of small drops of DNA cholesteric phase (spherulites) under crossed polarizers (Fig. 15) reveals the intricacies of orientational packing of DNA, where its local orientation is set by a compromise between interaction forces and macroscopic geometry of a spherulite. It is thus only at these low densities that the chiral character of the DNA

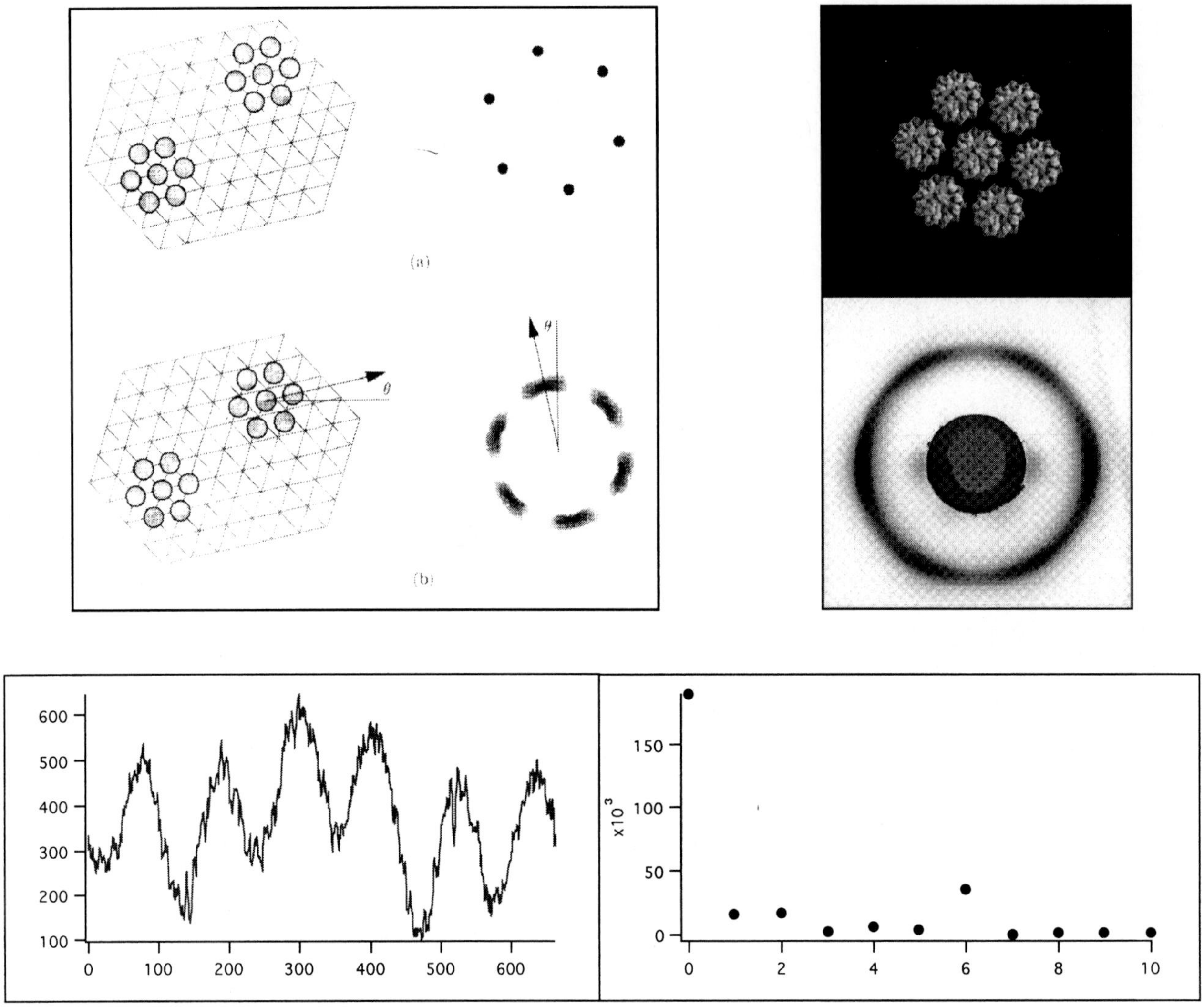

Figure 14 Bond orientational or hexatic order. With a real crystal, if one translates part of the crystal by a lattice vector, the new position of the atoms completely coincides with those already there. (Adapted from Ref. 67.) In a hexatic phase the directions to the nearest neighbors (bond orientations) coincide (after rotation by 60°), but the positions of the atoms don't coincide after displacement in one of the six directions! Consequently a real crystal gives a series of very sharp Bragg peaks in x-ray scattering (upper half of box), whereas a hexatic gives hexagonally positioned broad spots. The pattern of x-ray scattering by high-density DNA samples gives a fingerprint of a hexatic phase. The densitogram of the scattering intensity (right) shows six pronounced peaks that can be Fourier decomposed with a marked sixth order Fourier coefficient (left), another sign that the scattering is due to long-range bond orientational order (63).

finally makes an impact on the symmetry of the mesophase. It is not yet fully understood why the chiral order is effectively screened from the high-density DNA mesophases.

At still smaller DNA densities, the predominance of the chiral interactions in the behavior of the system remains. Recent work on the behavior of low-density DNA mesophases indicates (68) that the cholesteric part of the phase diagram might end with a sequence of blue phases, which would emerge as a consequence of the loosened packing constraints coupled to the chiral character of the DNA molecule. At DNA density of about 10 mg/mL the cholesteric phase line would end with DNA reentering the isotropic liquid solution, where it remains at all subsequent densities, except perhaps at very small ionic strengths (69).

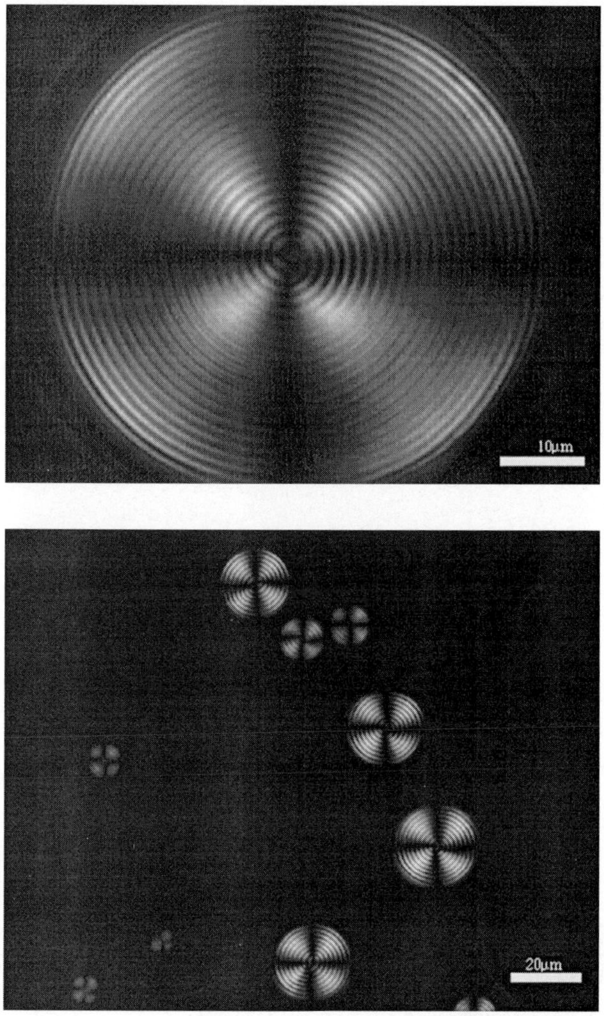

Figure 15 Texture of small drops of DNA cholesteric phase (spherulites) in a PEG solution under crossed polarizers at two different magnifications. These patterns reveal the intricacies of DNA orientational packing when its local orientation is set by a compromise between interaction forces and the macroscopic geometry of a spherulite. The change from a bright to a dark stripe indicates that the orientation of the DNA molecule has changed by 90 degrees.

G. DNA Equation of State

The free energy of the DNA cholesteric mesophase appears to be dominated by the large elastic shape fluctuations of its constituent DNA molecules (70), which leave their imprint in the very broad x-ray diffraction peak (55). Instead of showing the expected exponential decay characteristic of screened electrostatic interactions (71), where the decay length is equal to the Debye length, it shows a fluctuation-enhanced repulsion similar to the Helfrich force existing in the flexible smectic multilamellar arrays (41). Fluctuations not only boost the magnitude of the existing screened electrostatic repulsion but also extend its range through a modified decay length equal to four times the Debye length. The factor-of-four enhancement in the range of the repulsive force is a consequence of the coupling between the bare electrostatic repulsions of exponential type and the elastic shape fluctuations described through elastic curvature energy that is proportional to the square of the second derivative of the local helix position (42). In the last instance it is a consequence of the fact that DNAs in the array interact via an extended, soft-screened electrostatic potential and not through hard bumps as assumed in the simple derivation in Chapter 2.

The similarity of the free energy behavior of the smectic arrays with repulsive interactions of Helfrich type and the DNA arrays in the cholesteric phase, which can as well be understood in the framework of the Helfrich-type enhanced repulsion, satisfies a consistency test for our understanding of flexible supermolecular arrays.

IV. LIPID MESOPHASES

A. Aggregation of Lipids in Aqueous Solutions

Single-molecule solutions of biological lipids exist only over a negligible range of concentrations; virtually all interesting lipid properties are those of aggregate mesophases such as bilayers and micelles. Lipid molecules cluster into ordered structures to maximize hydrophilic and minimize hydrophobic interactions (72,73). These interactions include negative free energy contribution from the solvation of polar heads and van der Waals interactions of hydrocarbon chains, competing with positive contributions such as steric, hydration, and electrostatic repulsions between polar heads. The ''hydrophobic effect,'' which causes segregation of polar and nonpolar groups, is said to be driven by the increase of the entropy of the surrounding medium.

Intrinsic to the identity of surfactant lipids is the tension between water-soluble polar groups and lipid-soluble hydrocarbon chains. There is no surprise, then, that the amount of water available to an amphiphile is a parameter pertinent to its modes of packing and to its ability to incorporate foreign bodies.

These interactions, therefore, force lipid molecules to self-assemble into different ordered microscopic structures, such as bilayers, micelles (spherical, ellipsoidal, rod-like, or disk-like), which can, especially at higher concentrations, pack into macroscopically ordered phases, such as lamellar, hexagonal, inverted hexagonal, and cubic. The morphology of these macroscopic phases changes with the balance between attractive van der Waals and ion correlation forces versus electrostatic, steric, hydration, and undulation repulsion (74).

B. The Lipid Bilayer

The workhorse of all lipid aggregates is the bilayer (Fig. 16) (73). This sandwich of two monolayers, with nonpolar hydrocarbon chains tucked in toward each other and polar groups facing water solution, is only about 20–30 Å thick. Yet it has the physical resilience and the electrical resistance to form the plasma membrane that divides ''in'' from ''out'' in all biological cells. Its mechanical properties have been measured in terms of bending and stretching moduli. These strengths together with measured interactions between bilayers in multilamellar stacks have taught us to think quantitatively about the ways in which bilayers are formed and maintain their remarkable stability.

With some lipids, such as double-chain phospholipids, when there is the need to encompass hydrocarbon compo-

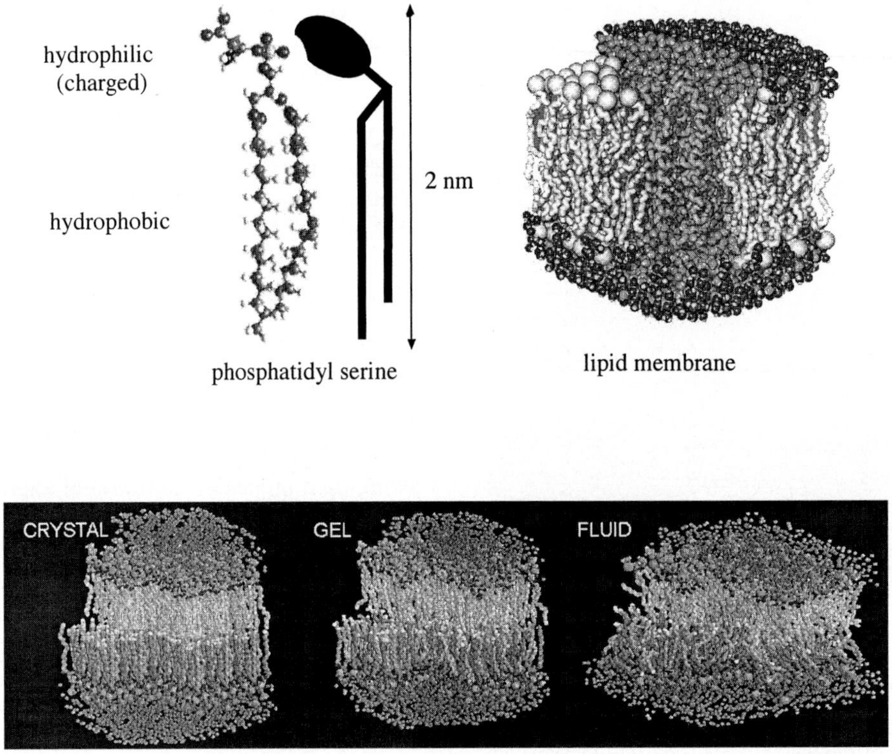

Lipid	Bending rigidity [10-19 J]	Area compression [mN/m]
DMPC	1.15	145
SOPC	2.0	200
EYPC	1.15	
SOPC:CHOL	2.46	700
Red Blood Cell	2.0 - 4.0	450

Figure 16 The lipid bilayer. A lipid molecule has a hydrophilic and a hydrophobic part (shown here is the phosphatidylserine molecule with a charged headgroup). At high enough densities lipid molecules assemble into a lipid bilayer. Together with membrane proteins, the lipid bilayer is the underlying structural component of biological membranes. The degree of order of the lipids in a bilayer depends drastically on temperature and goes through a sequence of phases (see main text): crystalline, gel, and fluid. The table at bottom gives sample values of bilayer bending rigidity and area compressibility for some biologically relevant lipids and one well-studied cell membrane. (Adapted from Ref. 110.)

nents voluminous compared with the size of polar groups, the small surface-to-volume ratio of spheres, ellipsoids, or even cylinders cannot suffice even at extreme dilution. Bilayers in this case are the aggregate form of choice. These may occur as single ''unilamellar'' vesicles, as onion-like multilayer vesicles, or multilamellar phases of indefinite extent. In vivo, bilayer-forming phospholipids create the flexible but tightly sealed plasma-membrane matrix that defines the inside from the outside of a cell. In vitro, multilayers are often chosen as a matrix of choice for the incorporation of polymers. Specifically, there are tight associations between positively charged lipids that merge with negatively charged DNA in a variety of forms (see below).

The organization of lipid molecules in the bilayer itself can vary (73). At low enough temperatures or dry enough conditions, the lipid tails are frozen in an all-*trans* conformation that minimizes the energy of molecular bonds in the alkyl tails of the lipids. Also, the positions of the lipid heads along the surface of the bilayer are frozen in 2D positional order, making the overall conformation of the lipids in the bilayer crystalline (L_C). The chains can be either oriented perpendicular to the bilayer surface (L_β and $L_{\beta'}$) or tilted (crystalline phase L_C or ripple phase P_β). Such a crystalline bilayer cannot exist by itself, but assembles with others to make a real 3D crystal.

Upon heating, various rearrangements in the 2D crystalline bilayers occur; first the positional order of the headgroups melts leading to a loss of 2D order($L_{\beta'}$) and tilt (L_β), then at the gel-liquid crystal phase transition the untilted or rippled (P_β phase) bilayer changes into a bilayer membrane with disordered polar heads in two dimensions and conformationally frozen hydrocarbon chains, allowing them to spin around the long axes of the molecules, the so-called L_α phase. At still higher temperatures the thermal disorder finally destroys the ordered configuration of the alkyl chains, leading to a fluid-like bilayer phase. The fluid bilayer phase creates the fundamental matrix that according to the fluid mosaic model (72) contains different other ingredients of biological membranes, e.g., membrane proteins, channels.

Not only bilayers in multilamellar arrays but also liposome bilayers can also undergo such phase transition; electron microscopy has revealed fluid, rippled, and crystalline phases in which spherical liposomes transform into polyhedra due to very high values of bending elasticity of crystallized bilayers (75).

The fluid phase of the lipid bilayer is highly flexible. This flexibility makes it prone to pronounced thermal fluctuations, resulting in large excursions away from a planar shape. This flexibility of the bilayer is essential for understanding the zoo of equilibrium shapes that can arise in closed bilayer (vesicles) systems (76). Also, just as in the case of flexible DNA, it eventually leads to configurational entropic interactions between bilayers that have been crammed together (41). Bilayers and linear polyelectrolytes thus share a substantial amount of fundamentally similar physics, which allows us to analyze their behavior in the same framework.

C. Lipid Polymorphism

Low-temperature phases (77) are normally lamellar with frozen hydrocarbon chains, tilted (crystalline phase L_C or ripple phase P_β) or nontilted (L_β and $L_{\beta'}$ form 3, 2, or 1D crystalline or gel phases) with respect to the plane of the lipid bilayers. Terminology from thermotropic liquid crystal phenomenology (50) can be used efficiently in this context: these phases are smectic and SmA describes 2D fluid with no tilt while a variety of SmC phases with various indices encompass tilted phases with various degrees of 2D order. Upon melting, liquid crystalline phases with one- (lamellar L_α), two- (hexagonal II), or three-dimensional (cubic) positional order can form. The most frequently formed phases are micellar, lamellar, and hexagonal. Normal hexagonal phase consists of long cylindrical micelles ordered in a hexagonal array, while in the inverse hexagonal II phase water channels of inverse micelles are packed hexagonally with lipid tails filling the interstices. In excess water, such arrays are coated by a lipid monolayer. The morphology of these phases can be maintained upon their (mechanical) dispersal into colloidal dispersions. Despite the fact that energy has to be used to generate dispersed mesophases, relatively stable colloidal dispersions of particles with lamellar, hexagonal, or cubic symmetry can be formed.

Many phospholipids found in lamellar cell membranes after extraction, purification, and resuspension prefer an inverted hexagonal geometry (Fig. 13) (77). Under excess water conditions, different lipids will assume different most-favored spontaneous radii for the water cylinder of this inverted phase (78). An immediate implication is that different lipids are strained to different degrees when forced into lamellar packing. Lamellar-inverted hexagonal phase transitions occur with varied temperature, hydration, and salt concentration (for charged lipids), which form in order to alleviate this strain (Fig. 17).

In the presence of an immiscible organic phase, emulsion droplets can assemble (79). In regions of phase diagram, which are rich in water, oil-in-water emulsions and microemulsions can be formed, while in oil-rich regions these spherical particles have negative curvature and are therefore water-in-oil emulsions. The intermediate phase between the two is a bicontinuous emulsion that has zero

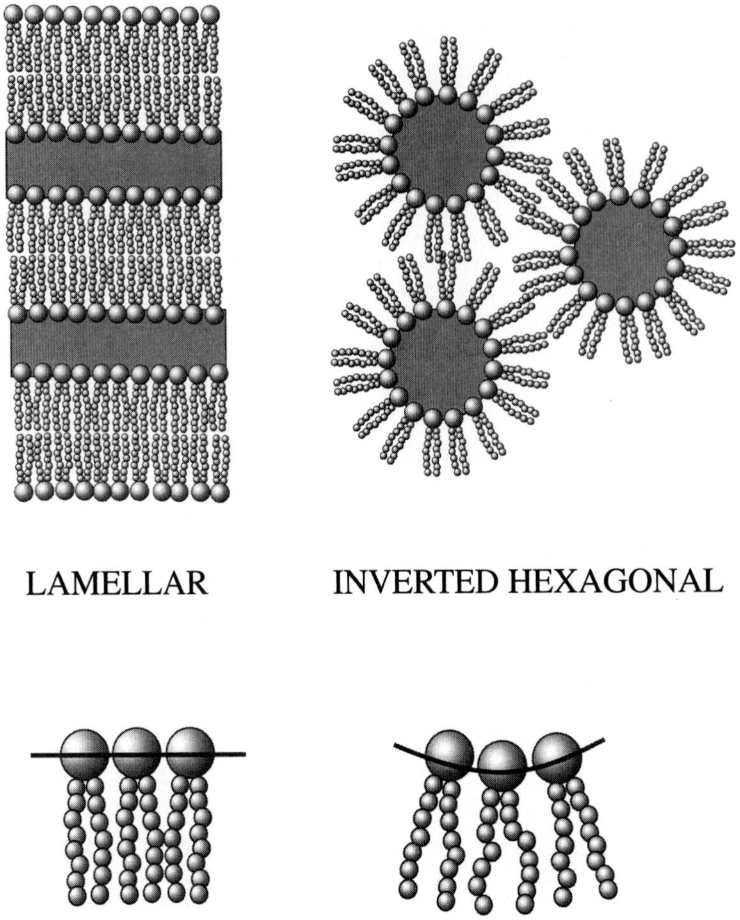

Figure 17 Different lipids are strained to different degrees when forced into lamellar packing. Relaxation of this strain contributes to the conditions for lamellar–to–inverted hexagonal phase transitions that depend on temperature, hydration, and salt concentration (for charged lipids). In the inverted hexagonal phase the lipid/aqueous solution interface is curved, thus relaxing the stresses developed in the tail region of the lipids.

average curvature and an anomalously low value of the surface tension (usually brought about the use of different cosurfactants) between the two immiscible components. Only microemulsions can form spontaneously (analogously to micelle formation), while for the formation of a homogeneous emulsion some energy has to be dissipated into the system.

The detailed structure of these phases as well as the size and shape of colloidal particles are probably dominated by (a) the average molecular geometry of lipid molecules, (b) their aqueous solubility and effective charge, (c) weaker interactions such as intra- and intermolecular hydrogen bonds, and (d) stereoisomerism as well as interactions within the medium. All of these depend on the temperature, lipid concentration, and electrostatic and van der Waals interactions with the solvent and solutes. With charged lipids, counterions, especially anions, may also be important. Ionotropic transitions have been observed with negatively charged phospholipids in the presence of metal ions leading to aggregation and fusion (80). In cationic amphiphiles it was shown that simple exchange of counterions can induce micelle-vesicle transition. Lipid polymorphism is very rich, and even single-component lipid systems can form a variety of other phases, including ribbon-like phases, coexisting regions, and various stacks of micelles of different shapes.

D. Forces in Multilamellar Bilayer Arrays

Except for differences in dimensionality, forces between bilayers are remarkably similar to those between DNA.

At very great separations between lamellae, the sheet-like structures flex and ''crumple'' because of (thermal) Brownian motion (41). Just as an isolated flexible linear polymer can escape from its one linear dimension into the three dimensions of the volume in which it is bathed, so can two-dimensional flexible sheets. In the most dilute solution, biological phospholipids will typically form huge floppy closed vesicles; these vesicles enjoy flexibility while satisfying the need to keep all greasy nonpolar chains comfortably covered by polar groups rather than exposed at open edges. For this reason, in very dilute solution, the interactions between phospholipid bilayers are usually space wars of collision and volume occupation. This steric competition is always seen for neutral lipids; it is not always true for charged lipids (74).

Especially in the absence of any added salt, planar surfaces emit far-ranging electrostatic fields (27) that couple to thermally excited elastic excursions to create very long-range repulsion (44,83). As with DNA, this repulsion is a mixture of direct electrostatic forces and soft collisions mediated by electrostatic forces rather than by actual bilayer contact. In some cases electrostatic repulsion is strong enough to snuff out bilayer bending when bilayers form ordered arrays with periodicities as high as hundreds of Å (82).

Almost always bilayers align into well-formed stacks when their concentration approaches ~50–60 wt%, and their separation is brought down to a few tens of Å. In this region charged layers are quite orderly with little lamellar undulation. In fact, bilayers of many neutral phospholipids often spontaneously fall out of dilute suspension to form arrays with bilayer separations between 20 and 30 Å. These spontaneous spacings are thought to reflect a balance between van der Waals attraction and undulation-enhanced hydration repulsion (74). One way to test for the presence of van der Waals forces has been to add solutes such as ethylene glycol, glucose, or sucrose to the bathing solutions. It is possible then to correlate the changes in spacing with changes in van der Waals forces due to the changes in dielectric susceptibility through the relation as described above (83). More convincingly, there have been direct measurements of the work to pull apart bilayers that sit at spontaneously assumed spacings. This work of separation is of the magnitude expected for van der Waals attraction (84).

Similar to DNA, multilayers, of charged or neutral lipids, subjected to strong osmotic stress reveal exponential variation in force versus bilayer separation (74). Typically at separations between dry ''contact'' and 20 Å, exponential decay constants are 2–3 Å in distilled water or in salt solution, whether phospholipids are charged or neutral. Lipid bilayer repulsion in this range is thought to be due to the work of polar group dehydration sometimes enhanced by lamellar collisions from thermal agitation (85). Normalized per area of interacting surface, the strength of hydration force acting in lamellar lipid arrays and DNA arrays is directly comparable.

Given excess water, neutral lipids will usually find the above-mentioned separation of 20–30 Å at which this hydration repulsion is balanced by van der Waals attraction. Charged lipids, unless placed in solutions of high salt concentration, will swell to take up indefinitely high amounts of water. Stiff charged bilayers will repel with exponentially varying electrostatic double-layer interactions, but most charged bilayers will undulate at separations where direct electrostatic repulsion has weakened. In that case, similar to what has been described for DNA, electrostatic repulsion is enhanced by thermal undulations (86).

E. Equation of State of Lipid Mesophases

Lipid polymorphism shows much less universality that DNA. This is, of course, expected since lipid molecules come in many different varieties (73) with strong idiosyncrasies in terms of the detailed nature of their phase diagrams. One thus can not achieve the same degree of generality and universality in the description of lipid phase diagram and consequent equations of state as was the case for DNA.

Nevertheless, recent extremely careful and detailed work on phosphatidylcholines (PCs) by J. Nagle and his group (87) points strongly to the conclusion that at least in the lamellar part of the phase diagram of neutral lipids, the main features of the DNA and lipid membrane assembly physics indeed is the same (85). This statement, however, demands qualification. The physics indeed is the same, provided one first disregards the dimensionality of the aggregates—one dimensional in the case of DNA and two dimensional in the case of lipid membranes—and takes into account the fact that while van der Waals forces in DNA arrays are negligible, they are essential in lipid membrane force equilibria. One of the reasons for this state of affairs is the large difference between the static dielectric constant of hydrophobic lipid tails and the aqueous solution bathing the aggregate.

We have already pointed out that in the case of DNA arrays, quantitative agreement between theory, based on hydration and electrostatic forces augmented by thermal undulation forces, and experiment has been obtained and extensively tested (7,42). The work on neutral lipids (85) claims that the same level of quantitative accuracy can be achieved in lipid membrane assemblies if one takes into account hydration and van der Waals forces, again augmented by thermal undulations. Of course the nature of the fluctuations in the two systems is different and is set by the dimensionality of the fluctuating aggregates—one versus two dimensional.

The case of lipids adds an additional twist to the quantitative link between theory and experiments. DNA in the line hexatic as well as cholesteric phases (where reliable data for the equation of state exist) is essentially fluid as far as positional order is concerned and thus has unbounded positional fluctuations. Lipid membranes in the smectic multilamellar phase, on the other hand, are quite different in this respect. They are not really fluid as far as positional order is concerned but show something called quasi-long-range (QLR) order, meaning that they are in certain respects somewhere between a crystal and a fluid (50,67). The quasi-long-range positional order makes itself recognizable through the shape of the x-ray diffraction peaks in the form of persistent (Caille) tails (67). In a crystal one would ideally expect infinitely sharp peaks, broadened only because of finite accuracy of the experimental setup. Lipid multilamellar phases, however, show peaks with very broad and extended tails that are one of the consequences of QLR positional order. It is this property that allows us to measure not only the average spacing between the molecules but also the amount of fluctuation around this average spacing. Luckily the theory predicts that too, and without any free parameters (all of them being already determined from the equation of state) the comparison between predicted and measured magnitude in positional fluctuations of membranes in a multilamellar assembly is more than satisfactory (85).

In sum, the level of understanding of the equation of state reached for DNA and neutral lipid membrane arrays is pleasing.

V. DNA-CATIONIC LIPID COMPLEXES

A. The Nature of DNA-Lipid Interactions

DNA-lipid interactions retain all the characteristics of the DNA-DNA as well as lipid-lipid interactions described above. One obviously has hydration repulsion, electrostatic interaction, the sign of which depends on the sign of the lipid charges, as well as the ubiquitous van der Waals forces. The strengths of all these are well known. However, the tight binding of DNA to cationic lipid bilayers brings forth additional facets of the lipid DNA interactions, specific for this strong adsorption problem, that have not been addressed before.

To understand the specifics of the DNA–cationic lipid interactions, consider first DNA adsorption to an isolated positively charged surface (88). We must compare free energies of free DNA plus that of bare surface with the free energy of the state in which the DNA is bound to the surface. The driving force of adsorption comes from direct electrostatic attraction leading to charge neutralization as well as from the entropy increase of the counterions released from between the negative DNA and the positive surface. These counterions lower their electrostatic energy by accumulating near a charged body, but their translational entropy is reduced compared to that of ions far away (89). When DNA binds to a positively charged surface, counterions of both DNA and the surface are released into the bulk solution while DNA charge is neutralized by that of the positive surface. The net entropic change is the gain from released counterions minus the comparatively negligible conformational entropy loss of the bound DNA. The consequence of ion release is strongest when the surface charge density is high enough to neutralize all the charges on the DNA molecule.

DNA adsorbed to an immobilized surface still retains some flexibility in the plane of the surface and can thus interact with its neighbors through fluctuation interactions of the type that we already described in three-dimensional DNA assemblies. In the case of intercalation of DNA between the bilayers in a multilamellar lipid system, the fluctuations of DNA perpendicular to the planes of the bilayers are of course coupled to the membrane fluctuations themselves. Also there is the possibility that DNAs intercalated between different bilayers can still feel each other (90,91). All this adds to the difficulty in understanding the behavior of intercalated DNA.

B. Adsorption Studies of DNA

Experimentally, DNA adsorbed on cationic (DPTAB) as well as zwitterionic (DPPC) lipid bilayers was visualized using atomic force microscopy (AFM) as shown in Figure 18. DNA not only adsorbs to these surfaces but upon adsorption also condenses into nematically ordered two-dimensional structures. This two-dimensional ordering is characterized by a very low number of crossing defects (one DNA strand crossing another). Most DNAs remain in a locally parallel conformation throughout the sample. This is presumably an effect of the interplay between very strong (electrostatic neutralization) adsorption energies and the high stiffness of the DNA molecules. The average spacing between DNA molecules at zero added salt corresponds approximately to charge neutrality. Assuming an area per lipid of 70 Å^2 and a DNA linear charge density of 1 e^-/1.7 Å suggests an average spacing of 76 Å^2/1.7 Å = 45 Å (vs. 43 Å measured at zero salt). Similar experiments on varying charge densities that were prepared on a mixture of neutral and charged lipid showed that DNA slightly overcharges the surface (92). If the surface was initially

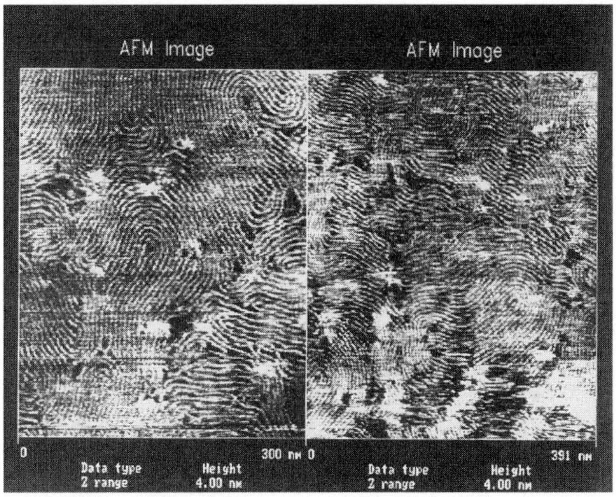

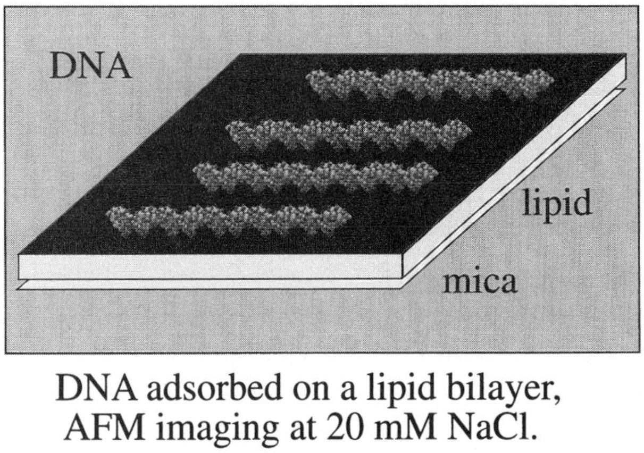

Figure 18 DNA adsorbed onto a cationic lipid bilayer deposited onto a mica surface. An AFM image shows the strikingly ordered arrangement of the DNA on the surface. There are very few defects in patterns that spread over large domains. Changes in DNA-DNA separation as a function of the bathing solution ionic strength still elude explanation. (Courtesy J. Yang.)

positively charged, then after DNA adsorption it will be weakly negatively charged.

The exact equilibrium spacing between DNA molecules deposited on a cationic lipid surface also depends on the ionic strength of the bathing solution. Yang and Feng (93) measured this dependence for NaCl salt and obtained an increase in the separation between adsorbed DNA strands ranging from 43 Å in zero salt conditions and going all the way to almost 60 Å in 1 M salt. This dependence is in itself rather surprising because the addition of salt should screen the electrostatic interactions, leading consequently to smaller interaxial separations for larger ionic strengths. Although there is no shortage of theories trying to come to grips with these perplexing results, no meaningful consensus has yet emerged. This remains one of the most surprising facts of DNA adsorption studies.

Also, by combining deposition of negative DNA layers with polycations (e.g., polyallylamine, polyethilenimin, polylysine, polyarginine) (94), one can create films with alternating negative and positive polyelectrolytes. Although the possible benefits of such complexes in DNA transfection studies are obvious, we shall not discuss them explicitly.

C. DNA-Lipid Complexes

When cationic lipid and DNA are mixed, complexes of different nature and symmetry can form (for a review see Ref. 95) and have indeed been observed in different studies. DNA–cationic liposome complexes were first examined under the electron microscope. Tight association of intact cationic liposomes and DNA was assumed in the early studies (96) without any unequivocal experimental proof. Electron microscopy and the inability of DNA to interact with intercalating agents was used by Gershon et al. (97) as proof that DNA-lipid interaction reorganizes the liposomes that eventually encapsulate DNA in their interior. Small added amounts of cationic lipid liposomes bind to DNA as beads-on-a-string. When more cationic lipids are added, DNA is completely encapsulated by a single lipid bilayer. At high liposome-to-DNA ratios, larger complexes form. Similar conclusions were also drawn by others (95). Later Sternberg et al. (98), basing their conclusion on freeze fracture electron microscopy, claimed that DNA is not only encapsulated within a liposome but is actually coated with a bilayer of cationic lipid. There were also claims that DNA could be hexagonally packed in the complex but unfortunately without any firm experimental evidence (99). All these structural models have only very indirect links to any direct structural probes that might unequivocally reveal the nature of the packing of DNA in the complexes.

D. Direct Structural Characterization of DNA-Lipid Complexes

The equilibrium DNA–cationic lipid phase diagram was investigated only recently by explicit structural small angle x-ray scattering studies. X-ray scattering probes local order in the DNA-lipid complex and allows one to deduce the symmetry of the packing, through analysis of the position of the diffraction peaks, as well as the range of the order, by studying the shape of each peak. In this respect it is of course the definitive method to study the structure of the complexes. X-ray scattering was first used as a probe to characterize the nature of the DNA-lipid complex by Lasic et al. (100).

In this study DODAB-cholesterol liposomes were rapidly mixed with DNA, and the ensuing complexes were studied by x-ray scattering as well as cryomicroscopy. Both methods confirmed the structural model where DNA is intercalated between lipid bilayers (Fig. 19). X-ray diffraction revealed a succession of peaks that are a fingerprint of lamellar phase. The fundamental repeat distance was 64.4 Å. On this structure DNA scattering was superimposed as a separate peak corresponding to the interaxial separation of 36 Å (Fig. 20). Cryomicroscopy results were completely consistent, showing structures with fundamental periodicities of ~6.5 and 3.5 nm within particles of diameter below 0.5 μm. These in vitro results were later systematically studied by in vivo delivery studies of DNA–cationic lipid complexes (101). For these complexes, prepared with small liposomes, cryomicroscopy showed that complexes have a novel morphology and that DNA is condensed on the interior of invaginated liposomes between lipid bilayers. This structure is of course completely consistent with the intercalated DNA-lipid multilayers observed in in vitro studies.

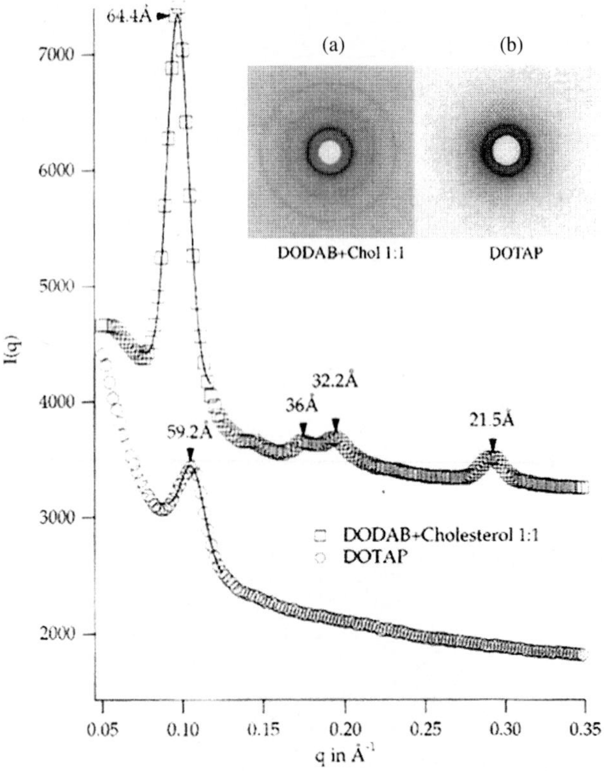

Figure 20 X-ray scattering from DODAB-cholesterol-DNA complexes. Three peaks (at 64.4, 32.2, and 21.5 Å) indicate the lamellar phase of the lipid subphase, whereas the peak at 36 Å corresponds to the intercalated DNA (see Fig. 19). The DNA peak also indicates that DNA between the lipid bilayers itself is at least partly ordered. The scattering pattern from cholesterol-free bilayers shows no intercalation of DNA.

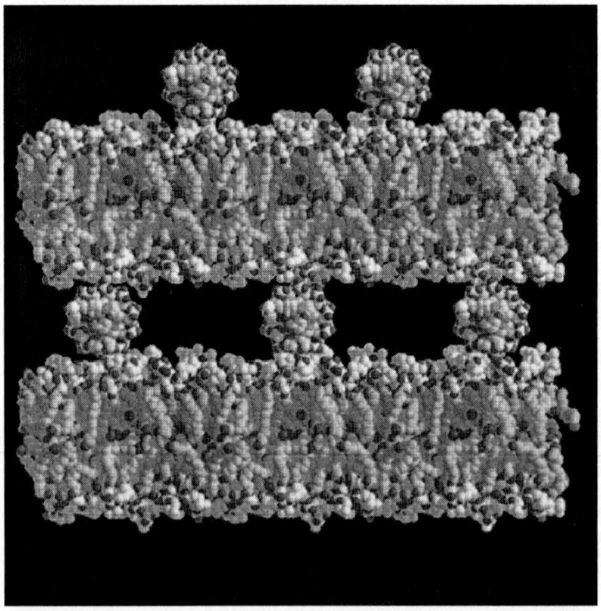

Figure 19 A model of DNA intercalated between cationic lipid bilayers. Cationic DODAB-cholesterol liposomes were rapidly mixed with DNA that intercalated between the cationic lipid membranes in the liposome. X-ray diffraction as well as cryomicroscopy confirmed that DNA is indeed intercalated between lipid bilayers. (Courtesy M. Hodošček.)

X-ray diffraction studies on DNA lipid complexes were given further impetus by the beautiful work of Safinya and coworkers (102,103). They systematically studied the diffraction of DNA–cationic lipid complexes when one varies the charge on the lipid bilayers by changing the lipid: DNA ratio. A systematic variation in the spacing between intercalated DNA molecules was found that followed the amount of charge present in the lipid subphase (102). Also, detailed analysis of the form of the DNA diffraction peak revealed a very peculiar anisotropic nature of correlations between the DNA chains intercalated between different bilayers (104). Furthermore, it was shown that the intercalated lamellar phase of the DNA–cationic lipid complexes is not the only, and maybe even not the most relevant one in connection with transfection in vivo. Koltover et al. (103) realized that if DOPE or the cosurfactant hexanol are added to the cationic DOTAP lipid, the DNA–cationic lipid

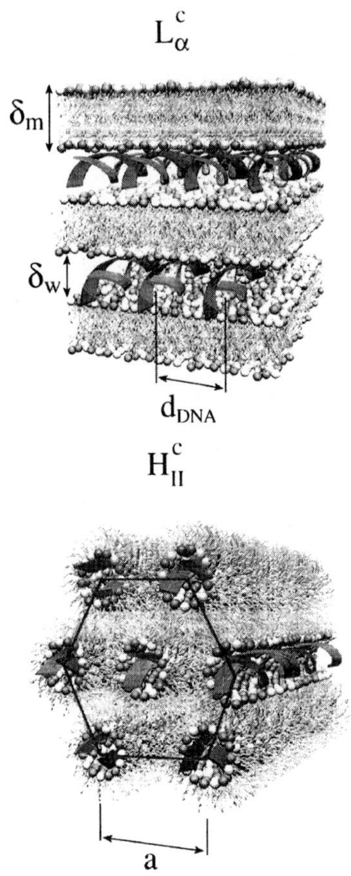

Figure 21 The structure of DNA–cationic lipid complexes in lamellar and inverted hexagonal phases. It seems that the lipids dictate the packing symmetry of the DNA–cationic lipid complex. While lipids can exist in both lamellar as well as inverted hexagonal phases (Fig. 13), lamellar packing of DNA by itself does not occur. These models of DNA packing in DNA–cationic lipid complexes demonstrate the power of x-ray scattering as a structural probe. (Adapted from Refs. 102, 103.)

shows the fingerprint of an inverted hexagonal phase (Fig. 21). In this phase, similarly to the hexagonal packing of DNA in concentrated solutions, DNA is arranged on the vortices of a hexagon, while lipids fill the space in between with their headgroups directed towards the charges on DNA. From the standpoint of the lipid this structure could also be called an inverted hexagonal phase, which is also well known for lipids in concentrated solutions. The way this transition comes about involves of course the two ''helpers'': DOPE and hexanol. DOPE is well known to make inverted hexagonal phases in solution because it is a conically shaped molecule that prefers strong negative curvatures. Hexanol, on the other hand, is a cosurfactant that drastically diminishes the curvature modulus of the bilayer and thus allows it to wrap tightly around each DNA molecule.

The inverted hexagonal DNA–cationic lipid phase was found to be more efficient in transfection because it is less stable and readily fuses with membranes of anionic vesicles, thus releasing the trapped DNA (103). These results point strongly to a close connection between transfection efficiency and the structure of the DNA–cationic lipid complex. If this connection is further corroborated, there is hope that our knowledge regarding the polymorphism of DNA, lipids, and DNA-lipid complexes might prove essential in engineering the structure of DNA vectors that will yield a programmed release of DNA in transfection.

A detailed electrostatic calculation based on the ideas of the DLVO theory of colloid stability has been performed for both cases to give the free energy change upon complexation (105). Depending on surface charge density, complexation free energies are on the order of 6–10 kT/bp. Again, the driving force of complexation is due to the release of counterions into the bulk. If the link between transfection efficiency and the structure of the DNA–cationic lipid complexes withstands the test of time, theoretical estimates of the complexation energies are very important since they can provide much needed guidance in the search for appropriate formulations of successful transfection vehicles.

We might add at the end that the two DNA–cationic lipid complexes described above do not in any way exhaust all structural possibilities. The seminal work of Ghirlando (106) shows that one can expect a much richer structural phase diagram for DNA condensation induced by cationic surfactants, including lipids. The lamellar intercalated and inverted hexagonal phases might only be the tips of a much richer iceberg. One might also safely expect to find (107) structural phases were the lipid hexagonal phase, characterized by hexagonal columnar packing of cylindrical lipid micelles, will be intercalated with a DNA hexagonal columnar crystal (Fig. 22) or even cubic micellar phase intercalated with a cubic or hexagonal DNA packing. There is no way to say offhand whether these hypothetical structures might not introduce new twists into a rational theory of in vivo genome delivery.

E. Colloidal Properties of DNA-Lipid Complexes

To use DNA–cationic lipid complexes in nonviral gene therapy, the complexes must be small enough to escape from blood vessels and then to diffuse through tissue. At the same time these complexes have to be stable enough in

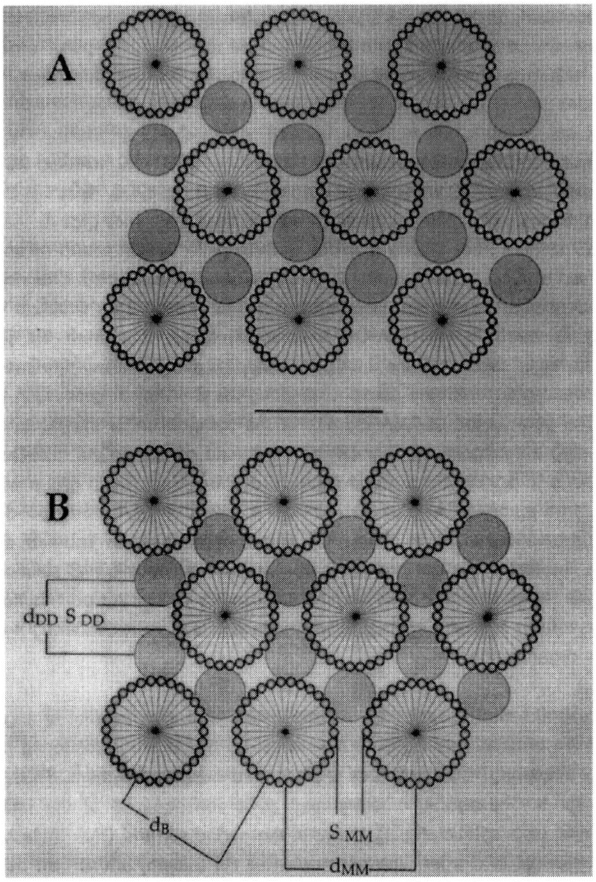

Figure 22 Lamellar and inverted hexagonal symmetries might not be the only possibilities for DNA–cationic lipid packing. Other structures of the DNA cationic surfactant assemblies have been seen. Here are two interpenetrating hexagonal lattices, one composed of DNA molecules and the other of cylindrical surfactant micelles at two different densities (A and B). (From Ref. 106, courtesy R. Ghirlando.)

serum to protect the DNA from nucleases and the immune system.

Colloidal properties of complexes can be determined by:

Capillary electrophoresis determining the electrostatic zeta-potential of the particles
Dynamic light scattering (DLS) for diffusion constants and consequently particle size
Single molecule counting devices that measure individual particle sizes from the flow of dilute suspensions through a small hole

Small size and solution stability can be achieved by preparing metastable overcharged complexes. Stable suspensions of complexes for in vivo transfection can be prepared by extruding small vesicles from cationic lipid–helper lipid mixtures, which are then mixed with plasmid DNA (101). This procedure resulted in 100 nm complexes containing only few plasmid DNAs. Empirically, a ratio of 2 to 10 cationic charges per anionic DNA charge has been found to be optimal for efficient transfection. The excess positive charge inhibits aggregation into larger complexes. Even though larger complexes are thermodynamically more favorable, the electrostatic energy barrier between particles can be high enough to stabilize a suspensions of virus-size complexes for months. In most cases helper lipids like DOPE or cholesterol that mix with the cationic lipid improve efficiency. As discussed earlier, they do this most probably by being able to match better the surface charge density to the charge density on DNA.

Typically colloidal interactions are taken to be nonspecific. Using these concepts when dealing with a complex system like a cell requires caution. Most of a cell's interactions with its environmental are very specific. Therefore it is not surprising that endocytosis and transport to the nucleus depend more on the particular chemical composition than on the structure of the complexes. More studies of these specific mechanisms are needed to design better delivery systems.

VI. RETROSPECT AND PROSPECT

Structural elucidation of DNA–cationic lipid complexes and realization of the extent to which they share the structural features of pure DNA or pure lipid polymorphism have advanced notably in the past few years. Some old questions have been answered and new questions raised. It is these new questions that challenge our knowledge of the intricacies of interactions between macromolecules.

The DNA-lipid complexes found so far are only a sample of the much wider set of structures that will be seen on a full DNA-lipid phase diagram. We argue that this larger set of possibilities should be approached by firmly established methods to measure the energies of these structures at the same time that they are determined and located on a phase diagram. Built on principles of direct molecular interactions, recognizing the consequences of thermal agitation, this line of observation and analysis can lead to an understanding of the energetic whys and preparative hows of complex structures.

Forces so delineated are already knowledgeably applied in new preparations. Precisely how the structure of DNA–lipid aggregates will affect their efficacy in transfection remains to be seen. So far the ideas we have are too general and have been learned from studying analytically tractable but technically inadequate preparations. General principles do not lead to specific results. Molecules are too interesting to allow easy success in clinical design. Still, there is little doubt of a practical link between the energy and structure of these complexes and their viability in a technological application.

Even the present general understanding of forces, even the cartoon ideas of the directions in which forces act in macromolecular complexes can tutor the bench scientist on how to improve preparations. There is enough known for a healthy iteration between experimental attempt and theoretical reason. Experimental successes and failures become the data for molecule force analyses. Various DNA-lipid assemblies reflect the various actions of competing forces. Molecular theorists can define and delineate these forces as they act to create each form; they can provide a logic to design variations in preparation. Basic scientists and clinicians are already in a position to help each other to improve their ways.

REFERENCES

1. Bloomfield VA, Crothers DM, Tinoco I. Nucleic Acids: Structures, Properties and Functions. Mill Valley: University Science Books (Sausalito, CA), 1998.
2. Vologotskii AV. Topology and Physics of Circular DNA (Physical Approaches to DNA). Boca Raton: CRC Press, 1992.
3. Strey HH, Podgornik R, Rau DC, Parsegian VA. Colloidal DNA. Curr Op Coll Interf Sci 1998; 3:534–539.
4. Podgornik R, Strey HH, Parsegian VA. DNA-DNA Interactions. Curr Op Struc Biol 1998; 8:309–313.
5. Kabanov VA, Flegner P, Seymour LW. Self-Assembling Complexes for Gene Delivery. New York: John Wiley and Sons, 1998.
6. Lasic DD. Liposomes in Gene Delivery. Boca Raton, FL: CRC Press, 1997.
7. Podgornik R. Rau DC, Parsegian VA. Parametrization of direct and soft steric-undulatory forces between DNA double helical polyelectrolytes in solutions of several different anions and cations. Biophys J 1994; 66:962–971.
8. Livolant F, Leforestier A. DNA mesophases. A structural analysis in polarizing and electron microscopy. Mol Cryst Liq Cryst 1992; 215:47–56.
9. Derjaguin BV, Churaev NV, Muller VM. Surface Forces. New York: Plenum Pub Corp, 1987.
10. Bloomfield VA. DNA condensation. Curr Op Struc Biol 1996; 6:334–341.
11. Leikin S, Parsegian VA, Rau DC, Rand RP. Hydration forces. Annu Rev Phys Chem 1993; 44:369–395.
12. Darnell J, Lodish H, Baltimore D. Molecular Cell Biology. 2d ed. New York: Scientific American Books, 1990.
13. Cerritelli ME, Cheng N, Rosenberg AH, McPherson CE, Booy FP, Steven AC. Encapsidated conformation of bacteriophage T7 DNA. Cell 1997; 91:271–280.
14. Safinya CR, Koltover I, Rädler J. DNA at membrane surfaces: an experimental overview. Curr Op Colloid Interf Sci 1998; 1:69–77.
15. Mahanty J, Ninham BW. Dispersion Forces. London: Academic Press, 1976.
16. Safran SA. Statistical Thermodynamics of Surfaces, Interfaces and Membranes. New York: Addison Wesley, 1994.
17. Eisenberg D, Kauzmann W. The Structure and Properties of Water. Oxford: Clarendon Press, 1969.
18. Parsegian VA, Rand RP, Fuller NL, Rau DC. Osmotic stress for the direct measurement of intermolecular forces. Methods Enzymol 1986; 127:400–416.
19. Marčelja S, Radić N. Repulsion of interfaces due to boundary water. Chem Phys Lett 1976; 42:129–130.
20. Rand RP, Parsegian VA. Hydration forces between phospholipid bilayers. Biochim Biophys Acta 1989; 988: 351–376.
21. Kornyshev AA, Leikin S. Fluctuation theory of hydration forces: the dramatic effects of inhomogeneous boundary conditions. Phys Rev A 1998; 40:6431–6437.
22. Rau DC, Parsegian VA. Direct measurement of the intermolecular forces between counterion-condensed DNA double helices. Evidence for long range attractive hydration forces. Biophys J 1992; 70:246–259.
23. Parsegian VA. Long-range physical forces in the biological milieu. Ann Rev Biophys Bioeng 1973; 2:221–255.
24. Bernal JD, Fankuchen I. X-ray and crystallographic studies of plant virus preparations. J Gen Physiol 1942; 25: 111–165.
25. Verwey EJW, Overbeek JTG. Theory of the Stability of Lyophobic Colloids. New York: Elsevier, 1948.
26. Hill TL. Statistical Mechanics. Principles and Selected Applications. New York: Dover, 1956.
27. Andelman D. Electrostatic properties of membranes: the Poisson-Boltzmann theory. In: Lipowsky R, Sackmann E, eds. Structure and Dynamics of Membranes. Vol. 1B. Amsterdam: Elsevier, 1995:603–642.
28. Landau LD, Lifshitz EM. The Classical Theory of Fields. 4th ed. Oxford: Pergamon Press, 1986.
29. McLaughlin S. Electrostatic potential at membrane solution interfaces. Curr Top Membrane Transp 1985; 4: 71–144.
30. Brenner SL, McQuarrie DA. Force balances in systems of cylindrical polyelectrolytes. Biophys J 1973; 13:301–331.
31. Parsegian VA, Rand RP, Fuller NL, Direct osmotic stress measurements of hydration and electrostatic double-layer forces between bilayers of double-chained ammonium acetate surfactants. J Phys Chem 1991; 95:4777–4782.
32. Kjellander R. Ion-ion correlations and effective charges in electrolyte and macroion systems. Ber Bunsenges Phys Chem 1996; 100:894–904.
33. Hunter RJ. Foundations of Colloid Science. New York: Oxford University Press, 1987.
34. Parsegian VA. Long range van der Waals forces. In: Olphen H, Mysels KL, eds. Physical Chemistry: Enriching Topics from Colloid and Interface Science. La Jolla: Theorex 1975:27–72.
35. Landau LD, Lifshitz EM. Statistical Physics Part 2. Oxford: Pergamon Press, 1986.

36. Parsegian VA, Rand RP. Interaction in membrane assemblies. In: Lipowsky R, Sackmann E, eds. Structure and Dynamics of Membranes. Vol. 1B. Amsterdam: Elsevier, 1995:643–690.
37. Parsegian VA. Non-retarded van der Waals between anisotropic long thin rods at all angles. J Chem Phys 1972; 56: 4393–4397.
38. Brenner SL, Parsegian VA. A physical method for deriving the electrostatic interaction between rod-like polyions at all mutual angles. Biophys J 1974; 14:327–334.
39. Parsegian VA, Fuller N, Rand RP. Measured work of deformation and repulsion of lecithin bilayers. Proc Natl Acad Sci 1979; 76:2750–2754.
40. Lipowsky R. Generic interactions of flexible membranes. In: Lipowsky R, Sackmann E, eds. Structure and Dynamics of Membranes. Vol. 1B. Amsterdam: Elsevier, 1995: 521–596.
41. Helfrich W. Steric interactions of fluid membranes in multilayer systems. Z Naturforsch 1978; 33a:305–315.
42. Strey HH, Parsegian VA, Podgornik R. Equation of state for polymer liquid crystals: theory and experiment. Phys Rev E 1998; 59:999–1008.
43. Seifert U, Lipowsky R. Morphology of Vesicles. In: Lipowsky R, Sackmann E, eds. Structure and Dynamics of Membranes. Vol. 1A. Amsterdam: Elsevier, 1995: 403–446.
44. Podgornik R, Parsegian VA. Thermal-mechanical fluctuations of fluid membrans in confined geometries: the case of soft confinement. Langmuir 1992; 8:557–562.
45. Podgornik R, Parsegian VA. Charge-fluctuation forces between rodlike polyelectrolytes: pairwse summability reexamined. Phys Rev Lett 1998; 80:1560–1563.
46. Ha BJ, Liu AJ. Counterion-mediated attraction between two like charged rods. Phys Rev Lett 1997; 79:1289–1292.
47. Saenger W. Principles of Nucleic Acid Structure. New York: Springer-Verlag, 1984.
48. Rhodes D, Klug A. Helical periodicity of DNA determined by enzyme digestion. Nature 1980; 286:573–578.
49. Rill RL. Liquid crystalline phases in concentrated DNA solutions. In: Pifa-Mrzljak G, ed. Supramolecular Structure and Function. New York: Springer, 1988:166–167.
50. De Gennes PG, Prost J. The Physics of Liquid Crystals. 2d ed. Oxford: Oxford University Press, 1993.
51. Hagerman PJ. Flexibility of DNA. Ann Rev Biophys Biophys Chem 1988; 17:265–286.
52. Pruss GJ, Drlica K. Dna supercoiling and prokaryotic transcription. Cell 1989; 56:521–523.
53. Grosberg AY, Khokhlov AR. Statistical Physics of Macromolecules (AIP Series in Polymers and Complex Materials). New York: American Institute of Physics, 1994.
54. Rau DC, Lee BK, Parsegian VA, Measurement of the repulsive force between polyelectrolyte molecules in ionic solution: hydration forces between parallel DNA double helices. PNAS 1984; 81:2621–2625.
55. Strey HH, Parsegian VA, Podgornik R. Equation of state for DNA liquid crystals: fluctuation enchanced electrostatic double layer repulsion. Phys Rev Lett 1997; 78: 895–898.
56. Reich Z, Wachtel EJ, Minsky A. In vivo quantitative characterization of intermolecular interaction. J Biol Chem 1995; 270:7045–7046.
57. Barrat JL, Joanny JF. Theory of polyelectrolyte solutions. In: Prigogine I, Rice SA, eds. Advances in Chemical Phsyics. New York: John Wiley and Sons, 1995:1–66.
58. Lyubartsev AP, Nordenskiold L. Monte Carlo simulation study of ion distribution and osmotic pressure in hexagonally oriented DNA. J Phys Chem 1995; 99:10373–10382.
59. Oosawa F. Polyelectrolytes. New York: Marcel Dekker, 1971.
60. Rouzina I, Bloomfield VA. Macro-ion attraction due to electrostatic correlation between screening counterions. J Phys Chem 1996; 100:9977–9989.
61. Podgornik R, Strey HH, Rau DC, Parsegian VA. Watching molecules crowd: DNA double helices under osmotic stress. Biophys Chem 1995; 26:111–121.
62. Lindsay SM, Lee SA, Powell JW, Weidlich T, Demarco C, Lewen GD, Tao NJ, Rupprecht A. The origin of the A to B transition in DNA fibers and films. Biopolymers 1988; 17:1015–1043.
63. Podgornik R, Strey HH, Gawrisch K, Rau DC, Rupprecht A, Parsegian VA. Bond orientational order, molecular motion, and free energy of high-density DNA mesophases. Proc Natl Acad Sci USA 1996; 93:4261–4266.
64. Strandberg D. Bond-Orientational Order in Condensed Matter Systems. New York: Springer, 1992.
65. Durand D. Doucet J, Livolant F. A study of the structure of highly concentrated phases of DNA by x-ray diffraction. J Phys II France 1992; 2:1769–1783.
66. Kamien RD. Liquids with chiral bond order. J Phys II France 1996; 6:461–475.
67. Chaikin PM, Lubensky TC. Principles of Condensed Matter Physics. Cambridge: Cambridge University Press, 1995.
68. Leforestier A, Livolant F. DNA Liquid-crystalline blue phases—electron-microscopy evidence and biological implications. Mol Cryst Liquid Cryst 1994; 17:651–658.
69. Wang L, Bloomfield VA. Small-angle x-ray scattering of semidilute rodlike DNA solutions: polyelectrolyte behavior. Macromolecules 1991; 24:5791–5795.
70. Podgornik R, Rau DC, Parsegian VA. The action of interhelical forces on the organization of DNA double helices: fluctuation enhanced decay of electrostatic double layer and hydration forces. Macromolecules 1989; 22: 1780–1786.
71. Frank-Kamenetskii MD, Anshelevich VV, Lukashin AV. Polyelectrolyte model of DNA. Sov Phys Usp 1987; 4: 317–330.
72. Tanford C. The Hydrophobic Effect. Formation of Micelles and Biological Membranes. New York: John Wiley and Sons, 1980.
73. Cevc G, Marsh D. Phospholipid Bilayers: Physical Principles and Models (Cell Biology: A Series of Monographs, Vol. 5) New York: John Wiley & Sons.
74. Parsegian VA, Evans EA. Long and short range intermolecular and intercolloidal forces. Curr Opin Coll Interf Sci 1996; 1:53–60.
75. Duzgunes N, Wilshut L, Hong K, Fraley R, Perry C, Friends DS, James TL, Papahadjopoulos D. Physicochem-

ical characterization of large unilamellar phospholipid vesicles prepared by reverse-phase evaporation. Biochim. Biophys. ACTA 1983; 732:289–299.
76. Seifert U. Configurations of fluid membranes and vesicles. Adv Phys 1997; 46:13–137.
77. Small DM. The Physical Chemistry of Lipids. From Alkanes to Phospholipids. New York: Plenum Press, 1986.
78. Gruner SM, Parsegian VA, Rand RP. Directly measured deformation energy of phospholipid H2 hexagonal phases. Faraday Disc 1986; 81:213–221.
79. Daoud M, Williams CE. Soft Matter Physics. New York: Springer, 1999.
80. Lasic DD. Liposomes: From Physics to Applications. Amsterdam: Elsevier, 1993.
81. Parsegian VA, Podgornik R. Surface-tension suppression of lamellar swelling on solid substrates. Colloids Surf A Physicochem Eng Asp 1997; 129–130:345–364.
82. Roux D, Safinya CR. A synchrotron x-ray study of competing undulation and electrostatic interlayer interactions in fluid multimembrane lyotropic phases. J Phys-Paris 1988; 49:307–318.
83. Leneveu DM, Rand RP, Gingell D, Parsegian VA, Apparent modification of forces between lecithin bilayers. Science 1976; 191:399–400.
84. Parsegian VA. Reconciliation of van der Waals force measurements between phosphatidylcholine bilayers in water and between bilayer coated mica surfaces. Langmuir 1993; 9:3625–3628.
85. Gouliaev N, Nagle JF. Simulations of interacting membranes in soft confinement regime. Phys Rev Lett 1998; 81:2610–2613.
86. Rand RP, Parsegian VA. Hydration forces between phospholipid bilayers. Biochim Biophys Acta 1989; 988: 351–376.
87. Petrache HI, Gouliaev N, Tristram-Nagle S, Zhang R, Suter RM, Nagle JF. Interbilayer interactions from high-resolution x-ray scattering. Phys Rev E 1998; 57: 7014–7024.
88. Fang Y, Yang J. Two-dimensional condensation fo DNA molecules on cationic lipid membranes. J Phys Chem 1997; 101:441–449.
89. Bruinsma R. Electrostatics of DNA-cationic lipid complexes: isoelectric instability. Eur Phys J B 1998; 4:75–88.
90. O'Hern CS, Lubensky TC. Sliding columnar phase of DNA lipid complexes. Phys Rev Lett 1998; 80: 4345–4348.
91. Golubovic L, Golubovic M. Fluctuations of quasi-two-dimensional smectics intercalated between membranes in multilamellar phases of DNA cationic lipid complexes. Phys. Rev. Lett. 1998; 80:4341–4344.
92. Melghani MS, Yang J. Stable adsorption of DNA on zwitterionic lipid bilayers (preprint, 1999).
93. Fang Y, Yang J. Two-dimensional condensation of DNA molecules on cationic lipid membranes. J Phys Chem B 1996; 101:441–449.
94. Lvov Y, Decher G, Sukhorukhov G. Assembly of thin films by means of successive deposition of alternate layers of DNA and poly(allylamine). Macromolecules 1993; 26: 5396–5399.
95. Lasic DD, Papahadjopoulos D, Podgornik R. Polymorphism of lipids, nucleic acids, and their interactions. In: Kabanov AV, Felgner PL, Seymour LW, eds. Self-assembling complexes for gene delivery: from laboratory to delivery. Chichester: J. Wiley, 1998:3–26.
96. Felgner PL, Ringold GM. Cationic liposome-mediated transfection. Nature 1989; 337:387–388.
97. Gershon H, Ghirlando R, Guttman SB, Minsky A. Mode of formation and structural features of DNA-cationic liposome complexes used for transfection. Biochemistry 1993; 32:7143–7151.
98. Sternberg B, Sorgi FL, Huang L. New structures in complex-formation between DNA and cationic liposomes visualized by freeze-fracture electron-microscopy. FEBS Lett 1994; 356:361–366.
99. Lasic DD, Barenholz Y. Handbook of Nonmedical Applications of Liposomes: From Gene Delivery and Diagnostics to Ecology. Boca Raton, FL: CRC Press, 1996:43–57.
100. Lasic DD, Strey H, Stuart MCA, Podgornik R, Frederik PM. The structure of DNA-liposome complexes. J Am Chem Soc 1997; 119:832–833.
101. Templeton NS, Lasic DD, Frederik PM, Strey HH, Roberts DD, Pavlakis GN. Improved DNA:liposome complexes for increased systemic delivery and gene expression. Nature Biotechnol 1997; 15:647–652.
102. Radler JO, Koltover I, Salditt T, et al. Structure of DNA-cationic liposome complexes: DNA intercalation in multilamellar membranes in distinct interhelical packing regimes. Science 1997; 275:810–814.
103. Koltover I, Salditt T, Radler JO, et al. An inverted hexagonal phase of cationic liposome-DNA complexes related to DNA release and delivery. Science 1998; 281:78–81.
104. Salditt T, Koltover I, Radler O, et al. Self-assembled DNA-cationic-lipid complexes: two-dimensional smectic ordering, correlations, and interactions. Phys Rev E 1998; 58: 889–904.
105. Harries D, May S, Gelbart WM, Ben-Shaul A. Structure, stability and thermodynamics of lamellar DNA-lipid complexes. Biophys J 1998; 75:159–173.
106. Ghirlando R. DNA condensation induced by cationic surfactants. Ph.D. dissertation. The Weizmann Institute of Science, Rehovot, Israel, 1991.
107. Ghirlando R. DNA Condensation induced by cationic surfactants. Ph.D. dissertation. The Weizmann Institute of Science, Rehovot, Israel, 1991.
108. Kleinschmidt AK, Lang D, Jacherts D, Zahn RK. Darstellung und langen messungen des gesamten desoxyribonuclein-saure inhaltes von T2-bakteriophagen. Biochim Biophys ACTA 1962; 61:857–864.
109. Kessel RG, Kardon RH. Tissues and Organs. San Francisco: W.H. Freeman and Co, 1979.
110. Heller H, Schaefer M, Schulten K. Molecular dynamics simulation of a bilayer of 200 lipids in the gel and in the liquid-crystal phases. J Phys Chem 1993; 97:8343–8360.

12

Bioorganic Colloids: Macromolecules, DNA, Self-Assembled Particles, and Their Complexes

Danilo D. Lasic
Liposome Consultations, Newark, California

Nancy Smyth Templeton
Baylor College of Medicine, Houston, Texas

I. GENERAL INTRODUCTION TO COLLOIDS

Colloids are systems in which one phase is dispersed in another continuous phase, normally—but not necessarily—in a different aggregate state. The dimensions of the dispersed phase are typically in the range of several to a few thousand nanometers. In gene delivery aqueous colloidal dispersions are encountered because DNA plasmids, liposomes, and their complexes as well as viral constructs are formed, depending on thermodynamic conditions and kinetic parameters, stable colloidal dispersions, or unstable precipitates (cakes). Because of the didactic nature of this book, we shall briefly introduce colloidal systems relevant in gene delivery.

A. Brief History

While stable emulsions (milk and milk product–based mixtures) and lyophobic suspensions (aqueous suspensions of insoluble hydrophobic pigments) have been known since the Stone Age, it was realized only some 200 years ago that some opalescent solutions behave differently than do regular solutions. In addition to slight turbidity, it was, for instance, found that solutions of gelatin, albumin, or silicic acid pass through parchment membrane much more slowly than salt or sugar solutions. Due to this glue-like property, T. Graham called them colloids (*colla* meaning glue in Greek) in 1861. The colloidal state, had been studied earlier by Bergman (silicic acid, 1779), Berzelius (arsenic sulfide, 1833), and Faraday (colloidal gold, 1857). Following Faraday's work, Tyndall in 1869 explained the turbidity of colloids by scattering of light by particles. Continuing work of Raleigh (scattering of light as a function of particle size in 1871), Gouy (electric potential, 1888, and explanation of Brownian motion discovered in 1827), Ostwald, and many others resulted in rapid development of the field. We must not forget the theoretical contributions of Einstein (theory of Brownian motion, 1905) and Perrin, who also determined Avogadro's number from a diffusion of gamboge and mastic to be between 5.5 and 8×10^{23}. Svedberg and Brillouin later also used colloidal gamboge and gold and obtained 6×10^{23} in 1911 and 1912, respectively. Studying colloidal electrolytes, McBain in the 1910s established the structure of the micelle, the idea of which was at first hotly disputed. The micelle is an example of a self-assembled colloidal particle, as opposed to dispersed solids or gels. In the period between World Wars I and II, it was established that colloidal solutions contain particles smaller than the resolution power of the optical microscope (0.2 m) and larger than ~5 nm, which classified many protein and polymer solutions as colloidal, as indeed their properties, e.g., viscosity, surface tension, electrophoretic mobility, and sedimentation coefficient, indicated. In the 1940s the DLVO theory of colloidal stability was established (by Derjaguin and Landau in 1943 and Verwey and Overbeek in 1948), which postulated that in the case of electrostatic repulsion exceeding ubiquitous van der Waals attraction, colloidal systems can be stable. Obviously many systems, such as uncharged soot particles or lecithin liposomes, do not obey this law. Work in the last several decades added several new forces, such as repulsive hydration, and steric and undulation forces, which could explain the stability of particles. Attractive forces due to hydrophobic interaction and ion-correlation forces are also better understood. While inorganic colloidal particles have been introduced in novel sizes, shapes, and compositions since the beginning of the century, the development of polymer chemistry resulted in many organic colloids, such as latex particles, microspheres, micellar block copolymers, and dendrimers. Emulsions were studied as well as self-assembled colloidal particles. Although lecithin sols—as colloidal solutions have been sometimes called—have been studied for more than a century, it was Bangham in the early 1960s who discovered liposomes and recognized their unique properties. Following this short historical introduction, we shall introduce suspensions of biological colloids and their applications in drug and gene delivery.

B. Aqueous Colloidal Suspensions

Colloidal suspensions are, by definition, dispersions of small particles with at least one—typically the largest—dimension in the size range from 1 nm to 1 μm in a continuous medium. While the continuous medium can be gas (e.g., fog, smoke), liquid (e.g., milk, wine), or solid (e.g., clay, butter), we shall discuss only liquid systems and, among those, mostly the ones in which water is the continuous phase. They are distinguished from normal solutions by their ability to scatter light, apparent lack of osmotic pressure and freezing point depression, slow diffusion rate as well as sedimentation in a centrifugal field and normally relatively high viscosity.

Colloids can be either lyophilic and lyophobic. The former are formed spontaneously (albeit often very slowly, e.g., dissolution of large DNA molecules or liposomes by some detergents) and typically consist of large macromolecules in a solvent (proteins, starch in water) or micelles (soaps, detergents). Lyophobic colloids consist of aggregates of insoluble substances produced either by specific chemical reactions (quick precipitation, mixing melt or fusing metal into an aqueous phase, swelling, agitation, etc.) or by downsizing or milling (homogenization or colloidal mill) of larger particles in aqueous phase or normal suspensions. The best known examples range from historically important systems of silver iodide, iron hydroxides, carbon black, platinum, and gold to the now widely used silica, titania, as well as emulsions and liposomes.

Aqueous colloidal systems are important in many scientific disciplines as well as in biological processes, which support life. Biological colloids include (lipo)proteins, nucleic acids and other macromolecules, suspensions of cells, cell organelles, and viruses in vitro as well as cells in blood, synaptic, and many other (secretory, trafficking, etc.) vesicles in vivo. Additionally, intake into cells, secretion from cells, and inter- and intracellular communication often occur via different lipid vesicles.

In contrast to other systems, such as solids, crystals, and solutions, lyophobic colloidal systems are typically not in a thermodynamically stable state. They are kinetically trapped states rather than in a thermodynamic equilibrium. Therefore their characteristics, such as stability and size distribution, depend on, in addition to thermodynamic factors (including concentration, temperature, ionic strength, acidity, and presence of impurities), also on kinetic factors, such as the preparation path. This kinetic component is the reason why the preparation of colloidal systems is often characterized by low reproducibility. Now, however, we understand the importance of the sequence of operations and can carefully control the energy (and power) intake in each step, resulting in reproducible and scale-invariant preparations of colloidal suspensions, such as liposomes or emulsions.

Apart from the theoretical importance of understanding colloids, they offer numerous applications. Inorganic colloidal particles from metals, metal oxides, silica, silicates, and ceramics are used in coating, ceramic, metal, semiconductor, computer, and many other industries. Organic colloids can be solid, semi-solid, or fluid. Solid organic colloids such as latex particles and polymers are used in diagnostics, coating, pharmacological, food, paper, and some other industries, while semi-solid or fluid particles, such as micelles, liposomes, emulsions, and microemulsions, are also used in the cosmetics industry, in diagnostics, and as drug-delivery vehicles.

Micelles, liquid crystals, and liposomes are self-assembling colloids, meaning that amphiphilic molecules self-aggregate into ordered structures. Several other self-assembling particles, which have different local symmetry as compared to liposomes or micelles, as will be mentioned below, are simply dispersed liquid crystals in excess water. Because, additionally, different lipid structures and symmetries, as opposed to lamellar symmetry of liposomes, might be important in biological processes, such as cell fusion, we shall briefly introduce liquid crystals. They are normally considered colloidal systems, despite the fact that some of their dimensions can be macroscopic.

Liquid crystals are systems that are simultaneously characterized by some properties of liquids and solids. Similarly to liquids, they can flow, form droplets, and take on the shape of the container. However, the molecules possess some short- as well as long-range order. While in liquids there is no orientational and translational (positional) order, liquid crystals can have at least orientational order (and possibly translational order in one or two dimensions), resulting in anisotropy of optical, mechanic, and electromagnetic properties (1).

Lyotropic liquid crystals are anisotropic phases of amphiphiles at higher concentrations in water mixtures. At higher concentrations lipid-based colloidal systems as well as nucleic acids (above ca 500 base pairs in length) form lyotropic liquid crystalline phases (see Chapter 11). These phases are often characterized by a long-range orientational order at translational (positional) disorder. At higher concentrations translational order in one or two dimensions may occur. Liposomes and some other lipid colloidal particles are simply dispersions of lyotropic phases in excess water.

C. Colloidal Particles in Living Systems

The functioning of living systems is based not only on the order, organization, compartmentalization, and accompanying information but also on rapid diffusion of this information and the molecules supporting it between various compartments and through barriers separating them. Therefore, the organization in living systems is based on liquid crystalline rather than on crystalline systems, where the diffusion is too slow to be of interest for biological systems. Both polar lipids and DNA in aqueous mixtures form different liquid crystalline phases. The most important biological colloids are lipid membranes and colloidal DNA. In vitro, both of these systems, however, typically form smaller particles, such as liposomes and DNA plasmids.

Nonliving nature can create large, well-ordered systems, such as monocrystals meters long which are nonetheless characterized by a rather simple structure. On the other hand, living nature can create much more complex organizations of complex macromolecules on colloidal scale. These include self-assembly of lipid molecules into structures with complex topology and the ability to compartmentalize space (1,2) as well as molecules of nucleic acids, which can store and duplicate information and also use it for spatially and temporally controlled function, molecular construction, and action (3–5).

Lipid bilayers and other lipid phases as well as DNA and its liquid crystalline behavior are the best known examples of super- and supramolecular organization in biology. In addition to structural and dynamic information about lipid bilayers, DNA also contains genetic information, which is stored in a sequence of bases. The aim of molecular biotechnology is to manipulate this genetic information in the test tube and express the genes in exogenous cells and organisms. While in living systems lipid bilayers and DNA form lyotropic liquid crystals, in the test tube such systems can be fragmented or diluted into finite particles, which behave as classical colloids.

In general one can distinguish between solid (and semisolid) particulate, macromolecular, and self-assembled colloidal particles. Solid particles are typically small organic or inorganic systems. In gene delivery they can be used as a substrate for DNA adsorption in the gene gun. For gene delivery by nonviral vectors, however, only the latter two systems are interesting and will be further discussed below. Obviously, also viral gene-delivery systems form colloidal suspensions. First we shall briefly describe the colloidal behavior of dissolved macromolecules in aqueous suspensions.

II. MACROMOLECULAR COLLOIDS

Due to their size, many natural and synthetic molecules, such as proteins and polymers, form colloidal suspensions when dissolved in aqueous phase. Below we shall briefly describe a few such systems.

A. Macromolecules

In aqueous macromolecular suspensions interactions with the solvent are typically much more important than in the case of small molecules, and therefore their behavior is far from ideal. In a good solvent (stronger attractive interactions between polymer and solvent molecules than intra- and interpolymer interactions), polymer stretches and uncoils. At higher concentrations and in worse solvents, polymers start to coil, and eventually, in a bad solvent, they phase separate (flocculate) and eventually precipitate. Solutions of polymers are normally characterized by thermodynamic, x-ray and light scattering, sedimentation, viscosity, and hydrodynamic measurements. Complex theories have been developed to describe their behavior (6,7). Nevertheless, the apparent anomaly of their colligative properties, so puzzling some 75 years ago, can be now easily explained by large molecular masses of macromolecules. Examples of macromolecular colloids are aqueous suspensions of polyethylene, polystyrene, polyoxyethylene, and, in biological systems, globular proteins, polysaccharides, polypeptides and nucleic acids (DNA, RNA, antisense oligonucleotides, ribozymes).

B. Polyelectrolytes

Polyelectrolytes are charged polymers. Charged groups on the polymer chain influence its conformation. Typically, polyelectrolytes are, because of repulsion between charges on the polymer backbone, more extended than noncharged polymers and can at higher concentrations form ordered phases, especially if they are rather rigid. Their colloidal behavior, structure, conformation, and interaction characteristics, which all strongly depend on ionic conditions in the solution, can be studied in addition to the above-mentioned methods by zeta potential measurements and polyion dynamics in electric fields. Examples of negatively charged polyelectrolytes are polystyrene-sulfonic acid, polyglutamic acid, and nucleic acids, while examples of positively charged include polyamines, polyethyleneimine, polyvinyl pyridine, and others. While theoretical and experimental studies mostly concentrate on linear homopolymers, block copolymers, branched polymers, and starburst (dendritic) structures are becoming increasingly important in various applications. Theoretical description of polyelectrolytes is based mostly on electrostatic forces. Their interactions with oppositely charged colloidal particles or polyelectrolytes are becoming very important for drug and gene delivery. However, little theoretical or experimental work has been done to parallel gene-transfection experiments (which start with mixing of DNA, ribozymes, or antisense oligonucleotides with cationic liposomes or polymers and measuring gene expression after administration) with the physicochemical properties of the complexes.

C. Nucleic Acids

DNA is a biopolyelectrolyte that contains the complete information (''blueprint'') that specifies structural and temporal synthesis of all the proteins and RNA molecules, thus determining the activity and individuality of every given organism (with the exception of some RNA viruses that never produce DNA in any part of their life cycle) during its life (4). This information, which is coded in a sequence of bases (primary structure), is maintained by replication and executed by transcription (synthesis of RNA) followed by translation (subsequent protein synthesis from RNA). A strand of DNA consists of a string of deoxyriboses with attached bases [guanine (G), adenosine (A), cytosine (C), and thymine (T)] bridged by a phosphate.

In aqueous suspensions DNA forms a double helix (a secondary structure in which H bonds pair A-T and G-C), which exhibits an A, B, C, or Z conformation, depending on ionic conditions, concentration, and sequence. In standard solvents and conditions, mostly the B conformation occurs (10.4 base pairs form a pitch with a length of 0.34 nm per base pair with diameter of 2 nm). This molecule, defined as a tertiary structure, can be further linear, circular (self-closed), nicked (self-closed with one strain broken), or supercoiled (like wrapped and wound elastic band), which significantly reduces its dimensions (8–10).

Rigidity of polymers is expressed as persistence length (i.e., length of an arc, which can bend 180 degrees at thermal energy). The DNA double helix is rather rigid because the persistence length is around 50 nm. This depends on the primary structure and can decrease upon strong interaction of the polymer with counterions or adsorbed proteins. Sharp turns observed in some systems very likely harbor a nicked string.

DNA molecules in living cells can have contour lengths of the order of centimeters, and yet they fit into a small cell. In the cell nucleus (diameter 5–8 μm) they are tightly packed in chromosomes that contain several packing orders of chromatin, a nucleohistone complex in which DNA is tightly wrapped around spherical basic (positively charged) proteins. Similarly, DNA in a colloidal suspension can be condensed by addition of condensing agents, such as multivalent cations (e.g., Co^{3+}), polycations (spermine^{4+}), cationic polypeptides (polylysine), cationic polymers, and vesicles. Typically, condensed structures are, depending on the condensing agent, either small toroids (outer diameter ~70–100 nm, inner diameter ~30 nm smaller) or rodlike particles of equal diameter (bunch of DNA fibers) and volume. DNA condensates can be also disordered. In the case of univalent cationic lipid liposomes, an intercalated lamellar phase with two-dimensionally condensed DNA was observed. Minimal base pair content of a condensed ordered particle is around 30–50 kb and can be fulfilled by one or many plasmids. In the process of DNA condensation, the hydrodynamic volume of the macromolecule can be reduced up to a millionfold. Several articles report very small spherical DNA condensates, possibly containing a single DNA plasmid. Because of DNA rigidity, such reports must be critically addressed for possible artifacts. Also, as will be shown below, it seems that in many cases lipids condense DNA into two-dimensional condensates rather than three-dimensional tori or rodlike particles.

III. PLASMID DESIGN, GENE DELIVERY, AND GENE EXPRESSION

Recombinant DNA technology allows production of specific proteins in different host organisms. A gene for a particular protein is ligated into a specifically designed plasmid and inserted into cells of host species, which can range from bacteria and plants to mammals. The cells then start to synthesize the encoded protein, which is either harvested from these cells or excreted in some body fluids or fruits. In addition to the synthesis of proteins, plasmids themselves can be multiplied and harvested in such a process. Typically, 1–10 mg of purified plasmid can be purified from 1 L of bacterial broth.

While general DNA interactions and condensation are largely independent of primary, secondary, and even tertiary DNA structure, on the other hand, gene expression critically depends on the primary structure and function of various sequences ligated into the plasmid. The basic elements used in the creation of expression vectors have been comprehensively reviewed (11).

Points to consider in achieving expression of a cDNA of interest include the required level of expression, regulated or inducible expression, and the cell types or tissues that will be transfected. Typically, each plasmid contains various functional sequences such as tissue-specific promoters, promoters + enhancer, hybrid or synthetic introns, and translation-enhancing sequences (and possibly cassettes for autonomous replication and nuclear retention, DNA insertion and recombination) upstream of the complementary DNA (cDNA or exon that encodes the desired protein) and the untranslated region (polyadenylation signals, downstream (Fig. 1).

The major classes of promoter + enhancer regions used to provide gene expression include viral, cellular, and inducible (11). The most commonly used viral promoter + enhancer region is the human cytomegalovirus (CMV) immediate-early gene promoter + enhancer. This regulatory region provides the highest levels of gene expression in virtually all cell types and tissues of most species. The simian virus 40 (SV40) promoter + enhancer is also often used; however, the level of gene expression produced is far less than that produced by the CMV promoter + enhancer. Other viral enhancers sometimes used include those from polyoma virus, retroviruses, papilloma virus, hepatitis B virus, human immunodeficiency virus (HIV), and the gibbon ape leukemia virus (11).

Gene expression produced by some cellular promoters and enhancers can be induced or repressed (11). The metallothionein (MT) promoter and the mouse mammary tumor virus (MMTV) promoter are the most frequently used inducible promoters. The MT promoter is induced by heavy metals such as zinc, cadmium, and copper or by the phorbol ester 12-0-tetradecanoyl phorbol-13-acetate (TPA). A tightly regulated MT promoter containing only two copies of the highly conserved 17 bp metal-regulatory element produces a 10- to 20-fold increase in gene expression upon induction (12). Other promoters that can be tightly regulated include the tetracycline-responsive promoters (13) and promoters for steroid hormone receptors.

Gene expression can be increased by including a functional intron in the expression vector. The increase in mRNA produced can range from 10- to 100-fold, and artificial introns are highly functional. These introns are usually placed immediately downstream of the promoter + enhancer region. Placement of an appropriate 3′ untranslated region (UTR) immediately downstream of the cDNA coding region is crucial. The 3′ UTR includes sequences for the polyadenylation signal (poly A). Derivatives of the SV40 poly A sequences are usually used for construction of gene expression vectors. The 3′ UTR provides for mRNA stability and efficient transport of mRNA to the cytoplasm and can increase the efficiency of mRNA translation. In addition, sequences for an internal ribosome entry site (IRES) are used to increase the efficiency of mRNA translation. IRES sequences are placed immediately upstream of the 5′ end of the cDNA coding region. The IRES sequence from the encephalomyocarditis virus (EMCV) is frequently used. The inverted terminal repeats (ITRs) can bind proteins that mediate attachment to the nuclear matrix (14). In addition, ITRs can provide for enhanced gene expression and efficient transcription (15). DNA ends, such as ITRs and telomeres, can be protected from degradation by protein attachments to the ends. Finally, efficient nuclear transport can be mediated by nuclear localization signals (NLSs), which are provided as peptides or proteins that contain NLSs or DNA sequences that can bind appropriate endogenous proteins.

After construction and amplification of plasmids, they must be delivered to the appropriate cells in order to induce gene expression (i.e., synthesis of the encoded protein by the cell machinery). The delivery of these large molecules

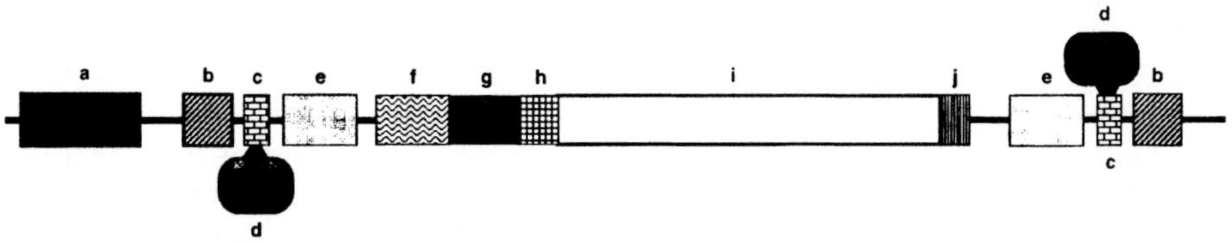

Figure 1 A segment of the hypothetical plasmid, which induces gene expression. Normally not all the sequences are included. (a) Autonomous replication/nuclear retention sequences; (b) sequences for homologous recombination; (c) site-specific integration part; (d) site-specific recombination; (e) tissue-specific promoter; (f) promoter enhancer region; (g) hybrid or synthetic introns; (h) translation-enhancing sequences; (i) cDNA; (j) 3′ untranslated region, including a polyadenylation signal.

seems to be the most difficult challenge in gene therapy and is discussed in most of this book as well as elsewhere in this chapter.

Reporter genes are often used to measure the efficiency of gene transfer in vivo and in vitro. Protein products encoded by most of these genes can be readily assayed by enzyme-linked immunoassay (ELISA) kits that are commercially available, and several other procedures exist that are used for in vivo and in vitro detection of reporter gene products. Reporter genes that are commonly used include chloramphenicol acetyl transferase (CAT), β-galactosidase (β-Gal), luciferase (Luc), human growth hormone (hGH), and the green fluorescent protein (GFP). Typically, initial experiments are performed using reporter genes to measure the efficacy of gene expression from DNA constructs. After gene expression has been demonstrated in the appropriate cells or tissues at an adequate level, the cDNA of interest is substituted for the reporter gene. Recently, however, many researchers bypass the reporter genes by the direct detection of therapeutic mRNA by highly automated PCR techniques. These plasmids are nowadays delivered into cells using either mechanical methods (direct injection, osmotic shocks, electroporation, gene gun) or polymeric (16,17) or lipid DNA carriers (18–20).

IV. SELF-ASSEMBLING COLLOIDAL PARTICLES

Polar lipids are molecules containing hydrophilic and hydrophobic parts. Therefore, these molecules form ordered structures in aqueous solutions because contact of nonpolar with polar phases is not energetically favored. In aqueous mixtures lipids give rise to structurally rich phase diagrams (Fig. 2). The richness of different phases (as shown in Fig. 2) depends on the molecular geometry and interaction properties of lipid molecules. In living systems, predominantly a lamellar phase, along with an isotropic micellar phase, is present. For instance, each cell membrane is actually a piece of a fully swollen lamellar phase self-enclosed into a spherical bag (with various distortions), which supports numerous proteins associated within to carry out their functions. The phase diagram shown in Figure 2 can be applied to many different lipid-water systems, including diacyl chain cationic lipids. In the case of cationic lipids mostly lamellar phases are present, which upon dilution give rise to liposomes. In the case of some univalent lipids, however, an inverse hexagonal phase can also be formed, which gives rise upon dilution and sonication to a stable colloidal dispersion of hexasomes, typically in the size range of 100–150 nm.

A useful parameter to describe the shape of the repeating units in liquid crystalline phases or macroscopically isotropic solutions of colloidal particles is the so-called packing parameter (Fig. 3) (21). Briefly, in the cases where the cross section of the hydrophobic part (b) is similar to the area of the polar head (a) of the lipid, these molecules pack into flat bilayers (i.e., with zero curvature, c = 0). For b > a we observe the formation of inverse structures with negative curvature, such as inverse micelles and inverse hexagonal (II) phase, while for a > b we observe normal micelles (c > 0), which can form isotropic phases or pack

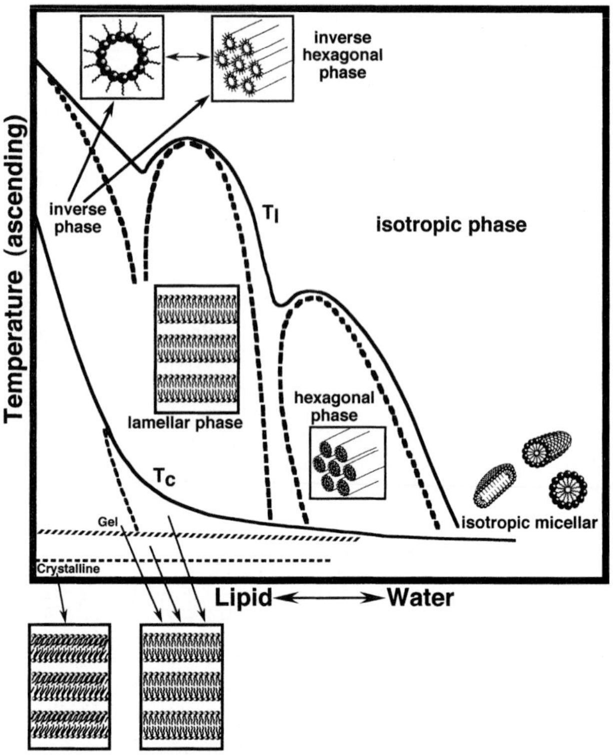

Figure 2 Lipid polymorphism. A general phase diagram of structures into which polar lipids self-assemble in aqueous mixtures at different conditions. The polar part of lipid molecules is schematically shown as an open circle and the nonpolar part as a (hydrocarbon) tail. In aqueous solutions these molecules self-assemble into various structures, which can organize themselves macroscopically into different phases or form isotropic colloidal solutions, as shown schematically. Below T_c the hydrocarbon chains are frozen, while above T_c they melt (i.e., exhibit rapid motion). In the case of diacyl lipids, liposomes can be found as metastable structures on the right side of the diagram (above 75 wt% of water). In the case of cationic lipids, mostly lamellar phase (and occassionally inverted hexagonal phase) is found in the phase diagram at higher lipid concentrations. At lower concentrations, lamellar phase in excess water and dispersed liposomes typically coexist. (Computer drawing courtesy of S. Hansen.)

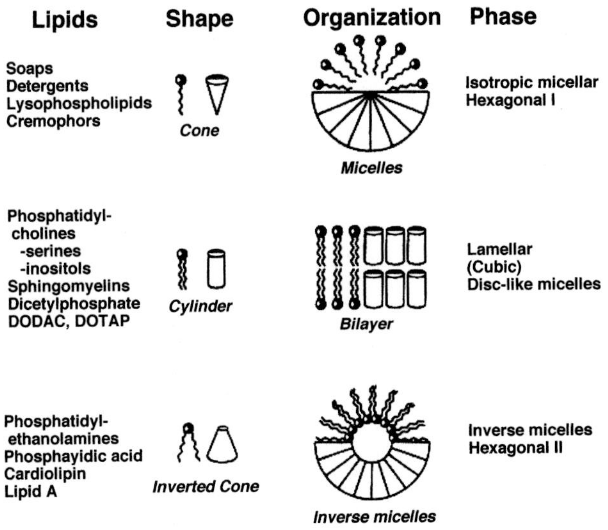

Figure 3 Schematic presentation of packing characteristics of lipids and structures formed (21). Cone-like amphiphiles, where the polar head (circle) is larger than the cross section of the nonpolar hydrocarbon tail (wavy line), pack into normal micelles. When the areas are similar, these molecules pack into bilayers and consequently form liposomes. For the case where hydrocarbon chains are very bulky (inverted cone), molecules pack into inverse phases. (Computer drawing courtesy of S. Hansen.)

into liquid crystalline phases, such as the hexagonal I phase. Cubic phases are typically different three-dimensional (D) networks of minimal surfaces often defined by zero mean curvature.

Figure 2 shows the morphology of various lipid phases and particles. These are mostly thermodynamically stable phases, which can form macroscopically ordered liquid crystalline phases or stable colloidal dispersions. The morphology of these phases changes with lipid concentration and temperature. In specific conditions, however, these macroscopic phases can be fragmented into (meta)stable colloidal particles: hexagonal phase yields hexasomes, cubic phase cubosomes, and lamellar phase various types of liposomes.

A. Micelles

As shown above, amphiphiles with relatively small hydrophobic parts can form particles with high radii of curvature, such as micelles. With increasing lipid concentration and/or with decreasing (a : b) ratio, spherical micelles grow into rodlike micelles, and at higher lipid concentrations these micelles form lyotropic liquid crystals (see Figs. 2 and 3).

Micelles are lyophilic colloids, which form spontaneously upon dissolution of surfactant in the aqueous phase. Although they are thermodynamically stable phases, their structures are in a dynamic equilibrium. A fraction of molecules is always dissolved in solution as monomers, and their concentration is referred to as critical micelle concentration (cmc) (22). It has important consequences on the solubilizing power of any particular detergent and its ability to denaturate various proteins. The exchange time for a molecule between the free and micellar state is typically in the microsecond time scale, which makes micelles extremely unstable upon application, which is associated with the sample dilution and the presence of absorbing moieties. Although micelles containing cationic surfactants can complex DNA, the association complex is rather unstable (especially in the case of univalent amphiphiles) and therefore they are in general not used for gene transfection. Additionally, single-chain lipids are normally strong detergents and therefore quite toxic (especially cationic ones, which are frequently used in disinfectants).

B. Liposomes or Lipid Vesicles

Liposomes are spherical particles in which the membrane, composed from the lipid bilayer, encapsulates part of the solvent in the interior. They can have one (unilamellar, U) or many (multilamellar, M) (concentric) layers and can be small (S) or large (L) vesicles (V). Therefore, with respect to their geometry, one can distinguish between SUV (0.02–0.1 μm), LUV (0.1–0.5 μm), and LMV (0.1–10 μm). With respect to surface characteristics, we distinguish between neutral, negative, and positively charged liposomes, which can be coated with polymers and contain various ligands on their surface (1).

With respect to structure and composition, liposomes resemble cell membranes. The typical composition includes lecithin (phosphatidylcholines) and kephalins (phosphatidylethanolamines) containing negatively charged lipids, such as phosphatidylserine and phosphatidylinositol. In addition to ceramides, such as sphingomyelin, sterols (cholesterol, ergosterol, sitosterol, etc.) are also included. A recent surge in gene transfection applications resulted in the synthesis of hundreds of novel cationic lipids, which are, either alone or in (equimolar) mixtures with fusogenic lipid dioleoyl phosphatidylethanolamine (DOPE) or stabilizing lipid cholesterol, used for DNA complexation and delivery. DOPE is lipid with $b > a$ and therefore tends to form inverse hexagonal phases. Bilayers containing this lipid are therefore stressed, and under certain conditions they can counteract the property utilized in transfection. Table 1 shows the most commonly used cationic lipids in liposome formulations, and Table 2 lists

Table 1 Some Cationic Lipids

Abbreviation	Chemical name
DODAB	Dioctadecyldimethylammonium bromide
DOTMA	*N*-[1-(2,3-Dioleoyloxy)propyl]-*N,N,N*-trimethylamm onium chloride
DOTAP	1,2-Dioleoyloxy-3-(trimethylammonio)propane
DMRIE	1,2-Dimyristoyloxypropyl-3-dimethylhydroxyethylammonium bromide
DOSPA	2,3-Dioleoyloxy-*N*-[2-sperminecarboxamido)ethyl]-*N,N*-dimethyl-1-propanaminium tfa
GAP-DLRIE	(±)-*N*-(3-Aminopropyl)-*N,N*-dimethyl-2,3-bis(dodecyl oxy)-1-propanaminium bromide
DORI	1,2-Dioleoyloxypropyl-3-dimethylhydroxyethylammonium bromide
EDMPC	1,2-Dimyristoyl-*sn*-glycero-3-ethylphosphocholine chloride
DOGS	Dioctadecylamidoglycospermine
DC-Chol	3 β-[*N*-(*N'*,*N'*-Dimethylaminoethane)carbamoyl] cholesterol
BGTC	Bis-guanidinium-tren-cholesterol
DPPES	Dipalmytoylphosphatidylethanolamidospermine
ELMPC	1,2-Dilauroyl-*sn*-glycero-3-ethylphosphocholine chloride
EOMPC	1,2-Dioleoyl-*sn*-glycero-3-ethylphosphocholine chloride
DODAC	Dioleoyldimethylammonium chloride
DOTIM	1-[2-(Oleoyloxy)-ethyl]-2-oleoyl-3-(2-hydroxyethyl) imidazolinium chloride
DOSPER	1,3-Di-oleoyloxy-2 (6-carboxy spermyl) propylamide 4 acetate
SAINT-n	A series of dialkyl pyridinium—alkyl halides

some commercially available liposomal transfection agents.

A lipid bilayer can be in a fluid or solid state. Bilayers containing uniform and saturated hydrocarbon chains exhibit phase transition from low-temperature, rigid (ordered, crystalline, gel, i.e., two-dimensional solid) state into a fluid phase (disordered, liquid crystalline or two-dimensional fluid) at temperature T_c. Bilayer permeability and fusogenic ability increase drastically in the high-temperature phase. Addition of cholesterol in the bilayer can eliminate this phase transition, and an ordered fluid phase is stable over a wide temperature range. Such bilayers are characterized by enhanced mechanical stability and are almost exclusively used in liposomal drug delivery.

Table 2 Some Commercially Available Liposomal Transfection Reagents

Name	Composition	Producer
Lipofectin	DOTMA:DOPE 1/1 w/w	Gibco BRL
DOTAP	DOTAP	Roche
Lipofectamine	DOSPA:DOPE 3/1 w/w	Gibco BRL
Transfectam	DOGS	ProMega
LipofectAce	DODAB/DOPE ½.5 w/w	Gibco BRL
DC-Chol	DC-Chol:DOPE 3/2 w/w	Sigma
DOTAP:Chol	DOTAP:Chol 1/1 m/m	Sigma
Transfectall	Cholesteryl-spermidine	Apollon
Clonfectin	Dimiristoyl-amidine	Clontech

Liposomes are used extensively in basic research as a model for biological membranes and, due to their biocompatibility, colloidal character (small size), and ability to encapsulate active substances as well as biodegradability and, in general, absence of toxicity and immunogenicity, in applications from drug and gene delivery to diagnostics and cosmetics.

1. Liposome-Preparation Methods

Liposome properties, including stability, reactivity, and interaction characteristics, can be rationally designed by selecting liposome composition (Table 3). Lipids are normally mixed in the organic phase (chloroform, methylene chloride, methanol), which is evacuated either by rotary evaporation, lyophilization (most often from tertiary butanol), or spray-drying. Dry lipid film, cake, or powder can be hydrated by the addition of an aqueous phase during agitation. An alternative hydration method is injection of an organic lipid solution into the aqueous phase followed by removal of organic solvent by dialysis (ethanol, propylene glycol) or evaporation (ether, Freons). This normally results in the formation of large multilamellar vesicles. In the case of highly charged lipid bilayers, a larger fraction of unilamellar liposomes with larger encapsulated volume is formed. Typically size distribution ranges from very

Table 3 Methods for Hydration of Cationic Lipids

Method	Pros	Cons
Thin film hydration	Easy and effective	Traces of organic solvents; not easy to scale up
Lyophilized cake from *t*-butanol	Easy and scalable	Some lipids may not be very soluble
Ethanol injection	Easy and scalable	Some lipids may not be very soluble
Spray-dried powder from an organic solvent	Scalable	Complex equipment
Direct lipid powder hydration	Easy and no organic solvents	Can be used only in single component liposomes
Supercritical CO_2 expansion in air/liquid	Elegant	Not adequately tested for lipid mixtures

small unilamellar vesicles to large multilamellar liposomes in the 1–10 μm size range, possibly with some liposomes that can be observed by the naked eye. These liposomes are too heterogeneous and have too small internal volumes for many applications and are therefore sized down. In a small-scale setting, this can be done by sonication or extrusion. The size distribution of sonicated vesicles is relatively broad around the minimal size characteristic for a particular lipid mixture. For egg lecithin the liposome minimal size varies from 25 to 30 nm. Addition of cholesterol increases liposome size. For liposomes containing long and saturated fatty acid chains, this size is around 50–85 nm, with the addition of cholesterol reducing the size. These samples, however, typically contain some very large particles, which must be removed by centrifugation or filtration before use. Extrusion is a method of choice to prepare liposomes with narrow size distributions. For pore sizes from 1 to 0.2 μm repeated extrusions produce liposomes smaller than filter pore sizes, while for smaller sizes the liposome size slowly approaches filter pore size after repeated extrusions. For lipid concentrations around 100 mM and liposome sizes around 100 nm, typically few extrusions through 0.6, 0.4-, and 0.2-μm membranes have to be followed by 5–10 extrusions through 1-μm, and possibly through 0.08-μm filters. For large-scale applications homogenization is normally used, while for tighter size distributions large-scale extrusion is performed. Homogenization also produces vesicles of minimal size, which is determined by the bending elasticity of the membrane. Like in sonication, these samples are contaminated with a few percent of larger liposomes or lipid particles. Careful optimization of homogenization improves sample homogeneity, and so does final extrusion.

Cationic liposomes are prepared by similar methods as described above (10). Most frequently, cationic liposomes contain around 50% neutral lipids, such as dioleoyl phosphatidyl ethanolamine (DOPE) or cholesterol (Chol). None of the current formulations includes antioxidants; with the development of pharmaceutical formulations this will likely change. Because of high surface charge and because they are typically prepared in solutions of low ionic strength (distilled water, 10% sucrose or 5% dextrose), they swell and upon agitation relatively small (250–400 nm) and oligolamellar liposomes are formed. Some lipid mixtures, such as DOTAP:cholesterol (1:1), however, do not swell easily, and swelling at elevated temperatures with agitation/stirring and occasional brief sonication is recommended (Table 4).

While all of these liposomes can be stable in the test tube, they interact rapidly or are quickly adsorbed upon

Table 4 Methods for Size Reduction of Large Multi/Oligolamellar Vesicles

Method	Pros	Cons
Shaking/Vortexing	Quite effective at high σ and low ι	Heterogeneous vesicles, some oligolamellar
Bath sonication	Easy and clean	Not scalable, makes only small SUV
Tip sonication	High energy, very small	Not scalable, tip contamination, makes only small SUV
Extrusion	Very tight size distribution; control of size distribution	More work demanding
Homogenization	Easy	Makes only small SUV
Very high shear mixing	Easy; good dispersal at high σ and low ι	Heterogeneous size distribution

σ = Surface charge; ι = ionic strength.

application. To prevent such nonspecific interactions, liposomes are coated by inert hydrophilic polymers, such as polyethylene glycol (PEG). Because stability is increased due to steric repulsion of the surface-grafted polymers, these liposomes are called sterically stabilized liposomes. Because of their invisibility to the body's immune system they are sometimes referred to as stealth liposomes.

2. Liposome Stability and Interaction Characteristics

As mentioned earlier, like all lyophobic colloids, liposomes are in general metastable structures. We can distinguish between physical, colloid, chemical, and biological stability of liposomes (1).

Physical and colloidal stability in general deal with the constancy of size distribution. In addition to typical lyophobic colloids, where the size distribution instability is mainly due to aggregation or Ostwald ripening, liposomes can fuse and leak the entrapped or associated molecules. Cationic liposomes, however, are normally characterized by high surface charge, and therefore aggregation is greatly reduced due to strong electrostatic repulsion. In low ionic strength media such liposomes can maintain their size distribution for years.

Chemical stability is another obstacle in liposome applications. By optimizing pH, addition of antioxidants, and chelators, however, suspensions can be stable within specification limits (5% lipid degradation) for at least a year when stored in liquid form at 4°C. Freezing or lyophilization (in the presence of appropriate cryoprotectants, such as 10% sucrose) can greatly extend their stability.

Liposome interactions with the surroundings are based on attractive electrostatic, van der Waals, hydrophobic, and hydrogen-bonding interactions. As mentioned above, repulsive interactions, such as steric shielding by surface-grafted polymer, can reduce the above interactions and rate of reactions, which give rise to liposome instability. The simplest interaction is entrapment of noninteractive molecules in the liposome interior. Similarly, hydrophobic molecules can be associated with the bilayers or dissolved in the hydrophobic part of the liposome while charged molecules can bind to oppositely charged liposomes. Drugs or other ligands can be also grafted to the liposome surface by covalent linkage to a lipid, by a specific interaction between functionalized lipid and ligand (avidin-biotin), or inserted hydrophobically via hydocarbon tail. Positively charged liposomes interact with negatively charged species and have been used to complex DNA to enhance its delivery into cells for gene expression.

Interaction of liposomes and cells involves simple adsorption, lipid exchange, as well as endocytosis and fusion. In some cases it has been speculated that cationic liposomes can induce simple (and reversible) cell membrane poration (10).

In biological systems liposomes are recognized as foreign particulates and are therefore quickly cleared by the immune system (1,23). Positively charged particles additionally exhibit strong attractive interaction with the milieu, which is in general negatively charged (cell walls, endothelial and mucosal surfaces, cell surfaces) and are typically adsorbed very quickly after administration. In some cases, however, opsonization (coating by plasma proteins) is so fast that it neutralizes the positive charge before adhesion to the blood vessel walls, blood cells, or even coagulation with blood components. Coating of such particles with inert hydrophilic polymers, such as PEG, can protect the coated particles and greatly extends their blood circulation times. Liposomes normally contain 5 mol% of lipid with covalently attached PEG with a molecular weight of 2000 daltons. While these lipids are typically introduced in the liposome in the beginning of preparation procedure, it was shown that they can be also transferred into liposomes by incubating conventional liposomes with PEG-lipid micelles at elevated temperatures (24). Such stabilization is especially useful for DNA-lipid complexes because PEGylated cationic liposomes do not interact with DNA because of its the protective polymer sheath.

3. Liposome Characterization

To characterize liposomes and perform quality control, several different parameters must be measured (Table 5) (25). In addition to general parameters, such as turbidity,

Table 5 Characteristics of Cationic Liposomes and Major Quality-Control Parameters

Parameter	Comment
Lipid composition	HPLC, TLC
Lipid concentration(s)	HPLC, colorimetric assays
Degradation products	HPLC, TLC, NMR
Active agent concentration	HPLC, spectrophotometry, ELISA
Vesicle size distribution	Dynamic light scattering, microscopy
Agent encapsulation efficiency	Separation and analysis
pH	Typically around 6–6.5
Osmolality	Around 290 mOsm/kg
Zeta potential	
Sterility and bioburden	Often problem of DNA
Pyrogenicity and endotoxin	Often problem of DNA

The same parameters can be used to characterize DNA-lipid complexes. In addition to the DNA stability parameters, the fraction of unreacted DNA and liposomes has to be determined.

pH, conductivity, osmolality, concentrations of lipids, solutes, encapsulated agents and degradation products (chemical stability, quality control), and percentage of encapsulated drug, physical characterization of liposomes includes size distribution and zeta potential measurements. In the case of DNA delivery, DNA: lipid mass and charge ratios are important as well. For stable and commercializable formulations, these values must remain within 5–10% of specification limits over prolonged periods of time (1–2 years).

C. Emulsions

Emulsion droplets can be formed in ternary systems water-polar lipid-oil. To improve dispersal (decrease interface tension and bending elasticity), cosurfactants such as glycerol, pentanol, and decanol are added. In regions of the phase diagram that are rich in water, oil-in-water emulsions and microemulsions (by definition the surface has a positive curvature, $c > 0$) can be formed, while in oil-rich regions these spherical particles have negative curvature ($c < 0$) and are water-in-oil emulsions. The intermediate phase between the two is a bicontinuous emulsion, which has zero average curvature. Emulsions are prepared by high-energy treatment (sonication, extrusion, homogenization) of appropriate mixtures. Microemulsions, however, can form spontaneously (analogously to micelle formation). The reason for this is that by selecting appropriate surfactant and co-surfactant, the bending elasticity of the surface is very low and the elastic bending energy needed to curve the interfacial films is comparable to the available thermal energy. This is the so-called entropic stabilization. Emulsions and microemulsions can also be made from cationic surfactants.

Typical oils used in the formation of emulsions are soybean and olive oils and, more recently, Capmul or Miglyol. Detergents like Tween, Span, Brij, and others, lecithins, and PEG lipids can be used as emulsifiers, and co-solubilizers (e.g., pentanol, glycerol, or decanol) can be added.

In gene delivery, emulsions containing castor oil, detergent, lecithin, and DC-Chol were tried. Nonionic detergents, such as Tween 80, Brij, and Span, were used. Compared to DC-Chol/Chol liposomes, higher stability upon storage and higher transfection efficiency in the presence of serum was found. The optimal charge ratio was 6–8 : 1 (DC-Chol : DNA, w/w). It seems, however, that liposomal systems exceed the transfection efficiency of these systems, which do not seem to have been further pursued (26).

Fine structure of amphiphilic colloidal particles as well as their size and shape are probably determined by the detailed molecular geometry of lipid molecules, their aqueous solubility and protolytic activity (pK in the case of weak bases or acids and degree of dissociation of salts, both of which give rise to effective charge), and weaker interactions such as intra- and intermolecular hydrogen bonds, stereoisomerism, as well as interactions within the medium. Obviously they depend on the temperature, lipid concentration, and electrostatic and electrodynamic interactions with the solvent and solutes. In the case of charged lipids, the effects of counterions, especially anions, may also be important. Like the shape parameter (a/b), a very useful quantity to describe surfactants is hydrophilic-lipophilic balance (HLB), which classifies surfactant with respect to its relative amphiphilicity and is applicable especially in formulating emulsions.

V. COLLOIDAL PARTICLES IN DRUG AND GENE DELIVERY

Before we describe the use of cationic liposomes in gene delivery, we shall very briefly introduce the status of lipid colloidal particles, such a micelles, liposomes and emulsions, in drug delivery in the clinic (27).

Chemotherapy, especially in the case of very potent drugs, is often limited by the toxic side effects of the drug. Pharmacokinetics and biodistribution, however, can be changed by encapsulating active substances into colloidal particles, and the safety as well as activity may be significantly increased. Among micelles, mixed micelles, emulsions, and polymeric particulate systems (microspheres and nanospheres), liposomes are becoming the most widely used drug-carrier system.

Several compounds with poor aqueous solubility are formulated into micelles. The best known example is amphotericin B, which is formulated in deoxycholic acid micelles. Such systems, however, are inherently unstable upon administration due the cmc phenomenon and the presence of the sink for detergent molecules (dilution and adsorption). Therefore, their main purpose is simply to solubilize the drug and they do not act as drug carriers. Emulsions and especially microemulsions are also very unstable, especially with respect to the retention of the dissolved drug molecules. While there are many emulsions in topical delivery and as parenteral nutrition supplements and oxygen-carrying vehicles, serious trials for systemic drug delivery are only beginning. One example is prostaglandin or its pro-drug in oil-in-water emulsion.

Phospholipid-based liposomes are biocompatible, biodegradable, and in general nonimmunogenic and can be therefore used as a drug-delivery system. Liposomes offer enhanced drug solubilization of difficult-to-dissolve drugs (minoxidil, amphotericin B), protection of the encapsulated drug against degrading enzymes (cytosine arabinose, antisense oligonucleotides), decrease of toxicity due to site avoidance (reduced cardiotoxicity of anthracyclines and nephro- and neurotoxicity of amphotericin) as well as drug targeting. Conventional liposomes are cleared by the cells of the body's immune system, located mostly in the liver and spleen, and therefore encapsulated molecules can be targeted to these cells. On the other side, small and stable and, especially, polymer-coated (long-circulating) liposomes are not cleared by those cells and therefore accumulate at sites where the vascular system is leaky. This often happens in tumors and other sites of trauma, such as sites of infection and inflammation.

This passive targeting is achieved mostly after intravenous administration. Subcutaneous administration at specified locations can be used to deliver conventional liposomes to the lymph nodes, while intramuscular administration can serve as drug depot in a vehicle with controllable release characteristics. In general, however, liposomal drugs can be administered by many different routes. While oral delivery is still in the early phases and topical transdermal delivery is still plagued by irreproducibility, nebulized liposomal aerosols are clearly an excellent system for this promising port of entry. In addition to delivery of antiasthmatic drugs and antibiotics, this may apply also to DNA-lipid complexes. Obviously, direct injections into tumors and other localized sites are possible.

After two decades of research, several products are on the market, including antifungal drugs in conventional liposomes and doxorubicin in sterically stabilized (stealth) liposomes. While conventional liposomes largely reduce toxicity and increase drug accumulation in the organs of the reticuloendothelial system, sterically stabilized liposomes achieve passive tumor targeting. These liposomes were shown to accumulate in several solid tumors and resulted in increased activity of the drug at reduced toxicity.

For this reason sterically stabilized DNA-lipid complexes may be a very important vehicle to deliver DNA and antisense oligonucleotides to tumors and sites of infection and inflammation. In general these complexes, which can be formulated in liquid, solid, aerosolized, or semisolid (cream, gel) form, can be administered by the same routes as liposomes.

While liposomal drugs concentrate mostly on cancer and infectious diseases, the spectrum of applications of DNA-liposome complexes seems to be much wider. In the treatment of cancer, researchers envision various combinations from direct tumor injections of suicide, antigen, and tumor-suppressor genes and genes for cytokines, to systemic treatments with different genes and targeting of endothelial cells to stop angiogenesis. Alternatively, the growth of tumor cells in cancer or smooth muscle cells in cardiovascular disorders can be turned down by the delivery of appropriate antisense oligonucleotides and ribozymes. Other administration routes include injection into hepatic artery, oral, and topical administration. Genes include ones for immunomodulation and immunotherapy: a promising possibility is also genetic immunization in which genes encoding for selected immunogenic portions of pathogens are delivered subcutaneously, intramuscularly, or orally. Other diseases on the list are neurological disorders, acquired immunodeficiency syndrome (AIDS), cardiovascular diseases, and inflammation. In the cardiovascular area, DNA plasmids encoding vascular endothelial growth factors (VEGF) can sprout the growth of new blood vessels in ischemic areas (28). Inhalation of gene-lipid aerosol might be important in the treatment of cancer, infections (tuberculosis), asthma and other inflammations and genetic diseases, such as cystic fibrosis. While this is definitively an early period, some promising results have been already achieved, as shown below and elsewhere in this book.

VI. INTERACTIONS OF MICELLES AND LIPOSOMES WITH NUCLEIC ACIDS

In simple solutions and solids, thermodynamic parameters can quantitatively explain their behavior. However, both isotropic suspensions of DNA and liposomes are colloidal solutions and therefore, during their interaction, kinetic factors are, in addition to thermodynamics, also very important (1,10,27). While there is not much interaction between DNA and neutral or anionic liposomes or micelles, interaction with cationic particulates can change the morphology of both reactants.

Oppositely charged micelles and emulsion droplets can also interact with nucleic acids, and the complexes have shown some transfection activity. Unfortunately, none of the systems have been physicochemically and structurally characterized. Although the cmc of detergent molecules must be drastically reduced in these complexes, we can expect that such DNA-micellar complexes are not too stable in the systems, which provide sinks for free detergent molecules, as well as due to the toxicity of single-chain cationic detergents. For this reason, we believe micelles of single charged lipid-DNA complexes have not yet been tried in gene transfection. However, liposomes made from a cationic detergent and DOPE and complexed with DNA were shown to transfect cells in vitro. However, the levels of expression were relatively low, and toxicity was rather high, and we are not aware of any other recent trials (29). Some multivalent cationic detergents (such as DOGS), however, form micelles, which were shown to be effective transfection systems in vitro (20).

In in vitro assays gene expression is normally significantly reduced in the presence of serum. In order to overcome this problem, complexation with cationic emulsions, instead of with liposomes, has been tried. DNA-emulsion complexes were stabilized by nonionic surfactants. The emulsion consisted of castor oil, cationic lipids, and nonionic surfactants. It has been shown that the presence of surfactants with PEGylated polar heads reduces the size of the droplets and increases transfection efficiency in vitro, including in the presence of serum. It remains to be seen if the difference was due to the substitution of liposomes by an emulsion or to the presence of the PEGylated surface, which can prevent coagulation and precipitation of the complexes. Other studies have indicated that higher excesses of cationic charge also increase transfection. This probably indicates that this charge is used for neutralization of certain plasma components and that after these compounding factors are neutralized and prevented from coagulating DNA-lipid or polymer complexes, DNA complexes can transfect cells. Emulsion-based systems require large surpluses of cationic lipid to prevent aggregation and might also therefore have some toxicity problems. It has not been proven that lipid-coated DNA resides in the interior of the oil droplet (26).

Liposomes seem to be the most effective lipid-based nonviral gene-delivery system (30,31). Nowadays, however, not many researchers are aware that liposomes were used for DNA encapsulation in the late 1970s. Early studies used anionic liposomes to encapsulate DNA molecules. Although some transfection activity has been reported and the proof of concept established, the procedure was rather cumbersome and the transfection levels were very low (32). Although the researchers have also used positively charged liposomes, they have overlooked their potential for almost quantitative DNA encapsulation and improvement in DNA transfection.

In contrast to negatively charged and neutral liposomes, there is a strong electrostatic interaction between cationic liposomes and DNA. Reaction of the two oppositely charged systems can result in partial or complete condensation of DNA, liposome disintegration, and restructuring into novel structures. These can be thermodynamically stable particles or many particles trapped in various kinetic traps (i.e., particles with random and irreproducible morphologies), which are a simple consequence of local conditions, such as local concentrations of reactants and their fluctuations (10).

VII. THE STRUCTURE OF CATIONIC LIPOSOME-DNA COMPLEXES

We have characterized DNA-cationic liposome interactions and the structure of the resulting colloidal particles as a function of thermodynamic parameters, such as concentrations, temperature, ionic strength, surface charge (pK), and pH. Phase diagrams of DNA-lipid complexes in the phase space of DNA and cationic liposome concentration were determined (10). As expected, higher reactant concentrations and ionic strengths and charge ratios close to unity resulted in more precipitation. Additionally, however, a strong kinetic component has been noticed. It was found that kinetics of mixing as well as the order of mixing of the two solutions can give rise to irreversible and path-dependent flocculation or precipitation. Qualitative explanations as to the rate and order of mixing have been postulated. Briefly, in the phase diagram DNA-cationic liposomes, precipitation occurs around the electrical neutrality diagonal. To prepare stable complexes on either side of the diagonal, mixing should be performed in such a way that the solubility gap should not be crossed; this means that the minor component, with respect to the charge, must be added to the major one. Also, it was shown that quick dispersal assures the least precipitation. This was qualitatively explained by the formation of a very large number (''sudden burst'') of small crystallization/nucleation embrii, which give rise to many small complexes as opposed to a growth closer to thermodynamic equilibrium, which results in the formation of fewer, larger, particles (10).

A very interesting observation was that an excess of DNA solution can dissolve multilamellar vesicles, i.e., upon adding DNA to a turbid solution of large multi(oligo)-lamellar vesicles, the turbidity disappears. This probably indicates that DNA can dissolve and disintegrate large cationic liposomes. The structure of such solutions has not yet been determined. Preliminary analyses, however, point to DNA helices (partially) coated by lipid tubes.

The interaction of oppositely charged colloidal solutions has been investigated extensively (33,34). However, most studies involved the determination of simple precipitation boundaries without detailed studies of particle structure. The same is the case for DNA and cationic liposomes. Few electron microscopic studies of DNA-lipid complexes have been published (35–38). They report on undefined colloidal aggregates, occasionally surrounded by a halo of thin fibers. Detailed analyses established that spherical structures are aggregated liposomes and the thin fibers are lipid-coated DNA helices (35). Simultaneous presence of fibrilar and globular structures clearly indicates that these phases are not at thermodynamic equilibrium.

Following these and other studies, several models of DNA-lipid aggregates have been postulated. (Fig. 4), none of which has been substantiated by more than one independent measurement. We can, however, group the published information into two groups: dense, condensed aggregates (37–39), and heterogeneous systems containing spherical aggregates and fibrilar structures (35,40,41).

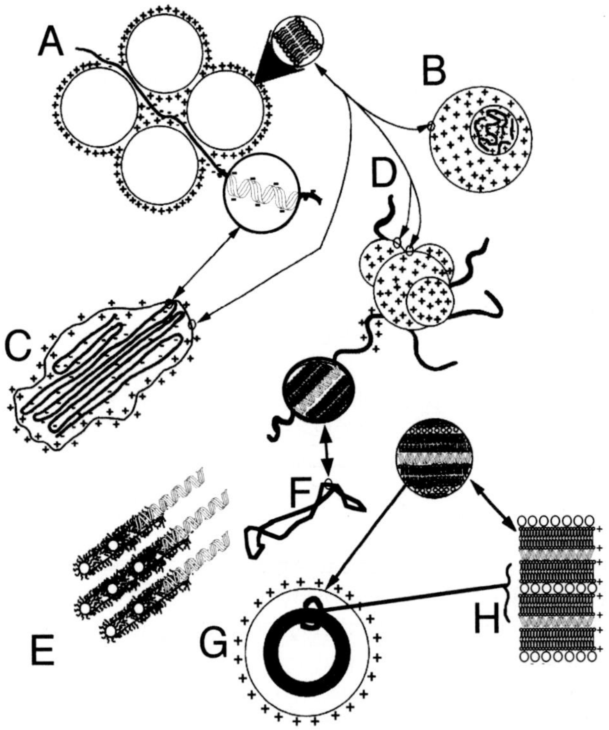

Figure 4 Schematic presentation of various DNA-lipid complex models (A) Stoichiometric model in which DNA is adsorbed between cationic liposomes (18). (B) Model of condensed DNA coated by cationic lipid (20). (C) During interaction, DNA induces liposome fusion and in the process condenses and becomes encapsulated in a lipid bilayer. (D) Aggregated liposomes with attached fibers of DNA encapsulated by a bilayered lipid cylinder (35). (E) Model of hexagonally packed DNA in the hex II phase (81). (F) Model of coated DNA helices (10,35). (H) Model of intercalated lamellar phase in which DNA is condensed two-dimensionally between stacked bilayers (37–39). (G) Model of two-dimensional condensed DNA encapsulated in cationic liposome (44). (Computer drawing courtesy of S. Hansen.)

If complete neutralization and condensation occurs, however, DNA tends to form dense aggregates, which are often characterized by lamellar symmetry. Such a structure was characterized by x-ray scattering and high-resolution cryo-electron microscopy (37,38). Recent work (37,38, 39,42) has shown that such a structure is a rather general phenomenon observed by a variety of cationic lipids and liposomes. Other recent work has shown that such complexes can be stabilized by replacing DOPE with cholesterol (10,43,44), condensation with spermidine, inclusion of PEGylated phospholipids, while retaining transfection activity in vivo (45).

Because dense and condensed phases of lipids and DNA belong to different symmetry classes, their interaction changes the symmetry of at least one reactant (46). An exception might be phases containing large fractions of DOPE or other lipids with the tendency to form hexagonal phases in which educts and product may have local hexagonal ordering.

In general, however, studies show random aggregates with few structures, which have been observed in several unrelated experiments and also in different lipid systems. The most often observed are lamellar aggregates and fibrilar structures. We must be aware, that they might be simply the two limiting cases of lipid bilayers adsorbing the DNA and DNA double helices coating themselves with lipids in the regions where (the excess of) DNA charge dictates the restructuring. In the case of a large excess lipid more random structures of liposomes with adsorbed DNA and their aggregates may be observed. Depending on the local conditions during mixing of DNA and liposomes, obviously different structures may co-exist in the sample. Obviously quick mixing and good dispersal result in more homogeneous complexes while very slow addition of one component into other should result in a precipitation because large structures can form at local high densities of one reactant. As a thermodynamically stable structure intercalated lamellar phase has been observed. In this particular phase cationic lipid bilayers sandwich two dimensionally condensed DNA. Several theoretical models have been tried to describe this structure as well (47–49). Various studies have hypothesized different structure of cationic liposome-DNA complexes, some of which are shown in Figure 4.

If we view the intercalated DNA-lipid lamellar phase as an equilibrium structure, all these structures represent relatively stable kinetic traps bridging the two limiting structures: intercalated lamellar phase and lipid-wrapped DNA coils. In practice, DNA-lipid complexes can be stable in liquid form for months and in freeze-dried form for years. However, due to the random nature of local conditions (concentration fluctuations in general and relative concentrations at the boundaries of one phase diluting in the other in particular), we believe that the structure of complexes is inherently heterogeneous with respect to the structure, size and shape. A sample can therefore contain the whole spectrum of structures between the two limiting structures. Therefore, the spectrum of the observed structures can also be an artifact of the experimental method: small-angle x-ray scattering does not detect random structures, freeze fracture electron microscopy can miss stacks of lamellae, and cryo electron microscopy may not visualize fibrilar structures.

VIII. DNA DELIVERY INTO CELLS

As stated above, the major problem is not the construction and manufacturing of plasmids, but their efficient delivery into the appropriate cells. We have mentioned very briefly mechanic as well as viral and nonviral delivery systems.

Several viral systems are currently used for DNA delivery in vitro and in vivo, as described elsewhere in this book. These viruses include retroviruses such as the Moloney murine leukemia virus (MoMLV) and the human immunodeficiency virus (HIV), adenoviruses (Ad), adeno-associated virus (AAV), herpes simplex virus (HSV), Epstein-Barr virus (EBV), Sindbis virus, bovine and human papilloma viruses (BPV and HPV), hepatitis B virus (HBV), vaccinia virus, and polyoma virus SV40. Each virus has evolved its own mechanism for delivery that primarily involves viral-encoded proteins. These viral delivery systems are extensively described in other chapters. Nonviral systems include DNA complexes with polymers and liposomes. The former are described in chapters by Wagner and Behr in this volume, while here we shall very briefly describe some results of DNA delivery by cationic liposomes, especially the type that has achieved the highest reported levels of expression (44).

Cationic liposome technology has provided some of the best characterized nonviral DNA delivery systems. Cationic liposomes have been used extensively for in vivo DNA delivery, and efficient gene expression has been demonstrated after intravenous injection (43,50,51). Furthermore, many authors claim that no toxic effects have been observed in in vivo experiments using DNA-lipid complexes. In addition, therapeutic cDNAs have been delivered by cationic liposomes in human gene therapy trials, and no toxicity has been observed (52–55). Moreover, efficacy has been demonstrated for melanoma patients injected in their tumor nodules with DNA-lipid complexes that delivered the HLA-B7 gene (52,56).

For many gene therapy applications it is essential to achieve high localized expression of a cDNA of interest. Receptor-mediated gene transfer, provided by molecular conjugate vectors (57), has been used to achieve this goal. Commonly used conjugate vectors include the asialoglycoprotein to target gene delivery to hepatocytes (58). Asialoglycoproteins are internalized by high-affinity receptors that exist on the surface of hepatocytes. In addition, transferrin-polylysine DNA complexes have been used for gene delivery by the receptor-mediated endocytosis pathway (59,60). Delivery to respiratory epithelial cells has been accomplished by using the immunoglobulin A (IgA) transcytosis pathway (61). Other ligands used for receptor-mediated endocytosis have been reviewed (62) and include insulin (63), epidermal growth factor (EGF) (64), and lectins (65). Folate as well as receptors expressed on tumor cells, such as HER-2, have been also used.

Most DNA-delivery systems cannot mediate transfection into all cells in vivo. This presents a major barrier to the cure of certain cancers that require delivery of therapeutic genes to 100% of tumor cells. Strategies that use suicide genes to produce a bystander effect have been developed for effective treatment of such tumors, and DNA delivery to 100% of cells is not necessary. In these systems a small portion of tumor cells (1–10%) expresses a suicide gene product. The toxic effect is transmitted to the neighboring tumor cells that do not express the suicide gene, and killing of 100% of tumor cells has been accomplished (66,67). The strategies most widely used include the use of herpes simplex virus thymidine kinase (HSV-TK) and cytosine deaminase, which activate subsequently introduced prodrugs.

The use of HSV-TK was initially described for the treatment of brain tumors (62). Ganciclovir is a drug that can be administered intravenously after the HSV-TK gene has been delivered to tumor cells. Ganciclovir interacts only with the HSV-TK enzyme; therefore, it is toxic to cells that express HSV-TK. HSV-TK converts ganciclovir into nucleotide-like precursors that block DNA synthesis and kill cells. This toxic effect is diffusible to the surrounding tumor cells that do not express HSV-TK, and these cells are also killed.

Another suicide approach utilizes the conversion of the nontoxic prodrug 5-fluorocytosine (5FCyt) to the toxic 5-fluorouracil (5FUra). This conversion is mediated by cytosine deaminase. This strategy uses tumor-specific antigen promoters to express the cytosine deaminase gene (67). For example, the carcinoembryonic antigen (CEA) promoter is active in human colorectal carcinoma cells and is totally inactive in normal colorectal cells. After delivery of vectors containing the cytosine deaminase gene expressed by the CEA promoter to colorectal carcinoma cells, 5FCyt is administered. 5FUra is produced only in cells that express cytosine deaminase. This system provides a powerful bystander effect because 5FUra is highly diffusible to surrounding tumor cells.

While in recombinant DNA technology and genetic engineering nucleic acids are introduced into cells by physical and chemical methods (osmotic shock, membrane permeabilization, electroporation, calcium phosphate precipitation), the delivery of genes into appropriate cells in vivo for applications in gene therapy involves at present mostly synthetic viral constructs or lipid-based systems. Among polymers, micelles, mixed micelles, emulsions, and liposomes, the latter seem to have shown the most promise.

IX. LIPOSOMAL TRANSFECTION IN VIVO

A. A Brief Overview

Gene delivery by cationic liposomes in vivo was first described in 1989 (68). Intravenous (iv), intratracheal (it), and intraperitoneal (ip) administration of Lipofectin containing marker gene was tried. Gene expression persisted in the lung up to a week upon iv and its administration, while they did not observe any expression in organs of the reticuloendothelial system. Similar experiments were performed in rats (69). Gene expression after delivery of aerosolized complexes (CAT marker gene and DOTMA/DOPE liposomes) to the lung after pulmonary application and after tail vein injection into mice have been reported (43,70).

These and several other studies that mainly used marker genes were followed by gene therapy studies in model animals. Correction of ion transport defect in cystic fibrosis transgenic mice by administering cystic fibrosis transmembrane conductance regulator gene (CFTR) in mice has been reported (71). Lipofectin-based DNA-lipid complexes were delivered to airways and deep alveoli via intratracheal instillation. The authors concluded that this approach should be efficacious in humans (71). Seven years later, however, this prediction has yet to be fulfilled.

Cancer immunotherapy is one of the primary interests of preclinical work. Therapeutic DNA, normally injected directly into the tumor, encodes the foreign major histocompatibility antigen, which after expression triggers autoimmune attack. Results showed hindered tumor growth and complete tumor regression in a few cases (72). In an analogy to the treatment with recombinant proteins, other treatments include gene transfer for cytokine genes, which can help to combat neoplastic tissue growth or inflammation, and genes for various blood factors and proteins involved in cholesterol removal from blood circulation in order to prevent hypertension and arteriosclerosis. As stated before, VEGF-encoded plasmids may be useful in the growth of new blood vessels, while restenosis can be prevented by local delivery (possibly intraarterially by a catheter) of appropriate antisense oligonucleotides or ribozymes.

Early work, as we have seen above, concentrated on optimizing liposomes (composition, charge, size distribution), plasmids, DNA: lipid ratio and concentrations, few neutral lipids and several different cationic lipids (20,73–76). While the majority of plasmids used were reporter genes, several expressions of therapeutic genes have also been observed, in several cases with some biological effects.

In the next stage researchers turned mostly to the improvements of cationic lipids (50,77–81). Perhaps the most methodical work from this period is the systematic analysis of almost 100 novel cationic lipids by Genzyme (78). The main message of their work was that in vivo cholesterol was a better hydrophobic anchor than diacyl lipids and vice versa for in vitro transfection. While no clear dependence on the number of positive charges has been established, the work showed that the orientation of the attachment of positive charges is important. Namely, the highest transfection was observed for a lipid which had spermine attached via a nonterminal tertiary amine, forming a T-like conformation. Such conformation might allow better interaction of DNA with the bilayer due to parallel alignment of polycationic charges and bilayer.

Structure-activity studies have been performed mostly in vitro (75,78,80,81). When studying cationic cholesterol derivatives, it was noted that tertiary amine gave the best transfection at the lowest toxicity (80). For multivalent cholesterol derivatives it was shown that the site and the angle of the attachment of the polyamine was important. Molecules having perpendicular arrangement between the long axis of sterol and the direction of polyamine were found to be more active than the parallel ones (78). The sterol hydrophobic anchor was found to be more effective for in vivo gene delivery, while for in vitro systems diacyl chains were found to give rise to higher gene expression. In the case of diacyl lipids it was discovered that dioleoyl and dimyristoyl chains give rise to the highest expression (74,78,81). This is hardly surprising, because for both interaction of DNA with liposome as well as of DNA-lipid complexes with cells, fluid membranes are necessary. With respect to polar heads and number of charges, no clear conclusions have been reported. Studies of DOTMA-like molecules have shown that decorating polar head with hydroxyethyl group and with beta amines increased transfection efficiencies in vitro (79).

The importance of neutral lipid was also carefully studied. While for in vitro transfection DOPE seems to be a superior choice (76,77,80), many recent experiments show that for systemic delivery, the use of cholesterol can result in much higher transfection (43,44). Based on these observations, neutral lipid has to be optimized for each delivery route. For instance, it is not known which lipid is better for pulmonary delivery, in which, similarly to the transfection in cell cultures, even the optimal complex size is still not known.

B. Novel Lipids

Many researchers are still trying to synthesize a novel lipid, which would "magically" improve expression and reduce toxicity. The philosophy of the search for magic cationic lipids, so prevalent in the early 1990s, with numerous anecdotal but unsubstantiated results being rumored in the nonviral gene-delivery community, still exists, although on a smaller scale. Obviously, with rational synthesis, one can generate less toxic cationic lipids. However, early claims of several groups that they synthesized lipids, that targeted specific organs upon systemic administration and achieved high transfection levels have never been confirmed. Many cationic lipids have been synthesized, which have shown improved transfection in some cell lines and altered conditions (82–86). It is the opinion of this author that less toxic lipids can be synthesized but that none of the lipids alone will achieve high, durable, and targetable expression. With existing lipids, subtle changes in the molecular geometry giving rise to specific interactions with particular cells are offset by much stronger nonspecific electrostatic interactions of the whole complexes. Interactions with nucleic acid, however, depend on the number of charges, their pK values, stereochemistry, and possible hydrogen bonding and hydrophobic interactions with DNA. These might be important in the complexation/condensation and decomplexation/decondensation of DNA, rather than in the delivery of complexes to specific cells. Some of the lipids, however, can give rise to very unstable complexes: in such a case, aggregation/agglutination upon injection can lead to changed biodistribution and safety profile. Again, however, these changes are due to colloidal behavior of complexes, rather than the molecular geometry of lipids. Also, cationic lipids will always bear some safety risks because of their reactivity. In the longer run, the improved transfection efficiency will be probably obtained by colloidal changes rather than on the molecular level.

Obviously there are differences in expression levels in various organs following administration of different lipids. But these differences can usually be explained by differences in the stability of complexes and their colloidal behavior rather than by specific interactions due to a particular lipid. The differences observed are due to the ability of lipids to complex or condense DNA into more or less stable complexes. The origin of these is based in their charge density, pK values, cmc values, size, as well as the possible presence of other interactive groups in the polar head region. All this can lead to different colloidal behavior during complex formation and its administration rather than to some specific interactions upon administration (82–86).

The cationic lipid synthesis efforts generated much data but no clear (quantitative) structure-activity relationships (QSAR). Therefore some researchers concentrated on the optimization of the complexes by using existing lipids. Improvement of complexes can be based on their size reduction and DNA compaction, coating of complexes to reduce nonspecific interactions, and eventual attachment of targeting ligands and fusigenic elements in order to improve uptake into cytosol.

C. Complex Optimization

The lack of the appearance of ''magic'' lipids and further work on complex characterization led several groups to work on optimization of colloidal properties of the complexes. These include control over size distribution, surface charge, surface coatings, and attachment of targeting ligands and/or fusigenic groups.

D. DNA Precondensation

DNA condensation in the complexes has been shown by small-angle x-ray scattering, cryoelectron microscopy, and analytical ultracentrifugation (10,37–39). In the case of fluorescent labeled DNA, the coiled/globular-compacted phase transition was also observed. In between the two states a coexistence region of both structures was found, in agreement with numerous electron micrographs, which show coexistence region of condensed and uncondensed DNA with a bimodal size distribution (87). It was speculated that tight, compact complexes are a necessary condition for effective in vivo gene delivery because in these complexes DNA was well protected (10). These qualitative arguments were confirmed by recent studies, which have shown that lamellar complexes were the most effective in transfection in vitro (88). Analogously to previous work with liposomes, it was shown that DNA transforms also micelles into lamellar aggregates (88).

During complex characterization studies it was realized that DNA must be compacted in order to form small and stable complexes. Many different agents that can compact DNA are known, and various combinations of these were used to prepare better defined complexes (80).

Often cationic lipids do not condense DNA well, and fibrillar structures are formed at higher lipid-to-DNA ratios. Several authors have reported improved transfection upon precondensing DNA with polymers, polyamines, or proteins (45,89). Some researchers are using various basic proteins, such as histones. Their use, however, is hampered by cumbersome protein preparation and immunogenicity upon repeated administrations. For this reason, people are using shorter polypeptides, either prepared synthetically or representing short sequences from natural basic proteins (90). Typical sequences used are KTPKKAKKP (from human histone H1) or synthetic ones, such as K_n ($n = 10–18$).

During the preparation of DOTAP/Chol liposomes, a special liposome shape and subsequently interaction with DNA has been observed (44). Liposomes prepared by a special extrusion technique were shown to contain a large fraction of invaginated liposomes. These liposomes have a large excess of surface area and, therefore, during interaction with DNA can form liposomes with encapsulated two-dimensionally condensed DNA. These complexes were shown to be very efficient gene-delivery vehicles, as will be briefly described below.

E. Targeting of DNA-Lipid Complexes

In analogy with the developments in liposomal drug delivery, several groups are trying to improve transfection and gene expression by targeting of DNA-lipid complexes.

For in vivo targeting many different ligands have been tried. Macrophages express manose receptors and hepatocytes galactose. Complexes can contain various sugars to affect cell targeting. Galactose, lactose, and their oligomers, possibly synthesized in di- or tri-antenary conformation, were used to improve targeting to hepatocytes, while mannosylated complexes have shown enhanced uptake by macrophages. Sugar can be part of the lipid, cationic lipid, neutral lipid, compacting polycation, or polymer. For instance, it has been shown that mannosylated polylysine complexes exploited endocytosis by mannose receptor in the cultured macrophages as well as in vivo, resulting in enhanced expression in cells and in liver and spleen of animal models (91).

To target DNA-lipid complexes to asialoglycoprotein receptor expressed on liver parenchymal cells, galactosylated cationic lipids were synthesized. They were based on cholesterol as hydrophobic anchor, and longer spacer arm was shown to increase transfection in vitro (92). Hepatocytes can also be targeted by asialofetuin-labeled liposomes. The uptake occurs via endocytosis through asialoglycopreotein receptor (93). Sevenfold enhanced transfection in the liver has been observed by asialofetuin-targeted DOTAP/Chol liposomes (44).

Rapidly growing cancer cells express various receptors to satisfy the increased demand for nutrients. Transferrin and folic acid receptors are perhaps the best known examples. Cationic liposome-transferrin complexes mediated p53 sensitization of squamous cells up to 10 times more efficiently than untargeted liposomes alone (94). Rapidly growing cells express folate receptor, and DNA or antisense oligonucleotides can be targeted by the use of folate ligand. To decrease nonspecific interactions and increase targeting ability, folate can be bound to the far end of the (polyethylene) glycol polymer. This is a rather stable molecule and can be synthesized and used as a normal lipid, thus simplifying the preparation procedure (95).

Fusigenic peptides or transferrin were used in negatively charged ternary complexes of DNA and cationic liposomes, and expression levels of reporter gene (pCMVLuc) were 10-fold higher as compared to liposome-DNA complexes (96).

In order to enhance DNA entry into cells, several fusigenic components can be built in the complex. These include fusigenic proteins (human influenza virus hemagglutinin), metastable bilayers, as well as larger parts or whole viruses. An example of the latter approach are the HVJ (Sendai virus)-cationic liposome conjugates. Hemagglutinating virus of Japan (HVJ) is a member of the mouse paramyxovirus family, and its fusigenic envelope proteins enhance the delivery of encapsulated/associated material into cells. The system, however, will require further modifications to achieve sufficient gene expression in vivo (97).

Human epidermal growth factor receptors (HER 2) are another potential target (27). These are membrane tyrosin kinases, which are overexpressed in various epithelial tumors. Downregulating them may stop tumor growth or angiogenesis (vascular endothelial growth factor), while in the ischemic tissue their upregulation may improve vascularization in infarction areas. HER2 targeting was tried with DNA-polymer complexes as well as with cationic lipid-DNA sterically stabilized complexes. Humanized antibody (rhuMAbHER2)-polylysine-DNA(luciferase gene pRSVLuc) complexes were shown to express luciferase gene up to 180-fold more than untargeted complexes (98).

F. PEG Coating of Complexes

Pharmacokinetic and biodistribution data indicate that the biological fate of complexes depends mostly on the nonspecific electrostatic interactions. Obviously, there is a need to decrease nonspecific interactions of cationic particles and shift their biodistribution to other cells. Apart from direct injections, PEGylation of DNA-lipid complexes and attachment of targeting ligands are evidently the solutions for systemic administration.

If complexes are small and they need to be targeted to sites with increased vascular permeability (100), one can use small PEG-coated DNA-lipid complexes. These can deliver the cargo into tumors, sites of infections, and inflammations. While the payload can be accumulated in the target tissue, it still remains in the intercellular space and not inside the cells. For this reason appropriate ligands, which target endocytotic surface receptors, should increase the efficiency of the treatment. Endocytosis is, however, deleterious to the nucleic acids, and fusogenic liposomes might be a better choice. Practice, however, still lags behind these theoretical concepts, as does our understanding of DNA migration into the cell nucleus. Obviously several entry mechanisms operate simultaneously, including cationic lipid-mediated poration, what can explain transfection results in several studies (10).

The anticipated problem is the reactivity of sterically stabilized cationic liposomes with DNA. Due to the presence of the polymer shield, DNA does not interact or complex with these liposomes. There are two possible solutions to this problem: either reduce the density of the polymer cloud or attach polymer coating after complexation reaction. This can be done by incubation of DNA-lipid complexes with PEG-lipid micelles. Yet another possibility is to use precondensed DNA and encapsulate it into normal stealth liposomes or interact these condensates with cationic sterically stabilized liposomes, similarly to the aftercoating of normal liposomes (10). Cationic lipid-DNA particles can be solubilized by detergents and upon detergent removal complexes can be prepared.

Another problem is internalization and nuclear entry of DNA (101). Sterically stabilized liposomes typically do not interact with cells, and therefore the polymer coating should be shed off to increase internalization, either by endocytosis or membrane poration by the positively charged lipids. Endocytosis, however, is not desired, because nucleic acids are degraded in endosomes. While the positive transfection data indicate that some of the DNA escapes this fate, rational design calls for different approaches. In a more futuristic scenario, targeting ligands and fusogenic proteins may be expressed on the DNA-lipid complex surface or hidden in a metastable steric shield to increase direct entry of DNA into the cytoplasm. Indeed, recent data have shown that transfection of cells in the culture start only when metastable PEG-lipid is removed from the complex (102).

An additional benefit of PEG-coating is increased stability of particles because many DNA-lipid complexes are notorious for their instability.

Sterically stabilized complexes were shown to transfect cells in culture in the presence of plasma, which typically neutralizes cationic complexes. The incorporation of PEG-surfactant into the complexes also increased transfection in vivo (103). These data can be understood by the fact that steric stabilization decreased interactions with plasma proteins that neutralize normal cationic complexes. Enhanced gene expression in vivo was also reported for precondensed DNA entrapped into DNA-lipid complexes stabilized by PEG-PE. Complexes were coated by polymer by addition of PEG-PE after their formation (45).

Similarly, DNA-lipid complexes for the nebulization were stabilized by inclusion of 1.67 mol% of ^{5000}PEG-DMPE into the complexes. Complexes were shown to have increased stability, could be prepared at higher concentrations, and had the same transfection activity. Complexation of DNA with cationic lipid was achieved due to the fact that PEG coating was not very dense (104).

The beneficial effect of PEG coating on pharmacokinetics and biodistribution can be used also to deliver antisense oligonucleotides and ribozymes (10). Furthermore, targeting ligands can be attached. To improve binding, they are usually attached to the far end of PEG chains (27,95).

Not only lipid and polymer delivery systems, but also viruses can be improved by steric stabilization. For instance, it was shown that complexation of adenoviruses with polyethylene glycol conjugated lipids improved the infectivity due to polymer shielding of neutralizing antibodies. In vitro 50-fold higher concentration of immune plasma was required to neutralize transfection of adenovirus coated with cationic lipid and PEG-lipid, as compared to virus alone (105). Similarly, arterial gene transfer of adenoviral vectors was improved by the use of Poloxamer 407, a PEG block-copolymer with similar steric stabilizing properties as PEG-lipids. Adenovector was diluted in a poloxomer solution as compared to the buffer, and resulting complexes expressed galactosidase reporter gene over threefold more efficient in transfecting balloon injured smooth muscle cells in rat carotid arteries (106).

As discussed elsewhere in this book and this chapter, there are other nonviral and nonliposomal gene-delivery systems (31,34,107). Among various polymers, dendrimers, and especially linear or branched cationic polymers, it seems that polyethylenimine (PEI) is the most widely used. Unfortunately, there are not many comparisons with lipid-based systems, especially not in vivo. Systemic administration data suggest that lipid-based delivery systems are more efficient for systemic administration, possibly due to the fact that lipids can better coat and protect plasmid. Additionally, lipids are self-assembling and can therefore dissolve, disperse, and be excreted or metabolized better than polymers. However, in vitro data or direct localized injections can show quite different results. For instance, PEI (molecular weight 25 kDa) was shown to be the only system, in comparison with DOTAP and DOGS, a polycationic lipid, that could elicit gene expression in rat kidney upon injection into left renal artery and also showed dose-dependent expression (108). On the other hand, however, the size of PEI-DNA complexes was found to be critical for gene expression in mouse central nervous system, and linear, 22 kDa PEI was found to give rise to the smallest and most stable complexes, which also yielded the highest expression in mouse central nervous system (109).

Genes and their formulations can be administered by all techniques used to deliver drugs, from systemic, topical (nasal, intratracheal instillation, inhalation of nebulized aerosol), parenteral (subcutaneous and intramuscular injection as well as intravenously or intraarterialy, possibly via a catheter or slow release collar/stint) to oral. In the latter the complex can be delivered directly into intestine in special capsules that protect it during their passage through deleterious environments.

While the majority of pulmonary studies center on cystic fibrosis, it is quite likely that the treatment of other indications, such as gene therapy for lung inflammatory diseases or cancer, will become a reality much sooner. For instance, very broad and less sophisticated is the area of inflammations where obviation of host immune response may lead to clinical therapies. Immunosuppression may involve downregulation of certain cytokines or activators of T cells or simply expressing antielastase gene to circumvent elastase-mediated lung damage and emphysema (110).

Medical applications at present are rarely based on slow, sustained release of DNA into the surrounding area. One can approach such systems from lipid-DNA, polymer-DNA, or mixed lipid-polymer-DNA systems. However, there are numerous other possibilities, from mechanic and osmotic pumps, DNA-lipid complexes encapsulated in capsules for oral delivery, polymerized liposomes to conventional slow-release systems. DNA can be incorporated into any inert matrix and implanted into the appropriate location. Along those lines, gelatin microspheres (200–700 nm) containing 25–30 wt% of DNA between cross-linked gelatin matrix were prepared. The efflux rate was approximately 2% DNA/day, and the possibility of coentrapping endolysolytic agent chloroquine and conjugation of transferrin onto microspheres was investigated (111).

Gene expression can also be improved by improving other steps in the transfection, such as increasing targeting of cell nucleus. A threefold increase in gene expression was reported for complexes containing nuclear localization signal peptide derived from the SV40 virus in the conglomerate of peptide, cationic and neutral lipid, and plasmid (112).

DNA delivery can also be used indirectly in the treatment of certain diseases, such as cancer. For instance, bone marrow cells can be transfected to express more factors that stimulate the formation of new blood cells (113). Additionally, certain cells can be protected from damage by chemotherapy or radiotherapy. For instance, overexpression of human manganese superoxide dismutase delivered by plasmid-liposomes into mice lungs decreases the effects of lung radiation damage if injected before irradiation (114).

Gene expression experiments are not simple. They involve many different branches of science, from colloid science, organic chemistry to molecular biology, biochemistry, and histology. Therefore, prudent work of specialized researchers is required to generate reproducible results.

Historically, many gene-expression experiments are plagued by poor reproducibility. This was especially true at first, and numerous data presented were in fact artifacts of experimental procedures rather than of successful gene transfection. In addition to questionable staining and other analytical procedures, one could understand certain results as consequences of reversible physical damage rather than of successful transfection. Examples include damaged vasculature upon too quick injections of too large volumes or transfection of infiltrating macrophages in the lungs flooded with DNA-lipid complex dispersion in intratracheal studies. Although one hears about the influence of injection rates, volumes applied, tonicity shocks, vertical vs. horizontal intramascular injection, etc., few data have been published. An exception is a study in which it was shown that false-positive reading of β-galactosidase are in fact due to microinfarctions in the heart rather then effective gene expression (115). More work is required in order to understand gene transfection, expression, and its quantization and to prevent observations of artifacts.

The mechanism of gene expression is still poorly understood. In vitro the main bottle-neck seems to be the entry of uncondensed DNA into cell nuclei. In vitro experiments with ethidium bromide labeling of DNA entry in the cell and green fluorescent protein transgene to measure expression have shown that more than 90% of HeLa cells with DOTAP:DOPE-green fluorescent protein complex were transfected. However, in only 30% of these cells did gene expression occur. It took more than 3 hours to measure the first expressed protein, and after 1 day each cell contained more than 100,000 plasmids, and cells where gene expression occurred, more than 2 million GFP molecules (116).

X. RECENT DEVELOPMENTS AND FUTURE DIRECTIONS

This book testifies that there are many different approaches to the construction of artificial viruses. Each of them has some pros and cons, and it is very likely that ultimately a system merging beneficial properties of several delivery systems will be constructed. Viruses as DNA-delivery vehicles have several problems including insertional mutagenesis and risk of cancer due to random integration into the host cell chromosomes, risk of viral infection and replication after recombination events that reconstitute wild-type viral functions, host immune response and inflammation upon readministering viral vectors, exorbitant cost and time involved in producing adequate virus titers, and difficulty in redirecting host cell tropism for targeted delivery to different cell types. Use of nonviral systems can avoid these problems; however, the transfection efficiencies of nonviral systems have been inadequate. In the mid-1990s, several laboratories reported high levels of gene expression in animals after injection of nonviral vectors (43, 67–86,117,118). However, the levels of gene expression were not high enough to achieve therapeutic efficacy for most diseases. Recently we reported the use of highly efficient liposomes that increased gene delivery and expression by two orders of magnitude in all organs (44). Below we shall briefly discuss this system because many data indicate that at present it is the most effective nonviral system. These improved liposomes and nucleic acid–liposome complexes are characterized by good shelf-life stability and can be frozen or lyophilized to increase stability. They have extended half-life in the circulation (see below), are stable in serum, have broad biodistribution, efficiently encapsulate all types of nucleic acids, can be made targetable to specific organs and cell types, are able to penetrate through tight barriers in several organs, and have been optimized for nucleic acid:lipid ratio and colloidal suspension in vivo. MRI data of complexes containing Gd-labeled chelating lipids showed a 5-hour half-life in the circulation of DOTAP:Chol:Gd-chelatelipid-DNA liposome complexes in rats and rabbits after tail vein injections (Bednarsky, M., Lasic, D., Templeton, N. S. unpublished). This rather unexpected result may be a consequence of fast-coating of small complexes with plasma proteins, which shield their charge and protect them from opsonins. In contrast to other complexes, these do not seem to have sharp edges and spikes, which catalyze attractive interactions.

DOTAP/Cholesterol liposomes can efficiently encapsulate nucleic acids of any size, including small oligonucleotides or large mammalian artificial chromosomes. We have encapsulated DNA, RNA, ribozymes, DNA-RNA hybrids, proteins with low isoelectric points, and mixtures of nucleic acid and protein. These complexes have been injected into mice, rats, rabbits, pigs, and nonhuman primates. Furthermore, we have demonstrated efficacy in various animal models of disease including cancer (119), restenosis (120), and AIDS.

In porcine models for restenosis, a reduction of 51% to 30% occlusion of the arteries was achieved by introducing ribozymes directed against the proliferating cell nuclear antigen (PCNA) encapsulated in DOTAP:Chol liposomes (119). In cancer therapy, p53 can be expressed in all cells of the lung after intravenous delivery and in all cells of a subcutaneous tumor after direct injection of p53 DNA-liposome complexes. Efficacy was demonstrated in both models by complete elimination of all metastatic tumors in the lung (about 800 colonies eliminated per lung) and by apoptosis of all cancer cells in the subcutaneous tumor (119).

In extensive toxicity studies, no toxicity has been found, even at the highest doses in mice, i.e., 200 μL tail vein injection containing 100 μg DNA and and 4 mM DOTAP:Chol (119). In some cases, however, the observed toxicity seemed to correlate more with particular DNA plasmids in the complex rather than with the adverse effects of cationic liposomes, which were not observed. Also, large volumes (9 mL) of complexes were injected into the saphenous vein of rhesus macaques, 12 inches high and 4.5–5.5 kg in weight, were well tolerated, and no toxicity was observed. In addition, no toxicity was found in pigs during restenosis studies. The pigs were injected by cardiovascular surgeons, reinforcing our observations that DNA-complex administration requires very skilled administration. Obviously, high-quality DNA (purity, absence of endotoxins) and sterility are necessary. Starting with sterile DNA and sterilized liposomes (sterile filtration through 0.2-μm filters), complex formation and handling should be done under sterile conditions to avoid sepsis.

Further improvements in our nonviral delivery system are required for optimal use in humans to treat diseases. The primary goal is to deliver small amounts of nucleic acids efficiently and noninvasively, thereby decreasing the dose required for efficacy. This goal can be achieved by improving the targeting efficiency to specific organs. We now have the technology for adding specific ligands either by ionic interactions or by covalent attachments to DOTAP/cholesterol-DNA complexes. These ligands include monoclonal antibodies, Fab fragments, peptides, peptide mimetics, small molecule drugs, proteins, and parts of proteins (Fig. 5). We can also size-fractionate our complexes before adding ligands to produce a homogeneous population of complexes prior to injection. Furthermore, we can change the charge on the surface of these complexes using polysaccharides or PEG-lipids in order to avoid nonspecific charge interactions with nontarget cells.

A second goal is to increase the persistence of gene expression for applications that require sustained expression. This can be accomplished by making improvements in the design of plasmid vectors. Using our improved liposomal formulations, we have achieved more efficient delivery than lentiviral and adenoviral vectors. Adult rhesus macaques were injected in the saphenous vein with DOTAP:cholesterol liposomes complexed to SIVmac239 DNA that had been propagated in *Escherichia coli*. These monkeys were highly infected with SIV within one month postinjection (120). High levels of SIV RNA were detected in the serum 4 days postinjection with DNA-liposome com-

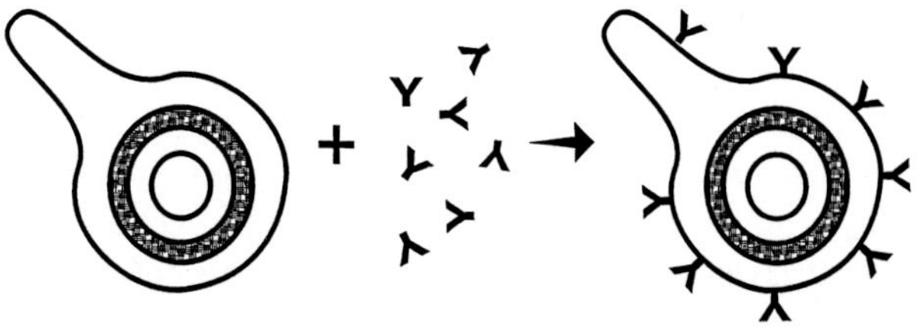

Figure 5 Cross sections of nucleic acid:DOTAP:Chol liposome complexes (left) that can also be coated with ligands (right). Ligands can be attached to the surface of preformed nucleic acid:liposome complexes by ionic interactions or through covalent attachments.

plexes, and after 14 days RNA levels were higher than that ever produced by SIV. Furthermore, the CD4 counts dropped to abnormal levels in less than 28 days postinjection with SIV DNA-liposome complexes. To assess the efficacy of vaccines, adult rhesus macaques are injected in the saphenous vein with SIV during challenge experiments. All monkeys injected with SIV that become infected, including the controls, showed drops in CD4 counts only several months or even years postinjection. Therefore, the liposomes delivered DNA more efficiently than SIV. Other studies in mice showed far greater numbers of transfected cells in the lung using our improved liposomes to deliver plasmids encoding galactosidase versus adenovirus (119). Therefore, nonviral delivery is not limited by the ability to deliver nucleic acids. It seems that limitations lie in the nucleic acids that are delivered. Viral sequences that confer persistent gene expression have been incorporated into plasmid vectors to achieve long-term gene expression. For example, sequence elements such as AAV inverted terminal repeats (ITRs) can be added to nonintegrating vectors for attachment to the nuclear matrix, thereby ensuring plasmid persistence in the nucleus. Other strategies use sequences that confer autonomous replication so that plasmids can be passed on to daughter cells after cell division. Plasmids can also be designed to provide specific integration or homologous recombination into the host chromosomes. These sequences can be used to correct host chromosome mutations or to eliminate harmful sequences in the chromosome. These strategies also have the ability to achieve persistent expression of genes encoding a normal protein.

Specific promoters and enhancers can also be used in plasmid vectors to avoid the rapid elimination of gene expression in certain tissues and cell types. The major problem involves promoter shut-off, particularly in plasmids that utilize viral promoters such as the human cytomegalovirus (CMV) major immediate-early promoter. Gfi-1–binding sites exist in the CMV promoter that bind repressors of gene expression present in certain cell types such as T cells (121). Transient expression can be shut off in less than 24 hours posttransfection as a result of this repression. Therefore, many investigators have placed tissue-specific promoters and enhancers in their plasmid vectors to provide for sustained gene expression. However, many of these tissue-specific elements do not provide significant levels of gene expression. Several recent reports demonstrate high levels of sustained expression by using the CMV enhancer followed by potent, nonviral promoters. For example, sustained, high-level gene expression was produced in all cells of a transgenic mouse throughout its lifetime using the CMV enhancer + the β-actin promoter (122). β-Actin is an abundant protein found in all cells; therefore, the promoter for this gene would not be shut off as would a viral promoter. Cells, particularly those involved in immune surveillance, possess mechanisms to eliminate viral gene expression. In summary, proper design of plasmids used for delivery of cDNAs is critical.

Since the beginning of transfection studies, the activity of DNA-lipid complexes as measured by gene expression (i.e., synthesis of the encoded protein) increased more than 1000-fold (50). In nonviral gene delivery, we can anticipate two major areas of development: (1) on the molecular biology level, modification of DNA sequences to improve nuclear targeting, entry, and persistence, as well as (2) increased transcription and translation activity. More futuristic approaches deal with self-replication and homologous recombination. On the colloidal level, rational buildup of complexes has begun. From generating liposomes, which can effectively encapsulate DNA and be tagged with ligand to the construction of the structure on the core of nucleic acids. Condensed or complexed DNA molecule(s) by a lipid, peptide, protein, or polymer can be coated with various lipid or polymer coating, which can bear various ligands with specific functions, such as targeting or fusogenic ability. Additionally, several proteins, such as HMG (high-mobility group) nonhistone chromosomal proteins, transcription factors, and protein nuclear localization factors, can be used for activation of chromatin and to enhance import and transcription of transgene (101).

In conclusion, lipids and DNA exhibit rich polymorphism, which is also reflected in (and governs) their interactions. Furthermore, it is this polymorphism that makes lipid-DNA systems effective for gene delivery. While the majority of researchers are trying to improve transfection by synthesizing novel cationic lipids, we believe that the colloidal properties of DNA-lipid complexes are at least as important. This claim can be strengthened by the fact that despite a decade of work, no clear (molecular) structure-transfection activity correlations, especially for in vivo applications, have been found (52–55). Moreover, in some cases enhanced transfection can be related simply to detergent activity of the lipids. On the other hand, some clear colloidal structure–transfection activity relationships have been found (10,42,44,45).

In this chapter we have discussed the colloidal properties of lipids, DNA, and their complexes, which are a consequence of various attractive and repulsive interactions, as well as liquid crystalline behavior of both reactants. We believe that by the improved understanding of thermodynamics, kinetics, and stability of these complexes, better transfection delivery vehicles will be possible (123).

REFERENCES

1. Lasic DD. Liposomes: From Physics to Applications. Amsterdam: Elsevier, 1993.

2. Lasic DD, Barenholz Y, eds. Handbook of Nonmedical Applications of Liposomes. Vol. I–IV. Boca Raton, FL: CRC Press, 1996.
3. Bloomfield VA, Crothers DM, Tinoco I. Physical Chemistry of Nucleic Acids. New York: Harper & Row, 1974.
4. Watson JD, Toose J, Kurtz DT. Recombinant DNA. New York: Scientific American Books, 1983.
5. Sinden RR. DNA Structure and Function. San Diego: Academic Press, 1994.
6. Flory P. Principles of Polymer Chemistry. Ithaca, NY: Cornell University Press, 1971.
7. de Gennes PG. Scaling Concepts in Polymer Physics. Ithaca, NY: Cornell University Press, 1979.
8. Bloomfield VA. DNA condensation. Curr Op Struct Biol 1996; 6:334–341.
9. Lehninger L. Principles of Biochemistry. New York: Worth Publ., 1982.
10. Lasic DD. Liposomes in Gene Delivery. Boca Raton, FL: CRC Press, 1997.
11. Kriegler M. Gene transfer. In: Gene Transfer and Expression: A Laboratory Manual. New York: W. H. Freeman and Company, 1990:3–81.
12. Culotta VC, Hamer DH. Fine mapping of a mouse metallothionein gene metal response element. Mol Cell Biol 1989; 9:1376–1380.
13. Gossen M, Bujard H. Tight control of gene expression in mammalian cells by tetracycline-responsive promoters. Proc Natl Acad Sci USA 1992; 89:5547–5551.
14. Schaack J, Ho WY-W, Freimuth P, Shenk T. Adenovirus terminal protein mediates both nuclear matrix association and efficient transcription of adenovirus DNA. Genes Dev 1990; 4:1197–1208.
15. Miralles VJ, Cortes P, Stone N, Reinberg D. The adenovirus inverted terminal repeat functions as an enhancer in a cell-free system. J Biol Chem 1989; 264:10763–10772.
16. Boussif O, Lezoulach F, Zanta MA, Schermann D, Demeneix B, Behr JP. A versatile vector for gene and oligonucleotide transfer into cells. 1995; 92:7297–7301.
17. Kabanov AV, Kabanov VA. Interpolyelectrolyte and block ionomer complexes for gene delivery. Adv Drug Del Rev 1998; 30:49–60.
18. Felgner PL, Gadek TR, Holm M, Roman R, Chan HS, Wenz M, Northrop JP, Ringold M, Danielsen H. Lipofection: a highly efficient lipid-mediated DNA transfection procedure. Proc Natl Acad Sci USA 1987; 84:7413–7417.
19. Gao X, Huang L. A novel cationic liposome reagent for efficient transfection of mammalian cells. Biochem Biophys Res Comm 1991; 179:280–285.
20. Behr JP. Synthetic gene transfer vectors. Acc Chem Res 1993; 26:274–278.
21. Israelachvili JN. Intermolecular and Surface Forces. New York: Academic Press, 1985.
22. Tanford C. The Hydrophobic Effect. New York: J. Wiley, 1980.
23. Lasic DD, Martin FJ, eds. Stealth Liposomes. Boca Raton, FL: CRC Press, 1995.
24. Uster P, Allen TM, Daniel B, Mendez C, Newman M, Zhu G. Insertion of poly(ethylene) glycol derivatized phospholipid into pre-formed liposomes results in prolonged in vivo circulation time. FEBS Lett 1996; 386:243–246.
25. Barenholz Y, Lasic DD. An overview of liposome scale-up and quality control. In: Lasic DD, Barenholz Y, eds. Handbook of Nonmedical Applications of Liposomes. Boca Raton, FL: CRC Press, 1996:23–30.
26. Liu F, Yang J, Huang L, Liu D. Effect of non-ionic surfactants on the formation of DNA/emulsion complexes and emulsion mediated gene transfer. Pharm 1996; 13: 1642–1648.
27. Lasic DD, Papahadjopoulos D, eds. Medical Applications of Liposomes. Amsterdam: Elsevier, 1998.
28. Isner JM, Walsh K, Rosenfeld R. Clinical protocol: arterial gene therapy for restenosis. Hum Gene Ther 1996; 7: 989–1011.
29. Pinnaduwage P, Schmitt L, Huang L. Use of quaternary ammonium detergent in liposome mediated DNA transfection of mouse L-cells. Biochim. Biophys Acta 198 9; 985: 33–37.
30. Miller AD. Cationic liposomes in gene therapy. Curr Res Mol Ther 1998; 1:494–502.
31. Kabanov AV, Felgner PL, Seymour LW. Self-Assembling Complexes in Gene Delivery. Chichester: Wiley, 1998.
32. Nicolau C, Papahadjopoulos D. Liposomes in gene delivery—a perspective. In: Lasic DD, Papahadjopoulos D, eds. Medical Application of Liposomes. Amsterdam: Elsevier, 1998:347–352.
33. Li Y, Xia J, Dubin PL. Complex formation between polyelectrolyte and oppositively charged micelles. Macromolecules. 1994; 27:7049–7055.
34. Kabanov AV, Kabanov VA. DNA complexes with polycations for delivery of genetic material into cells. Bioconj Chem 1995; 6:7–20.
35. Sternberg B, Sorgi F, Huang L. New structures in complex formation between DNA and cationic liposomes visualized by freeze-fracture electron microscopy. FEBS Lett 1994; 356:361–366.
36. Gustaffson J, Almgrem M, Karlsson G, Arvidson G. Complexes by cationic lipids and DNA as visualized by cryo transmission electron microscopy. Biochim Biophys Acta 1995; 1235:305–317.
37. Lasic DD, Strey HH, Podgornik R, Frederik P. Recent developments in medical applications of liposomes: sterically stabilized and cationic liposomes. 4th European Symp. Control. Drug Del., Book of Abstracts, Nordwijk aan Zee, April 1996, pp. 61–65.
38. Lasic DD, Strey H, Podgornik R, Frederik PM. The structure of DNA-liposome complexes. J Am Chem Soc 1997; 119:832–833.
39. Raedler J, Koltover I, Salditt T, Safinya C. The structure of DNA-liposome complexes. Science 1997; 275:810–814.
40. Sternberg B. Liposomes as models for membrane structures and structural transformations. In: Lasic DD, Barenholz Y, eds. Handbook of Nonmedical Applications of

Liposomes. Vol. IV. Boca Raton, FL: CRC Press, 1996: 271–298.
41. Zuidam N, Barenholz Y. Electrostatic parameters of cationic liposomes commonly used in gene delivery. Biochim Biophys Acta 1997; 1329:211–222.
42. Lasic DD, Podgornik R, Frederik P, Strey H, Yie J. (In preparation).
43. Zhu N, Liggitt D, Liu Y, Debs R. Systemic gene expression after intravenous DNA delivery in adult mice. Science 1993; 261:209–211.
44. Templeton NS, Lasic DD, Frederik PM, Strey HH, Roberts DD, Pavlakis G. Improved DNA:liposome complexes for increased systemic delivery and gene expression. Nature Biotech 1997; 15:647–652.
45. Hong K, Zheng W, Baker A, Papahadjopoulos D. Stabilization of cationic complexes by polyamines and PEG-phospholipid conjugates for efficient in vivo delivery. FEBS Lett 1997; 400:233–237.
46. Lasic DD, Papahadjopoulos D, Podgornik R. Polymorphism of lipids, nucleic acids and their intreactions. In: Kabanov AV, et al., eds. Self-Assembling complexes in Gene Delivery. Chichester: Wiley, 1998:3–26.
47. Dan NL. Multilamellar structures of DNA complexes with cationic liposomes. Biophys J 1997; 73:1842–1846.
48. Podgornik R, Strey H, Parsegian VA. Colloidal DNA. Curr Op Colloid Interface Sci 1998; 3:534–539.
49. Harries D, May S, Gelbart WM, BenShaul A. Structure, stability and thermodynamics of lamellar DNA-lipid complexes. Biophys J 1998; 75:159–173.
50. Felgner PL. Improvement in cationic liposomes for in vivo gene delivery. Hum Gene Ther 1996; 7:1791–1793.
51. Tsukamoto M, Ochiya T, Yoshida S, Sugimura T, Terada M. Gene transfer and expression in progeny after intravenous DNA injection into pregnant mice, Nature Genet 1995; 9:243–248.
52. Nabel EG, Gordon D, Yang Z-Y, Xu L, San H, Plautz GE, Wu B-Y, Gao X, Huang L, Nabel GJ. Gene transfer in vivo with DNA-liposome complexes: lack of autoimmunity and gonadal localization. Hum Gene Ther 1992; 3:649–656.
53. Nabel GJ, Nabel EG, Yang Z-Y, Fox BA, Plautz GE, Gao X, Huang L, Shu S, Gordon D, Chang AE. Direct gene transfer with DNA-liposome complexes in melanoma: expression, biologic activity, and lack of toxicity in humans, Proc Natl Acad Sci USA 1993; 90:11307–11311.
54. Caplen NJ, Gao X, Hayes P, Elaswarapu R, Fisher G, Kinrade E, Chakera A, Schorr J, Hughes B, Dorin JR, Porteous DJ, Alton EWFW, Geddes DM, Coutelle C, Williamson R, Huang L, Gilchrist C. Gene therapy for cystic fibrosis in humans by liposome-mediated DNA transfer: the production of resources and the regulatory process. Gene Ther 1994; 1:139–147.
55. Caplen NJ, Alton EWFW, Middleton PG, Dorin JR, Stevenson BJ, Gao X, Durham SR, Jeffrey PK, Hodson ME, Coutelle C, Huang L, Porteous DJ, Williamson R, Geddes DM. Liposome-mediated CFTR gene transfer to the nasal epithelium of patients with cystic fibrosis. Nature Med 1995; 1:39–46.
56. Nabel GJ, Chang A, Nabel EG, Plautz G, Fox BA, Huang L, Shu S. Immunotherapy of malignancy by in vivo gene transfer into tumors. Hum Gene Ther 1992; 3:399–410.
57. Michael SI, Curiel DT. Strategies to achieve targeted gene delivery via the receptor-mediated endocytosis pathway. Gene Ther 1994; 1:223–232.
58. Wu GY, Wu CH. Receptor-mediated in vitro gene transformation by a soluble DNA carrier system. J Biol Chem 1987; 262:4429–4432.
59. Wagner E, Zenke M, Cotten M, Beug H, Birnsteil ML. Transferrin-polycation conjugates as carriers for DNA uptake into cell. Proc Natl Acad Sci USA 1990; 87: 3410–3414.
60. Zenke M, Steinlein P, Wagner E, Cotten M, Beug H, Birnstiel ML. Receptor-mediated endocytosis of transferrin-polycation conjugates: an efficient way to introduce DNA into hematopoietic cells. Proc Natl Acad Sci USA 1990; 87:3655–3659.
61. Ferkol T, Kaetzel CS, Davis PB. Gene transfer into respiratory epithelial cells by targeting the polymeric immunoglobulin receptor. J Clin Invest 1993; 92:2394–2400.
62. Miller N, Vile R. Targeted vectors for gene therapy. FASEB J 1995; 9:190–199.
63. Rosenkranz AA, Yachmenev SV, Jans DA, Serebryakova NV, Murav + ev VI, Peters R, Sobolev AS. Receptor-mediated endocytosis and nuclear transport of a transfecting DNA construct. Exp Cell Res 1992; 199:323–329.
64. Chen J, Gamou S, Takayanagi A, Shimizu N. A novel gene delivery system using EGF receptor-mediated endocytosis. FEBS Lett 1994; 338:167–169.
65. Batra RK, Wang-Johanning F, Wagner E, Garver RI, Curiel DT. Receptor-mediated gene delivery employing lectin-binding specificity. Gene Ther 1994; 1:255–260.
66. Culver KW, Ram Z, Wallbridge S, Ishii H, Oldfield EH, Blaese RM. In vivo gene transfer with retroviral vector-producer cells for treatment of experimental brain tumors. Science 1992; 256:1550–1552.
67. Huber BE, Austin EA, Richards CA, Davis ST, Good SS. Metabolism of 5-fluorocytosine to 5-fluorouracil in human colorectal tumor cells transduced with the cytosine deaminase gene: significant antitumor effects when only a small percentage of tumor cells express cytosine deaminase. Proc Natl Acad Sci USA 1994; 91:8302–8306.
68. Brigham KL, Meyrick B, Christman B, Magnuson M, King G, Barry L. In vivo transfection of murine lungs with a functional prokaryotic gene using a liposome vehicle, Am J Med Sci 1989; 298:278–281.
69. Hazinski TA, Ladd PA, DeMateo CA. Localization and induced expression of fusion genes in the rat lung. Am J Respir Cell Mol Biol 1991; 2:206–209.
70. Stribling R, Brunette E, Gaensler K, Debs R. Aerosol gene delivery in vivo. Proc Natl Acad Sci USA 1992; 89: 11277–11281.
71. Hyde SC, Gill DR, Higgins FC, MacVinish LJ, Cuthbert AW, Ratcliff R, Evans M, Colledge WH. Correction of the ion transport defect in cystic fibrosis mice with gene therapy. Nature 1993; 362:250–255.

72. Plautz GE, Yang ZY, Wu BJ, Gao X, Huang L, Nabel GJ. Immunotherapy of malignancy by in vivo gene transfer into tumors. Proc Natl Acad Sci USA 1990; 90:465–469.
73. Leventis R, Silvius JR. Interactions of mammalian cells with lipid dispersions containing novel metabolizable cationic amphiphiles. Biochim Biophys Acta 1990; 1023: 124–132.
74. Felgner JH, Kumar R, Sridhar R, Wheeler C, Tsai YJ, Border R, Ramsay P, Martin M, Felgner PL. Enhanced gene delivery and mechanism studies with novel series of cationic lipid formulations. J Biol Chem 1994; 269: 2550–2561.
75. Farhood H, Bottega R, Epand RM, Huang L. Effect of cholesterol derivatives on gene transfer and protein kinase C activity. Biochim Biophys Acta 1992; 1111:239–246.
76. Solodin I, Brown CS, Bruno MS, Ching-Yi C, Eun-Hyun J, Debs R, Heath TD. A novel series of amphiphilic imidazolinium compounds for in vitro and in vivo gene delivery. Biochemistry 1995; 34:13537–13544.
77. Byk G, Sherman D. Novel cationic lipids for gene delivery and gene therapy. Exp Opin Ther Patents 1998; 8: 1125–1141.
78. Lee ER, Marshall JM, Siegel CS, Jiang C, Yew NS, Nichols MR, Nietupski JB, Ziegler JR, Lane MB, Wang KX, Wan NC, Scheule RK, Harris DJ, Smith AE, Cheng SH. Detailed analysis of structures and formulations of cationic lipids for efficient gene transfer to the lung. Human Gene Ther 1996; 7:1701–1717.
79. Wheeler CJ, Sukhu L, Yang G, Tsai Y, Bustamante C, Felgner P, Norman J, Manthorpe M. Converting an alcohol to an amine in a cationic lipid dramatically alters the co-lipid requirement, cellular transfection activity and the ultrastructure of DNA-cytofectin complexes. Biochim Biophys Acta 1996; 1280:1–11.
80. Farhood H, Huang L. Delivery of DNA, RNA and proteins by cationic liposomes. In: Lasic DD, Barenholz Y, eds. Liposomes: From Gene Therapy to Diagnostics and Ecology. Boca Raton, FL: CRC Press, 1996:31–42.
81. Felgner PL, Tsai YJ, Felgner JH. Advances in the design and application of cytofectin formulations. In: Lasic DD, Barenholz Y, eds. Liposomes: From Gene Therapy to Diagnostics and Ecology.
82. Walker S, Sofia MJ, Karakla R, Kogan N, Weirich L, Longley CB, Brucker K, Axelrod HL, Midha S, Kahne D. Cationic facial amphiphiles: a promising class of transfection agents. Proc Natl Acad Sci USA 1996; 93:1585–1590.
83. Lewis JG, Lin K, Kothavale A, Flanagan WM, Mateucci MD, dePrince R, Mook RA, Hendren R, Wagner RW. Proc Natl Acad Sci USA 1996; 93:3176–3181.
84. Oudrhiri N, Vigneron JP, Peuchmaur M, Leclerc T, Lehn JM, Lehn P. Gene transfer by guanidinium-cholesterol cationic lipids into airway epithelial cells in vitro and in vivo. Proc Natl Acad Sci USA 1997; 94:1651–1656.
85. Van der Woude I, Wagenaar A, Meekel A, ter Beest MBA, Ruiters M, Engberts JBFN, Hoekstra D. Novel pyridinium surfactants for efficient, nontoxic in vitro gene delivery. Proc Natl Acad Sci 1997; 94:1160–1165.
86. Byk G, Dubertret C, Escriouu V, Frederic M, Jaslin G, Rangara R, Pitard B, Crouzet J, Wils P, Schwartz B, Scherman D. Synthesis, activity and structure-activity relationship studies of novel cationic lipids for DNA transfer. J Med Chem 1998; 41:224–235.
87. Melnikov SM, Melnikova YS, Lofroth JE. Single molecule visualization of interaction between DNA and oppositely charged mixed liposomes. J Phys Chem 1998; 102: 9367–9369.
88. Pitard B, Aguerre O, Airiau M, Lachages AM, Boukni-kachvili T, Byk G, Dubertret C, Herviou C, Scherman D, Mayaux JF, Crouzet J. Virus sized self-assembling lamellar complexes between plasmid DNA and cationic micelles promote gene transfer. Proc Natl Acad Sci USA 1997; 41: 14412–14417.
89. Gao X, Huang L. Potentiation of cationic liposome-mediated gene delivery by polycations. Biochemistry 1996; 35:1027–1036.
90. Schwartz B, Ivanov MA, Pitard B, Ranara R, Byk B, Wils P, Crouzet J, Scherman D. Synthetic DNA compacting peptides derived from human sequence enhance cationic lipid mediated gene transfer in vitro and in vivo. Gene Ther 1999; 6:283–292.
91. Ferkol T, Peralse JC, Mularo F, Hanson RW. Receptor mediated gene transfer into macrophages. Proc Natl Acad Sci USA 1995; 93:101–105.
92. Kawakami S, Yamashita F, Nishikawa M, Takakura Y, M Hashida. Asialoglycoprotein receptor-mediated gene transfer using novel galactosylated cationic liposomes. Biochem Biophys Res Comm 1998; 252:78–83.
93. Hara T, Kuwasawa H, Aramaki Y, Takada S, Koioke K, Ishidata K, Kato H, Tsuchiya S. Effects of fusogenic and DNA binding amphiphilic compounds on the receptor mediated gene transfer into hepatic cells by asialofetuin labeled liposomes. Biochim Biophys Acta 1996; 1278: 51–58.
94. Xu L, Pirrolio KF, Chang EH. Transferrin liposome mediated p53 sensitization of squamous cell carcinoma of the head and neck to radiation in vitro. Hum Gene Ther 1997; 6:467–475.
95. Wang S, Lee RJ, Causchon G, Gorenstein DG, Low PS. Delivery of antisense oligonucleotides against HEGF receptor into cultured KB cells with liposomes conjugated to folate via PEG. PNAS 1995; 92:3318–3322.
96. Simoes S, Slepushkin V, Gaspar R, Pedroso da Lima MC, Duzgunes N. Gene delivery by negatively charged ternary complexes of DNA and cationic liposomes and fusigenic peptides or transferrin. Gene Ther 1998; 5:955–964.
97. Yonemitsu Y, Alton EW, Komori K, Youshuzumi T, Sugimachi K, Kaneda Y. Liposome mediated gene transfer: current status and future perspectives. Int J Oncol 1998; 12:1277–1285.
98. Foster BJ, Kerr JA. HER2 targeted gene transfer. Hum Gene Ther 1997; 8:719–727.
99. Lasic DD, Papahadjopoulos D. Liposome revisited. Science 1995; 267:1275–1276.

100. Lasic DD. Doxorubicin in sterically stabilized liposomes. Nature 1996; 380:561–562.
101. Boulikas T, ed. Gene Therapy and Molecular Biology. From Basic Mechanisms to Clinical Applications. Palo Alto: Gene Therapy Press, 1998.
102. Wheeler JJ, Palmer I, Ossanlau M, Maclahlan I, Zhang Y, Hope MJ, Scherrer P, Cullis PR. Stabilized plasmid-lipid particles: construction and characterization. Gene Ther 1999; 6:271–281.
103. Liu F, Qi H, Huang L, Liu D. Factors controlling the efficiency of cationic lipid mediated transfection in vivo via iv administration. Gene Ther 1997; 4:517–523.
104. Eastman SJ, Lukason M, Toussignant J, Murray H, Lane MD, StGeorge J, Akita G, Cherry M, Cheng S, Scheule RK. A concentrated and stable aerosol formulation of cationic lipid: DNA complexes giving high level gene expression in mouse lung. Hum Gene Ther 1997; 8: 765–773.
105. Chilon M, Lee JH, Fasbender A, Walsh JM. Adenovirus complexed with PEG and cationic lipids is shielded from neutralizing antibodies. Gene Ther 1998; 5:995–1002.
106. Feldman LJ, Pastore CJ, Aubilly N, Kearny M, Perricaudet M, Steg PG, Isner JM. Improved efficiency of arterial gene transfer by use of poloxamen 407 as a vehicle for adenoviral vectors. Gene Ther 1997; 4:189–198.
107. Kabanov VA, Szoka F, Seymour LW. Interply electrolyte complexes for gene delivery: polymer aspects of gene delivery. In: Kabanov AV, et al., eds. Self-Assembling Complexes in Gene Delivery. Chichester: Wiley, 1998: 197–218.
108. Boletta A, Benigin A, Lutz J, Remuzzi G, Soria MC, Monaco L. Nonviral gene delivery to the rat kidney with polyethylenimine. Human Gene Ther 1997; 8:1243–1251.
109. Goula D, Remy JS, Erbachre P, Wasowitz M, Levi G, Abdallah B, Demeneix BA. Size, diffusability and transfection performance of linear PEI/DNA complexes in mouse central nervous system. Gene Ther 1998; 5: 712,717.
110. Sellanave JM, Porteous DJ, Chasleu. Gene therapy for lung inflammatory diseases: not so far away? Thorax 1997; 52: 742–744.
111. Le VLT, August JT, Leong KW. Controlled gene delivery by DNA-gelatin nanospheres. Hum Gene Ther 1998; 9: 1709–1717.
112. Aronsohn AI, Hughes JA. Nuclear localization signal peptides enhance cationic lipid mediated gene delivery. J Drug Targ 1998; 5:163–169.
113. Kessler PD, Podsakoff GM, Chen X, McQuiston SA, Colosi PC, Matelis LA, Kurtzman GJ, Byrne BJ. Gene delivery to skeletal muscle results in a sustained expression and systemic delivery of a therapeutic protein. Proc Natl Acad Sci 1996; 93:14082–14087.
114. Epperly M, Bray J, Kraeger S, Zwacka R, Engelhardt J, Travis E, Greenberger J. Prevention of late effects of irradiation lung damage by manganese superoxide dismutase gene therapy. Gene Ther 1998; 5:196–208.
115. Wright MJ, Rosenthal E, Stewart L, Wrigham LM, Miller AD, Latchman DS, Marber MS. Beta galactosidase staining following intracoronary infusion of cationic liposome in the in vivo rabbit heart is produced by microinfarction rather then effective gene transfer: a cautionary tale. Gen Ther 1998; 5:301–308.
116. Tseng WC, Haselton FR, Giorgio TD. Transfection by cationic liposomes using simultaneous single cell measurements of plasmid delivery and transgene expression. J Biol Chem 1997; 272:25641–25647.
117. Thierry AR, Rabinovich P, Peng B, Mahan LC, Bryant JL, Gallo RC. Characterization of liposome-mediated gene delivery: expression, stability and pharmacokinetics of plasmid DNA. Gene Ther 1997; 4:226–237.
118. Tsukamoto M, Ochiya T, Yoshida S, Sugimura T, Terada M. Gene transfer and expression in progeny after intravenous DNA injection into pregnant mice. Nature Genetics 1995; 9:243–248.
119. Ramesh R, Saeki T, Wu Z, Templeton NS, Zhang S, Wilson DR, Branch C, Roth JA. Inhibition of tumor growth following liposome-mediated p53 delivery. 2nd Annual Meeting of the American Society of Gene Therapy, Washington, D.C., 1999.
120. Templeton NS, Alspaugh E, Antelman D, Barber J, Csaky KG, Fang B, Frederik P, Honda H, Johnson D, Litvak F, Machemer T, Ramesh R, Robbins J, Roth JA, Sebastian M, Tritz R, Wen SF, Wu Z. Non-viral vectors for the treatment of disease. Keystone Symposia on Molecular and Cellular Biology of Gene Therapy, Salt Lake City, 1999.
121. Zweidler-McKay PA, Grimes HL, Flubacher MM, Tsichlis PN. Gfi-1 encodes a nuclear zinc finger protein that binds DNA and functions as a transcriptional repressor. Mol Cell Biol 1996; 16:4024–4034.
122. Okabe M, Ikawa M, Kominami K, Nakanishi T, Nishimune Y. 'Green mice' as a source of ubiquitous green cells. FEBS Lett 1997; 407:313–319.
123. Meyer O, Kirpotin D, Hong K, Sterneberg B, Park JW, Woodle MC, Papahadjopoulos D. Cationic liposomes coated with PEG as carriers for oligonucleotides. J Biol Chem 1998; 273:15621–15627.
124. Woodle MC, Leserman L. Liposomal antisense oligonucleotide therapeutics. In: Lasic DD, Papahadjopoulos D, eds. Medical Applications of Liposomes. Amsterdam: Elsevier, 1998:429–450.
125. Lasic DD. Liposomes. Science & Medicine, 1996; 3: 34–43.

13

Synthetic Virus Systems for Systemic Gene Therapy

Ian MacLachlan, Pieter Cullis, and Roger W. Graham
Inex Pharmaceuticals Corporation, Burnaby, British Columbia, Canada

I. INTRODUCTION

In the early 1980s the concept of treating disease through correction of aberrant gene function rose to the attention of both the scientific community and the general public. At the time techniques for gene transfer were underdeveloped, but in the following years efficient methods for gene transfer were established and preclinical studies demonstrated the feasibility of correcting disease phenotypes both in vitro and in vivo. These early proof of principal experiments successfully capped the first, ''conceptual phase'' (1) of the development of gene therapy and helped to ensure a position for the field in both the medical and popular lexicon. It is generally agreed that the second, translational phase of the development of gene therapy has been considerably less successful. The first human gene marking study performed at the National Institutes of Health (NIH) in 1989 was followed within a year by the first sanctioned therapeutic study (2). In the following decade hundreds of gene therapy clinical trials were initiated worldwide. Today each new advance in medicine is, almost without exception, accompanied by proposals for genetic intervention in associated disease states. In spite of this enthusiasm, gene therapy has been a clinical disappointment. Although numerous reports describe successful gene transfer and prolonged expression of therapeutic transgenes, most clinical trials have failed to demonstrate a therapeutic benefit to treating patients with gene therapy. This was officially recognized in 1995 when the director of the NIH, Harold Varmus, struck two independent committees to review both the scientific and the regulatory aspects of the field. The outcome of this analysis was the consensus that most of the failures of gene therapy could be attributed to the ''discordant combination of overinterpreted clinical concepts and immature technology, including poor vector design'' (3). This conclusion resulted in a shift in emphasis and expectations for the field, culminating in a recent refocusing on the design and implementation of vector systems for gene therapy as well as a reevaluation of appropriate disease targets. Once regarded as an experimental treatment for inherited genetic disorders, gene therapy is now considered a candidate for front-line therapy of acquired diseases such as cancer. Because the future success of gene therapy will be measured by the ability to compete with the clinical utility of conventional therapeutics, the areas of medicine thought to be most suited to gene therapy are those that have failed to respond to existing treatments (4). The advantage of gene therapy over conventional therapy, and hence its promise, is the ability to regulate gene function and achieve prolonged and specific activity.

In oncology, the holy grail is systemic administration of gene therapy to impact metastatic disease, the primary determinant of survival in most cancers. A defining attribute of metastatic disease is its disseminated nature. As such, treatment with local or regional therapeutics is unlikely to affect clinical outcome or overall disease progression. In the case of intracavitary administration (intrapleural or intraperitoneal), the surface of the tumor mass is coated by the vector, but intratumoral delivery is not achieved. It is increasingly apparent that relevant gene-delivery systems for oncology applications must be able to access distal disease sites following systemic administration. For this reason a number of investigators have chosen to focus on the development of gene-transfer systems that will have utility in this context (5–8).

Gene-transfer systems are based on one of two predominant platforms—viral or nonviral. Although recognized as being very efficient gene-transfer agents, viral vectors are limited by their inability to access disease sites upon systemic administration. Until significant progress has been made in improving the pharmacology and toxicology of viral vectors, their utility will be limited to local or regional administration in clinical application. Nonviral gene-transfer systems offer specific clinical and commercial advantages as potential therapeutics. Because nonviral systems use synthetic or highly purified components, they are chemically defined and free of adventitious agents. Nonviral systems do not contain adjuvants or undescribed molecular sequences inherent in many viral gene-transfer systems. Nonviral systems can be manufactured under controlled conditions which are not constrained by the biological considerations as cell growth and viability that define viral scale-up processes. In spite of these advantages, progress in the development of systemic nonviral vectors has been slow.

In this chapter we will discuss recent progress in nonviral gene therapy with an emphasis on developments that specifically attempt to address the limitations of current vector systems and their inability to overcome the first barrier to systemic gene delivery—delivery to the disease site and the target cell. Other important barriers to transfection include cytoplasmic delivery, endosomal release, and nuclear delivery. It is unlikely that one single approach will overcome all of these barriers. In fact, properties that are required for systemic disease site targeting have been shown to inhibit intracellular delivery and nuclear uptake. This supports the concept of a modular solution for systemic gene therapy, a vector with individual components fulfilling different functions in the transfection process. An ideal artificial virus would incorporate the most beneficial attributes from both viral and nonviral gene systems. Refinement of gene therapies can be viewed as the convergence of ''top-down'' deconstruction of viral systems and ''bottom-up'' engineering of nonviral systems. A number of investigators have chosen to address the limitations of viral systems by removing viral sequences from viral vectors in an attempt to reduce their undesirable characteristics. In this chapter we describe the status of the development of lipid-based systems with virus-like qualities and the potential to rationally incorporate other virus functions.

II. DESIRED PROPERTIES OF A SYNTHETIC GENE-DELIVERY SYSTEM FOR THE TREATMENT OF SYSTEMIC DISEASE

A. Definition of an Appropriate Vector

An objective inherent in all pharmaceutical development is to minimize the risks associated with treatment while maximizing the benefit to patient health. The most important risk to patients is the toxicity associated with the administration of poorly tolerated compounds or cytotoxic agents. Toxicity is often exacerbated by attempts to increase efficacy by escalating the administered dose. The differential between the minimum dose at which a therapeutic benefit is obtained and the maximum dose that can be safely administered to the patient is known as the ''therapeutic window.'' Any reduction in toxicity or increase in potency results in a concomitant increase and improvement in the therapeutic window of a given drug. Toxicity is often the result of preferential accumulation of therapeutic agents in nontarget tissue. One strategy for reducing toxicity involves optimization of drug delivery to maximize delivery to the target site. Therapeutics designed for systemic administration must be capable of bypassing numerous obstacles to effective drug delivery. Drug distribution will be determined by physical and biochemical properties including stability, size, charge, hydrophobicity, interaction with serum proteins, and interaction with nontarget cell surfaces. In the context of an oncology application, effective therapeutics must be able to overcome obstacles associated with heterogeneous cell populations that are often proliferating rapidly at different stages of the cell cycle and do not conform to the patterns of organization established during the development of normal tissue. In particular, tumor growth is associated with changes in vascular organization and permeability that have the potential to affect drug delivery. Normal vascular endothelium is characterized by intact intracellular junctions, which permit only the passage of small molecules. However, the capillaries in tumors develop in a less organized fashion, leaving fenestrae or gaps in the endothelial layer ranging in size from 30 to 500 nm, (9). A few normal tissues, most importantly liver and spleen, have similar fenestrations in the vascular epithelium, which directly expose the underlying endothelial cells to material in the circulation. Importantly, these tissues are often the sites of drug accumulation upon systemic administration.

In conventional pharmacology in vivo studies are initiated once a drug formulation has been developed that exhibits the properties required to ensure effective drug delivery and pharmaceutical viability. Progress in gene therapy has been driven primarily by the pursuit of vectors that are

Table 1 Target Attributes of Carrier Systems for Systemic Gene Therapy

Attribute	Target value	Effect
Toxicity	Low	Facilitates dose escalation
Stability	$>$ 6 months	Facilitates QC
Size	$<$100 nm	Disease site targeting and extravasation and endocytosis
Surface charge	Neutral or shielded	Disease site targeting and extravasation
Serum half-life	$>$ 3 hours	Disease site targeting
Immunogenicity	Moderate	Multiple dosing
Manufacturability	Reproducible and scalable	Clinical utility

effective in vitro transfection reagents. Acknowledgment of the properties required for effective systemic gene transfer and pharmaceutical viability may require a strategic reevaluation of systemic vector development (Table 1). We propose the following definition of an ideal carrier for systemic gene therapy. The ideal synthetic vector for systemic gene therapy will have the following properties:

1. It must be safe and well tolerated upon systemic administration.
2. It must have appropriate pharmacokinetic attributes to ensure delivery to disease sites.
3. It must deliver intact DNA to target tissue and mediate transfection of that tissue.
4. It must be nonimmunogenic.
5. It must be stable upon manufacture so that large batches can be prepared with uniform reproducible specifications.

B. Barriers to Transfection

DNA is generally limited by poor pharmacokinetic attributes, which limit delivery to disease sites upon systemic administration. Once at the target cell, DNA is again limited in its ability to traverse the numerous biological barriers to transfection. Nucleic acids clearly require pharmaceutical enablement in the form of appropriate carriers, which are able to confer protection from degradation and facilitate delivery and uptake at the disease site. In order to achieve delivery to a disease site, an appropriate systemic carrier must overcome a number of pharmacological barriers. When in the blood compartment an effective gene-delivery system must be able to confer stability to the nucleic acid payload in spite of the presence of serum nucleases and other enzymatic activities that have the potential to degrade carrier components. Indiscriminate interaction with lipoproteins or serum proteins can cause aggregation before a carrier reaches the disease site. Systemic carriers encounter several nontarget cells in the blood compartment, such as blood cells and vascular endothelium, which may be only moderately differentiated from target cells. In addition, systemic delivery systems have a greater potential for inducing toxicity through interaction with complement and coagulation pathways. This is especially true for systems that contain large polyanionic molecules such as plasmid DNA. Other barriers to gene delivery include the microcapillary beds of so-called first-pass organs (lung and liver), the phagocytic cells of the reticuloendothelial system, and filtration by kidney glomeruli. The critical parameters that must be measured and optimized to ensure the performance of systemic gene delivery systems are stability, circulation lifetime, biodistribution, and toxicity profile.

Accessing target cell populations requires extravasation from the blood compartment to the disease site. Carriers may leave the blood compartment by passing between endothelial cells or in some cases by transcytosis through specialized endothelial cell systems. Carriers of appropriate size pass through the fenestrated epithelium of tumor neovasculature. Delivery from the blood compartment is followed by diffusion through tissue. In the case of solid tumors, this is often an inefficient process. Although the disorganized nature of tumor growth would intuitively imply accessibility in practice, this is not always true. Tumor growth is often characterized by an underdeveloped lymphatic drainage, which leads to a build-up of hydrostatic pressure unfavorable to extravasation. Other physical barriers to extravasation include large areas of fibrosis and necrosis, which must be bypassed to access actively dividing target cell populations.

Although a prerequisite, delivery of a gene therapy vector to a target cell in no way guarantees transfection. Once at the cell surface, gene therapy vectors are confronted with a number of physical and biochemical barriers, each of which must be overcome in order to effect transfection and transgene expression. The first physical barrier to transfection is the plasma membrane. The plasma membrane is a

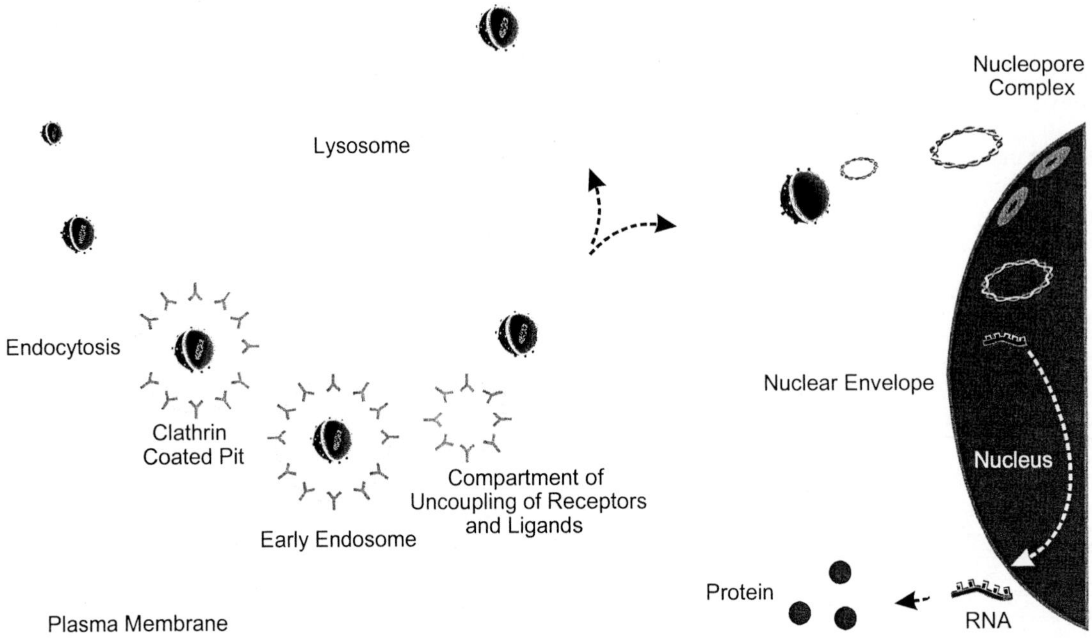

Figure 1 Physical and biochemical barriers to transfection. Most intracellular delivery is thought to occur through endocytosis via cell surface clathrin-coated pits. Endocytic vesicles undergo a series of morphological changes, which define the various stages of intracellular processing. Internalized vesicles or primary endosomes are differentiated from tubulovesicular early endosomes, multivesicular late endosomes, and lysosomes. Late endosomes have a significantly lower luminal pH than early endosomes and contain multivesicular bodies, carrier vesicles, and the prelysosomal compartment. Lysosomal maturation is accompanied by a further decrease in internal pH, a destabilization of the lysosomal membrane, and an increase in fusogenicity. Untargeted nonviral vectors rely on diffusion to facilitate interaction with the nuclear envelope, the final physical barrier to transfection.

discontinuous phospholipid bilayer containing intercalated amphipathic membrane proteins (10). The external surface of the plasma membrane is protected by a carbohydrate coating, or glycocalyx, formed by the posttranslational glycosylation of transmembrane proteins. This carbohydrate layer may be up to 100 nm thick (11). The luminal side of the plasma membrane is supported by an actin-rich cytoskeletal matrix of microfilaments and microtubules. Although early models of lipid-mediated transfection invoked a putative fusion event between the plasma membrane and the membrane of the lipid vesicle, it is now generally agreed that the majority of intracellular delivery occurs through endocytosis.

Endocytosis is a complex process by which cells take up extracellular material by translocation across the cell surface membrane (12). This process is known to occur through the activity of cell surface clathrin-coated pits, invaginations in the plasma membrane which are subsequently pinched off into the cytoplasm (Fig. 1). When this occurs, internalized material remains on the exoplasmic side of the internalized vesicle, without direct access to the cytoplasm. The contents of the internalized vesicles are enriched in ligands such as low-density lipoproteins and transferrin (12). In contrast, the fluid content of the vesicle has the same composition as the extracellular medium. The nonspecific uptake of extracellular material through the internalization of coated vesicles is referred to as bulk uptake or fluid phase endocytosis.

Endocytic vesicles undergo a series of morphological changes, which define the various stages of intracellular processing. Internalized vesicles or primary endosomes are differentiated from tubulovesicular early endosomes, multivesicular late endosomes, and lysosomes. According to the maturation model of endocytosis, these organelles are transient entities which undergo successive remodeling to form the organelles associated with each subsequent stage of the pathway (13). This occurs by progressive addition or subtraction of individual organelle components at a rate that maintains the appearance of a homeostatic complement of organelles at each stage of maturation. The first such change occurs within 5 minutes of uptake as internalized vesicles undergo a series of changes and form the tubulovesicular early endosome or compartment of uncoupling of receptor and ligand (CURL) (14). In this compartment sorting of receptors and ligands occurs. Early endosomes are transiently fusogenic (15). Late endosomes are differentiated from early endosomes both morphologically and biochemically. Late endosomes have a significantly lower luminal pH than early endosomes and contain multivesicular bodies, carrier vesicles, and the prelysosomal compartment. Lysosomal maturation is accompanied by a further decrease in internal pH, a destabilization of the lysosomal membrane and an increase in fusogenicity. Although the process of endocytosis has been well characterized, the processing and release of internalized nonviral vectors and/or their payload DNA is not well understood.

Following endosomal release, plasmid DNA spends an indeterminate residency time in the cytoplasm prior to gaining entry to the nucleus. Unlike viral systems, which have evolved specific mechanisms to traverse this barrier, untargeted nonviral vectors rely on diffusion to facilitate interaction with the nuclear envelope. However, the cytoplasm is a highly organized space containing networks of cytoskeletal elements and membrane-bound organelles, which have the potential to interact with and accumulate vector systems that arrive at the cytosol intact. In particular, mitochondria have been shown to preferentially accumulate polycationic compounds. Until recently the cytoplasmic degradation of plasmid DNA has not been thought to be limiting transfection. However, recent results suggest that this assumption may be incorrect. The turnover of plasmid DNA in the cytoplasm can be measured by quantitative single-cell video analysis (16). When plasmid DNA is delivered by direct microinjection into the cytosol of mammalian cells, it is rapidly degraded by divalent-cation–dependent cytosolic nucleases. This finding is a partial explanation for the strikingly low efficiency of the nuclear translocation process and may have implications for vector design. Vector systems which either protect the DNA payload from degradation following endosome release or effectively minimize the cytoplasmic residency time would be expected to yield improved transfection efficiencies.

The nuclear envelope presents the final physical barrier to transfection. Evolution has led to the development of the nuclear envelope as a means of organizing and maintaining the integrity of the large genome of eukaryotic cells. The nuclear envelope also effectively isolates and protects genetic material from any adventitious elements, such as viruses or transposons, which may enter the cytoplasm of the cell. Appropriately designed gene therapy vectors must overcome this barrier. For this reason an understanding of the systems that mediate the nuclear import of plasmid DNA is essential. The importance of the nuclear envelope in the transfection process is underscored by the finding that nonviral transfection occurs more readily in mitotic cells (17,18). This implies that the nuclear uptake of DNA is limited by the presence of an intact nuclear envelope, which is destabilized during mitosis. Strategies to overcome this barrier can take one of two forms, either targeting transfection reagents to cell populations with a high degree of mitotic activity, such as tumor tissue, or enhancing the low level of transfection that occurs in the absence of nuclear envelope breakdown.

III. PROPERTIES OF CURRENTLY AVAILABLE GENE-DELIVERY SYSTEMS

A. Viral Vectors

Although viral vectors have shown considerable promise in local and regional applications, the utility of viral vectors for systemic gene therapy remains limited (Table 2). This limitation is primarily due to the inability of viral vectors to overcome the first barrier to transfection—delivery to the target cell. Upon systemic administration most viral vectors are rapidly cleared by the organs of the reticuloendothelial system. The resulting gene expression is usually confined to the liver, a significant disadvantage unless the liver is the target organ (19). An additional disadvantage to the use of viral vectors in systemic gene therapy is the strong host immune response elicited by viral components.

Table 2 Relevant Properties of Viral Vectors for Systemic Gene Therapy

Virus	Size (nm)	Integration competent?	Mitosis requirement?	Intravenous transfection	Ref.
Adenovirus	70–90	No	No	Liver, lung	120
Adeno-associated virus	18–26	Yes (in replicating cells)	Yes (S phase)	Liver	121,122
Retrovirus	80–100	Yes	Yes	Liver	123
Vaccinia virus	200–400	No	No	Liver	124
Herpes simplex virus	120–200	No	No	Liver	124

Intravenous administration in particular elicits a powerful immune response (20). This immune response serves to both eliminate the vector and decrease expression of the transduced gene. For this reason many of successful preclinical studies performed in immunodeficient hosts have failed to translate to successful clinical protocols. Strategies to overcome this limitation include the transient suppression of host immunity (21) or modification of viral vectors in an effort to decrease their immunogenicity (22). Although recent results indicate the potential for development of viral vectors that are relatively nonimmunogenic, the most serious limitation of viral vector systems is their inability to access distal disease sites upon systemic administration. Until significant progress has been made in improving the pharmacokinetics and biodistribution of viral vectors, their utility is likely to be limited to local or regional applications.

B. Nonviral Vectors

The majority of nonviral vectors can be distinguished on the basis of their composition as belonging to one of three main classes: lipoplex, polyplex, or lipopolyplex. Polyplex vectors are defined as cationic polymer–nucleic acid complexes formed by the addition of nucleic acid to cationic polymer, lipoplex vectors are cationic lipid–nucleic acid complexes formed by the addition of nucleic acid to preformed liposomes, and lipopolyplex vectors are complexes that contain both polycationic polymers and cationic lipids (23).

Polyplex-mediated transfection has become an established approach since polylysine-DNA complexes were first shown to be capable of transfecting mammalian cells (24). In spite of early in vitro success, systemic utility has been elusive because of rapid clearance by the reticuloendothelial system and dose-limiting pulmonary and hepatic toxicities. In an attempt to address these limitations, some investigators have chosen to focus on the development of polyplex systems that are either less toxic or are capable of condensing plasmid DNA into smaller, more stable particles than are currently available or incorporation of targeting ligands in an attempt to redirect the distribution of these systems. (These systems are discussed in more detail in Chapter 7.)

Although lipid-mediated systemic gene delivery and expression was reported by Zhu et al. in 1993 (7), progress in developing lipoplex systems capable of delivering plasmid DNA to distal disease sites has also been slow. Early studies on the biodistribution and pharmacokinetics of DC-Chol:DOPE lipoplex (25,26) determined that cationic liposomes were cleared from the circulation within minutes of intravenous administration. The majority of lipid label accumulates immediately in the lung, with the remainder being distributed in the spleen, heart, and liver. Lipoplex vectors are cleared rapidly because the lungs, the first major organ encountered upon intravenous administration, have a large capillary bed with internal diameters $<$ 10 μm. Large cationic lipoplexes interact electrostatically with the pulmonary epithelium, and deposition presumably ensues. Attempts to overcome the inappropriate pharmacokinetics of lipoplex systems by escalating the delivered dose typically lead to dose-limiting toxicities (27).

Despite alterations in plasmid:liposome charge ratios or the nature of the cationic lipid or co-lipids in lipoplex systems, their pharmacokinetic limitations have not been overcome. This may be the result of strategies that have relied too heavily on empirical derivation of ''systemically active'' formulations in the absence of appropriate pharmacological analysis or an understanding of the effect of these modifications on the ability of the delivery system to overcome the biological barriers to transfection. Although several factors contribute to clearance, size and surface charge are thought to be most critical. The sizes of nonviral gene-transfer systems are determined by the physical chemistry of the self-assembly process. Lipoplex formation occurs spontaneously upon addition of plasmid DNA to cationic liposomes. Although theoretically it should be possible to standardize this process, in practice the process generates a heterogeneous mixture of complexes of lipid and plasmid DNA that range in size from 100 to 1000 nm in diameter, which often tends to aggregate over time. In such cases, this necessitates the preparation of lipoplex systems immediately before use, precluding the manufacture of large-scale batches or effective quality control over the final product. Due to the heterogeneous and unstable nature of lipoplex, it is difficult to determine which fraction represents the active form responsible for mediating transfection. The physical characteristics of the formulation change further upon intravenous administration and exposure to blood components by dissociation, aggregation, and/or fusion with blood cells (28–31).

In an effort to address some of these issues, investigators have pursued a strategy that involves precondensation of plasmid DNA with protamine sulfate or other polycationic agents prior to the addition of cationic liposomes (8,31,32). Plasmid condensation results in the formation of a DNA core that presumably becomes coated with a lipid shell. The resulting lipopolyplex systems are complexes that contain both polycationic polymers and cationic lipids. Precondensing DNA with protamine sulfate results in an increase in protection from serum nucleases in vitro and improved gene expression following systemic administration, however, due to the large size and charged nature of these particles the majority are rapidly cleared by the lung where the bulk of the gene expression is observed (32).

In summary, nucleic acids clearly require pharmaceutical enablement in the form of appropriate carriers, which are able to deliver intact DNA to disease sites without causing undue toxicity. Viral and nonviral gene-transfer systems suffer from common pharmacological issues, which limit their utility as systemic delivery agents. Attempts to address these issues through manipulation of the virology or molecular biology of these systems have met with limited success. The issues for nucleic acid drugs are similar to those faced by many low molecular weight chemotherapeutic drugs. The pharmacology of these toxic agents has been successfully enhanced by encapsulation within liposomes. Application of this approach to DNA should overcome a number of the limitations of first-generation delivery systems. In the following sections we will describe the benefits of encapsulation for the chemotherapeutic vincristine and discuss progress in the development of formulations that completely encapsulate plasmid DNA.

IV. CURRENT STATUS OF LIPID-BASED DRUG-DELIVERY SYSTEMS

As an example of the successful implementation of liposome carrier technology in an oncology application we will elaborate on the use of a liposomal carrier for vincristine. Vincristine is an plant alkaloid that effects growth arrest of mitotic cells by binding to and inhibiting tubulin polymerization. It is approved for use against lymphoblastic leukemia, lymphoma, and a number of childhood sarcomas and is often used in combination with other drugs. Evidence suggests that there is a correlation between antitumor efficacy and the duration of exposure to vincristine. One of the attractive features of vincristine is the relative lack of bone marrow toxicity common among many antineoplastic agents. The dose-limiting toxicity of vincristine is neurological, primarily peripheral and autonomic neuropathy (33,34). These qualities combine to make vincristine an attractive target for liposomal encapsulation.

Vincristine has been encapsulated in liposomes through a pH-dependent remote loading procedure. Briefly, liposomes are formed by rehydration of lipid films in low-pH buffer. Vincristine is then added to the preformed liposomes. Finally the pH of the liposome-drug mixture is raised. The pH differential between the external compartment and the interior aqueous space effectively draws the cationic vincristine molecule into the liposome. Entrapment efficiencies of greater than 98% can be achieved (35). Vincrisitine-containing liposomes composed of sphingomyelin and cholesterol (SM/Chol) were found to have mean diameters of 120–130 nm as measured by quasielastic light scattering (36). When the lipid and drug pharmacokinetics of vincristine-SM/Chol liposomes were evaluated in mice, the half-life for removal of vincristine-loaded liposomes from the circulation was 18.9 hours. Vincristine leakage from SM/Chol liposomes in vivo was also slow with 25% of the trapped drug remaining in the liposomes after 72 hours in the circulation. The half-life of vincristine derived from vincristine-loaded SM/Chol liposomes was 12.1 hours (Fig. 2a). This compares favorably with the behavior of free vincristine, which is rapidly removed from the circulation. To determine if the pharmacokinetic attributes of liposomal vincristine affect the ability of vincristine to accumulate in tumor tissue, SCID mice bearing solid A431 tumors were injected intravenously with either free or liposomal vincristine. Improved circulation half-life correlates with an increase in the accumulation of vincristine in distal subcutaneous A431 tumors (Fig. 2b). Free vincristine levels peak at 0.5 hour after injection at 0.856 μg/g tumor and decreased to 0.32 μg/g tumor at 24 hours after injection, while liposomal delivery resulted in 3.2 and 2.8 μg/g tumor at 24 and 48 hours, respectively (Fig. 2b). This represents a 10-fold increase in drug concentration at later time points.

The antitumor efficacy of vincristine correlates with vincristine accumulation at the tumor site (Fig. 2c). A431 tumor–bearing mice that received no treatment required termination 10 days after tumor cell inoculation when the tumor volume reached 10% of the total body weight. Treatment with free vincristine results in a slight inhibition in tumor growth and increase in short-term survival (Fig. 2c). Liposomal formulation results in a significant improvement in antitumor efficacy. Mice treated with liposomal vincristine demonstrate complete tumor regression and an improved survival, a significant improvement over the performance of free vincristine.

The clinical utility of liposomal vincristine has been evaluated in a phase I clinical trial (37). Twenty-five patients with confirmed malignancies were treated with multiple doses of liposomal vincristine. Pharmacokinetic data were collected that suggest that liposomal encapsulation confers dramatically improved pharmacokinetics and serum half-life, supporting the preclinical data collected in animal studies. Based on the successful phase I study, a phase II clinical trial for pancreatic cancer and a separate phase II clinical trial for lymphoma have been initiated.

This example shows that lipid formulation can affect the pharmacology of small molecule drugs in a number of ways. Drugs that have limited serum half-lives can be enhanced by formulation in liposome carriers (38–41). Likewise, drugs that degrade rapidly in the presence of serum components can often be stabilized by liposomal formulation. Drugs that are specific to one phase of the

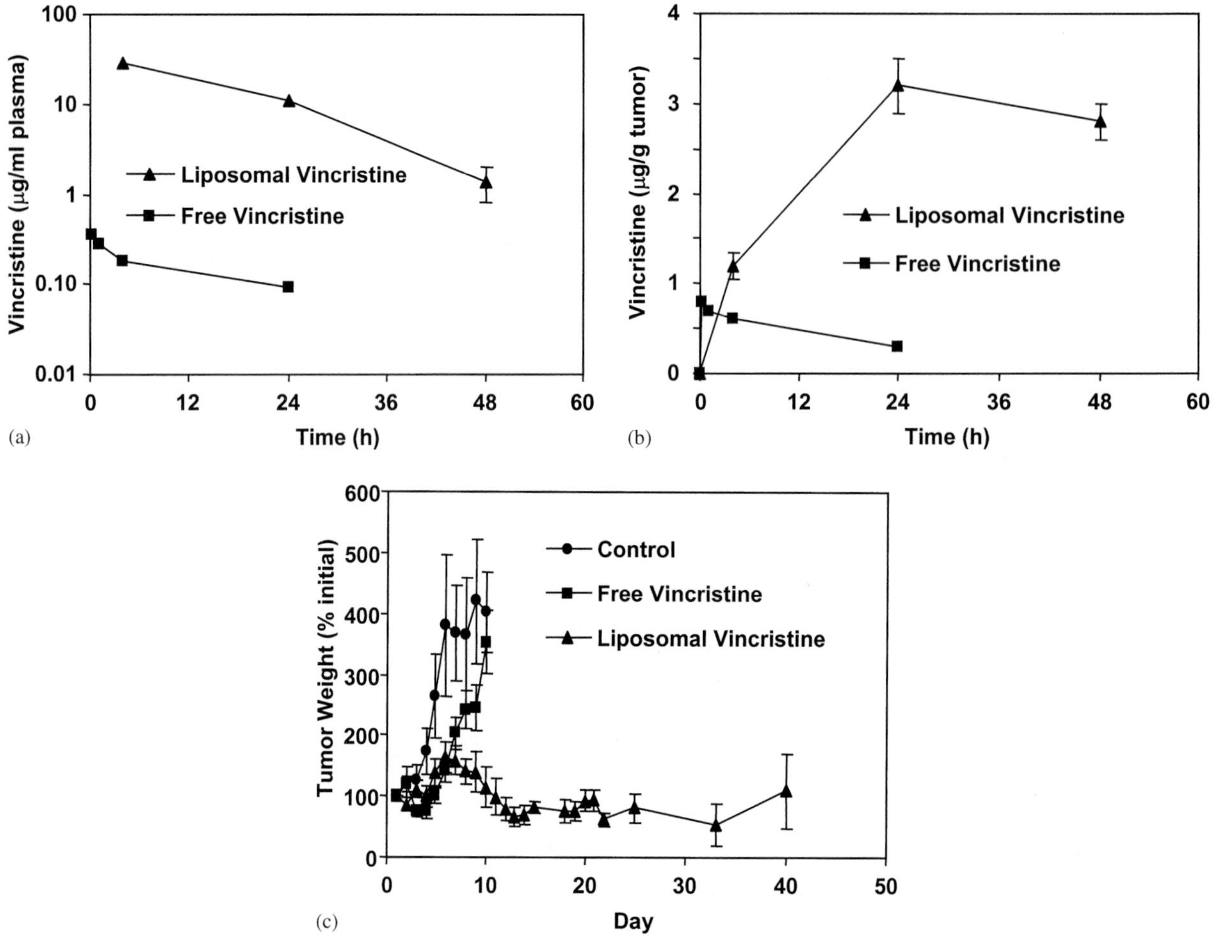

Figure 2 Pharmacology of liposomal vincristine. (a) Pharmacokinetics of liposomal vincristine. Female SCID mice were injected subcutaneously in the hind flank with 2×10^6 A431 cells. Fourteen days after tumor seeding, 2.0 mg/kg free or liposomal vincristine was administered through the tail vein. Blood was collected at the indicated time points by cardiac puncture. Plasma was isolated from whole blood and analyzed for ^{3}H-vincristine by liquid scintillation. (b) Accumulation of vincristine in distal tumors following systemic administration. Tumors and other organs were removed and frozen at -70°C prior to homogenization and analysis for ^{3}H-vincristine by liquid scintillation. (c) Efficacy of liposomal vincristine: inhibition of tumor growth. Tumors were seeded as in (a). Fourteen days after tumor seeding, a single dose corresponding to 2.0 mg/kg free or liposomal vincristine was administered through the tail vein. Animals received no treatment (circle), free vincristine (square), or sphingomyelin:cholesterol formulated vincristine (triangle). Error bars indicate SEM for six tumors.

cell cycle can be modified with liposomal formulation such that they are bioavailable through the entire cell cycle (41). An additional benefit of liposomal encapsulation of conventional drugs is the reduction in acute toxicity that often accompanies the shift in biodistribution associated with lipid formulation. Many chemotherapeutics suffer from toxicity resulting from the pooling of systemically administered drugs in organs such as the kidney, liver, or spleen. Liposomal formulations can be engineered to bypass the reticuloendothelial system and thereby avoid the pooling in nontarget organs, which is often the cause of the acute toxicity associated with systemic drug administration. The redirected biodistribution of liposomal drugs can be extended further. Appropriately designed liposomal carriers are able to take advantage of the phenomenon of ''disease site targeting.'' The changes in vascular permeability associated with tumor growth and inflammatory disorders favor the local accumulation of liposomes with small size and long circulation lifetimes. Delivery systems that aim to take advantage of this unique physiology should have circula-

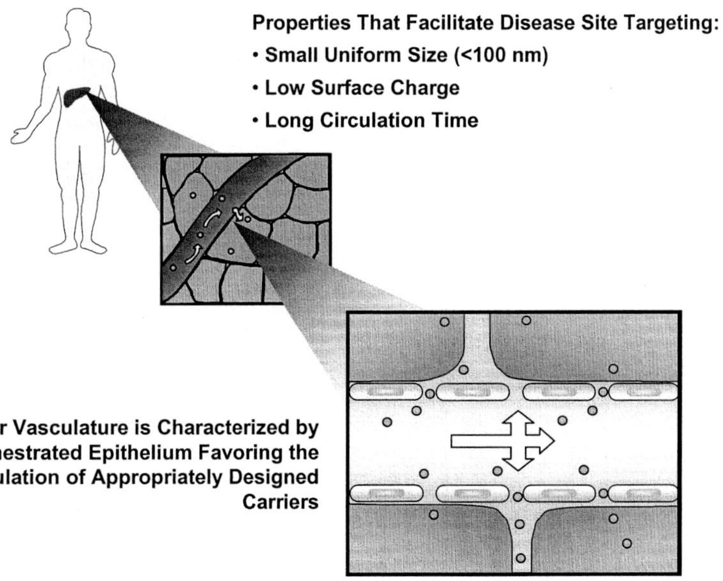

Properties That Facilitate Disease Site Targeting:
• Small Uniform Size (<100 nm)
• Low Surface Charge
• Long Circulation Time
Tumor Vasculature is Characterized by Fenestrated Epithelium Favoring the Accumulation of Appropriately Designed Carriers

Figure 3 Systemic delivery and disease-site targeting. Accessing target cell populations requires delivery from the blood compartment to the disease site. Delivery from the blood compartment is followed by extravasation through tissue. The changes in vascular permeability associated with tumor growth and inflammatory disorders favor the local accumulation of liposomes with small size and long circulation lifetimes. Delivery systems with circulation times of hours or longer with homogeneous small size (≤100 nm) can take advantage of this unique physiology. This is small enough to exit the fenestrated epithelia of tumor neovasculature and well within the size limit for receptor-mediated endocytosis and intracellular delivery.

tion times of hours or longer in murine models and exhibit a homogeneous small size with a mean diameter of ≤100 nm (Fig. 3). This is small enough to exit the fenestrated epithelia of tumor neovasculature and well within the size limit for receptor-mediated endocytosis and intracellular delivery. The benefits of disease site targeting can be profound. In the case of delivery of chemotherapeutic drugs to distal tumor sites, for example, encapsulation in small long-circulating liposomes results in 50- to 100-fold enhancements in the amount of drug delivered to the disease site (36,40,41).

This approach has also been applied to other small-molecule drugs which are either undergoing clinical trial or have been approved for use (Table 3). One of these is the antineoplastic anthracycline doxorubicin (42). Doxorubicin is indicated for a variety of nonhematological tumors. The clinical utility of doxorubicin is limited by cumulative myocardial toxicity, which can result in congestive heart failure during or even years after treatment with the drug. Preclinical and clinical studies show that liposomal doxorubicin has a reduced myocardial toxicity, enhanced antitumor activity, and an improved therapeutic index (38, 39,42). In a similar manner, the toxicity of another anthracycline, daunorubicin, has been partially ameliorated through liposomal encapsulation (43). Liposomal formulations of both daunorubicin and doxorubicin are currently approved for use against AIDS-related Kaposi's sarcoma (Table 3). *cis*-Platinum (cisplatin) is a heavy metal–containing DNA cross-linking agent used against a wide variety of malignancies including ovarian, lung, testicular, bladder, and cervical cancers. Cisplatin is subject to a dose-limiting renal toxicity (44), which is significantly reduced upon liposomal encapsulation (45,46). Other examples of liposomal drugs currently under investigation are summarized in Table 3.

V. METHODS OF ENCAPSULATING PLASMID DNA

In order to capitalize on the pharmacology and disease-site targeting demonstrated by liposomal drug carriers, it is necessary to completely entrap plasmid DNA within the contents of a liposome. Unlike small-molecule drugs, plasmid DNA cannot be "loaded" into preformed liposomes using pH gradients or other similar strategies. A number of investigators have evaluated alternative approaches to entrapping plasmid DNA. Lipid encapsulation of high molecular weight DNA was first demonstrated in

Table 3 Liposomal Drugs in Clinical Development

Drug	Indication	Investigator	Status	Ref.
Amikacin (Mikasome)	Urinary tract infection	NeXstar	Phase II	
Amphotericin B (AmBisome)	Antifungal	NeXstar	Approved	125
Annamycin	Breast cancer	Aronex Pharmaceuticals Inc.	Phase II	
Cisplatin (SPI-77)	Ovarian cancer	Sequus Pharmaceuticals Inc.	Phase II	126
Cyclophosphamide	Non-Hodgkin's lymphoma	Case Western Reserve University	Phase II	
Daunorubicin (DaunoXome)	Kaposi's sarcoma	NeXstar Pharmaceuticals Inc.	Approved	43
Doxorubicin (Doxil)	AIDS-related Kaposi's sarcoma	Sequus Pharmaceuticals Inc.	Approved	127,
	Leukemia and non-Hodgkin's lymphoma		Phase I/II	128
	Cancers of gynecological origin and carcinoma of the liver or bile ducts		Phase III	
Doxorubicin (Evacet)	Breast cancer	The Liposome Company	NDA	
Doxorubicin (LED)	Solid tumors	Neopharm	Phase I/II	
Lurtotecan (NX-211)	Ovarian cancer, solid tumors	NeXstar	Phase I	
Mitoxantrone	Breast cancer	University Hospital of Zurich	Phase II	129
Nystatin (Nyotran)	Antifungal	Aronex Pharmaceuticals Inc.	NDA	130
Paclitaxel (LEP)	Solid tumors	Neopharm	Phase I	
Trans-retinoic Acid (Atragen)	Leukemia	Aronex Pharmaceuticals Inc.	NDA	
	Non-Hodgkin's lymphoma		Phase II	
	Renal cell and bladder cancer		Phase I/II	
Tretinoin (Atragen, L-ATRA)	Acute promyelocytic leukemia	Aronex Pharmaceuticals Inc.	Phase II	131
Vincristine (ONCO-TCS)	Lymphoma	Inex Pharmaceuticals Corp.	Phase II	37

the late 1970s, prior to the development of cationic lipid–containing lipoplex (47–49). Although previous attempts to encapsulate plasmid DNA yielded mostly large multilamellar vesicles with poor transfection efficiency (50–52), recent improvements in formulation technology have resulted in the production of cationic lipid–containing particles with much greater transfection potential. Many of these methods are summarized in Table 4. Plasmid DNA has been encapsulated by reverse-phase evaporation (53–56), either injection (57,58), detergent dialysis in the absence of PEG stabilization (55,58), lipid hydration-dehydration techniques (52,59,60), sonication (61–63), and others (64,65). The two approaches that have shown the most promise differ conceptually in that one relies on a spontaneous internalization of plasmid DNA in preformed liposomes (6), while the other, detergent dialysis, is a process in which unilamellar vesicles containing plasmid DNA are formed upon removal of detergent from a DNA:lipid solution (5). We will briefly describe the invaginated liposome approach (covered in detail in Chapter 12) and then describe in detail the detergent dialysis approach.

Templeton et al. have described a novel formulation of stable complexes composed of DOTAP, cholesterol, and plasmid DNA (6). DOTAP:cholesterol liposomes (1:NO1) were formed by hydration of a lipid film, sonication, and extrusion through a series of filters of decreasing size. Particular attention was paid to optimization of conditions in order to maximize the colloidal properties of the resulting delivery system. Extrusion of the large unilamellar liposomes with excess surface area results in the formation of unique vase-like structures. Upon addition of plasmid DNA, plasmid is condensed in a space formed by invagination or complete circling and fusion of two lipid bilayers. Systemic administration of these particles results in high levels of reporter gene expression in the lung and other organs, a portion of which can be redirected to the liver by the incorporation of the targeting ligand, succinylated asialofetuin. This work clearly demonstrates the advantages of protective encapsulation of the plasmid DNA payload and reduction in surface charge upon incorporation of a targeting ligand, two concepts that support the concept of an artificial virus for systemic gene delivery.

Novel encapsulation methods have been developed in an effort to improve the clearance properties of encapsulated plasmid systems containing high ratios of cationic lipid and associated surface charge. It is of interest to extend these procedures to generate plasmid-containing cationic liposomes stabilized in a manner analogous to liposomal drug formulations, which have been shown to facilitate disease-site targeting (66). In particular, lipo-

Table 4 Procedures for Encapsulating Plasmid in Lipid-Based Systems

Procedure	Lipid composition	Length of DNA	Trapping efficiency[a] (%)	DNA-to-lipid ratio[a]	Diameter	Ref.
Reverse-phase evaporation	PS or PS:Chol (50:50)	SV40 DNA	30–50	<4.2 μg/μmol	400 nm	53
Reverse-phase evaporation	PC:PS:Chol (40:10:50)	11.9 kb plasmid	13–16	0.23 μg/μmol	100 nm to 1 μm	54
Reverse-phase evaporation	PC:PS:Chol (50:10:40)	8.3 kb, 14.2 kbp plasmid	10	0.97 μg/μmol	ND	55
Reverse-phase evaporation	EPC:PS:Chol (40:10:50)	3.9 kb plasmid	12	0.38 μg/μmol	400 nm	56
Ether injection	EPC:EPG (91:9)	3.9 kb plasmid	2–6	<1 μg/μmol	0.1–1.5 μm; Aug = 230 nm	58
Ether injection	PC:PS:Chol (40:10:50) PC:PG:Chol (40:10:50)	3.9 kb plasmid	15	15 μg/μmol	ND	57
Detergent dialysis	EPC:Chol:stearylamine (43.5:43.5:13)	sonicated genomic DNA (approximately 250,000 MW)	11	0.26 μg/μmol	50 nm	97
Detergent dialysis, extrusion	DOPC:Chol:oleic acid or DOPE:Chol:oleic acid (40:40:20)	4.6 kb plasmid	14–17	2.25 μg/μmol	180 nm (DOPC) 290 nm (DOPE)	104
Lipid hydration	EPC:Chol (65:35) or EPC	3.9 kb, 13 kb plasmid	ND	ND	0.5–7.5 μm	59
Dehydration-rehydration, extrusion (400 or 200 nm filters)	Chol:EPC:PS (50:40:10)	ND	ND	0.83 μg/μmol (200 nm) 1.97 μg/μmol (400 nm)	142.5 nm (200 nm filter) 54.6 nm (400 nm filter, ultracentrifugation)	60
Dehydration-rehydration	EPC	2.96 kb, 7.25 kb plasmid	35–40	2.65–3.0 μg/μmol	1–2 μm	52
Sonication (in the presence of lysozyme)	asolectin (soybean phospholipids)	1.0 kb linear DNA	50	0.08 μg/μmol	100–200 nm	61
Sonication	EPC:Chol:lysine-DPPE (55:30:15)	6.3 kb ssDNA 1.0 kb dsRNA	60–95 ssDNA 80–90 dsRNA	13 μg/μmol ssDNA; 14 μg/μmol dsRNA	100–150 nm	62
Spermidine-condensed DNA, sonication, extrusion	EPC:Chol:PS (40:50:10) EPC:Chol:EPA (40:50:10) or EPC:Chol:CL (50:40:10)	4.4 kb, 7.2 kb plasmid	46–52	2.53–2.87 μg/μmol	400–500 nm	63
Ca^{2+}-EDTA entrapment of DNA-protein complexes	PS:Chol (50:50)	42.1 kbp bacteriophage	52–59	22 μg/μmol	ND	65
Freeze-thaw, extrusion	POPC:DDAB (99:1)	3.4 kb linear plasmid	17–50	ND	80–120 nm	64
SPLP	DOPE:PEG-Cer: DODAC (84:10:6)	4.4 to 10 kb plasmid	60–70	62.5 μg/μmol	75 nm (QELS); 65 nm (freeze-fracture)	5

ND = not determined.
[a] Some values calculated based on presented data.

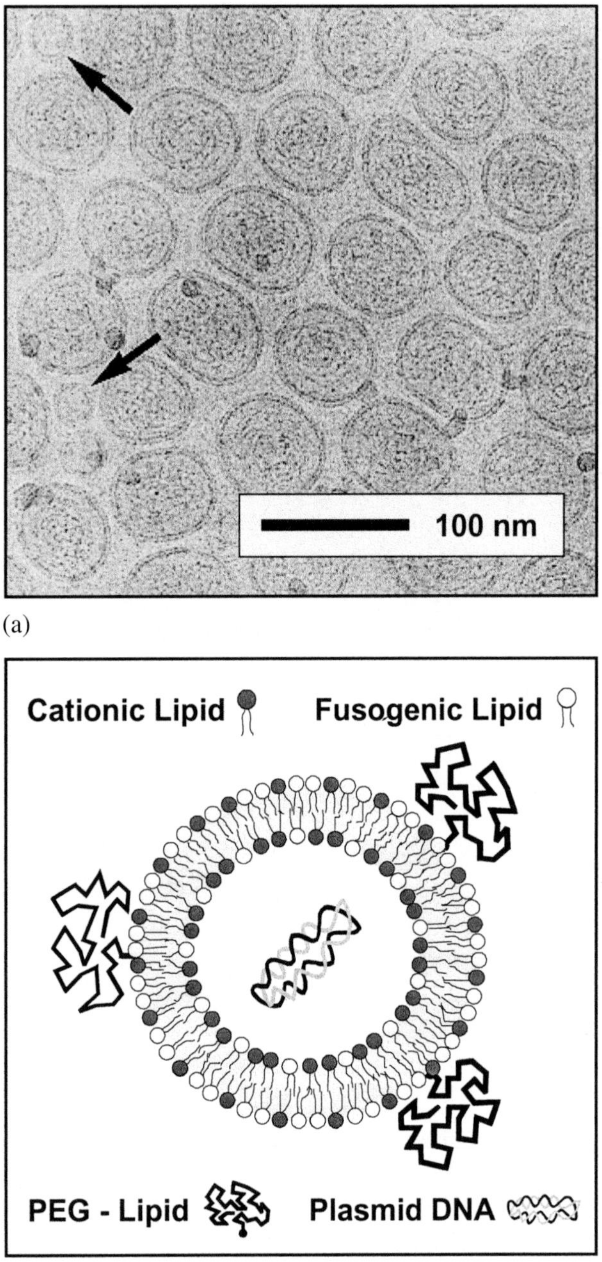

Figure 4 Structural model of SPLP. (a) Cryo-electron microscopy of SPLP. SPLP were prepared from DOPE:DODAC:Peg-CerC$_{20}$ and pCMVLuc and purified employing DEAE column chromatography and density gradient centrifugation. Arrows indicate the presence of residual ''empty'' vesicles formed during the detergent dialysis but not removed by the density gradient centrifugation purification step. (b) Structural schematic of SPLP. SPLP are formed with neutral fusogenic lipid, cationic lipid, PEG-ceramide, and plasmid DNA. The process results in the formation of small (approximately 70 nm diameter) particles containing one plasmid surrounded by a lipid bilayer.

somes that incorporate PEG conjugates in the lipid bilayer have been shown to yield long circulation lifetimes (67–69). PEG conjugates are thought to sterically stabilize liposomes by forming a protective layer, which shields the hydrophobic lipid layer (70). This prevents the association of serum proteins and resulting uptake by the reticuloendothelial system (71,72). This approach has been investigated with a view towards improving the stability and pharmacokinetics of lipoplex (73). However, lipoplex incorporating PEG-phosphatidylethanolamine demonstrate an improved stability at the expense of transfection activity.

A method of encapsulating plasmid in small, PEG-coated lipid vesicles has recently been described (5). In this method hydrophobic and hydrophilic carrier components are simultaneously solubilized in a single detergent-containing phase. Particle formation occurs spontaneously upon removal of the detergent by dialysis. Under appropriate conditions thermodynamics favor the formation of small (approximately 70 nm in diameter) stabilized plasmid lipid particles (SPLP) containing one plasmid/vesicle in combination with plasmid-trapping efficiencies approaching 70% (Fig. 4). The SPLP protocol results in stable particles with low levels of cationic lipids, high levels of fusogenic lipids, and high DNA-to-lipid ratios. SPLP can be concentrated to achieve plasmid DNA concentrations > 1 mg/mL. These attributes compare favorably with the previously reported plasmid encapsulation processes summarized in Table 4. The SPLP method yields the highest plasmid DNA-to-lipid ratio (62.5 μg/μmol) of any of these methods and is remarkably stable when compared to other encapsulated systems. The stability of SPLP facilities a thorough characterization of their physical properties. In particular it is possible to monitor the efficiency of the encapsulation process and the degree to which plasmid DNA is protected from exogenous nuclease activity. Although the SPLP process results in the formation of empty lipid vesicles and unencapsulated DNA in addition to SPLP, free plasmid DNA can be removed by ion-exchange chromatography while density gradient centrifugation effectively removes empty vesicles. The plasmid-to-lipid ratio of pure SPLP, 65 μg/μmol, corresponds to one plasmid per SPLP (5). This is achieved without the use of extreme conditions, which have the potential to compromise the integrity of plasmid DNA.

Several parameters have been shown to be critical for SPLP formation (5,74). Ionic strength, cationic lipid, and PEG lipid content must be optimized to maximize plasmid entrapment and minimize aggregation (Fig. 5). Entrapment is a sensitive function of cationic lipid content (5). The first stage of dialysis is proposed to result in the formation of macromolecular intermediates, possibly lamellar lipid sheets or micelles. Plasmid DNA is recruited by electro-

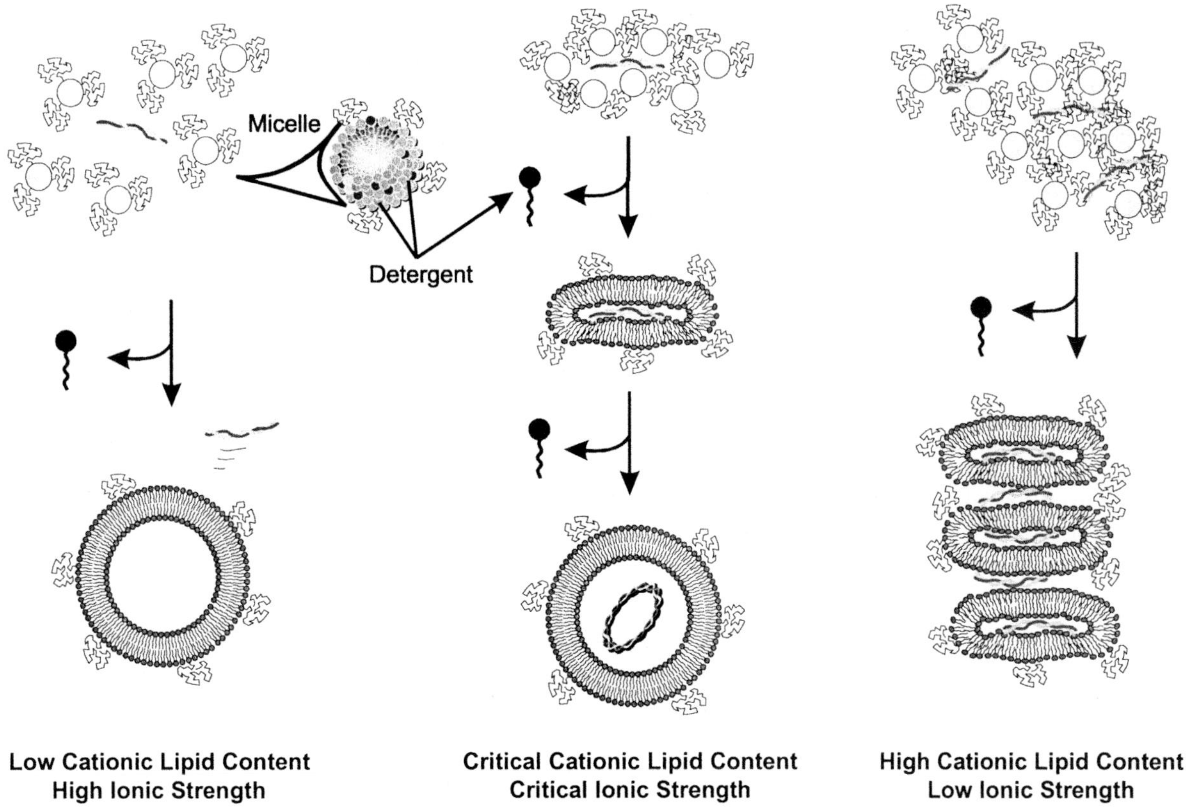

Figure 5 Critical parameters for SPLP formation. Dialysis is proposed to result in the formation of macromolecular intermediates, possibly lamellar lipid sheets or micelles. If the cationic lipid content is too low, plasmid fails to associate with these intermediates, favoring the formation of empty vesicles. If the cationic lipid concentration is too high, the surface charge on the lipid intermediate attracts excess plasmid DNA leading to the formation of polydisperse aggregates. At optimal cationic lipid concentrations, plasmid DNA is proposed to associate with the lipid intermediates in such a way as to reduce the net positive charge on the lipid surface. Association of further lipid leads to the formation of vesicles containing encapsulated plasmid. The electrostatic interaction between plasmid DNA and cationic lipids is also affected by the ionic strength of the dialysis buffer. However, at buffer concentrations above the optimal range, the positive charge on lipid intermediates is shielded to such an extent that formation of empty vesicles is favored. Likewise, if the ionic strength is suboptimal, large plasmid-lipid aggregates are formed.

static attraction. If the cationic lipid content is too low, plasmid fails to associate with these intermediates, favoring the formation of empty vesicles. If the cationic lipid concentration is too high, the surface charge on the lipid intermediate attracts excess plasmid DNA leading to the formation of polydisperse aggregates. At optimal cationic lipid concentrations plasmid DNA is proposed to associate with the lipid intermediates in such a way as to reduce the net positive charge on the lipid surface. Association of further lipid leads to the formation of vesicles containing encapsulated plasmid (5). Initial experimentation determined that the optimal cationic lipid content was 6–7% when formulation was attempted in HBS buffer. However, the electrostatic interaction between plasmid DNA and cationic lipids is also affected by the ionic strength of the dialysis buffer. Polyvalent buffers such as citrate can be used to shield the positive charge on cationic lipids to facilitate the formulation of SPLP containing higher concentrations of cationic lipid (74). However, at citrate concentrations above the optimal range, the positive charge on lipid intermediates is shielded to such an extent that formation of empty vesicles is favored. Likewise, if the ionic strength is suboptimal, large plasmid-lipid aggregates are formed. By careful manipulation of ionic strength SPLP can be formed containing up to 30 mol% cationic lipid (74). In a similar manner, selective replacement of individual lipid components can be achieved without sacrificing small uniform size and encapsulation efficiency.

VI. PHARMACOLOGY OF ENCAPSULATED PLASMID DNA

The properties of small size, serum stability, low levels of cationic lipid (approximately 6 mol%), and the presence of the PEG coating suggest that SPLP should exhibit extended circulation lifetimes and disease-site–targeting properties following intravenous administration. A direct test of the pharmacokinetic properties of SPLP particles is shown in Figure 6a (75). SPLP were formulated containing trace amounts of ^{3}H-cholesteryl hexadecyl ether (CHE), a nonexchangeable lipid marker routinely used to label liposomes or vesicle preparations (76). SPLP were administered intravenously to mice bearing distal hind-flank tumors. Blood was drawn at the indicated time points and subjected to analysis for ^{3}H-CHE lipid by liquid scintillation analysis. SPLP are cleared from serum gradually with a measured serum half-life of between 3 and 6 hours (75,77). The serum half-life of unprotected plasmid DNA is known to be less than 5 minutes (28,77). SPLP accumulate in distal tissue following intravenous administration. SPLP accumulate primarily in the tumor and liver, bypassing the capillaries of the lung. Twenty-four hours after tail vein injection, the tumor and liver have accumulated 1–3 and 5–10% of the total injected lipid dose, respectively. The ability of SPLP to bypass the lung, unique among cationic lipid–containing gene-delivery systems, is thought to correlate with the properties required for disease-site targeting, small uniform size, and surface charge shielding. The stability of SPLP protects plasmid DNA and facilitates intratumoral delivery of intact plasmid following systemic administration (75). In contrast, intact DNA is not delivered to the tumor at any of the time points assayed following intravenous administration of naked plasmid DNA.

The observation that SPLP are able to transfect mammalian cells in vitro demonstrates that SPLP plasmid DNA retains biological activity through the formulation process. Furthermore, SPLP are capable of overcoming the barriers to transfection, intracellular delivery and nuclear uptake, when applied directly to cells. SPLP containing reporter gene constructs have been shown to be transfection competent in vivo when applied either regionally (74) or systemically (5). SPLP are capable of mediating reporter gene expression in distal tumors following systemic administration (77). This supports the concept of the artificial virus in that the properties required for disease-site targeting, stability and low surface charge, are not necessarily incompatible with those needed to facilitate intracellular delivery and transfection. This suggests that SPLP containing plasmid coding for an appropriate therapeutic transgene may be capable of mediating an antitumor effect following systemic administration. There are a number of reports of antitumor efficacy following systemic administration of lipoplex or lipopolyplex systems containing therapeutic plasmids, however, supporting pharmacokinetic and accumulation data have not been reported. Furthermore, it is increasingly apparent that some disease models are responsive to nonspecific effects associated with the delivery of vector components or plasmid DNA. For this reason the choice of therapeutic transgene and appropriate controls is critical to ensure the collection of meaningful data. One strategy that allows for partial differentiation between gene specific and nonspecific effects is the use of suicide genes. Transfection of mammalian cells with suicide genes sensitizes them to a nontoxic prodrug. Transfection in the absence of prodrug treatment has no specific therapeutic benefit. To test the therapeutic potential of SPLP, SPLP were manufactured containing plasmid DNA coding for the herpes simplex virus thymidine kinase (HSV-TK) and evaluated for antitumor efficacy upon systemic administration. Mice bearing MCA-207 tumors were treated with five tail vein injections of either TK-SPLP or a frameshift mutant control over the course of 10 days in combination with daily intraperitoneal administration of the prodrug ganciclovir. Those animals treated with TK-SPLP in combination with ganciclovir demonstrated the greatest antitumor response (Fig. 6c.). Four out of eight animals demonstrated complete tumor regression. Upon tumor rechallenge, three of these four animals failed to develop new MCA-207 tumors, a possible indication of adaptive tumor immunity. The long-term effects of SPLP-mediated systemic suicide gene therapy are even more pronounced than the results of short-term tumor growth–inhibition studies (Fig. 6d). In a larger study 60% of the animals treated with TK-SPLP in combination with ganciclovir remained tumor-free after 60 days, while only 15% of the animals treated with TK-SPLP alone survived for this period.

Although these results support the conclusion that SPLP can mediate antitumor effects upon delivery of a therapeutic gene, it is important to control for nonspecific effects associated with systemic administration of plasmid DNA. Figure 6c shows that some antitumor effect is obtained when TK-SPLP are administered in the absence of prodrug treatment. Here a frameshift control plasmid was used to assist in differentiating between gene-specific and nonspecific effects. Cells transfected with the frameshift control plasmid do not produce TK protein. This plasmid serves as a control for the nonspecific effects associated with systemic delivery of bacterial DNA containing unmethylated CpG dinucleotides, which can induce activation and proliferation of B, NK, CD4$^+$ T cells, and macrophages (78–82). This nonspecific immune activation must be taken into consideration when interpreting studies that rely on plasmid DNA as a therapeutic agent. Those animals that

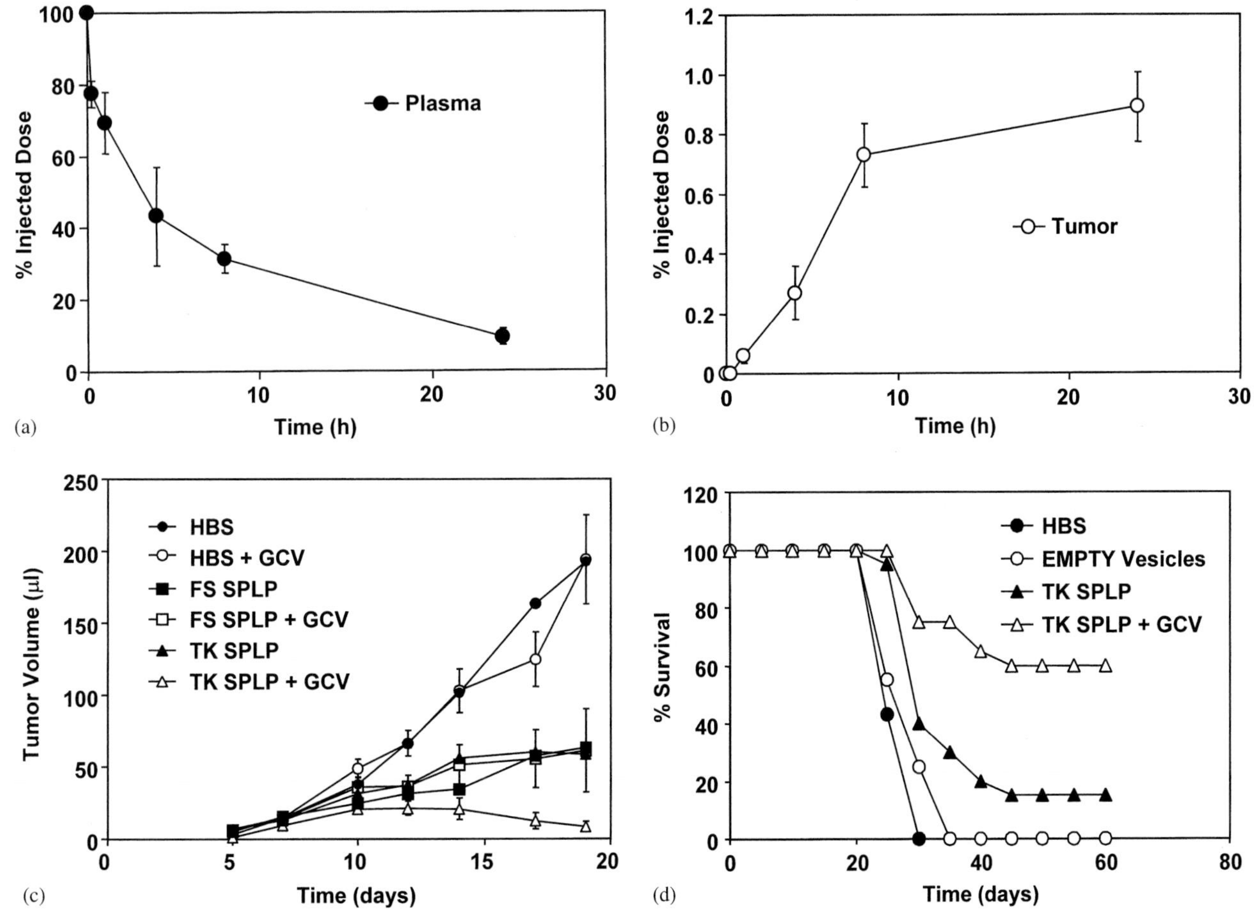

Figure 6 Pharmacology of SPLP. (a) Pharmacokinetics of SPLP. Female C57BL/6 mice were injected subcutaneously in the hind flank with 1×10^5 MCA-207 murine fibrosarcoma cells in a total volume of 50 μL PBS. Fourteen days after tumor seeding, 100 μg of SPLP DNA was administered through the tail vein in a total volume of 200 μL HBS. Blood was collected at the indicated time points by cardiac puncture. Plasma was isolated from whole blood and analyzed for ^{3}H-CHE by liquid scintillation. (b) Accumulation of SPLP in distal tumors following systemic administration. Tumors and other organs were removed and frozen at $-70°$C prior to homogenization and analysis for ^{3}H-CHE by liquid scintillation. (c) Efficacy of systemically administered SPLP: inhibition of tumor growth. Tumors were seeded as in (a). Starting 5 days after tumor seeding, SPLP were administered through the tail vein once every other day for a total of five treatments. Animals were also treated twice daily with intraperitoneal injection of 200 μL of PBS with or without 1.0 mg ganciclovir. Animals were treated with HBS alone (closed circle), HBS with ganciclovir (open circle), SPLP formulated pCMV-FS-TK alone (closed square), SPLP formulated pCMV-FS-TK with ganciclovir (open square), TK-SPLP alone (closed triangle), or TK-SPLP with ganciclovir (open triangle). Error bars indicate SEM for those groups of eight mice treated with ganciclovir. (d) Efficacy of systemically administered SPLP: survival. Tumors were established as in (d). Animals were treated with HBS alone (closed circle), empty SPLP (open circle), TK-SPLP alone (closed triangle), or TK-SPLP with ganciclovir (open triangle). $N > 20$ in all groups.

received the frameshift SPLP either alone or in combination with ganciclovir demonstrated an inhibition of tumor growth, which corresponded with that observed when animals were treated with TK-SPLP in the absence of prodrug therapy. These results suggest that some nonspecific antitumor efficacy results from the systemic delivery of plasmid DNA, yet support the gene-specific gain in antitumor efficacy associated with the intratumoral delivery of biologically active plasmid DNA in combination with prodrug therapy. It is notable that systemic TK-SPLP administration in combination with prodrug treatment results in little or no toxicity in murine models. This may be a reflection of the preferential accumulation of SPLP in tumor tissue or the low transfection potential in organs such as the liver, which accumulate SPLP yet are not readily transfected due to their low level of mitotic activity. The use of HSV-TK confers an additional level of selectivity in that it only affects cells that are actively undergoing cell division. It remains to be seen if other antitumor strategies are less tolerable when applied systemically.

VII. ENGINEERING FUTURE GENERATIONS OF SYNTHETIC VIRUS

A. The Role of Cationic Lipids in Promoting Intracellular Delivery

The factors affecting intracellular delivery of nonviral vectors are poorly understood. It is believed that both polycations and cationic lipids function by surrounding plasmid DNA with a net positive charge, which in turn enables binding of the DNA complex to anionic cell surface molecules. Increasing our understanding of this process is important not only to improve the efficiency of gene transfer but also to facilitate control of the site of transfection. One approach to elucidating the mechanism of nonviral gene delivery is to identify the molecules on the cell surface that interact with and are responsible for the uptake of cationic gene-transfer agents. Obvious candidates for interaction with cationic vectors would be the most abundant anionic cell surface molecules: sulfated proteoglycans and sialic acids. Proteoglycans appear to enhance polyplex-mediated transfection both in vitro (83) and in vivo (84). In vitro treatment of HeLa cells with sodium chlorate, an inhibitor of proteoglycan sulfation, reduced polylysine-mediated gene expression by 69%. Mutant, proteoglycan-deficient CHO cells yield less than 2% of the reporter gene expression of wild-type cells transfected with polylysine. Both mutant and sodium chlorate–treated cells demonstrated a reduction in the uptake of polylysine DNA complex measured at 37°C and a reduction in binding of DNA to the surface of cells at 4°C (83). Cationic lipoplex systems also rely on proteoglycans to facilitate intracellular delivery. Raji cells lack proteoglycans and as such are poorly transfectable by lipoplex. When stably transfected with cDNA coding for the proteoglycan syndecan-1, Raji cells are rendered transfectable by DOTIM-cholesterol lipoplex (84). Inhibition of the interaction between the positively charged lipoplex and negatively charged cell surface molecules by pretreatment with polyanionic compounds also inhibits lipoplex-mediated transfection. In vitro treatment of B16 murine melanoma cells with the anionic polysaccharide fucoidan inhibited cationic lipoplex-mediated transfection while having no effect on electroporation or adenoviral transfection. Anionic cell surface proteins are also implicated in transfection following intravenous administration of cationic lipoplex. Treatment of mice with fucoidan prior to lipoplex administration dramatically inhibits transfection of the lung, the primary target tissue for this vector, but has little effect on the more moderate levels of transfection observed in the heart liver and spleen (84). Intravenous administration of heparinase I, an enzyme specific for the cleavage of heparan sulfate proteoglycans, also inhibited cationic lipoplex-mediated transfection of lung, spleen, and heart. This supports the concept that intact proteoglycans are required for the efficient delivery of cationic lipoplex to cells in vivo.

The precise role of proteoglycans in the transfection process remains to be determined. Proteoglycans may interact with cationic vectors directly and be internalized as a complex, or they may serve to anchor cationic vectors for presentation to secondary receptors that in turn undergo specific receptor-mediated endocytosis. Given that the basis of the interaction between proteoglycans and cationic vectors appears to be electrostatic, differences in charge and charge density between vector systems should yield differences in transfection efficiency. This has certain implications for the design of vector systems for systemic gene therapy.

B. The Role of Helper Lipids in Promoting Intracellular Delivery

The majority of cationic lipids require the addition of a fusogenic helper lipid for efficient in vitro gene transfer (85–88). Fusogenic liposomes are thought to facilitate the intracellular delivery of complexed plasmid DNA by fusing with the membranes of the target cell. Inclusion of lipids that preferentially form nonbilayer phases, such as unsaturated phosphatidylethanolamines like DOPE, promote destabilization of the lipid bilayer and concomitant fusion (89). However, certain cationic lipids can function in the absence of fusogenic helper lipids either alone (86,87) or in the presence of the nonfusogenic lipid cholesterol (90). This would suggest that these lipids may have properties that promote transfection through a mechanism that does not require membrane fusion. Recent results which suggest that lipoplex-containing fusogenic lipids are actually less effective than nonfusogenic lipoplex when delivered intravenously bring into question the specific role of fusogenic helper lipids in the transfection process and whether this role is conserved between lipoplex and systems that fully encapsulate plasmid DNA.

Membrane fusion events may occur at a number of different stages in the gene-delivery process, at either the plasma membrane, endosome, or nuclear envelope. In order for fusion with the plasma membrane to occur, lipid particles must first bypass the glycocalyx. Fusion of lipoplex systems with the plasma membrane would be expected to be a particularly inefficient method of introducing

DNA into the cytosol since these systems are topographically challenged. The original model for lipoplex formation suggests that it occurs by the electrostatic interaction between performed cationic liposomes and plasmid DNA, which become attached to the surface of the liposome (91). Lipoplex fusion events are expected to resolve with plasmid DNA, formerly attached to the liposome surface, deposited on the outside surface of the plasma membrane. Encapsulated systems differ from lipoplex in this respect. Upon fusion with the plasma membrane, encapsulated carriers deliver their contents into the cytosol. The major mode of lipoplex-mediated transfection may be either the inefficient translocation of plasmid DNA following fusion of the cationic liposome with the membrane of the target cell or postendocytic fusion of lipoplex that are taken up intact by endocytosis (92). Again, encapsulated systems have an advantage over lipoplex in that fusion with endosomal compartments would be expected to deliver the DNA payload to the cytosol. However, even in the absence of a fusion-induced translocation event, fusion of lipoplex systems with endosomal compartments results in a destabilization and disruption of the endosomal membrane.

In spite of attempts to elucidate the role of fusogenic lipids in facilitating intracellular delivery of plasmid DNA, it remains to be determined at which stage in the gene-transfer process membrane fusion occurs. Two factors confound investigators attempting to address this issue. First, attempts to modulate transfection efficiency by effecting the fusogenicity of lipoplex have the potential to affect fusion with the plasma membrane or the endosomal membrane, either of which would be expected to have an affect on gene expression. Second, attempts to follow the fate of plasmid DNA as it travels through the cell to the nucleus have been limited by technical difficulties. This has precipitated an investigative approach by which the process of lipoplex uptake and intracellular trafficking is biochemically dissected in an attempt to identify the critical barriers to transfection. An example of this approach is the transient inhibition of endocytosis by treating cells with cytochalasin-B, an inhibitor of actin polymerization (85). Actin polymerization is required in order to establish the formation of microfilaments that mediate the cytoskeleton-controlled lateral membrane movements that precede endocytosis. When cells in culture are pretreated with cytochalasin-B prior to exposure to cationic lipoplex, transfection is inhibited. This observation supports a major role for endocytosis in lipoplex-mediated transfection. Another approach utilizes fluorescently labeled liposomes to track the fate of lipids upon delivery to the cell. Fusion of labeled liposomes with the plasma membrane results in the transfer of lipid label to the membrane. Treatment of cells with DOTAP:DOPE lipoplex containing rhodamine PE results in the accumulation of fluorescent label in endocytic granules, which become visible at early time points, well before plasma membranes become fluorescent (85). This is additional evidence in support of an endocytic uptake mechanism for lipoplex systems and implies that the role of fusogenic lipids in intracellular delivery is limited. The benefits of incorporating fusogenic lipids in lipoplex systems may be manifest at the level of enhancing fusion and release from endosomal compartments. It remains to be seen if this is also true with encapsulated gene-delivery systems.

Attempts to address the in vivo role of fusogenic lipids in cationic liposome–mediated gene delivery have had confounding results. It has been suggested that lipoplex containing fusogenic lipids are actually less effective than nonfusogenic lipoplex when delivered intravenously. A number of investigators have reported that replacement of fusogenic DOPE with the nonfusogenic lipid cholesterol yields higher levels of gene expression upon systemic administration. It is important to distinguish the effect of fusogenic lipids on gene delivery from the effect on the transfection process. The enhanced gene expression observed upon incorporation of cholesterol in lipoplex formulations may be a result of either an increase in transfection efficiency or improved pharmacokinetics and delivery to the target cell. Fusogenic formulations are more likely to interact with the vascular endothelium, blood cells, and lipoproteins while in the blood compartment. Incorporation of cholesterol in cationic lipoplex may simply render them less promiscuous and thereby improve delivery to the target cell. The implication is that there may be an advantage to transiently shielding the fusogenic potential of systemic carriers. Encapsulated systems provide a platform that may facilitate this approach.

C. Dissociating PEG

Although PEG-containing SPLP are promising with respect to their ability to deliver intact plasmid DNA to disease sites, improvements are required in order to increase levels of gene expression. In particular, SPLP exhibit relatively low transfection efficiencies in vitro (5). This is mainly due to the ability of the PEG coating to inhibit cell association and uptake of PEG-containing liposomes (88,93,94). An ideal carrier would incorporate PEG-lipid conjugates that have the ability to dissociate from the carrier in the blood and transform the SPLP from a stable particle to a transfection-competent entity at the target site (Fig. 7). The feasibility of this approach has been confirmed (5). PEG-ceramide molecules differing in the length of the ceramide acyl chain ($CerC_{14}$ or $CerC_{20}$) were incorporated into SPLP, and the resulting particles were assayed for in vitro transfection activity. SPLP containing PEG-

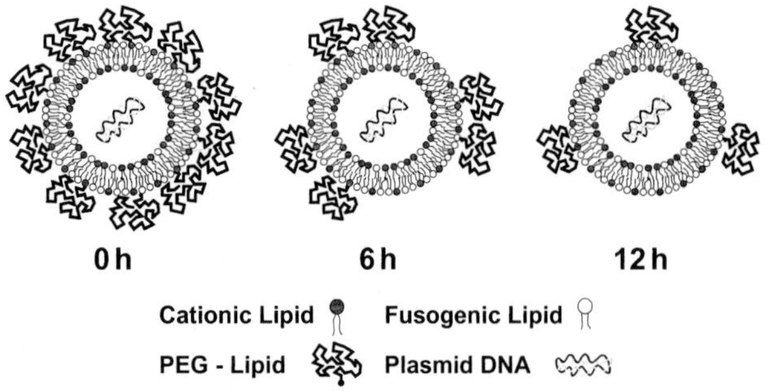

Figure 7 Dissociating PEG coatings for systemic carrier systems. PEG-containing systems exhibit relatively low transfection efficiencies in vitro due to the ability of the PEG coating to inhibit cell association and intracellular delivery. The use of diffusible PEG-ceramides facilitates the formulation of stable particles, which become increasingly fusogenic as the PEG-ceramide dissociates from the particle. This approach may help to resolve the two conflicting demands imposed upon carriers for systemic gene therapy. First, the carrier must be stable and circulate long enough to facilitate accumulation at disease sites. Second, the carrier must be capable of interacting with target cells in order to facilitate intracellular delivery.

$CerC_{20}$ demonstrated little if any transfection activity in vitro, consistent with the stability of the PEG in the particle. When the transfection properties of SPLP containing PEG-$CerC_{20}$ were compared to SPLP containing PEG-$CerC_{14}$, the SPLP containing the shorter-acyl-chain PEG exhibited substantially higher levels of activity than those containing PEG-$CerC_{20}$. This increase in transfection activity correlated with a more rapid dissociation rate when the rate of PEG-ceramide dissociation from egg phosphatidylcholine vesicles was measured in vitro. The use of diffusible PEG-ceramides facilitates the formulation of stable particles containing a high percentage (79–84 mol%) of the fusogenic lipid DOPE. As the PEG-ceramide dissociates from the particle, it is expected to become increasingly fusogenic. This approach may help to resolve the two conflicting demands imposed upon carriers for systemic gene therapy. First, the carrier must be stable and circulate long enough to facilitate accumulation at disease sites. Second, the carrier must be capable of interacting with target cells in order to facilitate intracellular delivery. The use of PEG coatings that dissociate from the carrier at the disease site is a potential solution to this problem.

D. Active Targeting

Active targeting is distinguished from passive disease-site targeting, which results in the accumulation of appropriately designed carriers in disease sites such as tumor tissue. Active targeting refers to processes that aim to increase the accumulation, retention, or internalization of targeted carriers through the addition of cell-specific ligands to the carrier surface. Targeting has been successfully applied to liposomal drug formulations and generally has the effect of improving the therapeutic index of the liposomal drug. Gene-delivery systems stand to benefit from targeting in two ways: through improving the accumulation and binding of formulations to target cells and by facilitating intracellular delivery through endocytosis. Targeting has been achieved through the use of molecules as diverse as antibodies (95,96), proteins (97–100), vitamins (101), and glycolipids (102,103). Liposomal systems modified to include antibodies directed against cell-surface proteins exhibit increased transfection in vitro when compared to untargeted controls (100,104). Targeting of liposomal systems to the asialoglycoprotein receptor has been achieved through the use of either asialofetuin (98) or simple galactosylated lipids (105). Likewise, the addition of transferrin to lipoplex systems results in an increase in both uptake and gene expression in vitro (106). In vitro studies demonstrate the potential advantage of targeted gene delivery at the level of increasing intracellular delivery but do not address the issue of enhanced accumulation at disease sites. It is unlikely that addition of targeting ligands to gene-transfer systems that are rapidly removed from the circulation will result in delivery exceeding that achieved by systems that display passive disease-site targeting. For this reason a number of investigators have pursued approaches involving the addition of targeting ligands to sterically stabilized systems containing PEG lipids, hoping that active and passive targeting effects will be at least additive. In one case PEG lipids were modified to contain folate, a ligand for the cell surface folate receptor (101). PEG lipids were used in the formation of anionic liposomes, which were added to precondensed polyplex. The resulting lipopolyplex demonstrated a significant increase in intracellular delivery when applied to KB cells, yet only a modest increase in gene expression in vitro. Nonetheless, this study demonstrates the potential for the application of targeting technology to sterically stabilized systems. It remains to be seen if encapsulated systems containing targeting ligands can achieve disease-site targeting following systemic administration. The benefits of active targeting may be outweighed by the deleterious effect on serum clearance rates and increased immunogenicity that often accompanies the addition of targeting ligands.

E. Endosomal Release

A variety of approaches can be considered for enhancing the endosomal release of internalized liposomes. We have already described the use of fusogenic lipids, which are thought to facilitate endosome release. Another strategy involves the incorporation of specific lipids, which render the liposome pH sensitive such that it becomes more fusogenic in low pH compartments such as the late endosome and lysosome (101,104). Alternatively, nonfusogenic liposomes can be rendered fusogenic by the addition of viral coat proteins, which promote intracellular delivery and endosomal release. The uptake and endosomal release of lipoplex are enhanced when associated with intact replication-deficient adenovirus (107,108). An extension of this approach has been used to form ''virosomes'' consisting of the major envelope glycoprotein, hemagglutinin, embedded in a phospholipid-cholesterol bilayer derived from the viral envelope (109,110). Sendai virus may be directly fused with preformed lipoplex to yield virosomes with improved in vitro transfection characteristics (111,112). This approach has also been applied to encapsulated systems. Virosomes containing the F (fusion) protein of Sendai virus, but devoid of hemagglutinin, were prepared by a detergent dialysis process, which results in the encapsulation of plasmid DNA within the lipid envelope. Virosomes prepared in this manner were found to mediate increased gene expression when compared to lipoplex systems (113). Sendai virus F protein is known to effect transfection through two independent mechanisms. Galactosylated F protein is a ligand for the cell surface asialoglycoprotein receptor. F protein also behaves as a membrane fusogen. The fusogenic activity of F protein–containing liposomes can be abrogated by a brief heat treatment without affecting the galactose-mediated endocytic pathway. Heat treatment results in a substantial decrease in the overall transfection efficiency but at the same time increases the rate of virosome accumulation in the endosomal compartments of the cell. Unlike cationic lipoplex, the preferred route of entry for F protein–coated virosomes appears to be direct fusion with the plasma membrane. This result has implications for other encapsulated gene-delivery systems. It implies that there may be significant advantages to increasing the fusogenicity of encapsulated systems such that they fuse with the plasma membrane and deliver their contents to the cytosol, bypassing the lysosomal degradation pathway. However, the addition of viral proteins to lipid-delivery systems is likely to increase their immunogenicity and thus compromise their utility in applications that require repeat administration. A number of peptide derivatives of fusogenic proteins have been described, which may provide a strategy to enhance the fusogenicity of encapsulated systems without the generation of a compromising immune response (114).

F. Nuclear Delivery

The kinetics of gene expression resulting from cytoplasmic injection of plasmid DNA-polyethylenimine polyplex is similar to that observed when the polyplex is administered to cell culture medium, implying that nuclear uptake is the rate-limiting step in the transfection process (115). In an effort to improve upon existing gene-delivery technology, a number of investigators have directed their attention to ''the last 200 nm'' (11) and the factors affecting the nuclear uptake and expression of gene-therapy vectors. The last stages of the transfection process are generally regarded as the least efficient, and in practice this may be due to the fact that compositions optimized for stability outside the cell may contain components that inhibit transport into the nucleus and/or inhibit transcription. Pollard et al. (115) determined that cationic lipids inhibit transgene expression when reporter plasmids were injected directly into the nucleus of COS-7 cells in association with cationic liposomes. Polycations had no such effect. In contrast, polyethylenimine was found to enhance nuclear uptake and gene expression when polyplex were injected into the cytoplasm. Nuclear uptake of polyplex DNA was independent of charge ratio, implying that nuclear uptake is mediated by DNA compaction rather than net positive charge. These results suggest that neither lipoplex or polyplex systems are capable of simultaneously maximizing gene delivery and gene expression.

Attempts to improve the nuclear uptake must take into consideration the physical constraints of the nucleopore complex that mediates the uptake of plasmid DNA. When fully condensed by monovalent detergent counterions, a 5.5 kb supercoiled plasmid DNA molecule becomes a sphere of about 25 nm in diameter (117). The passive diffusion channel of the nuclear pore complex has an internal diameter of 9 nm (116). The diameter of the activated nuclear pore complex through which active transport occurs and therefore the size limit for signal-mediated nuclear import is 25 nm. Clearly there may be an advantage to invoking active transport mechanisms for the uptake of plasmid DNA. Wolff et al. recently described results obtained using plasmid DNA covalently modified to contain multiple copies of the SV-40 large T antigen nuclear localization signal peptide (NLS) (118). NLS sequences bind to the nucleopore component protein importin alpha-triggering activation of the nucleopore complex (116). Wolff observed a significant enhancement in nuclear uptake upon treatment of digitonin-permeabilized cells with NLS plasmid conjugates (118). When these same conjugates were injected directly into the cytoplasm of normal cells no increase in nuclear uptake was observed. J. P. Behr has constructed a model that may explain these findings (119). His interpretation of these results is that multiple copies of NLS sequences may actually be inhibitory to nucleopore-mediated DNA uptake. In a separate study cells were treated with linearized restriction fragments, which had been capped with hairpin-loop oligonucleotides. One of these oligonucleotides was covalently modified to contain a single copy of the SV-40 large T antigen NLS or a mutant NLS. Transfection results were compared to those obtained using uncapped linear DNA. NLS-specific transfection enhancements of 10–1000 times were observed in a variety of cell types when plasmid DNA contained a single copy of NLS peptide (119). Behr proposes a model whereby plasmid DNA is rapidly incorporated into chromatin-like structures upon entry into the nucleus. The initial nucleopore interaction is specific and can be NLS mediated, whereas the remaining events are driven by interactions with histones and basic nuclear matrix proteins. The inclusion of multiple copies of NLS peptides on a single plasmid may inhibit nuclear translocation by enabling competing interactions with multiple nucleopores. The implication of these findings with respect to the uptake of supercoiled plasmid DNA are not known, however, there appears to be considerable potential for improving the nuclear uptake of supercoiled plasmids through attachment of NLS peptides. It remains to be seen if this can be accomplished in a manner that is compatible with formulation and systemic gene delivery.

VIII. CONCLUSION

There is clear rationale for the development of a synthetic virus that can be used for systemic administration. First-generation delivery systems have been developed that possess the minimum set of viral functions necessary to transfect eukaryotic cells in vitro and in vivo, namely the ability to protect DNA from nuclease digestion long enough to facilitate association with cells and transit the membrane systems blocking entry to the nucleus. The efficiency, reproducibility, and pharmacology of these systems do not as yet justify their clinical utilization for treatment of systemic diseases. The ability to capitalize on advances in the molecular biology of gene expression systems and fulfill the promise of sustained high-level regulated gene expression will require careful consideration of the pharmacology and formulation of systemically administered gene-delivery systems. Assessment of the performance of the first-generation systems indicates that there are a number of critical physiological barriers that limit their effectiveness. The next generation of delivery systems must balance the often contradictory requirements of formulation stability and bioavailability. Lessons from the formulation of conventional chemotherapeutic drugs suggest that optimal formulations that encapsulate therapeutic payloads can provide significant improvements in pharmacology, yielding increases in potency and reduced toxicity. The recent development of a number of encapsulated systems should improve the pharmacology of gene drugs and provide a platform for the systematic incorporation of additional viral functions designed to confer cellular tropism and maximize potency through enhanced intracellular delivery and gene expression. Ultimately, the goal is to develop synthetic gene-delivery systems with real clinical utility, systems that can be prescribed and administered in a manner analogous to conventional drugs.

REFERENCES

1. Friedmann T. Gene Therapy: Fact and Fiction in Biologies New Approaches to Disease. Plainview: Cold Spring Harbor Laboratory Press, 1994:124.
2. Anderson WF, Blaese RM, Culver K. The ADA human gene therapy clinical protocol. Hum Gene Ther 1990; 1: 331–362.
3. Friedmann T. Human gene therapy—an immature genie, but certainly out of the bottle. Nature Med 1996; 2: 144–147.
4. Mulligan RC. The basic science of gene therapy. Science 1993; 260:926–932.
5. Wheeler JJ, Palmer L, Ossanlou M, et al. Stabilized plasmid lipid particles: construction and characterization. Gene Ther 1999; 6:271–281.
6. Templeton NS, Lasic DD, Frederik PM, Strey HH, Roberts DD, Pavlakis GN. Improved DNA:liposome complexes for increased systemic delivery and gene expression. Nature Biotech 1997; 15:647–652.
7. Zhu N, Liggitt D, Liu Y, Debs R. Systemic gene expression after intravenous DNA delivery into adult mice. Science 1993; 261:209–211.
8. Li S, Huang L In vivo gene transfer via intravenous administration of cationic lipid-protamine-DNA (LPD) complexes. Gene Ther 1997; 4:891–900.
9. Dvorak HF, Nagy JA, Dvorak JT, Dvorak AM. Identification and characterization of the blood vessels of solid tumors that are leaky to circulating macromolecules. Am J Pathol 1988; 133:95–109.
10. Singer SJ. A fluid lipid-globular protein mosaic model of membrane structure. Ann NY Acad Sci 1972; 195:16–23.
11. Ito S. The enteric surface coat on cat intestinal microvilli. J Cell Biol 1965; 27:475–491.
12. Goldstein JL, Brown MS, Anderson RGW, Russell D, Schneider W. Receptor mediated endocytosis: concepts emerging from the LDL receptor system. Annu Rev Cell Biol 1985; 1:1–39.
13. Murphy RF, Schmid J, Fuchs R. Endosome maturation: insights from somatic cell genetics and cell free analysis. Biochem Soc Trans 1993; 21:716–720.

14. Geuze HJ, Slot JW, Strous GJ, Lodish HF, Schwartz AL. Intracellular site of asialoglycoprotein receptor-ligand uncoupling: double-label immunoelectron microscopy during receptor-mediated endocytosis. Cell 1983; 32: 277–287.
15. Dunn KW, Maxfield FR. Delivery of ligands from sorting endosomes to late endosomes occurs by maturation of sorting endosomes. J Cell Biol 1992; 117:301–310.
16. Lechardeur D, Sohn KJ, Haardt M, et al. Metabolic instability of plasmid DNA in the cytosol: a potential barrier to gene transfer. Gene Ther 1999; 6:482–497.
17. Wilke M, Fortunati E, Van den Brocek M, Hoogeveen AT, Scholte BJ. Efficacy of a peptide-based gene delivery system depends on mitotic activity. Gene Ther 1996; 3: 1133–1142.
18. Mortimer I, Tam P, MacLachlan I, Graham RW, Saravolac EG, Joshi PB. Cationic lipid mediated transfection of cells in culture requires mitotic activity. Gene Ther 1999; 6: 403–411.
19. Gao GP, Yang Y, Wilson JM. Biology of adenovirus vectors with E1 and E4 deletions for liver-directed gene therapy. J Virol 1996; 70:8934–8943.
20. Peeters MJTFDV, Patijin GA, Lieber A, Meuse L, Kay MA. Adenovirus-mediated hepatic gene transfer in mice: comparison of intravascular and biliary administration. Hum Gene Ther 1996; 7:1693–1699.
21. Scaria A, St George JA, Gregory RJ, et al. Antibody to CD40 ligand inhibits both humoral and cellular immune responses to adenoviral vectors and facilitates repeated administration in mouse airway. Gene Ther 1997; 4: 611–617.
22. Ilan Y, Droguett G, Chowdhury NR, et al. Insertion of the adenoviral E3 region into a recombinant viral vector prevents antiviral humoral and cellular immune responses and permits long-term gene expression. Proc Natl Acad Sci USA 1997; 94:2587–2592.
23. Felgner PL. Nomenclature for synthetic gene delivery systems. Hum Gene Ther 1997; 8:511–512.
24. Wu GY, Wu CH. Receptor-mediated in vitro gene transformation by a soluble DNA carrier system. J Biol Chem 1987; 262:4429–4432.
25. Rosengarten O, Horowitz AT, Tzemach D, Huang L, Gabizon A. In vitro cytotoxicity and pharmacokinetics of cationic liposomes in mice. Cancer Gene Ther 1994; 1:321.
26. Litzinger DC, Brown JF, Wala I, et al. Fate of cationic liposomes and their complex with oligonucleotide in vivo. Biochim Biophys Acta 1996; 1281:139–149.
27. Huang L, Li S. Liposomal gene delivery: a complex package. Nature Biotech 1997; 15:620–621.
28. Thierry AR, Rabinovich P, Peng B, Mahan LC, Bryant JL, Gallo RC. Characterization of liposome-mediated gene delivery: expression, stability and pharmacokinetics of plasmid DNA. Gene Ther 1997; 4:226–237.
29. Song YK, Liu F, Liu D. Enhanced gene expression in mouse lung by prolonging the retention time of intravenously injected plasmid DNA. Gene Ther 1998; 5: 1531–15337.
30. Song YK, Liu D. Free liposomes enhance the transfection activity of DNA/lipid complexes in vivo by intravenous administration. Biochim Biophys Acta 1998; 1372: 141–150.
31. Sternberg B, Hong K, Zheng W, Papahadjopoulos D. Ultrastructural characterization of cationic liposome-DNA complexes showing enhanced stability in serum and high transfection activity in vivo. Biochim Biophys Acta 1998; 1375:23–25.
32. Gao X, Huang L. Potentiation of cationic liposome-mediated gene delivery by polycations. Biochemistry 1996; 35:1027–1036.
33. McLeod JG, Penny R. Vincristine neuropathy: an electrophysiological and histological study. J Neurol Neurosurg Psychiatry 1969; 32:297–304.
34. Sandler SG, Tobin W, Henderson ES. Vincristine-induced neuropathy: a clinical study of fifty leukemic patients. Neurology 1969; 19:367–374.
35. Mayer LD, Bally MB, Loughrey H, Masin D, Cullis PR. Liposomal vincristine preparations which exhibit decreased drug toxicity and increased activity against murine L1210 and P388 tumors. Cancer Res 1990; 50:575–579.
36. Webb M, Harasym T, Masin D, Bally M, Mayer L. Sphingomyelin-cholesterol liposomes significantly enhance the pharmacokinetic and therapeutic properties of vincristine in murine and human tumour models. Br J Cancer 1995; 72:896–904.
37. Gelman KA, Tolcher A, Diab AR, et al. Phase I study of liposomal vincristine. J Clin Oncol 1999; 17:697–705.
38. Mayer LD, Tai LCL, Ko DSC, et al. Influence of vesicle size, lipid composition, and drug-to-lipid ratio on the biological activity of liposomal doxorubicin in mice. Cancer Res 1989; 49:5922–5930.
39. Embree L, Gelmon K, Lohr A, et al. Chromatographic analysis and pharmacokinetics of liposome-encapsulated doxorubicin in non-small cell lung cancer patients. J Pharm Sci 1993; 82:627–634.
40. Mayer L, Nayar R, Thies R, Boman N, Cullis P, Bally M. Identification of vesicle properties that enhance the antitumour activity of liposomal vincristine against murine L1210 leukemia. Cancer Chemother Pharmacol 1993; 33: 17–24.
41. Boman N, Bally M, Cullis P, Mayer L, Webb M. Encapsulation of vincristine in liposomes reduces its toxicity and improves its anti-tumor efficacy. J Liposome Res 1995; 5:523–541.
42. Lasic D. Doxorubicin in sterically stabilized liposomes. Nature 1996; 380:561–562.
43. Gill P, Wernz J, Scadden D, et al. Randomized phase III trial of liposomal daunorubicin versus doxorubicin, bleomycin and vincristine in AIDS-related Kaposi's sarcoma. J Clin Oncol 1996; 14:2353–2364.
44. Loeher PJ, Einhorn LH. Drugs five years later: cisplatin. Ann Intern Med 1984; 100:704–713.
45. Steerenberg PA, Storm G, de Groot G, Bergers JJ, Claessen A, de Jong WH. Liposomes as a drug carrier system

for cis-diaminedichloroplatinum(II). I. Binding capacity, stability and tumor growth inhibition in vitro. Int J Pharmaceutics 1987; 40:51–62.
46. Potkul RK, Gondal J, Bitterman P, Dretchen KL, Rahman A. Toxicities in rats with free versus liposomal encapsulated cisplatin. Am J Obstet Gynecol 1991; 164:652–658.
47. Mannino RJ, Allebach ES, Strohl WA. Encapsulation of high molecular weight DNA in large unilamellar phospholipid vesicles. FEBS Lett 1979; 101:229–232.
48. Mukherjee AB, Orloff S, Butler JD, Triche T, Lalley P, Schulman JD. Entrapment of metaphase chromosomes into phospholipid vesicles (lipochromosomes): carrier potential in gene transfer. Proc Natl Acad Sci USA 1978; 75: 1361–1365.
49. Hoffman RM, Margolis LB, Bergelson LD. Binding and entrapment of high molecular weight DNA by lecithin liposomes. FEBS Lett 1978; 93:365–368.
50. Scaefer-Ridder M, Wang Y, Hofschneider PH. Liposomes as gene carriers: efficient transformation of mouse L cells by thymidine kinase gene. Science 1982; 215:166–168.
51. Nicolau C, Le Pape A, Soriano P, Fargette F, Juhel MF. In vivo expression of rat insulin after intravenous administration of the liposome-entrapped gene for rat insulin. Proc Natl Acad Sci USA 1983; 80:1068–1072.
52. Baru M, Axelrod JH, Nur I. Liposome-encapsulated DNA-mediated gene transfer and synthesis of human factor IX in mice. Gene 1995; 161:143–150.
53. Fraley R, Subramani S, Berg P, Papahadjopoulos D. Introduction of liposome-encapsulated SV-40 DNA into cells. J Biol Chem 1980; 255:10431–10435.
54. Soriano P, Dijkstra J, Legrand A, et al. Targeted and non-targeted liposomes for in vivo transfer to rat liver cells of plasmid containing the preproinsulin I gene. Proc Natl Acad Sci USA 1983; 80:7128–7131.
55. Nakanishi M, Uchida T, Sugawa H, Ishiura M, Okada Y. Efficient introduction of contents of liposomes into cells using HVJ (Sendai virus). Exp Cell Res 1985; 159: 399–409.
56. Cudd A, Nicolau C. Intracellular fate of liposome encapsulated DNA in mouse liver: analysis using electron microscope autoradiography and subcellular fractionation. Biochim Biophys Acta 1985; 845:477–491.
57. Nicolau C, Rottem S. Expression of beta-lactamase activity in *Mycoplasma capricolum* transfected with the liposome-encapsulated *E. coli* pBR32 plasmid. Biochem Biophys Res Commun 1982; 108:982–986.
58. Fraley RT, Fornari CS, Kaplan S. Entrapment of a bacterial plasmid in phospholipid vesicles: potential for gene therapy. Proc Natl Acad Sci USA 1979; 76:3348–3352.
59. Lurquin PF. Entrapment of plasmid DNA by liposomes and their interactions with plant protoplasts. Nucleic Acids Res 1979; 6:3773–3784.
60. Alino SF, Bobadilla M, Garcia-Sanz M, Lejarreta M, Unda F, Hilario E. In vivo delivery of human alpha 1-antitrypsin gene to mouse hepatocytes by liposomes. Biochem Biophys Res Commun 1993; 192:174–181.
61. Jay DG, Gilbert W. Basic protein enhances the incorporation of DNA into lipid vesicles: model for the formation of primordial cells. Proc Natl Acad Sci USA 1987; 84: 1978–1980.
62. Puyal C, Milhaud P, Bienvenue A, Philippot JR. A new cationic liposome encapsulating genetic material. A potential delivery system for polynucleotides. Eur J Biochem 1995; 228:697–703.
63. Ibanez M, Gariglio P, Chavez P, Santiago R, Wong C, Baeza I. Spermidine-condensed DNA and cone-shaped lipids improve delivery and expression of exogenous DNA transfer by liposomes. Biochem Cell Biol 1997; 74: 633–643.
64. Monnard PA, Oberholzer T, Luisi P. Entrapment of nucleic acids in liposomes. Biochim Biophys Acta 1997; 1329: 39–50.
65. Szelei J, Duda E. Entrapment of high molecular mass DNA molecules in liposomes for the genetic transformation of animal cells. Biochem J 1989; 259:549–553.
66. Allen TM, Chong A. Large unilamellar liposomes with low uptake into the reticuloendothelial system. FEBS Lett 1987; 223:42–46.
67. Klibanov AL, Maruyama K, Torchilin VP, Huang L. Amphipathic polyethyleneglycols effectively prolong the circulation time of liposomes. FEBS Lett 1990; 268: 235–237.
68. Papahadjopoulos D, Allen TM, Gabizon A, et al. Sterically stabilized liposomes: improvements in pharmacokinetics and anti-tumor therapeutic efficacy. Proc Natl Acad Sci USA 1991; 88:11460–11464.
69. Needham D, McIntosh TJ, Lasic DD. Repulsive interactions and mechanical stability of polymer grafted lipid membranes. Biochim Biophys Acta 1992; 1108:40–48.
70. Semple S, Chonn A. Protein-liposome interactions in relation to clearance. J Liposome Res 1996; 6:33–60.
71. Senior J, Delgado C, Fisher D, Tilcock C, Gregoriadis G. Influence of surface hydrophilicity of liposomes on their interaction with plasma protein and their clearance from the circulation: studies with poly(ethylene glycol)-coated vesicles. Biochim Biophys Acta 1991; 1062:77–82.
72. Gabizon A, Paphadjopoulos D. Liposome formulations with prolonged circulation time in blood and enhanced uptake by tumors. Proc Natl Acad Sci USA 1988; 85: 6949–6953.
73. Hong K, Zheng W, Baker A, Papahadjopoulos D. Stabilization of cationic liposome-plasmid DNA complexes by polyamines and poly(ethylene glycol)-phospholipid conjugates for efficient in vivo gene delivery. FEBS Lett 1997; 400:233–237.
74. Zhang YP, Sekirov L, Saravolac EG, et al. Stabilized plasmid lipid particles for regional gene therapy: formulation and transfection properties. Gene Ther 1999; 6: 1438–1447.
75. MacLachlan I, Tam P, Lee D, et al. A gene specific increase in the survival of tumor bearing mice following systemic non-viral gene therapy. (In Press.)

76. Stein Y, Halperin G, Stein O. Biological stability of [3H]cholesteryl esther in cultured fibroblasts and intact rat. FEBS Lett 1980; 111:104–106.
77. Monck M, Tam P, Lee D, et al. Stabilized plasmid lipid particles for systemic gene therapy. (In Press.)
78. Sato Y, Roman M, Tighe H, et al. Non-coding bacterial DNA sequences necessary for effective intradermal gene immunization. Science 1996; 273:351–354.
79. Stacey KJ, Sweet MJ, Hume DA. Macrophages ingest and are activated by bacterial DNA. J Immunol 1996; 157: 2116–2122.
80. Klinman DM, Yi AK, Beaucage SL, Conover J, Kreig AM. CpG motifs present in bacterial DNA rapidly induce lymphocytes to secrete interleukin 6, interleukin 12 and interferon gamma. Proc Natl Acad Sci USA 1996; 93: 2879–2883.
81. Ballas ZK, Rasmussen WL, Krieg AM. Induction of NK activity in murine and human cells by CpG motifs in oligonucleotides and bacterial DNA. J. Immunol 1996; 157: 1840–1845.
82. Yi AK, Chace JH, Cowdery JS, Krieg AM. IFN-gamma promotes IL-6 and IgM secretion in response to CpG motifs in bacterial DNA and oligonucleotides. J Immunol 1996; 156:558–564.
83. Mislick KA, Baldeschwieler JD. Evidence for the role of proteoglycans in cation mediated gene transfer. Proc Natl Acad Sci USA 1996; 93:12349–12354.
84. Mounkes LC, Zhong W, Cipres-Palacin G, Heath TD, Debs RJ. Proteoglycans mediate cationic liposome-DNA complex-based gene delivery in vitro and in vivo. J Biol Chem 1998; 273:26164–26170.
85. Hui SW, Langner M, Zhao YL, Ross P, Hurley E, Chan K. The role of helper lipids in cationic liposome-mediated gene transfer. Biophys J 1996; 71:590–599.
86. Felgner JH, Kumar R, Sridhar CN, et al. Enhanced gene delivery and mechanism studies with a novel series of cationic lipid formulations. J Biol Chem 1994; 269: 2550–2561.
87. Gao X, Huang L. Cationic liposome-mediated gene transfer. Gene Ther 1995; 2:710–722.
88. Farhood H, Serbina N, Huang L. The role of dioleoylphosphatidylethanolamine in cationic liposome mediated gene transfer. Biochim Biophys Acta 1995; 1235:289–295.
89. Hui SW, Stewart TP, Boni LT, Yeagle PL. Membrane fusion through point defects in bilayers. Science 1981; 212:921–923.
90. Liu Y, Liggitt D, Zhong W, Tu G, Gaensler K, Debs R. Cationic liposome mediated intravenous gene delivery. J Biol Chem 1995; 270:24864–24870.
91. Felgner P, Gadek T, Holm M, et al. Lipofection: a highly efficient lipid-mediated DNA transfection procedure. Proc Natl Acad Sci USA 1987; 84:7413–7417.
92. Wrobel I, Collins D. Fusion of cationic liposomes with mammalian cells occurs after endocytosis. Biochim Biophys Acta 1995; 1235:296–304.
93. Holland J, Hui C, Cullis P, Madden T. Poly(ethyleneglycol)-lipid conjugates regulate the calcium-induced fusion of liposomes composed of phosphatidylethanolamine and phosphatidylserine. Biochemistry 1996; 35:2618–2624.
94. Xu Y, Szoka FC. Mechanism of DNA release from cationic liposome/DNA complexes used in cell transfection. Biochemistry 1996; 35:5616–5623.
95. Ahmad I, Longnecker M, Samuel J, Allen TM. Antibody-targeted delivery of doxorubicin entrapped in sterically stabilized liposomes can eradicate lung cancer in mice. Cancer Res 1993; 53:1484–1488.
96. Wang CY, Huang L. Highly efficient DNA delivery mediated by pH sensitive immunoliposomes. Biochemistry 1989; 28:9508–9514.
97. Stavridis JC, Deliconstantinos G, Psallidopoulos MC, Armenakas NA, Hadjiminas DJ, Hadjiminas J. Construction of transferrin-coated liposomes for in vivo transport of exogenous DNA to bone marrow erythroblasts in rabbits. Exp Cell Res 1986; 164:568–572.
98. Hara T, Aramaki S, Takada S, Koike K, Tsuchiya S. Receptor-mediated transfer of pSV2CAT DNA to a human hepatoblastoma cell line HepG2 using asialofetuin-labeled cationic liposomes. Gene 1995; 159:167–174.
99. Kikuchi A, Sugaya S, Ueda H, et al. Efficient gene transfer to EGF receptor overexpressing cancer cells by means of EGF-labeled cationic liposomes. Biochim Biophys Res Commun 1996; 227:666–671.
100. Kao GY, Chang LJ, Allen TM. Use of targeted cationic liposomes in enhanced DNA delivery to cancer cells. Cancer Gene Ther 1996; 3:250–256.
101. Lee RJ, Huang L. Folate-targeted, anionic liposome-entrapped polylysine-condensed DNA for tumor cell-specific gene transfer. J Biol Chem 1996; 271:8481–8487.
102. Blom M, Anderson L, Carlsson A, Herslof B, Zhou L, Nilsson A. Pharmacokinetics, tissue distribution and metabolism of intravenously administered digalactosyldiacylglycerol and monogalactosyldiacylglycerol in the rat. J Liposome Res 1996; 6:737–753.
103. Sasaki A, Murahashi N, Yamada H, Morikawa A. Synthesis of novel galactosyl ligands for liposomes and the influence of the spacer on accumulation in the rat liver. Biol Pharm Bull 1995; 18:740–746.
104. Wang CY, Huang L. pH-sensitive immunoliposomes mediate target cell-specific delivery and controlled expression of a foreign gene in mouse. Proc Natl Acad Sci USA 1987; 84:7851–7855.
105. Remy J, Kichler A, Mordvinov V, Schuber F, Behr JP. Targeted gene transfer into hepatoma cells with lipopolyamine-condensed DNA particles presenting galactose ligands: a stage toward artificial viruses. Proc Natl Acad Sci USA 1995; 92:1744–1748.
106. Cheng P. Receptor ligand-facilitated gene transfer: enhancement of liposome-mediated gene transfer and expression by transferrin. Hum Gene Ther 1996; 7:1010–1017.
107. Meunier-Durmort C, Ferry N, Hianque B, Delattre J, Forest C. Efficient transfer of regulated genes in adipocytes and hepatoma cells by the combination of liposomes and replication-deficient adenovirus. Eur J Biochem 1996; 237:660–667.

108. Kreuzer J, Denger S, Reifers F, et al. Adenovirus-assisted lipofection: efficient in vitro gene transfer of luciferase and cytosine deaminase to human smooth muscle cells. Atherosclerosis 1996; 124:49–60.
109. Bron R, Oritz A, Dijkstra J, Stegmanm T, Wilschut J. Preparation, properties and applications of reconstituted Influenza virus envelopes (virosomes). Methods Enzymol 1993; 220:313–331.
110. Bron R, Oritz A, Wilschut J. Cellular cytoplasmic delivery of a polypeptide toxin by reconstituted Influenza virus envelopes (virosomes). Biochemistry 1994; 33:9110–9117.
111. Dzau VJ, Mann MJ, Morishita R, Kaneda Y. Fusogenic viral liposome delivery for gene therapy in cardiovascular diseases. Proc Natl Acad Sci USA 1996; 93:11421–11425.
112. Yanagihara I, Inui K, Dickinson G, et al. Expression of full-length human dystrophin cDNA in mdx mouse muscle by HVJ-liposome injection. Gene Ther 1996; 3:549–553.
113. Ramani K, Bora RS, Kumar M, Tyagi SK, Sarkar DP. Novel gene delivery to liver cells using engineered virosomes. FEBS Lett 1997; 404:164–168.
114. Wyman T, Nicol F, Zelphati O, Scaria P, Plank C, Szoka F. Design, synthesis, and characterization of a cationic peptide that binds to nucleic acids and permeabilizes bilayers. Biochemistry 1997; 36:3008–3017.
115. Pollard H, Remy JS, Loussouarn G, Demolombe S, Behr JP. Polyethylenimine but not cationic lipids promotes transgene delivery to the nucleus in mammalian cells. J Biol Chem 1998; 273:7507–7511.
116. Ohno M, Fornerod M, Mattaj IW. Nucleocytoplasmic transport: the last 200 nanometers. Cell 1998; 92:327–336.
117. Blessing T, Remy JS, Behr JP. Monomolecular collapse of plasmid DNA into stable virus-like particles. Proc Natl Acad Sci USA 1998; 95:1427–1431.
118. Sebestyen MG, Ludtke JJ, Bassik MC, et al. DNA vector chemistry: the covalent attachment of signal peptides to plasmid DNA. Nature Biotech 1998; 16:80–85.
119. Zanta MA, Belguise-Valladier P, Behr JP. Gene delivery: a single nuclear localization signal peptide is sufficient to carry DNA into the cell nucleus. Proc Natl Acad Sci USA 1999; 96:91–96.
120. Stratford-Perricaudet LD, Makeh I, Perriccaudet M, Briand P. Widespread long-term gene transfer to mouse skeletal muscles and heart. J Clin Invest 1992; 90: 626–630.
121. Russell DW, Miller AD, Alexander IE. Adeno-associated virus vectors preferentially transduce cells in S phase. Proc Natl Acad Sci USA 1994; 91:8915–8919.
122. Koeberl DD, Alexander IE, Halbert CL, Russell DW, Miller AD. Persistent expression of human clotting factor IX from mouse liver after intravenous injection of adeno-associated virus vectors. Proc Natl Acad Sci USA 1997; 94:1426–1431.
123. Miller DG, Adam MA, Miller AD. Gene transfer by retrovirus vectors occurs only in cells that are actively replicating at the time of infection. Mol Cell Bio 1990; 10: 4239–4242.
124. Jolly D. Viral vector systems for gene therapy. Cancer Gene Ther 1994; 1:51–64.
125. Walsh T, Yeldandi V, McEvoy M, et al. Safety, tolerance, and pharmacokinetics of a small unilamellar liposomal formulation of amphotericin B (AmBisome) in neutropenic patients. Antimicrob Agents Chemother 1998; 42: 2391–2398.
126. Newman M, Colbern G, Working P, Engbers C, Amantea M. Comparative pharmacokinetics, tissue distribution, and therapeutic effectiveness of cisplatin encapsulated in long-circulating, pegylated liposomes (SPI-077) in tumor-bearing mice. Cancer Chemother Pharmacol 1999; 43:1–7.
127. Northfelt D, Dezube B, Thommes J, et al. Pegylated-liposomal doxorubicin versus doxorubicin, bleomycin, and vincristine in the treatment of AIDS-related Kaposi's sarcoma: results of a randomized phase III clinical trial. J Clin Oncol 1998; 16:2445–2451.
128. Muggia F. Clinical efficacy and prospects for use of pegylated liposomal doxorubicin in the treatment of ovarian and breast cancers. Drugs 1997; 54(suppl):22–29.
129. Rentsch K, Schwendener R, Pestalozzi B, Sauter C, Wunderli-Allenspach H, Hanseler E. Pharmacokinetic studies of mitoxantrone and one of its metabolites in serum and urine in patients with advanced breast cancer. Eur J Clin Pharmacol 1998; 54:83–89.
130. Wallace T, Paetznick V, PA C, Lopez-Berstein G, Rex J, Anaissie E. Activity of liposomal nystatin against disseminated *Aspergillus fungimatus* infection in neutropenic mice. Antimicrob Agents Chemother 1997; 41: 2238–2243.
131. Parthasarathy R, Sacks P, Harris D, Brock H, Mehta K. Interaction of liposome-associated all-trans-retinoic acid with squamous carcinoma cells. Cancer Chemother Pharmacol 1994; 34:527–534.

14

Gene Therapy Applications of Ribozymes

Bruce A. Sullenger and Lynn Milich
Duke University Medical Center, Durham, North Carolina

I. INTRODUCTION

Since their discovery in the early 1980s, RNA enzymes, or ribozymes, have been the subject of much investigation. Numerous studies have been performed to elucidate the biochemistry of how certain RNA molecules can fold into complex tertiary structures to form active sites and perform catalysis. Other studies have focused upon identifying the roles that RNA enzymes play in cell biology. More recently, even more attention has been focused on the study of ribozymes because it was recognized that these RNA enzymes can potentially be quite useful for a variety of gene therapy applications.

The first discovered ribozyme was the self-splicing group I intron from *Tetrahymena thermophila.* The reaction mediated by this RNA enzyme has now been extensively characterized, and the mechanism by which it excises itself from precursor ribosomal RNAs (pre-rRNA) without the aid of proteins is well understood (1–3). The second ribozyme to be recognized was the RNA subunit of RNase P. RNase P catalyzes the removal of upstream sequences on precursor tRNAs to produce mature 5′ ends on tRNA molecules in a wide variety of cell types (3,4).

Several other catalytic RNA motifs have been discovered that are naturally associated with plant and human pathogens. The hammerhead and hairpin ribozymes are derived from satellite RNAs from plant viroid and virusoids and the hepatitis delta virus ribozyme is derived from a short, single-stranded RNA virus found in some patients with hepatitis B virus. Each of these small RNA enzymes catalyzes a self-cleavage reaction that is believed to play a major role in the replication of these single-stranded RNA pathogens (5).

All of these self-cleaving ribozymes have been reengineered so that they can cleave other target RNA molecules in *trans* in a sequence-specific manner (6). This ability to specifically cleave targeted RNAs has led to much speculation about the potential utility of *trans*-cleaving ribozymes as inhibitors of gene expression (7–11). In addition, the group I self-splicing ribozyme from *Tetrahymena* can be reengineered to perform splicing upon a targeted RNA molecule in *trans.* It has been argued that such *trans*-splicing ribozymes may prove to be effective at repairing mutant cellular transcripts by cleaving off mutant nucleotides and ligating on functional RNA sequences (12–14).

The purpose of this chapter is not to provide an extensive review of the enzymology of ribozymes or to catalog the published results demonstrating that ribozymes may become useful reagents for gene therapy applications. Both of these topics have been extensively reviewed elsewhere (2–14). Moreover, we will not discuss the use of synthetic ribozymes and will leave the description of various gene transfer and expression systems that can be employed to deploy ribozymes to the other chapters in this book. Rather, we will attempt to present a focused account of the potential utility of catalytic RNAs for gene therapy by first presenting an overview of the basic biochemistry of well-characterized ribozymes and then discussing how *trans*-cleaving and *trans*-splicing ribozymes may be employed for a variety of gene therapy applications. Our hope is that this approach will enhance the reader's understanding of the potential utility of ribozymes for both gene inhibition and genetic repair.

II. CATALYTIC RNAs

Five classes of catalytic RNAs have been extensively characterized. Each class of ribozyme adopts a characteristic secondary and tertiary structure that is required to assemble a catalytic center and perform catalysis (Fig. 1) (6). In addition, these classes of ribozymes differ in size, and the mechanism that each employs to perform catalysis varies. Hammerhead, hairpin, and the hepatitis delta virus (HDV) ribozymes are only 30–80 nucleotides in length and form cleavage products with 2′,3′-cyclic phosphate and 5′-hydroxyl termini. By contrast, catalytic RNAs derived from group I introns and RNase P are typically greater than 200 nucleotides in length, and both cleave target RNAs to generate products with 3′-hydroxyl and 5′-phosphate termini. Each of these classes of ribozyme will be discussed in more detail below.

A. The Group I Intron from *Tetrahymena thermophila*

The intervening sequence (IVS) found in nuclear precursor rRNA transcripts from *T. thermophila* is one of the most well-characterized catalytic RNAs. This IVS is a member of a growing family of group I introns that have common structural and functional features. The *Tetrahymena* intron is naturally 413 nucleotides long and is found in the middle of the 26S rRNA gene. The IVS is transcribed as part of the rRNA precursor and excises itself by performing a cleavage and a ligation reaction to form a functional rRNA without the aid of proteins (1,15). Prior to the discovery of this self-splicing reaction, RNA was thought to be only a carrier of genetic information or a scaffold for protein binding and not able to perform catalysis on it own.

1. The Self-Splicing Reaction of the *Tetrahymena* Group I Intron

Comparative sequence analysis of several group I introns (16,17) as well as mutational analyses (18–26) have been employed to develop a phylogenetically conserved prediction of the secondary structure of group I introns consisting of a set of paired regions, P1–P9. More recently, x-ray crystallography and chemical probing studies have revealed that the *Tetrahymena* intron adopts a particular three-dimensional structure using several tertiary interactions (27–34) and contains a catalytic core surrounded by a close-packed layer of RNA helices (32–34). Several studies have shown that this folded RNA structure participates directly in self-splicing (35,36).

The *Tetrahymena* intron excises itself and ligates together its flanking exons by performing two consecutive transesterification reactions (2,15). The first step of splicing is a cleavage reaction initiated by a free guanosine that is bound by the intron. This guanosine serves as a nucleophile attacking the 5′ splice site and is covalently attached to the 5′ end of the intron (Fig 2a). The recognition element that defines the exact site of guanosine attack is a G-U wobble base pair that is highly conserved among group I introns. The G-U base pair is part of a short duplex called P1. The P1 duplex includes base pairing between the last six nucleotides of the 5′ exon and sequences within the intron called the internal guide sequence (IGS) or the 5′ exon–binding site. In the second step of splicing, the newly generated 3′-hydroxyl group, at the 3′ end of the cleaved 5′ exon, attacks the phosphorus atom at the 3′ splice site, resulting in the ligation of the 5′ and 3′ exons and the excision of the intron. The excised group I intron maintains its ability to make and break phosphodiester bonds. However, because the group I intron is not regenerated in its original form following self-splicing, this catalytic RNA is not a true enzyme in the strictest sense (37). Subsequently shortened forms of the *Tetrahymena* group I intron, which lack exon sequences, were generated that fulfill the definition of a true enzyme in that they can perform multiple turnover reactions without being modified in the process (38).

2. The *Trans*-Cleaving Reaction of the *Tetrahymena* Ribozyme

Shortened versions of the intervening sequence from *Tetrahymena* that lack the first 19 or 21 nucleotides (called L-19 or L-21) can catalyze the cleavage of oligonucleotide substrates with multiple turnover (38). Moreover, the rate enhancement achieved by this shortened form of the intron is within the range of values achieved by protein enzymes, such as EcoRI, that catalyze sequence-specific cleavage of nucleic acids. The catalytic mechanism employed by the shortened form of the *Tetrahymena* ribozyme in this *trans*-cleavage reaction is quite similar to that used by the full-length intron in the cleavage step of self-splicing, with a few exceptions (39). First, the 5′ exon sequences preceding the IGS have been removed in the shortened form of the intron. Therefore, the ribozyme must bind to a target RNA that is present in *trans* (Fig 2b). As in the case of the self-splicing reaction, a wobble G-U base pair is required at the cleavage site and the IGS of the ribozyme must be complementary to the sequence found on the substrate RNA just 5′ of the reactive uridine residue (40). For the wild-type IGS (5′-GGAGGG-3′) binding would occur at nucleotides 5′-CCCUCU-3′ within the substrate RNA. Cleavage occurs just 3′ of the uridine residue on the substrate RNA at the reconstructed G-U base pair (Fig. 2b).

As noted, substrate recognition and *trans*-cleavage require base pairing between the IGS on the ribozyme and the RNA substrate. Substrate specificity can be manipulated by

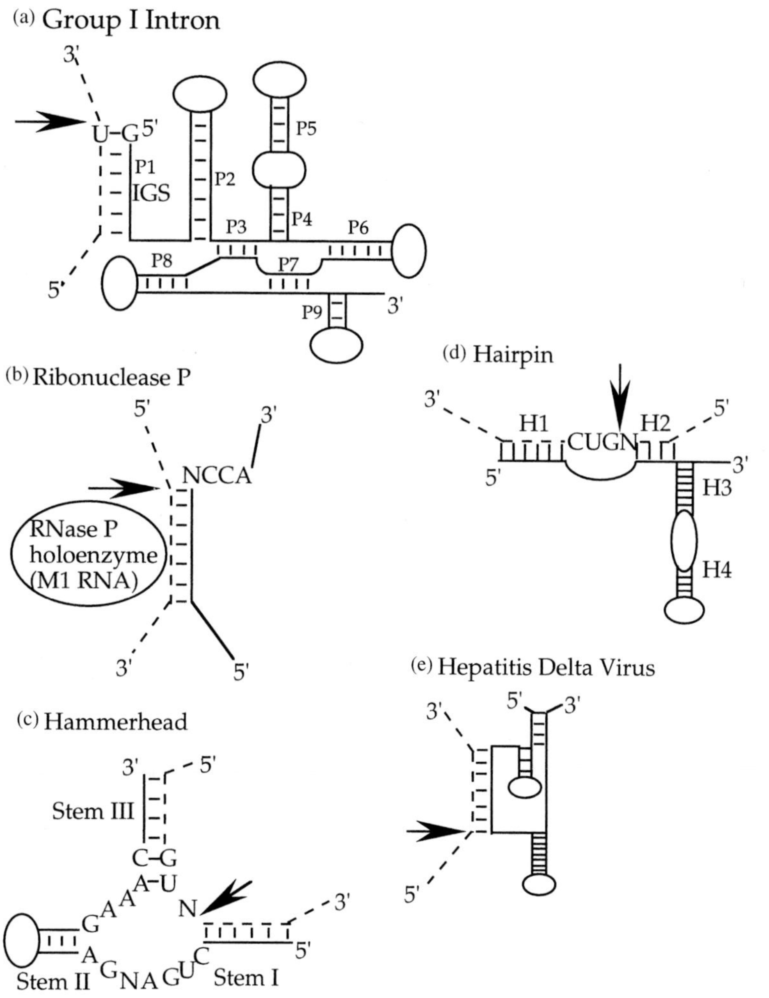

Figure 1 Secondary structures of five classes of ribozymes. All five ribozymes, shown in solid black lines, have been engineered to cleave specific target RNAs, shown as dashed lines. The base pairing formed between the ribozymes and their target RNAs are shown, and the site of cleavage of the substrate RNAs is indicated by an arrow. (a) The group I ribozyme P1 through P9 represent the conserved based paired regions found in group I introns. The internal guide sequence (IGS) is shown paired to a target RNA. The substrate is cleaved just 3′ of the conserved G-U wobble base pair. (b) RNase P holoenzyme contains an RNA subunit as well as a protein cofactor. The substrate for RNase P cleavage is indicated bound to an external guide sequence (EGS) just 5′ of a free 5′-NCCA-3′ sequence. Cleavage of the targeted RNA occurs just across from the end of the EGS-target duplex. (c) The hammerhead ribozyme is shown bound to a target RNA through base-pairing interactions formed by stems I and III. The single-stranded regions encompass the catalytic core of the ribozyme. Cleavage of the substrate RNA occurs at an unpaired residue positioned between stems I and III. (d) The hairpin ribozyme binds its target RNA through two base-pairing regions called helix 1 (H1) and helix 2 (H2). Cleavage of the target RNA occurs between the N and G nucleotides on the substrate as indicated. (e) The HDV ribozyme forms seven or eight base pairs with its target RNA, and cleavage occurs just 5′ of this base-pairing interaction.

altering the sequence of the ribozyme's IGS to make it complementary to any target RNA molecule (40–42). Moreover, no specific sequence requirements exist for the IGS except that it must contain a guanosine residue at the reaction site. Thus, by altering the guide sequence of the L-21 version of the *Tetrahymena* catalytic RNA, a ribozyme can be created that can be employed to recognize and cleave a target RNA following any uridine residue (Fig. 2b).

The L-21 form of the *Tetrahymena* ribozyme binds to a six-nucleotide-long substrate RNA 10^3- to 10^4-fold tighter than would be predicted by base pairing binding energy

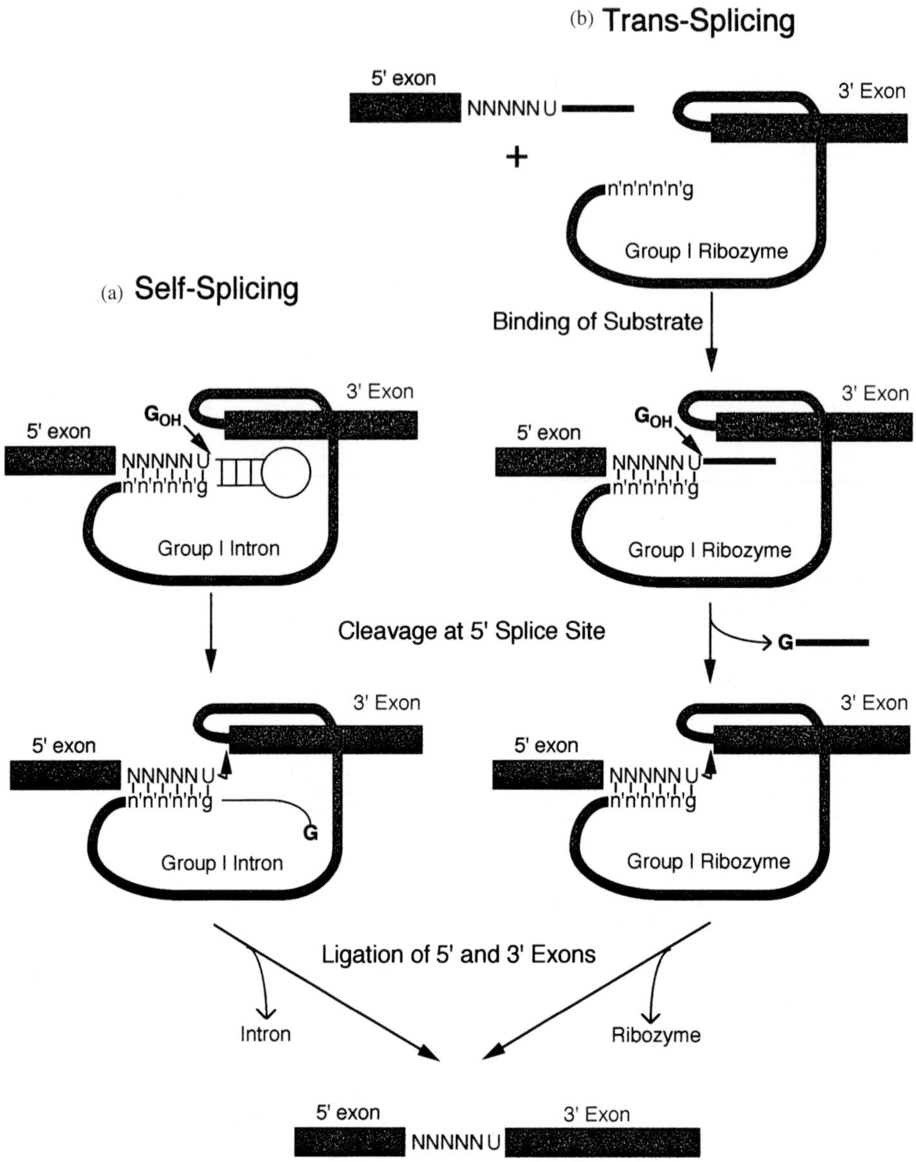

Figure 2 Group I ribozyme–mediated self- and *trans*-splicing. (a) Self-splicing is initiated by the attack of the 5′ splice site by an intron-bound guanosine. This cleavage occurs just 3′ of the uridine shown that is involved in a G-U wobble base pair. The group I intron holds onto the 5′ cleavage product via base pairs formed between the internal guide sequence of the ribozyme and the 3′ end of the 5′ exon. In the second step of splicing, the intron attaches the cleaved 5′ exon onto the 3′ exon and liberates itself. (b) During *trans*-splicing, the ribozyme binds to a sequence in a target RNA (5′-NNNNNU-3′) via base pairing through its internal guide sequence (5′-gn′n′n′n′n′-3′). The ribozyme cleaves the target RNA at the reactive uridine, releases the downstream cleavage product, and ligates a 3′ exon onto the upstream cleavage product.

alone (43–45). Studies on the L-21 ribozyme, as well as the self-splicing form of the intron, suggest that tertiary interactions contribute to the ribozyme-substrate binding energy. Specific tertiary interactions have been identified that involve 2′-hydroxyl groups on the ribose backbone of the substrate and the intron (46–49). This tight binding between the ribozyme and RNA substrate limits the substrate specificity of the *Tetrahymena* ribozyme because both matched substrates, which are only six nucleotides long, and substrates that form single base pair mismatches with the IGS serve as excellent substrates for the ribozyme (44,45). Under conditions of saturating guanosine and 10 mM $MgCl_2$, such RNA substrates are bound so tightly that the ribozyme goes on to cleave essentially every RNA that it binds. Therefore, the substrate specificity of this ribozyme will probably have to be improved if it is to become useful for gene therapy because any six-nucleotide sequence would be expected to be present in many cellular RNAs. Fortunately, several logical approaches exist that can potentially be employed to enhance the substrate specificity of the *Tetrahymena* ribozyme (50,51).

If the specificity of the group I ribozyme proves very difficult to improve, then trans-cleaving ribozymes derived from group II introns may represent an alternative catalytic RNA motif that may be able to achieve the high levels of substrate specificity that might be required for gene therapy applications. At least some of these group II autocatalytic RNAs which are present in organelles of plants, lower eukaryotes, and prokaryotes, do not appear to form additional tertiary interactions with their substrates (52). Thus, group II introns may be particularly adept at recognizing only the intended RNA sequence in the pool of cellular transcripts.

3. The *Trans*-Splicing Reaction of the *Tetrahymena* Ribozyme

In addition to performing a trans-cleavage reaction, the *Tetrahymena* ribozyme can also mediate targeted trans-splicing by employing intermolecular cleavage and ligation reactions (41,53). During trans-splicing, a ribozyme with a 3′ exon attached to its 3′ end recognizes a target RNA (5′ exon) by complementary base pairing as in trans-cleavage (Fig 2B). The ribozyme then cleaves its target RNA as usual at a site immediately 3′ of a conserved G-U base pair formed between a guanosine nucleotide at the 5′ end of the IGS and a uridine nucleotide within the substrate RNA. The sequences downstream of the cleavage site (3′ cleavage product) are then released by the ribozyme. The 3′ end of the 5′ cleavage product is then attached to the 3′ exon, that is originally appended to the ribozyme, to generate the ligated product (Fig 2B).

As with the trans-cleavage reaction, targeted trans-splicing is very malleable. In principle any uridine residue in an RNA molecule can be targeted for trans-splicing by simply making the nucleotides in the ribozyme's IGS complementary to the nucleotides which precede an available uridine residue in a targeted RNA. No specific sequence requirements for the 3′ exon are know to exist for this splicing reaction. Thus essentially any RNA sequence can be employed as a 3′ exon in this reaction and spliced onto a targeted 5′ exon as long as the 3′ exon sequences do not inhibit the ribozyme from folding into a catalytically competent conformation.

B. The RNase P Ribozyme

RNase P, unlike the other four ribozymes discussed in this chapter, is the only catalytic RNA that is naturally a true enzyme. RNase P is found in both prokaryotic and eukaryotic cells, where it catalyzes the removal of the 5′ leader sequences from the variety of precursor tRNAs (3,4). This catalytic RNA is naturally part of a ribonucleoprotein (RNP), and in the case of RNase P isolated from *Escherichia coli* the RNP consists of a 377-nucleotide RNA subunit (M1) and a 119-amino-acid protein (Fig. 1b). Although it was initially thought that the holoenzyme was required to perform catalysis in vitro, M1 RNA preparations from *E. coli* (54) as well as in vitro transcribed versions of M1 RNA (55) are able to cleave tRNA precursors with multiple turnover in the presence of high concentrations of magnesium in the test tube. RNase P cleaves substrate RNA by hydrolysis to generate 5′-phosphate and 3′-hydroxyl termini. While the RNA subunit of RNase P alone is catalytic, the protein cofactor facilitates the RNA-processing reaction and allows it to proceed efficiently under physiologically relevant conditions (55).

When processing its natural pre-tRNA substrate, RNase P removes the 5′ leader sequences from the end of the precursor transcript. Cleavage occurs specifically and accurately just 5′ of the first nucleotide in the mature tRNA, even though only a small degree of sequence conservation exists between different pre-tRNA species. This observation suggested that some facet of the three-dimensional structure of the precursor tRNAs is the feature of the transcript recognized by RNase P. Mutagenesis studies supported this hypothesis because disruption of tRNA folding was shown to decrease the rate of RNase P–mediated cleavage of substrate RNAs. However, the full tertiary structure of tRNA is not required for RNase P recognition and RNA processing (56). Rather, the ribozyme appears to recognize a short RNA duplex similar to the acceptor stem of a tRNA just upstream of an unpaired CCA sequence found on the 3′ end of partially processed tRNA transcripts (56). The structure recognized by RNase P can be approximated by a short RNA fragment, termed the external guide sequence or EGS, that is complementary to a substrate (Fig. 1b). RNase P will cleave single-stranded 5′ leader sequences adjacent to any double-stranded RNA duplex as long as the unpaired CCA nucleotides are present at the 3′ end of the EGS (Fig. 1b) (56). Thus, through the use of EGS oligonucleotides, RNase P can in principle be targeted to cleave any target RNA.

C. The Hammerhead Ribozyme

The hammerhead ribozyme is a catalytic RNA motif originally derived by comparing the self-cleavage domains from a number of naturally occurring viroid and satellite RNAs that replicate in plants (5). The self-cleaving consensus domain consists of a highly conserved catalytic region and three helices and has been shown to have sequence-specific ribonuclease activity (Fig. 1c). Subsequently, a hammerhead domain of less than 60 nucleotides was shown to be sufficient for cleavage (57,58), and two separate oligonucleotides that assembled into a hammerhead structure were shown to mediate a *trans*-cleavage reaction (59,60).

Crystallographic studies of the hammerhead ribozyme have demonstrated that the tertiary structure of the hammerhead appears to be ''Y-shaped'' or like that of a ''wishbone'' (61,62). Helices I and II are in close juxtaposition, while helix III is at the bottom of the molecule. However, all three are A-form helices. As shown in Figure 1c, the minimal structural requirements for hammerhead-catalyzed cleavage include two single-stranded regions that contain nine highly conserved nucleotide sequences, three helices, and the nucleotides GUN immediately 5′ of the cleavage site in the substrate RNA. Results of mutagenesis and kinetic studies suggest that the conserved residues comprise the catalytic core of the ribozyme and are required for cleavage (63,64). Helices I and III, which flank the cleavage site, are formed by base pairing with the substrate. This base-pairing interaction is extremely important not only because it holds the ribozyme and substrate together but because it precisely positions the ribozyme relative to the cleavage site. The most efficient cleavage has been observed with GUC, GUA, or GUU at the cleavage site, although some cleavage also occurs after CUC, UUC, and AUC. The hammerhead catalyzes transesterification of the 3′,5′-phosphodiester bond at the cleavage site, which results in the production of RNA with 2′,3′-cyclic phosphate and 5′-hydroxyl termini.

Much effort has been focused on developing hammerhead ribozymes into useful therapeutic agents. The hammerhead's small size and simple secondary structure, containing helices I and III, which can be made to base pair with virtually any substrate RNA, has allowed a great number of investigators to design hammerhead ribozymes to target any RNA molecule for cleavage and destruction (discussed in detail below). In particular, efforts have been directed at optimizing the interaction between the ribozyme and its substrate since both the length and base composition of complementary helices I and III can affect substrate specificity, ribozyme-substrate affinity, and rate of reaction turnover.

D. The Hairpin Ribozyme

As is the case for the hammerhead ribozyme, the hairpin ribozyme represents a catalytic RNA motif that is derived from RNA associated with a plant pathogens (5). This small catalytic RNA was discovered in the 359-nucleotide-long negative strand satellite RNA of tobacco ringspot virus [(−)sTRSV], which was shown to mediate a self-catalyzed cleavage reaction as part of its replication pathway (57,65).

A minimal catalytic domain for this RNA molecule has been identified (66,67), which consists of a 50-base RNA catalyst that efficiently cleaves an RNA substrate containing 14 bases of satellite RNA sequence (68). Features of secondary structure within this domain, defined from minimum-energy RNA-folding calculations and supported by mutagenesis studies, include four helices, two of which are formed by base pairing between the RNA catalyst and the substrate (Fig. 1d) (69). These two helices form part of the substrate recognition site and flank a four-base loop within the substrate (5′-AGUC-3′) containing the cleavage site. For the wild-type (−)sTRSV, cleavage occurs between the nucleotides, A and G, by transesterification generating a 5′ fragment with 2′,3′-cyclic phosphate termini and a 3′ fragment with a 5′-hydroxyl terminus. *Trans*-cleavage has also been observed in vitro with multiple turnover when substrate RNAs are added to the hairpin ribozyme as separate transcripts (68,69).

The hairpin catalytic RNA motif can be designed to target a great variety of RNA molecules for cleavage since only two sequence requirements exist for this reaction. First, to maintain catalytic activity complementary base pairing between the ribozyme and substrate must occur. Single base pair mismatches at the 10 positions included in the two flanking helices can result in the loss of catalytic activity (69), although single base pair mismatches distal to the cleavage site appear to be tolerated (70). In addition, it has been noted that the composition of base-paired substitutions in these helices can have a wide range of affects on the kinetic properties of the ribozyme (69), suggesting that base pair substitutions should be optimized for each application. The second sequence requirement for the hairpin cleavage reaction involves the nucleotides that compose the target site. Optimal substrate cleavage occurs with the nucleotides GUC immediately 3′ of the cleavage site. The guanosine residue appears to be essential and is believed to be directly involved in catalysis (71). Moreover, catalytic activity has been shown to vary widely when nucleotide substitutions are made at the other 3 positions (71).

E. The Hepatitis Delta Virus Ribozyme

Hepatitis delta virus (HDV) is a 1700-nucleotide, covalently closed circular RNA that is associated with hepatitis B virus infection in certain patients. This animal RNA virus undergoes autocatalytic self-cleavage as part of its replication cycle (5). A minimal self-cleaving RNA motif has been determined for the HDV catalytic RNA (72,73), which includes approximately 85 nucleotides from both the genomic (74) and antigenomic RNAs (75). Features of secondary structure were proposed based on nuclease probing and/or site-directed mutagenesis and were found to be similar for both the genomic and antigenomic self-cleaving sequence elements (75). More recently, x-ray crystal structure studies have been employed to determine the three-dimensional structure of the genomic HDV ribozyme (76). Such analysis demonstrates that the ribozyme forms four stems, two of which (stems I and II) generate a tertiary interaction called a pseudoknot (Fig. 1e) (75,76). Stems II, III, and IV appear to be important for stabilizing the catalytic form of the ribozyme, while formation of stem I is required for efficient cleavage (75).

The self-cleavage reaction mediated by the HDV ribozyme occurs by transesterification and is dependent on divalent cations. Cleavage products have 5′-hydroxyl and 2′,3′-cyclic phosphate termini. The rate of HDV self-cleavage in vitro using either in vitro transcribed HDV RNA or HDV RNA isolated from infected tissue appears to be very slow. However, addition of urea or formamide has been shown to increase the rate of cleavage as much as 50-fold, suggesting that these denaturants may be mimicking a viral or cellular RNA binding or unwinding factor, which facilitates cleavage in vivo (77). A derivative of the catalytic RNA motif from HDV has been engineered to catalyze cleavage reactions in *trans* with multiple turnover (78,79). Target site recognition is dependent on the formation of seven to eight base pairs formed between the target RNA and the HDV ribozyme 3′ of the cleavage site (79).

III. THERAPEUTIC APPLICATIONS OF *TRANS*-CLEAVING AND *TRANS*-SPLICING RIBOZYMES

Ribozymes have the potential to become useful therapeutic agents, and currently they are being developed for a wide variety of clinical applications. The vast majority of effort has been expended in the development of *trans*-cleaving hammerhead and hairpin ribozymes as inhibitors of viral gene expression. In particular, these ribozymes have been targeted to cleave and destroy HIV-1 RNAs to inhibit viral replication in infected cells. The effectiveness of ribozymes as inhibitors of cellular gene expression in both prokaryotes and eukaryotes has been examined, and in a number of studies hammerhead ribozymes have been used to reveal particular gene functions. *Trans*-cleaving ribozymes are also being developed to target transcripts encoding oncogenes such as the *bcr*/*abl* and c-Ha-*ras*. As mentioned earlier, new ribozyme applications are being developed for the group I *trans*-splicing ribozyme from *T. thermophila*, which can be used to repair defective cellular RNAs and to revise viral transcripts to give them antiviral activity. In the following section, we will discuss the therapeutic applications of *trans*-cleaving and *trans*-splicing ribozymes. Because so much effort has been devoted to developing trans-cleaving ribozymes that target HIV-1 RNA, a more a detailed summary of the work performed in this area will be presented.

A. Inhibition of Gene Expression by *Trans*-Cleaving Ribozymes

1. Inhibition of HIV Replications by Ribozymes

Several different approaches have been described that employ RNA molecules to render cells resistant to HIV replication, including the use of antisense RNA and RNA decoys (80). Although these and other approaches have been reported to be effective in suppressing HIV replication in infected cells, ribozymes have two theoretical advantages compared with other RNA-based HIV-inhibition strategies: (1) cleavage of viral transcripts results in the direct, irreversible inactivation of the target RNA, and (2) fewer ribozymes may be required to inhibit a given target gene effectively because a single ribozyme can catalyze multiple cleavage reactions and thus destroy multiple viral transcripts. However, like many other antivirals, ribozymes may also be sensitive to HIV sequence heterogeneity, and effective inhibition may require the use of a combination of these strategies.

Ribozymes may be able to cleave viral target RNAs at a number of stages in the viral life cycle. Potential RNA targets include incoming genomic RNAs, early viral mRNAs, late viral mRNAs, and full-length genomic RNAs that are being encapsidated into virion (Fig. 3). Although cleavage of incoming RNAs would prevent viral integration and therefore be highly effective in protecting cells, the fact that HIV genomic RNAs are encapsidated within a viral core may make these transcripts difficult to access by ribozymes. Moreover, the viral polymerase may initiate reverse transcription before the ribozyme can base pair with and cleave the target sequence setting up a race between the ribozyme and the reverse transcriptase machinery. Nevertheless, several reports suggest that ribozymes may be able to inhibit the initial step of the viral life cycle by cleaving incoming HIV genomic RNAs. However, in most these HIV-inhibition studies, cleavage of incoming genomic RNAs has been assessed only semi-quantitatively. Differences in the amount of proviral DNA (81) or gag mRNA (82) in ribozyme-expressing cells and controls cells has been only analyzed by PCR amplification reactions, which were not internally controlled. Unfortunately, no

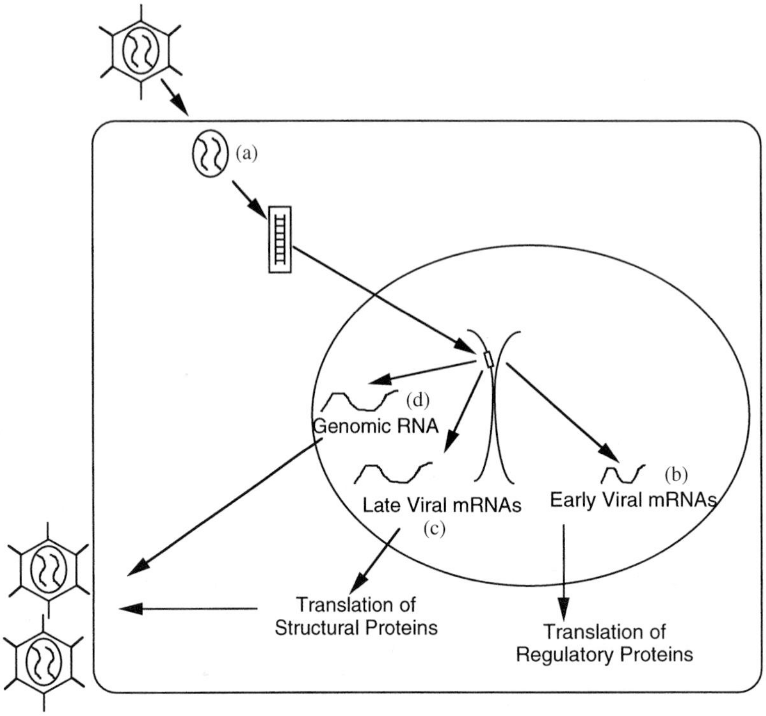

Figure 3 HIV RNAs in the context of the viral life cycle. *Trans*-cleaving ribozymes can potentially inhibit HIV replication by cleaving and destroying viral RNA at a number of steps in the HIV life cycle. (a) Viral genomic RNAs can be targeted prior to reverse transcription into dsDNA and proviral integration. (b) During early gene expression, messenger RNAs encoding regulatory proteins are made. (c) During late gene expression, mRNAs encoding structural proteins are produced. (d) Full-length genomic RNAs are expressed for packaging into viral particles budding from the cell surface.

system has been developed to date that allows for the direct detection of cleavage products of incoming HIV genomic RNAs in mammalian cells.

Early viral transcripts may prove to be the most attractive targets for conferring resistance to HIV-1 (Fig. 3). Viral RNAs expressed at this stage of the HIV-1 life cycle, such as those encoding tat, rev, and nef proteins, are not very abundant. Thus, fewer catalytic RNAs may be required to be protective. Cleavage of early transcripts that inhibit the expression of regulatory proteins such as rev should also result in the inhibition of late gene expression.

Ribozyme-mediated cleavage of late viral transcripts may not be effective in inhibiting HIV replication. Although these RNAs may be accessible for ribozyme cleavage, their shear abundance would probably require that extremely high levels of ribozyme be expressed to reduce their levels in infected cells. In addition, the detrimental affects mediated by early viral regulatory proteins would not be inhibited even if late viral gene function was eliminated. An alternative strategy may be to target highly conserved sequences in the long terminal repeats present in all viral RNAs. This approach could result in the inhibition of both early and late gene expression.

As mentioned above, much work has been performed to develop ribozymes for HIV gene therapy strategies. Hammerhead and hairpin ribozymes are particularly well suited for this purpose because of their small size, their simple secondary structure, and the ease with which they can be manipulated to target specific HIV substrate RNAs for cleavage. In the first application of this approach to inhibit HIV replication, an anti-*gag* hammerhead ribozyme was generated that specifically cleaved gag-encoding RNAs in vitro and inhibited HIV-1 replication in a human T-cell line (82). Subsequently, such *trans*-cleaving ribozymes have been designed to target a variety of highly conserved sequences throughout the HIV-1 genome and have been shown to inhibit HIV replication to varying degrees in a number of tissue culture studies (for extensive review, see Refs. 83 and 84). Moreover, certain *trans*-cleaving ribozymes have been shown to be able to inhibit the replication of diverse viral strains as well as clinical isolates in primary T-cell cultures (81,83–85). Comparisons between catalytically active and inactive forms of these anti-HIV ribozymes have demonstrated that maximal inhibition of virus replication is usually associated with catalytic activity and not simply due to the antisense property of these anti-HIV ribozymes (86–88).

To assess the activity of ribozymes in more clinically relevant settings, human peripheral blood lymphocytes have been stably transduced with a hairpin ribozyme targeting U5 region of the HIV-1 genome. These cells were shown to resist challenge by both HIV-1 molecular clones and clinical isolates (89). More recently, macrophage-like cells that differentiated from hematopoietic stem/progenitor cells from fetal cord blood and were stably transduced with a hairpin ribozyme targeted at the 5′ leader sequence resisted infection by a macrophage-tropic virus (90). Transduction of pluripotent hematopoietic stem cells with HIV-resistance genes may represent an avenue to continually generate cells that are resistant to HIV infection (see Chapter 19). Such stem cells differentiate into monocytes and macrophages, the major targets of HIV-1 infection.

The generation of sequence variants during HIV-1 replication has posed a major problem for immunization strategies and anti-HIV-1 drug therapies designed to suppress viral replication in infected patients. Frequent substitution of amino acids within the variable domains of the HIV-1 *env* gene has resulted in the emergence of neutralization escape mutants both in cell culture and in vivo. Similarly, the rapid emergence of resistant viral strains has limited the effectiveness of both nucleoside and nonnucleoside analog reverse transcriptase inhibitors. Selection for variants resistant to anti-HIV-1 ribozymes is also likely to occur since a single point mutation at the cleavage site on the substrate RNA could inhibit ribozyme-mediated cleavage of viral transcripts. Unlike small molecule drugs, which require substitutions at the protein level, even a silent point mutation can generate a ribozyme-resistant strain. The affect of single point mutations at the cleavage site of hairpin (5′N∧GHY3′, where H = U, C, or A; and Y = C or U) and hammerhead (5′NUX∧3′, where X = C, U, or A) ribozymes has not been studied, but the more stringent sequence requirement at the cleavage site of the hairpin ribozyme could enhance its sensitivity to mutations. Approaches that have been suggested to overcome sequence heterogeneity among HIV isolates include the development of multitargeted ribozymes that cleave a given RNA at multiple sites and target either single or multiple ribozymes to highly conserved sequences within the HIV genome.

In summary, several studies have suggested that ribozymes can inhibit HIV replication in cell culture experiments when cells are challenged with very low innocula of HIV. It remains to be tested if this first generation of ribozymes can also inhibit virus replication in HIV-infected patients under conditions of active viremia and where a multitude of quasi-species of the virus preexist. Ultimately, this question will be answered as ribozymes begin to be evaluated in clinical trials in HIV-infected individuals (91,92).

2. *Trans*-Cleavage of mRNAs Encoding Dominant Oncogenes

Neoplastic transformation is often associated with the expression of mutant oncogenes. Because ribozymes can be designed to inhibit the expression of specific gene products, their potential as antineoplastic agents is currently being evaluated. For example, hammerhead ribozymes have been reported to be able to suppress the tumorigenic properties of cells harboring an activated human *ras* gene (93–95). More recently, the *bcr/abl* fusion transcript has been the target of many ribozyme studies (96–99). This abnormal mRNA is transcribed from the Philadelphia chromosome, which is present in 95% of patients with chronic myelogenous leukemia (CML) and in many patients with acute lymphocytic leukemia (ALL). In vitro experiments have shown that the 8500-nucleotide-long *bcr/abl* transcript was efficiently cleaved by an anti-*bcr/abl* ribozyme. In CML blast crisis cell lines, expression of ribozymes targeted at *bcr/abl* mRNA was reported to be able to reduce the production of p210*bcr/abl* and *bcr/abl* transcripts and reduce cell proliferation.

B. RNA Revision by *Trans*-Splicing Ribozymes

Recently, it has been argued that ribozymes may also be able to alter the sequence of targeted RNAs, not just destroy them, and that such RNA revision may be useful for treating a variety of diseases via gene therapy (12). As described earlier, the *Tetrahymena* group I ribozyme can catalyze a *trans*-splicing reaction (20,53). Such targeted *trans*-splicing can potentially be used to repair mutant transcripts and to alter viral RNAs to give them antiviral activity.

In the targeted *trans*-splicing reaction, the *Tetrahymena* ribozyme recognizes and binds to its substrate RNA (the 5′ exon) by base pairing between the IGS and a sequence in the substrate. Following cleavage, the ribozyme splices its 3′ exon onto the cleaved substrate RNA (Fig. 2c). Since the ribozyme cleaves after the sequence N_5U, the only sequence requirement for the substrate is to have a uridine residue preceding the cleavage site. Thus, any uridine nucleotide in an RNA molecule can in principle serve as a target for the ribozyme if the target sequence is accessible for ribozyme binding. Moreover, because there are no sequence requirements for the 3′ exon in the *trans*-splicing reaction (2), almost any sequence can be spliced onto the 5′ target transcript.

The lack of sequence requirements for the 3′ exon suggests that it could be manipulated so that *trans*-splicing can be employed to replace a defective portion of an RNA transcript with a functional sequence (Fig. 4). *Trans*-splicing ribozymes could be designed that would cleave defective transcripts upstream of point mutations or small insertions or deletions. A 3′ exon consisting of the wild-type sequence could then be spliced onto the cleaved target, resulting in a corrected mRNA. *Trans*-splicing ribozymes can be employed to repair defective RNA messages. In the first example of this application, the group I ribozyme from *T. thermophila* was reengineered to repair truncated *lacZ* transcripts via targeted *trans*-splicing in *E. coli* (100) and in mammalian cells (101). In both settings, the ribozyme was shown to be able to splice restorative sequences onto mutant *lacZ* target RNAs with high fidelity and thus maintain the open reading frame for translation of the repaired transcripts. In a subsequent study, the efficiency of RNA repair was monitored and the ribozyme was shown to be able to revise up to 50% of the truncated *lacZ* transcripts when ribozyme and *lacZ* substrate–encoding plasmids were cotransfected into mammalian fibroblasts (102).

More recently, two groups have demonstrated that group I ribozymes can be employed to amend faulty transcripts that are associated with common genetic diseases. Phylactou et al. demonstrated that a *trans*-splicing ribo-

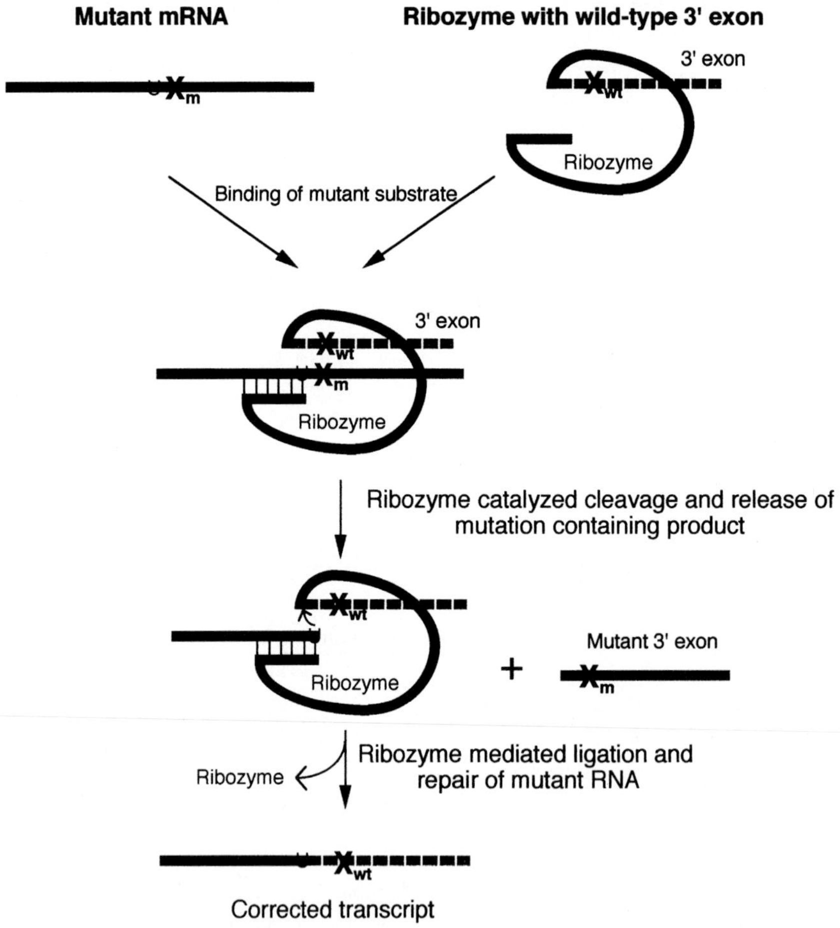

Figure 4 Ribozyme-mediated repair of mutant transcripts. A *trans*-splicing ribozyme binds to a mutant RNA transcript that contains a point mutation, deletion, or insertion. The IGS on the ribozyme recognizes a uridine residue 5′ of the mutation (indicated by X_m). The ribozyme cleaves the mutant RNA and releases the downstream, mutation-containing cleavage product. Next, the ribozyme ligates the wild-type sequence (X_{wt} and dashed line) of the target RNA onto the upstream cleavage product to yield a repaired transcript.

zyme could be employed to amend transcripts associated with myotonic dystrophy (103), while Lan et al. employed this RNA repair approach to correct mRNAs associated with sickle cell disease (104). In the myotonic dystrophy case, a *trans*-splicing ribozyme was employed to shorten the trinucleotide repeat expansion found in the 3′ untranslated region of the human myotonic dystrophy protein kinase transcript in cell culture studies (103). In the sickle cell experiments, *trans*-splicing was employed to convert sickle-β-globin transcripts into γ-globin encoding mRNAs in erythrocyte precursors isolated from patients with sickle cell disease (104). In both studies, sequence analysis of the amended RNAs demonstrated that the ribozyme had accomplished such repair with high fidelity forming the proper splice junctions between the targeted transcript and the corrective sequences.

These results demonstrate that a *trans*-splicing group I ribozyme can be employed to repair pathogenic transcripts in clinically relevant, cellular settings. However, as with the development of almost every novel therapeutic approach, several technical issues must be addressed before ribozyme-mediated repair of mutant RNAs can become useful in the clinic. First, it remains to be determined if repair of any pathogenic transcript can proceed efficiently enough in primary human cells to be therapeutically beneficial. In the case of sickle cell disease, conversion of as little as 5–10% of the sickle β-globin transcripts into mRNAs encoding γ-globin is expected to greatly reduce cell sickling and thus the severity of the disease. Whether this relatively modest level of repair can be achieved in erythrocyte precursors from individuals with sickle cell disease is unclear, but results demonstrating that 50% of the mutant *lacZ* transcripts expressed in mammalian cells can be revised by ribozymes (102) are at least encouraging in this regard. Second, the specificity of *trans*-splicing may have to be increased because in mammalian cell experiments the *Tetrahymena* group I ribozyme was shown to react not only with intended *lacZ* target RNAs but also with other cellular transcripts (101). Such limited reaction specificity is fully anticipated from knowledge about the energetics of substrate binding by this ribozyme. This biochemical knowledge is now being utilized to redesign the ribozyme to enhance its specificity (51).

In summary, the ability to employ *trans*-splicing ribozymes to revise genetic instructions embedded in targeted RNAs represents a broad new approach to genetic therapy. Because defective RNAs can only be repaired in the cells in which they are present and only when they are expressed, RNA repair may become an effective means of recapitulating the natural expression pattern of therapeutic genes. Moreover, RNA repair may be especially useful in the treatment of genetic disorders associated with the expression of dominant or deleterious mutant RNAs and proteins. In these cases, RNA repair should simultaneously engender wild-type protein production and eliminate production of the deleterious gene product. For these reasons, the concept of RNA repair is likely to continue to attract increased interest from gene therapists.

IV. CONCLUSION

Trans-cleaving and *trans*-splicing ribozymes, either alone or in combination with other therapeutic agents, have the potential to restore genetic information or to eliminate it. The information presented in this chapter describes how ribozymes can be employed to mediate repair of defective transcripts or the destruction of pathogenic RNAs. Although the results from the first generation of therapeutic ribozyme experiments are in general quite encouraging, the long-term utility of catalytic RNAs is still unclear. Many factors may limit the efficacy of ribozymes in the clinic. Thus, it will be essential to evaluate RNA catalysis in clinically relevant settings and to use the knowledge gained from such experiments to aid in the design of therapeutic ribozymes. Once adequately developed, catalytic RNAs should become new and useful weapons in the wars being waged on a great number of devastating diseases.

REFERENCES

1. Kruger K, Grabowski PJ, Zaug AJ, Sands J, Gottschling DE, Cech TR. Self-splicing RNA: autoexcision and autocyclization of the ribosomal RNA intervening sequence of *Tetrahymena*. Cell 1982; 31:147–157.
2. Cech TR. Self-splicing of group I introns. Annu Rev Biochem 1990; 59:543–568.
3. Cech TR. Structure and mechanism of the large catalytic RNAs: group I and group II introns and ribonuclease P. In: Gesteland RF, Atkins JF, eds. The RNA World. Cold Spring Harbor, NY: Cold Spring Harbor Press, 1993: 239–269.
4. Altman S. Ribonuclease P: an enzyme with a catalytic RNA subunit. Advances Enzymol Related Areas Mol Biol 1989; 62:1–36.
5. Symons RH. Small catalytic RNAs. Annu Rev Biochem 1992; 61:641–671.
6. Cech TR. Ribozyme engineering. Curr Opin Struct Biol 1992; 2:605–609.
7. Rossi JJ, Sarver N. Catalytic antisense RNA (ribozymes): their potential and use as anti-HIV-a therapeutic agents. Advances Exp Med Biol 1992; 312:95–109.
8. Poeschla E, Wong-Staal F. Antiviral and anticancer ribozymes. Curr Opin Oncol 1994; 6:601–606.
9. Zaia JA, Chatterjee S, Wong KK, Elkins D, Taylor NR, Rossi JJ. Status of ribozyme and antisense-based develop-

mental approaches for anti-HIV therapy. Ann NY Acad Sci 1992; 660:95–106.
10. Thompson JD, Macejak D, Couture L, Stinchcomb DT. Ribozymes in gene therapy. Nat Med 1995; 1:277–278.
11. Rossi JJ. Ribozymes, genomics and therapeutics. Chem Biol 1999; 5:33–37.
12. Sullenger BA. Revising messages traveling along the cellular information superhighway. Chem Biol. 1995; 2: 249–253.
13. Rossi JJ. Ribozymes to the rescue: repairing genetically defective mRNAs. Trends Genet 1998; 14:295–298.
14. Sullenger BA. RNA repair as a novel approach to genetic therapy. Gene Ther 1999; 6:461–462.
15. Cech TR, Zaug AJ, Grabowski PJ. In vitro splicing of the ribosomal RNA precursor of *Tetrahymena:* involvement of a guanosine nucleotide in the excision of the intervening sequence. Cell 1981; 27:487–496.
16. Michel F, Jacquier A, Dujon B. Comparison of fungal mitochondrial introns reveals extensive homologies in RNA secondary structure. Biochemie 1982; 64:867–881.
17. Davies RW, Waring RB, Ray JA, Brown TA, Scazzocchio C. Making ends meet: a model for RNA splicing in fungal mitochondria. Nature 1982; 300:719–724.
18. Weiss-Brummer B, Holl J, Schweyen RJ, Rodel G, Kaudewitz F. Processing of yeast mitochondrial RNA: involvement of intramolecular hybrids in splicing of cob intron 4 RNA by mutation and reversion. Cell 1983; 33:195–202.
19. Perea J, Jacq C. Role of the 5′ hairpin structure in the splicing accuracy of the fourth intron of the yeast cob-box gene. EMBO J 1986; 4:3281–3288.
20. Been MD, Cech TR. One binding site determines sequence specificity of *Tetrahymena* pre-rRNA self-splicing, trans-splicing, and RNA enzyme activity. Cell 1986; 47: 207–216.
21. Waring RB, Towner P, Minter SJ, Davies RW. Splice-site selection by a self-splicing RNA of *Tetrahymena.* Nature 1986; 321:133–139.
22. Burke JM, Irvine KD, Kaneko KJ, Kerker BJ, Oettgen AB. Role of conserved sequence elements 9L and 2 in self-splicing of the *Tetrahymena* ribosomal RNA precursor. Cell 1986; 45:167–176.
23. Williamson CL, Desai NM, Burke, JM. Compensatory mutations demonstrate that P8 and P6 are RNA secondary structure elements important for processing of a group I intron. Nucleic Acids Res 1989; 17:675–689.
24. Williamson CL, Tierney WM, Kerker BJ, Burke JM. Site-directed mutagenesis of core sequence elements 9R′, 9L, 9R and 2 in self-splicing *Tetrahymena* pre-rRNA. J Biol Chem 1987; 262:14672–14682.
25. Flor PJ, Flanegan JB, Cech TR. A conserved base pair within helix P4 of the Tetrahymena ribozyme helps to form the tertiary structure required for self-splicing. EMBO J 1989; 8:3391–3399.
26. Ehrenman K, Schroeder R, Chandry PS, Hall DH, Belfort M. Sequence specificity of the P6 pairing for splicing of the group I td intron of phage T4. Nucleic Acids Res 1989; 17:9147–9163.
27. Latham JA, Cech, TR. Defining the inside and outside of a catalytic RNA molecule. Science 1989; 245:276–282.
28. Celander DW, Cech TR. Visualizing the higher order folding of a catalytic RNA molecule. Science 1991; 251: 401–407.
29. Murphy FL, Cech TR. An independently folding domain of RNA tertiary structure within the *Tetrahymena* ribozyme. Biochemistry 1993; 32:5291–5300.
30. Wang Y-H, Murphy FL, Cech TR, Griffith JD. Visualization of a tertiary structural domain of the *Tetrahymena* group I intron by electron microscopy. J Mol Biol 1994; 236:64–71.
31. Laggerbauer B, Murphy FL, Cech TR. Two major tertiary folding transitions of the *Tetrahymena* catalytic RNA. EMBO J 1994; 13:2669–2676.
32. Cate JH, Gooding AR, Podell E, Zhou K, Golden BL, Kundrot C, Cech TR, Doudna JA. Crystal structure of a group I ribozyme domain: principles of RNA packing. Science 1996; 273:1678–1685.
33. Cate JH, Gooding AR, Podell E, Zhou K, Golden BL, Szewczak AA, Kundrot CE, Cech TR, Doudna JA. RNA tertiary structure mediation by adenosine platforms. Science 1996; 273:1696–1699.
34. Golden BL, Gooding AR, Podell ER, Cech TR. A preorganized active site in the crystal structure of the *Tetrahymena* ribozyme. Science 1998; 282:259–264.
35. Wang J-F, Downs WD, Cech TR. Movement of the guide sequence during RNA catalysis by a group I ribozyme. Science 1993; 260:504–508.
36. Downs WD, Cech TR. A tertiary interaction in the *Tetrahymena* intron contributes to selection of the 5′ slice site. Genes Dev 1994; 8:1198–1211.
37. Zaug AJ, Grabowski PJ, Cech TR. Autocatalytic cyclization of an excised intervening sequence RNA is a cleavage-ligation reaction. Nature 1983; 301:578–583.
38. Zaug AJ, Cech TR. The intervening sequence RNA of *Tetrahymena* is an enzyme. Science 1986; 231:470–475.
39. Cech TR, Herschlag D, Piccirilli JA, Pyle AM. RNA catalysis by a group I ribozyme: developing a model for transition state stabilization. J Biol Chem 1992; 267: 17479–17482.
40. Zaug AJ, Been MD, Cech TR. The *Tetrahymena* ribozyme acts like an RNA restriction endonuclease. Nature 1986; 324:429–433.
41. Been MD, Cech TR. One binding site determines sequence specificity of *Tetrahymena* pre-rRNA self-splicing, trans-splicing, and RNA enzyme activity. Cell 1986; 46: 207–216.
42. Murphy FL, Cech TR. Alteration of substrate specificity for the endoribonucleolytic cleavage of RNA by the *Tetrahymena* ribozyme. Proc Natl Acad Sci USA 1989; 86: 9218–9222.
43. Pyle AM, McSwiggen JA, Cech TR. Direct measurement of oligonucleotide substrate binding to wild-type and mutant ribozymes from *Tetrahymena.* Proc Natl Acad Sci USA 1990; 87:8187–8191.

44. Herschlag D, Cech TR. Catalysis of RNA cleavage by the *Tetrahymena* thermophila ribozyme. 1. Kinetic description of the reaction of an RNA substrate complementary to the active site. Biochemistry 1990; 29:10159–10171.
45. Herschlag D, Cech TR. Catalysis of RNA cleavage by the *Tetrahymena* thermophila ribozyme. 2. Kinetic description of the reaction of an RNA substrate that forms a mismatch at the active site. Biochemistry 1990; 29:10172–10180.
46. Pyle AM, Murphy FL, Cech TR. RNA substrate binding site in the catalytic core of the *Tetrahymena* ribozyme. Nature 1992; 358:123–128.
47. Bevilacqua PC, Kierzek R, Johnson KA, Turner DH. Dynamics of ribozyme binding of substrate revealed by fluorescence-detected stopped-flow methods. Science 1992; 258:1355–1358.
48. Strobel SA, Cech TR. Tertiary interactions with the internal guide sequence mediate docking of the P1 helix into the catalytic core of the *Tetrahymena* ribozyme. Biochemistry 1993; 32:13593–13604.
49. Knitt DS, Narlikar GJ, Herschlag D. Dissection of the role of the conserved G-U pair in group I RNA self-splicing. Biochemistry 1994; 33:13864–13879.
50. Herschlag D. Implications of ribozyme kinetics for targeting the cleavage of specific RNA molecules in vivo: more isn't always better. Proc Natl Acad Sci USA 1991; 88: 6921–6925.
51. Zarrinkar PP, Sullenger BA. Optimizing the substrate specificity of a group I intron ribozyme. Biochemistry 1999; 38:3426–3432.
52. Griffin EA Jr, Qin Z, Michels WJ Jr, Pyle AM. Group II intron ribozymes that cleave DNA and RNA linkages with similar efficiency, and lack contacts with substrate 2′-hydroxyl groups. Chem Biol 1995; 2:761–770.
53. Inoue T, Sullivan FX, Cech TR. Intermolecular exon ligation of the rRNA precursor of *Tetrahymena:* oligonucleotides can function as 5′ exons. Cell 1985; 43:431–437.
54. Guerrier-Takada C, Gardiner K, Marsh T, Pace N, Altman S. The RNA moiety of ribonuclease P is the catalytic subunit of the enzyme. Cell 1983; 35:849–857.
55. Guerrier-Takada C, Altman S. Catalytic activity of an RNA molecule prepared by transcription in vitro. Science 1984; 223:285–286.
56. Forester AC, Altman S. External guide sequences for an RNA enzyme. Science 1990; 249:783–786.
57. Buzayan JM, Gerlach WL, Bruening G. Non-enzymatic cleavage and ligation of RNA complementary to a plant virus satellite RNA. Nature 1986; 323:349–353.
58. Forster AC, Symons RH. Self-cleavage of virusoid RNA is performed by the proposed 55-nucleotide active site. Cell 1987; 50:10–16.
59. Uhlenbeck OC. A small catalytic oligoribonucleotide. Nature 1987; 328:596–600.
60. Hasseloff J, Gerlach WL. Simple RNA enzymes with new and highly specific endoribonuclease activities. Nature 1988; 334:585–591.
61. Pley HW, Flaherty KM, McKay DB. Three-dimensional structure of a hammerhead ribozyme. Nature 1994; 372: 68–74.
62. Scott WG, Finch JT, Klug A. The crystal structure of an all-RNA hammerhead ribozyme: a proposed mechanism for RNA catalytic cleavage. Cell 1995; 81:991–1002.
63. Ruffner DE, Stormo GD, Uhlenbeck OC. Sequence requirements of the hammerhead RNA self-cleavage reaction. Biochemistry 1990; 29:10695–10702.
64. Fedor MJ, Uhlenbeck OC. Substrate sequence effects on hammerhead RNA catalytic efficiency. Proc Natl Acad Sci USA 1990; 87:1668–1672.
65. Gerlach WL, Buzayan JM, Schneider IR, Bruening G. Satellite tobacco ringspot virus RNA: biological activity of DNA clones and their in vitro transcripts. Virology 1986; 151:172–185.
66. Haseloff J, Gerlach WL. Sequences required for self-catalyzed cleavage of the satellite RNA of tobacco ringspot virus. Gene 1989; 82:43–52.
67. Feldstein PA, Buzayan JM, Bruening G. Two sequences participating in the autolytic processing of satellite tobacco ringspot virus complementary RNA. Gene 1989; 83: 53–61.
68. Hampel A, Tritz R. RNA catalytic properties of the minimum (−)sTRSV sequence. Biochemistry 1989; 28: 4929–4933.
69. Hampel A, Tritz R, Hicks M, Cruz P. ''Hairpin'' catalytic RNA model: evidence for helices and sequence requirements for substrate RNA. Nucleic Acids Res 1990; 18: 299–304.
70. Joseph S, Berzal-Herranz A, Chowrira BM, Butcher SE. Substrate selection rules for the hairpin ribozyme determined by in vitro selection, maturation and analysis of mismatched substrates. Genes Dev. 1993; 7:130–138.
71. Chowrira BM, Berzal-Herranz A, Burke JM. Novel guanosine requirement for catalysis by the hairpin ribozyme. Nature 1991; 354:320–322.
72. Kuo MY, Sharmeen L, Dinter-Gottlieb G, Taylor J. Characterization of self-cleaving RNA sequences on the genome and antigenome of human hepatitis delta virus. J Virol 1988; 62:4439–4444.
73. Wu HN, Lin YJ, Lin FP, Makino S, Chang MF, Lai MM. Human hepatitis delta virus RNA subfragments contain an autocleavage activity. Proc Natl Acad Sci USA 1989; 86: 1831–1835.
74. Perrotta AT, Been MD. The self-cleaving domain from the genomic RNA of hepatitis delta virus: sequence requirements and the effects of denaturant. Nucleic Acids Res 1990; 18:6821–6827.
75. Perrotta AT, Been MD. A pseudoknot-like structure required for efficient self-cleavage of hepatitis delta virus RNA. Nature 1991; 350:434–436.
76. Ferre-D'Amare AR, Zhou K, Dounda JA. Crystal structure of a hepatitis delta virus ribozyme. Nature 1998; 395: 567–574.
77. Rosenstein SP, Been MD. Self-cleavage of hepatitis delta virus genomic strand RNA is enhanced under partially denaturing conditions. Biochemistry 1990; 29:8011–8016.
78. Branch AD, Robertson HD. Efficient trans cleavage and a common structural motif for the ribozymes of the human

hepatitis δ agent. Proc Natl Acad Sci USA 1991; 88: 10163–10167.
79. Perotta AT, Been MD. Cleavage of oligoribonucleotides by a ribozyme derived from the hepatitis δ virus RNA sequence. Biochemistry 1992; 31:16–21.
80. Sullenger BA, Gallardo HF, Ungers GE, Gilboa E. Overexpression of TAR sequences renders cells resistant to human immunodeficiency virus replication. Cell 1990; 63: 601–608.
81. Yamada O, Yu M, Yee J-K, Kraus G, Looney D, Wong-Staal F. Intracellular immunization of human T cells with a hairpin ribozyme against human immunodeficiency virus type 1. Gene Ther 1994; 1:38–44.
82. Sarver N, Cantin EM, Chang PS, Zaia JA, Ladne PA, Stephens DA, Rossi JJ. Ribozymes as potential anti-HIV agents. Science 1990; 247:1222–1225.
83. Yu M, Poeschla E, Wong-Staal F. Progress towards gene therapy for HIV infection. Gene Ther 1994; 1:13–26.
84. Rossi JJ. Controlled, targeted, intracellular expression of ribozymes; progress and problems. TIBTECH 1995; 13: 301–306.
85. Yu M, Ojwang J, Yamada O, Hampel A, Rapapport J, Looney D, Wong-Staal F. A hairpin ribozyme inhibits expression of diverse strains of human immunodeficiency virus type 1. Proc Natl Acad Sci USA 1993; 90: 6340–6344.
86. Homman M, Tzortzakaki S, Rittner K, Sczakiel G, Tabler M. Incorporation of the catalytic domain of a hammerhead ribozyme into antisense RNA enhances its inhibitory effect on the replication of human immunodeficiency virus type 1. Nucleic Acids Res 1993; 21:2809–2814.
87. Yamada O, Kraus G, Leavitt MC, Yu M, Wong-Staal F. Activity and cleavage site specificity of an anti-HIV-1 hairpin ribozyme in human T cells. Virology 1994; 205: 121–126.
88. Zhou C, Bahner JC, Larson GP, Zaia JA, Rossi JJ, Kohn DB. Inhibition of HIV-1 in human T-lymphocytes by retrovirally transduced anti-tat and rev hammerhead ribozymes. Gene 1994; 149:33–39.
89. Leavitt MC, Yu M, Yamada O, Kraus G, Looney D, Poeschla E, Wong-Staal F. Transfer of an anti-HIV-1 ribozyme gene into primary human lymphocytes. Hum Gene Ther 1994; 5:1115–1120.
90. Yu M, Leavitt MC, Maruyama M, Yamada O, Young D, Ho AD, Wond-Staal F. Intracellular immunization of human fetal cord blood stem/progenitor cells with a ribozyme against human immunodeficiency virus type 1. Proc Natl Acad Sci USA 1995; 92:669–703.
91. Wong-Staal F, Poeschla EM, Looney DJ. A controlled, phase 1 clinical trial to evaluate the safety and effects in HIV-1 infected humans of autologous lymphocytes transduced with a ribozyme that cleaves HIV-1 RNA. Hum Gene Ther 1998; 9:2407–2425.
92. Law P, Lane TA, Gervaix A, Looney D, Schwarz L, Young D, Ramos S, Wong-Staal F, Recktenwald D, Ho AD. Mobilization of peripheral blood progenitor cells for human immunodeficiency virus-infected individuals. Exp Hematol 1999; 27:147–154.
93. Bos JL. *Ras* oncogene in human cancer: a review. Cancer Res 1989; 49:4682–4689.
94. Koizumi M, Kamiya H, Ohtsuka E. Ribozymes designed to inhibit transformation of NIH3T3 cells by the activated c-Ha-*ras* gene. Gene 1992; 117:179–184.
95. Kashani-Sabet M, Funato T, Tone T, Jiao L, Wang W, Yoshida E, Kashfinn BI, Shitara T, Wu AM, Moreno JG, Traweek ST, Ahlering TE, Scanlon KJ. Reversal of the malignant phenotype by an anti-ras ribozyme. Antisense Res Dev 1992; 2:3–15.
96. Wright L, Wilson SB, Milliken S, Biggs J, Kearney P. Ribozyme-mediated cleavage of the bcr/abl transcript expressed in chronic myeloid leukemia. Exp Hematol 1993; 21:1714–1718.
97. Shore SK, Nabissa PM, Reddy EP. Ribozyme-mediated cleavage of the BRCABL oncogene transcript: in vitro cleavage of RNA and in vivo loss of P210 protein kinase activity. Oncogene 1993; 8:3183–3188.
98. Lange W, Cantin EM, Finke J, Dolken G. In vitro and in vivo effects of synthetic ribozymes targeted against BCR/ABL mRNA. Leukemia 1993; 7:1786–1794.
99. Snyder DS, Wu Y, Wang JL, Rossi JJ, Swiderski P, Kaplan BE, Forman SJ. Ribozyme-mediated inhibition of bcr-abl gene expression in a Philadelphia chromosome-positive cell line. Blood 1993; 82:600–605.
100. Sullenger BA, Cech TR. Ribozyme-mediated repair of defective mRNA by targeted trans-splicing. Nature 1994; 371:619–622.
101. Jones JJ, Lee S-W, Sullenger BA. Tagging-ribozyme reaction sites to follow trans-splicing in mammalian cells. Nat Med 1996; 2:643–648.
102. Jones JJ, Sullenger BA. Evaluating and enhancing ribozyme reaction efficiency in mammalian cells. Nat Biotech 1997; 15:902–905.
103. Phylactou LA, Darrah C, Wood MJ. Ribozyme-mediated trans-splicing of a trinucleotide repeat. Nat Genetics 1998; 18:378–381.
104. Lan N, Howery RP, Lee S-W, Smith CA, Sullenger BA. Ribozyme-mediated repair of sickle β-globin mRNAs in erythrocyte precursors. Science 1998; 280:1593–1596.

15

Antisense Oligonucleotide–Based Therapeutics

C. Frank Bennett, Madeline Butler, P. Dan Cook, Richard S. Geary, Arthur A. Levin, Rahul Mehta, Ching-Leou Teng, Hemant Deshmukh, Lloyd Tillman, and Greg Hardee
Isis Pharmaceuticals, Inc., Carlsbad, California

I. INTRODUCTION

Antisense oligonucleotides are short synthetic oligonucleotides, usually between 15 and 25 bases in length, designed to hybridize to RNA through Watson-Crick base pairing (Fig. 1). Upon binding to the target RNA, the oligonucleotide prevents expression of the encoded protein product in a sequence-specific manner. Because the rules for Watson-Crick base pairing are well characterized (1), antisense oligonucleotides represent, in principal, a simple method for rationally designing drugs. In practice, exploitation of antisense oligonucleotides for therapies has presented a unique set of challenges, some anticipated and others unanticipated. Nevertheless, antisense oligonucleotides are showing promise as therapeutic agents broadly applicable for the treatment of human diseases. Currently there is one approved antisense product on the market and 11 agents in clinical trials, several of which are in advance stages of development (Table 1). In this chapter we will summarize the properties of antisense oligonucleotides in terms of their application as therapeutic agents. As expected, there is significantly more information regarding first-generation phosphorothioate oligodeoxynucleotides, which thus serve as a benchmark for comparison with some of the newer modified oligonucleotides.

II. ANTISENSE MECHANISM OF ACTION

Antisense oligonucleotides are small synthetic oligonucleotides designed to bind to mRNA through Watson-Crick hybridization. Upon binding to RNA, the oligonucleotide may inhibit expression of the encoded gene product either through inducing cleavage of the RNA by RNase H or other RNases or by occupancy of critical regulatory sites on the RNA (Fig. 2). Several studies have documented that phosphorothioate oligodeoxynucleotides promote cleavage of the targeted RNA by a mechanism consistent with RNase H cleavage (2–5). RNase H is an ubiquitously expressed enzyme that cleaves the RNA strand of an RNA-DNA heteroduplex (6). If the antisense oligonucleotide utilizes DNA chemistry, it will direct RNase H to specifically cleave the target RNA upon binding. There are other RNase present in cells that may be exploited in a similar manner, such as RNase L (7) or a novel double-stranded RNase (8).

It should be noted that not all oligonucleotides designed to hybridize to a target RNA effectively inhibit target gene expression (9–11). This is thought to be due to the inaccessibility of some regions of the RNA to the oligonucleotide because of secondary or tertiary structure or to protein interactions with the RNA. At this time, there are no good predictive algorithms for predicting antisense oligonucleotide-binding sites on a target RNA. In our experience, we have found active oligonucleotides that work through an RNase H–dependent mechanism can hybridize to any region on the mRNA or pre-mRNA. Thus some serendipity is still involved in the process of identifying and optimizing potent and effective antisense inhibitors.

Early on it was thought that occupancy of the RNA (the receptor for the antisense oligonucleotide) by the oligonucleotide would be sufficient to block translation of the RNA, i.e., translation arrest (12). Subsequent studies have documented that oligonucleotides are not efficient at block-

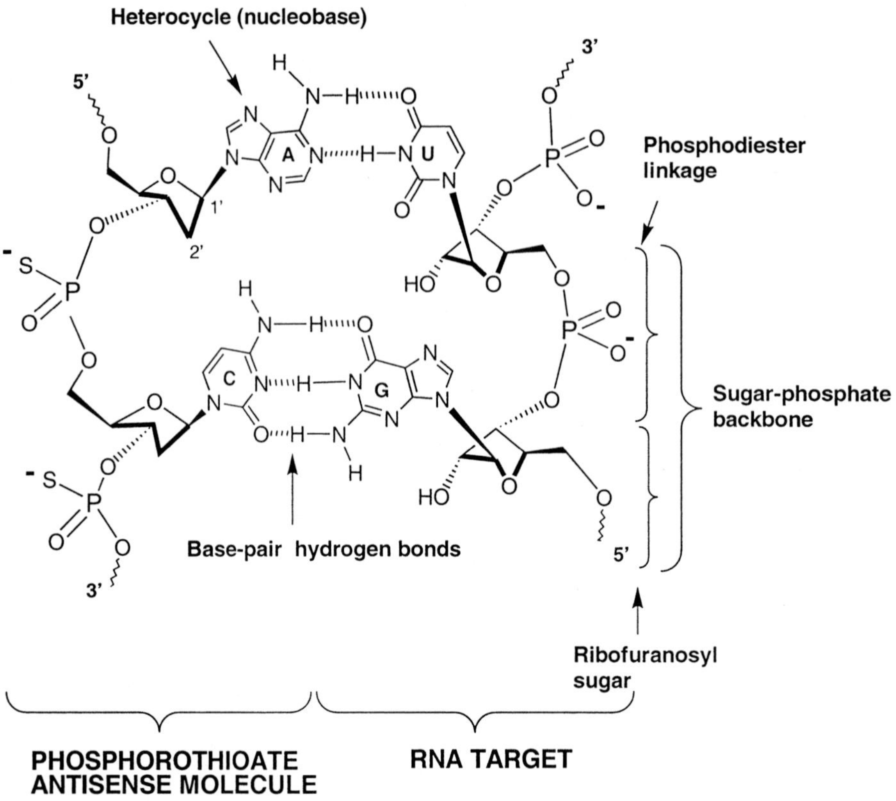

Figure 1 Phosphorothioate antisense oligodeoxynucleotide targeting an RNA receptor. Watson-Crick base-pairing rules are indicated: nucleobase adenosine hydrogen bonds to nucleobase uracil, nucleobase cytosine hydrogen bonds to nucleobase guanine.

ing translation of mRNA if they bind 3′ to the AUG translation initiation codon. Furthermore, we have found that only certain sites in the 5′-untranslated region of a mRNA are effective target sites for an antisense oligonucleotide. In particular the 5′-terminus of a transcript appears to be a good target site for oligonucleotides for some molecular targets in that occupancy of this region prevents assembly of the ribosome on the RNA (13). It should be noted that occupancy of the receptor (RNA) and steric blocking of factor binding by high-affinity oligonucleotides can be an efficient mechanism for blocking gene expression. For the example cited above the steric blocking oligonucleotide was approximately 10-fold more potent than an oligonucleotide that supports RNase H activity. These results suggest that catalytic turnover of the target RNA is not the rate-limiting step for antisense oligonucleotides.

Another process by which noncatalytic oligonucleotides can alter gene expression is through regulating RNA processing. Most mammalian RNAs undergo multiple post-or co-transcriptional processing steps, including addition of a 5′-cap structure, splicing, and polyadenylation. Because antisense oligonucleotides localize to the cell nucleus (14–17), they have the potential of regulating these processes. Several studies have been published documenting that antisense oligonucleotides can be used to regulate RNA splicing (18–22). Oligonucleotides can be used to modulate alternative splicing by promoting use of cryptic splice sites, as exemplified for β-thalassemia (18,19), or by enhancing use of an alternative splice site. Finally, oligonucleotides can regulate RNA function by sterically preventing factors from binding or changing the structure of the RNA such that it is no longer recognized by the factor. Thus there are multiple mechanisms by which oligonucleotides can be utilized to inhibit or modulate expression of a target gene product.

III. ANTISENSE OLIGONUCLEOTIDE CHEMISTRY

The most advanced oligonucleotide chemistry used for antisense drugs involves phosphorothioate oligodeoxynucleotides. Phosphorothioate oligodeoxynucleotides differ

Table 1 Antisense Oligonucleotides Approved or Currently in Clinical Development

Oligonucleotide	Molecular target	Disease indication	Chemistry	Route of administration	Status	Sponsor
Vitravene (fomivirsen, ISIS 2922)	Human cytomegalovirus IE-2 gene	CMV retinitis	Phosphorothioate oligodeoxynucleotide	Intravitreal	Marketed	ISIS Pharmaceuticals/ Ciba Vision
ISIS 2302	ICAM-1	Crohn's disease, renal transplantation	Phosphorothioate oligodeoxynucleotide	Intravenous	Phase II/III	ISIS Pharmaceuticals/ Boehringer Ingelheim
G3139	BCL-2	Cancer	Phosphorothioate oligodeoxynucleotide	Intravenous	Phase II	Genta
Gem-231	Protein kinase A	Cancer	Phosphorothioate 2′-O-methyl/ oligodeoxynucleotide chimera	Intravenous	Phase II	Hybridon
ISIS 3521/CGP 64128A	Protein kinase C-α	Cancer	Phosphorothioate oligodeoxynucleotide	Intravenous	Phase II	Novartis/ISIS Pharmaceuticals
ISIS 5132/CGP 69846A	c-*raf* kinase	Cancer	Phosphorothioate oligodeoxynucleotide	Intravenous	Phase II	Novartis/ISIS Pharmaceuticals
ISIS 2503	ha-*ras*	Cancer	Phosphorothioate oligodeoxynucleotide	Intravenous	Phase II	ISIS Pharmaceuticals
IN-3001	c-myb	Cancer	Phosphorothioate oligodeoxynucleotide (liposome formulation)	Intravenous	Phase I	Inex Pharmaceuticals
GPI-2A	HIV *gag* gene	HIV	Phosphorothioate oligodeoxynucleotide	Intravenous	Phase I	Novopharm Biotech
GEM-132	Human cytomegalovirus UL36 and UL37	CMV retinitis	Phosphorothioate 2′-O-methyl/ oligodeoxynucleotide chimera	Intravitreal	Phase I	Hybridon
ISIS 13312	Human cytomegalovirus IE-2 gene	CMV retinitis	Phosphorothioate 2′-O-methoxyethyl/ oligodeoxynucleotide chimera	Intravitreal	Phase I	ISIS Pharmaceuticals
GEM-92	HIV *gag* gene	HIV	Phosphorothioate 2′-O-methyl/ oligodeoxynucleotide chimera	Intravenous	Phase I	Hybridon

from natural DNA in that one of the nonbridging oxygen atoms in the phosphodiester linkage is substituted with sulfur (Fig. 1). Phosphorothioate oligodeoxynucleotides are commercially available and easily synthesized, support RNase H activity, exhibit acceptable pharmacokinetics for systemic and local delivery, and have not exhibited major toxicities that would prevent their use in humans. Significant resources have been applied to identify chemical modifications to further improve upon the properties of phosphorothioate oligodeoxynucleotides. The primary objectives of this effort are similar to those of medicinal chemistry efforts for other types of pharmacological agents, i.e., to increase potency, decrease toxicity, enhance pharmacokinetics, and decrease costs.

A dimer of an oligonucleotide depicting subunits that may be modified to enhance oligonucleotide drug properties is depicted in Figure 3. These subunits are composed of heterocycles, carbohydrates, phosphodiesters, and sugar-phosphates (a four-atom linkage or backbone). Modifications can be performed on these subunits as can modifications that relate to how these units are connected (connection sites). Complete removal of the sugar-phosphate backbone with appropriate replacements and attaching, or conjugating, drug-enhancing moieties at various positions in the subunits are also important modifications. Finally, prodrug modifications may be employed to enhance drug properties. Most of the positions available in a G-C or A-T dimer (approximately 26 positions for each dimer) that

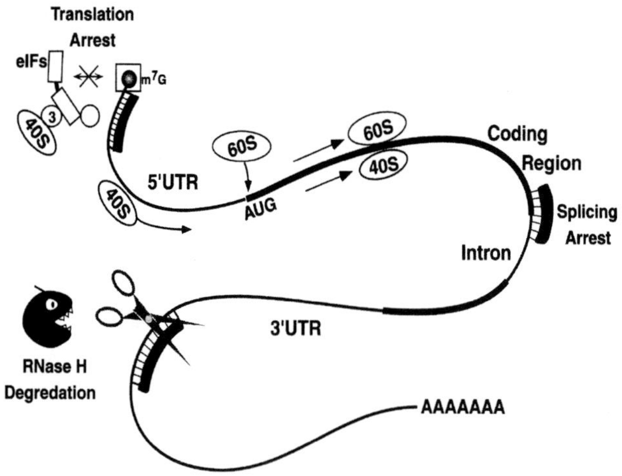

Figure 2 Antisense mechanisms of action. Cartoon depicts three different mechanisms by which an antisense oligonucleotide can inhibit expression of a targeted gene product by hybridization to the mRNA or pre-mRNA that codes for the gene product.

do not directly interfere with Watson-Crick base pair hydrogen bonding (Fig. 1) have been modified.

The nucleobases or heterocycles of nucleic acids provide the recognition points for the Watson-Crick base pairing rules, and any oligonucleotide modification must maintain these specific hydrogen-bonding interactions. Thus, the scope of heterocyclic modifications is quite limited. These heterocyclic modifications can be grouped into three structural classes—enhanced base stacking, additional hydrogen bonding, and a combination of these—with the primary objective being to enhance hybridization resulting in increased affinity (Fig. 4). Modifications that enhance base stacking by expanding the π-electron cloud are represented by conjugated, lipophilic modifications in the 5-position of pyrimidines, such as propynes, hexynes, azoles, and simply a methyl group (23–26) and the 7-position of 7-deazapurines including iodo, propynyl, and cyano groups (27–30). Investigators have continued to build out of the 5-position of cytosine by going from the propynes to five-membered heterocycles to the most recently reported, tricyclic fused systems emanating from the 4,5-positions of cytosine clamps (Fig. 4) (31–34). A second type of heterocyle modification is represented by the 2-amino-adenine (Fig. 4), where the additional amino group provides another hydrogen bond in the A-T base pair analogous to the three hydrogen bonds in a G-C base pair. Heterocycle modifications providing a combination of effects are represented by 2-amino-7-deaza-7-modified A (30) (Fig. 4) and the tricyclic cytosine analog having hydrogen-bonding capabilities in the major groove of heteroduplexes (33) (Fig. 4). Furthermore, N2-modified 2-amino adenine oligonucleotides have exhibited interesting binding properties (35,36). All of these modifications are positioned to lie in the major or minor groove of the heteroduplex, do not affect sugar conformation of the heteroduplex, provide little nuclease resistances, but will generally support an RNase H cleavage mechanism.

Modifications in the ribofuranosyl moiety have provided the most value in the quest to enhance oligonucleotide drug properties (Fig. 5). In particular, certain 2′-O-modifications have greatly increased binding affinity, nuclease resistance, and altered pharmacokinetics and are potentially less toxic (37). Preorganization of the sugar into a 3′-endo pucker conformation is responsible for the increased binding affinity (38–40). More recently, the 2′-O-(dimethylaminooxyethyl) (Fig. 5) has shown a combination of binding affinity and nuclease resistance superior at this stage to all other 2′-modifications (41).

It is now well known that uniformly 2′-O-modified oligonucleotides do not support an RNase H mechanism (42). The 2′-O-modified oligonucleotide-RNA heteroduplex has been shown to present a structural conformation that is recognized by the enzyme, but cleavage is not supported (43–45). The lack of activity of 2′-O-modified oligonucleotides has led to the development of a chimeric oligonucleotide strategy (42,46–48). This approach focuses on the design of high-binding, nuclease-resistant antisense oligonucleotides that are "gapped" with a contiguous sequence of 2′-deoxy phosphorothioates (Fig. 6). On hybridization to target RNA, a heteroduplex is presented that supports an RNase H–mediated cleavage of the RNA strand. The stretch of the modified oligonucleotide-RNA heteroduplex that is recognized by RNase H may be placed anywhere

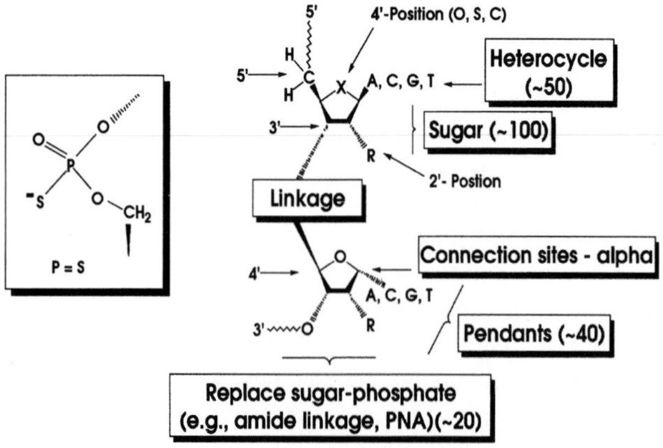

Figure 3 Positions that have been chemically modified for antisense oligonucleotides.

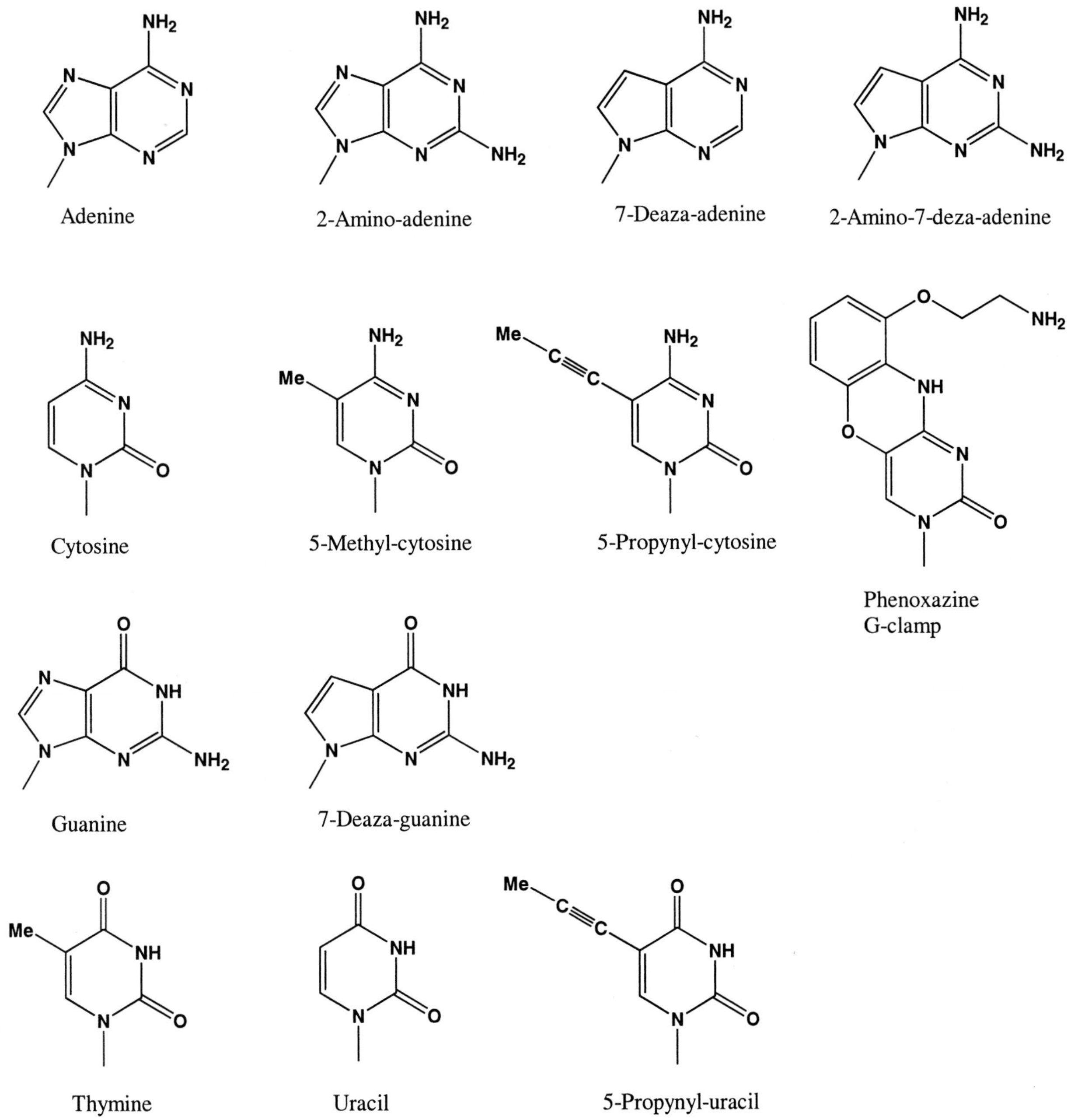

Figure 4 Examples of different heterocycle modifications that support antisense activity.

within the modified oligonucleotide. The modifications in the flanking regions of the gap should not only provide nuclease resistance to exo- and endonucleases, but also not compromise binding affinity and base-pair specificity. Several types of structures have been successfully developed (Fig. 6). The major nucleolytic activity appears to involve a 3′-exonuclease, therefore protecting the 3′-end of the oligonucleotide will confer greater nuclease resistance to the oligonucleotide.

In addition to heterocycle and sugar modification, discussed above, oligonucleotides have been modified extensively on the phosphate backbone; phosphate substitutions have been identified as well as sugar phosphate substitutions. Finally, various pendant groups have been attached

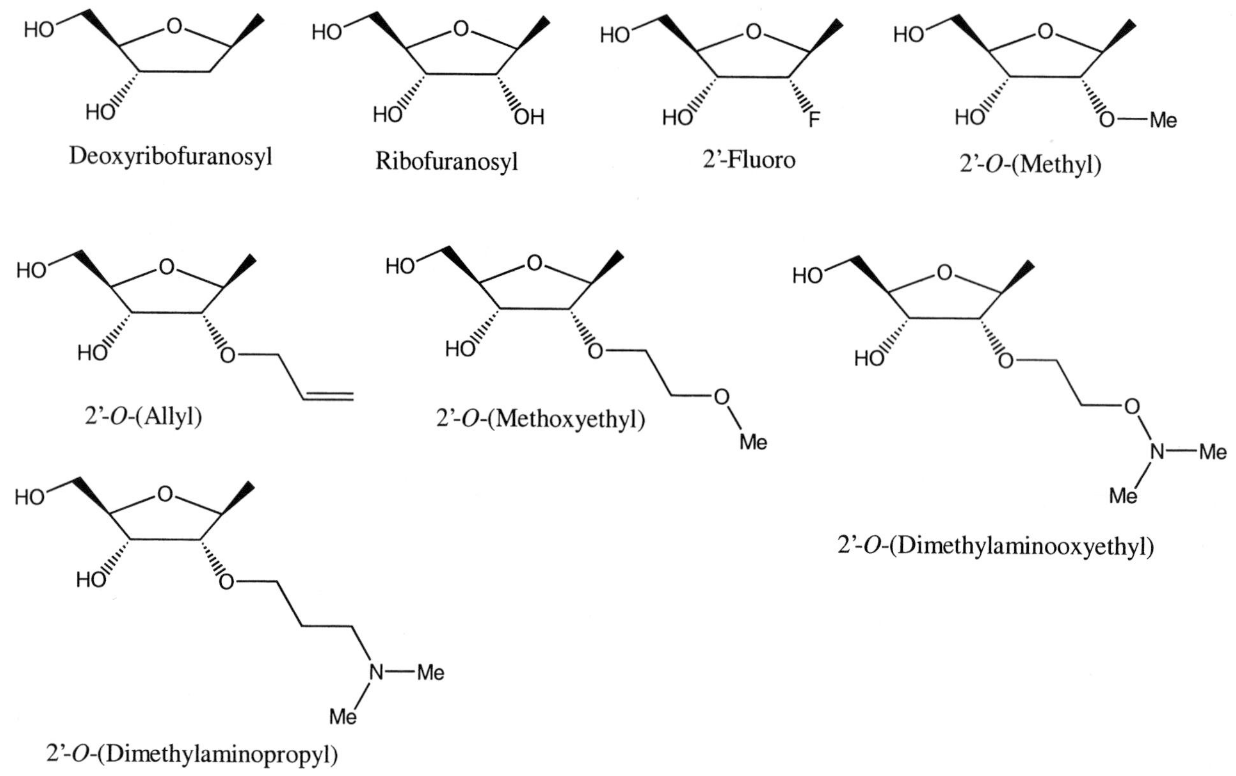

Figure 5 Examples of different sugar modifications that support antisense activity.

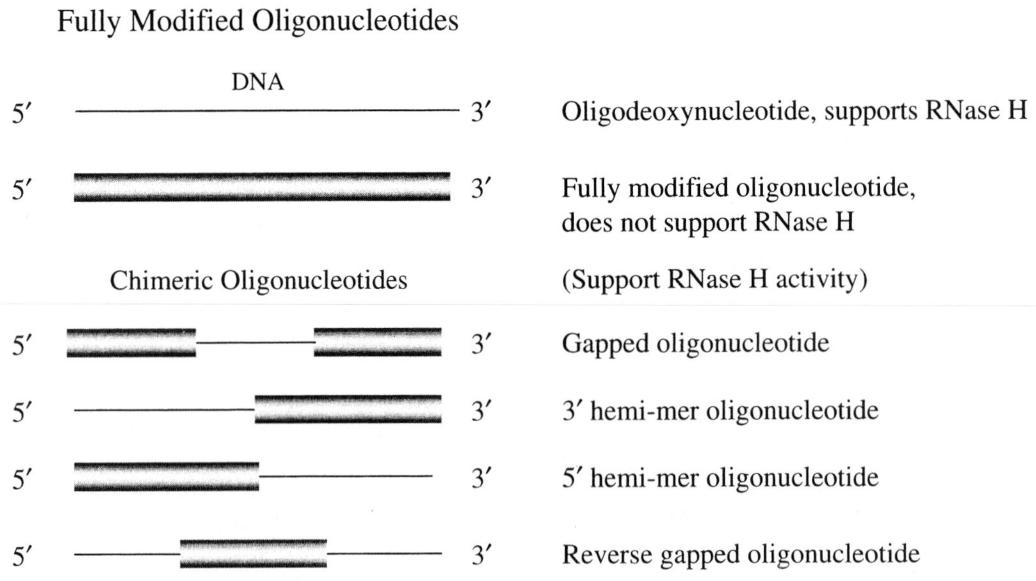

Figure 6 Examples of different oligonucleotide structures.

Table 2 Attributes of Various Modified Oligonucleotides

Attribute	Examples
Increased affinity for RNA	2′-O-Methyl, 2′-fluoro, 2′-O-methoxyethyl, 2′-O-(dimethylaminooxyethyl), 5-methyl cytosine, 5-propynyl, phenoxazine G-clamp, peptide nucleic acid, MMI bis-methoxy, others
Increased nuclease resistance	2′-O-Methoxyethyl, peptide nucleic acid, MMI bis-methoxy, chiral methylphosphonate bis-methoxy, 2′-O-(dimethylaminooxyethyl), others
Altered tissue distribution	2′-O-Methoxyethyl, peptide nucleic acid, MMI bis-methoxy, chiral methylphosphonate bis-methoxy, cholesterol conjugate, others
Decreased toxicity	2′-O-Methyl, 2′-O-methoxyethyl, 5-methyl cytosine, MMI bis-methoxy, chiral methylphosphonate bis-methoxy, others

to oligonucleotides such as cholesterol, folic acid, fatty acids, etc. to alter pharmacokinetic properties. The reader is referred to several recent reviews that discuss chemistry of oligonucleotides in more detail (37,49). It should be noted that no single modification covers all the desired properties for a modified oligonucleotide. Modification have been identified that increase hybridization affinity of the oligonucleotide for its target RNA, increase nuclease resistance, decrease toxicity, and alter the pharmacokinetics (Table 2). Furthermore, the ideal oligonucleotide will differ for different applications. Therefore, it is important to be able to mix and match properties of different oligonucleotide modifications for specific applications.

IV. PHARMACOKINETICS OF OLIGONUCLEOTIDES

A. Cellular Pharmacokinetics

Cellular uptake of phosphorothioate oligonucleotides has been documented to occur in most mammalian cells (50–57). Cellular uptake of oligonucleotides is time and temperature dependent. It is also influenced by cell type, cell culture conditions and media, and the length/sequence of the oligonucleotide itself (58). No obvious correlation between the lineage of cell, whether the cells are transformed or virally infected, and uptake has been identified. Cellular uptake appears to be an active process, i.e., oligonucleotide will accumulate in greater concentration intracellularly than in the medium and is energy dependent. Despite the fact that mammalian cells in culture will readily accumulate oligonucleotides, it has been necessary to further facilitate cytosolic delivery for many, but not all cells with transfection agents such as cationic lipids, dendrimers, and fusogenic peptides (16,59–63). In the absence of these facilitators, it has been difficult to demonstrate true antisense effects in cultured cells although there are some exceptions. However, in vivo this is not the case. It has become apparent that in vitro cell-uptake studies do not predict in vivo cell uptake and pharmacokinetics of oligonucleotides (58,64–68). Our understanding of cellular and subcellular uptake has evolved as superior analytical tools have been developed. These advances include development of immunohistochemical techniques utilizing oligonucleotide-specific antibodies (68) and in situ perfusion of whole organs followed by cell sorting and subcellular separation techniques coupled with capillary gel electrophoresis (66).

Our understanding of cellular and subcellular distribution and pharmacokinetics of oligonucleotides in whole animals is emerging. In our laboratories (66,68) we have utilized more specific tools for qualification and even quantification of intact oligonucleotide. Phosphorothioate oligonucleotides rapidly distribute to whole tissue with distribution half-lives range from 30 to 60 minutes in vivo. Approximately half of the oligonucleotide associated with the liver (as an example) is intracellular in both parenchymal and nonparenchymal cells by 4 hours after intravenous administration (66). The other half of the organ-associated oligonucleotide appears to be associated with extracellular matrix, interstitium, or loosely bound to the cell membrane. Consistent with this observation, others have shown that phosphorothioates have been localized to connective tissue and can bind to various proteins within these matrices such as laminin and fibronectin (68–70). Some of this matrix-associated oligonucleotide will diffuse to cells over time or be lost to efflux from the organ (68). It is likely that both of these processes are functioning up to 24 hours after administration of oligonucleotide. By 24 hours after injection of phosphorothioate oligonucleotide, very little is seen to be associated with extracellular matrix (Fig. 7) (68). Thus, it is likely that whole organ pharmacokinetic evaluation after 24 hours will parallel cellular clearance kinetics.

Although the in vitro studies fail to predict which cell types will take up oligonucleotides in vivo, the general trend of variability from cell type to cell type continues to be observed in vivo (Fig. 7). Based upon these results one would not expect to uniformly inhibit expression of a targeted gene product within a tissue or whole organism, resulting in differential sensitivity of different tissues and cells within tissue to the antisense effect. Subcellular distribution has been shown to be broad, and the extent of cytosolic and nuclear distribution differs between cells (66). In general the total number of oligonucleotide molecules is

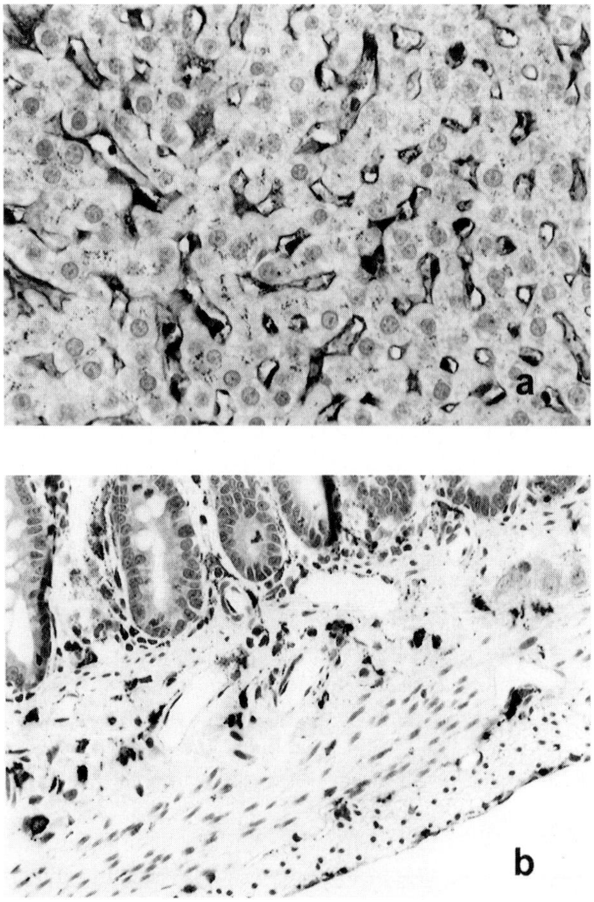

Figure 7 Distribution of an oligonucleotide in rodent tissues. A second-generation 2′-O-methoxyethyl chimeric oligonucleotide was administered to a rat by intravenous injection. Twenty-four hours after injection, liver (a) and large intestine (b) were collected fixed in formalin and stained with an oligonucleotide-specific monoclonal antibody followed by horseradish peroxidase-conjugated anti-mouse antibody (68). Oligonucleotide staining is brown. Tissue was counterstained with hematoxylin to provide structural detail in the tissue. In both panels, it is apparent that the oligonucleotide accumulates within certain cells in the tissues (i.e., Kupffer cells and sinusoidal endothelial cells in liver) to a greater extent than other cell types.

greatest in the cytosol. However, because of the much smaller volume of the nucleus, the nucleus may often contain a higher concentration of oligonucleotide than the cytosol.

Nuclease metabolism has been shown to account for the clearance of phosphorothioate oligonucleotide from organs of distribution. Within the cells, the pattern of metabolites appears to be quite similar between cell types and the subcellular compartments (membrane associated, cytosolic, and nuclear). Increasing doses from 5 to 50 mg/kg only moderately decreased metabolism intracellularly, consistent with whole organ data (66).

Several studies have suggested that active uptake processes including receptor-mediated endocytosis and pinocytosis are involved in uptake of oligonucleotides in vivo. At very low doses (< 1 mg/kg), competition of binding for scavenger receptors in vivo altered the whole organ distribution of oligonucleotides in liver but not kidney (71,72). However, distribution studies conducted in scavenger receptor knockout mice did not show significantly altered intracellular and whole-organ distribution of phosphorothioate oligonucleotides (M. Butler et al., unpublished).

Distribution in the kidney has been more thoroughly studied, and drug has been shown to be present in Bowman's capsule, the proximal convoluted tubule, the brush border membrane, and within renal tubular epithelial cells (73). These data suggested that the oligonucleotides are filtered by the glomerulus and then reabsorbed by the proximal convoluted tubule epithelial cells. Moreover, the authors identified a specific protein in the brush border that may mediate uptake. In separate studies, other investigators have shown that although some oligonucleotide is taken up from the tubular lumen brush border, the distribution to the tubule epithelial cells is predominantly from the capillary serosal side (74). The uptake from capillary circulation may not be receptor mediated. In summary, it is likely that multiple processes are involved in the uptake of oligonucleotides into cells in vivo. Additional research will be required to further elucidate these mechanisms.

B. Whole Animal Oligonucleotide Pharmacokinetics

1. Phosphorothioate Oligodeoxynucleotides

The plasma pharmacokinetics of phosphorothioate oligodeoxynucleotides are characterized by rapid and dose-dependent clearance (30–60 min half-life) driven primarily by distribution to tissue and secondarily by metabolism. Urinary and fecal excretion are minor pathways for elimination of phosphorothioate oligonucleotides. Dose-dependent clearance from plasma is predominantly a function of saturable tissue distribution (75,76). Metabolism has been shown to be unchanged in plasma over a large dose range (1–50 mg/kg) and after repeated administration up to one month (77), suggesting that metabolism is neither inhibited nor induced by repeat administration.

The plasma pharmacokinetics are quite similar between animals and humans, and they scale from one species to the next on the basis of body weight, not surface area (77–79). For example, it is possible to show that, when dosed on the basis of body weight, the concentrations of oligonucleotides in plasma administered by a 2-hour constant intravenous infusion are similar between humans and monkeys. Thus it has been possible to predict plasma concentrations in humans from nonclinical pharmacokinetic data.

Phosphorothioate oligonucleotides bind to circulating plasma proteins (including albumin and α_2 macroglobulin). The apparent affinity for human serum albumin is low (10–30 μM). Therefore, plasma protein binding provides a repository for these drugs, preventing rapid renal excretion. Because serum protein binding is saturable at high concentrations, intact oligonucleotide may be found in urine in increasing amounts as dose rate and/or amount is increased (64,77,80).

Phosphorothioate oligonucleotides are rapidly and extensively absorbed after intradermal, subcutaneous, intramuscular, or intraperitoneal administration (65,75,81,82) (J. Leeds, unpublished observations). Nonparenteral absorption has been characterized for pulmonary and oral routes of administration. Estimates of bioavailability range from 3–20% following intranasal dosing to $< 1\%$ by the oral route (83). Although it is likely that permeability in the intestine is low, stability of these compounds in the intestine (prior to absorption) may be a rate-limiting factor for oral absorption. The metabolic half-life of a 20-mer phosphorothioate oligonucleotide in the rat intestine (in vivo) is less than 1 hour.

Phosphorothioates are broadly distributed to all peripheral tissues. The highest concentrations of oligonucleotides are found in the liver, kidney, spleen, lymph nodes, and bone marrow, with no measurable distribution to the brain (84). Many other tissues take up smaller amounts of oligonucleotide resulting in lower tissue concentrations. Phosphorothioate oligonucleotides are primarily cleared from tissues by nuclease metabolism. Rate of clearance differs between tissues with the spleen, lymph nodes, and liver generally clearing more rapidly than kidney. In general the clearance rates result in half-lives of elimination ranging from 2 to 5 days in rodents and primates (65,76).

In summary, pharmacokinetic studies of phosphorothioate oligonucleotides demonstrate that they are well absorbed from parenteral sites, distribute broadly to all peripheral tissues, do not cross the blood-brain barrier, and are eliminated primarily by slow metabolism. In short, once-a-day or every-other-day systemic dosing should be feasible. In general, the pharmacokinetic properties of this class of compounds appear to be largely driven by chemistry rather than sequence. Additional studies are required to determine whether there are subtle sequence-specific effects on the pharmacokinetic profile of this class of drugs.

2. Second-Generation Oligonucleotides

The plasma pharmacokinetics of 2′-O-methyl-, 2′-O-propyl-, or 2′-O-methoxyethyl-modified oligonucleotides do not differ significantly from their-deoxy congeners (85–87). Since metabolism plays only a minor role in the plasma distribution kinetics, this modification is expected to do very little to alter the distribution and excretion kinetics. Early studies in our laboratory indicate that the binding affinity to serum albumin may be somewhat lessened by 2′-ribose sugar modifications, but the overall capacity of the plasma proteins to bind these oligonucleotides is not significantly changed (Table 3). Therefore, urinary excretion remains a minor route of elimination, and these compounds are broadly distributed to peripheral tissues.

Several of the 2′-ribose sugar modification produces enough of an increase in nuclease resistance that it is possible to produce relatively stable oligonucleotides with phosphodiester linkages (Table 2). Thus this modification allows for elimination or reduction in the number of sulfurs contained in the internucleotide bridge, but these compounds are less stable than their 2′-modified phosphorothioate congeners (88). In addition, as sulfur is removed, plasma protein binding is greatly decreased and rapid removal from plasma by filtration in the kidney increases significantly. This pharmacokinetic characteristic may limit the use of phosphodiester second-generation modified oligonucleotides intended for treatment of systemic disease. Alternatively, this pharmacokinetic profile may be ideal for locally administered oligonucleotides since it limits the accumulation of systemically absorbed drug.

Absorption for parenterally administered modified oligonucleotides is consistently rapid and nearly complete. Some of the second-generation modified oligonucleotides have exhibited improved intestinal permeability (85) as

Table 3 Serum Albumin Affinity, Whole Plasma Fraction Bound to Proteins (F_b), and Fraction of Dose Excreted in Urine ($f_{excreted}$, 0–24 h) Following Intravenous Administration of 3 mg/kg—Comparison of First- and Second-Generation Chemistries

Compound	Chemistry	Kd (μM)	F_b (%)	$f_{excreted}$
ISIS 2302	PS ODN	17.7	99.2	0.003
ISIS 11159	PS 2′-MOE	29.3	95.5	0.032
ISIS 16952	PO 2′-MOE	>500	79.6	0.45

PS ODN = Phosphorothioate oligodeoxynucleotide; PS 2′-MOE = 2′-O-methoxyethyl ribose modified phosphorothioate (all nucleotides were modified); PO 2′-MOE = 2′-O-methoxyethyl ribose modified phosphodiester (all nucleotides were modified).

Table 4 Summary of Observed Organ Clearance Half-Lives Comparing Second- and First-Generation Chemistries

	Half-life (days)	
Organ	2′-Modified phosphorothioate oligonucleotide	Phosphorothioate oligodeoxynucleotide
Kidney cortex	21.7	5.0
Kidney medulla	10.4	3.1
Liver	7.7	2.8
Spleen	8.1	3.3
Lymph nodes	16.5	0.9
Bone marrow	11.5	1.3

well as significantly improved stability in the intestine (O. Khatsenko et al., unpublished). It is likely this combination of improved biochemical characteristics that has led to the observation of improved oral bioavailability (85) for this class of oligonucleotide compounds.

The distribution pattern of the 2′-ribose modified phosphorothioate oligonucleotides are similar to first-generation phosphorothioates and similarly not altered by changes in sequence. Kidney, liver, spleen, bone marrow, and lymph nodes are the major sites of distribution. The most exciting difference in pharmacokinetics is, not surprisingly, manifested in prolonged terminal elimination half-lives from tissues of distribution. The elimination half-lives appear to be increased nearly 5- to 10-fold, suggesting that once-weekly systemic dosing may be feasible (Table 4).

In summary, pharmacokinetic studies of 2′-modified ribose phosphorothioate oligonucleotides demonstrate that they are well absorbed from parenteral sites, may have improved oral absorption attributes, and distribute broadly to all peripheral tissues. Although stability has been greatly enhanced, nuclease metabolism is likely the primary mechanism for ultimate elimination of these modified oligonucleotides. In short, once-a-week systemic dosing should be feasible, and oral administration may be possible in the near future. Additional studies are required to determine whether there are substantial sequence-specific effects on the pharmacokinetic profile of this class of drugs.

V. TOXICOLOGY OF OLIGONUCLEOTIDES

Phosphorothioate oligodeoxynucleotides have been examined extensively in a full range of acute, chronic, and reproductive studies in rodents, lagomorphs, and primates. At high doses, there is a distinctive pattern of toxicity that is common to all phosphorothioate oligodeoxynucleotides (89–96). The remarkable similarity in toxicity to different phosphorothioate oligodeoxynucleotides suggests that for this class of antisense compounds, toxicity is independent of sequence and is the result of non–antisense-mediated mechanisms. The most probable mechanism of the observed toxicities is the binding of oligodeoxynucleotides to proteins. These non–antisense-mediated pathways are thought to be responsible for most, if not all, of the toxicities associated with the administration of these compounds to laboratory animals. This conclusion is strengthened by studies in which few or no differences in toxicity are observed between pharmacologically active and inactive sequences. Different patterns of toxicity exist between rodents and primates. Understanding the mechanisms behind these differences is crucial to understanding which species best predict the potential human effects. A comparison of the toxicological profiles of phosphorothioate oligodeoxynucleotides with that of the next generation of phosphorothioate oligodeoxynucleotides suggests that some of the chemical class-related toxicities of phosphorothioate oligodeoxynucleotides can be ameliorated by chemical modification.

A number of phosphorothioate oligodeoxynucleotides have been examined in one or more of the following battery of genotoxicity assays: Ames test, in vitro chromosomal aberrations, in vitro mammalian mutation (HGPRT locus and mouse lymphoma), in vitro unscheduled DNA synthesis tests, and in vivo mouse micronucleus. In all of these assays the results were negative, and there was no evidence of mutagenicity or clastogenicity of these compounds (76).

A. Acute Toxicities

In rodents, the acute toxicity of phosphorothioate oligodeoxynucleotides has been characterized as part of an effort to determine the maximum tolerated dose for in vivo genotoxicity assays. The doses of three phosphorothioate oligodeoxynucleotides required to produce 50% lethality (LD_{50}) were estimated to be approximately 750 mg/kg (76).

In primates, the acute dose-limiting toxicities are a transient inhibition of the clotting cascade and the activation of the complement cascade (89,97–99). Both of these toxicities are thought to be related to the polyanionic nature of the molecules and the binding of these compounds to specific protein factors in plasma.

Prolongation of clotting times following administration of different phosphorothioate oligodeoxynucleotides is characterized by a concentration-dependent prolongation of activated partial thromboplastin times (aPTT) (94,99–101). The prolongation of aPTT is highly transient and directly proportional to plasma concentrations of oligodeoxynucleotide, therefore parallels the plasma drug concentration curves with various dose regimens. As drug is cleared from plasma, the inhibition diminishes such that there is complete reversal within hours of dosing. With repeated administration, there is no evidence of residual inhibition. Prolongation of aPTT has been observed in all species examined to date, including human, monkey, and rat. The mechanism of prolongation of aPTT by phosphorothioate oligodeoxynucleotides is thought to be a result of the interaction of the oligonucleotides with proteins. It is well known that polyanions are inhibitors of clotting, and phosphorothioate oligodeoxynucleotides may act through similar mechanisms. If these oligonucleotides inhibit the clotting cascade as a result of their polyanionic properties, then binding and inhibition of thrombin would be a likely mechanism of action. However, the greater sensitivity of the intrinsic pathway to inhibition by phosphorothioate oligodeoxynucleotides suggests that there are other clotting factors specific to this pathway that may be inhibited as well. Recent data suggest that there is a specific inhibition of the tenase complex as well as binding to thrombin (J. Sheehan et al., unpublished).

In clinical trials with ISIS 2302, normal volunteers and patients were dosed with 2 mg/kg infused over 2 hours. This regimen produced total oligonucleotide concentrations of 10–15 μg/mL and a concomitant increase in aPTT of approximately 50% (102), which correlates well with in vitro human and animal data (76). The transient and reversible nature of aPTT prolongation, combined with the relatively small magnitude of the change, makes these effects clinically insignificant for the current treatment doses and regimens.

Activation of the complement cascade by phosphorothioate oligodeoxynucleotides has the potential to produce the most profound acute toxicological effects. In primates, treatment with high doses over short infusion times resulted in marked hematological effects and marked hemodynamic changes, when are thought to be secondary to complement activation. Hematological changes are characterized by transient reduction in neutrophil counts, presumably due to margination, followed by neutrophilia with abundant immature, nonsegmented neutrophils (98,103). In a small fraction of monkeys, complement activation was accompanied by marked reductions in heart rate, blood pressure, and subsequently cardiac output. In some animals, these hemodynamic changes were lethal (89,98,104).

There is an association between cardiovascular collapse and complement activation. That is, all monkeys demonstrating some degree of cardiovascular collapse or hemodynamic changes had markedly elevated levels of complement split products. However, the converse is not true, in that only a fraction of the animals with activated complement had cardiovascular functional changes (76). Thus, this observation suggests that there may be sensitive subpopulations or predisposing factors within individual animals that make them susceptible to the physiological sequelae of complement activation. Because of these observed hemodynamic changes, primate studies to monitor for these effects have become part of the normal evaluation of these compounds (105,106). Although complement activation at high doses is consistent and predictable between animals, there is currently little appreciation for the variability in the severity of the associated hemodynamic changes. While the split product Bb can be used to monitor complement activation, C5a (complement split product) is the most biologically active split product. Preliminary data obtained relating response to complement split product levels indicate that C5a levels are elevated more significantly in some of the more affected animals (76).

The goal of toxicity studies is to characterize the toxicity of compounds and to establish a framework upon which clinical safety studies can be designed. In this regard, it is useful to examine the relationship between plasma concentrations of oligonucleotides and the activation of complement. When Bb concentrations were plotted against the concurrent plasma concentrations of oligodeoxynucleotides in primates, it was apparent that complement was only activated at concentrations of phosphorothioate oligodeoxynucleotides that exceed a threshold value of 40–50 μg/mL (98). Bb levels remained unchanged from control values at plasma concentrations below the threshold. Remarkably, this threshold concentration is similar for three 20-mer phosphorothioate oligodeoxynucleotides and for an 8-mer phosphorothioate oligodeoxynucleotide that forms a tetrad complex (79). Recent data demonstrate that human serum may be less sensitive to activation than monkey serum, suggesting a species difference in sensitivity. Regardless of small differences, it is clear that clinical dose regimens should be designed to avoid plasma oligodeoxynucleotide concentrations that exceed 40–50 μg/mL. To this end, the similarities in plasma pharmacokinetics between monkeys and humans have allowed the design of dose regimens that achieve desired plasma concentration profiles.

The most direct approach for staying below the plasma thresholds for complement activation is to reduce the dose rate by substituting prolonged infusions for bolus injections. In clinical trials with phosphorothioate oligodeoxynucleotides, the drugs are administered either as 2-hour infusions or as constant 24-hour infusions. At a rate of infusion of 2 mg/kg over 2 hours, the Cmax was 8–15 μg/mL, still well below the threshold for complement activation (107). Phosphorothioate oligodeoxynucleotides have been administered by intravenous infusion to more than 500 patients and volunteers as part of clinical trials without any significant indication of activation of the alternative complement cascade.

B. Modified Oligonucleotides

Chemical modifications to phosphorothioate oligodeoxynucleotides may reduce the potential to activate complement. In one study, cynomolgus monkeys were administered an intravenous infusion over a 10-minutes period with a 5, 20, or 50 mg/kg dose of a 17-mer phosphodiester oligodeoxynucleotide, Ar177, that had phosphorothioate caps on the 3′ and 5′ termini (99,108). This oligonucleotide is known to have a complex secondary structure. In this experiment, although there was a dose-related increase in plasma concentrations of Bb, the magnitude of the increases were small in comparison to the known activity of full-phosphorothioate oligodeoxynucleotides (99). Whether this diminished potential to activate the complement cascade is related to the reduction of phosphorothioate linkages or whether it is due to the complex secondary structure of this particular oligodeoxynucleotide was not established by these experiments. Some insight into this question was obtained in a second series of experiments performed with oligonucleotides that contained 2′-O-methoxyethyl modifications of the ribose sugar in 12 of the 20 nucleotides (76). Cynomolgus monkeys were treated by 10-minutes intravenous infusion with single doses of 1, 5, or 20 mg/kg of this 20-mer oligonucleotide that was either fully modified phosphorothioate linkages (ISIS 13650) or had phosphodiester wings and a central region of phosphorothioate linkages (nine linkages, ISIS 12854). The termini of both compounds contained six 2′-modified nucleotides. A third unmodified phosphorothioate oligodeoxynucleotide, ISIS 1082, was included as a positive control. The unmodified compound produced marked increases in Bb and severe cardiovascular effect at the dose of 5 mg/kg (30- to 60-fold over baseline). At 5 mg/kg the aPTT values were 41 and 33 seconds for the fully phosphorothioate and partially phosphorothioate 2′-modified oligonucleotides, respectively. In contrast, the unmodified phosphorothioate oligodeoxynucleotide produced an aPTT of 72 seconds at the same dose. These data suggest that reduction in the number of phosphorothioate linkages reduced the inhibitory effects on aPTT and the activation of the complement cascade. However, the more important difference was that both 2′-O-methoxyethyl compounds were markedly less potent in activating complement than an unmodified oligodeoxynucleotide (D. K. Monteith, P. L. Nicklin, and A. A. Levin, unpublished observations). Although the safety profile of phosphorothioate oligodeoxynucleotides has proven satisfactory, the acute safety profile of the next generation of oligonucleotides may be improved by modification of the 2′ position of the ribose sugar with an alkoxy such as 2′-O-methyl or 2′-O-methoxyethyl and by reductions in phosphorothioate linkages.

C. Toxicological Effects Associated with Chronic Exposure

One of the characteristic toxicities observed with repeated exposure of rodents to phosphorothioate oligodeoxynucleotides is a profile of effects that can be described as immune stimulation. The profile is characterized by splenomegaly, lymphoid hyperplasia, and diffuse multiorgan mixed mononuclear cell infiltrates (76). The severity of these changes is dose dependent and most notable at doses equal to or exceeding 10 mg/kg. The mixed mononuclear cell infiltrates consisted of monocytes, lymphocytes, and fibroblasts and were particularly notable in liver, kidney, heart, lung, thymus, pancreas, and periadrenal tissues (93,96,109,110).

Although immune stimulation in rodents is thought to be a class effect of phosphorothioate oligodeoxynucleotides and not dependent on hybridization, sequence is an important factor in determining immunostimulatory potential (111–113). Immunostimulatory motifs have been described in the literature and involve palindromic sequences and CpG (cytosine-guanosine) motifs.

Among the most remarkable features of oligodeoxynucleotide-induced immune stimulation are the species differences. Rodents are highly susceptible to this generalized immune stimulation, whereas primates appear to be relatively insensitive to the effect at equivalent doses. Even 6 months of treatment of cynomolgus monkeys with 10 mg/kg of a 20-mer oligodeoxynucleotide, ISIS 2302, given every other day produced only a relatively mild increase in B-cell numbers in spleen and lymph nodes of the primates with no change in organ weights. The mixed monocellular infiltrates in liver and other organs that are so characteristics of the response in rodents are absent even after long-term exposure in monkeys (76). It is known that rodents are more susceptible to the stimulatory effects of lipopolysaccharides, and much of the immune stimulation produced by oligodeoxynucleotides shares characteristics with lipopolysaccharide stimulation. Assuming results obtained in monkeys can be used to predict stimulation in humans, then the immunostimulatory effects may not be a prominent adverse effect in humans. In clinical trials with ISIS 2302, there are no indications of immune stimulation with intravenous doses of 2 mg/kg administered for 1 month.

It is evident that there are both species and sequence differences involved in immune stimulation and that specific sequences should, if possible, be excluded from oligodeoxynucleotides. In long-term toxicity studies in rodents, the constant cell proliferation associated with immune stimulation may have promoter-like effects and may thus complicate the interpretation of rodent carcinogenicity studies. At this time there are no reports of toxicity studies longer than 6 months, and the long-term sequelae of immune stimulation in rodents are at present merely speculation. More importantly, immune stimulation following systemic administration of phosphorothioate oligodeoxynucleotides does not appear to be clinically relevant.

Morphological changes in the bone marrow of mice were observed after 2 weeks of treatment (3 doses/week) with 100–150 mg/kg phosphorothioate oligodeoxynucleotides. There was reduction in number of megakaryocytes that was accompanied by a reduction of approximately 50% in circulating platelet counts (96). Reductions in platelets have been observed in rats treated with 21.7 mg/kg ISIS 2105 given every other day (95), but they were not observed in primates administered 10 mg/kg. Similarly, a reduction in platelets was observed in mice, but not in monkeys treated for 4 weeks with ISIS 2302 at doses of 100 and 50 mg/kg every other day, respectively. Similar observations were made for ISIS 5132 with reductions in platelets at 20 and 100 mg/kg in mice and no observed effect in monkeys up to 10 mg/kg (110). These data suggest that the mouse may be more sensitive to these subchronic effects on platelets than nonhuman primates. However, in acute studies in primates, transient reductions in platelets are occasionally observed. These transient reductions in platelets occur acutely during 2-hour infusions at doses of 10 mg/kg, reverse after completion of the infusion, and have not been associated with any measurable change in platelet number 24–48 hours after subchronic or chronic treatment regimens (76). Thrombocytopenia has been reported in AIDS patients treated with GEM 91, a 27-mer phosphorothioate oligodeoxynucleotides (114).

Tissue distribution studies have shown that the liver and kidney are major sites of deposition of phosphorothioate oligodeoxynucleotide. In toxicity studies with phosphorothioate oligodeoxynucleotides, a variety of hepatic changes have been observed. The immune-mediated cellular infiltrates in rodent livers were discussed above. With high-dose administration of oligodeoxynucleotides in all species examined, there was a hypertrophic change in Kupffer cells accompanied by inclusions of basophilic material that was observed with hematoxylin and eosin staining. These basophilic granules have been identified as inclusions of oligodeoxynucleotide (68). Furthermore, it was demonstrated that the presence of these inclusions was related to dose.

Hepatocellular changes were not a prominent feature of toxicity in primates. In cynomolgus monkeys, 50 mg ISIS 2302 per kg administered every other day for 4 weeks by intravenous injection produced no morphological indication of liver toxicity, although there was a slight (1.5-fold) increase in AST in this group (103). Following subcutaneous doses of ISIS 3521 and ISIS 5132 of up to 80 mg/kg every other day for four doses, there was Kupffer cell hypertrophy and periportal cell vacuolation but no indication of necrosis and only a very slight increase in ALT (76). After 4 weeks of alternate-day dosing with 10 mg/kg via 2-hour intravenous infusion of either ISIS 3521 or ISIS 5132, there were no alterations in AST or ALT, suggesting that at clinically relevant doses of these compounds, there was no evidence for hepatic pathology or tansaminemia. In clinical trials with ISIS 2302, ISIS 3521, and ISIS 5132 at doses of 2 mg/kg administered by 2-hour infusion on alternate days for 3–4 weeks, there was no indication of hepatic dysfunction, nor was there any evidence of transaminemia.

Like Kupffer cells in the liver, renal proximal tubule epithelial cells take up oligodeoxynucleotide, as demonstrated by autoradiographic studies and immunohistochemistry as discussed previously (68,69,115,116), and by the use of special histological stains (103). The appearance of basophilic inclusions is dose dependent in proximal tubule cells. Significant renal toxicity can be induced by extremely high doses. Doses of 80 mg/kg in rats and monkeys have induced both histological and serum chemistry changes in the kidney (D. K. Monteith, unpublished observations). At clinically relevant doses, however, there was no indication of renal dysfunction. In 4-week or 6-month toxicity studies with phosphorothioate oligodeoxynucleotides, we observed a much more subtle type of morphological change in the kidney. At a dose of 10 mg/kg on alternate days, there was a decrease in the height of the brush border and enlarged nuclei in some proximal tubule cells. These changes have been characterized as minimal to mild tubular atrophic and regenerative changes. At doses of ≤ 3 mg/kg, these changes were only infrequently observed, if at all.

An important aspect of dose-dependent effects is characterization of exposure concentrations and their relationship to morphological changes. To assess exposure, concentrations of oligodeoxynucleotides have been measured in the renal cortex obtained in subchronic and chronic toxicity studies. Renal concentrations increase with increasing doses. The concentration of total oligodeoxynucleotide in the renal cortex associated with minimal to mild (although not clinically relevant) renal tubular atrophy or regenerative changes is approximately 100 μg/g of tissue. The cortex concentrations of total oligodeoxynucleotide that are associated with moderate degenerative changes after subcutaneous doses of 40–80 mg/kg are greater than 2000 μg/g. At a clinically relevant dose of 3 mg/kg every other day, the steady-state concentration of total oligodeoxynucleotide in the kidney is in the range of 400–500 μg/g, thus demonstrating a significant margin of safety between the clinical doses and those doses associated with even the most minimal morphological renal changes. Application of clearance and steady-state pharmacokinetic models suggests that continued administration of oligodeoxynucleotide at this dose should never achieve the renal concentrations associated with dysfunction (77). These models have been confirmed in 6-month chronic toxicology studies where tissue concentrations measured at the end of 6 months of every-other-day dosing was no different than levels observed after 4 weeks of dosing at a similar or equivalent dose.

D. Chemical Modification of Oligodeoxynucleotides

Chemical modifications of oligodeoxynucleotides have been shown to reduce the potency of immune stimulation. The simplest modification with remarkable activity for reducing the immunostimulatory effects of oligodeoxynucleotides is the replacement of cytosine with 5-methyl cytosine. The methylation of a single cytosine residue in a CpG motif reduced [^{3}H] uridine incorporation and IgM secretion by mouse splenocytes. Methylation of a cytosine not in a CpG motif did not reduce the immunostimulatory potential (112). In our experience with mice, when sequences with 5-methyl cytosine are compared with the same sequence without methylation, the methylated sequence has a lower potency for inducing immune stimulation, as determined by spleen weights (117).

Substitution of methylphosphonate linkages for phosphorothioate linkages on each of the 3′ and 5′ termini have also been reported to reduce the proliferative effects and the secretion of IgG and IgM compared to the full phosphorothioate analog (118). This suggests that that this modification can also be used to ameliorate immune stimulation. The addition of 2′-O-methyl substituents also reduced immunostimulatory potential (118). The relative contribution of the uridine substitution and the 2′-methoxy substitution could not be differentiated in this experiment. The effect of 2′-alkoxy modifications on immunostimulatory potential needs further investigation. Finally, the effects of chemical modifications of phosphorothioate oligonucleotides on renal and hepatotoxicity are currently being investigated.

VI. OLIGONUCLEOTIDE FORMULATIONS

A. Physical-Chemical Properties

Due to the presence of a mixture of diastereisomers, phosphorothioate oligodeoxynucleotides are amorphous solids possessing the expected physical properties of hygroscopicity, low-bulk density, electrostatic charge pick-up, and poorly defined melting point prior to decomposition. Their good chemical stability allows storage in the form of a lyophilized powder, spray-dried powder, or concentrated, sterile solution; more than 3 years of storage is possible at refrigerated temperatures.

Due to their polyanionic nature, phosphorothioate oligodeoxynucleotides are readily soluble in neutral and basic conditions. Drug-product concentrations are limited (in select applications) only by an increase in solution viscosity. The counterion composition, ionic strength, and pH also influence the apparent solubility. Phosphorothioate oligodeoxynucleotides have an apparent pKa in the vicinity of 2 and will come out of solution in acidic environments, i.e., the stomach. This precipitation is readily reversible with increasing pH or by acid-mediated hydrolysis.

Instability of phosphorothioate oligodeoxynucleotides have been primarily attributed to two degradation mechanisms: oxidation and acid-catalyzed hydrolysis. Oxidation of the (P = S) bond in the backbone has been observed at elevated temperatures and under intense UV light, leading to partial phosphodiesters (still pharmacologically active), and are readily monitored by anion-exchange HPLC. Under acidic conditions, hydrolysis reactions followed by chain-shortening depurination reactions have been documented by length-sensitive electrophoretic techniques.

B. Parenteral Injections

Given the excellent solution stability and solubility possessed by phosphorothioate oligodeoxynucleotides, it has been relatively straightforward to formulate the first-generation drug products in support of early clinical trials. Simple, buffered solutions have been successfully used in clinical studies by intravenous intradermal, and subcutaneous injections. Recently the intravitreal route was approved for the first antisense drug application.

C. Topical Delivery for Diseases of the Skin

The barrier properties of human skin have been an area of multidisciplinary research for a long time. Skin is one of the most difficult biological membranes to penetrate, primarily due to the presence of stratum corneum (SC). Stratum corneum is composed of corneocytes laid in a brick-and-mortar arrangement with layers of lipid. The corneocytes are partially dehydrated, anuclear, metabolically active cells completely filled with bundles of keratin with a thick and insoluble envelope replacing the cell membrane (119). The primary lipids in the SC are ceramides, free sterols, free fatty acids, and triglycerides (120), which form lamellar lipid sheets between the corneocytes. These unique structural features of SC provide an excellent barrier to penetration by most molecules.

Therefore, as the primary barrier to transport of molecules to the skin, physical alteration in the stratum corneum can result in improved skin penetration. Tape stripping and abrasion by repeated brushing reduced the SC barrier sufficiently to allow penetration of naked plasmid DNA and produced gene expression in skin at a level comparable to that after intradermal injection of naked plasmid DNA (121). Other studies have also shown an increase in oligonucleotide penetration upon physical removal of the SC barrier (122,123).

1. Altering the Thermodynamic Properties of the Molecules

Increasing lipid partitioning to improve skin penetration has been evaluated using two techniques that alter the thermodynamic properties of oligonucleotide molecules. A complex of phosphorothioate oligonucleotide with hydrophobic cations such as benzalkonium chloride resulted in increased penetration through isolated hairless mouse skin explained on the basis of greater partitioning in lipid phase (122). Chemical modification of oligonucleotides to eliminate the negative charges also resulted in a size-dependent increase in the penetration of oligonucleotide into the skin when used with chemical penetration enhancers such as ethanol and dimethyl sulfoxide (123).

2. Electrical Field for Alteration of Skin Permeability

Iontophoresis, which involves application of electric field across the skin to induce electrochemical transport of charged molecules, has been studied extensively for transdermal delivery of phosphorothioate oligonucleotides (124). Transdermal delivery was shown to be size dependent with steady-state flux values ranging from 2 to 26 pmol/cm^2 in isolated hairless mice skin. Steady-state flux also depended on the sequence, not just the base composition, of the oligonucleotide. Molecular structure, therefore, is a key contributor to iontophoretically assisted transport of oligonucleotides (125,126). Electroporation, a technique using much higher voltage than iontophoresis to cause formation of transient aqueous pathway in skin lipids, provides therapeutic levels ($> 1\ \mu$M) of oligonucleotides in the viable tissues of the skin (127).

3. Formulations for the Alteration of Skin Permeability

Chemical penetration enhancers have recently been studied for increasing transdermal delivery of oligonucleotides or other polar macromolecules. Chemically induced transdermal penetration results from a transient reduction in the resistance of the SC barrier properties. The reduction may be attributed to a variety of factors, such as opening of intercellular junctions due to hydration (128), solubilization of SC lipids (129,130), or increased lipid bilayer fluidization (131). Types of chemicals known to be penetration enhancers include alkyl esters (132), phospholipids (133), terpenes (134), nonionic surfactants (135), and laurocapram (Azone) (136). Combination of various surfactants and co-solvents can be used to achieve skin penetration with therapeutically relevant concentration of phosphorothioate oligonucleotides in the viable epidermis and dermis (R. Mehta et al., unpublished). The topical formulations produced significantly higher epidermal and dermal levels of oligonucleotide than those achieved by an intravenous injection at highest tolerated doses. This suggests that the topical route is more efficient in reaching all layers of the skin than systemic administration of phosphorothioate oligonucleotides.

Liposomes have been studied to transport oligonucleotides into the skin. They can increase the fluidity of skin lipid layers (similar to chemical enhancers) to facilitate transdermal permeation and can also carry encapsulated molecules through the appendageal pathway (137,138). Mixture of a phosphorothioate oligodeoxynucleotide with a suspension of anionic or neutral lipids resulted in a slight increase in accumulation in epidermis and dermis (R. Mehta, unpublished). Using a combination of different delivery techniques and formulations, it appears to now be feasible to deliver a therapeutically relevant amount of antisense oligonucleotide to the skin. In addition, preliminary results in our laboratory show a dose-dependent pharmacological effect consistent with the antisense mechanism of action of an ICAM-1 antisense oligonucleotide, ISIS 2302. Studies are also underway to assess the pharmacology and tissue kinetics of ISIS 2302 in human disease models.

D. Oral Delivery

Of the numerous barriers proposed by Nicklin and others (82) to the oral delivery of oligonucleotides, our experience has confirmed that two stand out as critical: instability in the gastrointestinal (GI) tract and low permeability across the intestinal mucosa. Given the formidable nature of these two barriers, it is not surprising that oral delivery of oligonucleotides has been considered impossible or at best difficult—as is the case with proteins, which has necessitated the latter's nonenteral administration in order to achieve systemic concentrations considered therapeutic. Nevertheless, progress has been made to address and/or understand each of these barriers with respect to oligonucleotides. (P = S)-oligonucleotides have a distinct advantage over proteins in that the former does not rely on secondary structure for activity. This provides freedom from concern over secondary structure destabilization and allows for (P = S)-oligonucleotides structural modifications to address both presystemic and systemic metabolism.

Natural DNA and RNA are rapidly digested by the ubiquitous nucleases found within the gut. As a consequence, oligonucleotides need to be stabilized in order to achieve a reasonable GI residence time to allow for absorption to occur. Surprisingly, phosphorothioate oligodeoxynucleotides were found to be rapidly degraded by nucleases found in the GI tract, therefore additional protection from nuclease degradation is required to achieve significant oral bioavailability. Oligonucleotides that are uniformly modified or modified on the 3′ end (gapmers or 3′-hemimers) (Fig. 6) with nuclease-resistant modification have the potential to exhibit increased oral bioavailability. This was demonstrated for both backbone modifications (methylphosphonates) and for sugar-modified (2′-O-methyl) oligonucleotides (85,139). We have found that 2′-O-methoxyethyl modified oligonucleotides also exhibit increased oral absorption compared to phosphorothioate oligodeoxynucleotides (unpublished data).

The physicochemical properties of phosphorothioate oligodeoxynucleotides present a significant barrier to their GI absorption into the systemic circulation or the lymphatics. These factors include their large size and molecular weight (i.e., up to 6.5 kDa for 20-mers), hydrophilic nature (log $D_{o/W}$ approximating −3.5) and multiple ionization pk_as (e.g., unpublished titration data, using a Sirius GlpKa instrument on a 20-mer sequence, noted over 17 pk_as for phosphorothioate oligodeoxynucleotide and over 32 pk_as) for the 2′-O-methoxyethyl hemi-mer form. The use of formulations can improve upon gastrointestinal permeability. Oligonucleotide drug formulations designed to improve oral bioavailability need to consider the mechanism of oligonucleotide absorption—either paracellular via the epithelial tight junctions or transcellular by direct passage through the lipid membrane bilayer. By using paracellular and transcellular models appropriate for water-soluble hydrophilic macromolecules, it was determined that oligonucleotides predominantly traverse GI epithelium via the paracellular route. In this regard, formulation design considerations involve the selection of those penetration enhancers (PEs) facilitate paracellular transport and meet other formulation criteria, including suitable biopharmaceutics, safety considerations, manufacturability, physical and chemical stability, and practicality of the product configuration (i.e., regarding production costs, dosing regimen, and patient compliance). Work is in progress optimizing oligonucleotide chemistry with various permeation enhancers. Preliminary data are encouraging and support continued investment of resources in this endeavor.

E. Liposome Formulations

Liposome formulations of antisense oligonucleotides offer several potential advantages over saline phosphorothioate oligodeoxynucleotides including (a) decreased toxicity, (b) tissue alteration and cellular distribution, and (c) a more convenient dose schedule for the patient. Interesting progress has been reported regarding the passive targeting of oligonucleotides to specific tissues using liposome-encapsulated therapeutics. Accumulation at sites of infection, inflammation, and tumor growth have been attributed to increased circulation times of the se materials and the leaky vasculatures associated with these processes (140,141). One caution regarding these observations is worth noting. Since the mononuclear phagocyte system (MPS) is largely responsible for clearing these materials from circulation, misleading data regarding circulation time may be obtained in species with less-evolved systems (e.g., rodents).

Cationic liposomes bind to oligonucleotides due to the electrostatic interaction between positively charged head groups on lipids and negatively charged phosphates on oligonucleotides. Using the technique of complexation, all the oligonucleotide can be entrapped and purification is not required. The utility of in vivo delivery of oligonucleotides using cationic lipid is limited due to sequestration of material in lung and the RES system (142,143). Additionally, interaction of the complex with blood components leads to serum sensitivity and cytotoxicity (144,145).

There are few examples of oligonucleotide delivery by anionic or charge-neutral liposomes. Oligonucleotides encapsulated into cardiolipin-containing anionic liposomes were shown to be taken up 7–18 times more in human T leukemia and ovarian carcinoma cells in vitro. The intracellular release of oligonucleotides was also facilitated and the majority of oligonucleotide was delivered into liposomes (146,147). Methylphosphonate analogs were incorporated into DPPC-containing liposomes and targeted against the Bcr-abl neogene found in chronic myelogenous leukemia (CML). The liposomal-encapsulated oligonucleotides inhibited the growth of CML cells (148). Cellular uptake of oligonucleotides against epidermal growth factor (EGF) encapsulated in DPPC:CHOL liposome containing folate was 9 times higher than nonfolate liposomes and 16 times higher than unencapsulated liposomes (149). There are two limitations to intracellular delivery of oligonucleotides by anionic or neutral liposomes; not all cells take up particulate matter, and these liposomes have low encapsulation efficiency.

There is only one report of using anionic liposomes in vivo to deliver oligonucleotides. Ponnappa et al. described liposomes consisting of DPPC:CHOL:DMPG targeted towards Kupffer cells (150). In this study, greater than 65%

of the liver associated oligonucleotide was found in Kupffer cells.

Conjugation of antibodies to liposomes have been used for targeting of oligonucleotides to specific targets (151). Problems with the approach include the inhibition of cellular uptake by the high molecular weight antibody, cost, and poor encapsulation efficiency.

The primary mechanism for cell internalization of neutral liposomes is by endocytosis with the vesicles and their contents delivered to lysozomes (152). pH-sensitive liposomes have been designed to fuse with the endosomes at low endosomal pH and empty their content into cytosol. These pH-sensitive liposomes have been used to deliver antisense oligonucleotides. pH-sensitive liposomes composed of oleic acid: DOPE:Chol encapsulating antisense oligonucleotide targeted against friend retrovirus inhibited the viral spreading, whereas free oligonucleotide and non–pH-sensitive liposomes were ineffective (153,154). pH-sensitive liposomes encapsulating the anti-env oligonucleotide were found to inhibit viral spread at low concentration in infected Dunni cells (155). The major limitation of pH-sensitive liposomes in vivo is their instability in plasma (156,157). This problem was overcome by adding PEG-PE to the formulation (158). PEG-PE is thought to coat the surface of liposomes, thereby preventing the interaction of liposomes with blood components. This reduced interaction leads to increased stability and plasma half-life of liposomes. The pH-sensitive liposomes composed of CHEMS-:DOPE:PEG-PE when injected intravenously into rats had similar pharmacokinetics parameters as non–pH-sensitive sterically stabilized liposomes. The regular pH-sensitive liposomes without PEG-PE were cleared rapidly from the circulation.

Looking past the question of uptake, a novel approach to releasing endosomal contents into the cytoplasm after uptake has been reported (159). A 58 kDa protein isolated from *Listeria monocytogenes* was incorporated into pH-sensitive fluorescent dye. As soon as the endosome began to acidify, the liposome/endosome contents were released into the cytosol. As with the other delivery systems mentioned above, the eventual usefulness of a particular approach will be determined in the near future as we further define the mechanisms and governing restrictions for the inter- and intracellular trafficking of oligonucleotides.

VII. CLINICAL EXPERIENCE WITH ANTISENSE OLIGONUCLEOTIDES

Twelve different antisense oligonucleotides are currently in clinical trials or approved for use in humans (Table 1). Like any other class of drugs, it can be expected that there will be failures in the clinic for a variety of reasons, such as lack of efficacy, marketing consideration, and toxicity. It is hoped that because of the generic pharmacokinetics and chemical class-specific toxicity that the failure rates for antisense oligonucleotides will be lower than for other classes of agents. However, this remains to be seen.

A. Use of Antisense Oligonucleotides as Antiviral Therapy

The most advanced antisense product is Vitravene™ (fomivirsen, ISIS 2922), which is marketed in the United States for the treatment of patients with CMV retinitis. Fomivirsen was identified from a screen of a series of phosphorothioate oligodeoxynucleotides targeting human cytomegalovirus (HCMV) DNA polymerase gene or RNA transcripts of the major immediate-early regions 1 and 2 (IE1 and IE2) (160). Fomivirsen is a 21-mer phosphorothioate oligodeoxynucleotide targeting the coding region of the immediate early 2 gene. Fomivirsen inhibits viral protein expression, as measured by an ELISA detecting a HCMV late protein product, in fibroblasts with an EC_{50} value of 0.1 μM. Noncomplementary phosphorothioate oligodeoxynucleotides exhibit an EC_{50} value of 2 μM, 20-fold higher than fomivirsen. In a plaque reduction assay, fomivirsen exhibited an IC_{70} value of 0.1 μM, while a control oligonucleotide exhibited an IC_{70} value of 2 μM. These data suggest that HCMV infection of human dermal fibroblast can be inhibited nonspecifically by higher concentrations of phosphorothioate oligodeoxynucleotides, however, fomivirsen is approximately 20-fold more effective than nonspecific oligonucleotides. Fomivirsen reduced IE1 and IE2 proteins in infected cells, as did control oligonucleotides at 10-fold higher concentrations. As the IE1 and IE2 gene products arise from a common pre-mRNA, these results suggest that the oligonucleotide hybridizes to the pre-mRNA. Deletion of sequences from the 5′ and/or 3′ end of the oligonucleotides reduced antiviral activity, while introduction of mismatches in the interior of the oligonucleotide did not significantly reduce antiviral activity, although they did reduce hybridization to the target RNA. These data suggest that the antiviral activity of fomivirsen may not be due entirely to an antisense effect. To address this issue in more detail, U373 cells permanently transfected with the IE72 or IE55 polypeptides (derived from the IE1 and IE2 genes, respectively) were treated with fomivirsen (161). Fomivirsen reduced IE55 but not IE72 protein or RNA levels in a sequence-specific manner, suggesting that reduction of IE55 expression occurs by an RNase H-dependent mechanism. Because the construct used to express IE72 protein does not contain the fomivirsen-binding site, these data would support the idea that fomivirsen reduces IE55 expression by an antisense mechanism of action. The antiviral activity of fomivirsen was not due to immune stimulation by the CpG motifs in the oligonucleotide (112), as methylation of all of the cytosines or only two cytosines in the CpG motifs did not reduce antiviral activity. These studies in aggregate suggest that fomivirsen is a potent inhibitor of CMV replication that is capable of inhibiting viral gene expression by an antisense mechanism of action, but that it also may inhibit viral replication by a nonantisense mechanism of action at higher concentrations. Whether both mechanisms of action are operational in the clinic remains to be elucidated.

Fomivirsen is approved for the local treatment of CMV retinitis in patients with acquired immunodeficiency syndrome (AIDS) who are intolerant of or have a contraindication to other treatments of CMV retinitis. The recommended dose is 330 μg every other week for two doses and then a maintenance dose administered every 4 weeks given as an intravitreal injection. The most frequently observed adverse event reported for fomivirsen is ocular inflammation (uveitis) including iritis and vitritis. Ocular inflammation has been reported to occur in approximately 25% of patients. Topical corticosteroids have been useful in treating the ocular inflammation. Open-label, controlled clinical studies have been performed evaluating the safety and efficacy of fomivirsen in newly diagnosed CMV retinitis patients. Based upon assessment of fundus photographs, the median time to progression was approximately 80 days for patients treated with fomivirsen compared to 2 weeks for patients not receiving treatment. Although the market for CMV retinitis is relatively small, this drug represents an important validation for the technology.

ISIS 13312 is a second-generation chimeric derivative of ISIS 2922 containing 2′-O-methoxylethyl modifications on the 5′ and 3′ ends with a central DNA gap. As previously discussed, 2′-O-methoxyethyl–modified oligonucleotides exhibit increased potency, longer duration of action, and decreased immune stimulation compared to phosphorothioate oligodeoxynucleotides (13,87). By maintaining a central DNA gap, the oligonucleotide still supports RNase H hydrolysis of the target mRNA. The longer duration of action is especially attractive for an intravitreal product, in that less frequent administration should be possible. Phase I clinical trials have been initiated for ISIS 13312.

Gem 132, a second-generation chimeric molecule targeting the HCMV UL36 gene product, is a 20-mer oligonucleotide containing two 2′-O-methyl nucleosides on the 5′ end of the molecule and four 2′-O-methyl nucleosides on the 3′ end, with the center 14 residues being oligodeoxynucleotides (162). The 2′-O-methyl residues also confer increased hybridization affinity and increased nuclease resistance, while the center oligodeoxynucleotide residues support RNase H activity. Gem 132 is being evaluated in CMV retinitis patients as both an intravenous infusion and a direct intravitreal injection. In healthy volunteers, single 2-hour infusions of GEM 132 were administered at doses ranging form 0.125 to 0.5 mg/kg. Similar to phosphorothioate oligodeoxynucleotides, the plasma pharmacokinetics of GEM 132 were nonlinear with respect to dose. As a single dose up to 0.5 mg/kg, GEM 132 was well tolerated in normal volunteers, with headache being the most frequently reported side effect (163).

Gem 91, a 25-mer phosphorothioate oligodeoxynucleotide, was designed to hybridize to a conserved region of the *gag* region of HIV RNA (164). GEM 91 inhibits viral replication in short-term viral assays in a concentration-dependent manner, while a four- to fivefold higher concentration of a random mixture of 25-mer phosphorothioate oligodeoxynucleotides (complexity = 4^{25} unique molecules) was required to inhibit viral replication to a similar extent (165). Other studies have demonstrated that acute HIV viral assays are particularly sensitive to the nonantisense effect of phosphorothioate oligodeoxynucleotides (166–169). In chronic HIV assays, GEM91 suppressed viral replication for greater than 30 days, while the random mixture of oligodeoxynucleotides only suppressed viral replication for 10 days. GEM 91 was found to be effective against several viral isolates in primary lymphocytes and macrophages and exhibited selectivity in comparison to the random mixture. Because a random mixture of 4^{25} sequences was used as a control, it is difficult to conclude that GEM 91 inhibits viral replication in a sequence-specific manner. Based upon these data, it is likely that at least part of the antiviral activity exhibited by GEM 91 is due to a nonantisense effect.

Phase I/II clinical studies were initiated for GEM 91 in the United States and France (162). The study performed in the United States was a randomized double-blind placebo-controlled dose-escalating study in which GEM 91 was administered as a continuous intravenous infusion for 2 weeks, while in the French study GEM 91 was given as a 2-hour intravenous infusion every other day for 28 days. Dose levels up to 4.4 mg/kg/day were achieved in the continuous infusion trials, while dose levels of 3.0 mg/kg/day were reported for the intermittent infusion trial. Plasma half-lives for GEM 91 were biphasic with mean half-lives of 0.18 and 26.7 hours (162,170). Hybridon recently announced the termination of clinical studies with GEM 91 based on lack of efficacy as measured by viral burden and the development of thrombocytopenia in some of the patients.

B. Use of Antisense Oligonucleotides for Cancer Therapy

Preclinical studies with OL(1)p53, a 20-mer phosphorothioate oligodeoxynucleotide complementary to a portion in exon 10 of the p53 mRNA, inhibited proliferation of acute myelogenous leukemia cells in cell culture (80,171). Correspondingly, OL(1)p53 was found to reduce the level of p53 in leukemic cells, while a reverse sequence control failed to do so (80). A phase I study was conducted at the University of Nebraska Medical center in which OL(1)p53 was infused at doses ranging from 0.05 to 0.25 mg/kg/h for 10 days into patients with hematological malignancies. There were no apparent toxicities that could be directly attributed to the oligonucleotide. Two patients experienced a transient increase in hepatic transaminase concurrent with administration of the drug. In contrast to observations made with other phosphorothioate oligodeoxynucleotides, 17–59% of intact drug was detected in urine in this group of patients. There was an inverse correlation between plasma concentrations of oligonucleotide and cumulative leukemic growth of long-term marrow cultures. However, this correlation was not observed clinically as there were no morphological complete responses. These results provide evidence that OL(1)p53 was tolerated in leukemic patients. OL(1)p53 is no longer in active development.

Overexpression of *bcl-2* gene is common in several cancers, in particular non-Hodgkin's lymphoma, and may contribute to decreased sensitivity to chemotherapeutic agents (172,173). An 18-mer phosphorothioate antisense oligodeoxynucleotide targeting the translation initiation codon of the *bcl-2* gene was shown to inhibit the growth of lymphoma cells in SCID mice (174). Webb et al. conducted a phase I clinical trial of this oligonucleotide (Genta 3139) at the Royal Marsden Hospital in London (175). Genta 3139 was administered as a daily subcutaneous infusion for 14 days to patients with BCL-2–positive non-Hodgkin's lymphoma. The dose of the drug given ranged from 4.6 to 73.6 mg/m^2. Other than local inflammation at the site of infusion, no treatment-related side effects were noted. In two patients, tomography scans revealed reductions in tumor size with one complete response. In two additional patients the number of circulating lymphoma cells decreased during treatment. Reduced levels of bcl-2 protein expression in circulating lymphoma cells were detected in two out of five patients. These findings again demonstrate that phosphorothioate oligodeoxynucleotides can be safely administered to patients and also provide preliminary efficacy data with a bcl-2 antisense oligonucleotide. The bcl-2 antisense oligonucleotide is currently in phase II trials for the treatment of prostate tumor and lymphoma.

Downregulation of C-myb transcription factor occurs during differentiation of hematopoietic cells, and C-myb protein expression appears to be necessary for the proliferation of these cells in vitro (176). Inhibition of the colony-forming ability of normal bone progenitor cells has been demonstrated using phosphorothioate oligodeoxynucleotides targeting c-myb (177). This oligonucleotide also reduced the growth of primary AML and CML cultures and proliferation of a T-cell leukemia cell line (177,178). A phosphorothioate oligodeoxynucleotide version of the c-myb oligodeoxynucleotide inhibited the growth of K562 erythroleukemia cells in SCID mice and prolonged survival of animals treated with the oligonucleotide (179). Based upon preclinical activity, an ex vivo bone marrow–purging study was initiated at the University of Pennsylvania with eight patients. Human stem cells were incubated with the c-myb antisense oligonucleotide for 24 hours prior to marrow cryopreservation. Patients were reinfused with their marrow following chemotherapy. One patient failed to engraft and four of six patients had normal leukocyte counts 3 months after engraftment. In follow-up, one patient was in hematological remission at 18 months, a second had 80% normal metaphases at 2 years, and a third exhibited a minor response. In a parallel study, 17 CML patients (4 in chronic stage and 13 with blast crisis) received systemic infusions of the C-myb phosphorothioate oligodeoxynucleotide continuously for 7 days followed by a one-week drug-free period. No drug-related toxicities were reported, and one patient with CML in blast crisis appeared to revert to the chronic stage, surviving for 14 months (180). These preliminary results suggest that the C-myb phosphorothioate oligodeoxynucleotide may have utility for the treatment of hematological malignancies.

Protein kinase C (PKC) was originally identified as a serine/threonine kinase involved in mediating intracellular responses to a variety of growth factors, hormones, and neurotransmitters (181). Molecular cloning studies have revealed that PKC exists as a family of at least 11 closely related isozymes, which are subdivided on the basis of certain structural and biochemical similarities (181–183). Considerable experimental evidence exists for a role of PKC in some abnormal cellular process, such as inflammation, tumor promotion, and carcinogenesis (184). Antisense oligonucleotides have been identified that target individual members of the PKC family, both as research tools and as potential drugs (10,185–188). Antisense oligonucleotides that specifically inhibit expression of PKC-α either in mouse or in human cell lines have been used to identify cellular processes governed by this PKC isozyme (10,188–190).

The effects of the human specific PKC-α phosphorothioate oligodeoxynucleotide ISIS 3521/CGP 64128A on the growth of human tumor xenografts in nude mice have been examined. Analysis of PKC-α expression in the tumor tissue by immunohistochemistry revealed positive staining present in the cytoplasm and occasionally in the nuclei of tumor cells in animals treated with either saline or a scrambled control phosphorothioate oligodeoxynucleotide.

In contrast, tumors treated with ISIS 3521/CGP 64128A showed much reduced staining for PKC-α. In a second series of independent studies, ISIS 3521/CGP 64128A has been used to suppress the growth of U-87 glioblastoma tumor cells in nude mice (191). This cell line was chosen for study as it has previously been shown to be sensitive to growth inhibition by transfection with an antisense PKC-α cDNA. ISIS 3521/CGP 64128A reduced the growth of these tumor cells when implanted both subcutaneously and intracranially while the scrambled control compound failed to inhibit tumor growth. This resulted in a doubling in median survival time of the animals with intracranially implanted tumors, with 40% long-term survivors of the treated animals. Levels of both ISIS 3521/CGP 64128A and the scrambled control oligodeoxynucleotide within tumor tissue were determined by capillary gel electrophoresis and found to both be about 2 μM after 21 daily intraperitoneal doses of 20 mg/kg oligodeoxynucleotide. ISIS 3521/CGP 64128A also reduced the expression of PKC-α in the tumor tissue, but not PKC-ε or PKC-ζ.

Based on the available biological evidence implicating PKC in the pathogenesis of certain solid tumor types and the broad spectrum of antitumor activity of ISIS 3521/CGP 64128A in the nude mouse xenograft implant model, a phase I clinical trial was initiated by Novartis in collaboration with ISIS Pharmaceuticals, Inc. A variety of tumors were evaluated in the trial, which was recently completed. ISIS 3521/CGP 64128A was administered as a continuous 21-day infusion, then rested for 7 days. The cycle could be repeated if the treatments were tolerated and the tumor did not progress (192). In a preliminary report of the trial, one patient with colon cancer had stabilization of previous rising CEA for 4 months on treatment and one ovarian cancer patient had stabilization of an enlarging abdominal mass for 4 months. There were no grade 3 or grade 4 toxicities reported. One patient displayed transient thrombocytopenia and one patient exhibited leukopenia. Based upon promising clinical results in phase I studies and safety profiles, phase II studies of ISIS 3521/CGP64128A have been initiated as well as phase I studies in combination with standard chemotherapeutic agents.

The *raf* family of gene products also encode for serine/threonine-specific protein kinases that play a pivotal role in mitogenic signaling events (193–196). There are three known isozymes of *raf* kinase: A-*raf*, B-*raf*, and C-*raf*. C-*raf* kinase associates with *ras* and transmits signals downstream of *ras* genes in the MAP kinase pathway. In addition, C-*raf* kinase has been shown to associate with *bcl*-2 and may also play a function in regulating apoptosis (197). These data suggest that inhibitors of C-*raf* kinase may be of value in regulating abnormal cell proliferation such as cancer.

A series of phosphorothioate oligodeoxynucleotides were designed and tested for inhibition of C-*raf* mRNA levels in A549 lung carcinoma cells (11). Reductions in C-*raf* mRNA levels were observed following treatment with only a small subset of the oligodeoxynucleotides targeting various regions of the C-*raf* kinase mRNA (198). Furthermore, for those oligonucleotides that did cause reduced C-*raf* mRNA levels, the degree of activity varied greatly. The most potent antisense inhibitor identified from this screen was ISIS 5132 (CGP 69846A), which targets the 3′-UTR of the C-*raf* message. The sequence requirements for inhibiting C-*raf* mRNA and protein expression have been examined thoroughly in vitro by comparing the dose-dependent effects of ISIS 5132 with a series of ''mismatched oligonucleotides'' containing between one and seven mismatches within the ISIS 5132 sequence (198). As expected for Watson-Crick–based hybridization, affinity decreased (measured by thermal melts) as the number of mismatches contained within the ISIS 5132 sequence increased. No cooperative binding was observed for oligonucleotides containing more than six mismatches. The IC_{50} for ISIS 5132–mediated reduction of C-*raf* mRNA levels in A549 tumor cell in culture is approximately 100 nM (11). Inhibition of C-*raf* mRNA levels gradually diminished as the number of mismatches within the ISIS 5132 sequence was increased. Incorporation of a single mismatch resulted in a two-fold loss in potency. No activity was observed for oligodeoxynucleotides containing more than four mismatches. In addition to sequence specificity, the effects of ISIS 5132 on other targets were examined to demonstrate the target specificity. ISIS 5132 failed to inhibit the expression of the structurally and functionally related A-*raf* kinase and B-*raf* kinase isozymes, nor did ISIS 5132 inhibit the expression of the housekeeping gene glyceraldehyde-3-phosphate-dehydrogenase (11,198,199).

The effects of antisense inhibitors targeted to C-*raf* kinase on downstream signaling events as well as on cellular proliferation have been examined (11,198–200). Inhibiting the expression of a single *raf* kinase isozyme can abrogate the MAP kinase phosphorylation cascade in response to specific growth factors and cytokines. C-*raf* protein levels were reduced by treating serum-starved A549 cells with ISIS 5132 for 48 hours, after which cells were stimulated with epidermal growth factor (EGF) or phorbol ester followed by quantitative measurements of MAP/ERK kinase activity. Reduction in C-*raf* protein levels by ISIS 5132 almost completely inhibited stimulation of MAP kinase activity by EGF but had no effect on MAP kinase stimulation by phorbol ester (201). The mismatched control ODN had no effect on MAP kinase stimulation by either agent. These results are consistent with a direct role of C-*raf* in mediating MAP kinase stimulation in response to EGF and demonstrates that activation of MAP kinase by phorbol ester, which requires the activity of protein kinase C (181), occurs independent of C-*raf* in A549 cells. These results also demonstrate that inhibition of a single *raf* kinase isozyme in the MAP kinase pathway is capable of abrogating MAP kinase stimulation almost completely despite the fact that levels of other *raf* kinase family members (A-*raf* and B-*raf*) are unchanged.

As discussed above, C-*raf* kinase plays a central role within the mitogen-activated protein kinase signal transduction pathway. The identification of mutations in *ras* gene products, which bind to C-*raf* kinase, resulting in transformation of cells, combined with the finding that C-*raf* kinase is overexpressed in some lung carcinomas suggest that inhibition of C-*raf* kinase expression may be beneficial in the treatment of some cancers. Isis Pharmaceuticals, Inc. and Novartis have also initiated two phase I studies for ISIS 5132/CGP69846A targeting human C-*raf* kinase. The study designs are similar to the ISIS 3521/CGP64128A trials in which the drug is administered either as a continuous 21-day infusion or as 2-hour infusions three times weekly for 21 days. Based upon safety and efficacy, a phase II trial for ISIS 5132/CGP69846A has also been initiated.

The discovery of viral oncogenes in the mid-1960s was a major breakthrough in understanding the molecular origins of cancer and directly led to the identification of the first human oncogene, *ras*, in 1982, (202). An antisense oligonucleotide targeting ha-*ras* gene product has begun clinical trials. ISIS 2503 targets the AUG translation initiation codon for the ha-*ras* gene product (203). Although the frequency of mutations in human cancers is significantly higher for the ki-*ras* gene product, we have found that antisense oligonucleotides targeting the ha-*ras* gene exhibit broader antitumor effects when evaluated in human tumor xenograft models. In fact the ha-*ras* antisense oligonucleotide was effective against human tumor xenografts known to contain a mutation in the ki-*ras* gene. A multicenter phase I trial against a broad spectrum of cancers has been completed. Patients received ISIS 2503 as a continuos intravenous infusion for 2 weeks followed by a one-week drug-free period. Patients will repeat the cycle as long as they tolerate the drug or tumors fail to respond to therapies. In a second study, the drug was administered on a more convenient schedule—a weekly 24-hour infusion of ISIS 2503. Similar to the PKC-α and C-*raf* kinase antisense oligonucleotides, the drug was tolerated and exhibited enough encouraging activity to warrant continuing phase II trials. Thus, a first-generation phosphorothioate oligodeoxynucleotide targeted to normal ha-*ras* is the first selective inhibitor of *ras* function to enter clinical trials.

Alterations in cellular cAMP concentrations have been associated with changes in cellular proliferation states. Two isoforms of the major cAMP receptors, cAMP-dependent protein kinases I and II, are distinguished by different regulatory subunits (RI and RII). Increased expression of the RI subunit of PKA I correlates with cellular proliferation and cellular transformation, while a decrease in the RI subunit and an increase in the RII subunit correlates with growth inhibition and cellular differentiation (204,205). To directly address the role of the RI subunit in cell growth and differentiation, an antisense oligonucleotide targeting the RI subunit was designed. This oligonucleotide at concentration of 15–30 μM inhibited growth of several human cell lines without signs of cytotoxicity (206–208). As expected, the phosphorothioate oligodeoxynucleotide was more effective than the phosphodiester version. A single injection of the RI subunit phosphorothioate oligodeoxynucleotide suppressed growth of a human colon carcinoma xenograft for a week (207). Tumors exhibited normal growth rates when treated with a control oligonucleotide. Examining levels of PKA-I activity in the tumor xenografts provided further support for an antisense mechanism. The antisense oligonucleotide–treated tumors exhibited loss of enzyme activity 24 hours after treatment. More recently a second-generation 2-O-methyl chimeric oligonucleotide targeting human PKA RI subunit has been described (209). This oligonucleotide was more effective than the first-generation oligonucleotide in suppressing growth of human tumor xenografts. Clinical trials have been initiated with a 2′-O-methyl chimeric PKA RI subunit antisense oligonucleotide (GEM 231) in the treatment of solid tumors.

C. Use of Antisense Oligonucleotides for the Treatment of Inflammatory Diseases

In addition to targeting gene products implicated in viral replication or cancer, antisense oligonucleotides have been used to inhibit the expression of gene products, which may have utility for the treatment of inflammatory diseases. Intercellular adhesion molecule 1 (ICAM-1) is a member of the immunoglobulin gene family expressed at low levels on resting endothelial cells and can be markedly upregulated in response to inflammatory mediators such as TNF-α, interleukin 1, and interferon-γ on a variety of cell types. ICAM-1 plays a role in the extravasation of leukocytes from the vasculature to inflamed tissue and activation of leukocytes in the inflamed tissue (210–212). ISIS 2302 was identified out of a screen of multiple first-generation phosphorothioate oligodeoxynucleotides targeting various regions of the human ICAM-1 (2,213). ISIS 2302 inhibits ICAM-1 expression by an RNase H–dependent mechanism of action (213). ISIS 2302 will selectively inhibit ICAM-

1 expression in a variety of cell types (213–215). Both sense and a variety of scrambled control oligonucleotides fail to inhibit ICAM-1 expression, including a two-base mismatch control (213–215). Treatment of endothelial cells with ISIS 2302 blocked adhesion of leukocytes, demonstrating that blocking expression of ICAM-1 will attenuate adhesion of leukocytes to activated endothelial cells (213). ISIS 2302 also blocked a one-way mixed lymphocyte reaction when the antigen-presenting cell was pretreated with ISIS 2302 to downregulate ICAM-1 expression prior to exposure to the lymphocyte (T. Vickers et al., unpublished). Thus, ISIS 2302 is capable of blocking leukocyte adhesion to activated endothelial cells and costimulatory signals to T lymphocytes, and both activities were predicted based on previous studies with monoclonal antibodies to ICAM-1.

To test the pharmacology of the human-specific antisense oligonucleotide, we have used experimental models in which immunocompromised mice contain human tissue xenografts. In one model we were able to demonstrate a role for ICAM-1 in metastasis of human melanoma cells to the lung of mice (214). A second study addressed the role of ICAM-1 in production of cytotoxic dermatitis (lichen planus) in SCID mice containing human skin xenografts (216). Upon engraftment of the human tissue, heterologous lymphocytes injected into the graft migrate into the epidermis (epidermaltropism) and produce a cytotoxic interaction between effector lymphocytes and epidermal cells. Systemic administration of ISIS 2302 inhibited ICAM-1 expression in the human graft, decreased the migration of lymphocytes into the epidermis, and prevented subsequent lesion formation. A sense control oligodeoxynucleotide failed to attenuate the responses. These data demonstrate that an ICAM-1 antisense oligonucleotide administered systemically can attenuate an inflammatory response in the skin.

ISIS 3082 and ISIS 9125 are 20-base phosphorothioate oligodeoxynucleotides that hybridize to an analogous region in the 3′-untranslated region of murine and rat ICAM-1 mRNA, respectively. Similar to ISIS 2302, ISIS 3082 and ISIS 9125 selectively inhibit ICAM-1 expression in mouse or rat cells by an RNase H–dependent mechanism (217). Rodent ICAM-1 antisense oligonucleotides have demonstrated activity in a mouse heterotopic heart transplant model (217), a mouse pancreatic islet transplant model (218), and rat heart and kidney transplants (231). The murine ICAM-1 antisense oligonucleotide has also shown activity in mouse models of pneumonia, colitis, and arthritis (109,219). Haller et al. independently used an ICAM-1 antisense oligonucleotide to decrease acute renal injury following ischemia in rats (220).

ISIS 2302, which targets human ICAM-1, is being developed jointly by Isis Pharmaceuticals, Inc. and Boehringer Ingelheim for the treatment of a variety of inflammatory disorders. Safety and pharmacokinetics of ISIS 2302 was established in a phase I study performed at Guy's hospital in normal volunteers (107). Volunteers were infused either over a 2-hour period with escalating single doses or as multiple doses given of ISIS 2302 or saline in a double-blinded trial. Brief dose-dependent increases in aPTT were seen at the time of peak plasma concentration, and clinically insignificant increases in C3a were seen after repeated 2.0 mg/kg doses. C5a, blood pressure, and pulse were unaffected by administration of ISIS 2302. No other adverse events or laboratory abnormalities related to the administration of the drug were noted. The C_{max} was linearly related to dose and occurred at the end of infusion. Plasma half-life was approximately 53 minutes. Nonlinear changes in AUC and volume of distribution were noted with increasing dose, suggesting that oligonucleotide disposition might have a saturable component. These data suggest that ISIS 2302 was well tolerated in normal volunteers and that the pharmacokinetics in humans was similar to that observed in nonhuman primates and rodents.

Small phase IIa studies (20–40 patients in each trial) have been initiated in rheumatoid arthritis, psoriasis, Crohn's disease, ulcerative colitis, and renal transplant. With the exception of the psoriasis study, the trials are placebo-controlled and double-blinded in which the drug is administered as a 2-hour intravenous infusion. As of this writing only the Crohn's disease trial has been completed. In that study, conducted by Dr. Bruce Yacyshyn at the University of Edmonton, patients were administered 0.5, 1.0, and 2.0 mg/kg of ISIS 2302 every other day for a total of 26 days. The response of the patients was not dose-dependent, probably due to the narrow dose range investigated and the small number of patients in the lower-dose groups (three each). Therefore, all ISIS 2302–treated patients were analyzed as one group. Complete response, defined as Crohn's disease activity index (CDAI) score $<$ 150, was observed in 7 of 15 patients treated with ISIS 2302 and 0 of 4 placebo patients (221). At the end of the study (6 months) five of the seven patients were still in remission and one patient had a CDAI score of 156. During the treatment phase of the study, steroid doses were fixed; afterwards the physician was allowed to adjust steroid dose based upon symptoms. There was a statistically significant decrease in steroid use in patients treated with ISIS 2302 compared to placebo-treated patients at the end of the study. Other than an expected increase in aPTT and mild facial flushing at the end of infusion in one patient, the drug was well tolerated. Based upon these promising data, a large multicenter phase IIb trial of ISIS 2302 in Crohn's disease has been initiated. Thus ICAM-1 antisense oligonucleotides may have therapeutic utility for the treatment of Crohn's disease.

VIII. CONCLUSION

As is to be expected with first-generation technology, undesirable properties have been identified for phosphorothioate oligodeoxynucleotides (222,223). Despite these limitations, it is possible to use phosphorothioate oligodeoxynucleotides to selectively inhibit the expression of a targeted RNA in cell culture and in vivo. The pharmacokinetics of phosphorothioate oligodeoxynucleotides are similar across species and do not appear to exhibit major sequence-specific differences. When dosed at high levels it is possible to identify toxicities in rodents and primates. However, at doses currently under evaluation in the clinic, phosphorothioate oligodeoxynucleotides have been well tolerated. In addition there is evidence that phosphorothioate oligodeoxynucleotides provide clinical benefits to patients with viral infections, cancer, and inflammatory diseases.

Extensive medicinal chemistry efforts have been successfully focused on identifying improved antisense oligonucleotides, which address some of these issues. There are at least four way in which chemistry can add value to first-generation drugs: by increasing potency, decreasing toxicity, altering pharmacokinetics, and lowering costs. For example, numerous modified oligonucleotides have been identified that have a higher affinity for target RNA than phosphorothioate oligodeoxynucleotides (49,87,224–227). Oligonucleotide modifications have been identified that exhibit increased resistance to serum and cellular nucleases, enabling use of oligonucleotides that do not have phosphorothioate linkages. The tissue distribution of oligonucleotides may be altered with either chemical modifications or formulations (85,139,142,228,229). Preliminary data also suggest that oral delivery of antisense oligonucleotides may be feasible (85). Finally, a number of modified oligonucleotides have been described that potentially exhibited less toxicity than first-generation phosphorothioate oligodeoxynucleotides (90,92,118,230). However, because experience with these modified oligonucleotides is rather limited, it remains to be seen whether they will have a distinct toxicity profile.

Formulations of first- or second-generation oligonucleotides appear to further broaden the utility of the technology. In particular, nonparenteral formulation offers significant advantages for the treatment of chronic non–life-threatening disease. Topical formulations are showing promise in preclinical models of inflammatory diseases. Studies examining oral delivery of oligonucleotides suggest that this route of administration may be feasible, which would dramatically increase the utility of the technology.

In conclusion, first-generation phosphorothioate oligodeoxynucleotides have proven to be valuable pharmacological tools for the researcher and have produced new therapies for the patient. Identification of improved second- and third-generation oligonucleotides with novel formulation should better therapies for patients.

REFERENCES

1. Watson JD, Crick FHC. Nature 1953; 171:737.
2. Chiang M-Y, Chan H, Zounes MA, Freier SM, Lima WF, Bennett CF. J Biol Chem 1991; 266:18162–18171.
3. Monia BP, Lesnik EA, Gonzalez C, Lima WF, McGee D, Guinosso CJ, Kawasaki AM, Cook PD, Freier SM. J Biol Chem 1993; 268:14514–14522.
4. Giles RV, Spiller DG, Tidd DM. Antisense Res Dev 1995; 5:23–31.
5. Condon TP, Bennett CF. J Biol Chem 1996; 271: 30398–30403.
6. Crouch RJ. New Biol 1990; 2:771–777.
7. Torrence PF, Maitra RK, Lesiak K, Khamnei S, Zhou A, Silverman RH. Proc Natl Acad Sci USA 1993; 90: 1300–1304.
8. Wu H, Macleod RA, Lima WF, Crooke ST. J Biol Chem 1998; 273:2532–2542.
9. Chiang MY, Chan H, Zounes MA, Freier SM, Lima WF, Bennett CF. J Biol Chem 1991; 266:18162–18171.
10. Dean NM, McKay R, Condon TP, Bennett CF. J Biol Chem 1994; 269:16416–16424.
11. Monia BP, Johnston JF, Geiger T, Muller M, Fabbro D. Nature Med 1996; 2:668–675.
12. Helene C, Toulme J-J. Biochim Biophys Acta 1990; 1049: 99–125.
13. Baker BF, Lot SF, Condon TP, Cheng-Flournoy S, Lesnik E, Sasmor HM, Bennett CF. J Biol Chem 1997; 272: 11994–12000.
14. Chin DJ, Green GA, Zon G, Szoka FC, Jr., Straubinger RM. New Biol 1990; 2:1091–1100.
15. Leonetti JP, Mechti N, Degols G, Gagnor C, Lebleu B. Proc Natl Acad Sci USA 1991; 88:2702–2706.
16. Bennett CF, Chiang MY, Chan H, Shoemaker JE, Mirabelli CK. Mol Pharmacol 1992; 41:1023–1033.
17. Lorenz P, Baker BF, Bennett CF, Spector DL. Mol Biol Cell 1998; 9:1007–1023.
18. Dominski Z, Kole R. Proc Natl Acad Sci USA 1993; 90: 8673–8677.
19. Dominski Z, Kole R. Mol Cell Biol 1994; 14:7445–7454.
20. Sierakowska H, Sambade MJ, Agrawal S, Kole R. Proc Natl Acad Sci USA 1996; 93:12840–12844.
21. Hodges D, Crooke ST. Mol Pharmacol 1995; 48:905–918.
22. Taylor JK, Dean NM. Curr Opin Drug Disc Dev 1999; 2: 147–151.
23. Froehler BC, Jones RJ, Cao X, Terhorst TJ. Tetrahedon Lett 1993; 34:1003–1006.

24. Gutierrez AJ, Terhorst TJ, Matteucci MD, Froehler BC. J Am Chem Soc 1994; 116:5540–5544.
25. Guiterrez AJ, Froehler BC. Tetrahedron Lett 1996; 37: 3959–3962.
26. Lin KY, Pudlo JS, Jones RJ, Bischofberger N, Matteucci MD, Froehler BC. Bioorg Med Chem Lett 1999; 4: 1061–1064.
27. Buhr CA, Wagner RW, Grant D, Froehler BC. Nucleic Acids Res 1996; 24:2974–2980.
28. Seela F, Thomas H. Helv Chim Acta 1995; 78:94.
29. Seela F, Ramzaeva N, Zulauf M. Nucleosides Nucleotides 1997; 16:963–966.
30. Balow G, Mohan V, Lesnik EA, Johnston JF, Monia BP, Acevedo OL. Nucleic Acids Res 1998; 26:3350–3357.
31. Flanagan WM, Wagner RW, Grant D, Lin KY, Matteucci MD. Nat Biotechnol 1999; 17:48–52.
32. Lin K-Y, Jones RJ, Matteucci M. J Am Chem Soc 1995; 117:3873–3874.
33. Lin K-Y, Matteucci MD. J Am Chem Soc 1998; 120: 8531–8532.
34. Flanagan WM, Wolf JJ, Olson P, Grant D, Lin K-Y, Wagner RW, Matteucci MD. Proc Natl Acad Sci USA 1999; 96:3513–3518.
35. Ramasamy KS, Zounes M, Gonzalez C, Freier SM, Lesnik FA, Cummins LL, Griffey RH, Monia BP, Cook PD. Tetrahedron Lett 1999; 35:215–218.
36. Manoharan M, Ramasamy KS, Mohan V, Cook PD. Tetrahedron Lett 1996; 37:7675–7678.
37. Cook D. In: Crooke ST, ed. Antisense Research and Application. Berlin: Springer, 1998:51–102.
38. Egli M, Usman N, Rich A. Biochemistry 1993; 32: 3221–3237.
39. Tereshko V, Portmann S, Tay EC, Martin P, Natt F, Altmann K-H, Egli M. Biochemistry 1998; 37:10626–10634.
40. Egli M. Antisense Nucleic Acid Drug Dev 1998; 8: 123–128.
41. Prakash TP, Kawasaki AM, Vasquez G, Fraser A, Casper M, Cook PD, Manoharan M. Nucleosides Nucleotides. In press.
42. Inoue H, Hayase Y, Iwai S, Ohtsuke E. FEBS Lett 1987; 215:327–330.
43. Lima WF, Crooke ST. J Biol Chem 1997; 272: 27513–27516.
44. Lima WF, Mohan V, Crooke ST. J Biol Chem 1997; 272: 18191–18199.
45. Lima WF, Crooke ST. Biochemistry 1997; 36:390–398.
46. Lamond AI, Sproat BS. FEBS Lett 1993; 325:123–127.
47. Monia BP, Lesnik EA, Gonzalez C, Lima WF, McGee D, Guinosso CJ, Kawasaki AM, Cook PD, Freier SM. J Biol Chem 1993; 268:14514–14522.
48. Yu D, Iyer RP, Shaw DR, Liziewicz J, Li Y, Jiang Z, Roskey A, Agrawal S. Bioorg Med Chem 1996; 4: 1685–1692.
49. Matteucci M. Perspectives Drug Dis Des 1996; 4:1–16.
50. Crooke RM, Graham MJ, Cooke ME, Crooke ST. J Pharm Exp Ther 1995; 275:462–473.
51. Krieg AM. Clin Chem 1993; 39:710–712.
52. Stein CA, Tonkinson JL, Zhang L-M, Yakubov L, Gervasoni J, Taub R, Rotenberg SA. Biochemistry 1993; 32: 4855–4861.
53. Wu-Pong S, Weiss TL, Hunt CA. Pharm Res 1992; 9: 1010–1017.
54. Loke SL, Stein CA, Zhang XH, Mori K, Nakanishi M, Subasinghe C, Cohen JS, Neckers LM. Proc Natl Acad Sci USA 1989; 86:3474–3478.
55. Beltinger C, Saragovi HU, Smith RM, LeSauteur L, Shah N, DeDionisio L, Christensen L, Raible A, Jarett L, Gewirtz AM. J Clin Invest 1995; 95:1814–1823.
56. Iversen PL, Zhu S, Meyer A, Zon G. Antisense Res Dev 1992; 2:211–222.
57. Gao W-Y, Storm C, Egan W, Cheng Y-C. Mol Pharmacol 1993; 43:45–50.
58. Crooke RM, Graham MJ, Cooke ME, Crooke ST. J Pharmacol Exp Ther 1995; 275:462–473.
59. Delong R, Stephenson K, Loftus T, Fisher M, Alahari S, Nolting A, Juliano RL. J Pharm Sci 1997; 86:762–764.
60. Bongartz J-P, Aubertin A-M, Milhaud PG, Lebleu B. Nucleic Acids Res 1994; 22:4681–4688.
61. Leonetti JP, Degols G, Lebleu B. Bioconjug Chem 1990; 1:149–153.
62. Wyman TB, Nicol F, Zelphati O, Scaria PV, Plank C, Szoka FC, Jr. Biochemistry 1997; 36:3008–3017.
63. Benimetskaya L, Takle GB, Vilenchik M, Lebedeva I, Miller P, Stein CA. Nucleic Acids Res 1998; 26: 5310–5317.
64. Agrawal S, Temsamani J, Tang JY. Proc Natl Acad Sci USA 1991; 88:7595–7599.
65. Cossum PA, Sasmor H, Dellinger D, Truong L, Cummins L, Owens SR, Markham PM, Shea JP, Crooke S. J Pharmacol Exp Ther 1993; 267:1181–1190.
66. Graham MJ, Crooke ST, Monteith DK, Cooper SR, Lemonidis KM, Stecker KK, Martin MJ, Crooke RM. J Pharmacol Exp Ther 1998; 286:447–458.
67. Dean NM, McKay R. Proc Natl Acad Sci USA 1994; 91: 11762–11766.
68. Butler M, Stecker K, Bennett CF. Lab Invest 1997; 77: 379–388.
69. Plenat F, Klein-Monhoven N, Marie B, Vignaud J-M, Duprez A. Am J Pathol 1995; 147:124–135.
70. Benimetskaya L, Tonkinson JL, Koziolkiewicz M, Karwowski B, Guga P, Zeltser R, Stec W, Stein CA. Nucleic Acids Res 1995; 23:4239–4245.
71. Bijsterbosch MK, Manoharan M, Rump ET, De Vrueh RLA, van Veghel R, Tivel KL, Biessen EAL, Bennett CF, Cook PD, van Berkel TJC. Nucleic Acids Res 1997; 25: 3290–3296.
72. Steward A, Christian RA, Hamilton KO, Nicklin PL. Biochem Pharmacol 1997; 56:509–516.
73. Rappaport J, Hanss B, Kopp JB, Copeland TD, Bruggeman LA, Coffman TM, Klotman PE. Kidney Int 1995; 47: 1462–1469.
74. Sawai K, Takenori M, Takakura Y, Hashida M. Antisense Res Dev 1995; 5:279–287.

75. Phillips JA, Craig SJ, Bayley D, Christian RA, Geary R, Nicklin PL. Biochem Pharmacol 1997; 54:657–668.
76. Levin AA, Monteith DK, Leeds JM, Nicklin PL, Geary RS, Butler M, Templin MV, Henry SP. In: Crooke ST, ed. Antisense Research and Applications. Heidelberg: Springer-Verlag, 1998:169–216.
77. Geary RS, Leeds JM, Henry SP, Monteith DK, Levin AA. Anticancer Drug Des 1997; 12:383–393.
78. Leeds JM, Henry SP, Truong L, Zutshi A, Levin AA, Kornbrust D. Drug Metab Dispos 1997; 25:921–926.
79. Leeds JM, Henry SP, Bistner S, Scherrill S, Williams K, Levin AA. Drug Metab Dispos 1998; 26:670–675.
80. Bishop MR, Iversen PL, Bayever E, Sharp JG, Greiner TC, Copple BL, Ruddon R, Zon G, Spinolo J, Arneson M, Armitage JO, Kessinger A. J Clin Oncol 1996; 14: 1320–1326.
81. Cossum PA, Truong L, Owens SR, Markham PM, Shea JP, Crooke ST. J Pharmacol Exp Ther 1994; 269:89–94.
82. Nicklin IL, Craig SJ, Phillips JA. In: Crooke ST, ed. Antisense Research and Application. Berlin: Springer, 1998: 141–168.
83. Nicklin PL, Bayley D, Giddings J, Craig SJ, Cummins LL, Hastewell JG, Phillips JA. Pharm Res 1998; 15:583–591.
84. Agrawal S, Temsamani J, Galbraith W, Tang J. Clin Pharmacokinet 1995; 28:7–16.
85. Agrawal S, Zhang X, Lu Z, Zhao H, Tamburin JM, Yan J, Cai H, Diasio RB, Habus I, Jiang Z, Iyer RP, Yu D, Zhang R. Biochem Pharmacol 1995; 50:571–576.
86. Crooke ST, Graham MJ, Zuckerman JE, Brooks D, Conklin BS, Cummins LL, Greig MJ, Guinosso CJ, Kornbrust D, Manoharan M, Sasmor HM, Schleich T, Tivel KL, Griffey RH. J Pharmacol Exp Ther 1996; 277:923–937.
87. Altmann K-H, Dean NM, Fabbro D, Freier SM, Geiger T, Haner R, Husken D, Martin P, Monia BP, Muller M, Natt F, Nicklin P, Phillips J, Pieles U, Sasmor H, Moser HE. Chimia 1996; 50:168–176.
88. Agrawal S, Jiang Z, Zhao Q, Shaw D, Cai Q, Roskey A, Channavajjala L, Saxinger C, Zhang R. Proc Natl Acad Sci USA 1997; 94:2620–26225.
89. Galbraith WM, Hobson WC, Giclas PC, Schechter PJ, Agrawal S. Antisense Res Dev 1994; 4:201–206.
90. Henry SP, Zuckerman JE, Rojko J, Hall WC, Harman RJ, Kitchen D, Crooke ST. Anti-cancer Drug Des 1996; 12: 1–14.
91. Henry SP, Grillone L, Orr JL, Brunner RH, Kornbrust DJ. Toxicology 1997; 116:77–88.
92. Monteith DK, Henry SP, Howard RB, Flournoy S, Levin AA, Bennett CF, Crooke ST. Anti-Cancer Drug Des 1997; 12:421–432.
93. Henry SP, Taylor J, Midgley L, Levin AA, Kornbrust DJ. Antisense Nucleic Acid Drug Dev 1997; 7:473–481.
94. Henry SP, Novotny W, Leeds J, Auletta C, Kornbrust DJ. Antisense Nucleic Acid Drug Dev 1997; 7:503–510.
95. Henry SP, Grillone LR, Orr JL, Bruner RH, Kornbrust DJ. Toxicology 1997; 116:77–88.
96. Sarmiento UM, Perez JR, Becker JM, Narayanan R. Antisense Res Dev 1994; 4:99–107.
97. Henry SR, Giclas PC, Leeds J, Pangburn M, Auletta C, Levin AA, Kornbrust DJ. J Pharmacol Exp Ther 1997; 281:810–816.
98. Henry SP, Giclas PC, Leeds J, Pangburn M, Auletta C, Levin AA, Kornbrust DJ. J Pharmacol Exp Ther 1997; 281:810–806.
99. Wallace TL, Bazemore SA, Kornbrust DJ, Cossum PA. J Pharmacol Exp Ther 1996; 278:1306–1312.
100. Griffin LC, Toole JJ, Leung LLK. Gene 1993; 137:25–31.
101. Nicklin PL, Ambler J, Mitchelson A, Bayley D, Phillips JA, Craig SJ, Monia BP. Nucleosides Nucleotides 1997; 16:1145–1153.
102. Glover JM, Leeds JM, Mant TG, Amin D, Kisner DL, Zuckerman JE, Geary RS, Levin AA, Shanahan WR, Jr. J Pharmacol Exp Ther 1997; 282:1173–1180.
103. Henry SP, Bolte H, Auletta C, Kornbrust DJ. Toxicology 1997; 120:145–155.
104. Cornish KG, Iversen P, Smith L, Arneson M, Bayever E. Pharmacol Comm 1993; 3:239–247.
105. Black LE, Degeorge JJ, Cavagnaro JA, Jordan A, Ahn C-H. Antisense Res Dev 1994; 3:399–404.
106. Black LE, Farrelly JG, Cavagnaro JA, Ahn C-H, Degeorge JJ, Taylor AS, DeFelice AF, Jordan A. Antisense Res Dev 1995; 4:299–301.
107. Glover JM, Leeds LM, Mant TGK, Kisner DL, Zuckerman J, Levin AA, Shanahan WR, Jr. J Pharmacol Exp Ther 1997; 282:1173–1180.
108. Wallace TL, Bazemore SA, Kornbrust DJ, Cossum PA. J Pharmacol Exp Ther 1996; 278:1313–1317.
109. Bennett CF, Kornbrust D, Henry S, Stecker K, Howard R, Cooper S, Dutson S, Hall W, Jacoby HI. J Pharmacol Exp Ther 1997; 280:988–1000.
110. Monteith DK, Henry SP, Howard RB, Flournoy S, Levin AA, Bennett CF, Crooke ST Anticancer Drug Des 1997; 12:421–432.
111. Branda RF, Moore AL, Mathews L, McCormack JJ, Zon G. Biochem Pharmacol 1993; 45:2037–2043.
112. Krieg AM, Yi A-K, Matson S, Waldschmidt TJ, Bishop GA, Teasdale R, Koretzky GA, Klinman DM. Nature 1995; 374:546–549.
113. Yamamoto S, Yamamoto T, Kataoka T, Kuramoto E, Yano O, Tokunaga T. J Immunol 1992; 148:4072–4076.
114. Plenat F. Mol Med Today 1996; 2:250–257.
115. Oberbauer R, Schreiner GF, Meyer TW. Kidney Int 1995; 48:1226–1232.
116. Sands H, Gorey-Feret LJ, Cocuzza AJ, Hobbs FW, Chidester D, Trainor GL. Mol Pharmacol 1994; 45: 932–943.
117. Henry SP, Zuckerman JE, Rojko J, Hall WC, Harman RJ, Kitchen D, Crooke ST. Anticancer Drug Des 1997; 12: 1–14.
118. Zhao Q, Temsamani J, Iadarola PL, Jiang Z, Agrawal S. Biochem Pharm 1995; 51:173–182.
119. Holbrook KA, Wolff K. In: Fitzpatrick TB, et al., eds. Dermatology in General Medicine. New York: McGraw-Hill, 1993:97–145.

120. Lampe MA, Burlingame AL, Whitney J, Williams ML, Brown BE, Roitmen E, Elias PM. J Lipid Res 1983; 24: 120–130.
121. Yu WH, Kashani-Sabet M, Liggitt D, Moore D, Heath TD, Debs RJ. J Invest Dermatol 1999; 112:370–375.
122. Lee YM, Lee SH, Ko GI, Kim JB, Sohn DH. Arch Pharm Res 1996; 19:435–440.
123. Nolen HW, III, Catz P, Friend DR. Int J Pharm 1994; 107: 169–177.
124. Banga AK, Prausnitz MR. Trends Biotech 1998; 16: 408–412.
125. Brand RM, Haase K, Hannah TL, Iversen PL. J Invest Dermatol 1998; 111:1166–1171.
126. Brand RM, Wahl A, Iversen PL. J Pharm Sci 1998; 87: 49–52.
127. Regnier V, Le Doan T, Preat V. J Drug Targ 1998; 5: 275–289.
128. Roberts MS, Walker M. In: Walters CA, Hadgraft J, eds. Pharmaceutical Skin Penetration Enhancers. New York: Marcel Dekker, 1993:1–30.
129. Catz P, Friend DR. Pharm Res 1988; 6:s108.
130. Millns JL, Maibach HL. Arch Derm Res 1982; 272: 351–362.
131. Hadgraft J, Williams DG, Guy RH. In: Walters CA, Hadgraft J, eds. Pharmaceutical Skin Penetration Enhancers. New York: Marcel Dekker, 1993, pp 153–169.
132. Friend DR, Catz P, Heller J. J Controlled Rel 1989; 9: 33–41.
133. Martin GP. Pharmaceutical Skin Penetration Enhancers. In: Walters CA, Hadgraft J, eds. New York: Marcel Dekker, 1993:57–94.
134. Takayama K, Nagai T. Drug Dev Indust Pharm 1994; 20: 677–684.
135. Walters KA, Walker M, Olejnik O. J Pharm Pharmacol 1988; 40:525–529.
136. Michniak BB, Player MR, Chapman JM, Sowell JW. Int J Pharm 1993; 91:351–362.
137. Weiner N, Williams N, Birch G, Ramachandran C, Shipman C, Flynn G. Antimicrob Agents Chemother 1989; 33: 1217–1221.
138. Lieb LM, Flynn G, Weiner N. Pharm Res 1994; 11: 1419–1423.
139. Zhang R, Iyer RP, Yu D, Tan W, Zhang X, Lu Z, Zhao H, Agrawal S. J Pharmacol Exp Ther 1996; 278:971–979.
140. Lasic D, Needham D. Chem Rev 1995; 95:2601–2628.
141. Boman N, Bally M, Cullis P, Mayer L, Webb M. J Lipid Res 1995; 5:523–541.
142. Bennett CF, Zuckerman JE, Kornbrust D, Sasmor H, Leeds JM. and Crooke, ST. J Control Rel 1996; 41:121–130.
143. Litzinger DC, Brown JM, Wala I, Kaufman SA, Van GY, Farrell CL. and Collins D. Biochim Biophys Acta 1996; 1281:139–149.
144. Filion MC. and Phillips, NC. Int J Pharm 1998; 162: 159–170.
145. Senior JH, Trimble KR. and Maskiewicz R. Biochem Biophys Acta 1991; 1070:173–179.
146. Thierry AR. and Dritschilo, A. Nucleic Acids Res. 1992; 20:5691–5698.
147. Thierry AR, Rahman A. and Dritschilo, A. Biochem Biophys Res Commun 1993; 190:952–960.
148. Tari AM, Tucker SD, Deisseroth A, and Lopez-Berestein G. Blood 1994; 84:601–607.
149. Wang S, Lee RJ, Cauchon G, Gorenstein DG, Low PS. Proc Natl Acad Sci USA 1995; 92:3318–3322.
150. Ponnappa BC, Dey I, Tu G-c, Zhou F, Garver E, Cao Q-n, Israel Y. J Liposome Res 1998; 8:521–535.
151. Zelphati O, Zon G, Leserman L. Antisense Res Dev 1993; 3:323–338.
152. Zelphati O, Szoka F. J Controlled Rel 1996; 41:99–119.
153. Ropert C, Lavignon M, Dubernet C, Couvreur P, Malvy C. Biochem Biophys Res Comm 1992; 183:879–887.
154. Ropert C, Malvy C, Couvreur P. Pharm Res 1993; 10: 1427–1433.
155. De Oliviera MC, Fattal E, Ropert C, Malvy C, Couvreur P. J Controlled Rel 1997; 48:179–184.
156. Litzinger DC, Huang L. Biochim Biophys Acta 1992; 1113:201–207.
157. Chu CJ, Dijkstra J, Lai MZ, Hong K, Szoka FC. Pharm Res 1990; 7:824–834.
158. Slepushkin VA, Simoes S, Dazin P, Newman MS, Guo LS, Pedroso de Lima M, Duzgunes N. J Biol Chem 1997; 272:2382–2388.
159. Lee K, Oh Y, Portnoy D, Swanson J. J Biol Chem 1996; 271:7249–7252.
160. Azad RF, Driver VB, Tanaka K, Crooke RM, Anderson KP. Antimicrob Agents Chemother 1993; 37:1945–1954.
161. Anderson KP, Fox MC, Brown-Driver V, Martin MJ, Azad RF. Antimicrob Agents Chemother 1996; 40:2004–2011.
162. Kilkuskie RE, Field AK. Adv Pharmacol 1997; 40: 437–483.
163. Guinot P, Martin R, Bonvoisin B, Toneatt C, Bourque A, Cohen A, Dvorchik B, Schechter P. 4th Conference Retroviruses and Opportunistic Infections, 1997, Washington D.C. A742.
164. Agrawal S, Tang JY. Antisense Res Dev 1992; 2:261–266.
165. Lisziewicz J, Sun D, Weichold FF, Thierry AR, Lusso P, Tang J, Gallo RC, Agrawal S. Proc Natl Acad Sci USA 1994; 91:7942–7946.
166. Agrawal S, Ikeuchi T, Sun D, Sarin PS, Konopka A, Maizel J, Zamecnik PC. Proc Natl Acad Sci USA 1989; 86:7790–7794.
167. Lisziewicz J, Sun D, Metelev V, Zamecnik P, Gallo RC, Agrawal S. Proc Natl Acad Sci USA 1999; 90:3860–3864.
168. Stein CA, Tonkinson JL, Yakubov L. Pharmacol Ther 1991; 52:365–384.
169. Stein CA, Neckers M, Nair BC, Mumbauer S, Hoke G, Pal R. J AIDS 1991; 4:686–693.
170. Zhang R, Yan J, Shahinian H, Amin G, Lu Z, Liu T, Saag MS, Jiang Z, Temsamani J, Martin RR, Schechter PJ, Agrawal S, Diasio RB. Clin Pharmacol Ther 1995; 58: 44–53.
171. Bayever E, Iversen P. Hematol Oncol 1994; 12:9–14.

172. Reed JC, Cuddy M, Haldar S, Croce C, Nowell P, Makover D, Bradley K. Proc Natl Acad Sci USA 1990; 87: 3660–3664.
173. Reed JC. Curr Opin Oncol 1995; 7:541–546.
174. Cotter FE, Johnson P, Hall P, Pocock C, Al Mahdi N, Cowell JK, Morgan G. Oncogene 1994; 9:3049–3055.
175. Webb A, Cunningham D, Cotter F, Clarke PA, di Stefano F, Corbo M, Dziewanowska Z. Lancet 1997; 349: 1137–1141.
176. Westin EH, Gallo RC, Arya SE, Eva A, Souza LM, Baluda MA, Aaronson SA, Wong-Staal F. Proc Natl Acad Sci USA 1982; 79:2194–2199.
177. Calabretta B, Sims RB, Valtieri M, Caracciolo D, Szczylik C, Venturelli D, Ratajczak M, Beran M, Gewirtz AM. Proc Natl Acad Sci USA 1991; 88:2351–2355.
178. Anfossi G, Gewirtz AM, Calabretta B. Proc Natl Acad Sci USA 1989; 86:3379–3384.
179. Ratajczak MZ, Kant JA, Luger SM, Hijiya N, Zhang J, Zon G, Gewirtz AM. Proc Natl Acad Sci USA 1992; 89: 11823–11827.
180. Gewirtz AM. Anti-cancer Drug Des 1997; 12:341–358.
181. Nishizuka Y. Science 1992; 258:607–614.
182. Asaoka Y, Nakamura S, Yoshida K, Nishizuka Y. Trends Biochem Sci 1992; 17:414–417.
183. Dekker LV, Parker PJ. Trends Biochem Sci 1994; 19: 73–77.
184. Yuspa SH. Cancer Res 1994; 54:1178–1189.
185. Dean NM, McKay R. Proc Natl Acad Sci USA 1994; 91: 11762–11766.
186. Liao D-F, Monia BP, Dean N, Berk BC. J Biol Chem 1997; 272:6146–6150.
187. McKay RM, Cummins LL, Graham MJ, Lesnick EA, Owens SR, Winniman M, Dean NM. Nucleic Acid Res 1996; 24:411–417.
188. Levesque L, Dean NM, Sasmor H, Crooke ST. Mol Pharmacol 1996; 51:209–216.
189. Lee Y-S, Dlugosz AA, McKay R, Dean NM, Yuspa SH. Mol Carcinogen 1996; 18:44–53.
190. Levesque L, Crooke ST. J Pharmacol Exp Ther. 1998; 287:425–434.
191. Yazaki T, Ahmad S, Chahlavi A, Zylber-Katz E, Dean NM, Rabkin SD, Martuza RI, Glazer RI. Mol Pharmacol 1996; 50:236–242.
192. Sikic BI, Yuen AR, Halsey J, Fisher GA, Pribble JP, Smith RM, Dorr A. Proc Am Soc Clin Oncol 1997; 16:212a.
193. Rapp UR. Oncogene 1991; 6:495–600.
194. Williams NG, Roberts TM, Li P. Proc Natl Acad Sci USA 1992; 89:2922–2926.
195. Howe IR, Leevers SJ, Gomez N, Nakielny S, Cohen P, Marshall CJ. Cell 1992; 71:335–342.
196. Daum G, Eisenmann-Tappe I, Fries H-W, Troppmair J, Rapp UR. Trends Biol Sci 1994; 19:279–283.
197. Wang H-G, Miyashita T, Takayama S, Sato T, Torigoe T, Krajewski S, Tanaka S, Hovey L, Troppmair J, Rapp UR, Reed JC. Oncogene 1994; 9:2751–2756.
198. Monia BP, Sasmor H, Johnston JF, Freier SM, Lesnik EA, Muller M, Geiger T, Altmann K-H, Moser H, Fabbro D. Proc Natl Acad Sci USA 1996; 93:15481–15484.
199. Cioffi CL, Garay M, Johnson JF, McGraw K, Boggs RT, Hreniuk D, Monia BP. Mol Pharm 1997; 51:383–389.
200. Schulte TW, Blagosklonny MV, Romanova L, Mushinski JF, Monia BP, Johnston JF, Nguyen P, Trepel J, Neckers LM. Mol Cell Biol 1996; 16:5839–5845.
201. Monia BP. In: Stein C, Krieg A, eds. Applied Antisense Oligonucleotide Technology. New York: John Wiley and Sons. 1998, pp 245–261.
202. Chang EH, Furth ME, Scolnick EM, Lowy DR. Nature 1982; 297:479–483.
203. Monia BP, Johnston JF, Ecker DJ, Zounes M, Lima WF, Freier SM. J Biol Chem 1992; 267:19954–19962.
204. Lohmann SM, Walter U. In: Greengard P, Robison PA, eds. Advances in Cyclic Nucleotide and Protein Phosphorylation Research. Vol. 18 New York: Raven, 1984: 63–117.
205. Cho-Chung YS. Cancer Res 1990; 43:2736–2740.
206. Tortora G, Yokozaki H, Pepe S, Clair T, Cho-Chung YS. Proc Natl Acad Sci USA 1991; 88:2011–2015.
207. Nesterova M, Cho-Chung YS. Nature Med 1995; 1: 528–533.
208. Yokozaki H, Budillon A, Tortora G, Meissner S, Beaucage SL, Miki K, Cho-Chung YS. Cancer Res 1993; 53: 868–872.
209. Cho-Chung YS. In: Stein CA, Krieg AM, eds. Applied Antisense Oligonucleotide Technology. New York: Wiley-Liss, 1998:263–281.
210. Dustin ML, Springer TA. Annu Rev Immunol 1991; 9: 27–66.
211. Springer TA. Nature 1990; 346:425–434.
212. Butcher EC. Cell 1991; 67:1033–1036.
213. Bennett CF, Condon T, Grimm S, Chan H, Chiang M-Y. J Immunol 1994; 152:3530–3540.
214. Miele ME, Bennett CF, Miller BE, Welch DR. Exp Cell Res 1994; 214:231–241.
215. Nestle FO, Mitra RS, Bennett CF, Chan H, Nickoloff BJ. J Invest Dermatol 1994; 103:569–575.
216. Christofidou-Solomidou M, Albelda SM, Bennett FC, Murphy GF. Am J Pathol 1997; 150:631–639.
217. Stepkowski SM, Tu Y, Condon TP, Bennett CF. J Immunol 1994; 153:5336–5346.
218. Katz SM, Browne B, Pham T, Wang ME, Bennett CF, Stepkowski SM, Kahan BD. Transplant Proc 1995; 27: 3214.
219. Kumasaka T, Quinlan WM, Doyle NA, Condon TP, Sligh J, Takei F, Beaudet AL, Bennett CF, Doerschuk CM. J Clin Invest 1996; 97:2362–2369.
220. Haller H, Dragun D, Miethke A, Park JK, Weis A, Lippoldt A, Grob V, Luft FC. Kidney Int 1996; 50:473–480.
221. Yacyshyn BR, Bowen-Yacyshyn MB, Jewell L, Tami JA, Bennett CF, Kisner DL, Shanahan WR. Gastroenterology 1998; 114:1133–1142.
222. Stein CA. TIBTECH 1996; 14:147–149.
223. Crooke ST, Bennett CF. Ann Rev Pharmacol Toxicol 1996; 36:107–129.
224. Kawasaki AM, Casper MD, Freier SM, Lesnik EA, Zounes MC, Cummins LL, Gonzalez C, Cook PD. J Med Chem 1993; 36:831–841.

225. Wagner RW, Matteucci MD, Lewis JG, Gutierrez AJ, Moulds C, Froehler BC. Science 1993; 260:1510–1513.
226. Nielsen PE, Egholm M, Berg RH, Buchardt O. Science 1991; 254:1497–1500.
227. Milligan JF, Matteucci MD, Martin JC. J Med Chem 1993; 36:1923–1937.
228. Crooke ST, Graham MJ, Zuckerman JE, Brooks D, Conklin BS, Cummins LL, Greig MJ, Guinosso CJ, Kornbrust D, Manoharan M, Sasmor HM, Schleich T, Tivel KL, Griffey RH. J Pharmacol Exp Ther 1996; 277:923–937.
229. Zhang R, Lu Z, Zhao H, Zhang X, Diasio RB, Habus L, Jiang Z, Iyer RP, Yu D, Agrawal S. Biochem Pharm 1995; 50:545–556.
230. Boggs RT, McGraw K, Condon T, Flournoy S, Villiet P, Bennett CF, Monia BP. Antisense Nucleic Acid Drug Dev 1997; 7:461–471.
231. Stepkowski SM, Wang M-e, Condon TP, Cheng-Flournoy S, Stecker K, Graham M, Qu XQ, Tian L, Chen W, Kahan BD, Bennett CF. Transplantation 1998; 66:699–707.

16

Selectable Markers for Gene Therapy

Michael M. Gottesman, Thomas Licht,* Yi Zhou, Caroline Lee,† Tzipora Shoshani-Kupitz,‡ Peter Hafkemeyer,¶ Christine A. Hrycyna, and Ira Pastan
National Cancer Institute, National Institutes of Health, Bethesda, Maryland

I. INTRODUCTION

A. The Use and Choice of Selectable Markers

One of the major problems with current approaches to gene therapy is the instability of expression of genes transferred into recipient cells. Although in theory homologous recombination or use of artificial chromosomes can stabilize sequences with wild-type regulatory regions, such approaches to gene therapy are not yet feasible and may not be efficient for some time to come. In most high-efficiency DNA transfer in current use in intact organisms, selectable markers must be used to maintain transferred sequences; in the absence of selection the transferred DNAs or their expression are rapidly lost.

There are several different selectable markers that might be used for in vivo selection, including genes whose expression has been associated with resistance of cancers to anticancer drugs. Examples include (a) methotrexate resistance due to mutant dihydrofolate reductase (DHFR) (1), (b) Alkylating agent resistance due to expression of methylguanine methyltransferase (MGMT) (2), and (c) the expression of the multidrug transporting proteins P-glycoprotein (P-gp, the product of the *MDR*1 gene) (3) and multidrug-resistance associated protein (MRP) (4). In this chapter, we will detail our experience with the *MDR*1 gene.

The resistance of many cancers to anticancer drugs is due, in many cases, to the overexpression of the human multidrug resistance gene *MDR*1 (3,5) and perhaps to MRP (6). *MDR*1 encodes the multidrug transporter, or P-glycoprotein (P-gp). P-gp is a 12-transmembrane-domain glycoprotein composed of two homologous halves, each containing six transmembrane (TM) domains and one ATP binding/utilization site. P-gp recognizes a large number of structurally unrelated hydrophobic and amphipathic molecules, including many chemotherapeutic agents, and removes them from the cell via an ATP-dependent transport process.

*MDR*1 has many obvious advantages for use as a selectable marker in gene therapy. It is a cell surface protein that can be easily detected by FACS or immunohistochemistry. Cells expressing P-gp on their surfaces can be enriched using cell sorting or magnetic bead panning technologies. The very broad range of cytotoxic substrates recognized by P-gp makes it a pharmacologically flexible system, allowing the investigator to choose among many different selection regimens with differential toxicity for different tissues and different pharmacokinetic properties. Furthermore, as will be discussed in detail in this chapter, P-gp can be mutationally modified to increase resistance to specific substrates and alter inhibitor sensitivity. Hematopoietic cells appear to tolerate relatively high levels of P-gp expression without major effects on differentiated function (7).

Current affiliation:
* Technical University of Munich, Munich, Germany.
† National University of Singapore, Singapore.
‡ QBI Enterprises Ltd., Nes Ziona, Israel.
¶ University Hospital Freiburg, Freiburg, Germany.

B. Lessons from Transgenic and Knockout Mice

Two lines of evidence support the concept of using *MDR*1 as a selectable marker in human gene therapy. Transgenic mice expressing the *MDR*1 gene in their bone marrow are resistant to the cytotoxic effects of many different anticancer drugs (7–9). *MDR*1 transgenic bone marrow can be transplanted into drug-sensitive mice, and the transplanted marrow is resistant to cytotoxic drugs (10). Mice transplanted with bone marrow transduced with the human *MDR*1 cDNA and exposed to taxol show specific enrichment of the *MDR*1-transduced cells (11–13), and this transduced marrow can be serially transplanted and remains drug resistant (13).

Recently, the mouse *mdr*1a and *mdr*1b genes have been insertionally inactivated in mice (14–17). These animals, although otherwise normal, are hypersensitive to cytotoxic substrates of P-gp. This hypersensitivity is due in part to the abrogation of the *mdr*1a-based blood-brain barrier and to enhanced absorption and decreased excretion of *mdr*1 substrates. These studies demonstrate the critical role that P-gp plays in drug distribution and pharmacokinetics and argue that specific targeting of P-gp to tissues that do not ordinarily express it (as in gene therapy) will protect such tissues from cytotoxic *mdr*1 substrates.

II. SELECTABLE MARKERS IN HEMATOPOIETIC SYSTEMS

As noted above, studies on mice transgenic for human *MDR*1 established that constitutive overexpression of this gene protects animals from antineoplastic agents. Drugs could be administered safely at dose levels severalfold higher than to mice of the respective background strains (7,8). To demonstrate the specificity of this protection, verapamil, an inhibitor of P-glycoprotein, was coadministered, resulting in reversal of drug resistance (9). Similarly, mice transgenic for a mutated dihydrofolate reductase or an O^6-methylguanine DNA methyltransferase cDNA were protected from methotrexate or 1,3-bis(2-chloroethyl) nitrosourea (BCNU) toxicity, respectively (18–20).

Upon overexpression in target cells, drug-resistance genes may also protect them from environmental toxins such as carcinogens in addition to amelioration of anticancer chemotherapy (21). For instance, transfer of O^6-methylguanine methyltransferase increases repair of DNA damage in sensitive cells. In vitro and in vivo studies confirmed this aspect of the function of drug resistance genes (22,23). Liu et al. (24) showed that rapid repair of O^6-methylguanine-DNA adducts in transgenic mice protected them from *N*-methyl-nitrosourea–induced thymic lymphomas. This protection from carcinogens can be targeted to other organs like liver or skin by suitable promoter systems (25,26).

Chemoprotection exerted by overexpression of chemoresistance genes in hematopoietic organs of transgenic animals could be transferred by transplantation of bone marrow to normal recipients (10,27). These experiments provided a basis for gene therapy approaches with drug-resistance genes. Hence, drug-resistance genes that were initially studied because of their association with failure of anticancer chemotherapy are expected to serve as useful tools for gene therapy of cancer by protecting patients from the toxic side effects of chemotherapy. Protection of chemosensitive cells from toxic compounds may be particularly helpful in the case of the hematopoietic system because most cells in blood and bone marrow are highly susceptible to antineoplastic compounds. $CD34^+$ hematopoietic progenitor cells do not express glutathione-S-transferases (28), and only very low levels of endogenous *MDR*1 gene are expressed in myeloid and erythroid progenitor cells (29,30). These low expression levels are not capable of providing protection from the cytotoxicity of anticancer drugs. Conversely, the high susceptibility of normal hematopoietic cells to cytotoxic agents allows selection strategies exploiting drug-resistance genes if sufficient levels of resistance can be conferred.

Retroviral transduction with a full-length *MDR*1 cDNA promoted by long-terminal repeats (LTRs) of Harvey sarcoma virus protected normal, clonogenic hematopoietic precursors or erythroleukemia cells from anticancer drugs (31,32). Transduced cells were found to be resistant to multiple drugs including taxol, colchicine, and daunomycin. Murine hematopoietic stem cells originating from fetal liver (33) and peripheral blood following mobilization with the use of growth factors (34) or from bone marrow (35) were efficiently transduced with retroviral *MDR*1 vectors. In the latter study, it was shown that transplantation of transduced hematopoietic stem cells results in efficient expression of functional human P-glycoprotein in recipient mice. In spite of generally lower transduction frequencies, $CD34^+$ human progenitor cells could also be transduced with retroviruses conveying the multidrug-resistance gene (36,37). Pluripotent human hematopoietic progenitors or stem cells, respectively, are difficult to transduce with retroviruses (38). Fruehauf et al. (39) targeted immature, cobblestone area–forming progenitor cells. However, in this study significant vincristine resistance was achieved only in a small minority of the immature cell population.

Transplantation of *MDR*1-transduced murine bone marrow cells into W/W^V mice (11) or lethally irradiated normal syngeneic mice (12) resulted in significant gene expression in the bone marrow of recipient animals. Both investigators detected elevated levels of *MDR*1 expression after treatment of recipient mice with taxol, favoring the idea of a selective advantage in vivo of hematopoietic cells overexpressing the *MDR*1 transgene. This observation was in marked contrast to previous studies with selectable markers such as genes conferring resistance to neomycin, puromycin, or hygromycin. Because of their pharmacology or pharmacokinetics, such compounds cannot be used for selection in vivo.

Further support for the potential usefulness of drug resistance genes for selection in vivo was provided by experiments in which *MDR*1-transduced bone marrow was first transplanted into recipient mice (13). After taxol treatment of recipient mice, their bone marrow was then retransplanted into a second generation of recipient mice. In several cycles of retransplantation and taxol treatment of recipient animals, increasingly high levels of drug resistance were generated in vivo. Mice of the fifth and sixth generation survived doses of taxol that were lethal for mice that had not undergone bone marrow transplantation. Bunting et al. (40) have recently shown that transduction of murine bone marrow cells with pHaMDR1 retroviral vector enables ex vivo stem cell expansion, which might help account for the ability of transduced cells to survive multiple cycles of transplantation. In one study of *MDR*1-transduced progenitor cells expanded with growth factors for extended periods (up to 12 days), uncontrolled proliferation was observed (40). Thus, the safety of such procedures is currently being investigated.

Several of the drug-resistance genes have been used to protect hematopoietic cells from drugs used in anticancer treatment. As has been seen with *MDR*1, chemoprotection of hematopoietic progenitor cells and a selective advantage in vitro were demonstrated following transduction by mutated dihydrofolate reductase cDNAs, which confer resistance to methotrexate (1,41–44). Williams et al. (45), Cline et al. (46), and Vinh et al. (47) demonstrated protection of recipient animals from lethal doses of methotrexate. Retransplantation experiments performed with dihydrofolate reductase (48) gave results comparable to those obtained with *MDR*1 (17); both genes facilitate increased levels of resistance after several cycles of transplantation and drug treatment of recipient animals.

Resistance to another antimetabolite drug, cytosine arabinoside, which is a major component of treatment for acute leukemias, is conferred by cytidine deaminase. Hematopoietic cell were rendered resistant to cytosine arabinoside by transfer of this gene (49).

Different patterns of chemoresistance can be attributed to various drug-resistance genes. For instance, the *MRP*1 gene is genetically and functionally related to *MDR*1. Retroviral transfer of *MRP*1 resulted in resistance to doxorubicin, etoposide, and vincristine (4). However, since binding and transport of inhibitors to *MDR*1 may be different from *MRP*, transfer of this gene may be useful if naturally occurring resistance due to *MDR*1 overexpression in cancer cells has to be overcome to allow for effective chemotherapy of an *MDR*1-expressing cancer.

Resistance to alkylating agents is multicausative, and several genes may be useful as selectable markers. Retroviral transfer of a rat glutathione S-transferase Yc cDNA to hematopoietic cells conveyed moderate resistance to melphalan, mechlorethamine, and chlorambucil (50). Resistance to cyclophosphamide or 4-hydroperoxycyclophosphamide, respectively, could be conferred on hematopoietic cells by transfer of aldehyde dehydrogenase with the use of retroviral vectors (51,52). Leukemic or primary hematopoietic cells were rendered resistant to BCNU by retroviral transfer of a human O^6-alkylguanine-DNA alkyltransferase cDNA (2,53,54). Transplantation of transduced bone marrow cells rescued recipient animals from the toxicity of nitrosoureas (55). In particular, nitrosourea-induced severe immunodeficiency can be overcome by transduction of immature progenitor cells (56). Furthermore, resistance to nitrosoureas in combination with an inhibitor of O^6-alkylguanine-DNA alkyltransferase, a key enzyme involved in naturally occurring resistance to nitrosoureas, could be conferred by retroviral transfer of a mutated O^6-methylguanine DNA methyltransferase cDNA (20). This approach protected mice from lethal drug doses and allowed selection of transduced hematopoietic progenitor cells.

Based on experiments in tissue culture and animal models, early clinical trials on transfer of the *MDR*1 gene to hematopoietic progenitor cells have been conducted (57–59). Bone marrow or peripheral blood progenitor cells from patients suffering from advanced neoplastic diseases were retrovirally transduced and reinfused after high-dose chemotherapy (60–62). These studies revealed that transduction efficiencies using *MDR*1 vectors as detected in bone marrow or peripheral blood of patients tended to be low and varied from one patient to another. Thus, gene transfer procedures and selection strategies need to be improved to protect efficiently human hematopoietic cells from the cytotoxicity of drug treatment.

Improvements in vector design have been suggested by several groups. Using the multidrug resistance gene, Metz et al. (63) showed that retroviral vectors derived from Harvey viruses can be substantially shortened without reduction of gene transfer efficiency, thereby increasing the maximum size of the packaged gene of interest. By systematic analysis of the U3-region of various 5′-long-terminal repeats, Baum et al. (64) optimized *MDR*1 transfer to hematopoietic cells. Notably, transfer to immature hematopoietic progenitor cells, which are generally difficult to transduce, was improved (65). Other vector systems used for chemoresistance gene transfer to hematopoietic cells include adeno-associated virus vectors (66) or liposomes (67) (see Sections IV and V).

A different approach to improve the utility of selectable markers is to coexpress two drug-resistance genes, thereby conferring resistance to a broad range of cytotoxic agents. To this end, mutated dihydrofolate reductase has been coexpressed with *MDR*1 or with thymidylate synthase (68,69), and *MDR*1 has also been expressed with O^6-methylguanine-DNA-methyltransferase (70,71). Alternatively, a dominant-positive selectable marker gene can be coexpressed with a negative selectable marker such as thymidine kinase from herpes simplex virus (HSV-TK) (72,73). The latter approach allows selective elimination of transduced cells. Such an approach may increase the safety of gene transfer if cancer cells contaminating hematopoietic cell preparations are inadvertently rendered drug-resistant or if transduced cells become malignant (40). Selective killing of *MDR*1-HSV-TK transduced cells in vivo has been demonstrated (73). Thymidine kinase may not only facilitate selective killing of cancer cells but instead increase the efficacy of certain selectable marker genes. A bicistronic vector in which thymidine kinase was combined with dihydrofolate reductase displayed enhanced resistance as compared to a construct that contained a neomycin phosphotransferase instead of thymidine kinase (74). The authors concluded that thymidine kinase may be useful to salvage thymidine.

To increase the safety of gene therapy of cancer using drug-resistance genes, they may be combined with cDNAs that specifically eliminate cancer cells. This has been demonstrated for chronic myeloid leukemia (CML), which is characterized by a specific molecular marker, the BCR/ABL gene fusion. A vector has been constructed that combined a methotrexate-resistant dihydrofolate reductase with an anti-BCR/ABL antisense sequence (75). Transfer of this vector to CML cells led to the restoration of normal cellular function of BCR/ABL cDNA+ cells due to reduced levels of transcripts while conferring drug resistance.

In addition to improvement of gene therapy of cancer, drug-resistance genes may be helpful for gene therapy of nonmalignant diseases if increased gene expression is desired. In fact, there is considerable interest in using drug-selectable marker genes to introduce and enrich otherwise nonselectable genes in target organs. Gene therapy, although thought to bear the potential of curing genetically determined diseases, is frequently hampered by low gene expression in target organs. This is particularly true for hematopoietic disorders because the efficiency of gene transfer is often limited, and stable expression of transgenes in bone marrow has been found difficult to accomplish.

For instance, Gaucher disease is characterized by accumulation of a glucosylceramide in glucocerebrosidase-deficient hematopoietic cells. These patients suffer from skeletal lesions, severe hepatosplenomegaly, anemia, and disorders of the central nervous system. While it is possible to efficiently transduce a glucocerebrosidase cDNA to hematopoietic progenitor cells (76,77), expression levels tend to decrease after several weeks or months in vivo because of silencing or limited lifespan of the transduced cells' progeny. To increase expression of glucocerebrosidase in vivo, Aran et al. (78) constructed a transcriptional fusion between *MDR*1 and the glucocerebrosidase gene. Increased expression of the latter gene was achieved by selection with cytotoxic substrates of P-glycoprotein. Appropriate selection strategies allowed complete restoration of the underlying genetic defect in cells from Gaucher patients (79). Transduction of such bicistronic vectors into hematopoietic stem cells might allow treatment of patients by chemotherapeutic elimination of nontransduced cells that continue to synthesize or store glucosylceramide. Moreover, following chemotherapy the numbers of genetically corrected hematopoietic progenitor cells should increase in bone marrow to maintain physiological numbers of mature granulocytes, monocytes, and lymphocytes in peripheral blood.

Similarly, bicistronic vectors that facilitate coexpression of *MDR*1 and α-galactosidase A have been engineered (80). Defects of α-galactosidase A are the cause of Fabry disease, a globotriaosylceramide storage disorder that affects skin, kidneys, heart, and nervous system. Other applications for bicistronic fusions include immunological disorders such as chronic granulomatous disease and X-linked or adenosine deaminase (ADA) deficiency–related severe combined immunodeficiency (SCID) syndromes. For treatment of these diseases, vectors have been constructed that contain a gp91phox or an ADA cDNA (81–83). Further discussion of the use of bicistronic vectors can be found in Section III.

A different strategy to exploit the *MDR*1 gene as a drug-selectable marker for correction of ADA deficiency was described by Germann et al. (84). In this study, both genes were fused to a single cDNA encoding a bifunctional chimeric protein. This approach, however, cannot be used if the two proteins are physiologically located in different cellular compartments.

While such vectors are well characterized in vitro, their usefulness in vivo has still to be established. Animal models should facilitate development and optimization of selection strategies in live animals. However, detection of the function of transferred genes may be difficult if normal animals are utilized because of the activity of the respective endogenous gene product. To circumvent this difficulty, ''knockout'' animals whose genes has been inactivated by targeted disruption can serve as useful models. For instance, mice whose α-galactosidase genes have been disrupted may be helpful to characterize a bicistronic vector in which *MDR*1 is combined with the respective human gene for correction of Fabry disease (85). Another alternative is to use marking genes that are not physiologically expressed at high levels in normal tissues. To characterize bicistronic vectors containing *MDR*1, this gene has been coexpressed with a green fluorescent protein or β-galactosidase (86).

These model systems should help to improve protocols for efficient drug selection and to identify strategies for selection at limited systemic toxicity. For instance, addition of P-glycoprotein inhibitors at low concentration to cytotoxic drugs may increase the stringency of drug selection, thereby allowing use of anticancer drugs at low concentrations for selection (79).

III. BICISTRONIC VECTORS CONTAINING SELECTABLE MARKERS

Although co-expression of two proteins can be achieved through the use of separate promoters, the co-expression is frequently uncoupled due to promoter interference or shut-off of gene expression from one of the promoters, which causes the selected cells not to express the desired protein. To overcome this problem, the selectable marker may be expressed with the therapeutic gene as a translational or transcriptional fusion. A therapeutic protein can be directly linked to the carboxyl terminus of the multidrug transporter P-gp. The resulting fusion protein possesses functions of both P-gp and the target protein (87). Since P-gp is an integral membrane protein that functions on the cell plasma membrane, unless two proteins can be separated by a posttranslational proteolytic modification, the expressed target protein will be associated with the plasma membrane regardless of its normal cellular location. Thus, even though translational fusions guarantee protein co-expression, their potential is limited. On the other hand, transcriptional fusions, e.g., using bicistronic or polycistronic mRNA to encode more than one cDNA, may prove to be more generally applicable.

A. *MDR*1 Bicistronic Vectors Containing Internal Ribosome Entry Sites

A DNA segment corresponding to one polypeptide chain plus the translational start and stop signals for protein synthesis can be loosely defined as a cistron. An mRNA encoding only a single polypeptide is called monocistronic mRNA; if it encodes two or more polypeptide chains, it may be called bicistronic or polycistronic mRNA. Almost all eukaryotic mRNA molecules are monocistronic. Initiation of translation of eukaryotic mRNA is mediated by a cap-binding protein that recognizes a methylated guanosine cap at the 5′ terminus of mRNA. However, some viral mRNA molecules transcribed in eukaryotic cells are polycistronic. They can use a cap-independent mechanism to initiate translation in the middle of mRNA molecules. For picomavirus, this cap-independent internal initiation of translation is mediated through a unique internal ribosome entry site (IRES) within the mRNA molecule (88,89).

Identification of IRES sequences led to the development of bicistronic vectors that allow co-expression of two different polypeptides from a single mRNA molecule in eukaryotic cells (90,91). Using a bicistronic vector containing an IRES to co-express a target gene and a selectable marker has several advantages. First, since two polypeptides are translated from the same mRNA molecule, the bicistronic vector guarantees co-expression of a selectable marker and a second protein. Second, bicistronic mRNA allows two polypeptides to be translated separately. Thus, this system does not compromise the correct intracellular trafficking of proteins directed to different subcellular compartments. In addition, using a bicistronic vector, expression of a target gene is proportionate to the expression of a selectable marker. Hence, expression of a target protein can be achieved quantitatively by applying selections of different stringencies.

To demonstrate co-expression of a dominant selectable marker with a therapeutic gene using a bicistronic vector, our laboratory has co-expressed P-gp with glucocerebrosidase (78,79), α-galactosidase (80), adenosine deaminase (82), a subunit of the NAPH oxidase complex (81), the shared gamma chain of the interleukin receptors (83), and a hammerhead ribozyme targeted to the U5 region of HIV-1 LTR (92). In those experiments, *MDR*1 served as a selectable marker linked to the target gene by an IRES from encephalomyocarditis virus (EMCV) and constructed in a retroviral vector containing Harvey sarcoma virus LTR (93). Two configurations, in which *MDR*1 is placed either before or after the IRES, have been examined in some cases. As demonstrated in those experiments, P-gp and the target gene are co-expressed in the cells selected using cytotoxic P-gp substrates, such as colchicine or vincristine; the expressed target proteins are functional as detected using in vitro or ex vivo analysis. In one case, using subcellular fractionation, we have demonstrated that P-gp and glucocerebrosidase are translocated separately to the cell plasma membrane and lysosomes, indicating correct intracellular protein trafficking (98). The demonstration that a non-coding RNA, such as a hammerhead ribozyme, can function even though tethered to an mRNA encoding a functional *MDR*1 provides an additional powerful way to use bicistronic vectors (92).

Another approach to the use of *MDR*1-based bicistronic vectors is to develop ''suicide'' vectors for cancer gene therapy. Using *MDR*1 to protect bone marrow cells from cytotoxic drugs represents a promising approach to improve cancer chemotherapy. However, contaminating cancer cells may be inadvertently transduced with *MDR*1, or transduced bone marrow cells may accidentally develop new tumors. In those cases, overexpression of P-gp could cause multidrug resistance in inadvertently transduced tumor cells that contaminate bone marrow or in any transduced cells which later become malignant. A bicistronic ''suicide'' vector developed in this laboratory links P-gp expression with herpes simplex virus thymidine kinase expression (72,73). Thus the cells containing this vector can be eliminated through ganciclovir treatment.

A third approach is to link two drug-resistance genes together using a bicistronic vector system to extend the ability of the vector to confer drug resistance. Examples include the use of *MDR*1 with dihydrofolate reductase, which confers methotrexate resistance (94), and *MDR*1 plus MGMT, which confers resistance to certain alkylating agents (70,71).

Finally, bicistronic vectors can be used to introduce marker genes into selected cells. For example, *MDR*1 vectors containing green fluorescent protein or β-galactosidase have been constructed to determine the efficiency of expression of the target gene in transduced and *MDR*1 selected cells (86).

B. Efficiency of IRES-Dependent Translation

Using an IRES to generate a bicistronic mRNA ensures co-expression of two different proteins. However, IRES-dependent mRNA translation (or cap-independent translation) is less efficient than cap-dependent translation, so that the two proteins are not expressed in equal amounts. It has been shown that in a monocistronic vector, insertion of an IRES upstream from an open reading frame of either P-gp or dihydrofolate reductase (DHFR) reduces the translation efficiency by 2- to 10-fold (91,95). Using a bicistronic vector, expression of *neo* in the position downstream from the IRES is 25–50% of that observed when *neo* is in the upstream position (90). The asymmetrical expression pattern of the bicistronic vector results in a significant difference in *MDR*1-transducing titer between a configuration with P-gp placed before the IRES and a configuration in which P-gp is placed after the IRES. We have found that the apparent titer of a bicistronic vector containing *ADA-IRES-MDR*1 was only 7% of the titer of a bicistronic vector containing *MDR*1-*IRES-ADA* (82). Similar reductions in *MDR*1-transducing titer and in expression of the nonselected downstream gene was seen with *MDR*1–α-galactosidase bicistronic vectors too (80). The apparent *MDR*1-transducing titer of the retrovirus is based on the drug resistance conferred by expression of P-gp as the result of retroviral infection; thus the viral titer is proportional to the P-gp expression level. Insufficient expression of P-gp is unable to protect the cells from cytotoxic drug selection. To achieve P-gp expression at the same level, the lower efficiency of translation would have to be compensated for by a higher level of transcription, which can occur only in a minority of the cells in the transduced population. This may account for the apparent lower *MDR*1-transducing titer of bicistronic vectors with a configuration of P-gp placed after the IRES. On the other hand, when cells express P-gp at the same level (i.e., the cells survived vincristine or colchicine selection at the same concentration), ADA expressed from *ADA-IRES-MDR*1 is 15-fold higher than the ADA expressed from *MDR*1-*IRES-ADA*. This difference is probably due to a combination of the lower translation efficiency of ADA located downstream from the IRES and the high transcription level of *ADA-IRES-MDR*1 as the result of vincristine selection. A similar asymmetrical expression of P-gp and human α-galactosidase A is also observed in NIH3T3 cells, where the difference is about eightfold.

IRES-dependent translation is a complex process, in which mRNA containing IRES interacts with various cellular proteins. The efficiency of IRES-dependent translation can be affected by the cell type (96), IRES origin (97,98), and the size and structure of a particular mRNA molecule. We have found that the titer of retrovirus containing pHa-*MDR*1 was higher than pHa-*MDR*1-*IRES-ADA*, even though P-gp translation was cap-dependent in both cases. P-gp expressed from pHa-*MDR*1 was also at a higher level in a vincristine resistant cell population than the P-gp expressed from pHa-*MDR*1-*IRES-ADA*. A possible explanation for the relatively low retroviral titers observed is RNA instability or alternative splicing, since no DNA rearrangement was detected by Southern blot analysis of the transduced cells using a *MDR*1 probe.

C. Flexibility Using Bicistronic Vectors in Coordinating Expression of Selectable Markers and a Therapeutic Gene

Selectable bicistronic vectors provide great flexibility in coordinating expression of a selectable marker, such as P-gp, and a therapeutic gene. The low translation efficiency of the IRES results in asymmetrical expression of genes positioned before and after the IRES. This asymmetrical expression pattern makes it possible to alter the relative expression level of a therapeutic gene and P-gp to achieve maximum therapeutic effects while applying minimal selective pressure using a cytotoxic drug. By choosing different configurations, i.e., placing *MDR*1 before or after the IRES, we can select cells expressing a therapeutic gene at either a low level (*MDR*1 before IRES) or a high level (*MDR*1 after IRES).

In addition, expression of a therapeutic gene can also be achieved at a desired level by altering the selection conditions. The degree of multidrug resistance conferred by P-gp corresponds to the amount of P-gp expressed on the plasma membrane. Using a bicistronic vector, the expression of a target gene is proportional to the expression of P-gp, which is directly linked to the selection conditions. In a highly stringent selection, instead of increasing the concentration of cytotoxic drug, P-gp–reversing agents can also be applied in combination with low concentrations of cytotoxic drugs (99). P-gp–reversing agents, also known as chemosensitizers, are noncytotoxic hydrophobic compounds that interact with P-gp and cause a direct inhibition of P-gp function. In the presence of a P-gp–reversing agent, most P-gp–expressing cells are killed by the cytotoxic drug unless they express a large amount of P-gp to overcome the inhibitory effects. Using a combination of cytotoxic drug and chemosensitizer allows selection of cells expressing the therapeutic gene at a high level without need for a high concentration of cytotoxic drug. This strategy is especially desirable for an in vivo selection in which avoiding systemic toxicity is essential.

High expression of the target gene can be selected using cytotoxic drugs, cytotoxic drugs combined with chemosensitizers, or the vector configured to place the target gene placed before the IRES. However, those approaches also reduce the overall number of cells that can survive the selection. Nevertheless, using a minimum concentration of drug, the selectable bicistronic vector provides options for selecting a large population of cells with low expression of the target gene or a small population of cells with high expression of the target gene. Both options may be useful for gene therapy. For instance, ADA levels in normal individuals occur over a very broad range. Heterozygous carriers can be immunologically normal with as little as 10% of the normal amount of ADA (reviewed in Ref. 100). Expression of ADA at a low level in a large number of cells may prove sufficient to treat SCID. On the other hand, high ADA-expressing lymphoid cells, even though present as a small percentage of total cells, are also able to correct the SCID syndrome due to a beneficial bystander effect (101). In gene therapy applications, the choice of the approach depends on the therapeutic strategy for a specific disease. Experiments on animal models are essential to prove the concepts that underlie gene therapy using selectable markers such as *MDR*1.

IV. NONRETROVIRAL AND EPISOMAL VECTORS EXPRESSING SELECTABLE MARKERS: AAV, EBV, SV40

Efficient delivery of a therapeutic gene to the appropriate target cells and its subsequent maintenance and expression are important steps for successful gene therapy. Genes introduced into cells are rapidly lost unless there is a mechanism to retain these genes within the nucleus and to ensure that the genes are also replicated and partitioned into daughter cells during cell division. Long-term expression of the transgene within cells can be achieved either via the integration of the transferred DNA into the host genome or maintenance of the introduced DNA as an autonomously replicating extrachromosomal element or episome. In either case, inclusion of a drug-selectable marker, like the *MDR*1 gene, in the construct would ensure that rapidly dividing cells containing the transgene are given a selective growth advantage.

Delivery modalities can be viral or nonviral. Retroviral gene transfer, one of the most exploited systems for gene transfer into actively dividing cells, was discussed earlier in this chapter, while liposomal gene delivery will be in later sections. In this section, nonretroviral and/or episomal vectors expressing selectable markers will be described.

In addition to retroviruses, adeno-associated virus (AAV) can also facilitate integration of the transgene into the host genome. Unlike retroviruses, AAV was found to integrate preferentially into a specific site on chromosome 19 (102). AAV is a naturally defective, nonpathogenic, single-strand human DNA parvovirus. For productive infection and viral replication, coinfection with helper viruses (e.g., adenovirus, herpesvirus, or vaccinia virus) is required. In the absence of a helper virus, AAV establishes latency in the host by integrating itself into the host genome. AAV has a broad host range and is also able to infect both dividing and nondividing cells (103). Hence recombinant AAV (rAAV) vectors have been exploited as alternative vehicles for gene therapy.

AAV-based vectors (104) are simple to construct, requiring only that the viral inverted terminal repeat (ITR) (145 nucleotides) is upstream from the gene of interest. Other important viral genes like *rep* (involved in replication and integration) and *cap* (encoding structural genes) can then be supplied in *trans*. One disadvantage with such rAAV vectors is that site-specific integration of the gene of interest into the host genome is not observed (66). This is probably because the *rep* gene, which is important for mediating site specific integration in the absence of helper viruses, is not included in the construct with the gene of interest. Nonetheless, rAAV has been successfully applied to the delivery of various genes into a variety of tissues and persistence of transgene expression in these nondividing tissues was reported (105–110). Baudard et al. (66) demonstrated that in rapidly dividing cells, continuous selective pressure is necessary to sustain gene expression in cells. *MDR*1 was used as the selectable marker in this study. Being among the smallest DNA animal viruses (~20 nm in diameter), another disadvantage of the AAV system is its limited packaging capacity since it can accomodate only approximately 4.7 kb of the gene of interest. As such, a small and efficient promoter would be required to drive the expression of large genes. One such promoter is the AAV p5 promoter, which together with the ITR forms a 263-base-pair cassette capable of mediating efficient expression in a CF bronchial epithelial cell line (105,106). Baudard et al. further demonstrated that the reduction of the p5 promoter-ITR cassette to 234 bp was also able to promote efficient gene expression (66).

Vectors that facilitate extrachomosomal replication have some advantages. High gene expression is often observed in such vectors. This could be a result of vector amplification, promotion of nuclear localization and retention, as well as transcriptional activation by viral genes involved in episomal replication. Selective pressure using selectable markers like the *MDR*1 gene, however, is necessary to maintain these episomes in actively dividing cells. Thus, another potential advantage of using episomally replicating vectors is that since they are not integrated into the cells, one could potentially extinguish expression at will by withdrawing selective pressure to replicating cells. Episomally replicating vectors can be easily created by the inclusion into the vector design of replicons, which can be derived from DNA viruses like the simian virus 40 (SV40) (111), Epstein-Barr virus (EBV) (112), and the BK virus (113–115). Such replicons usually comprise a viral origin of replication as well as a viral gene product that is important for maintaining extrachromosomal replication.

SV40 is a 5.2 kb DNA papovavirus that was discovered as a harmless contaminant in early preparations of the Salk polio vaccine (116,117). One of the advantages of using SV40 as a gene-delivery vehicle is its ability to infect a wide variety of mammalian cells, including human ones. It is, however, unable to replicate its DNA in rodent cells, hence no progeny virions can be produced in these cells. Nonetheless, infection of SV40 in murine cells can result in the integration of viral DNA into the host chromosome (118). SV40 delivery systems can be generated by replacing the late or early region with a foreign gene. Recombinant viral particles are then propagated using either wild-type or temperature-sensitive mutant of SV40 as helper or via a viral producer cell line, COS7, that stably expresses an origin-defective SV40 mutant and is capable of supporting the lytic cycle of SV40. It was demonstrated that when the large T-antigen gene, whose gene product is responsible for episomal replication, was replaced with a reporter gene, replication-deficient recombinant SV40 viruses can be produced and can mediate gene transfer in vivo. Reporter gene expression was detectable for about 3 months without selection (119,120).

Present SV40 vectors have most of the viral coding sequences removed retaining only the packaging sequences, the polyadenylation signal, and the early promoter of the virus, thus increasing the capacity for transgene DNA to ~5.3 kb (121,122). These vectors, however, do not have a mechanism to maintain the transferred DNA episomally in the target cells. In this system, SV40 pseudovirions comprising largely nonviral DNA are packaged, using wild-type SV40 as helper, in COS cells which harbor the SV40 large T-Ag. Rund et al. demonstrated very efficient delivery (> 95%) of the drug-selectable marker, *MDR*1, into various murine and human cell types including primary human bone marrow cells (122). Although such pseudovirions can transfer the gene of interest to a variety of cells including hematopoietic cells with reasonable efficiency, its clinical applicability is currently limited by the contamination (~90%) of viral preparations with wild-type SV40. Recently, the same group developed an in vitro method of preparing helper-free SV40 vectors (123). SV40 viral capsid proteins, VP1, VP2, and VP3 are overexpressed in *Spodoptera frugiperda* (Sf9) insect cells, where they accumulate in the nucleus. Incubation of vector DNA with nuclear extracts from these insect cells leads to the formation of particles capable of infecting target cells resulting in transgene expression. Such in vitro assembly allows larger DNA (> 7 kb) to be packaged quite efficiently. However, the present method of generating infectious particles is at least a log less efficient than when wild-type SV40 is used as a helper virus to produce infectious pseudovirions. Fang et al. reported a different packaging system for SV40 vectors (124) where the vector carrying the gene of interest contains only one viral gene, namely, the SV40 origin of replication. Instead of using wild-type SV40 viruses as helper to package the recombinant vector, recombinant adenoviruses expressing SV40 capsids were used to package these plasmids containing SV40 replication origins in COS-7 cells. The helper adenovirus can be effectively heat-inactivated without adverse effect on the infectivity of the recombinant SV40 viruses due to the differential heat sensitivity of these two viruses.

Episomal replication in SV40 virus requires the SV40 replication origin as well as the large T antigen (T-Ag), which activates the replication origin. Such episomal replication can generate more than 10^5 copies per cell of recombinant plasmids (125). Safety modified SV40-based episomal vectors have recently been explored as potential gene therapy vectors (116). In this strategy, the gene of interest is inserted into a vector containing an SV40 replication origin as well as a mutant SV40 large T antigen that is deficient in binding human tumor suppressor gene products yet retains replication competence. When these vectors are delivered into cells via electroporation or into HT1376 tumor explants in nude mice using liposomes, extrachromosomal replication can be observed both in vitro and in the tumor explants. High gene expression for about one week was also found using these vectors under no selective pressure. It would be interesting to determine if episomal gene maintenance and more sustained gene expression is possible by including selectable markers like the *MDR*1 gene or if the extremely high replication potential of these vectors become too toxic for the host cells as they overwhelm the cellular machinery to support their replication.

Episomal vectors based on EBV are also being developed for gene therapy purposes. EBV is a human B-lymphotropic herpesvirus that resides asymptomatically in more than 90% of the adult human population by establishing latency and maintaining its genome episomally (127). The life cycle of EBV comprises two phases, a lytic and a latent phase. During the lytic phase, EBV DNA replicates via a rolling circle intermediate to achieve a 1000-fold increase in copy number. The origin of replication, Ori Lyt, and the transacting element ZEBRA are required for the lytic replication. Rolling circle replication results in the formation of linear head-to-tail concatamers. The presence of the EBV terminal repeat (TR) sequence causes cleavage of the concatemerized DNA to molecules of about 150–200 kbp, which are then packaged into virions. Upon infection into a permissive cell, the viral DNA circularizes by ligation of TR. Latency is established in the cells by episomal replication of the circular DNA.

Episomal replication in EBV is maintained by two elements interacting to ensure that the viral genome is retained within the nucleus, efficiently replicated, and partitioned into daughter cells. Although the copy numbers of episomal viral DNA varies from 1 to 800, only 4–10 episomal copies per cell are usually observed using vectors containing EBV OriP and EBNA-1 (128). Unlike other episomal vector systems, very low rates of spontaneous mutation have been observed with EBV-based episomal vectors (129). The *cis*-acting element responsible for episomal replication is a 1.8 kb OriP, while the *trans*-acting element is EBNA-1. OriP comprises two distinct sequence motifs, the dyad symmetry motif (DS), from which replication is initiated, and the family of repeats (FR), which serves as a replication fork barrier. Interaction of EBNA-1 with DS initiates bidirectional replication, while binding of EBNA-1 to FR enhances transcription from the episome and terminates DNA replication. EBNA-is reported not to be oncogenic nor immunogenic. It evades the host immune system via the presence of the repeat motif, Gly-Ala, which was found to interfere with antigen processing and MHC class I–restricted presentation (130). These EBV episomal vectors replicate once per cell cycle (131) and are capable of stably maintaining human genomic inserts of sizes between 60 and 330 kb for at least 60 generations (132).

Vos et al. (133) developed a helper-dependent infectious recombinant EBV to evaluate the feasibility of using such a vector system to correct hereditary syndromes in B lymphocytes already harboring the EBV virus latently. The EBV-containing target B lymphocytes will supply EBNA-1 in *trans* for the episomal maintenance of the transgene. Hence only minimal *cis*-EBV elements for episomal replication (OriP), viral amplification (Ori Lyt), and packaging (TR) are included in their construct. The hygromycin resistance gene was included as a selectable marker in their vector. Infectious virions are generated by the producer cell line HH514. They demonstrated successful transfer of such infectious virions carrying the therapeutic gene, Fanconi anemia group C (FA-C) cDNA, into HSC536, a FA-C patient cell line. Upon selection with hygromycin, long-term (at least 6 months) correction of the Fanconi phenotype in vitro was observed, as determined by cellular resistance to the cross-linking agent, diepoxybutane. They also observed that in the absence of selective pressure, their episomal vector is retained in rapidly dividing cells at a rate of 98% per cell division translating to a half-life of 30 days in cells doubling every 20 hours.

Our laboratory has been exploring the use of EBV episomal vectors containing only the OriP and EBNA-1 and carrying the selectable marker *MDR*1 as potential gene therapy vectors. Using the liposome formulation, DOGS/DOPE (1:1) (134), we successfully delivered the vector to various cultured cells as well as human $CD34^+$ stem cells. *MDR*1 was found to be expressed at a higher level in the episomal vector compared to its nonepisomal counterpart, and more drug colonies were obtained upon selection. Episomal plasmids could be recovered in drug selected cells for many weeks (C. Lee et al., unpublished, data).

Other episomally replicating vectors can be derived from BPV viruses (135) or BK virus (114). Unfortunately, BPV vectors cannot be reliably maintained as episomes as they exhibit high spontaneous mutation rate (~1%), frequently undergoing integration, deletion, recombination, and rearrangements (136). Furthermore, BPV has a limited host range and BPV vectors cannot be efficiently maintained in human cells. Not too much is known about BK virus–derived episomal vectors. Nonetheless, successful stable maintenance of episomal gene expression was reported in human transitional carcinoma cells using BK-based vectors but not EBV-based vectors probably due to the differential tropism of BK and EBV viruses for human uroepithelial cells (113).

Various chimeric viruses have been developed to improve the efficiency of gene transfer as well as the maintenance of gene expression within target cells. These chimeric virus systems attempt to combine the favorable attributes of each vector system and overcome the limitations associated with each system. The episomal replication ability of EBV was exploited to produce both rapid and long-term high-titer recombinant retroviruses (up to 10^7 IU/mL) for efficient gene transfer into human hematopoietic progenitor cells (137,138). A novel adenoviral/retroviral chimeric vector was also reported in which an adenoviral delivery system was utilized to efficiently deliver both the retroviral vector and its packaging components, thereby inducing the target cells to function as transient retroviral producers capable of infecting neighboring cells. This system capitalizes on the superior efficiency of adenoviruses to deliver genes in vivo and the integrative ability of retroviruses to achieve stable gene expression (139). An EBV/HSV-1 amplicon vector system was also described that combines the efficiency of HSV-1 virus to transfer DNA into various mammalian cells, including the postmitotic neuronal cells and the ability of EBV to maintain genes episomally. This vector system contains the HSV-1 origin of DNA replication (oriS) and a packaging signal, which allow replication and packaging of the amplicon into HSV-1 virions in the presence of HSV-1 helper functions as well as EBV oriP and EBNA-1 (140). Another report describes the use of a similar HSV-1 amplicon system for efficient gene transfer, but AAV was included in their vector to achieve stable expression. This HSV/AAV hybrid vector contains OriS and packaging sequences from HSV-1, a transgene cassette that is flanked by AAV ITRs as well as an AAV rep gene residing outside the transgene cassette to mediate amplification and genomic integration of ITR-flanked sequences (141). A HVJ-liposome vector system developed by Kaneda et al. (see Ref. 142) was utilized to improve the efficiency of liposome-mediated transfer of an EBV-episomally maintained transgene (143,144). This system exploits the fusigenic properties of the hemagglutinating virus of Japan (HVJ or Sendai virus) since envelope proteins of inactivated HVJ were found to mediate liposome–cell membrane fusion and facilitate cellular uptake of packaged plasmid DNA, bypassing endocytosis and lysosomal degradation.

One of the limitations of using viral episomal systems is the limited host range of such vectors. Although EBV episomal vectors replicate well in various human and primate cells, they are unable to replicate in rodent cells, limiting their utility in gene therapy since testing of these vectors in rodent models is not easy. Nonetheless, it was found that large fragments of human genomic DNA (10–15 kb) can mediate autonomous replication if there is also a mechanism to retain them in the nucleus (145). Such vectors based on a human origin of replication were also found to be capable of replicating in rodent cells (146), probably due to the common host factors that drive their replication. A hybrid class of vectors was thus developed that employs a human origin of replication to mediate vector replication as well as EBV FR and EBNA-1 gene product to provide nuclear retention functions (see Ref. 147). EBNA-1 binding to the FR of the vector DNA causes the adherence of this complex to the chromosomal scaffold in a noncovalent fashion, thus retaining the vector DNA in the nucleus (148). These vectors were reported to replicate somewhat in synchrony with chromosomal DNA once per cell cycle. Maintenance of these vectors within cells is related to the frequency of cell division (147). Such vectors have been reported to persist in cells for at least 2 months under no selective pressure (145,149).

Ultimately, the development of a true mammalian artificial chromosome (MAC) without dependence on viral elements will be the key to obtaining stable episomal replication without dependence on selective pressure. Functional elements in mammalian cells important for maintaining DNA episomally as a minichromosome include a replication origin to promote autonomous replication, telomeres to protect ends of linear DNA and replicate DNA termini, and a centromere to facilitate correct segregation of the construct during mitotic division. Various mammalian chromosomal DNA replication initiation sites have been identified (reviewed in Ref. 150) and found to comprise a 0.5–11 kb primary origin of bidirectional replication (OBR) flanked by an initiation zone of about 6–55 kb. These sequences show characteristics of DNA unwinding, a densely methylated island, attachment sites to the nuclear matrix and some palindromic sequences.

Vectors utilizing human genomic sequences that promote extrachromosomal vector replication have already been successfully applied, as mentioned above. Telomeres required for the stability and integrity of the eukaryotic chromosome have been well characterized. In mammalian cells, the telomeric tracts comprise 2–50 kb of tandem TTAGGG repeats. Human centromeres, necessary for proper chromosome segregation at mitosis and meiosis, have been localized cytogenetically as primary constrictions of the chromosomes. They are thought to consist of up to several megabases of highly repetitive DNA belonging to the alpha satellite DNA family (151) and are attached to microtubules (152). Until recently, the functional isolation of the centromere has been a great hurdle in the progress towards the construction of a MAC. The group of Willard et al. developed the first generation of human artificial microchromosomes (HAC) by creating synthetic alpha satellite arrays ~1 Mb in size (153). They found that such a HAC about 6–10 Mb in size is mitotically and cytogenetically stable for up to 6 months in culture in the absence of selective pressure. Nonetheless, the technical challenge of assembling a MAC is still formidable because cloning and manipulating such large constructs are not trivial using conventional bacterial cloning systems and transfer to mammalian cells is difficult.

V. USE OF LIPOSOMES TO DELIVER VECTORS WITH SELECTABLE MARKERS

Liposome-mediated gene transfer appears to be a safe and noninvasive method of DNA delivery into cells. Since high efficiency and stable expression have not yet been achieved using liposomal methods, the use of the human *MDR*1 gene as a selectable marker may allow for the selection and enrichment of the recipient cells and may be useful in the future for the long-term maintenance of the cationic liposome:DNA complex.

Previous studies in our laboratory have shown that a liposomal delivery system can mediate successful *MDR*1 transfection of mouse bone marrow cells and in vivo expression of functional P-gp in hematopoietic cells (67). The introduction via liposomes into hematopoietic cells of an *MDR*1 gene driven by Harvey murine sarcoma virus long-terminal repeat sequences (Ha-MSV-LTR) was achieved either "directly" by intravenous administration into mice or "indirectly" by adoptive transplantation of previously in vitro transfected bone marrow cells. In these studies, using a cationic liposome complex consisting of dioctadecylamidoglycyl spermidine (DOGS) and dioleoylphosphosphatidyl ethanolamine (DOPE), *MDR*1 transfection was detected in up to 30% of unselected and 66% of vincristine preselected murine bone marrow cells as demonstrated by drug resistance in an in vitro colony-forming unit assay. Although transfection into human bone marrow cells is likely to be much less efficient, the potential of obtaining drug-selectable mouse bone marrow progenitor cells after gene transfer using such a liposome delivery system may eventually make it possible to protect cancer patients undergoing chemotherapy from bone marrow toxicity of anticancer drugs.

Liposome-mediated gene transfer can also be used for in vivo delivery of AAV-*MDR*1–based vectors. Recently, drug-selected coexpression of both P-gp and glucocerebrosidase (GC) was achieved with an AAV vector containing the *MDR*1-IRES-GC fusion delivered to NIH 3T3 cells by lipofection (66). Moreover, a single intravenous injection of this bicistronic vector complexed with cationic liposomes into recipient mice allowed detection of GC and *MDR*1 sequences by PCR in all organs tested 7 weeks later.

For nonintegrating DNA vectors such as EBV-based systems (see Section IV) and the AAV system (66), liposome-based gene delivery usually results in transient transgene expression due to the episomal nature of the transfected plasmid and loss of the plasmid when the cells proliferate (154,155). Use of a selectable marker such as *MDR*1 may make it possible to maintain nonintegrated episomal forms in proliferating cells (see Section IV). Since only cells carrying such episomal *MDR*1-based vectors would survive the selection, this advantage should be useful for gene therapy with episomal *MDR*1 vectors in vivo. Combining liposomes with AAV- or EBV-based vectors and *MDR*1 as a selectable marker may make it possible to expand the population of expressing cells by *MDR*1 drug selection.

We are developing a gene therapy model to treat Fabry disease (85) using intravenous injections of a pHa-aGal-IRES-MDR bicistronic vector complexed to cationic liposomes into α-galactosidase A–deficient mice (T. Shoshani et al., unpublished results). Both human α-Gal and *MDR*1 were detectable in the lungs of the recipient Fabry mice by Southern blot analysis 7 days after injection. Reverse transcriptase polymerase chain reaction (RT-PCR) analysis of total RNA extracted from the kidneys of recipient Fabry mice showed the presence of both human α-Gal and *MDR*1 mRNA. The expression in the kidneys was specific to the α-galactosidase A–deficient mice, where renal tubule cells may be damaged by an accumulation of glycosphingolipids. In situ hybridization analysis localized the mRNA expression to the renal distal tubule epithelial cells. Higher RNA expression was obtained in Fabry mice that were injected three times every third day. The repeated administration is tolerated by the recipient mice, and no toxic effects were obtained. Current efforts are aimed at determining whether this therapy can reduce the levels of glycosphingolipid globotriaosylceramide (GL3) in the Fabry mice. It remains to be determined whether selection in vivo will allow expansion of cell populations expressing human α-Gal by repeated administration of cytotoxic *MDR*1 substrates.

VI. ENGINEERING MDR VECTORS TO IMPROVE EFFICIENCY OF DRUG SELECTION

One of the goals of gene therapy is to modify cells genetically such that they can supply a useful or necessary function to the cell (3). One of the most promising applications of the *MDR*1 gene in therapeutic vectors as a selectable marker in vivo is the protection of bone marrow cells during intensive chemotherapy. During chemotherapy, the *MDR*1 gene is transduced or transfected into drug-sensitive bone marrow cells and selected for by exposure to MDR agents. The untransfected/untransduced cells will necessarily be killed and those containing the *MDR*1 gene will expand. The efficacy of this therapy depends on the interaction between P-gp and the selecting agent employed. Thus, it is important to be able to distinguish between the endogenous P-gp and the exogenously introduced molecule. Furthermore, it obviously would be beneficial to create a P-gp molecule that would confer very high levels of resistance to certain drugs giving an advantage to transduced cells/tissues compared to wild-type P-gp. Studies of a number of mutations made in P-glycoprotein have suggested that it should be possible to construct mutant ''designer'' transporters useful for *MDR*1-based gene therapy.

One of the hallmark characteristics of the multidrug transporter is its extremely broad substrate specificity. Over the past several years, the identification of specific domains and amino acid residues involved in substrate recognition has contributed to our present understanding of the mechanism of action of P-gp. The major sites of interaction have been shown to reside in transmembrane domains (TM) 5 and 6 in the N-terminal half of the protein and in TMs 11 and 12 in the C-terminal half and the loops that conjoin them (156–160). For the purposes of chemoprotection, the design of a P-gp that has increased resistance to chemotherapeutic agents compared to the endogenous P-gp would be most useful because increased doses of the agent could be administered without harming the bone marrow cells expressing the exogenous P-gp molecule. To date, a number of these types of mutations have been described.

Mutations in TM domains of P-gps from both rodent and human have demonstrated significant alterations in substrate specificity (3,161). An F338A mutation in hamster P-gp enhances resistance to vincristine, colchicine, and daunorubicin but has little impact on resistance to actinomycin D (162,163). An F339P mutation in the same molecule only increases actinomycin D resistance. However, the double F338A/F339P mutant demonstrates an increased level of resistance to actinomycin D and vincristine but a lowered level of resistance to colchicine and daunorubicin (162,163). Of these mutants, the F338A may prove most useful because it confers increased resistance to a wider range of chemotherapeutic agents. In human P-gp, however, a homologous mutation at F335 confers greater resistance to colchicine and doxorubicin but causes a severe reduction in resistance to vinblastine and actinomycin D (164,165). Additionally, cells expressing a Val→Ala mutation at position 338 also exhibit preferential resistance to colchicine and doxorubicin but are severely impaired for vinblastine (165). Resistance to actinomycin D, however, is unaffected. Alanine scanning of TM 11 in mouse P-gp encoded by *mdr*1a revealed that two mutants, M944A and F940A, show an increase in resistance to doxorubicin and colchicine while maintaining wild-type levels of resistance to vinblastine and actinomycin D (166). For certain treatment protocols, it is conceivable that increased resistance to certain agents would be desirable and the reduction in levels of resistance to other compounds would not be problematic, especially if a well-defined chemotherapy regimen was being employed.

Although the majority of residues that increase resistance to various chemotherapeutic agents reside in the TM domains, a number of residues in the putative cytoplasmic loops also have been implicated in defining drug-resistance profiles for cytotoxic drugs. The best characterized of these mutations is the G185V mutant that confers an increased resistance to colchicine and etoposide but decreased resistance to actinomycin D, vinblastine, doxorubicin, vincristine, and taxol (167–170). Interestingly, and perhaps relevant clinically, when this mutation is made in conjunction with an Asn→Ser mutation at residue 183, increased resistance to actinomycin D, vinblastine, and doxorubicin is achieved without loss of the increase in colchicine resistance (168). Mutations of Gly-141, 187, 288, 812, or 830 to Val in human P-gp increase the relative resistance of NIH3T3 cells to colchicine and doxorubicin but do not alter resistance to vinblastine (171). Only the mutations at positions 187, 288, and 830 confer decreased resistance to actinomycin D to cells in culture.

Due to its broad substrate specificity, P-gp not only interacts with chemotherapeutic compounds but also with reversing agents and inhibitors. In combination chemotherapies, reversing agents increase the efficacy of cytotoxic agents in *MDR*1-expressing cancers. Two of the most potent reversing agents currently in use or in clinical trials are cyclosporin A and its nonimmunosuppressive analog PSC833. Recently, a number of mutants have been described that affect sensitivity to these agents. Cells expressing a human P-gp containing a deletion at Phe335 or Phe334 are substantially resistant to cyclosporin A and PSC-833 (172) (C. A. Hrycyna, I. Pastan, and M. M. Gottesman, unpublished data). A similar phenotype has been observed for a transporter containing five mutations in the region including TM 5 and TM6, namely Ile299Met, Thr319Ser, Leu322Ile, Gly324Lys, and Ser351Asn (173). Additionally, in hamster P-gp, the substitution of an alanine at position 339 with proline results in a transporter that confers lowered sensitivity to cyclosporin A (163). From these studies, it appears that TM6 plays an important role in the recognition of cyclosporin A and its analogs. The decreased sensitivity to these reversing agents observed in cells expressing the TM6 mutations could help protect bone marrow stem cells transduced with the mutant *MDR*1 gene from the toxic effects of chemotherapy given with reversing agents to sensitize MDR1-expressing tumors.

The *cis* and *trans* isomers of flupentixol, a dopamine receptor antagonist, have also been shown to inhibit drug transport and reverse drug resistance mediated by P-gp (174,175). The substitution of a single phenylalanine residue at position 983 with alanine (F983A) in TM 12 affects inhibition of P-gp–mediated drug transport by both isomers of flupentixol (P. Hafkemeyer, S. Dey, I. Pastan, and M. M. Gottesman, unpublished data). Both isomers were found to be less effective at reversing P-gp mediated drug transport of daunorubicin and bisantrene. However, the inhibitory effects of other reversing agents such as cyclosporin A were not affected. The reduced sensitivity of the F983A mutant to this compound coupled to the apparent lack of clinical toxicity of (*trans*)-flupentixol (174) suggests that this mutant may be useful in combining *MDR*1 gene therapy with chemotherapy including *trans*-flupentixol as a chemosensitizer. This approach, in theory, should allow for effective treatment at lower doses of chemotherapeutic agents while maintaining bone marrow protection.

Presently, the use of *MDR*1 gene therapy in bone marrow chemoprotection protocols is in clinical trials. In the future, with the generation of higher-resolution structures of human P-gp, it should be feasible to model and synthesize new more effective cytotoxic drugs or modulators capable of blocking P-gp function clinically. However, until that time, the analysis of spontaneously occurring or engineered mutants coupled to our knowledge of the current battery of anticancer and reversing agents offers a great opportunity to begin designing second-generation vectors for use in these trials.

VII. CONCLUSIONS AND FUTURE PROSPECTS

We have argued in this review that drug-selectable marker genes may be helpful for gene therapy in two ways: first, to protect bone marrow progenitor cells (and other sensitive cells) from the cytotoxicity of anticancer drugs, thereby allowing safe chemotherapeutic treatment at reduced risk of severe side effects, and second, to enrich the expression of otherwise nonselectable genes in drug-sensitive cells to overcome low or unstable gene expression in vivo. Given the current instability of expression of genes from existing vectors, especially episomal vectors, such selectable markers may be an essential component of gene therapy protocols.

We are still in the early stages of vector development, and until transduction efficiencies into human tissues such as bone marrow are improved, long-term human gene therapy will not be feasible. The combination of more efficient gene transfer targeted vector systems and effective, relatively nontoxic selection systems to maintain gene expression will make long-term correction of human genetic defects feasible.

REFERENCES

1. Flasshove M, Banerjee D, Leonard JP, Mineishi S, Li MX, Bertino JR, Moore MA. Retroviral transduction of human CD34+ umbilical cord blood progenitor cells with a mutated dihydrofolate reductase cDNA. Hum Gene Ther 1998; 9:63–71.
2. Wang G, Weiss C, Sheng P, Bresnick E. Retrovirus-mediated transfer of the human O^6-methylguanine-DNA methyltransferase gene into a murine hematopoietic stem cell line and resistance to the toxic effects of certain alkylating agents. Biochem Pharmacol 1996; 51:1221–1228.
3. Gottesman MM, Hrycyna CA, Schoenlein PV, Germann UA, Pastan I. Genetic analysis of the multidrug transporter. Annu Rev Genet 1995; 29:607–649.
4. D'Hondt V, Caruso M, Bank A. Retrovirus-mediated gene transfer of the multidrug resistance-associated protein (MRP) cDNA protects cells from chemotherapeutic agents. Hum Gene Ther 1997; 8:1745–1751.
5. Gottesman MM, Pastan I. Biochemistry of multidrug resistance mediated by the multidrug transporter. Annu Rev Biochem 1993; 62:385–427.
6. Deeley RG, Cole SP. Function, evolution and structure of multidrug resistance protein (MRP). Semin Cancer Biol 1997; 8:193–204.
7. Mickisch GH, Licht T, Merlino GT, Gottesman MM, Pastan I. Chemotherapy and chemosensitization of transgenic mice which express the human multidrug resistance gene in bone marrow: efficacy, potency and toxicity. Cancer Res 1991; 51:5417–5424.
8. Galski H, Sullivan M, Willingham MC, Chin K-V, Gottesman MM, Pastan I, Merlino GT. Expression of a human multidrug resistance cDNA (MDR1) in the bone marrow of transgenic mice: resistance to daunomycin induced leukopenia. Mol Cell Biol 1989; 9:4357–4363.
9. Mickisch GH, Merlino GT, Galski H, Gottesman MM, Pastan I. Transgenic mice which express the human multidrug resistance gene in bone marrow enable a rapid iden-

tification of agents which reverse drug resistance. Proc Natl Acad Sci USA 1991; 88:547–551.

10. Mickisch GH, Aksentijevich I, Schoenlein PV, Goldstein LJ, Galski H, Staehle C, Sachs DH, Pastan I, Gottesman MM. Transplantation of bone marrow cells from transgenic mice expressing the human MDR1 gene results in long-term protection against the myelosuppressive effect of chemotherapy in mice. Blood 1992; 79:1087–1093.
11. Sorrentino BP, Brandt SJ, Bodine D, Gottesman M, Pastan I, Cline A, Nienhuis AW. Selection of drug-resistant bone marrow cells in vivo after retroviral transfer of human MDR1. Science 1992; 257:99–103.
12. Podda S, Ward M, Himelstein A, Richardson C, DelaFlor-Weiss E, Smith L, Gottesman MM, Pastan I, Bank A. Transfer and expression of the human multiple drug resistance gene into live mice. Proc Natl Acad Sci USA 1992; 89:9676–9680.
13. Hanania EG, Deisseroth AB. Serial transplantation shows that early hematopoietic precursor cells are transduced by MDR-1 retroviral vector in a mouse gene therapy model. Cancer Gene Ther 1994; 1:21–25.
14. Schinkel AH, Smit JJ, van Tellingen O, Beijnen JH, Wagenaar E, van Decemter L, Mol CA, van der Valk MA, Robanus-Maandag EC, te Riele HP, et al. Disruption of the mouse mdrla P-glycoprotein gene leads to a deficiency in the blood-brain barrier and to increased sensitivity to drugs. Cell 1994; 77:491–502.
15. Schinkel AH, Wagenaar E, Mol CA, van Deemter L. P-glycoprotein in the blood-brain barrier of mice influences the brain penetration and pharmacological activity of many drugs. J Clin Invest 1996; 97:2517–2524.
16. Schinkel AH, Mayer U, Wagenaar E, Mol CA, van Deemter L, Smit JJ, van der Valk MA, Voordouw AC, Spits H, van Tellingen O, Zijlmans JM, Fibbe WE, Borst P. Normal viability and altered pharmacokinetics in mice lacking mdr1-type (drug-transporting) P-glycoproteins. Proc Natl Acad Sci USA 1997; 94:4028–4033.
17. Smit JW, Schinkel AH, Weert B, Meijer DK. Hepatobiliary and intestinal clearance of amphiphilic cationic drugs in mice in which both mdr1a and mdr1b genes have been disrupted. Br J Pharmacol 1998; 124:416–424.
18. Isola LM, Gordon JW. Systemic resistance to methotrexate in transgenic mice carrying a mutant dihydrofolate reductase gene. Proc Natl Acad Sci USA 1986; 83: 9621–9625.
19. James RI, May C, Vagt MD, Studebaker R, McIvor RS. Transgenic mice expressing the tyr22 variant of murine DHFR: protection of transgenic marrow transplant recipients from lethal doses of methotrexate. Exp Hematol 1997; 25:1286–1295.
20. Davis BM, Reese JS, Koc ON, Lee K, Schupp JE, Gerson SL. Selection for G156A methylguanine DNA methyltransferase gene-transduced hematopoietic progenitors and protection from lethality in mice treated with O^6-benzylguanine and 1,3-bis(2-chloroethyl)-1-nitrosourea. Cancer Res 1997; 57:5093–5099.
21. Gottesman MM. Multidrug-resistance during chemical carcinogenesis: a mechanism revealed? J Natl Cancer Inst 1988; 80:1352–1353.
22. Ishizaki K, Tsujimura T, Yawata H, Fujio C, Nakabeppu Y, Sekiguchi M, Ikenaga M. Transfer of the *E. coli* O^6-methylguanine methyltransferase gene into repair-deficient human cells and restoration of cellular resistance to N-methyl-N-nitro-N-nitrosoguanidine. Mutat Res 1986; 166:135–141.
23. Zaidi NH, Pretlow TP, O'Riordan MA, Dumenco LL, Allay E, Gerson SL. Transgenic expression of human MGMT protects against azoxymethane-induced aberrant crypt foci and G to A mutations in the K-ras oncogene of mouse colon. Carcinogenesis 1995; 16:451–456.
24. Liu L, Allay E, Dumenco LL, Gerson SL. Rapid repair of O^6-methylguanine-DNA adducts protects transgenic mice from N-methylnitrosourea-induced thymic lymphomas. Cancer Res 1994; 54:4648–4652.
25. Nakatsuru Y, Matsukuma S, Nemoto N, Sugano H, Sekiguchi M, Ishikawa T. O^6-methylguanine DNA methyltransferase protects against nitrosamine-induced hepatocarcinogenesis. Proc Natl Acad Sci USA 1993; 90: 6468–6472.
26. Becker K, Gregel CM, Kaina B. The DNA repair protein-methylguanine-DNA methyltransferase protects against skin tumor formation induced by antineoplastic chloroethylnitrosourea. Cancer Res 1997; 57:3335–3338.
27. May C, Gunther R, McIvor RS. Protection of mice from lethal doses of methotrexate by transplantation with transgenic marrow expressing drug-resistant dihydrofolate reductase activity. Blood 1995; 86:2439–2448.
28. Czerwinski M, Kiem HP, Slattery JT. Human CD34+ cells do not express glutathione S-transferases alpha. Gene Ther 1997; 4:268–270.
29. Drach D, Zhao S, Drach J, Mahadevia R, Gattringer C, Huber H, Andreeff M. Subpopulations of normal and peripheral blood and bone marrow cells express a functional multidrug resistant phenotype. Blood 1992; 80: 2735–2739.
30. Klimecki WT, Futscher BW, Grogan TM, Dalton WS. P-glycoprotein expression and function in circulating blood cells from normal volunteer. Blood 1994; 83:2451–2458.
31. McLachlin JR, Eglitis MA, Ueda K, Kantoff PW, Pastan I, Anderson WF, Gottesman MM. Expression of a human complementary DNA for the human multidrug resistance gene in murine hematopoietic precursor cells with the use of retroviral gene transfer. J Natl Cancer Inst 1990; 82: 1260–1263.
32. DelaFlor-Weiss E, Richardson C, Ward M, Himelstein A, Smith L, Podda S, Gottesman M, Pastan I, Bank A. Transfer and expression of the human multidrug resistance gene in mouse erythroleukemia cells. Blood 1992; 80: 3106–3111.
33. Richardson C, Ward M, Podda S, Bank A. Mouse fetal liver cells lack amphotropic retroviral receptors. Blood 1994; 84:433–439.

34. Bodine DM, Seidel NE, Gale MS, Nienhuis AW, Orlic D. Efficient retrovirus transduction of mouse pluripotent hematopoietic stem cells mobilized into the peripheral blood by treatment with granulocyte colony-stimulating factor and stem cell factor. Blood 1994; 84:1482–1491.
35. Licht T, Aksentijevich I, Gottesman MM, Pastan I. Efficient expression of functional human MDR1 gene in murine bone marrow after retroviral transduction of purified hematopoietic stem cells. Blood 1995; 86:111–121.
36. Ward M, Richardson C, Pioli P, Smith L, Podda S, Goff S, Hesdorffer C, Bank A. Transfer and expression of the human multiple drug resistance gene in human $CD34^+$ cells. Blood 1994; 84:1408–1414.
37. Bertolini F, de Monte L, Corsini C, Lazzari L, Lauri E, Soligo D, Ward M, Bank A, Malavasi F. Retrovirus-mediated transfer of the multidrug resistance gene into human haemopoietic progenitor cells. Br J Haematol 1994; 88: 318–324.
38. Nolta JA, Dao MA, Wells S, Smogorzewska EM, Kohn DB. Transduction of pluripotent human hematopoietic stem cells demonstrated by clonal analysis after engraftment in immune-deficient mice. Proc Natl Acad Sci USA 1996; 93:2414–2419.
39. Fruehauf S, Breems DA, Knaan-Shanzer S, Brouwer KB, Haas R, Lowenberg B, Nooter K, Ploemacher RE, Valerio D, Boesen JJ. Frequency analysis of multidrug resistance-1 gene transfer into human primitive hematopoietic progenitor cells using the cobblestone area-forming cell assay and detection of vector-mediated P-glycoprotein expression by rhodamine-123. Hum Gene Ther 1996; 7: 1219–1231.
40. Bunting KD, Galipeau J, Topham D, Benaim E, Sorrentino BP. Transduction of murine bone marrow cells with an MDR1 vector enables ex vivo stem cell expansion, but these expanded grafts cause a myeloproliferative syndrome in transplanted mice. Blood 1998; 92:2269–2279.
41. Miller AD, Law M-F, Verma IM. Generation of a helper free amphotropic retrovirus that transduces a dominant acting methotrexate resistant dihydrofolate reductase gene. Mol Cell Biol 1985; 5:431–437.
42. Hock RA, Miller AD. Retrovirus-mediated transfer and expression of drug resistance genes in human haematopoietic progenitor cells. Nature 1986; 320:275–277.
43. Li M-X, Banarjee D, Zhao S-C, Schweitzer BI, Mineishi S, Gilboa E, Bertino J. Development of a retroviral construct containing a human mutated dihydrofolate reductase cDNA for hematopoietic stem cell transduction. Blood 1994; 83:3403–3408.
44. Zhao SC, Li M-X, Banerjee D, Schweitzer BI, Mineishi S, Gilboa E, Bertino JR. Long term protection of recipient mice from lethal doses of methotrexate by marrow infected with a double copy vector retrovirus containing a mutant dihydrofolate reductase. Cancer Gene Ther 1994; 1:27–33.
45. Williams DA, Hsieh K, DeSilva A, Mulligan RC. Protection of bone marrow transplant recipients from lethal doses of methotrexate by the generation of methotrexate resistant bone marrow. J Exp Med 1987; 166:210–218.
46. Cline MJ, Stang H, Mercola K, Morse L, Ruprecht R, Brown J, Salser W. Gene transfer in intact animals. Nature 1980; 284:422–425.
47. Vinh DB, McIvor RS. Selective expression of methotrexate-resistant dihydrofolate reductase (DHFR) activity in mice transduced with DHFR retrovirus and administered methotrexate. J Pharmacol Exp Ther 1993; 267:989–996.
48. Corey CA, DeSilva AD, Holland CA, Williams DA. Serial transplantation of methotrexate resistant bone marrow: protection of murine recipients from drug toxicity by progeny of transduced stem cells. Blood 1990; 76:337–343.
49. Momparler RL, Eliopoulos N, Bovenzi V, Letourneau S, Greenbaum M, Cournoyer D. Resistance to cytosine arabinoside by retrovirally mediated gene transfer of human cytidine deaminase into murine fibroblast and hematopoietic cells. Cancer Gene Ther 1996; 3:331–338.
50. Letourneau S, Greenbaum M, Cournoyer D. Retrovirus-mediated gene transfer of rat glutathione S-transferase Yc confers in vitro resistance to alkylating agents in human leukemia cells and in clonogenic mouse hematopoietic progenitor cells. Hum Gene Ther 1996; 7:831–840.
51. Magni M, Shammah S, Schiro R, Mellado W, Dalla-Favera R, Gianni AM. Induction of cyclophosphamide-resistance by aldehyde-dehydrogenase gene transfer. Blood 1996; 87: 1097–1103.
52. Moreb J, Schweder M, Suresh A, Zucali JR. Overexpression of the human aldehyde dehydrogenase class I results in increased resistance to 4-hydroperoxycyclophosphamide. Cancer Gene Ther 1996; 3:24–30.
53. Allay JA, Dumenco LL, Koc ON, Liu L, Gerson SL. Retroviral transduction and expression of the human alkyltransferase cDNA provides nitrosourea resistance to hematopoietic cells. Blood 1995; 85:3342–3351.
54. Moritz T, Mackay W, Glassner BJ, Williams DA, Samson L. Retrovirus-mediated expression of a DNA repair protein in bone marrow protects hematopoietic cells from nitrosourea-induced toxicity in vitro and in vivo. Cancer Res 1995; 55:2608–2614.
55. Maze R, Carney JP, Kelley MR, Glassner BJ, Williams DA, Samson L. Increasing DNA repair methyltransferase levels via bone marrow stem cell transduction rescues mice from the toxic effects of 1,3-bis(2-chloroethyl)-1-nitrosourea, a chemotherapeutic alkylating agent. Proc Natl Acad Sci USA 1996; 93:206–210.
56. Maze R, Kapur R, Kelley MR, Hansen WK, Oh SY, Williams DA. Reversal of 1,3-bis(2-chloroethyl)-1-nitrosourea-induced severe immunodeficiency by transduction of murine long-lived hemopoietic progenitor cells using O^6-methylguanine DNA methyltransferase complementary DNA. J Immunol 1997; 158:1006–1013.
57. O'Shaughnessy JA, Cowan KH, Nienhuis AW, McDonagh KT, Sorrentino BP, Dunbar CE, Chiang Y, Wilson W, Goldspiel B, Kohler D, Cottler-Fox M, Leitman SF, Gottesman MM, Pastan I, Denicoff A, Noone M, Gress R. Retroviral mediated transfer of the human multidrug resistance gene (MDR-1) into hematopoietic stem cells

during autologous transplantation after intensive chemotherapy for metastatic breast cancer. Hum Gene Ther 1994; 5:891–911.

58. Hesdorffer C, Antman K, Bank A, Fetell M, Mears G, Begg M. Human MDR1 gene transfer in patients with advanced cancer. Hum Gene Ther 1994; 5:1151–1160.
59. Deisseroth AB, Kavanagh J, Champlin R. Use of safety-modified retroviruses to introduce chemotherapy resistance sequences into normal hematopoietic cells for chemoprotection during the therapy of ovarian cancer: a pilot trial. Hum Gene Ther 1994; 5:1507–1522.
60. Hanania EG, Giles RE, Kavanagh J, Fu SQ, Ellerson D, Zu Z, Wang T, Su Y, Kudelka A, Rahman Z, Holmes F, Hortobagyi G, Claxton D, Bachier C, Thall P, Cheng S, Hester J, Ostrove JM, Bird RE, Chang A, Korbling M, Seong D, Cote R, Holzmayer T, Mechetner E, Heimfeld S, Berenson R, Burtness B, Edwards C, Bast R, Andreeff M, Champlin R, Deisseroth AB. Results of MDR-1 vector modification trial indicate that granulocyte/macrophage colony-forming unit cells do not contribute to posttransplant hematopoietic recovery following intensive systemic therapy. Proc Natl Acad Sci USA 1996; 93:15346–15351.
61. Hesdorffer C, Ayello J, Ward M, Kaubisch A, Vahdat L, Balmaceda C, Garrett T, Fetell M, Reiss R, Bank A, Antman K. Phase I trial of retroviral-mediated transfer of the human MDR1 gene as marrow chemoprotection in patients undergoing high-dose chemotherapy and autologous stem-cell transplantation. J Clin Oncol 1998; 16:165–172.
62. Cowan KH, Moscow JA, Huang H, Zujewski J, Shaughnessy JO, Sorrentino B, Hines K, Carter C, Schneider E, Cusack G, Noon M, Dunbar D, Stein S, Wilson W, Goldspiel B, Read EJ, Leitman SF, McDonagh K, Chow C, Abati A, Chiang Y, Chang YN, Gottesman MM, Pastan I, Nienhuis A. Paclitaxel chemotherapy following autologous stem cell transplantation and engraftment of hematopoietic cells transduced with a retrovirus containing the multidrug resistance cDNA (MDR1) in metastatic breast cancer patients. Clin Cancer Res 1999; 5:1619–1628.
63. Metz MZ, Best DM, Kane SE. Harvey murine sarcoma virus/MDR1 retroviral vectors: efficient virus production and foreign gene transduction using MDR1 as a selectable marker. Virology 1995; 208:634–643.
64. Baum C, Hegewisch-Becker S, Eckert HG, Stocking C, Ostertag W. Novel retroviral vectors for efficient expression of the multidrug resistance (mdr-1) gene in early hematopoietic cells. J Virol 1995; 69:7541–7547.
65. Eckert HG, Stockschläder M, Just U, Hegewisch-Becker S, Grez M, Uhde A, Zander A, Ostertag W, Baum C. High-dose multidrug resistance in primary human hematopoietic progenitor cells transduced with optimized retroviral vectors. Blood 1996; 88:3407–3415.
66. Baudard M, Flotte TR, Aran JM, Thierry AR, Pastan I, Pang MG, Kearns WG, Gottesman MM. Expression of the human multidrug resistance and glucocerebrosidase cDNAs from adeno-associated vectors: efficient promoter activity of AAV sequences and in vivo delivery via liposomes. Hum Gene Ther 1996; 7:1309–1322.
67. Aksentijevich I, Pastan I, Lunardi-Iskandar Y, Gallo RC, Gottesman MM, Thierry AR. In vitro and in vivo liposome-mediated gene transfer leads to human MDR1 expression in mouse bone marrow progenitor cells. Hum Gene Ther 1996; 7:1111–1122.
68. Galipeau J, Benaim E, Spencer HT, Blakley RL, Sorrentino BP. A bicistronic retroviral vector for protecting hematopoietic cells against antifolates and P-glycoprotein effluxed drugs. Hum Gene Ther 1997; 8:1773–1783.
69. Fantz CR, Shaw D, Moore JG, Spencer HT. Retroviral coexpression of thymidylate synthase and dihydrofolate reductase confers fluoropyrimidine and antifolate resistance. Biochem Biophys Res Commun 1998; 243:6–12.
70. Suzuki M, Sugimoto Y, Tsukahara S, Okochi E, Gottesman MM, Tsuruo T. Retroviral co-expression of two different types of drug-resistance genes to protect normal cells from combination chemotherapy. Clin Cancer Res 1997; 3:947–954.
71. Suzuki M, Sugimoto Y, Tsuruo T. Efficient protection of cells from the genotoxicity of nitrosureas by the retrovirus-mediated transfer of human O^6-methylguanine-DNA methyltransferase using bicistronic vectors with human multidrug resistance gene 1. Mutat Res 1998; 401: 133–141.
72. Sugimoto Y, Hrycyna CA, Aksentijevich I, Pastan I, Gottesman MM. Coexpression of a multidrug-resistance gene (MDR1) and herpes simplex virus thymidine kinase gene as part of a bicistronic messenger RNA in a retrovirus vector allows selective killing of MDR1-transduced cells. Clinical Cancer Res 1995b; 1:447–457.
73. Sugimoto Y, Sato S, Tsukahara S, Suzuki M, Okochi E, Gottesman MM, Pastan I, Tsuruo T. Co-expression of a multidrug resistance gene (MDR1) and herpes simplex virus thymidine kinase gene in a bicistronic vector Ha-MDR-IRES-TK allows selective killing of MDR1-transduced human tumors transplanted in mice. Cancer Gene Ther 1997; 4:51–58.
74. Mineishi S, Nakahara S, Takebe N, Banerjee D, Zhao SC, Bertino JR. Co-expression of the herpes simplex virus thymidine kinase gene potentiates methotrexate resistance conferred by transfer of a mutated dihydrofolate reductase gene. Gene Ther 1997; 46:570–576.
75. Zhao RC, McIvor RS, Griffin JD, Verfaillie CM. Gene therapy for chronic myelogenous leukemia (CML): a retroviral vector that renders hematopoietic progenitors methotrexate-resistant and CML progenitors functionally normal and nontumorigenic in vivo. Blood 1997; 90: 4687–4698.
76. Xu LC, Kluepfel-Stahl S, Blanco M, Schiffmann R, Dunbar C, Karlsson S. Growth factors and stromal support generate very efficient retroviral transduction of peripheral blood $CD34^+$ cells from Gaucher patients. Blood 1995; 86:141–146.
77. Havenga M, Fisher R, Hoogerbrugge P, Roberts B, Valerio D, van Es HH. Development of safe and efficient retroviral vectors for Gaucher disease. Gene Ther 1997; 4: 1393–1400.

78. Aran JM, Gottesman MM, Pastan I. Drug-selected coexpression of human glucocerebrosidase and P-glycoprotein using a bicistronic vector. Proc Natl Acad Sci USA 1994; 91:3176–3180.
79. Aran JM, Licht T, Gottesman MM, Pastan I. Complete restoration of glucocerebrosidase deficiency in Gaucher fibroblasts using a bicistronic MDR retrovirus and a new selection strategy. Hum Gene Ther 1996; 7:2165–2175.
80. Sugimoto Y, Aksentijevich I, Murray GJ, Brady RO, Pastan I, Gottesman MM. Retroviral co-expression of a multidrug resistance gene (MDR1) and human α-galactosidase A for gene therapy of Fabry disease. Hum Gene Therapy 1995; 6:905–915.
81. Sokolic RA, Sekhsaria S, Sugimoto Y, Whiting-Theobald N, Linton GF, Li F, Gottesman MM, Malech HL. A bicistronic retrovirus vector containing a picornavirus internal ribosome entry site allows for correction of X-linked CGD by selection for MDR1 expression. [Rapid Communication] Blood 1996; 87:42–50.
82. Zhou Y, Aran J, Gottesman MM, Pastan I. Co-expression of human adenosine deaminase and multidrug resistance using a bicistronic retroviral vector. Hum Gene Ther 1998; 9:287–293.
83. Kleiman SE, Pastan I, Puck JM, Gottesman MM. Characterization of an MDR1 retroviral bicistronic vector for correction of X-linked severe combined immunodeficiency. Gene Ther 1998; 5:671–676.
84. Germann UA, Chin K-V, Pastan I, Gottesman MM. Retroviral transfer of a chimeric multidrug resistance-adenosine deaminase gene. FASEB J 1990; 4:1501–1507.
85. Ohshima T, Murray GJ, Swaim WD, Longenecker G, Quirk JM, Cardarelli CO, Sugimoto Y, Pastan I, Gottesman MM, Brady RO, Kulkarni AB. α-Galactosidase A deficient mice: a model of Fabry disease. Proc Natl Acad Sci USA 1997; 94:2540–2544.
86. Aran JM, Gottesman MM, Pastan I. Construction and characterization of bicistronic vectors encoding the multidrug transporter and β-galactosidase or green fluorescent protein. Cancer Gene Ther 1998; 5:195–206.
87. Germann UA, Gottesman M, Pastan I. Expression of a multidrug resistance-adenosine deaminase fusion gene. J Biol Chem 1989; 264:7418–7424.
88. Pelletier J, Sonenberg N. Internal initiation of translation of eukaryotic mRNA directed by a sequence derived from poliovirus RNA. Nature 1988; 334:320–325.
89. Trono D, Pelletier J, Sonenberg N, Baltimore D. Translation in mammalian cells of a gene linked to the poliovirus 5′-noncoding region. Science 1988; 41:445–448.
90. Adam MA, Ramesh N, Miller AD, Osborne WA. Internal initiation of translation in retroviral vector carrying picornavirus 5′ nontranslated regions. J Virol 1991; 65: 4985–4990.
91. Kaufman RJ, Davies MV, Wasley LC, Michnick D. Improved vectors for stable expression of foreign genes in mammalian cells by use of the untranslated leader sequence from EMC virus. Nucleic Acids Res 1991; 19: 4485–4490.
92. Lee CGL, Jeang K-T, Martin MA, Pastan I, Gottesman MM. Efficient long term co-expression of a hammerhead ribozyme targeted to the U5 region of HIV-1 LTR by linkage to the multidrug-resistance gene. Antisense Nucleic Acid Drug Dev 1997; 7:511–522.
93. Pastan I, Gottesman MM, Ueda K, Lovelace E, Rutherford AV, Willingham MC. A retrovirus carrying an MDR1 cDNA confers multidrug resistance and polarized expression of P-glycoprotein in MDCK cells. Proc Natl Acad Sci USA 1988; 85:4486–4490.
94. Zhang S, Sugimoto Y, Shoshani T, Pastan I, Gottesman MM. A pHaMDR-DHFR bicistronic expression system for mutational analysis of P-glycoprotein. Methods Enzymol 1998; 292:474–480.
95. Sugimoto Y, Aksentijevich I, Gottesman M, Pastan I. Efficient expression of drug-selectable genes in retroviral vectors under control of an internal ribosome entry site. Bio/Technology 1994; 12:694–698.
96. Toyoda H, Koide N, Kamiyama M, Tobita K, Mizumoto K, Imura N. Host factors required for internal initiation of translation on poliovirus RNA. Arch Virol 1994; 138: 1–15.
97. Brown EA, Zajac A, Lemon S. In vitro characterization of an internal ribosomal entry site present within the 5′ nontranslated region of hepatitis A virus RNA: comparison with the IRES of encephalomyocarditis virus. J Virology 1994; 68:1066–1074.
98. Borman AM, Bailly J, Girard M, Kean K. Picornavirus internal ribosome entry segments: comparison of translation efficiency and the requirements for optimal internal initiation of translation in vitro. Nucleic Acid Res 1995; 23:3656–3663.
99. Aran JM, Germann UA, Gottesman MM, Pastan I. Construction and characterization of a selectable multidrug resistance-glucocerebrosidase fusion gene. Cytokines Mol Ther 1996; 2:47–57.
100. Blaese RM. Development of gene therapy for immunodeficiency: adenosine deaminase deficiency. Ped Res 1993; 33(suppl):S49–S55.
101. Kantoff PW, Kohn DB, Mitsuya H, Armentano D, Sieberg M, Zweibel JA, Eglitis MA, McLachlin JR, Wiginton DA, Hutton JJ, Horowitz SD, Gilboa E, Blease RM, Anderson WF. Correction of adenosine deaminase deficiency in human T and B cells using retroviral gene transfer. Proc Natl Acad Sci USA 1986; 83:6563–6567.
102. Kotin RM, Siniscalco M, Samulski RJ, Zhu XD, Hunter L, Laughlin CA, McLaughlin S, Muzyczka N, Rocchi M, Berns KI. Site-specific integration by adeno-associated virus. Proc Natl Acad Sci USA 1990; 87:2211–2215.
103. Flotte TR, Afione, SA, Zeitlin PL. Adeno-associated virus vector gene expression occurs in nondividing cells in the absence of vector DNA integration. Am J Respir Cell Mol Biol 1994; 11:517–521.
104. Flotte TR, Carter BJ. Adeno-associated virus vectors for gene therapy. Gene Ther 1995; 2:357–362.
105. Flotte TR, Afione SA, Conrad C, McGrath SA, Solow R, Oka H, Zeitlin PL, Guggino WB, Carter BJ. Stable in vivo

expression of the cystic fibrosis transmembrane conductance regulator with an adeno-associated virus vector. Proc Natl Acad Sci USA 1993; 90:10613–10617.

106. Flotte TR, Afione SA, Solow R, Drumm ML, Markakis D, Guggino WB, Zeitlin PL, Carter BJ. Expression of the cystic fibrosis transmembrane conductance regulator from a novel adeno-associated virus promoter. J Biol Chem 1993; 268:3781–3790.
107. Kaplitt MG, Leone P, Samulski RJ, Xiao X, Pfaff DW, O'Malley KL, During MJ. Long-term gene expression and phenotypic correction using adeno-associated virus vectors in the mammalian brain. Nat Genet 1994; 8:148–154.
108. Kessler PD, Podsakoff GM, Chen X, McQuiston SA, Colosi PC, Matelis LA, Kurtzman GJ, Byrne BJ. Gene delivery to skeletal muscle results in sustained expression and systemic delivery of a therapeutic protein. Proc Natl Acad Sci USA 1996; 93:14082–14087.
109. Snyder RO, Miao, CH, Patijn, GA, Spratt SK, Danos O, Nagy D, Gown AM, Winther B, Meuse L, Cohen LK, Thompson AR, Kay MA. Persistent and therapeutic concentrations of human factor 1X in mice after hepatic gene transfer of recombinant AAV vectors. Nat Genet 1997; 16:270–276.
110. Xiao X, Li J, McCown TJ, Samulski RJ. Gene transfer by adeno-associated virus vectors into the central nervous system. Exp Neurol 1997; 144:113–124.
111. Tsui LC, Breitman ML, Siminovitch L, Buchwald M. (1982). Persistence of freely replicating SV40 recombinant molecules carrying a selectable marker in permissive simian cells. Cell 1982; 30:499–508.
112. Yates JL, Warren N, Sugden B. Stable replication of plasmids derived from Epstein-Barr virus in various mammalian cells. Nature 1985; 313:812–815.
113. Cooper MJ, Miron S. Efficient episomal expression vector for human transitional carcinoma cells. Hum Gene Ther 1993; 4:557–566.
114. Milanesi G, Barbanti-Brodano G, Negrini M, Lee D, Corallini A, Caputo A, Grossi MP, Ricciardi RP. BK virus-plasmid expression vector that persists episomally in human cells and shuttles into *Escherichia coli.* Mol Cell Biol 1984; 4:1551–1560.
115. Sabbioni S, Negrini M, Rimessi P, Manservigi R, Barbanti-Brodano G. A BK virus episomal vector for constitutive high expression of exogenous cDNAs in human cells. Arch Virol 1995; 140:335–339.
116. Mortimer EA Jr, Lepow ML, Gold E, Robbins FC, Burton GJ, Fraumeni JF Jr. Long-term follow-up of persons inadvertently inoculated with SV40 as neonates. N Engl J Med 1981; 305:1517–1518.
117. Shah K, Nathanson N. Human exposure to SV40: review and comment. Am J Epidemiol 1976; 103:1–12.
118. Chia W, Rigby PW. Fate of viral DNA in nonpermissive cells infected with simian virus 40. Proc Natl Acad Sci USA 1981; 78:6638–6642.
119. Strayer DS. SV40 as an effective gene transfer vector in vivo. J Biol Chem 1996; 271:24741–24746.
120. Strayer DS., Milano J. SV40 mediates stable gene transfer in vivo. Gene Ther 1996; 3:581–587.
121. Daylot N, Oppenheim A. Efficient transfer of the complete human b-globin gene into human and mouse hematopoietic cells via SV40 pseudovirions. In: Beaudet AL, Mulligan R, Verma IM, eds. Gene Transfer and Gene Therapy. New York: Alan R. Liss, Inc, 1989:47–56.
122. Rund D, Dagan M, Dalyot-Herman N, Kimchi-Sarfaty C, Schoenlein PV, Gottesman MM, Oppenheim A. Efficient transduction of human hematopoietic cells with the human multidrug resistance gene 1 via SV40 pseudovirions. Hum Gene Ther 1998; 9:649–657.
123. Sandalon Z, Dalyot-Herman N., Oppenheim AB, Oppenheim A. In vitro assembly of SV40 virions and pseudovirions: vector development for gene therapy. Hum Gene Ther 1997; 8:843–849.
124. Fang B, Koch P, Bouvet M, Ji L, Roth JA. A packaging system for SV40 vectors without viral coding sequences. Anal Biochem 1997; 254:139–143.
125. Mellon P, Parker V, Gluzman Y, Maniatis T. Identification of DNA sequences required for transcription of the human alpha 1-globin gene in a new SV40 host-vector system. Cell 1981; 27:279–288.
126. Cooper MJ, Lippa M, Payne JM, Hatzivassiliou G, Reifenberg E, Fayazi B, Perales JC, Morrison LJ, Templeton D, Piekarz RL, Tan J. (1997). Safety-modified episomal vectors for human gene therapy. Proc Natl Acad Sci USA 1997; 94:6450–6455.
127. Kieff E, Liebowitz D. Epstein Barr virus and its replication. In: Fields BN, Knipe DM, eds. Virology. New York: Raven, 1990:1921–1958.
128. Margolskee RF. Epstein-Barr virus based expression vectors. Curr Top Microbiol Immunol 1992; 158:67–95.
129. Sarasin, A. Shuttle vectors for studying mutagenesis in mammalian cells. J Photochem Photobiol B: Biology 1989; 3:143–155.
130. Levitskaya J, Coram M, Levitsky V, Imreh S, Steigerwald-Mullen PM, Klein G, Kurilla MG, Masucci MG. Inhibition of antigen processing by the internal repeat region of the Epstein-Barr virus nuclear antigen-1. Nature 1995; 375: 685–688.
131. Haase SB, Calos, MP. Replication control of autonomously replicating human sequences. Nucleic Acids Res 1991; 19:5053–5058.
132. Sun TQ, Fernstermacher DA, Vos JM. Human artificial episomal chromosomes for cloning large DNA fragments in human cells [published erratum appears in Nat Genet 1994; 8:410]. Nat Genet 1994; 8:33–41.
133. Banerjee S, Livanos E, Vos JM. Therapeutic gene delivery in human B-lymphoblastoid cells by engineered non-transforming infectious Epstein-Barr virus. Nat Med 1995; 1: 1303–1308.
134. Lee CGL, Vieira WD, Pastan I, Gottesman MM. Delivery systems for the MDR1 gene. Gene Ther Mol Biol 1998; 1:241–251.
135. DiMaio D, Treisman R, Maniatis T. Bovine papillomavirus vector that propagates as a plasmid in both mouse

and bacterial cells. Proc Natl Acad Sci USA 1982; 79: 4030–4034.
136. Mecsas J, Sugden B. Replication of plasmids derived from bovine papilloma virus type 1 and Epstein-Barr virus in cells in culture. Annu Rev Cell Biol 1987; 3:87–108.
137. Grignani F, Kinsella T, Mencarelli A, Valtieri M, Riganelli D, Grignani F, Lanfrancone L, Peschle C, Nolan GP, Pelicci PG. High-efficiency gene transfer and selection of human hematopoietic progenitor cells with a hybrid EBV/retroviral vector expressing the green fluorescence protein. Cancer Res 1998; 58:14–19.
138. Kinsella TM, Nolan GP. Episomal vectors rapidly and stably produce high-titer recombinant retrovirus. Hum Gene Ther 1996; 7:1405–1413.
139. Feng M, Jackson WH Jr, Goldman CK, Rancourt C, Wang M, Dusing SK, Siegal G, Curiel DT. Stable in vivo gene transduction via a novel adenoviral/retroviral chimeric vector [see comments]. Nat Biotechnol 1997; 15:866–70.
140. Wang S, Di S, Young WB, Jacobson C, Link CJ Jr. A novel herpesvirus amplicon system for in vivo gene delivery. Gene Ther 1997; 4:1132–1141.
141. Fraefel C, Jacoby DR, Lage C, Hilderbrand H, Chou JY, Alt FW, Breakefield XO, Majzoub JA. Gene transfer into hepatocytes mediated by helper virus-free HSV/AAV hybrid vectors. Mol Med 1997; 3:813–825.
142. Dzau VJ, Mann MJ, Morishita R, Kaneda Y. Fusigenic viral liposome for gene therapy in cardiovascular diseases [comment]. Proc Natl Acad Sci USA 1996; 93: 11421–11425.
143. Hirai H, Satoh E, Osawa M, Inaba T, Shimazaki C, Kinoshita S, Nakagawa M, Mazda O, Imanishi J. Use of EBV-based Vector/HVJ-liposome complex vector for targeted gene therapy of EBV-associated neoplasms. Biochem Biophys Res Commun 1997; 241:112–118.
144. Satoh E, Osawa M, Tomiyasu K, Hirai H, Shimazaki C, Oda Y, Nakagawa M, Kondo M, Kinoshita S, Mazda O, Imanishi J. Efficient gene transduction by Epstein-Barr-virus-based vectors coupled with cationic liposome and HVJ-liposome. Biochem Biophys Res Commun 1997; 238:795–799.
145. Krysan PJ, Haase SB, Calos MP. Isolation of human sequences that replicate autonomously in human cells. Mol Cell Biol 1989; 9:1026–1033.
146. Krysan PJ, Calos MP. Epstein-Barr virus-based vectors that replicate in rodent cells. Gene 1993; 136:137–143.
147. Calos MP. The potential of extrachromosomal replicating vectors for gene therapy. Trends Genet 1996; 12:463–466.
148. Jankelevich S, Kolman JL, Bodnar JW, Miller G. A nuclear matrix attachment region organizes the Epstein-Barr viral plasmid in Raji cells into a single DNA domain. EMBO J 1992; 11:1165–1176.
149. Wohlgemuth JG, Kang SH, Bulboaca GH, Nawotka KA, Calos MP. Long-term gene expression from autonomously replicating vectors in mammalian cells. Gene Ther 1996; 3:503–512.
150. DePamphilis ML. Eukaryotic replication origins. In: DePamphilis ML, ed. DNA Replication in Eukaryotic Cells. Cold Spring Harbor, NY: Cold Spring Harbor Laboratory Press, 1996:983–1004.
151. Willard HF, Waye, JS. Hierarchical order in chromosome-specific human alpha satellite DNA. Trends Genet 1987; 3:192–198.
152. Bloom K. The centromere frontier: kinetochore components, microtubule-based motility, and the CEN-value paradox. Cell 1993; 73:621–624.
153. Harrington JJ, Van Bokkelen G, Mays RW, Gustashaw K, Willard HF. Formation of de novo centromeres and construction of first-generation human artificial microchromosomes [see comments]. Nat Genet 1997; 15: 345–355.
154. Philip R, Liggitt D, Philip M, Dazin P, Debs R. Efficient transfection of T lymphocytes in adult mice. J Biol Chem 1993; 268:16087–16090.
155. Philip R, Brunette E, Kilinski L, Murugesh D, McNally M, Ucar K, Rosenblatt J, Okarama TB, Lebkowski JS. Efficient and sustained gene expression in primary T lymphocytes and primary and cultured tumor cells mediated by adeno-associated virus plasmid DNA complexed to cationic liposomes. Mol Cell Biol 1994; 14:2411–2418.
156. Bruggemann EP, Currier SJ, Gottesman MM, Pastan I. Characterization of the azidopine and vinblastine binding site of P-glycoprotein. J Biol Chem 1992; 267: 21020–21026.
157. Greenberger LM. Major photoaffinity drug labeling sites for iodoaryl azidoprazosin in P-glycoprotein are within, or immediately C-terminal to, transmembrane domain-6 and domain-12. J Biol Chem 1993; 268:11417–11425.
158. Greenberger LM, Lisanti CJ, Silva JT, Horwitz SB. Domain mapping of the photoaffinity drug-binding sites in P-glycoprotein encoded mouse mdr1b. J Biol Chem 1991; 266:20744–20751.
159. Morris DI, Greenberger LM, Bruggemann EP, Cardarelli CO, Gottesman MM, Pastan I, Seamon KB. Localization of the forskolin labeling sites to both halves of P-glycoprotein: similarity of the sites labeled by forskolin and prazosin. Mol Pharmacol 1994; 46:329–337.
160. Zhang X, Collins KI, Greenberger LM. Functional evidence that transmembrane 12 and the loop between transmembrane 11 and 12 form part of the drug-binding domain in P-glycoprotein encoded by MDR1. J Biol Chem 1995; 270:5441–5448.
161. Gottesman MM, Pastan I, Ambudkar SV. P-glycoprotein and multidrug resistance. Curr Opin Genet Dev 1996; 6: 610–617.
162. Devine SE, Ling V, Melera PW. Amino acid substitutions in the sixth transmembrane domain of P-glycoprotein alter multidrug resistance. Proc Natl Acad Sci USA 1992; 89: 4564–4568.
163. Ma JF, Grant G, Melera PW. Mutations in the sixth transmembrane domain of P-glycoprotein that alter the pattern of cross-resistance also alter sensitivity to cyclosporin A reversal. Mol Pharmacol 1997; 51:922–930.
164. Loo TW, Clarke DM. Functional consequences of phenylalanine mutations in the predicted transmembrane domain of P-glycoprotein. J Biol Chem 1993; 268:19965–19972.

165. Loo TW, Clarke DM. Mutations to amino acids located in predicted transmembrane segment 6 (TM6) modulate the activity and substrate specificity of human P-glycoprotein. Biochemistry 1994; 33:14049–14057.
166. Hanna M, Brault M, Kwan T, Kast C, Gros P. Mutagenesis of transmembrane domain 11 of P-glycoprotein by alanine scanning. Biochemistry 1996; 35:3625–3635.
167. Choi K, Chen C-J, Kriegler M, Roninson IB. An altered pattern of cross-resistance in multidrug-resistant human cells results from spontaneous mutations in the mdr1 (P-glycoprotein) gene. Cell 1989; 53:519–529.
168. Currier SJ, Kane SE, Willingham MC, Cardarelli CO, Pastan I, Gottesman MM. Identification of residues in the first cytoplasmic loop of P-glycoprotein involved in the function of chimeric human MDR1-MDR2 transporters. J Biol Chem 1992; 267:25153–25159.
169. Kioka N, Tsubota J, Kakehi Y, Komano T, Gottesman MM, Pastan I, Ueda K. P-glycoprotein gene (MDR1) cDNA from human adrenal: normal P-glycoprotein carries Gly^{185} with an altered pattern of multidrug resistance. Biochem Biophys Res Commun 1989; 162:224–231.
170. Safa AR, Stern RK, Choi K, Agresti M, Tamai I, Mehta ND, Roninson IB. Molecular basis of preferential resistance to colchicine in multidrug-resistant human cells conferred by Gly to Val-185 substitution in P-glycoprotein. Proc Natl Acad Sci USA 1990; 87:7225–7229.
171. Loo TW, Clarke DM. Functional consequences of glycine mutations in the predicted cytoplasmic loops of P-glycoprotein. J Biol Chem 1994; 269:7243–7248.
172. Chen G. Duran GE, Steger KA, Lacayo NJ, Jaffrezou JP, Dumontet C., Dikic BI. Multidrug-resistant human sarcoma cells with a mutant P-glycoprotein, altered phenotype, and resistance to cyclosporins. J Biol Chem 1997; 272:5974–5982.
173. Shoshani T, Zhang S, Dey S, Pastan I, Gottesman MM. Analysis of random recombination between human *MDR*1 and mouse *mdr*1a cDNA in a pHaMDR-DHFR bicistronic expression system. Mol Pharmacol 1998; 54:623–630.
174. Ford JM, Prozialeck WC, Hait WN. Structural features determining activity of phenothiazines and related drugs for inhibition of cell growth and reversal of multidrug resistance. Mol Pharmacol 1989; 35:105–115.
175. Yang JM, Goldenberg S, Gottesman MM, Hait WN. Characteristics of P388/VMDRC.04, a simple, sensitive model for studying P-glycoprotein antagonists. Cancer Res 1994; 54:730–737.

17

Suicide Gene Therapy

Bert W. O'Malley, Jr.
The University of Maryland School of Medicine, Baltimore, Maryland

I. INTRODUCTION

Despite decades of scientific advancements and new developments in surgery, radiation therapy, and chemotherapy, human cancer continues to be a major and growing cause of death in the world today. For most solid tumors, surgical excision is the primary mode of treatment and is frequently combined with radiation or chemotherapy for maximal efficacy. Radiation is capable of destroying both normal and abnormal tissues but has a preferential effect on dividing malignant cells. Chemotherapy involves the use of cytotoxic drugs, which also have a preferentially effect on rapidly dividing cells. Chemotherapeutic drugs are often used in combination because tumors have shown greater susceptibility to multiple agents that attack tumor cells by different mechanisms. Progress with these standard modalities for treating cancer continues while a new field of cancer research and treatment is evolving at a rapid pace. This new field is ''gene therapy'' and is founded on the premise that specific genes can be introduced into tumor cells to cause either a direct or indirect antitumor effect.

At first consideration, cancer does not appear to be a suitable target for ''classic gene therapy.'' That is, the original concept of gene therapy stemmed from the observation that certain diseases are caused by the inheritance of a single defective gene. Such diseases with monogenic defects such as adenosine deaminase deficiency and Gaucher's disease could theoretically be treated by effective insertion and expression of a normal gene into the defective host cells or even the bone marrow stem cell population (1,2). On the other hand, our recent understanding of cancer is that it develops via a multistep process whereby a series of genetic alterations or mutations occur within one cell (3). This one cell then loses regulatory control and proliferates abnormally to produce a population of malignant cells that may also continue to mutate and lead to cancer spread or metastases. Given the complexity of this genetic progression of cancer and the still many unknown abnormalities within any given tumor type, the idea of replacing all the abnormal genes with normal copies using gene therapy would be prohibitive. Also, with the limitations of delivery vehicles or ''vectors'' currently available for gene therapy, it would be equally prohibitive to effectively deliver the normal genes to every defective cancer cell.

Cancer gene therapy, however, is moving in directions that attempt to circumvent these apparent limitations. On such direction is the development of prodrug or ''suicide gene therapy'' strategies, which involve specific gene transfer into tumor cells that enables intracellular conversion of a ''nontoxic'' prodrug into an active cytotoxic drug. Following effective suicide gene transfer and systemic or oral administration of the prodrug, an enzyme encoded by the therapeutic gene converts the prodrug into toxic anabolites or metabolites that inhibit or disrupt DNA synthesis. The tumor cells subsequently die via necrosis or apoptotic pathways. The most common suicide gene used in preclinical and human clinical investigation is the gene encoding herpes simplex virus thymidine kinase. A major advantage of many suicide gene therapy strategies is that not only are the tumor cells that have incorporated the gene destroyed, but surrounding ''nontransduced'' cells are also killed (4). The mechanism by which nontransduced neighboring tumor cells are killed is known as the ''bystander effect,'' which will be discussed in more detail later in the chapter. The many facets of the bystander effect significantly strengthen suicide gene therapy as a whole and add to its versatility.

Although the identification and selection of specific suicide genes that may induce both direct and/or indirect antitumor effects is a very important area in gene therapy research, equally important to the success of such strategies is the growing arena of vector or delivery vehicle development. The choice of delivery vehicle greatly influences the overall outcome and efficiency of the therapeutic strategy. Even with the beneficial bystander effect, the effects of suicide gene therapy are linearly related to the efficiency of gene transfer. New investigations and advances in both viral and nonviral gene therapy technologies should also prove valuable in overcoming many of the obstacles in the application of gene therapy to cancer.

This chapter will describe the various suicide gene therapy strategies for treating solid tumors and provide an overview of advantages and disadvantages of viral versus nonviral methods of delivering these genes. The two basic approaches for suicide gene delivery, in vivo and ex vivo, will also be reviewed and an update on the status of human clinical trials will be provided.

II. GENERAL PRINCIPLES AND SAFETY ISSUES

The principle of suicide gene therapy stems from the long history of drug discovery and development focusing on the treatment of microbial infections. The enyzmes encoded by suicide genes are important components in metabolic conversion pathways within bacteria, viruses, or fungi (5). The effect of a prodrug on human cells that have been transduced with a suicide gene therefore parallels the effect of an antibiotic on a human bacterial infection. The microbial origin of these enzymes provide two important safety and specificity features of suicide gene-prodrug therapy that are similar or identical to the features of antibiotic or antiviral therapy. First, the enyzmes and the associated metabolic pathway may be completely specific to microbial cells and not found in mammalian cells. Because mammalian cells lack the enzyme encoded by the suicide gene, systemic administration of the prodrug has no toxic effect on any human tissue or cell that has not been engineered to express the selected suicide gene (6). Second, certain mammalian cells may actually express the enyzme but the specific prodrug chosen may be a poor substrate for the mammalian form of the enzyme and an excellent substrate for the bacterial or viral form. Again in this scenario, administration of the prodrug would be harmless to the mammalian cell that has not been engineered to overexpress the nonmammalian enzyme. The prodrug is therefore similar to or may actually be a form of antibiotic or antiviral medicine. Systemic administrations of the prodrug will produce effects limited to cells expressing the suicide gene and the microenvironment surrounding these cells and would not cause significant systemic toxicity.

Another general safety feature for suicide gene therapy lies within the actual mechanism of cytotoxicity that results from the conversion of the prodrug to a toxic metabolite. Since the majority of these metabolites inhibit cellular nucleic acid synthesis pathways, the delivery of the suicide gene and administration of the prodrug would have a preferential cytotoxic effect on actively dividing cells. With respect to tumor cell populations versus normal mammalian cells, the tumor would be more susceptible to the effects of suicide gene therapy. Some suicide gene therapy systems do not show preference for dividing cells, which raises a safety issue. Surrounding normal tissue may be inadvertently injured after exposure and subsequent transduction by the suicide gene. Selection and application of gene-delivery techniques are therefore important in targeting the tumor while minimizing exposure of normal or systemic tissues to the suicide gene.

III. SUICIDE GENE THERAPY STRATEGIES

A key issue in the success of a suicide gene therapy strategy is the interaction between the enzyme produced and the prodrug administered. The selection of the enzyme and prodrug combination is influenced by certain variables critical to enyzme-substrate kinetics. Two important variables exist for the enzyme. The first is the speed of activation of the prodrug. The most effective suicide genes will express enzymes that rapidly activate the prodrug. Enzymes that are slower in their activation will be dependent on either higher concentrations of the prodrug or prolonged administration. Issues such as half-life and intracellular degradation and clearance mechanisms will also limit the presence of the prodrug. The second variable is the efficiency of prodrug activation. Enzymes that are highly efficient in converting the prodrug substrate into its toxic metabolite should prove advantageous because of known variances in the levels of effective gene transfer and gene expression (enzyme production) inherent to in vivo suicide gene transfer. Regarding the prodrug, it should be at least 100 times more cytotoxic than the preactivated form upon enzyme activation (7). Since many different types of prodrugs can be designed to achieve maximal activation, the most important and probably most limiting factor is the enzyme and therefore choice of suicide gene. Table 1 depicts the suicide gene and corresponding prodrug combinations under investigation for gene therapy application. Table 2 shows the

Table 1 Selected Suicide Gene Therapy Strategies

Gene/Enzyme	Prodrug	Initial toxic metabolite
Herpes simplex virus thymidine kinase (HSV-tk)	Ganciclovir (GCV)	Ganciclovir monophosphate
Cytosine deaminase (CD)	5-Fluorocytosine (5-FC)	5-Fluorouracil (5-FU)
Varicella zoster virus thymidine kinase (VZV-tk)	6-Methoxypurine arabinonucleoside (araM)	Adenine arabinonucleoside monophosphate
Escherichia coli nitroreductase (NTR)	5-(Aziridin-1-yl)-2,4-dinitrobenzamide (CB1954)	5-(Aziridin-1-yl)-4-hydroxyamino-2-nitrobenzamide
Cytochrome P450 B1 (CYP2B1)	Cyclophosphamide (CPA)	4-Hydroxy-cyclophosphamide (4-HCPA)
Carboxypeptidase G2 (CPG2)	Benzoic acid mustard gluconuride (CMDA)	Benzoic acid mustard

mechanisms of toxicity for selected genes presently being investigated in both preclinical and clinical studies.

Despite choosing a generally efficient enzyme-prodrug combination that proves successful with in vitro experimentation, there may not be a paralleled success after the transition to in vivo application against established tumors. In vivo efficacy may also vary among different types or classes of tumors for any one given enzyme-prodrug combination. An example of this is found within the herpes simplex virus thymidine kinase (HSV-tk) gene therapy strategy, the most widely used suicide gene in both preclinical investigation and human clinical trials. While HSV-tk has proven effective in many different solid tumors, it is generally less effective against hematopoietic malignancies (8). It has been hypothesized that HSV-tk is downregulated or lost more quickly in hematopoietic tumors such as leukemia, which results in ineffective or insufficient conversion of the prodrug to achieve antitumor effects (9).

A. Herpes Simplex Virus Thymidine Kinase

HSV-tk has shown the greatest potential to date for human application across a broad range of malignancies, and for this reason it is the most popular and widely studied suicide gene therapy strategy. The importance of HSV-tk gene transfer centers on its ability to render cells sensitive to the acyclic guanosine analog ganciclovir (GCV) (10,11). HSV-tk is a prototype ''suicide gene'' because it encodes a viral enzyme that is foreign to mammalian cells and will convert an inactive and relatively nontoxic prodrug to a toxic product. Upon effective HSV-tk gene transfer and expression, the prodrug GCV is monophosphorylated by the enzyme. Intracellular host kinases then metabolize this monophosphorylated nucleoside analog into di- and triphosphates (12). The triphosphate form of GCV is then incorporated into the replicating DNA chain in dividing cells and inhibits DNA polymerase. Inhibition of DNA polymerase results in chain termination, disruption of DNA synthesis, and cell death. The phosporylation of GCV impairs its ability to cross the cell membrane, and as a result the half-life increases by sixfold to 18–24 hours (13,14). The extended half-life of the phosphorylated GCV strengthens the overall anticancer effect of this HSV-tk strategy. With respect to sensitivity, viral thymidine kinase is approximately 1000 times more efficient in phosphory-

Table 2 Mechanisms of Cytotoxicity of Select Suicide Gene Therapy Strategies

Gene	Final toxic metabolite(s)	Direct cytotoxic effect	Bystander effect
HSV-tk	GCV-triphosphate	Disrupts DNA synthesis	Present
CD	5-FU-mono/tripohosphate	Disrupts DNA and RNA synthesis	Present
VZV-tk	ara-ATP	Disrupts DNA synthesis	Unknown
NTR	4-hydroxylamine metabolite of CB1954	Cross-links DNA (direct DNA breaks; disrupts synthesis)	Unknown
CYP2B1	Phosphoramide mustard DNA acrolein	Alkylation (cross links DNA) covalently links cellular proteins	Present
CPG2	Benzoic acid mustard	DNA alkylation (cross-links DNA)	Present

lating GCV than its mammalian counterpart (13). Since GCV is an excellent substrate for viral thymidine kinases and a poor substrate for mammalian thymidine kinases, concentrations can be achieved that are lethal to cells expressing HSV-tk but are nontoxic to normal mammalian cells (10,11,15).

Culver et al. demonstrated the first in vivo application of suicide gene therapy for cancer using retroviral-mediated HSV-tk gene transfer via fibroblast packaging cells injected into brain tumors in mice (16,17). Since this initial study, HSV-tk suicide gene therapy has been applied and investigated in multiple tumor types including thoracic, head and neck, and ovarian cancer (18–20). Critical to the tumor response described in these early studies was the observation that not all the tumor cells must express the HSV-tk gene for a complete or extensive tumoricidal effect. The term bystander effect has been attributed to the regression of noninfected surrounding tumor cells after HSV-tk delivery and GCV administration. There are both direct and indirect mechanisms driving the bystander effect that will be discussed in more detail later in the chapter. Briefly, the direct effect is an exchange of toxic metabolites between HSV-tk–infected tumor cells and neighboring noninfected cells (21,22). The indirect effect stems from antitumor immune responses, adding to the versatility of this suicide gene therapy strategy (23,24).

A potential disadvantage of the HSV-tk strategy is that it requires S-phase cell cycle activity and thus targets only dividing cells. At any given time, not all malignant cells within a tumor are cycling, and different tumor types display different rates of cell doubling both in vitro and in vivo. Conditions must therefore be worked out that provide adequate HSV-tk gene expression and administration of GCV over a long enough time to account for variability in cell cycling within a designated tumor. Although the bystander effect helps augment the antitumor effects, there is likely a threshold of HSV-tk transfer and expression and persistence of the enzyme that must be achieved to generate or sustain a significant therapeutic effect.

While a potential disadvantage, the requirement for cell division may also be an advantage for both safety and tumor targeting for the HSV-tk strategy. Normal mammalian cells in general divide at much slower rates than tumor cells within an established malignancy. This differential in S-phase activity allows for design of HSV-tk delivery and expression that would preferentially kill tumor cells while minimizing or eliminating direct toxicity to surrounding or systemic normal tissues that may incorporate the gene and express the enzyme.

B. Cytosine Deaminase

The enzyme cytosine deaminase (CD) is found in a variety of fungi and bacteria, but is not found in mammalian cells. In these microbes, CD is activated during nutritional stress and normally catalyzes the deamination of cytosine to produce uracil. CD is also capable of converting the nontoxic prodrug 5-fluorocytosine (5-FC) into the metabolite 5-fluorouracil (5-FU) (24–26). In a second metabolic conversion process, intracellular enzymes present in both microbial and mammalian cells then act on 5-FU to produce 5-fluorouridine 5′-triphosphate and 5-fluoro-2′-deoxyuridine 5′-monophosphate. These toxic phosporylated metabolites disrupt both RNA and DNA synthesis, resulting in direct cellular cytotoxicity. Because of the natural specificity of CD to fungi and relative lack of toxicity of 5-FC in human tissues at routine dosing, 5-FC has been developed as an antifungal agent. However, since 5-FU is also converted to toxic metabolites in mammalian cells, this compound has been developed and widely applied as a chemotherapeutic agent for cancer.

The original application of CD for cancer therapy involved implanting a capsule containing the enzyme into an established rat tumor, whereupon the enzyme diffused into the tumor cells. The animals were subsequently treated with 5-FC, which resulted in an antitumor response (27). Upon the cloning of the gene and building upon these early animal investigations, CD suicide gene therapy became a feasible strategy (24). Aside from the direct cytotoxicity with this system, a significant bystander effect has also been identified with this system. The CD system is different from the HSV-tk system and may have a bystander advantage because of the initial production of 5-FU. Since the initial conversion to a ''toxic metabolite'' (5-FC to 5-FU) does not involve phosporylation, the 5-FU produced within the cytoplasm may readily cross the cell membrane and enter surrounding tumor cells. Also, the phosphorylated toxic metabolites of 5-FU that disrupt DNA and RNA synthesis may also be transferred to surrounding cells via intercellular communication or similar mechanisms as reported for the HSV-tk system. In effect, the multiple conversion steps provide two possible means of bystander activity, which theoretically provide an enhanced overall antitumor and bystander effect as compared to the HSV-tk system. The full efficiency of the CD strategy and its bystander effect, however, has not been elucidated, and further preclinical investigations are needed to discern any significant bystander advantages.

The lack of natural CD within mammalian cells and safety of 5-FC dosing makes this enzyme-prodrug combination a natural choice for human cancer investigation. CD is presently the second most common suicide gene under preclinical and clinical investigation, but it has certain limitations that may affect successful application of this strategy. The toxicity of 5-FU is not S-phase cell-cycle specific, but it does depend on cell proliferation for its effect. As with the HSV-tk system, the CD strategy preferentially affects tumor cells that have a higher rate of proliferation. Although this provides some inherent safety and tumor-targeting specificity, heterogenous tumor cell populations with variable levels of cellular proliferation may reduce the overall therapeutic effect. In order to achieve substantial tumor cell toxicity, high doses of 5-FU at the cellular level are generally required. The need for high cellular levels of 5-FU requires both efficient CD gene transfer and expression followed by adequate systemic dosing of 5-FC. Another major limiting factor is that 5-FU is only active for a maximum of 10 minutes. Thus, prolonged systemic treatment with 5-FC after CD gene transfer is required to maintain the production of intracellular 5-FU. Possibly the most limiting factor is the complexity of the metabolic conversion pathway itself. A multistep complex pathway provides many opportunities for tumor cells to acquire resistance to the actual therapy (28).

C. Varicella Zoster Virus Thymidine Kinase

The varicella zoster virus is also capable of expressing a unique thymidine kinase (VZV-tk) whose substrate specificity is distinct from both mammalian cellular kinases and the HSV-tk enzyme. Upon gene transfer of VSV-tk into recipient cells, cytotoxicity is induced by administration of the prodrug 9-(b-D-arabinofuranosyl)-6-methoxy-9H-purine, also known as araM (29). VZV-tk enzyme initially phosphorylates araM, which is further metabolized by natural cellular enzymes (AMP deaminase, AMP kinase, nucleoside diphosphate kinase, and adenylosucinate synthestase lysase) into adenine arabinonucleoside triphosphate (araATP). ara-ATP is highly toxic, and therefore only small quantities of ara-M in the range of 1-100 μm are required to directly kill cells that contain the VZV-tk enzyme (29). As with GCV in the HSV-tk system, araM is an excellent substrate for VZV-tk but not mammalian nucleoside kinases. Normal mammalian cells are able to withstand over 1500 μm of ara-M exposure. The overall sensitivity of a transduced cell to the ara-M prodrug is directly proportional to the level of VZ-tk activity.

This system is still relatively new for preclinical investigation, and the presence of a bystander effect remains to be proven. The disadvantages of VZV-tk suicide gene therapy are similar to those of HSV-tk, and further experimentation is required to define the efficacy and safety rationale for selecting between these two strategies.

D. *Escherichia coli* Nitroreductase

The NTR enzyme activates the relatively nontoxic prodrug dintrophenylaziridine CB1954 through a reduction process that generates a 4-hydroxylamine metabolite. This intermediate molecule further reacts with intracellular thioesters such as acetyl-CoA to produce a highly cytotoxic alkylating agent that is 10,000 times more toxic than the original prodrug (30).

There are a few proposed mechanisms by which CB1954 mediates its cellular toxicity after reduction by NTR. The most commonly reported mechanism is through cross-linking DNA strands, causing disruption of synthesis and DNA breaks that are directly cytotoxic to both dividing and nondividing cells (31). Some investigators have reported increased apoptosis after delivery of NTR and CB1954 to targeted cells (32), which was presumed to be a result of the DNA alterations incurred. It appears that CD1954 acts more rapidly than other prodrugs such as GCV in the HSV-tk system with reports of cytolytic activity as early as 4 hours after prodrug administration (31,33). One explanation for this comparatively rapid response is that the NTR strategy does not require cells to be in the S phase of growth.

This lack of specificity for dividing cells may prove advantageous in achieving maximal antitumor efficacy, however, it raises a significant safety concern regarding normal surrounding tissues. A critical issue in the future application of this system will be the development of tumor-specific targeting so that normal somatic cells will not be exposed to the cytotoxic effects of the enzyme and prodrug. Another potential drawback to the CB1954/NTR system is that a bystander effect has not been identified to date (32). These two limitations may preclude the clinical application and benefit of this system until increased efficiency of gene transfer and tumor-specific targeting is achieved.

E. Cytochrome P450 2B1

The hepatic enzyme cytochrome P450 B1 (CYP2B1) will convert the inert lipophilic prodrug cyclophosphamide (CPA) into an effective anticancer agent (34). CPA is initially converted into 4-hydroxy-cyclophosphamide (4-HCPA), which is naturally unstable and will spontaneously decompose into two toxic metabolites: acrolein and phosphoramide mustard (PM). Acrolein will promote covalent links in cellular proteins, and PM induces DNA alyklation and results in DNA strand breaks during replication. The importance of acrolein in causing tumor cytotoxicity in vivo has yet to be proven, therefore the major anticancer metabolite appears to be PM. The cytotoxicity of PM affects both dividing and nondividing cells and so may prove useful for tumors that have low levels of S-phase activity such as the glioblastoma brain tumor (35).

Tumor cells usually express low levels of CYP2B1, but the liver expresses higher levels. Systemic exposure to

CPA at concentrations that would prove effective in killing tumor cells will result in high levels of toxic metabolites produced in normal liver tissue. These high levels of toxic metabolites not only injure normal liver tissue but also are released into the circulation. Systemic toxicity has therefore limited the ability to use these prodrugs alone as cancer chemotherapeutic agents. Gene transfer of the CYP2B1 gene and the resulting upregulated expression of the enzyme, however, will allow for administration of smaller systemic levels of CPA prodrug to maintain tumor cytotoxicity while minimizing systemic toxicity.

One important advantage of this system is that the intermediate metabolite 4-HCPA is lipophilic and so can pass through cellular membranes (36). Diffusion of these metabolites throughout the nontransduced tumor cells results in a strong bystander effect. Despite this apparent augmentation of overall antitumor effects, the free diffusion of 4-HCPA and the fact that the CYP2B1 gene therapy strategy does not require cell division also carries the disadvantage of possible toxicity in surrounding normal tissue.

F. Carboxypeptidase G2

The bacterial enzyme Carboxypeptidase G2 (CPG2) has no mammalian homolog and has been shown to activate the prodrug 4-[2-chloroethyl)(2-mesyloxyelhyl-O-amino)-]bensoyl-L-glutamic acid (CMDA), which is a derivative of a benzoic acid mustard. The CPG2 enzyme removes the glutamic acid moiety from the CMDA prodrug and releases a toxic benzoic acid mustard (37), which requires no further enzymatic or decomposition process. The benzoic acid mustard is a strong alkylating agent and cross-links DNA, thus imparting toxicity to both dividing and nondividing transduced cells.

The single-step process of converting CMDA to the toxic mustard metabolite offers an advantage over other suicide gene therapy strategies that have intermediate metabolites and multistep conversion processes within a targeted tumor cell. Should the cellular enzymes that are responsible for the second phase or multistep activation process become defective or deficient in the tumor cell, a significant resistance to the prodrug could develop (38). On the other hand, when the toxic metabolite is released directly from the initial step or prodrug cleavage, there is much less chance of developing resistance to the suicide gene therapy. Also, mustard alkylating agents such as benzoic acid mustard have the advantage that their cytotoxicity is dose related. This important factor further reduces the chance of resistance.

As mentioned with other suicide gene therapy strategies above, this broad killing is beneficial for tumors with significant number of cells in Go at the time of gene transfer and prodrug administration. However, there continues to exist the potential for direct toxicity to surrounding normal tissues that are transduced with this suicide gene.

A substantial bystander effect has been documented with the CPG2 strategy in vitro when as few as 3.7% of the tumor cells were expressing CPG2 (39). This is one of the strongest reported bystander effects and serves as an advantage for this strategy.

IV. THE BYSTANDER EFFECT

Although present to variable degrees for each suicide gene therapy strategy, the bystander effect provides a major advantage for these systems. The advantage of a bystander effect is obvious when considering that present gene transfer approaches provide relatively poor transduction efficiencies of tumors in vivo. Given that only a fraction of any targeted tumor can be effectively transduced, a supplemental antitumor effect that does not require exposure or uptake of the therapeutic gene is critical to the success of suicide gene therapy. As mentioned previously, the bystander effect is a phenomenon whereby neighboring nontransduced tumor cells are killed in conjunction with direct killing of transduced cells (Fig. 1). Multiple theories have been investigated and proposed as an explanation for this effect.

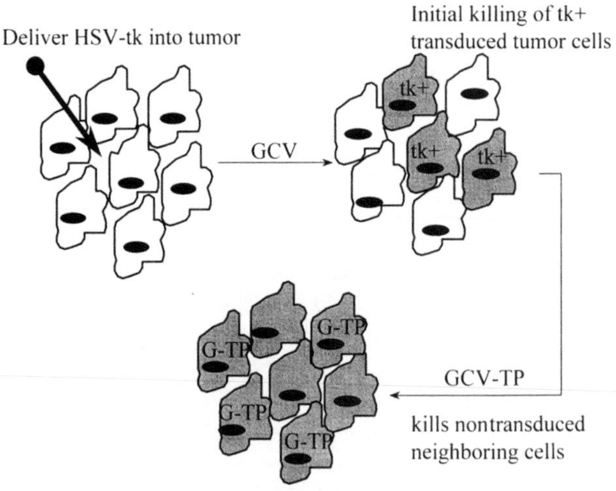

Figure 1 The bystander effect. The HSV-tk gene is delivered to a solid tumor resulting in effective transduction and gene expression in only a percentage of the tumor (shaded cells). Subsequent systemic treatment with ganciclovir (GCV) causes DNA disruption, cell death, and production of toxic metabolites. The toxic metabolites are then passed to surrounding nontransduced cells via gap junctions resulting in cell death.

A. Metabolic Cooperation and Gap Junctions

The most investigated and widely accepted theory to date is that toxic prodrug metabolites are passed between tumor cells through gap junctions. Gap junctions are small hexameric structures (2 nm) in the cell membrane which form part of a communication network between cells. This transfer of toxic metabolites via gap junctional intercellular communication is founded in the principle of ''metabolic cooperation,'' which was first described by Subak-Sharpe et al. in 1966 (40). Metabolic cooperation is the process whereby low molecular weight molecules (< 1000 daltons) are passed between cells that are in contact. Subsequent to these early studies, is was established that cells with gap junctions were ionically coupled and participated in metabolic cooperation (41). Cells that lacked gap junctions did not participate in this event.

The importance of cell contact in a suicide gene therapy system was identified by Moolten and colleagues, who demonstrated bystander killing of nontransduced cells after HSV-tk gene transfer and GCV administration in vitro (10). Although the GCV prodrug can readily and passively diffuse across a cell membrane, the toxic phosphorylated metabolite is not a permeable molecule. On the other hand, phosphorylated GCV is approximately 400 daltons in size and is well within the size limit for metabolic cooperation to occur via gap junctions (42). Subsequent to these early studies with the HSV-tk suicide gene therapy system, Bi et al. introduced the concept that the bystander effect was a result of metabolic cooperation (22). It was demonstrated that labeled phosphorylated GCV was able to enter adjacent contacting tumor cells and resulted in cell death. Gene transfer and expression of a much larger molecule such as β-galactosidase, however, was not transferred to nontransduced contacting tumor cells.

Gap junctional communication is believed to be mediated by a family of proteins called connexins, of which 12 genes have been cloned (43). Definitive proof that gap junctional intercelluar communication and connexin activity played a major role in the bystander effect came from the investigations of Mesril et al. (44). In their experiments, HeLa cells were chosen because they exhibit very little gap junctional communication and have no detectable expression of known connexin genes (45). Upon gene delivery of HSV-tk to cultured HeLa cells, only the actual HSV-tk–transfected cells were killed despite different levels of cell density or contact. When HeLa cells were transfected with a gene encoding the gap junctional protein connexin 43, both HSV-tk–positive and nontransfected surrounding cells in contact were killed. This effect was abrogated when HSV-tk–positive and negative HeLa cells were co-cultured without cell-cell contact.

B. Transfer of Toxic Metabolites via Apoptotic Vesicles

Another reported mechanism of bystander effect activity is the release of apoptotic vesicles by dying tumor cells after suicide gene therapy. Freeman and colleagues noted that HSV-tk–positive tumor cells exhibited characteristics of apoptosis when dying in culture (21). Microscopic analyses revealed cell shrinkage and detachments as well as chromatin condensation and vesicle formation. Further ultrastructural evaluation using transmission electron microscopy identified features consistent with apoptosis. Apoptotic vesicles released from HSV-tk and GCV-treated tumor cells could transfer the toxic phosphorylated GCV metabolite or even the HSV-tk gene itself. The mechanism of transfer would involve phagocytoses of these vesicles by surrounding viable tumor cells. This presumed transfer of apoptotic vesicles was demonstrated using a fluorescent tracking dye and fluorescence microscopy and flow cytometry. Nontransfected tumor cells were able to phagocytose the labeled apoptotic vesicles generated from dying HSV-tk–transfected cells. Further studies on the importance of this finding in mediating the extent of bystander activity are required before this principle is substantiated and accepted.

C. Local Antitumor Immune Responses

Although metabolic cooperation via gap junctions has been considered the major mechanism of the bystander effect, there is growing interest in the role of the immune system in this phenomenon (Fig. 2). A number of studies have reported the presence of an inflammatory infiltrate in dying or regressing tumors after both HSV-tk and CD gene therapy (46,47). Other investigations have described a lessened response to HSV-tk and GCV therapy for tumors grown in nude mice as compared to immunocompetent animals (23,48). The decreased effect in these athymic and therefore T-cell–deficient mice suggests that a T-cell–mediated immune response plays some role in tumor regression. In these studies, nude mice and sublethally irradiated mice failed to demonstrate subcutaneous tumor regression when the tumor cell population consisted of 50% HSV-tk transduced cells. The same experiments in immunocompetent mice, however, did show tumor rejection with the 50% proportion of HSV-tk–transduced cells.

More specific immune and cytokine analyses were subsequently performed using an intraperitoneal tumor model (49). Upon treatment of established tumors with HSV-tk transduced cells, the peritoneal exudate was analyzed for the presence of various cytokines. Expression of tumor necrosis factor-alpha (TNF-α), interleukin 1-alpha (Il-1α), and IL-6 was identified 24 hours after tumor treatment with HSV-tk positive cells. After 48 hours interferon gamma

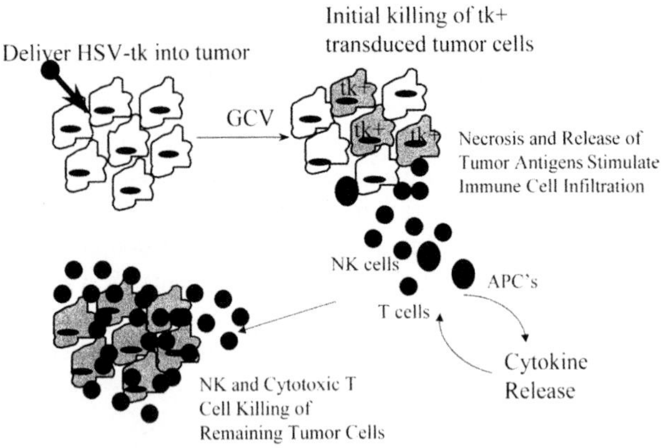

Figure 2 Immune component to the bystander effect. As tumor cells are killed by the suicide gene therapy, there is a release of cellular debris and tumor antigens within the local tumor environment. The cell necrosis and antigen load stimulates recruitment and activation of tumor-specific immune cells. The immune cells attack the local-regional tumor and also initiate a systemic response that may target and kill metastatic disease or prevent recurrence.

(INF-γ) was identified, and at 96 hours granulocyte-macrophage colony-stimulating factor (GM-CSF) was produced. There appeared to be a defined cascade of cytokine production that was specific to the HSV-tk–treated tumors. Immunohistochemical staining identified immune infiltrates consisting of macrophages and T lymphocytes that were predominantly in and surrounding regressing tumors subsequent to HSV-tk therapy. These representative studies as well as others have established a role for local immune responses in generating killing of both transduced and nontransduced tumor cells. The generation of an antitumor immune response against both transduced and nontransduced tumor cells greatly enhances the power of suicide gene therapy and its associated bystander effect.

D. Systemic Antitumor Immune Responses

There is increasing evidence that not only a direct local immune response but a systemic immune response is generated from suicide gene therapy. The development of a systemic immunity has been demonstrated for both the HSV-tk and CD strategies. In animal studies with HSV-tk–expressing tumor cells, administration of GCV resulted in both direct tumor cell killing and an ''initial'' protection against a second challenge of wild-type tumor cells (23,50). This effect could not be sustained, and eventually tumors grew at the site of second challenge. This initial antitumor immunity was not generated against a second local challenge of syngeneic but heterologous (antigen distinct) tumor cells. Using the same tumor strategy in T-cell–deficient nude mice, the antitumor effects and initial systemic immunity against a second site tumor challenge was greatly reduced. These findings again support the importance of a T-cell–mediated tumor-specific immune response. This initial systemic antitumor immunity has been documented in multiple tumor cell types for the HSV-tk strategy, although the extent and period of immune effect has been variable among studies.

Although most of the work centering on immune responses and suicide gene therapy has centered on HSV-tk therapy, the immune component of the bystander effect has also been identified in the cytosine deaminase scheme. Both fibrosarcoma and adenocarcinoma cells that were retrovirally transduced to express CD showed variable levels of resistance to second wild-type tumor challenges subsequent to systemic administration of the prodrug 5-FC (51). Second tumor challenges with antigen distinct tumor lines from the same murine background, however, displayed normal tumor growth indicating a tumor specificity to the immune response. These findings parallel the results noted in the HSV-tk system.

In the previous investigations, the fibrosarcoma and adenocarcinoma cell lines were generated via carcinogen induction. Subsequent studies have confirmed both a local and systemic protective immune responses after CD and 5-FC therapy in a spontaneously occurring mammary carcinoma (49). Antibody depletion against specific lymphocytes was performed in the animal tumor model system to further define specific components to these immune responses. Upon antibody depletion of CD8-positive T lymphocytes in vivo, a significantly decreased level of local tumor regression and even increased tumor growth was noted in CD-expressing tumors that were treated with 5-FC. Antibody depletion of granulocytes also appeared to limit the antitumor responses. Deletion of CD4 T lymphocytes had no significant effect on local tumor regression from the CD and 5-FC treatment. Interestingly, depletion of CD4-positive T lymphocytes dramatically reduced or in some cases eliminated the systemic immunity against a second local challenge of wild-type tumor. Depletion of CD8 T lymphocytes also appeared to limit the systemic antitumor bystander effects of a second challenge of wild-type tumor. Overall these studies support the ability of suicide gene therapy to generate some level of systemic immunity. The systemic protection, however, was present at variable levels, and only short-term systemic immunity was evaluated.

Although systemic immune responses can be generated against second tumor challenges after suicide gene therapy, could it be possible to induce regression of existing tumor metastases after treatment of the primary tumor? Original murine studies in multiple tumor types evaluating responses against an established subcutaneous wild-type tumor at a second site were not encouraging. Tumor killing and regression identified in subcutaneous flank tumors that expressed CD or HSV-tk did not induce a significant effect on wild-type (nontransduced) tumors growing on the opposite flank (21,26,51). This apparent lack of effect on the presence of established tumors at a distant site suggested that the immune bystander effect was not going to be effective against gross metastases present at the time of primary tumor therapy.

Further studies involving orthotopic metastases, however, have defined some role of this immune bystander effect in the treatment of metastatic disease. Consalvo et al. demonstrated regression of lung metastases in 20% of mice whose primary CD-expressing subcutaneous tumors regressed after 5-FC administration (47). Up to 90% regression of HSV-tk–negative liver metastases was also described after elimination of HSV-tk–expressing tumors growing intraperitoneal in a murine colon adenocarcinoma model (52). Immunohistochemical studies confirmed the presence of increased inflammatory infiltrates in these regressing metastases as compared to controls. These representative studies support the concept that a systemic antitumor immunity or bystander effect is capable of generating variable levels of tumor regression in distant metastases.

The issue has not been resolved as to why established second-site wild-type tumors are not affect by suicide gene therapy directed at the primary tumor but metastatic lung and liver tumors show some regression. Excluding possibilities such as natural antigenicity of various tumor types and inherent differences among animal tumor models, there are a few hypotheses to explain this somewhat contradictory finding. The first hypothesis is that anatomic location of second- site or metastatic disease is an important issue in generating effective immune-mediated regression after primary tumor therapy. The lung and liver have an increased number of cells from the reticuloendothelial system as compared to the subcutaneous tissues. The increased reticuloendothelial cells surrounding the metastases may facilitate or enhance antitumor immune activity generated from the initial primary tumor treatment. Also, this environment within the lung or liver may promote increased or more efficient antigen presentation. The second hypothesis may be related to gross tumor burden. Although in multiple animal models a second-site established tumor has not regressed after primary tumor treatment with suicide genes, an initial protection against repeat tumor challenges has been well documented. The second hypothesis is based on this finding. It is possible that the systemic immune response generated from the initial tumor treatment is not strong enough to manage the gross tumor burden of an established tumor but can handle the smaller tumorigenic doses given for a second challenge. Further experiments to evaluate this consideration of tumor burden or rate of cell division within the metastatic lung and liver models may help answer this question.

V. COMBINATION SUICIDE GENE AND CYTOKINE GENE THERAPY

Based on the initial immune responses generated after suicide gene therapy, there has been recent interest in combining this strategy with cytokine gene therapy. Cytokine gene therapy has arisen because of the growing opinion that tumor-specific antigens are expressed in many if not all human tumors, but the immune system fails to generate an adequate immune response against these antigens (53). Designing or discovering a means to augment baseline immune activity or generate tumor-specific responses would greatly enhance any cancer-treatment strategy. Systemic infusions of cytokines has demonstrated tumor regression in both animal tumor models and some human clinical trials, however, the severe toxicity associated with the high concentrations required to achieve antitumor efficacy significantly limits this strategy (54–56). Cytokine gene therapy may circumvent the toxicity of systemic infusions and provide both larger and sustained local concentrations of cytokine within the tumor environment. This augmentation of the immune response with cytokine production may also be synergistically enhanced by the addition of suicide gene therapy.

Upon treatment of a tumor with suicide gene, direct cytotoxicity and tumor cell death occurs. This tumor killing releases large amounts of tumor antigens as well as other cellular proteins and debris. As has been demonstrated previously, this results in variable levels of immune activity in and of itself. The suicide gene therapy not only reduces the gross tumor burden but also primes the local tumor immune environment for the beneficial effects of cytokine production. In addition, the actual suicide gene proteins themselves are thought to be immunogenic and may act as superantigens for both nonspecific and tumor-specific lymphocyte activation. By introducing high levels of local cytokine production using combined gene-transfer techniques, this overall antitumor immune response may be greatly magnified.

Pioneering this area have been Chen et al., who investigated the effects of combination HSV-tk and IL-2 gene therapy for colorectal cancer liver metastases (57). Upon injecting the liver metastases with a combination of HSV-tk and IL-2, a significantly increased level of tumor regression was noted as compared to either HSV-tk or IL-2 alone. A long-term survival benefit was not seen. The combination treatment did generate an initial systemic immunity against a second challenge of wild-type tumor at a distant site. This response was tumor specific but was not sustained. Immune studies revealed a predominantly CD8-positive T-lymphocyte response. Interestingly, the treatment of the liver metastases with HSV-tk alone did not demonstrate a significant effect with respect to protection against a second-site tumor challenge. When applied to a head and neck orthotopic squamous cell carcinoma model, the combination of HSV-tk and IL-2 gene therapy demonstrated both a synergistic antitumor response and increased survival as compared to single gene therapy (58). The combination of HSV-tk and IL-2 in this head and neck cancer model also generated an immediate systemic immunity and protection against a second-site challenge of wild-type tumor (53). Immunohistochemical analyses of local tumor environments revealed a predominance of CD8-positive T-cell infiltration, but CD4-positive T cells were also identified.

Further investigations with the combination of HSV-tk, IL-2, and GM-CSF have demonstrated both enhanced tumor regression and animal survival. Also, this triple combination has shown that systemic immunity can be sustained as long-term protection against second wild-type tumor challenges could be generated (59). It is hypothesized that the addition of GM-CSF not only stimulates antigen presentation cells within the local tumor environment, but also induces a long-term antitumor memory that is mediated by CD4-positive T cells (60).

VI. METHODS FOR SUICIDE GENE TRANSFER

There are two major areas of investigation regarding the application of suicide genes for the treatment of solid malignancies. The first area focuses on the development of suitable vehicles for introducing suicide genes into targeted tumor cells. The second area is the discovery and development of new suicide genes or gene combinations that will provide the greatest antitumor response while maintaining margins of safety. Regarding the area of gene transfer, two general classes of vehicles and transfer methods can be distinguished. DNA-mediated gene transfer involves the administration of DNA in the form of a circular double-stranded plasmid directly to the tumor. The vehicles for introducing therapeutic DNA into tumor cells are many. They include both mechanical methods and a more promising method that utilizes a wide variety of lipid or polymer formulations which are designed to maximize gene uptake and expression within the tumor cells. Viral-mediated gene transfer involves packaging a therapeutic gene into a replication-defective virus particle and utilizing the natural process of viral infection to introduce the gene. The purpose of viral-mediated gene transfer is to exploit the efficient and often complex mechanisms that viruses have evolved to introduce their viral genes into human cells during infections. DNA-mediated transfer, while less efficient than viral transfer, does not carry the risks of wild-type virus contamination and other known viral-associated toxicity. Furthermore, treatment-limiting immune responses are more prevalent with the use of viral vectors, in general, than DNA transfer systems, which may allow repeat gene delivery over a long period of time.

A. DNA-Mediated Gene Transfer

DNA-mediated gene transfer is commonly called transfection. The therapeutic gene is typically contained within a circular molecule of DNA (plasmid), which contains various additional genetic elements required to achieve expression of the gene product. Important components of these plasmids are special promoters and enhancers that direct gene expression. There may also be other specific elements that have been engineered to direct the processing and persistence of genetic material within the cell.

There are many methods for delivering plasmid DNA into tumor cells, but only a few are clinically applicable at present. A classic means of introducing DNA into cells in vitro is through electroporation, where cultured cells are exposed to DNA in the presence of a strong electrical pulse (61). The electrical pulse creates pores in the tumor cell membrane, allowing entry of DNA into the cell. A recent technical advance using a similar principle has been the development of the ''gene gun.'' This mechanical device uses electrical currents and magnetic properties to project gold-coated DNA vectors into the tumor cells (62). At present it is limited to cases where direct visualization and broad access to the tumor is possible.

It is possible to effectively introduce genes into muscle (63) or thyroid (64) simply by directly injecting DNA in saline solution into these tissues, whereupon the process of endocytosis enables cellular uptake. The use of saline as a gene-transfer vehicle, however, is extremely inefficient for solid tumors and generally not applicable for cancer suicide gene therapy. The state-of-the-art technology for DNA-mediated gene transfer into solid tumors is the use of liposomes or cationic lipid complexes. These lipid formulations are specifically designed to enhance DNA uptake and may be modified to provide higher levels of gene delivery to different histological tumor cell types, (65). The use of lipid or liposome formulation gene transfer is becoming a major focus for clinically applied cancer gene therapy.

There are two limiting factors with respect to DNA-mediated gene transfer in general. First, the overall efficiency of gene transfer is low with in vivo expression levels of 1–3% at best even with cationic lipid or polymer formulations. Although suicide gene therapy strategies do not require gene transfer into all or even a majority of tumor cells for effective killing, there is a correlation between levels of gene expression and antitumor effects. This correlation affects both the direct cytotoxicity and the bystander effect. In general, levels of transduction lower than 10% of the tumor population in vivo have very limited effects on either tumor regression or delay in tumor progression. The second limiting factor for DNA-mediated gene transfer is that the therapeutic gene usually resides or functions transiently in the targeted cell regardless of the formulation. Subsequent to DNA-mediated gene transfer the therapeutic genes are degraded and eliminated from the tumor cell over a short period of time. This factor may be less important for suicide gene therapy because the targeted tumor cells are generally killed within days to a week after initiating prodrug administration. It is also possible to perform repeat dosing with DNA-mediated gene transfer. Sugaya et al. reported antitumor effects of 10 serial DNA-mediated HSV-tk treatments for colon adenocarcinoma, with each injection providing only a maximal of 1–2% in vivo transduction efficiency (66).

Permanent incorporation of genes into cells occurs rarely after DNA-mediated gene transfer in cultured cells ($<1:10^5$ cells), however, this phenomenon has not been observed in vivo. Although the transient expression of the therapeutic gene may be a disadvantage in certain treatment schemes, there are also may advantages to this property. Because DNA vectors do no integrate into a host cells' chromosomes (i.e., in the case of normal tissue surrounding a tumor cell), they do not carry the risk of permanent alteration of a normal tissue's genome. The transient nature may also limit toxicity associated with any gene therapy system. The lack of significant immune responses against the DNA vector also allows repetitive administration of the therapeutic gene into persistent or recurrent tumors. The ability to perform repeat treatments may overcome the potential limiting aspect of transient gene expression.

B. Retrovirus-Mediated Gene Transfer

The majority of suicide gene therapy preclinical and human trial research to date has centered on the use of viruses as gene-delivery vehicles or vectors. The original prototypes for viral-mediated gene transfer are retroviral vectors derived from the Moloney murine leukemia virus (67,68). Retroviral vectors were chosen as vehicles because of several useful properties. First, ''defective'' virus particles can be constructed that contain therapeutic genes and are capable of infecting cells, but that contain no viral genes and express no pathogenic viral gene products. Second, retroviral vectors are capable of integrating the therapeutic genes they carry into the chromosomes of the target cell resulting in long-term gene expression. Third, modifications can be made in retroviral vectors and in the cell lines producing vectors, which result in enhanced safety features.

There are certain limitations to consider regarding the application of retroviruses in gene therapy for cancer. Retroviruses will only integrate into actively dividing cells. Since most tumors have heterogeneous populations of dividing and nondividing cells, many tumor cells that are exposed to the retrovirus vehicle may never take up the therapeutic gene. Moreover, the currently achievable viral titers (10^7) are relatively low, and the overall efficiency of retroviral infection of tumors in vivo is low. Because of this low level of in vivo transduction, the retrovirus must be delivered to the tumor via its murine or human packaging cell line. Also, serum complement can inactivate retroviruses that are produced from packaging cell lines that are not of human origin (69). Another important limitation is the variable receptivity of host cells to retroviral infection. And finally, under large-scale retrovirus production there is a risk of producing replication-competent viruses. These last two limitations are being addressed through modifications of the packaging cell lines (70,71).

C. Adenovirus-Mediated Gene Transfer

A recent focus of gene therapy has been the development of adenovirus vectors as powerful and effective vehicles for gene transfer. Adenoviral vectors differ from retroviral vectors in that they do not integrate their genes into the target cell's chromosome. Compared to retroviral vectors, adenoviral vectors can be produced at much higher titers (10^{11} or greater) and can efficiently transduce a wide variety of both dividing and nondividing cells in vitro and in vivo (72). Hematopoietic cells are the only cells that have demonstrated significant resistance to adenovirus infection thus far. Effective therapeutic gene expression is transient after adenovirus gene transfer and typically lasts for one to several weeks. There are both advantages and disadvantages to this last characteristic. While the safety of adenoviral vectors for gene therapy has not been studied as extensively as retroviral vectors, there is considerable experience with the use of attenuated adenovirus in animal models and in human subjects indicating a high margin of safety (73,74).

The disadvantages of the adenovirus system must be considered when designing and applying gene therapy strategies. Although the adenovirus vector is replication defective, it will express certain viral gene products or antigens that are capable of inducing an inflammatory response and subsequent lysis of the transduced cell (75). This inflammatory response could result in injury to normal surrounding tissues or even distant tissues that have been infected with the adenovirus vector. The generation of antibodies against the adenovirus vector may severely limit repeat adenovirus gene therapy treatments. Also, the transient level of gene expression may limit the desired therapeutic effect. As has been mentioned previously, transient gene expression may not be a significant disadvantage with a suicide gene therapy strategy. The potential disadvantages of transient gene expression and limiting inflammatory responses have been addressed with further manipulation of the adenovirus genetic backbone. New ''second-generation'' vectors, which remain for months in the target cell, express fewer viral proteins, and have greatly reduced inflammatory responses, are now available and under continued modification and development (76,77).

D. Other Viral Vectors

Other viruses exist that exhibit properties that may be useful to exploit for suicide gene therapy or other gene therapy strategies. The adeno-associated virus can provide a completely defective vector with the majority of the viral genome replaced by the therapeutic gene (78). As a result, this virus appears to generate fewer immune responses and has a longer period of therapeutic gene expression than the classic adenovirus vector. Unlike retrovirus, the adeno-associated virus integrates in a specific location on chromosome 19, thereby reducing the risk associated with randomly integrating vectors. Although a theoretical advantage, recombinant adeno-associated virus appears to have lost this predictable integration advantage (79). Another disadvantage of the adeno-associated virus is the requirement for wild-type ''helper virus'' in the vector production process. The ''safe'' recombinant vector must then be purified from the wild-type helper virus prior to amplification and in vivo application. Also, the viral titers are low for adeno-associated virus (10^4), in part because of the inefficient production process. Further investigation is required to define the role and safety of adeno-associated virus in clinical application.

The herpes simplex virus is capable of infecting cells and persisting indefinitely in a latent state. Vectors using the herpesvirus have been constructed, which are replication defective and capable of expressing recombinant genes for prolonged periods of time in animal models (80). These viruses are not completely defective and continue to express many viral proteins that can be cytopathic, a property that severely limits the herpesvirus for present gene therapy applications.

Other viruses, including the human papillomavirus, vaccinia virus, avipoxvirus, and baclovirus, are under investigation for gene therapy application. The improvements and continued refinements of presently available viral vectors as well as the development of new vectors should greatly expand the efficacy and applicability of suicide gene therapy.

VII. GENERAL STRATEGIES FOR SUICIDE GENE THERAPY

Two basic strategies exist for cancer gene therapy. The first conceived strategy is ''ex vivo'' gene therapy in which a tumor or fibrous tissue biopsy is taken from a cancer patient whereupon individual tumor cells or fibroblasts are isolated and grown in vitro (Fig. 3). Therapeutic genes are then inserted into these cells typically using retroviral vector infection in tissue culture. The cells are subsequently irradiated and then reimplanted into the original tumor site or distant to the tumor site by autologous transplantation. The level of irradiation is controlled so as not to immediately kill the cells but to prevent growth and allow only a short period of survival after reimplantation. This strategy has been more commonly applied to classic cancer vaccine and cytokine gene therapy strategies. Although this approach is feasible with suicide gene therapy, the predominant tumor response would come from a metabolic cooperation or immune bystander effect subsequent to prodrug administration and killing of the reimplanted transduced tumor cells. The inefficiency of such a system in general supports the predominant research and clinical focus on in vivo approaches for suicide gene therapy.

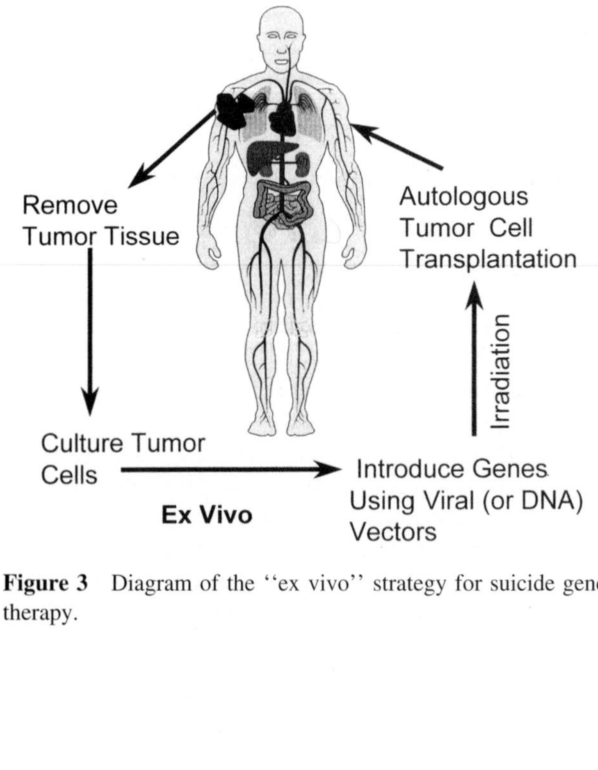

Figure 3 Diagram of the ''ex vivo'' strategy for suicide gene therapy.

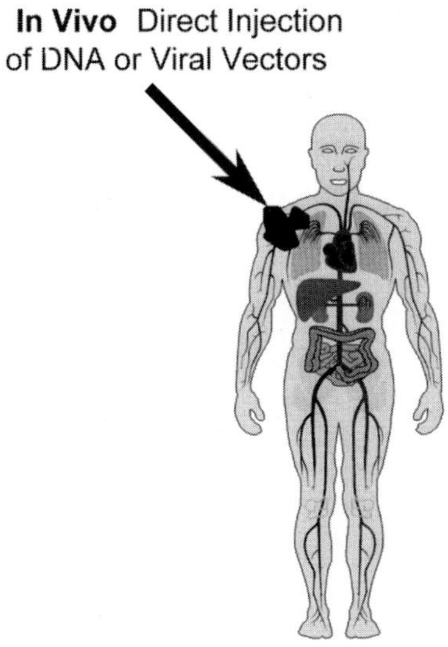

Figure 4 Diagram of the "in vivo" strategy for suicide gene therapy.

The second is basic strategy for cancer gene therapy is "in vivo" gene therapy where DNA, viral vectors alone, or packaging cell lines producing viral vectors are administered directly to a cancer patient (Fig. 4). The most common route of delivery is via direct injection of the delivery vehicle and gene or the packaging cell line into the tumor. Systemic injection is possible but with present technology results in limited exposure of the tumors to the vehicle. Tumors within tissues that have a large amount of blood flow or act as filters such as the lung or liver may prove more amenable to systemic delivery. As gene-transfer technology continues to advance, the development of vehicles with tumor- or tissue-specific receptor uptake or promotor activity may allow for systemic administration of the DNA or viral vector carrying the suicide gene.

VIII. CLINICAL TRIAL SUMMARY FOR SUICIDE GENE THERAPY STRATEGIES

An estimated 256 human gene therapy clinical trials had been either initiated or completed worldwide as of May 1997, and over 2200 patients have been enrolled (81). Gene therapy or marker gene transfer for malignancies comprised 195 of these trials. A summary of the progression of patient enrollment is depicted in Figure 5 and a breakdown of the trials by disease in Figure 6. With respect to gene therapy trials for malignancy, 167 of these were directed at solid tumors with the remaining trials targeting leukemia or myeloma.

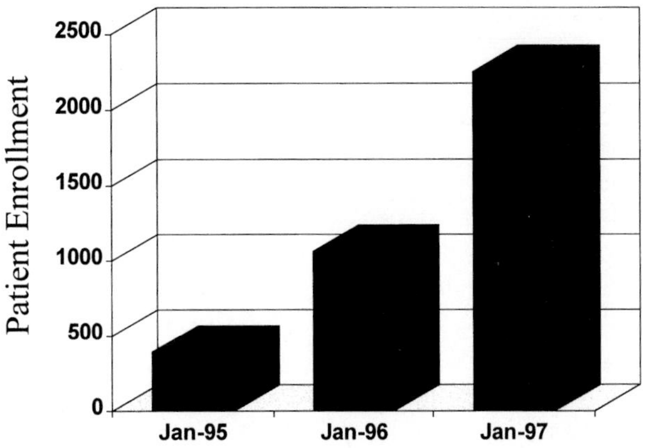

Figure 5 Trend for patient enrollment in gene therapy trials.

Of these 256 human trials, 29 involved HSV-tk gene delivery. Seven of these trials used the adenovirus and 22 trials used the retrovirus as the delivery vehicles (73,81). The adenovirus-based trials involved direct intratumor injections, whereas the retrovirus trials included both in vivo and ex vivo strategies of HSV-tk gene delivery. A summary of the HSV-tk trials, patient enrollment, and any reported responses and adverse events can be found in Table 3.

There are two phase I clinical trials under investigation that use the CD suicide gene therapy strategy. Adenovirus vector delivery of the CD gene to metastatic colon cancer followed by systemic infusion of 5-FC is the focus of one trial. Only one patient has been enrolled and there have been no responses or adverse events. The other CD trial centers on nonviral delivery of CD in a plasmid-lipid formulation to breast carcinoma. There have been four patients enrolled and no reported responses or adverse events.

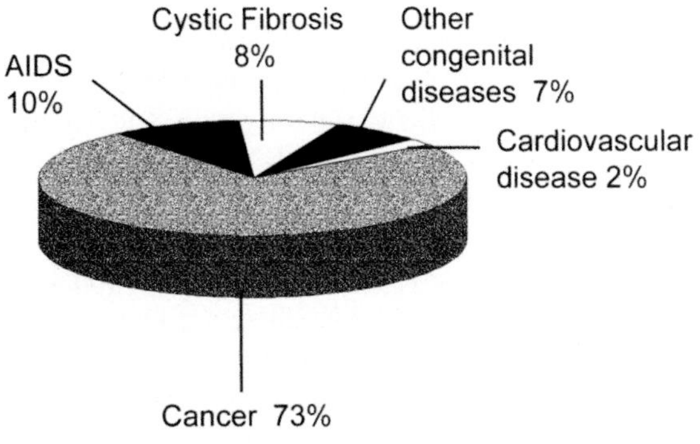

Figure 6 Diagram depicting the distribution of human gene therapy trials for general diseases.

Table 3 Summary of HSV-tk Gene Therapy Clinical Trials

Tumor target	Strategy	Delivery vehicle	# Patients	Biological responses	Adverse events	P.I.
Brain	In vivo	R	3	N/A	N/A	Raffel (USA)
Brain	In vivo	R	2	1 MR	Local edema	Kun (USA)
Brain	In vivo	R	20	2 CR 2 PR	Intratumor hemorrhage	Oldfield (USA)
Glioblastoma	In vivo	R	30	N/A	N/A	Berger (USA)
Glioblastoma	In vivo	Ad	3	None	None	Eck (USA)
Glioblastoma	In vivo	R	0	N/A	N/A	Favrol (France)
Glioblastoma	In vivo	R	0	N/A	N/A	Finocchiaro (Italy)
Glioblastoma	Ex vivo	R	0	N/A	N/A	Harsh (USA)
Glioblastoma	In vivo	R	9	1 PR 1 MR	Fever	Izquierdo (Spain)
Glioblastoma	In vivo	R	17	N/A	None	Klatzmann (France)
Glioblastoma	In vivo	R	13	N/A	N/A	Maria (USA)
Glioblastoma	In vivo	R	8	N/A	None	Mariani (Switzerland)
Glioblastoma	In vivo	R	4	1 MR	Seizure, confusion	Mulder (Netherlands)
Glioblastoma	In vivo	Ad	0	N/A	N/A	Grossman (USA)
Glioblastoma	In vivo	R	14	N/A	N/A	Van Gilder (USA)
Glioblastoma	In vivo	R	2	None	N/A	Fetell (USA)
Head and neck	In vivo	Ad	0	N/A	N/A	O'Malley (USA)
Hepatic mets	In vivo	Ad	0	N/A	N/A	Sung (USA)
Meningeal	In vivo	R	1	N/A	N/A	Oldfield (USA)
Melanoma	In vivo	R	8	N/A	None	Klatzman (France)
Melanoma	Ex vivo	R	3	N/A	N/A	Yee (USA)
Mesothelioma	In vivo	Ad	15	None	Fever ↑ LFTs	Albelda (USA)
Ovarian	In vivo	Ad	0	N/A	N/A	Alvarez (USA)
Ovarian	Ex vivo	R	16	2 CR	Fever, nausea	Freeman (USA)
Ovarian	Ex vivo (tk plus Her-2/neu cells)	R	0	N/A	N/A	Freeman (USA)
Ovarian	In vivo	R	0	N/A	N/A	Link (USA)
Ovarian	In vivo	R	0	N/A	N/A	Tanaka (Japan)
Prostate	In vivo	Ad	18	N/A	Thrombocytopenia	Scardino (USA)

LFTs, Liver function tests; A, adenovirus; R, retrovirus; CR, complete response; PR, partial response; MR, marginal response; SD, stable disease; N/A, not available.

The ongoing or completed clinical trials for suicide gene therapy and cancer overall have provided few important points for human gene therapy investigation. The first point is that retroviral, adenoviral, and DNA-mediated vectors are at present safe vehicles for gene transfer. There is no reported significant short- or long-term toxicity associated with retroviral gene therapy in human patients. Regarding adenovirus as a delivery vehicle, there are fewer of trials and data are limited, but the associated toxicity thus far has been both transient and relatively minor. Likewise, there have been no significant adverse events with DNA-mediated gene transfer in human trials. The second important point is that gene transfer and expression in human cancer cells in vivo is possible with both viral and nonviral strategies. The last point is that tumor responses or reports of regression must be interpreted cautiously since the majority of trials are phase I or phase I/II and are not well controlled for measuring outcomes.

At this early stage of human clinical trial investigation, the studies have focused on patients with advanced or incurable cancer. Although this patient population is a standard choice for establishing the safety of novel therapies, the greatest chance of eventual success with presently available suicide gene therapy strategies may be found in patients with less advanced disease. Another important potential for suicide gene therapy is in combination with immune therapies or standard therapy such as with surgery or radiation. As advancements in both preclinical development and clinical application continue, suicide gene therapy should achieve a role in the treatment of cancer.

REFERENCES

1. Anderson WF. Prospects for human gene therapy. Science 1984; 226:401–409.
2. Blaese RM, Anderson WF, Rosenberg SA, Culver KW. The ADA human gene therapy clinical protocol. Hum Gene Ther 1990; 327–362.
3. Cho and Vogelstein . . . . . . genetic progression colon cancer. ??, 1992.
4. Freeman SM, Koeplin DS, Abboud CN, et al. The bystander effect: tumor regression when a fraction of the tumor mass is genetically modified. Cancer Res 1993; 53:5274–5284.
5. . . . enzymes of sg's from . . . bacteria
6. Mullen CA. Metabolic suicide genes in gene therapy. Pharmacol Ther 1994; 63:199–207.
7. Connors TA. The choice of prodrugs for gene directed enzyme prodrug therapy of cancer. Gene Ther 1995; 2: 702–709.
8. Moolten FL, Wells JM. Curability of tumors bearing herpes thymidine kinase genes transferred by retroviral vectors. J Natl Cancer Inst 1990; 82:297–300.
9. Abe A, Takeo T, Emi N, Tanimoto M, Ueda R, Yee JK, Friedman T, Saito H. Transduction of a drug sensitive toxic gene into human leukemia cell lines with a novel retroviral vector. Proc Soc Exp Biol Med 1993; 203:354–359.
10. Moolten FL. Tumor chemosensitivity conferred by inserted herpes thymidine kinase genes: paradigm for a prospective cancer control strategy. Cancer Res 1986; 46:5276–5281.
11. Moolten FL. Drug sensitivity (''suicide'') genes for selective cancer chemotherapy. Cancer Gene Ther 1994; 4: 279–287.
12. Matthews T, Boehme R. Antiviral activity and mechanism of action of ganciclovir. Rev Infect Dis 1988; 10:s490–494.
13. Elion GB, Furman PA, Fyfe JA, et al. Selectivity of action of an antiherpetic agent, 9-(2-hydroxyethoxmethly) guanine. Proc Natl Acad Sci 1997; 74:5716–5720.
14. Elion GB. The chemotherapeutic exploitation of virus-specified enzymes. Adv Enzyme Reg 1980; 18:53–60.
15. St. Clair MH, Lambe CU, Furman PA. Inhibition by ganciclovir of cell growth and DNA synthesis of cells biochemically transformed with herpesvirus genetic information. Antimicrob Agents Chemother 1987; 31:844–889.
16. Culver KW, Ram Z, Wallbridge S, Ishii H, Olfield EH, Blaese RM. In vivo gene transfer with retroviral vector-producer cells for treatment of experimental brain tumors. Science 1992; 256:1550–1552.
17. Olfield EH, Ram Z, Culver KW, Blaese RM, DeVroom HL, Anderson WF. Gene therapy for the treatment of brain tumors using intra-tumoral transduction with the thymidine kinase gene and intravenous ganciclovir. Hum Gene Ther 1993; 4:39–69.
18. Smythe WR, Hwang HC, Amin KM, et al. Use of recombinant adenovirus to transfer the herpes simplex virus thymidine kinase (HSVtk) gene to thoracic neoplasms: an effective in vitro sensitization system. Cancer Res 1994; 54: 2055–2059.
19. O'Malley BWJ, Chen S, Schwartz MR, Woo SLC. Adenovirus-mediated gene therapy for human head and neck squamous cell cancer in a nude mouse model. Cancer Res 1995; 55:1080–1085.
20. Freeman SM, McCune C, Robinson W, et al. Treatment of ovarian cancer using a gene-modified vaccine. Hum Gene Ther 1995; 6:927–939.
21. Freeman SM, Abboud CN, Whartenby KA, Koeplin DS, Moolten FL, Abraham GN. The ''bystander effect'': tumor regression when a fraction of the tumor mass is genetically modified. Cancer Res 1999; 53:5274–5283.
22. Bi WL, Parysek LM, Warnick R, Stambrook PJ. In vitro evidence that metabolic cooperation is responsible for the bystander effect observed with HSV tk retroviral gene therapy. Hum Gene Ther 1993; 4:725–731.
23. Vile RG, Nelson JA, Castleden S, Chong H, Hart IR. Systemic gene therapy of murine melanoma using tissue specific expression of HSVtk gene involves an immune component. Cancer Res 1994; 54:6223–6224.
24. Austin EA, Huber BE. A first step in the development of gene therapy for colorectal carcinoma: cloning sequencing and expression of *E. coli* cytosine deaminase. Mol Pharmacol 1992; 43:380–387.
25. Mullen CA, Kilstrup M, Blaese M. Transfer of the bacterial gene for cytosine deaminase to mammalian cells confers lethal sensitivity to 5-fluorocytosine: a negative selection system. Proc Natl Acad Sci 1992; 89:33–37.
26. Huber BE, Austin EA, Good SS, Knick VC, Tibbels T, Richards CA. In vivo anti-tumor activity of 5-fluorocytosine on human colorectal carcinoma cells genetically modified to express cytosine deaminase. Cancer Res 1993; 53: 4619–4626.
27. Nishiyama T, Kawamura Y, Kawamoto K, et al. Antineoplastic effects in rats of 5-fluorocytosine in combination with cytosine deaminase capsules. Cancer Res 1985; 45: 1753–1761.
28. Pinedo HM, Peters GFJ. Fluorouracil: biochemistry and pharmacology. J Clin Oncol 1988; 6:1653–1644.
29. Huber BE, Richards CA, Krenitsky TA. Retroviral-mediated gene therapy for the treatment of hepatocellular carcinoma: an innovative approach for cancer therapy. Proc Natl Acad Sci 1991; 88:8039–8043.
30. Knox RJ, Friedlos F, Boland MP. The bioactivation of CB1954 and its use as a prodrug in antibody-directed enzyme prodrug therapy (ADEPT). Cancer Metastasis Rev 1993; 12:195–212.
31. Clark AJ, et al. Selective cell ablation in transgenic mice expressing *E. coli* nitroreductase. Gene Ther 1997; 4: 101–110.
32. Drabek D, Guy J, Craig R, Grosveld F. The expression of bacterial nitroreductase in transgenic mice results in specific

cell killing by the prodrug CB1954. Gene Ther 1997; 4: 93–100.
33. Bridgewater JA, et al. Expression of the bacterial nitroreductase enzyme in mammalian cells renders them selectively sensitive to killing by the prodrug CB1954. Eur J Cancer 1995; 31A:2362–2370.
34. Clarke L, Waxman DJ. Oxidation metabolism of cyclophosphamide: identification of the hepatic monooxygenase catalysts of drug activation. Cancer Res 1989; 49:2344–2350.
35. Wei MX, Tamiya T, et al. Experimental tumor therapy in mice using the cyclophosphamide-activating cytochrome P4502B1 gene. Hum Gene Ther 1994; 5:969–978.
36. Wei MX, Tamiya T, Rhee RJ, Breakefield XO, Chiocca EA. Diffusible cytotoxic metabolites contribute to the in vitro bystander effect associated with cyclophosphamide/cytochrome P450 2B1 cancer gene therapy paradigm. Clin Cancer Res 1995; 1:1171–1177.
37. Springer CJ, Antoniw P, Bagshawe KD, Searle F, Bisset GMF, Jarman M. Novel prodrugs which are activated to cytotoxic alkylating agents by cartoxypeptidase G2. J Med Chem 1990; 33:677–681.
38. Niculescu-Duvaz I, Springer CJ. Gene-directed enzyme prodrug therapy (GDEPT): choice of prodrugs. In: Bagshawe KD, ed. Gene-Directed Enzyme Prodrug Therapy (GDEPT): Choice of Prodrugs. Amsterdam: Elsevier Science B. V., 1996.
39. Marias R, Spooner RA, Light Y, Martin J, Springer CJ. Gene-directed enzyme prodrug therapy with a mustard prodrug/carboxypeptidase G2 combination. Can Res 1996; 56:4735–4742.
40. Subak-Sharpe JH, Burk RR, Pitts JD. Metabolic cooperation by cell to cell transfer between genetically different mammalian cells. Heredity 1966; 21:342–343.
41. Gilula NB, Reeves OR, Steinbach A. Metabolic coupling, ionic coupling, and cell contacts. Nature 1972; 235: 262–285.
42. Simpson I, Rose B, Lowenstein WR. Size limit of molecules permeating junctional membrane channels. Science 1977; 195:294–296.
43. Beyer EC. Int Rev Cytol 1993; 137C:1–37.
44. Mesnil M, Piccoli C, Tiraby G, Willecke K, Yamasaki H. Bystander killing of cancer cells by herpes simplex virus thymidine kinase gene is mediated by connexins. Proc Natl Acad Sci 1996; 93:1831–1835.
45. Mesnil M, Krutovskikh V, Piccoli C, Elfgang C, Traub O, Willecke K, Yamasaki H. Cancer Res 1995; 55:629–639.
46. Caruso M, Panis Y, Gagandeep S, Houssin D, Salzman JL, Klatzmann D. Regression of established microscopic liver metastases after in situ transduction of a suicide gene. Proc Natl Acad Sci 1993; 90:7024–7028.
47. Consalvo M, Mullen CA, Modesti A, et al. 5-Fluorocytosine induced eradication of murine adenocarcinomas engineered to express the cytosine deaminase suicide gene requires host immune competence and leaves an efficient memory. J Immunol 1995; 154:5302–5312.
48. Gagandeep S, Brew R, Green B, et al. Prodrug-activated gene therapy: involvement of an immunological component in the bystander effect. Cancer Gene Ther 1996; 3:83–88.
49. Ramesh R, Marrogi AJ, Munshi A, Abboud CN, Freeman SM. In vivo analysis of the ''bystander effect'': a cytokine cascade. Exp Haematol 1996; 24:829–838.
50. Barba D, Hardin J, Sadelain M, Gage FH. Development of anti-tumor immunity following thymidine kinase mediated killing of experimental brain tumors. Proc Natl Acad Sci 1994; 91:4348–4352.
51. Mullen CA, Coale MM, Lowe R, Blaese RM. Tumors expressing the cytisine deaminase suicide gene can be eliminated in vivo with 5-fluorocytosine and induce protective immunity to wild type tumor. Cancer Res 1994; 54: 1503–1506.
52. Misawa T, Chiang M, Scotzco L, et al. Induction of systemic responses against hepatic metastases by HSV1-TK ganciclovir treatment in a rat model. Cancer Gene Ther 1995; 2:332–337.
53. O'Malley BW, Jr., Sewell DA, Li D, Kosai K, Chen S, Woo SLC, Duan L. The role of Interleukin-2 in combination adenovirus gene therapy for head and neck cancer. Mol Endo 1997; 11:667–673.
54. Rosenberg SA, Lotze M, Maul LM. A progress report on the treatment of 157 patients with advanced cancer using lymphokine-activated killer cells and interleukin-2 or high-dose interleukin-2 alone. N Engl J Med 1987; 316:889–897.
55. West WH, Touer KW, Yanelli JR. Constant infusion of recombinant interleukin-2 in adoptive immunotherapy of advanced cancer. N Engl J Med 1987; 316:898–905.
56. West WH, Touer KW, Yanelli JR, et al. Constant infusion interleukin-2 in adoptive cellular therapy of cancer. Proc ASCI 1987; 6:929–933.
57. Chen S-H, Li Chen XH, Wang Y, Kosai K, Finegold MJ, Rich SS, Woo SLC. Combination gene therapy for liver metastasis of colon carcinoma in vivo. Proc Natl Acad Sci 1995; 92:2577–2581.
58. O'Malley BW, Jr., Cope KA, Chen S, Li D, Schwartz MR, Woo SLC. Combination gene therapy for oral cancer in a murine model. Cancer Res 1996; 56:1737–1741.
59. Chen SH, Kosai K, Xu B, Pham-Nguyen K, Contant C, Finegold MJ, Woo SL. Combination suicide and cytokine gene therapy for hepatic metastases of colon carcinoma: sustained antitumor immunity prolongs animal survival. Cancer Res. 1996; 56(16):3758–3762.
60. Dranoff G, Jaffe EM, Lazenby A, Golumbek P, Levitsky H, Brose K, Jackson V, Hirofumi H, Pardoll DM, Mulligan RC. Vaccination with irradiated tumor cells engineered to secrete murine granulocyte-macrophage colony-stimulating factor stimulates potent, specific, and long lasting anti-tumor immunity. Proc Natl Sci 1993; 90:3539–3543.
61. Chu G, et al. Nucleic Acids Res 1987; 15:1311–1326.
62. Yang NS, Burkholder J, Roberts B, Martinell B, McCabe D. In vivo and in vitro gene transfer to mammalian somatic cells by particle bombardment. Proc Natl Acad Sci 1990; 87:9568–9572.
63. Wolff JA, Malone RW, Williams P, Chong W, Acsadi G, Jani A, Felgner PL. Direct gene transfer into mouse muscle in vivo. Science 1990; 247:1465–1468.

64. Sikes ML, O'Malley BWJ, Finegold MJ, Ledley FD. In vivo gene transfer into rabbit thyroid follicular cells by direct DNA injection. Hum Gene Ther 1994; 5(7):837–884.
65. Felgner PL, Gadek TR, Holm M, et al. Lipofection: a highly efficient, lipid-mediated DNA-transfection procedure. Proc Natl Acad Sci 1987; 84:7413–7417.
66. Sugaya S, Fujita K, Kikuchi A, Ueda H, Takakuwa K, Kodama S, Tanaka K. Inhibition of tumor growth by direct intratumoral gene transfer of herpes simplex virus thymidine kinase gene with DNA-liposome complexes. Hum Gene Ther 1996; 7(2):223–230.
67. Miller AD. Retrovirus packaging cells. Hum Gene Ther 1990; 61:5–14.
68. Ledley FD. Human gene therapy. In: Jacobson GK, Jolly SO, eds. Biotechnology, A Comprehensive Treatise. Weinhim, 1989:399–461.
69. Habib NA, Ding S, El-Masry R, Dalla Serra G, Mikhail NE, Issi G, et al. Contrasting effects of direct p53 DNA injection in primary and secondary liver tumours. Tumor Targeting 1995; 1:295–298.
70. Markowitz D, Goff S, Bank A. Construction and use of a safe and efficient amphotropic packaging cell line. Virology 1988; 167:400–406.
71. Heinrish MC, Keeble WW, Grompe M, Bagby GC, Jr., Hoatlin ME. A gibbon ape leukemia virus (GALV) pseudotyped retroviral vector for gene therapy of Fanconi anemia complementation group C (FACC). Blood 1994; 84: 359a.
72. O'Malley BW, Jr., Ledley FD. Somatic gene therapy: methods for the present and future. Arch Otolaryngol Head Neck Surg 1993; 119:1100–1107.
73. Roth JA, Cristiano RJ. Gene therapy for cancer: What have we done and where are we going? J Natl Cancer Inst 1997; 89(1):21–39.
74. Crystal RG. Transfer of genes to humans: early lessons and obstacles to success. Science 1995; 270:404–410.
75. Yang Y, Nunes FA, Berencsi K, Futh EE, Gonczol E, Wilson JM. Cellular immunity to viral antigens limits E1-deleted adeno-viruses for gene therapy. Proc Natl Acad Sci 1994; 91:4407–4411.
76. Wang Q, Finer MH. Second generation adenovirus vectors. Nature 1996; 2(6):714–716.
77. Engelhardt JF, Ye X, Doranz B, Wilson JM. Ablation of E2A in recombinant adenoviruses improves transgene persistence and decreases response in mouse liver. Proc Natl Acad Sci 1994; 91:6196–6200.
78. Samulski RJ, Chang LS, Shenk T. Helper-free stocks of recombinant adeno-associated viruses: normal integration does not require viral gene expression. J Virol 1989; 63: 3822–3828.
79. Halbert CL, Alexander IE, Wolgamot GM, Miller AD. Adeno-associated virus vectors transduce primary cells much less efficiently than immortalized cells. J Virol 1995; 69(1473):1479.
80. Geller AI, Keyomarsi K, Bryan J, Pardee AB. An efficient deletion mutant packaging system for defective herpes simplex virus vectors: potential application to human gene therapy and neuronal physiology. Proc Natl Acad Sci 1990; 87: 8950–8954.
81. Marcel T, Grausz JD. The TMC worldwide gene therapy enrollment report, end 1996. Hum Gene Ther 1997; 8: 775–880.

18

Regulatory Aspects of Gene Therapy

Andra E. Miller and Stephanie L. Simek
Food and Drug Administration, Rockville, Maryland

I. U.S. OVERSIGHT OF GENE THERAPY

A. FDA Regulatory Authority

Since the beginning of recorded history, societies have been concerned about the purity of the food and drink available to the public. Regulation of food in the United States dates back to early colonial times. Federal controls over the drug supply started in 1848 when the state of California passed a pure food and drink law. In 1902 Congress made appropriations to establish food standards, and in the same year the Biologics Control Act was passed to license and regulate interstate sale of serum, vaccines, and other biologics used to prevent or treat disease in humans. The 1902 Act established federal inspection of licensed facilities, prohibition of false labeling, and the concept of a dating period during which a biological product would be medically used. In 1906 the Food and Drugs Act passed Congress and prohibited interstate commerce of misbranded and adulterated foods, drinks, and drugs. In 1938 the Federal Food Drug and Cosmetic (FD&C) Act was enacted, making the 1906 Food and Drug Act obsolete. The FD&C Act extended controls to cosmetics and therapeutic devices and also required predistribution clearance of new drugs based on safety. In addition, this act authorized standards of identity and quality for foods and drugs as well as authorizing factory inspections. In 1944 the Public Health Service Act (PHSA) was established and consolidated the major rule making authority for biological products under Sections 351 and 352. The PHSA requires that the product and the establishment meet standards to ensure continued safety, purity, and potency of the biologic.

Today the primary mission of the Food and Drug Administration (FDA) is to safeguard and promote the public health by promptly and efficiently reviewing clinical research and taking appropriate action on the marketing of regulated products. This is accomplished by upholding established regulatory principles, such as quality control, sound scientific rationale, and risk-benefit assessment. During the regulatory process, is important that these principles be applied in a way that will encourage early product development and not inhibit development of new clinical approaches. This is particularly challenging for the field of gene therapy where some of the risks are clearly undefined, while the potential benefit of these therapies may be great.

The Center for Biologics (CBER) is one of five centers comprising the FDA and is responsible for the regulation of biological products. The authority to regulate biologics is mandated by both the FD&C Act and the PHSA. These acts outline binding practices for the agency and the sponsor. The FD&C Act provides the legal interpretation that a "biologic product" is also a "drug," and section 351 of the PHSA makes provisions for the regulation of biological products through licensure of the establishment and the product. Under the PHSA a biologic is defined as "a virus, therapeutic serum, toxin, antitoxin, vaccine, blood, blood component or derivative, allergenic product, analogous product, or arsphenamine or derivative of arsphenamine (or any other trivalent organic arsenic compound), applicable to the prevention, treatment or cure of a disease or condition of human beings."

Regulations pertaining to the conduct of clinical investigations using biological products are outlined in title 21 of the Code of Federal Regulations (CFR). Regulations are interpretations of the laws that provide rules for daily business and are binding like laws. The regulations covered under 21 CFR 312 specify requirements necessary for submission of Investigational New Drug (IND) applications, while standards for licensure of a biologic product are described under 21 CFR 610. FDA's regulatory authority in the somatic cell and gene therapy area was established in the *Federal Register* notice of Oct. 14, 1993, entitled ''Application of Current Statutory Authorities to Human Somatic Cell Therapy Products and Gene Therapy Products.'' This document establishes that somatic cell and gene therapy products are biological products and as such are subject to the licensing provisions of the PHSA.

Besides the statutes and regulations by which the FDA governs its day-to-day interactions with industry and academia, the agency also issues guidance documents, which are not binding but rather describe CBER's policy and regulatory approach to specific product areas. Documents that present recommendations and give relevant guidance to somatic cell and gene therapy products are available (see Section V).

B. Status of Gene Therapy in the United States

As provided in the document ''Current Statutory Authorities to Human Somatic Cell Therapy Products and Gene Therapy Products,'' human gene therapy is defined as a medical intervention based on the administration of genetic material in order to modify or manipulate the expression of a gene product or to alter the biological properties of living cells. Cells may be modified ex vivo for subsequent administration or altered in vivo by gene therapy products given directly to the subject. Examples that fall under this definition include, but are not limited to, autologous bone marrow stem cells modified with a viral vector, intramuscular injection of a plasmid DNA vector, use of antisense oligonucleotides to block gene transcription, ribozyme technology, and use of sequence-specific oligonucleotides to correct a genetic mutation. Since submission of the first human gene therapy IND in 1989, 252 human gene therapy INDs have been submitted to the Office of Therapeutics, CBER for review (through 31 March, 1999). While more than half of these have involved ex vivo modification of cells using gene therapy vectors, since 1995 the number of INDs involving direct administration of gene therapy vectors has been increasing, and currently almost 45% of all INDs use direct vector administration. Overall, almost 90% of INDs submitted have involved expression or replacement of a gene with therapeutic intent and comprise indications as broad as cancer, HIV, cystic fibrosis, hemophilia, peripheral and arterial vascular disease, and arthritis. In approximately 20% of the INDs, nonviral plasmid vectors were used for gene delivery. Of the viral vector systems used, more than half of the INDs submitted have used retroviral vectors, about one quarter adenoviral vectors, and a small number adeno-associated or herpes virus vector systems.

For the area of gene therapy, CBER has applied a unique regulatory approach that has included an element of public process that is not typically used at the FDA. The goal of this public interaction has been to increase the community's understanding of the CBER review process and requirements, to allow deliberation of ethical and social issues that surround the area of gene therapy, to receive input into CBER gene therapy policy development, and to provide accurate information to the public about the progress of gene therapy clinical trials. Much of this process has been facilitated by the National Institutes of Health (NIH) and the Recombinant DNA Advisory Committee (RAC), but in addition the FDA has sponsored multiple forums with industry, trade groups, academia, and the public in order to foster public understanding in the area of gene therapy, which is essential for continued progress of the field.

C. FDA/RAC Oversight

Unlike other areas under clinical investigation that are regulated by the FDA, gene therapy clinical investigations are subject to the scrutiny of two federal agencies within the Department of Health and Human Services—the FDA and the NIH. Oversight of human gene therapy clinical trials at the NIH involves a public process of review and discussion conducted by the RAC that ensures public awareness of clinical trial registration and follow-up. As illustrated in Figure 1, the RAC meets quarterly for public discussion

RAC	FDA
– Public	– Confidential
– Quarterly Meetings	– Ad hoc Meetings
– Basic, Clinical, and Preclinical	– Basic, Clinical, and Preclinical
– Law, Ethics	– Regulatory, and Manufacturing, and Quality Control

Figure 1 Comparison of RAC and FDA considerations for review of human gene therapy proposals.

of proposals deemed novel. In contrast, FDA review of gene therapy INDs is confidential and conducted by agency reviewers on an ongoing basis.

The emphasis of the review by each group is complementary. Both NIH and FDA deliberate preclinical and clinical issues; however, the RAC's responsibilities extend beyond safety and efficacy to the consideration of the ethical, legal, and social implications of such research. The FDA provides careful and thorough review of product manufacturing related to product safety, purity, potency, and identity, whereas the RAC does not consider these manufacturing issues because of the proprietary nature of such information. Currently, information regarding human gene therapy clinical trials must be submitted to both the FDA and the NIH, however, there is an initiative underway to allow for a single submission, which would be shared by both groups.

1. RAC History

The RAC was established in 1975 as a result of public concern over the potential risks of the new field of recombinant DNA (rDNA) research. Scientists worldwide had voluntarily halted their research and met in Asilomar, California, to debate the future of the use of rDNA technology. The RAC evolved from these debates and met for the first time just after the Asilomar meeting. The RAC mission was to advise the NIH director and to review in public each experiment involving recombinant DNA research. Subsequently NIH established the Office of Recombinant DNA Activities (ORDA) now called Office of Biotechnology Activities (OBA) to provide administrative support to the RAC. Over the first few meetings the RAC set minimum standards for biological and physical containment of rDNA molecules. This was accomplished through public debate and with input from scientists and lay representatives, including ethicists and economists. Finally in 1976 the NIH Guidelines for Research Involving Recombinant DNA Molecules (NIH Guidelines) were published in the *Federal Register.* The NIH Guidelines provided for submission and review of rDNA experiments by the RAC and also provided for the element of public debate of rDNA research. The NIH Guidelines are not regulations, but establish their authority through the NIH funding process. Investigators receiving NIH funding or who are affiliated with an institution that has NIH funding must comply with the NIH Guidelines. In addition, they ask for voluntary compliance by non–NIH-funded investigators. This process has provided a precedent for the public discussion and consideration of gene therapy clinical trials conducted today.

In 1982 in response to the report of the President's Commission (entitled "Splicing Life: Social and Ethical Issues of Genetic Engineering with Human Beings"), the Human Gene Transfer Subcommittee (HGTS) to the RAC was established to review the application of rDNA technology to human gene therapies. The first human gene therapy protocol was approved after public discussion by this committee and separately by the FDA in 1990. Over time as public concern over rDNA experiments subsided and interest in gene therapy increased, the HGTS merged with the full RAC, and the combined group discussed and approved each gene therapy protocol prior to its initiation. In 1994, an accelerated review process was adopted for certain categories of clinical trails that had been routinely reviewed by the RAC and determined not to represent significant risk to human health and the environment. Under this mechanism, such protocols were subject only to written review by several RAC members outside of the quarterly meetings and OBA approval.

The RAC is currently composed of 15 members from the disciplines of science, medicine, law, and ethnics. They meet quarterly for the public review and discussion of novel gene-transfer protocols. They no longer approve or disapprove protocols; at this time their function is purely to provide a platform for public discussion of novel issues involved in gene therapy clinical trials. In addition the RAC sponsors the Gene Therapy Policy Conferences (GTPC), which provide a mechanism for in-depth discussion of a single issue. For this forum, a panel of experts is convened with the goal of reaching consensus and developing guidance in a particular area. GTPC discussions have focused on topics such as genetic enhancement, use of lentiviral vectors, and prenatal gene transfer.

2. Dual Submissions

As illustrated in Figure 2, there is a parallel path of submissions required prior to initiation of a gene therapy clinical trial. Sponsors of a gene therapy clinical trial must submit an IND application to CBER, FDA for review under a 30-day review cycle and may not proceed until the IND is found to be acceptable. Upon receipt of a gene therapy IND, CBER notifies OBA, NIH of the IND title, the date of submission, and the names of the investigators conducting the clinical trial to allow OBA to track compliance with their submission requirements. Prior to initiation of the clinical trial, the FDA requires Institutional Review Board (IRB) approval. In parallel, investigators who receive NIH funding must submit information as specified in Appendix M of the NIH Guidelines to OBA to determine if full RAC review is required. The OBA submission should be made prior to or concurrent with the IND submission. The OBA submission must be received no less than 8 weeks prior to the next scheduled RAC meeting. A gene therapy clinical trial will be judged as exempt from, or in need of, full RAC/public discussion based on the novelty of the vector, gene-delivery system, disease, and application of gene

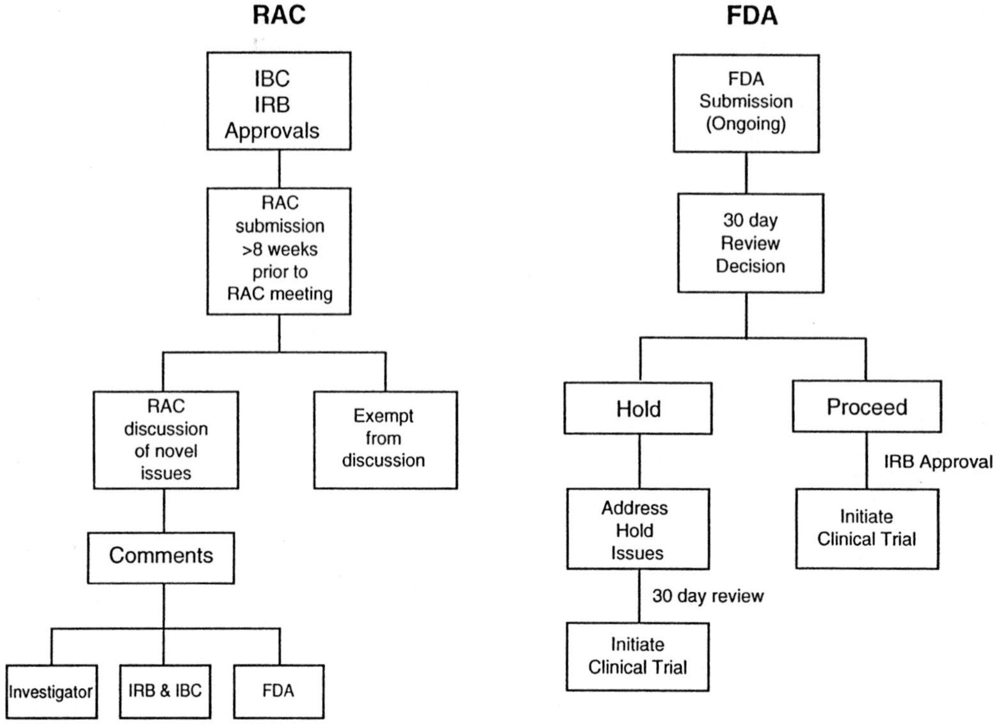

Figure 2 Overview of parallel processes for submission of documentation related to initiation of human gene therapy clinical trials to the RAC and the FDA. An effort is currently underway to allow for a single submission to be shared by both groups.

transfer. If discussion at the RAC meeting takes place, comments reflecting the discussion are forwarded to the investigator, the IRB, IBC, and FDA.

Due to timing and regulatory requirements, there are situations where the FDA decision to allow a clinical trial to proceed must be made before public discussion can occur. While there is presently no formal mechanism to put INDs on hold pending public discussion, FDA will request that sponsors have agreed to delay initiation of the clinical trial until the protocol can be presented for public consideration at the RAC. While the timing of the FDA and NIH review processes are often not ideal, the public aspect of review of gene therapy clinical trials is highly beneficial since it allows for consideration of societal and ethical issues surrounding the field of gene therapy and ensures the continued public acceptance and progression of the field.

II. THE IND PROCESS

As mandated under section 505 of the FD&C Act and section 351 of the PHSA, it is illegal to sell or distribute any biologic unless it is licensed or under an Investigational New Drug (IND) exemption (21 CFR 312.2). Submission of an IND to provide for this exemption allows clinical investigation of the product to proceed in order to determine safety, dosage, and effectiveness. This investigational process is usually divided into three phases, with each phase providing the next step in support of product licensure.

A. Definition of IND Phases

As illustrated in Figure 3, product development begins with the pre-IND stage and progresses through the investigational or IND stage (Phases I–III), where data are obtained to support product licensure. This is followed by the postlicensing stage (Phase IV), during which further studies are often performed. An IND may be submitted for one or more phases of an investigation, although in general the phases of a clinical study are conducted sequentially.

A Phase I trial includes the initial introduction of an investigational new drug into humans. The primary focus of a Phase I study is to monitor product safety in a specific patient population, although it should be noted that assessment of product safety remains a primary issue throughout

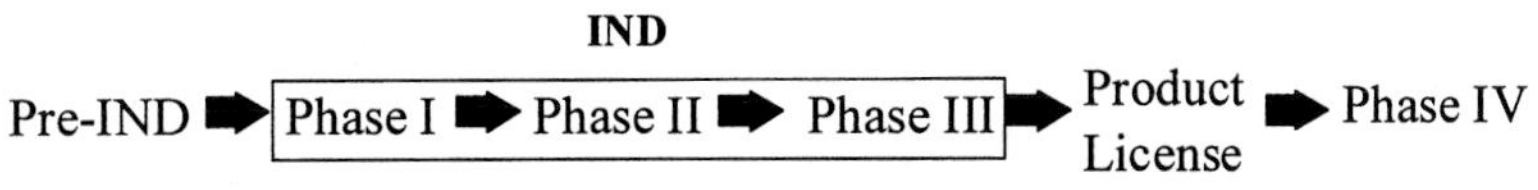

Figure 3 Phases of product development and approval.

product development. Phase I studies should be designed to determine the metabolic and pharmacological actions of the drug in humans, the side effects associated with increasing doses, and, if possible, to gain early evidence of product effectiveness. During the Phase I study the investigator should focus on obtaining sufficient information about the drug's pharmacokinetics and pharmacological effects that would permit for the design of well-controlled, scientifically valid, Phase II studies. In a Phase I study the product may also be assessed for structure-activity relationships as well as the mechanism of action in humans. The total number of subjects included in a Phase I gene therapy study varies but is typically between 10 and 40.

Phase II of an IND should include controlled clinical studies conducted to evaluate the effectiveness and dose ranging of the product for a particular indication in patients with the disease or condition under study. These studies should be designed to determine common short-term side effects and risks associated with the biological product. Phase II studies are typically well controlled, closely monitored, and conducted in a relatively small number of patients, usually involving no more that several hundred patients.

Phase III studies are expanded well controlled and uncontrolled studies that are performed after preliminary data for the effectiveness of the product have been obtained. These studies are intended to gather further information about product effectiveness and safety, which is needed to evaluate the overall benefit-risk relationship of the product and generally serve as the pivotal efficacy study to support licensure. Phase III studies usually include from several hundred to several thousand patients depending on the clinical indication and patient population.

Clinical evaluation of a biological product rarely ends with issuance of a biologics license. Phase IV or the postmarketing stage refers to the ongoing period of development after the product is licensed. Examples of postmarketing studies include clinical studies to extend claims or usage for the addition of a new patient population or indication, studies to demonstrate product comparability after manufacturing changes, and studies to validate surrogate clinical endpoints required in cases of expedited review and accelerated approval.

The FDA's primary objective when reviewing all phases of an IND is to assure the safety and rights of the patient and, later in Phase II and III, to help assure that the validity and quality of the scientific data used to evaluate the product is adequate to permit the evaluation of the product's effectiveness and safety.

B. Pre-IND Phase

An IND application and the application process can be bewildering to novice sponsors. Therefore, before IND submission, CBER encourages an early interaction, in the form of a pre-IND meeting, to discuss preclinical animal testing, product development, and clinical trial plans. While the central focus of the pre-IND meeting is to define what is needed to support the IND submission, another important goal is to create a dialog between CBER and the sponsor/investigator, which can be maintained throughout the process of product development. The pre-IND meeting is arranged at the request of the sponsor, but before CBER can grant a pre-IND meeting the sponsor will need to prepare a meeting package. Although the investigational plan does not have to be in its final form, the sponsor should be prepared to briefly describe all aspects of the proposed clinical study in the meeting package. This should encompass a description of the biological product, product manufacturing and testing schemes, established preclinical data, plans for additional preclinical studies, the proposed clinical protocol, and the general proof of concept behind the proposal. Most importantly, the pre-IND meeting should be used as a mechanism for focusing on unresolved issues relating to preclinical studies, clinical studies, or product development. It is recommended that questions be submitted with the pre-IND package addressing any concerns or potential problems with the investigational plan that would require guidance and/or discussion with the agency before submission of the IND. Past experience has proven that early identification and resolution of these issues will ultimately enhance and accelerate the product development process.

C. The IND Phase

Before submitting an IND, the sponsor must have generated enough preclinical data to ensure the safety of the proposed clinical trial. Preclinical data can be generated using either in vivo animal studies or in vitro studies to assess the product's activity, efficacy, pharmacology, pharmacokinetics, and toxicity. In addition, preclinical studies should be designed to identify potential target organs of toxicity and provide data to support clinical use of the product, such as safe starting dose, route of administration, and dosing regimen. Information to support the scientific rationale behind the proposal should also be provided. Issues specific for gene therapy that can be addressed with preclinical studies include aberrant localization or trafficking of vectors, level and persistence of gene expression, and germline alteration. The sponsor should also have a well-developed and controlled product-manufacturing scheme and have collected data regarding product characterization and consistency to support the manufacturing process. These data should also be used to support proposed specifications for product quality control and release.

Once these issues have been addressed, the next step is the preparation of the IND submission. For assistance in preparation of an adequate and complete IND, the sponsor should contact the Office of Communication, Training and Manufacturers Assistance (OCTMA) to request an IND submission package. The package contains forms to be submitted, copies of the IND regulations, informed consent and IRB regulations, information pertaining to GLP/GMP, and the essentials required for conducting adequate and well-controlled clinical trials.

Cover Sheet - Form FDA-1571

Table of Contents

Introductory Statement and General Investigational Plan

Investigator's Brochure

Required if product is supplied to clinical investigators other than the sponsor

Protocal

Chemistry, Manufacturing, and Control Information

Description of composition, manufacture, and control of the investigational product

Description of placebo

Labeling

Pharmacology and Toxicology Information

IRB approved Consent Form

Previous Human Experience with the Investigational Drug

Additional Information

Figure 4 Content and format of the IND submission as specified in 21CFR 312.23.

1. IND Submission

The content and format of an IND submission is specified in 21 CFR under part 312.23. This part lists, in order, the items that a sponsor (person responsible for conducting a clinical investigation) should submit in the IND (Fig. 4). The IND should be submitted to CBER in triplicate, and upon receipt the sponsor of a human gene therapy IND will be issued an acknowledgment letter containing the date of receipt, the assigned IND number, and a reminder of their responsibility for submission to OBA, NIH according to Appendix M of the NIH Guidelines. The IND receipt date begins the official review clock, and the IND review will take place over the next 30 calendar days. INDs automatically become effective 30 days after receipt unless FDA notifies the sponsor that the IND is subject to clinical hold. In CBER, where human gene therapy INDs are reviewed, the IND review team is composed of a product reviewer, a pharmacology/toxicology reviewer, a clinical reviewer, and a consumer safety officer, who handles administrative aspects of the IND review. The product reviewer is responsible for coordinating the review team and ensuring consistency within a product area. Consult reviewers are used on an ad hoc basis depending on the product and its application and could come from other offices in CBER or other centers within the Agency, depending on expertise.

At any point in the review process a reviewer may call the sponsor to request additional information or to discuss deficiencies in the IND. After each reviewer has completed his or her review, the team meets to discuss the file and make a final decision on the status of the application. The IND may also be discussed at office-level meetings for further input. The review decision is communicated to the sponsor by phone within the 30-day period, and this is followed by a letter giving the details of hold issues, review comments, or requests. The clinical trial may either proceed or be placed on clinical hold. Phase I INDs may be placed on clinical hold if (a) human subjects are exposed to unreasonable and significant risk of illness or injury, (b) the IND does not contain sufficient information to allow adequate assessment of the risk, (c) the information in the investigators brochure is misleading, erroneous, or materially incomplete, or (d) the clinical investigators are not qualified to conduct the study. In addition, Phase II and Phase III INDs may be put on hold if the protocol design is deficient to meet the objectives of the proposal. In order to proceed with the clinical study, the sponsor must correct the deficiencies identified during the review and submit the additional information or data in an amendment to the IND. Once this has been done the sponsor will be notified by phone that the clinical trial may proceed, followed by a written letter.

An annual report describing the progress of the investigation should be submitted to the IND within 60 days of the anniversary date on which the IND went into effect. 21 CFR part 312.33 should be consulted for details, but in general the annual report should provide information on the status of each study in progress or completed during the previous year. To this effect the annual report should include an update on the following: the number of subjects enrolled and their status, frequent and serious adverse experiences observed, summary of available study results, information relevant to understanding of the drug's action, results of additional preclinical studies performed during the year, manufacturing changes, and an investigational plan for the coming year. The annual report should also provide results of product characterization and lot release testing for all lots of product produced during the year under report. Annual reports for human gene therapy trials should include additional information relevant to gene therapy vectors, such as assessment of evidence of gene transfer and gene expression, biological activity, immune response, status of requests for autopsy, evidence of gene transfer and gonadal distribution upon autopsy, and results from assessment for evidence of infection by agents associated with the product.

2. Master File Submission

Another mechanism available for submission of information to the FDA is the Master File (MF). The procedures for submitting a MF are outlined in part 314.420 of 21 CFR. In contrast to the IND, which contains manufacturing, preclinical, and clinical information, the MF could contain product manufacturing, preclinical, or facilities information only. Submission of a MF allows the MF holder to incorporate the information by reference when the MF holder submits an IND or to permit the MF holder to authorize other sponsors to rely on the information to support an IND submission without disclosure of the information to that sponsor. There are five types of Master File submission; Type II, which provides information on the drug substance, drug substance intermediate, and materials used in their preparation, or the drug product, is generally most useful for biological product development. Type II MFs for biological products often contain product manufacturing and purification schemes, SOPs, lot release protocols, tests and specifications, descriptions of tissue culture media components, and other proprietary information needed to support an IND application. When granting written permission for a cross reference, a copy of the cross reference letter should be filed with the MF as well as the IND it is supporting and should identify by name, reference number, volume, and page number the information that each IND sponsor is authorized to incorporate. For example, in the case where retroviral vector supernatant is provided to an IND holder by a manufacturer and the method of manufacture is proprietary, the manufacturer could submit a MF documenting retroviral vector production and testing in support of the IND for review by the CBER staff. As product lots are produced, lot release protocols would be submitted to the product MF for CBER review.

Master files are often reviewed only in the context of an IND application. CBER will comment on the contents of the MF and ask for clarifying information in order to more adequately review an IND that cross-references the MF, however, a master file is neither approved nor disapproved. Importantly, the MF must contain complete information to support the decision for the associated IND to proceed.

III. REVIEW CONSIDERATIONS: EARLY PHASES

A. Continuum Approach

Product characterization and quality control of gene therapy products include issues and concerns common to most biological products such as demonstration of safety, development of methods for assessment of potency, determination of identify and purity, as well as product stability. In addition, development of specifications for each of these parameters is an important part of product development and characterization, with specifications being established and tightened over time as data become available. Another aspect common among biologics is control and regulation of not only the product, but also each step of the manufacturing process. Adherence to this approach, which is encompassed under current Good Manufacturing Practices (cGMPs), provides for quality and safety throughout the process and will lead to consistency of product lots.

In the area of gene therapy more than in other areas, a flexible approach to regulatory requirements has been attempted in order to find a balance between ensuring patient safety and fostering development of the field. In order to facilitate this process, a continuum approach to product characterization and compliance with cGMP has been adopted. The continuum approach involves a sliding scale of requirements, which increase as the study moves from Phase I toward Phase III (Fig. 5). Under the continuum approach, requirements for specific methods, fully validated assays, and full cGMP compliance are flexible. Requirements for licensure of a biological product, establishment standards, and current good manufacturing practices are specified in Parts 610, 210, and 211 of section 21 of the CFR. While it is recommended that products fully adhere to the CFR requirements by Phase III, the continuum approach can be applied to product characterization and cGMP compliance at early phases. The continuum approach applies at each step of manufacture of a gene ther-

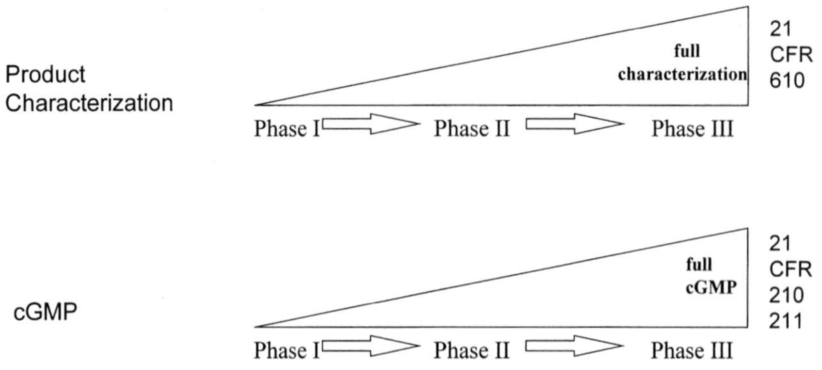

Figure 5 The continuum approach.

apy product beginning with vector development, establishment and characterization of cell banks, product manufacture and characterization, establishment of specifications for product release, and control of products used during manufacture (ancillary products). Control of each of these is important to assure product consistency and safety and is the focus of the Chemistry. Manufacturing, and Control (CMC) review.

B. CMC Review

Each step of product development, characterization, manufacture, and control should be described in the IND under the CMC section. Sufficient information is required in this section to assure the proper identification, quality, and safety of the investigational drug, although the amount of information needed will vary with the phase of the investigation. For Phase I trials, at minimum, product characterization should include a description of the product's physical, chemical, or biological characteristics, the method of manufacture, analytical methods used, and initial product specifications. In addition, data to establish product safety are essential. The emphasis of the review of an IND submission is on data, therefore in all cases data as opposed to conceptual information should be provided in support of the IND. Valid scientific principles should be applied throughout product development with regard to product safety, characterization, and quality control of the manufacturing process. During the review process a case-by-case approach is applied in order to ensure that requirements and recommendations are appropriate to a particular product and manufacturing method.

An early step in the development of a gene therapy product is construction of the initial gene therapy vector. The information supplied to the IND regarding the vector should include an explanation of the derivation of the vector, a description of the vector components and their sources, including the gene insert and regulatory elements, and a vector diagram. Ultimately, the final vector should be characterized, and all components required for its biological function should be verified using sequence analysis. However, for early phases of clinical development, sequencing limited to analysis of the gene insert, flanking regions, and any regions of the vector which are modified, in combination with restriction endonuclease analysis, is acceptable.

In general the next step in product development is the establishment of a clonal Master Cell Bank (MCB) to be used for vector production. MCB characterization includes testing to establish the properties and stability of the cells and is performed on a one-time basis. For the IND submission, information on the MCB history as well as culture and storage conditions should be included. Testing should be performed to establish vector integrity and identity, which includes cellular phenotype, cellular isoenzyme expression, genetic stability, and gene expression. Safety testing should be performed to demonstrate freedom from adventitious agents, including replication-competent virus (RCV). Analytical methods used should be summarized and initial specifications for qualification of the MCB established. Requirements for MCB testing and characterization would also apply to testing of Master Viral Banks (MVB).

The MCB is the first tier of a two-tier cell bank system; the second is the Working Cell Bank (WCB), which is derived from one or more vials of the MCB. The amount of information needed for characterization of the WCB is generally less extensive and includes demonstration of freedom from adventitious agents, limited testing for RCV, limited routine identity testing, and validation that aliquots can consistently be used for final product production.

Typically, vector production is initiated using one or more vials of the WCB. Safety testing and characterization of gene therapy vectors to be used for ex vivo modification of cells should be performed on each bulk production lot. For those vectors to be used for in vivo administration, testing should be performed on the bulk lot and on the final product after formulation and fill. During review of the IND, characterization of a gene therapy vector product with regard to its safety, potency, and purity is considered. Safety testing should include tests for sterility, mycoplasma, endotoxin, general safety, and RCV, as well as tests for adventitious virus. With regard to product potency, for early phase trials the level of gene expression will suffice as a measure of potency. However, analysis of biological activity is often more informative for assessment of product function, determination of dose, and interpretation of clinical trial outcomes. Purity of a gene therapy vector is typically established through determination of levels of residual materials such as cellular DNA, RNA and protein, noninfectious virus, and ancillary products. Product identity for a gene therapy vector product may be established through the physical or chemical characteristics of the product using in vitro, in vivo, or when appropriate molecular methods, but is not absolutely required at Phase I. As with testing of the MCB, analytical methods used should be summarized in the IND and initial specifications for qualification of the gene therapy vector product established. These are often presented in the form of a Certificate of Analysis.

To date the majority of gene therapy clinical trials have involved the genetic modification of autologous or allogeneic cells ex vivo. This has been accomplished using retroviral, adenoviral, and plasmid vectors. Information regarding the process of ex vivo modification of cells should be documented in the IND submission as follows: a description of the source of cells, results of donor screening (if applicable), method of cell collection and processing, culture conditions, and the procedure for ex vivo modification of cells. Safety testing and characterization of the ex vivo gene-modified cells should include assessment of sterility, mycoplasma, endotoxin, freedom from RCV, and potency. Analysis of phenotypic markers as well as confirmation of the integrity of the genetic insert may be used to confirm cell identity. Care should also be taken to assure patient specificity for autologous products using labeling and tracking systems. Additional parameters to be assessed include cell viability, transduction efficiency, longevity of gene expression, and the effects of irradiation or freeze/thaw on these parameters. Analytical methods used should be summarized in the IND and initial specifications for qualification of the ex vivo modified cells established.

For gene therapy vector products and ex vivo modified cell products, a stability program that assesses product safety, activity, and integrity should be established during early phases of investigation. The objectives of stability testing during early phases is to establish that the product is stable for the duration of the clinical trial and to begin to collect information needed to develop a final formulation. The submission to the IND should include a brief description of the stability study, the test methods used to monitor stability, and preliminary data if available.

The continuum approach provides flexibility to product manufacture, characterization, and testing during early phases of development. However, testing and assay validation should be performed in early phases to support data collection, development of specifications, and compliance with cGMP in preparation for Phase III studies.

C. Ancillary Products

Ancillary products are components used during manufacture that should not be present in the final product. Examples include growth factors, cytokines, monoclonal antibodies, cell separation devices, and media. The concern is that ancillary products can affect the safety, potency, and purity of the final product, especially with regard to the introduction of adventitious agents. Ideally, licensed or clinical grade ancillary products should be used for preparation of gene therapy products; however, these are often not readily available. Recommendations for the use of ancillary products that are not clinical grade during early phases of product development involve establishing a qualification program and specifications for the ancillary product. The qualification program should include adequate characterization including safety testing, functional analysis, and a demonstration of purity with regard to consistency of the purity profile for each ancillary product lot. The extent of testing required will depend on the point at which the ancillary product is used in the manufacturing process and the biological system used for production of the ancillary product, for example, eukaryotic expression system versus bacterial system. If there are known toxicities associated with the ancillary product, testing for residual levels of the ancillary product in the final product preparation should be performed. It should be noted that the use of ancillary products produced under full cGMP is recommended for Phase III trials.

D. Gene Therapy–Specific Safety Issues

Two concerns specific to the safe use of gene therapy vectors include the generation of replication competent virus and the risk of inadvertent modification of a recipient's germline. Because of their potential effect on the patient, the public health, and future generations, both of these issues need to be addressed during development of a gene therapy product and should be documented in the IND. Since RCV can arise from recombination events during manufacture, tests designed to detect RCV should be performed at multiple stages of manufacture and for each final lot. In addition, depending on the vector system in use, monitoring programs for patients who are the recipients of viral vectors are recommended. CBER Guidance should be consulted for determination of the appropriate testing and monitoring programs to employ.

For gene therapy vectors used for in vivo administration, data that demonstrate the extent to which a vector is able to disseminate out of the injection site and distribute to the gonads are necessary to assess the risk of inadvertent gene transfer to the germ cells, which may result in genetic changes in subsequent progeny. In general, these data should be obtained in the course of product development and be provided to the agency for review and comment. However, in cases where a novel vector, route of administration, or vector delivery system is proposed, preclinical studies to assess vector dissemination may be required prior to initiation of the Phase I study. Biodistribution data may be obtained from studies in animals, analysis of clinical samples, or a combination of preclinical and clinical sample analyses. Clinical data should be derived from peripheral blood cells and semen samples during the treatment and follow-up periods for the clinical trial and from gonadal tissues obtained at autopsy from consenting patients. The agency should be updated about the status of these studies at least at the time of each annual report in order to guide further product development. A statement explaining the risk for genetic alteration of sperm or eggs and possible outcome for a fetus and future child that could occur as a result of study participation should be included in the informed consent document. This statement should clearly explain the status of biodistribution studies to assess gonadal distribution for each particular clinical trial and the fact that the likelihood of an adverse outcome is currently unknown. In addition, the consent form should advise study participants to practice birth control for a suitable period of time.

IV. REVIEW CONSIDERATIONS: LATER PHASES

The previous sections have given an overview of the review process and CBER's expectations for product development as the clinical investigation proceeds through early phases. By Phase III, CBER recommends adherence to product standards and methods specified in the regulations and also that products are manufactured under full cGMP compliance. To better understand CBER's requirements for product licensure and establishment standards, a sponsor should be familiar with practices that are governed by law and specified in Parts 610, 210, and 211 of section 21 of the CFR. Part 610 provides information pertaining to product release requirements and general provisions for licensure and in some cases will provide information on specific assay methodology and Parts 210 and 211 explain the cGMPs.

Although the regulations by their nature proscribe requirements, there is a level of flexibility built into the regulations that allows for modification of required test methods or manufacturing processes. This is found under 21 CFR 610.9 and entitled ''Equivalent Methods and Processes.'' This provision is especially useful for gene therapy products, where conditions of the manufacturing process and many times the product itself make it difficult to perform standard assays. To apply this provision a sponsor should provide supporting evidence for why a specific method is not ideal for the gene therapy application and present data with appropriate controls to demonstrate that the modification will give assurances of the safety, purity, potency, and effectiveness of the biological product such that it will be equal to or greater than that provided by the specified method or process. Data to support the modification can be accumulated during the early IND phases and then validated in support of its use as an established method in Phase III.

For a product to meet the requirements for licensure it must be fully characterized prior to submission of the license application with regard to safety, purity, potency, and identity. Each of these will be discussed in the context of requirements for initiation of a Phase III trial and product licensure.

Demonstration of product safety requires the implementation of specific tests, which measure sterility, mycoplasma, endotoxin, and general safety of the product. Product safety also includes demonstration that the product is free from adventitious virus, which to support the Phase III study and product licensure includes in vitro and in vivo adventitious virus testing of the vector product and ex vivo modified cells and, when appropriate, testing for RCV. To ensure that each of these issues is adequately addressed for licensure, we recommend that the CFR-specified methods should be initiated by Phase II and that by Phase III these methods are optimized and validated. Testing for general safety is not as rigidly adhered to during Phase I and Phase II studies, but by Phase III the required standards should be in place. An exception is made for therapeutic DNA plasmid products (21CFR 610.10) and cellular therapy products (FR Notice, April 20, 1998), which have been exempted from this testing.

Potency is defined as the specific ability or capacity of the product to effect a given result. For Phase III, tests for potency should consist of quantitative in vitro or in vivo tests. A potency assay that reflects the relevant biological function of the product as opposed to an assay that measures just the level of gene product expression should be optimized and validated by Phase III. A valid potency assay is essential in order to interpret clinical trial results as well as to ensure consistent quality of the product after licensure.

Product identity can be demonstrated through the use of an assay or assays that are specific for each product in a manner that will adequately identify it as the designated product and distinguish it from any other product being processed in the same facility. At Phase I, a test for identity is not required, but it should be in place by Phase II, so that data can be collected, specifications determined, and the assay validated by Phase III.

Product purity is defined as freedom from extraneous material except that which is unavoidable in the manufacturing process. Testing for purity of a gene therapy product could involve assays for residual protein, DNA, RNA, solvents used during production and purification, or ancillary products used during manufacture such as cytokines, antibodies, or serum. As with all of the previously mentioned testing, a quantitative assay for purity should be in place by Phase III, with development of the assay being initiated much earlier in the investigational trial.

To complete product characterization in support of Phase III and product licensure, a stability testing program that includes assays that measure product integrity, potency, sterility, and, in the case of an ex vivo modified product, viability is needed. A stability protocol for study of both the bulk and final drug products should be defined so that stability data generated during Phase III will be appropriate to support licensure. In general the stability program should be initiated at Phase I so that by Phase II the objective of obtaining real-time data to support stability of the investigational formulation can be met. For Phase III, data collected should be used to support the proposed expiration-dating period of the final drug product as well as the container and closure system. In addition, stability testing of any product intermediates should be in place to support the validation of the duration and conditions of storage of the bulk product.

A. Current Good Manufacturing Practices

The second element to which the continuum approach applies is current good manufacturing practices (cGMP). cGMP is defined as a set of current, scientifically sound methods, practices, or principles that are implemented and documented during product development and production to ensure consistent manufacture of safe, pure, and potent products. Some major elements of cGMP include detailed record keeping, development of written procedures or SOPs, institution of quality control/assurance programs and assays, and equipment and process validation. cGMP also requires that a program be in place for the certification and training of personnel and for environmental monitoring. The approach to cGMP is also flexible at early stages of product development. The differences between Phase I and Phase III requirements are the degree to which each of the elements of cGMP are implemented. cGMPs play an integral part in the process of product development. As product development proceeds toward Phase III, so should the validation of the conditions under which the product is manufactured, controlled, and characterized.

B. Product Comparability

Changes in the manufacturing process, equipment, or facilities often occur during product development and can result in change in the biological product itself. A manufacturer must fully describe any change to a biological product in the IND or license application whether the change occurs prior to or after product approval. The manufacturing change should be assessed and the resulting product compared to the existing product to assure that the change does not alter the safety, purity, potency, or integrity of the final product. Determinations of product comparability may be based on a combination of in vitro or in vivo studies ranging from chemical, physical, and biological assays, assessment of pharmacokinetics, and/or pharmacodynamics and toxicity in animals to clinical testing. The type of study required would depend on the extent of change and phase of clinical development in which the change occurs. Product comparability should be demonstrated through side-by-side analyses of the old product and qualification lots of the new product. If a sponsor can demonstrate comparability with nonclinical data, additional clinical safety and/or efficacy trials with the new product generally will not be needed. FDA will determine if comparability data are sufficient to demonstrate that additional clinical studies are unnecessary. Examples of changes that would require a comparability study include any change in the manufacturing scheme or site, changes to the master cell bank, modification of the vector product, a change in fermentation, isolation, or purification, change in storage container, or product formulation. Additional guidance on product comparability requirements is available through CBER.

ACKNOWLEDGMENTS

We would like to thank Ms. Debra Knorr, OBA, NIH for critical reading of information pertaining to the RAC and

Ms. Jeanne Delasko, OTRR, CBER for providing accurate accounting of the numbers and types of gene therapy INDs submitted to CBER. Also we would like to thank Drs. Phil Noguchi and Joyce Frey Vasconcells OTRR, CBER for advice and editorial suggestions.

GUIDANCE DOCUMENTS AND OTHER REFERENCES

CBER Documents Relevant to Gene Therapy

All current and past regulatory documents can be obtained from the CBER Web site: *CBER info@CBER. FDA.Gov.*

Application of Current Statutory Authorities to Cell and Gene Therapy Products, *Federal Register*/Vol. 58, No. 1977 /Oct. 14, 1993. Rockville, MD.

Guidance for Human Somatic Cell Therapy and Gene Therapy. CBER, FDA, March 1998. Rockville, MD.

Points to Consider in the Characterization of Cell Lines to Produce Biologicals, CBER, FDA, 1993. Rockville, MD.

Points to Consider in the Production and Testing of New Drugs and Biologicals Produced by Recombinant DNA Technology, CBER, FDA, 1985 and Supplement: Nucleic Acid Characterization and Genetic Stability, CBER FDA, 1992. Rockville, MD.

Points to Consider in the Manufacture and Testing of Monoclonal Antibody Products for Human Use, CBER, FDA, 1997. Rockville, MD.

FDA Guidance Concerning Demonstration of Comparability of Human Biological Product. Including Therapeutic Biotechnology-Derived Products, CBER, FDA, 1996. Rockville, MD.

Guidance for Industry, Stability Testing of Drug Substances and Drug Products, Draft Guidance, FDA, CDER, CBER, FDA, June 1998. Rockville, MD.

Revisions to the General Safety Requirements for Biological Products; Companion Document to Direct Final Rule, *Federal Register*/Vol. 63, No. 75/ April 20, 1998. Rockville, MD.

Other References Useful for Gene Therapy

Additional information regarding gene therapy clinical trials and ORDA submission requirements can be found at the ORDA, NIH homepage: *http://www.nih.gov/od/orda/.*

Guidelines for Research Involving Recombinant DNA Molecules (NIH Guidelines), May 1999. Bethesda, MD.

International Conference on Harmonization; Guidance on Viral Safety Evaluation of Biotechnology Products Derived from Cell Lines of Human or Animal Origin, *Federal Register,* Sept. 24, 1998, Vol. 63, Number 185. Rockville, MD.

19

Gene Transfer into Hematopoietic Stem Cells

David M. Bodine
National Human Genome Research Institute, National Institutes of Health, Bethesda, Maryland

The goal of this chapter is to describe the properties of hematopoietic stem cells (HSC) and the most widely used methods to introduce novel genetic material into HSC. The purification, phenotype, and analysis of mouse and human HSC will be reviewed, as will animal models and human trials that demonstrate the potential of gene therapy. Finally, some of the problems that need to be solved before gene therapy becomes a common treatment for diseases of the hematopoietic system will be identified. The work described in this chapter comes from several different fields of study to which many authors and laboratories have contributed. The references cited should be considered to be representative, not complete.

I. PROPERTIES OF HEMATOPOIETIC STEM CELLS

The hematopoietic stem cell is the ultimate progenitor of all of the cells found in the peripheral blood. In mammalian systems, small numbers of HSC have been shown to be capable of extensive proliferation, generating millions of mature blood cells in regulated numbers each day. HSC are multipotent and differentiate into cells of the erythroid (red cell), megakaryocytic (platelets), myeloid (granulocytes and monocytes), and lymphoid (B- and T-cell) lineages. HSC can self-renew without differentiating, generating pluripotent progeny which themselves can proliferate and differentiate into mature blood cells (for reviews see Refs. 1–4). The ability of HSC to self-renew allows the transplantation of a small number of HSC to reconstitute the entire hematopoietic system of patients whose bone marrow had been destroyed (5,6).

The hematopoietic stem cell is especially attractive as a target for gene therapy of hematopoietic diseases (7–9). In theory, a small number of HSC could be exposed to gene transfer vectors ex vivo and returned to a myeloablated recipient. Repopulation of the recipient with gene corrected HSC would ensure a lifetime supply of modified peripheral blood cells of all lineages. If the transferred gene (transgene) were expressed at the appropriate levels in mature hematopoietic cells carrying the transgene, gene therapy could be the treatment of choice for many inherited and acquired hematopoietic diseases (8,9).

II. MOUSE HEMATOPOIETIC STEM CELLS

A. Transplantation Assays

The definitive assay for mouse hematopoietic stem cells is the repopulation of irradiated or stem cell–deficient W/W^v mice with transplanted hematopoietic cells (1,4). Repopulation by donor cells, as opposed to repopulation by residual host cells, is demonstrated by analysis of genetic markers that differ between the donor and recipient mouse. The genetic markers used include chromosomal translocations (10), isozyme polymorphisms (11,12), Y-chromosome–specific DNA sequences (13), cell surface markers (14), and combinations of these. Multilineage repopulation of lethally irradiated hosts is demonstrated by the detection of the host genetic marker in cells of the different hematopoietic lineages (3). Competitive repopulation assays are a powerful tool for identifying and purifying HSC. By injecting mixtures of genetically distinguishable hematopoietic cells, the relative ability of each population of cells to repopulate recipient animals can be quantified (15,16).

The repopulation of recipient mice with limiting numbers of bone marrow cells has shown that HSC are a rare population of cells. For example, one study transplanted bone marrow cells from female mice heterozygous for the X-linked isozyme marker phosphoglycerate kinase (Pgk) into stem cell–deficient W/W^v mice (11,17). Due to random inactivation of one X chromosome, individual HSC from heterozygous Pgk-a/b mice express either Pgk-a or Pgk-b. The peripheral blood cells of mice repopulated with large numbers of bone marrow cells contained an equal amount of Pgk-a and Pgk-b. In animals repopulated with successively fewer HSC, the contribution of a single HSC should be greater. As predicted, the peripheral blood cells of individual mice repopulated with limiting numbers of bone marrow cells contained high levels of either Pgk-a or Pgk-b. This work and related studies demonstrated that single HSC could repopulate a mouse but that repopulation required an average of 1×10^5 bone marrow cells (11,12,18). Limiting dilution assays have shown that the repopulating stem cell is more than 10-fold less common than the colony-forming unit–spleen (CFU-S) (19), a multipotent cell that forms a mixed colony in the spleen of irradiated mice. The HSC is also 10-fold less common than the cell that is required for the 30-day survival of irradiated mice (3).

B. Phenotype of Mouse Hematopoietic Stem Cells

The advent of fluorescence activated cell sorting (FACS) and monoclonal antibodies against specific markers expressed on the surface of hematopoioetic cells has made it possible to separate the rare HSC from the large number of more mature hematopoietic cells. Spangrude et al. (14) demonstrated that mouse HSC do not express antigens present on surface of mature cells of the different hematopoietic lineages. Lineage marker–negative (Lin-) cells represent less than 10% of bone marrow cells. Further enrichment of HSC was achieved by selecting Lin-cells expressing low levels of Thy-1.1 and the Sca-1 (stem cell antigen) marker. Lin- Thy-1.1lo Sca-1+ cells comprise less than 1% of Lin-cells and are highly enriched for HSC and other primitive progenitor cells, including CFU-S and radioprotective cells (14).

The Sca-1 marker is expressed in about 50% of all inbred mouse strains, and the Thy-1.1 allele is present in only a few inbred strains (20). The Sca-1 and Thy-1.1 markers are found together in only one strain of mice (21). Other groups have searched for other methods to isolate HSC. Several groups have shown that c-kit, the receptor for the hematopoietic growth factor SCF (stem cell factor), can be used to discriminate between HSC and more mature hematopoietic cells (22–25). In most strains of mice, Lin- cells expressing high levels of c-kit, (c-kit^{HI}) are highly enriched for HSC (22). In strains expressing Sca-1, the Lin- c-kit^{HI} cells are also Sca-1 positive (25). HSC are enriched using these markers to the point the injection of that an average of 30–50 cells will repopulate 100% of recipient mice (Fig. 1) (26).

The fluorescent dyes Hoechst 33342 and Rhodamine (Rho) 123 are pumped out of cells by p-glycoprotein (also referred to as the multiple drug resistance gene product—MDR). Cells that retain low levels of Hoechst 33342 Ho^{LO} and Rho 123 (Rho^{LO}) are enriched for HSC (27). Many groups have used the Rho 123 in combination with other markers to identify primitive hematopoietic cells (28,29). Other methods to enrich HSC have analyzed the blue and green fluorescence of bone marrow cells stained with Hoechst 33342. A rare ''side population'' of cells with low levels of blue and green fluorescence was highly enriched for HSC (30). The side population cells expressed c-kit and Sca-1, but were negative for other hematopoietic cell markers. Finally, a population of small, Lin-, hematopoietic cells that express high levels of aldehyde dehydrogenase (ALD) were shown to be highly enriched for HSC (31). Injection of as few as 10 small Lin-ALD–positive cells leads to the repopulation of 100% of recipient mice.

C. Sources of Mouse Hematopoietic Stem Cells

Repopulation assays have been used to demonstrate the location of repopulating hematopoietic stem cells in the mouse. During mouse development, hematopoiesis begins in the yolk sac at day 8.5 of the 21-day gestation period (17,32,33). Yolk sac hematopoiesis generates only nucleated erythrocytes containing embryonic hemoglobin. Yolk sac hematopoietic cells are capable of repopulating chemically ablated newborn mice (34,35) but do not repopulate adult animals (36). The first HSC capable of repopulating lethally irradiated adult mice are found in the aorta-gonad-mesonephros (AGM) region of mouse embryos at day 11.5 of gestation (36). AGM-region HSC are negative for lineage-specific markers and express c-kit (36). At day 12.5 of gestation, the fetal liver becomes the site of hematopoiesis, producing mature erythroid, myeloid, and lymphoid cells. Fetal liver HSC are lineage marker negative and express c-kit and the marker AA4.1 (37). The fetal liver is the site of mouse hematopoiesis from day 12.5 to day 17.5, after which the fetal spleen becomes the primary site of hematopoiesis (17). By the time of birth, the bone marrow has become the primary site of hematopoiesis. In adult animals, HSC are found in the bone marrow, spleen, and peripheral blood (38). Competitive repopulation assays have been used to estimate that approximately 80% of the HSC are

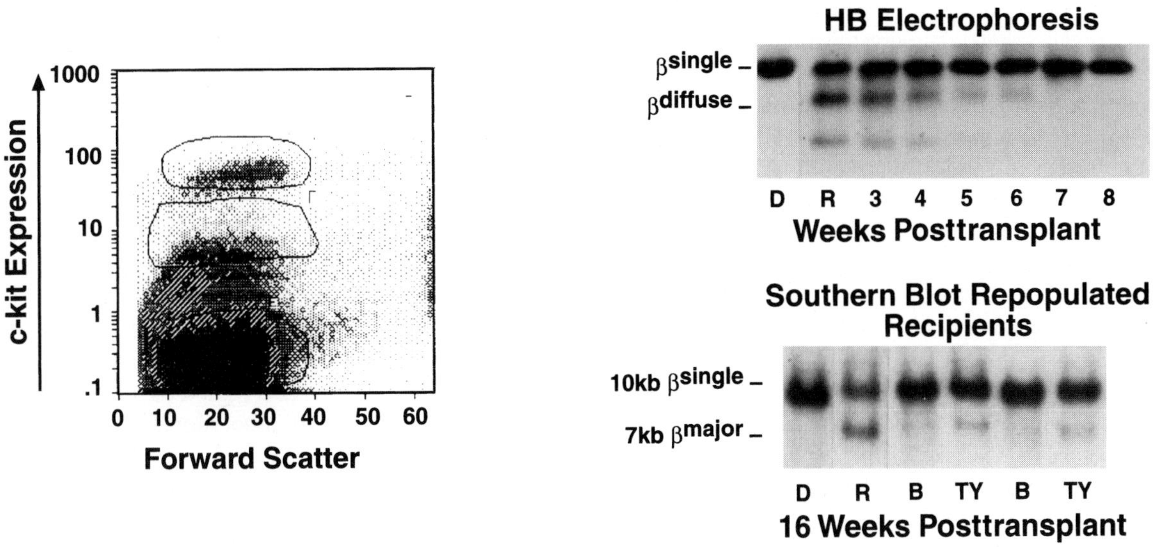

Figure 1 Mouse hematopoietic stem cells. Lineage negative (Lin-) bone marrow cells can be sorted into three populations based on the expression of the c-kit protein. The c-kit^{HI} population (left panel) contains the hematopoietic stem cells. The repopulation of recipient mice with donor cells is followed by polymorphisms in the B-globin gene. Injection of donor (D) Lin- c-kit^{HI} cells into irradiated or *W/W^v^* mice leads to repopulation of the recipient (R) with donor erythroid cells as demonstrated by the presence of 100% donor hemoglobin in the recipient after 8 weeks (top right). Southern blot analysis was used to demonstrate repopulation of the bone marrow (B) and thymus (TY) of recipient (R) with donor (D) cells (bottom panel). Phenotype: Lin- c-kit^{HI}. Assay: Repopulation of irradiated or W/W^v mice.

found in the bone marrow, 19% of the HSC reside in the spleen, and less than 0.5% of HSC are found in the peripheral blood (38,39).

The relative and absolute number of HSC in the peripheral blood of mice can be manipulated by treatment of animals with either hematopoietic growth factors or antitumor agents such as cyclophosphamide (CP). The redistribution of HSC and progenitor cells into the peripheral blood is termed mobilization (40). For example, in mice treated with granulocyte colony-stimulating factor (G-CSF) for 7 days, approximately 10% of the HSC are found in the bone marrow, 88% of the HSC reside in the spleen, and 2% of HSC are found in the peripheral blood (41–43). Mice treated with FLT3 ligand (FL) and G-CSF for up to 10 days showed greater than 200-fold increases in the repopulating ability of the peripheral blood compared to normal mice (44–46). Eight days after treatment with CP, the relative number of HSC in the peripheral blood is increased nearly 30-fold to a level similar to the HSC content of untreated bone marrow (47). Combinations of cytokines have even more pronounced effects, particularly in splenectomized mice. In untreated splenectomized mice, 99% of the HSC are found in the bone marrow. Treatment of splenectomized mice with G-CSF and SCF for 5 days causes a threefold increase in the total number of HSC, with 81% of the repopulating ability in the peripheral blood and 19% in the bone marrow (42,43). Similar results have been described with numerous other cytokines and cytotoxic drugs (44–47). An unexpected finding in mice treated with G-CSF and SCF was a greater than 10-fold increase in the repopulating ability of the bone marrow 14 days after cytokine treatment was discontinued (48).

III. HUMAN HEMATOPOIETIC STEM CELLS

A. Clinical Transplantation Models

The ability of human HSC to repopulate all hematopoietic lineages has been demonstrated by the success of bone marrow transplantation for the treatment of hematological diseases. Since the initial descriptions of successful bone marrow transplants (5,6), many improvements in the conditioning of the recipient and the management of histocompatibility differences between the donor and the recipient have been developed. These improvements have made bone marrow transplantation a common treatment for many inherited and acquired hematological diseases (49). Human HSC can be studied in selected patients transplanted with hematopoietic cells that can be genetically distinguished from recipient cells (50). Through the use of isozyme polymorphisms, DNA polymorphisms, and sex chromosome differences, it has been shown that the donor bone marrow can repopulate the lymphoid, myeloid, and erythroid lineages of human recipients (50). Analysis of transplant recipients infused with bone marrow from female donors heterozygous for the X-linked isozymes glucose-6-phosphate dehydrogenase (G-6-PD), phosphoglycerate kinase (PGK), or hypoxanthine phosphoribosyltransferase (HGPRT) has shown that human hematopoiesis can be reconstituted from a limited number of HSC (50).

Several sources of human HSC have been used successfully for transplantation. While bone marrow is the most common source of HSC, fetal liver, cord blood, and mobilized peripheral blood HSC are also used (for reviews see Refs. 51–53). Human HSC are mobilized into the peripheral blood by treating the donor with G-CSF or GM-CSF. Apheresis of the donor after 5–7 days of treatment gives a very high yield of cells, which generally exceeds the average number of stem and progenitor cells that can be harvested from bone marrow (53). Cord blood collected after delivery has also been shown to be a rich source of transplantable HSC. Recent work has shown that the HSC content of approximately 100 mL of cord blood is sufficient to repopulate 80 kg recipients (52).

B. In Vitro Assays for Human HSC

The development of in vitro assays for the most primitive human hematopoietic cells has greatly facilitated the study of human hematopoiesis. The long-term bone marrow culture (LTBMC) (54,55) and the ''extended'' LTBMC (56) define a primitive hematopoietic cell, which has the ability to differentiate into cells of various myeloid and lymphoid lineages. Cultures of bone marrow cells are initiated for the purpose of growing an adherent layer of stromal cells consisting of fibroblasts, endothelial cells, and macrophages. The stromal layers are then seeded with bone marrow cells to start the bone marrow culture. At biweekly intervals, a portion of the culture medium is replaced and the nonadherent cells in the aspirated medium can be analyzed for myeloid progenitor colony formation. Human long-term bone marrow cultures initiated by single cells generate myeloid colony-forming cells for periods of 40–60 days (57). After several weeks of culture, the standard LTBMC medium can be replaced with medium that supports the growth of lymphoid progenitor colonies. Following the medium change, the same culture will begin to produce lymphoid progenitor cells (58). The long-term maintenance and proliferation of multipotential hematopoietic cells in these cultures suggests strongly that these in vitro assays are good surrogates for the transplant experiments used to study mouse HSC (57).

Further support for these model systems is provided by the long-term culture-initiating cell (LTCIC) assay (55). In this assay, hematopoietic cells are enriched for HSC and single cells are cultured on preexisting stromal layers and analyzed for proliferation and colony formation for 40–60 days. The LTCIC assay demonstrates the presence of a rare hematopoietic cell capable of extensive proliferation and differentiation into multiple myeloid lineages (55). In mouse models, the behavior of purified murine HSC has been compared in both in vivo transplant models and in LTCIC. The number of LTCIC and the number of repopulating HSC were directly proportional (59). These studies suggest that human LTCIC assays are also recognizing the most primitive hematopoietic cells. In the extended LTCIC, hematopoietic cells are replated onto a ''fresh'' layer of stromal cells, which are cultured for an additional 40–60 days. The cells that have the capacity to generate colony-forming cells in the extended LTCIC assay have the most primitive phenotype, and the rate at which LTCIC are marked by transduction with retrovirus vectors closely resembles the rate at which human HSC are marked with retrovirus vectors (56).

C. Immune-Deficient Animal Models

Attempts to develop an in vivo transplantation assay for human hematopoietic stem cells have focused on immune-deficient sheep (reviewed in Ref. 60) or mice (61) as recipients for human hematopoietic cells. During development, the sheep hematopoietic system undergoes a rapid expansion between days 50 and 60 of gestation. The sheep immune system becomes functional between days 67 and 77 of gestation. The window between days 55 and 63 of gestation provides an opportunity to introduce human hematopoietic cells into fetal sheep. The transplantation of human cells during the ''expansion'' period facilitates engraftment, and the presence of human cells in the fetal sheep before the immune system becomes active induces tolerance to human antigens (Fig. 2) (60,62).

In a large series of sheep generated over the last 10 years, approximately 70% of the animals transplanted with human fetal liver cells had human hematopoietic cells in their peripheral blood and bone marrow. The human cells accounted for approximately 5% of the total number of peripheral blood and bone marrow cells, and all lineages were represented. Human cells were identified at all time points for periods of up to 4 years (63–65). To evaluate HSC self-renewal, bone marrow cells from primary animals are transplanted into preimmune fetuses. In approximately one third of the recipients, human cells were de-

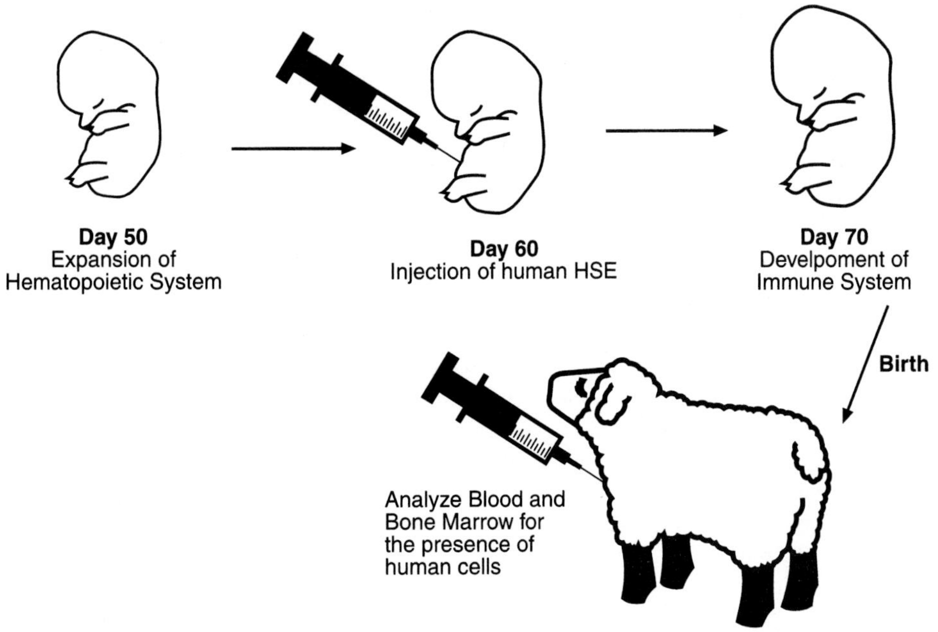

Figure 2 The fetal sheep model for the engraftment of human hematopoietic stem cells. The hematopoietic system of the developing sheep begins a rapid expansion around day 50 of gestation, but the immune system does not begin to develop until around day 70 of gestation. Injection of human hematopoietic cells around day 60 of gestation leads to engraftment and expansion of human cells that can be recovered from newborn and older sheep.

tected demonstrating self-renewal of the original engrafted cells (65,66).

The low percentage of human cells in the chimeric sheep can be increased by the injection of recombinant human cytokines. Injection of human interleukin-3 (IL-3) and granulocyte-macrophage colony-stimulating factor (GM-CSF) or stem cell factor (SCF) increased the number of human cells in the blood or marrow five- and twofold respectively (67,68).

Human bone marrow or cord blood HSC can also engraft into fetal sheep. Approximately 50% of recipient sheep transplanted with human marrow or cord blood cells show long-term persistence of human cells. The levels of human cells in sheep transplanted with either bone marrow or cord blood HSC were as good (bone marrow) or better (cord blood) than that seen in the recipients of human fetal liver cells (69–71). Approximately 80% of these recipients showed signs of graft-versus-host disease (GVHD), as might be expected from transplants including mature human T lymphocytes (69–71). The transplantation of T-cell–depleted bone marrow or cord blood prevented GVHD but was associated with lower levels of engraftment and a lower percentage of animals engrafted (72). These observations are nearly identical to what is observed in human bone marrow transplant recipients and validate the fetal sheep model as an assay for the most primitive human hematopoietic cells.

Although the fetal sheep model satisfies all of the criteria necessary as an animal model for human hematopoiesis, this model is not practical for most research laboratories. As a result, many groups have sought to develop animal models for human hematopoiesis that combine the advantages demonstrated in the fetal sheep model with the cost-effectiveness of a small animal model. These efforts have focused on either BNX mice or mice homozygous for the severe combined immunodeficiency (*scid*) mutation (reviewed in Refs. 73–75).

BNX mice are homozygous for three mutations causing immune deficiency in the mouse. The combination of the natural killer cell deficiency caused by the *bg* mutation, the lack of a thymus caused by the *nu* mutation, and the loss of some B-cell functions caused by the *xid* mutation renders BNX mice almost completely immune deficient. In the original report, human bone marrow cells were injected into sublethally irradiated BNX mice (76). The recipient mice contained low levels of human cells in the bone marrow and spleen (<1%), which could be detected by the presence of human repetitive DNA in these organs.

In addition, human colony-forming cells from the same tissues could be identified by their selective growth in medium supplemented with human IL-3 and GM-CSF. Since IL-3 and GM-CSF do not support the growth of mouse colony-forming cells, it was possible to rescue a low number of human progenitor cells for up to 8 weeks posttransplantation (76). The BNX model has been refined by the injection of human stromal cells engineered to produce human IL-3 along with human bone marrow cells (77). Human hematopoietic progenitors were recovered from the spleens and bone marrow of recipient mice for up to 9 months after transplantation. The co-injection of engineered human stromal cells improved the level of human cells in the bone marrow to approximately 6% (77).

The ability of a single cell to give rise to both lymphoid and myeloid progeny is a unique property associated with HSC. This property has been demonstrated in the BNX mouse model by transplanting human CD34+ umbilical cord blood cells transduced with a retrovirus containing a neomycin resistance (neo^r) gene (78). Following transplantation, a small number of human hematopoietic progenitor cells containing the neo^r provirus in the recipient animals were detected. If a myeloid progenitor cell and a T lymphocyte containing the neo^r provirus are derived from the same progenitor cell, the provirus should be integrated into exactly the same genomic site in each type of cell. DNA was extracted from human myeloid colonies grown in semisolid medium and from individual human T cells. The insertion site of the provirus was demonstrated using inverse PCR. Inverse PCR amplifies circular fragments generated by digestion of DNA with an enzyme that cuts once inside the provirus and at other random sites throughout the genome. Using primers specific to a single region of the provirus for PCR, the circular fragments can be amplified, generating a specific fragment for each proviral insertion that can be identified by its DNA sequence (79). Many insertion sites were detected in the myeloid colonies, four of which were shared by T-lymphocyte clones isolated from the same mouse. DNA sequence analysis demonstrated that the proviruses were integrated into the same spot in the genome. These studies provided the first and most definitive evidence that among the human cells that engraft into the BNX mouse are cells that have the properties associated with HSC (78).

Mice homozygous for the *scid* mutation lack functional B and T lymphocytes due to defects in V(D)J recombination and double-stranded break repair due to mutations in the gene encoding the catalytic subunit of DNA-PK, DNA-PK_{cs} (80). Improved levels of engraftment and proliferation of human bone marrow cells were transplanted into CB.17 *scid/scid* (SCID) mice. Human cells were detected in the bone marrow of transplanted CB.17 SCID mice at levels of 3% or higher for 8–10 weeks (81). Higher levels of human cells were detected in CB.17 SCID mice treated with human SCF and PIXY 321, a fusion molecule between human IL-3 and GM-CSF (81). Human myeloid and lymphoid cells were detected in the peripheral blood of transgenic SCID mice transplanted with human bone marrow cells for up to 24 weeks in a line of transgenic mice that expressed the human GM-CSF, IL-3, and SCF genes (82).

The meticulous work of Shultz and colleagues showed that the NOD strain of mice, which is susceptible to nonobese diabetes, was NK cell deficient (83). When the *scid* mutation was crossed onto this strain, the resulting NOD-SCID mouse was more immune deficient than any other strain carrying the *scid* mutation (83). A number of groups have demonstrated that NOD-SCID mice make superior hosts for engraftment of human hematopoietic cells (61).

NOD-SCID mice have been further engineered to provide the optimal microenvironment for human hematopoiesis. As noted above, engraftment of human cells in either BNX or SCID mice could be improved by the infusion of human cytokines. SCID mouse models containing pieces of human fetal thymus and fetal liver are implanted under the kidney capsule. Human T lymphocytes and myeloid cells are detected in the peripheral blood of transplanted SCID-hu animals for 6–12 months (84). Examination of the engrafted organs revealed the presence of multipotential myeloid and erythroid progenitor cells and a full complement of differentiating human T lymphocytes (84,85). Further refinement of the SCID-hu model implanted human fetal bone, thymus and spleen fragments (abbreviated BTS) into SCID mice. The SCID-hu BTS mouse can support human hematopoietic cells of all lineages for 36 weeks or more (86). The fetal bone fragments can be directly injected with purified hematopoietic cells, which can then be analyzed for their capacity to repopulate and proliferate (86).

D. Phenotype of Human HSC

The purification of human HSC has used strategies similar to those used to purify mouse HSC. Human hematopoietic cells expressing lineage markers have no ability to form colonies in vitro and are inactive in the LTCIC assay (87). All human hematopoietic colony-forming cells express the glycoprotein CD34. Human CD34+ cells from either bone marrow, mobilized peripheral blood, umbilical cord blood, or fetal liver are used for clinical transplantation, indicating that the CD34+ population contains HSC. Human HSC are distinguished from colony-forming cells on the basis of expression of the CD38 antigen (88). Colony-forming cells express CD38 (CD34+ CD38+), while the rare

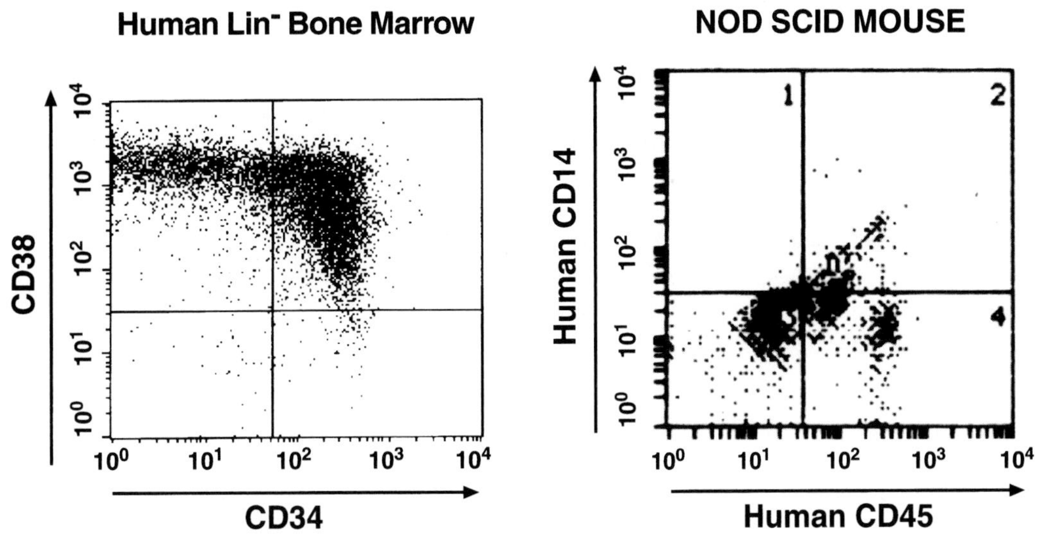

Figure 3 Human hematopoietic stem cells. Lineage-negative (Lin-) bone marrow cells can be sorted based on the expression of CD34 and CD38 (left panel). The Lin- CD34+ CD38− population (lower right) contains the hematopoietic stem cells. Human HSC can engraft and proliferate in immune-deficient NOD SCID mice. The right panel shows a FACS analysis of bone marrow cells collected from a NOD SCID from a mouse 10 weeks after injection with human Lin- CD34+ CD38− cells. The CD45+ cells are human cells, the CD14 staining identifies human monocytes. Phenotype: Lin- CD34+ CD38−. Assay: Repopulation of immune deficient mice.

CD34+ CD38-cells are the only cell type capable of generating extended LTCIC in vitro (56).

Human CD34+ cells engraft and proliferate in the BNX, SCID, and fetal sheep models (77,89–92). Recently, several lines of evidence have shown the existence of human CD34− HSC. Differential Hoechst staining of human bone marrow cells reveals a CD34− side population nearly identical to the side population of mouse cells containing HSC (93). Lin- CD34− CD38− bone marrow cells have been shown to engraft and proliferate in the fetal sheep (94) and NOD-SCID mouse models (Fig. 3) (5). These results indicate that at least some human HSC are CD34−, while others are CD34+. The difficulty in separating the repopulating CD34− CD38− cell from the large number of other CD34− cells may have prevented the injection of sufficient numbers of CD34− cells in previous studies.

IV. HEMATOPOIETIC STEM CELLS AS TARGETS FOR GENE THERAPY

A. Requirements for Effective Gene Therapy

The ability of the HSC to completely repopulate the entire hematopoietic system following transplantation makes it a particularly attractive target for gene therapy (7–9). Integration of new genetic material into the genome of HSC would ensure a continuous supply of modified hematopoietic cells in the transplant recipient. Potentially, this allows for a permanent correction of the defect. In contrast, gene transfer into progenitor cells, which do not have the ability to repopulate or self-renew, would be transient and would require periodic gene-transfer procedures to maintain a supply of corrected cells.

Successful gene transfer into hematopoietic stem cells requires several critical events. First, the new genetic material must be integrated into the genome of the hematopoietic stem cell (8,9). This will ensure transmission of the new genetic material to all progeny of the transduced target cell. Retrovirus and lentivirus vectors, which integrate into the host cell genome, are ideal gene-transfer vehicles for HSC. Conversely, adenovirus vectors, which do not integrate into the host cell genome, would not be effective for HSC gene therapy. If the gene-transfer vector does not integrate into the genome of the HSC, as the progeny of the HSC proliferate the number of vector-containing cells would be rapidly diluted with cells that do not carry the vector. Adeno-associated viruses (AAVs) have been shown to integrate into the genome of the target cell, and transduction of HSC with recombinant AAV vectors has been attempted (96–98). At the present time, the frequency of recombinant AAV integration into hematopoietic cell DNA has proven to be too low to predict that AAV-mediated gene transfer to HSC would be an efficient method of inserting new genes (99). Therefore, this chapter will focus on retrovirus and lentivirus-mediated gene transfer.

After integration, the transferred gene must be expressed at the appropriate levels in the appropriate cell type to correct the genetic defect. For some hematopoietic diseases, such as ADA deficiency, the expression of the ADA enzyme in hematopoietic cells of all lineages might have a beneficial effect. However, T lymphocytes must express the ADA gene at relatively high levels for gene therapy to be effective (9,100,101). For other diseases such as IL-2 receptor common chain deficiency (X-SCID), expression in lymphoid cells in essential (102), while expression in myeloid cells would have no beneficial effect on the disease (103).

B. Retrovirus-Mediated Gene Transfer

Currently, the delivery of new genetic material to primary hematopoietic cells has been achieved mainly through retroviral vectors (for reviews see Refs. 104, 105). Retrovirus particles contain an RNA genome that is reverse transcribed into DNA and integrated into the host cell genome (106,107). The Moloney murine leukemia virus (MMuLV) has a well-described genome and life cycle, and despite the fact that replication-competent MMuLV can cause leukemia in mice and monkeys, MMuLV were the first retroviruses to be adapted for gene therapy (108).

The development of MMuLV-based retrovirus vectors has been discussed in a previous chapter. As described, the ability of a retrovirus particle to transduce a target cell is determined by the gp70 envelope protein, which interacts with specific receptor molecules on the surface of target cells (109). Retroviruses are classified based on differences in their gp70 proteins. The gp70 envelope protein interacts with specific receptor molecules on the surface of target cells and determines which target cells can be transduced (109,110). The gp70 from ecotropic retroviruses binds to a murine basic cationic amino acid transport protein, mCAT (111,112). The three-amino-acid sequence of this protein that serves as the gp70-binding site is present only in the mouse protein and is not conserved in CAT from other mammals (113–115). The specificity of ecotropic gp70 binding restricts ecotropic retrovirus transduction to mouse cells. The gp70 from amphotropic retroviruses binds to a phosphate transporter protein, Pit-2 (116–118). The binding site for amphotropic gp70 is conserved among the different mammalian Pit-2 molecules, giving amphotropic viruses a broad host range that includes human cells. Up to now, most human gene therapy trials have involved amphotropic retroviruses (105).

Other retroviruses have been developed for gene transfer. The gp70 molecule from the Gibbon ape leukemia virus (GaLV) binds to a distinct phosphate channel protein known as Pit-1 (119,120). The Pit-1 and Pit-2 molecules are approximately 60% identical at the amino acid level (116,117). GaLV gp70 binds to a PiT-1 amino acid sequence that is present in most mammalian PiT-1 proteins with the exception of mouse PiT-1. The *env* region of GaLV retrovirus has been incorporated into packaging cells that produce recombinant virus particles with a GaLV envelope (121). These particles specifically use PiT-1 as a receptor and have been used to improve gene transfer into mature lymphocytes (122,123). The 10A1 virus is a laboratory recombinant whose envy protein binds to mouse PiT-1 and PiT-2. Recombinant 10A1 viruses enter mouse cells through interactions with either PiT-1 or PiT-2 and can also transduce human cells via the same receptors (124).

The vesicular stomatitus virus type G (VSV-G) infects almost all cell types regardless of species (125,126), presumably due to the fact that the VSV-G envelope recognizes a cell membrane phospholipid as a receptor (127). In contrast to other retroviruses, virus particles containing the VSV-G envelope can be agglutinated and concentrated to titers two orders of magnitude greater than can be obtained with other retroviruses (128–130).

A variety of recombinant MMuLV gene-transfer vectors have been described in previous chapters, each of which has advantages that may be exploited for gene-transfer applications (for review see Ref. 108). The LTR from different murine retroviruses express downstream transgenes differently in different cell types. Each LTR has its own advantages in terms of the level of expression and the cells in which the highest levels have been achieved. In general, MMuLV LTRs are most active in lymphoid cells, while the Harvey murine sarcoma virus (132), myeloproliferative sarcoma virus (MPSV), and mouse stem cell virus (MSCV) LTRs promote relatively high levels of transgene mRNA in both myeloid and lymphoid cells (133–135).

It is well documented that transgene expression in hematopoietic cells can be silenced over time (136). A detailed analysis of active and silent proviruses derived from the same hematopoietic stem cell identified site-specific methylation within the MMuLV LTR associated with the silencing of gene expression (136). Recent work indicates that mutation of the methylation sites improves the duration of gene expression in hematopoietic cells (137,138). Gene expression from the MSCV LTR promoter has also been shown to be resistant to silencing (139).

C. Lentivirus-Mediated Gene Transfer

MMuLV are dependent on cell division to become integrated into the genome of the host cell. This requirement limits gene transfer into HSC because HSC are usually quiescent or have a prolonged cell cycle (14,140–142). Lentiviruses, of which the human immunodeficiency viruses (HIV-1 and HIV-2) are the most familiar examples, have been shown to be able to integrate into the genome of nondividing cells (143). As described in previous chapters, this property is mediated by two virion proteins, matrix and *Vpr,* which promote the transport of the HIV preintegration complex to the nucleus using the host cell nuclear transport machinery (144,145).

A recombinant lentivirus packaging genome was constructed by deleting the HIV packaging signal (ψ) from an HIV-1 virus and blocking the *env* and *Vpu* reading frames with a frameshift mutation (146). Cells transfected with this construct expressed the HIV *gag* and *pol* genes. A recombinant HIV gene-transfer vector containing HIV LTRs surrounding an HIV ψ signal, a truncated and out-of-frame HIV *gag* region, a marker gene driven by a CMV promoter, and the Rev-responsive element, which promotes proviral gene expression, generated recombinant lentivirus particles (146). Compared to MMuLV vectors, the lentivirus vectors integrated into irradiated or cell cycle–arrested fibroblast cell lines at 5 to 20-fold greater efficiency (146). Related work by other groups has generated similar HIV-1– and HIV-2–based vector systems (147–149). These studies have confirmed high rates of transgene integration into nondividing cells, including primitive human hematopoietic progenitor cells.

To date, HIV vectors have been used only for marker gene transfer. It is clear that this vector system can be adapted to transfer other transgenes. It is also clear that there will be many safety concerns to address in the future in the design of HIV packaging and gene-transfer vectors. It appears that many of the modifications made to MMuLV vectors could be used to improve the safety of lentivirus vectors (146).

V. MOUSE MODELS FOR RETROVIRUS-MEDIATED GENE TRANSFER INTO HSC

A. Proof of Principle

Successful retrovirus-mediated gene transfer into HSC should provide transgene-containing peripheral blood cells to transplant recipients throughout life. In contrast, integration of a provirus into progenitor cells, which do not self-renew and have limited proliferative abilities, would result in transient production of transgene-containing cells. The initial attempts to introduce new genetic material into mouse HSC by retrovirus-mediated gene transfer used ecotropic retroviruses. The proof of principle experiments targeted a primitive hematopoietic progenitor cell, the colony-forming unit-spleen (CFU-S). CFU-S colonies contain mature cells of all mycloid lineages and are derived from single cells (150,151). The retroviruses used for these studies contained dominant selectable marker genes, either DHFR or neomycin phosphotransferase (neor). Mouse bone marrow cells were cultured on a monolayer of virus producing cells, often in medium conditioned with the hematopoietic growth factor interleukin-3 (IL-3). The cells recovered from these co-cultures were injected into lethally irradiated mice. Proviral DNA was identified in high molecular weight DNA extracted from individual spleen colonies. These studies established that primitive progenitor cells had been transduced without destroying the ability of those cells to differentiate (150–152).

Extensions of these experiments examined mice that had recovered from the bone marrow transplant. Southern blot analysis of proviral insertion sites in the bone marrow, spleen, and thymus revealed that a single HSC repopulated all three organs (151,153). Cells containing the unique proviral insertion site persisted in the peripheral blood, marrow, spleen, and thymus of these mice for periods of 12 months or more, with no changes observed after 90 days (13,154–156). These studies established that single HSC could be transduced without destroying the ability to repopulate the lymphoid and myeloid lineages.

In these early studies, less than 10% of recipient mice had long-term persistence of retrovirus marked cells. In the rare positive mice, 10% or less of the hematopoietic cells contained a provirus (13,155). A variety of protocols have been developed that improve the transduction of mouse HSC with ecotropic retroviruses, all of which share common elements. The best results are obtained when the donor animals are treated with 5-fluorouracil, a cell cycle–specific drug that is toxic to cycling cells like hematopoietic progenitor cells (140,157). The depletion of progenitor cells in the host may induce cycling of their more primitive precursors, which permits retroviral integration (153). Combining IL-3 with IL-6 and SCF in the culture medium extended the viability of PHSC in culture without significant loss of repopulating ability and improved gene transfer (155,156,158,159). Other cytokines, notably FLT3 ligand in combination with SCF, IL-6, and/or IL-3 (160,161), have had similar effects.

Many protocols include 48-hour "prestimulation" of bone marrow cells in medium containing cytokines prior to exposure to retrovirus particles (155,162). Recent experiments have shown that this prestimulation period appears to prevent the "loading" of retrovirus receptors with virus prior to the entry of HSC into cell cycle (141). Delaying the addition of virus until many HSC are competent for transduction optimizes the ability of the HSC to take up and integrate the provirus. Using the optimum combination

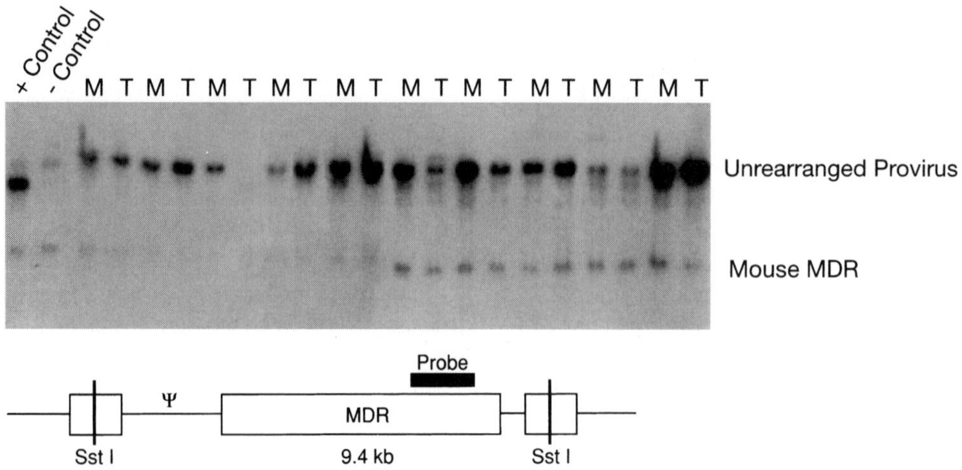

Figure 4 Transduction of mouse HSC. Mouse peripheral blood HSC were exposed to ecotropic retrovirus particles containing a human MDR gene (bottom). Sixteen weeks after transplantation DNA was extracted from the bone marrow (M) and thymus (T) of randomly selected mice and digested with the restriction enzyme Sst I for Southern blot analysis. Sst I digests the provirus in the LTR regions generating a 9.4 kb fragment if the provirus is intact. All of the mice analyzed in this experiment show relatively high levels of MDR proviral DNA in hematopoietic cells.

of hematopoietic growth factors and transduction protocols, most laboratories achieve gene transfer in 100% of transplanted mice, with a mean provirus copy number of between 0.2 and 0.5 copies per cell (Fig. 4).

B. Mouse Gene Therapy Models

Many different genes have been introduced into mouse HSC by retrovirus-mediated gene transfer and expressed in mature hematopoietic cells. These include the human ADA (162–164), glucocerebrosidase (165), and β-globin (13,155,166) genes. Mouse models exist for many inherited diseases of the lympho-hematopoietic system. Gene therapy using retrovirus-mediated gene transfer into HSC followed by transplantation has been evaluated in several of these models. The first successful correction of a mouse model for human disease was reported by Wolfe et al. (167), who introduced the β-glucuronidase gene into the HSC of the mouse model for Sly syndrome. The authors reported prolonged lifespans comparable to littermate controls and a reversal of the disease phenotype seen in untreated control animals. Subsequently, retrovirus-mediated gene transfer has been used to correct both the X-linked (gp91phox deficiency) and autosomal (p47phox deficiency) forms of chronic granulomatous disease (CGD) (168,169). Most recently the Jak3-deficient severe combined immune deficiency (SCID) mouse has been cured by the transplantation of retrovirus-transduced HSC (170).

VI. RETROVIRUS-MEDIATED GENE TRANSFER INTO HEMATOPOIETIC STEM CELLS FROM LARGER ANIMALS AND HUMANS

A. Demonstration of Stem Cell Transduction

The experiments using mouse models demonstrated that ecotropic retroviruses could introduce genes into HSC and documented the expression of transgenes in differentiated hematopoietic cells. Because ecotropic retroviruses can only transduce mouse cells, amphotropic retrovirus-mediated gene transfer into HSC of large animals was attempted. The original large animal gene-transfer protocols involved co-cultivation of rhesus monkey bone marrow cells on a layer of virus producer cells, similar to the successful strategies developed for mouse retrovirus-mediated gene transfer. Despite the use of similar protocols, the transduction of monkey HSC was more than 10-fold less frequent, with an average of less than 1% positive cells present in the best examples (171,172).

Safety concerns about the transduction of patient bone marrow cells with retroviral vectors were increased after the discovery that replication-competent virus emerging from producer cells could cause leukemia in severely immunosuppressed rhesus monkeys (173). These observations made it clear that only virus-containing media shown to be negative for replication-competent virus (and any other agents) could be used for patient studies. For most workers in the field, this meant transduction of hematopoietic cells in the absence of producer cells. This type of gene-transfer protocol has been used successfully in some mouse gene-transfer experiments (156,174) but has not been successful in other experiments (175).

An alternative procedure seeded populations of rhesus monkey CD34+ progenitor cells and HSC onto a previously established layer of bone marrow stromal cells that express SCF. The CD34+ cells were cultured for 96 hours in medium containing an amphotropic retrovirus containing the mouse ADA gene. The virus containing medium was replaced every 24 hours. After exposure to virus, the cells were collected and infused into the donor animal that had been irradiated while the CD34+ cells were in culture. The ADA provirus has been detected in 2% of mature blood cells of all lineages and bone marrow for a period of 6 years at the time of this writing (176,177). Mouse ADA was expressed at approximately 1–2% of the endogenous monkey ADA levels (176).

Another gene-transfer protocol was evaluated in a dog bone marrow transplant model. Bone marrow cells from the donor animal were used to establish a long-term bone marrow culture (LTBMC). LTBMC require regular replacement of media, which offers the opportunity for repeated exposure to virus-conditioned medium. At the end of 4 weeks in culture, the LTBMC was harvested and the cells used to transplant irradiated donor dogs. Gene-transfer efficiency using this protocol was similar to that observed in monkey models, with less than 1% of peripheral blood and bone marrow cells of the repopulated recipient containing the provirus (178–181). Transgene-marked hematopoietic cells were detected in the peripheral blood and bone marrow of these animals for periods of 5 years or more post transplantation (181).

B. Human Clinical Gene-Transfer Trials

Although the transduction of HSC in large animal models has been inefficient, the fact that marked cells could be detected in the recipient animals years after transplantation suggested that repopulating HSC were being marked. The ability to mark HSC even at a low level allowed specific experiments using retroviruses to mark the progeny of HSC to be developed. These studies have been described in detail in a previous chapter. As predicted from the large animal experiments, the frequency of marked cells in the peripheral blood of patients transplanted with transduced HSC has been less than 1% (182–186).

VII. PROBLEMS AND DIRECTIONS FOR THE FUTURE

A. Low Titer

The low level of gene transfer into human and large animal HSC can be attributed to a combination of factors. One consistent problem with retrovirus-mediated gene transfer appears to be the relatively low titer of retrovirus preparations. The titer of even the best preparations of retrovirus rarely exceeds 1 million particles per milliliter of conditioned medium, and the movement of retrovirus particles in solution is limited by Brownian motion (187). Thus, most HSC do not come in contact with retrovirus particles under standard culture conditions. To increase opportunities for HSC-retrovirus interactions, investigators have used "spinoculation" or centrifugation to move HSC through a large volume of retrovirus supernatant, effectively increasing the interaction with retrovirus particles (188). Other effects of "spinoculation" including conformational changes in the cell membrane are also possible (188). Alternatively, the cells may be immobilized on a filter through which large volumes of retrovirus containing supernatant can be drawn, allowing more opportunities for the interaction with retrovirus particles (189,190). Both of these procedures have been shown to improve gene transfer into hematopoietic progenitor cells and may ultimately prove useful for the transduction of human HSC.

Another approach to increasing the contact between virus particles and HSC involves the use of fibronectin-coated gene-transfer vehicles. It has been demonstrated that retrovirus particles and HSC bind specifically to a 35 kDa fragment of fibronectin (191). The co-localization of the target cell and the retrovirus particle increases the probability that a cell will be transduced. Human hematopoietic cell lines and human CD34+ progenitor cells are transduced with amphotropic retroviruses at higher frequencies on fibronectin-coated plates than in suspension culture. Furthermore, mouse HSC are transduced with ecotropic retroviruses at higher frequencies on fibronectin-coated plates than in suspension culture (175). The use of fibronectin in gene-transfer protocols may ultimately prove useful for the transduction of human HSC.

B. Selection of Transduced HSC In Vivo

Recognizing the inefficient transduction of human HSC by retroviral vectors, several groups have attempted to transfer drug resistance genes into HSC. These studies have a short-term goal of rendering bone marrow cells resistant to chemotherapeutic agents active against solid tumors and a long-term goal of providing a means to select for the rare transduced HSC. Selection for drug-resistant HSC and progeny would effectively amplify the number of transduced cells. If the retrovirus contained a therapeutic transgene along with the drug-resistance gene, the result would be a high level of marked cells. This concept has been shown to be feasible in mouse models using the p170 glycoprotein or multiple drug resistance (MDR) gene (192,193). However, in human clinical trials, no selection for transduced HSC has been observed (194,195). The reasons for this may be the initial low level of cells containing the MDR transgene compared to the mouse studies.

MDR selection of HSC may also be inefficient due to the high level of expression of the endogenous MDR genes in hematopoietic cells (30,132,196). Recent evidence also indicates that overexpression of MDR followed by extended in vitro culture can result in a myeloproliferative syndrome in mice (197). The DHFR gene has been considered to be a prime candidate for in vivo selection using methotrexate since the development of the first retroviral vectors. In mouse model systems, however, only mild resistance to methotrexate has been observed (198). Recent work has shown that trimetrexate (TMTX) given in combination with the nucleoside transport inhibitor nitrobenzylmercapt-purine riboside 5′-monophosphate (NBMPR-P) can efficiently select for HSC transduced with a retrovirus-containing DHFR (199). If these observations can be extended into the large animal models, TMTX/NBMPR-P selection may provide an efficient and valuable means to increase the relative frequency of transduced HSC.

C. Low Levels of Retrovirus Receptors

Many groups have focused on the question of why amphotropic retrovirus transduction of large animal and human HSC is low while ecotropic transduction of mouse HSC is relatively efficient. One hypothesis proposed that ecotropic receptor levels were relatively high on mouse HSC, but that amphotropic retrovirus receptor levels were low or absent on human and primate HSC. Initially this was not a concern, as amphotropic retroviruses had been used successfully to transduce mouse HSC (200). In addition, numerous studies had demonstrated that canine, monkey, and human hematopoietic progenitor cells could be efficiently transduced by amphotropic retrovirus vectors (105).

Using a semiquantitative RT-PCR assay, Orlic et al. (201) showed that the mRNA encoding the mouse ecotropic retrovirus receptor (mCAT) was easily detectable in mouse HSC, progenitor, and bone marrow cells. The mRNA encoding the amphotropic receptor (PiT-2) was easily detectable in human or mouse hematopoietic cell lines and primary hematopoietic progenitor cells. However, PiT-2 mRNA was nearly undetectable in mRNA isolated from mouse (Lin-c-kit^{HI}) (22) and human (Lin-CD34+ CD38-) (87) HSC. Further investigation identified and isolated a rare subpopulation of mouse HSC that had higher levels of Pit-2 mRNA. To correlate Pit-2 mRNA levels with transduction, PiT-2–positive and PiT-2–negative HSC were simultaneously transduced with genetically distinguishable retroviruses, one packaged by ecotropic packaging cells, the other by amphotropic packaging cells. More than 16 weeks after transplantation, greater than 90% of the animals in these experiments contained ecotropic proviral sequences in their hematopoietic cells. These results indicated that there was sufficient cell division to allow the integration of retroviral vectors in both Pit-2–positive and Pit-2–negative HSC. Consistent with the relatively high level of Pit-2 mRNA, more than 50% of mice repopulated with PiT-2–positive HSC also contained amphotropic proviral sequences. However, less than 10% of mice repopulated with PiT-2–negative HSC contained amphotropic proviral sequences (201). In animals repopulated with PiT-2–negative HSC, the relative number of ecotropic proviral sequences was 25-fold higher than the level of amphotropic proviral sequences. This 25-fold difference between ecotropic and amphotropic retrovirus transduction is similar to the relative difference in the levels of ecotropic receptor mRNA and Pit-2 mRNA in the Pit-2–negative HSC. The 25-fold difference is also similar to difference between the copy numbers observed between mice transplanted with HSC transduced by ecotropic retroviruses and large animal HSC transduced with amphotropic retroviruses (201). In summary, a major obstacle to gene therapy for human hematopoietic diseases is the low level of amphotropic retrovirus receptor on the surface of HSC (Fig. 5).

Significantly higher levels of PiT-2 mRNA were observed in G-CSF–mobilized peripheral blood HSC (Horowitz et al., personal communication) and in cord blood HSC that had been cyropreserved before analysis (202). While the significance of the latter observation has not been investigated, there is a large body of evidence that suggests that cytokine-mobilized peripheral blood HSC may be superior targets for amphotropic retrovirus-mediated gene transfer. In mouse models following mobilization of HSC with G-CSF and SCF, stem cells isolated from the bone marrow have 3- to 10-fold higher levels of PiT-2 (amphotropic retrovirus receptor) and PiT-1 (GaLV receptor) mRNA (202). Rhesus monkey HSC mobilized with G-CSF and SCF were transduced with amphotropic retrovirus vectors at a frequency that allowed detection of the provirus by Southern blot analysis (203,204).

The most encouraging levels of gene transfer into human HSC have been observed in patients transplanted with G-CSF–mobilized peripheral blood cells. Although

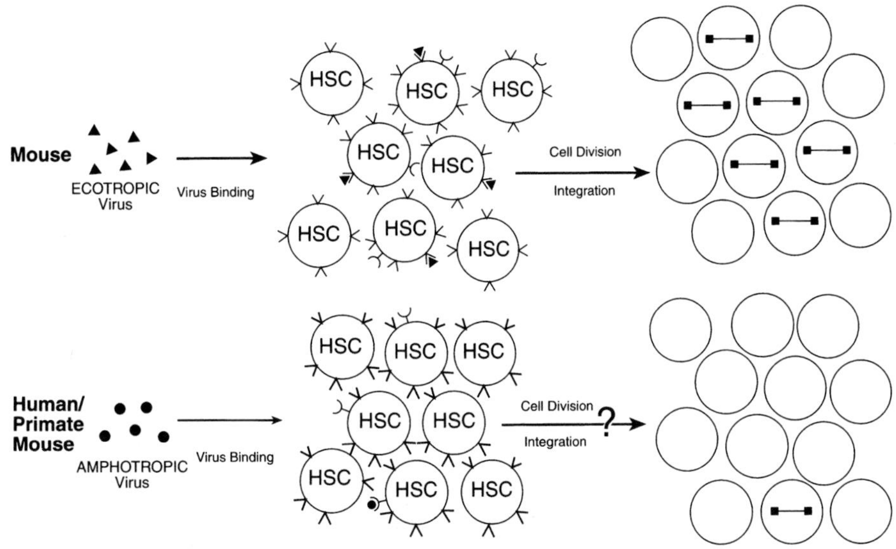

Figure 5 Comparison of transduction by ecotropic and amphotropic retrovirus particles. In the mouse (top), the high level of ecotropic retrovirus receptor allows many cells to bind a virus. Subsequent cell division allows these viruses to integrate into the genome. Amphotropic transduction of mouse primate or human HSC (bottom) is limited by low levels of amphotropic receptor expression on HSC. There are fewer opportunities for virus to bind to cells, and therefore any cell division that occurs is unlikely to result in a viral integration.

the use of G-CSF–mobilized peripheral blood HSC was only one of the differences between these studies and other related studies, two groups have described superior marking of human HSC from G-CSF–mobilized peripheral blood. G-CSF–mobilized peripheral blood HSC were more efficiently transduced than bone marrow HSC in a marking study (183) and in an ADA-deficient SCID gene therapy trial (186).

In mouse models, there is a transient increase in the number of bone marrow HSC number 14 days after the end of treatment with G-CSF and SCF (48). The increase in HSC number is accompanied by an increase in the level of PiT-1 and PiT-2 mRNA in HSC (202). Rhesus monkeys were treated for 5 days with G-CSF and SCF and allowed to recover for 10 days. At this time bone marrow CD34+ cells were collected and transduced with either amphotropic or GaLV retrovirus vectors before transplantation into irradiated recipients. In both studies gene transfer levels of 5–10% were detected by Southern blot analysis in repopulated animals (203–205). In a canine model system, dog bone marrow cells were collected 10 days after G-CSF and SCF treatment. These cells were transduced with a retrovirus containing the human IL-2 receptor gamma chain gene. An average of 30% of lymphocytes and myeloid cells in dogs repopulated with G-CSF and SCF-primed marrow expressed human IL-2 receptor gamma chain. Low (< 5%) and transient levels of gene transfer into untreated dog HSC were observed in parallel experiments (206).

The use of VSV-G pseudotyped retroviruses may eventually circumvent problems with low titer and low numbers of receptors. As noted previously, VSV-G particles can be efficiently concentrated to high titers without loss of activity (128,129). Since the VSV-G receptor is a membrane phosholipid (127), it would appear that there should be fewer problems with low receptor numbers. Problems associated with the toxicity of VSV-G *env* have slowed the development of VSV-G–mediated gene therapy (126), but recent work with concentrated and purified VSV-G vectors has shown great promise in model systems (129).

D. Quiescent HSC

Because MMuLV-based retroviral vectors require cell division to integrate into the host cell genome, another obstacle to retrovirus-mediated gene transfer is the fact that most HSC are quiescent. Although relatively efficient transduction of mouse HSC can be achieved with ecotropic MMuLV vectors, it is not clear that human HSC are as prone to enter the cell cycle during the time they are exposed to the virus. One approach to this problem has been to expose human HSC to retroviral vectors under culture conditions that would lower the levels of cell cycle inhibitors. A recent study showed that the level of the cell cycle inhibitor p15(INK)4B could be decreased in human CD34+ progenitor cells by culture in serum-free medium containing antibodies against TGF-β. In addition, antisense oligonucleotides inhibited the expression of a second cell cycle inhibitor P27(KIP-1) in CD34+ cells and promoted cell cycling (207). Human CD34+ CD38− HSC were cultured in serum-free medium containing SCF, Il-6, IL-3, FL, anti TGF-β antibodies and antisense p27(KIP-1) oligonucleotides for 12 hours and exposed to retrovirus vectors containing a neo gene for 12 hours. Parallel cultures of cells were cultured in the same cytokines minus the anti-TGF-β antibodies and antisense p27(KIP-1) oligonucleotides for 12 hours and then exposed to the same virus. Cells from both conditions were equally capable of engrafting and proliferating in the BNX mouse model. One year after transplantation, no neo transgenes were observed in the human hematopoietic cells derived from cells not exposed to the anti-TGF-β antibodies and antisense p27(KIP-1) oligonucleotides. In contrast, the neo transgene was detected in about 10% of cells derived from CD34+ CD38− HSC exposed to anti-TGF-β antibodies and antisense p27(kip-1) oligonucleotides (207). These results clearly show that cell-cycle induction can promote retrovirus-mediated gene transfer into HSC without damaging the ability of the HSC to repopulate BNX mice.

The gene-transfer problems relating to cell cycle may ultimately be overcome by the use of lentivirus-based vectors, which do not require cell division for integration. VSV-G pseudotyped lentivirus vectors have been shown to be greater than 20-fold more efficient at transducing freshly isolated human Lin- CD34+ CD38− HSC than MMuLV vectors (208). In addition, the expression level of the GFP reporter gene in lentivirus-transduced cells persisted for 5 weeks in culture, while expression of GFP from the MMuLV vector was lower and rapidly was silenced (208).

E. Summary

Improving the efficiency of gene transfer and the expression of the transferred genes are the critical basic research goals that will extend gene therapy from possibility to reality. Basic research into the biology of the PHSC has demonstrated low levels of retrovirus receptors and cell cycling as well as solutions to these problems. Basic research into retrovirus envelope proteins and backbones has led to new recombinant retrovirus vectors that are capable of transferring and expressing genes at higher rates. As clinical experience is acquired in the use of retrovirus vectors for marking human HSC, it is clear that therapeutic gene transfer to human HSC could soon be a practical method for the treatment of ADA deficiency and other immune disorders. I predict that success in treating these diseases by gene transfer to HSC will be rapidly expanded to the treatment of a wide variety of other inherited and acquired hematological diseases.

REFERENCES

1. Orlic D, Bodine DM. What defines a pluripotent hematopoietic stem cell (PHSC): will the real PHSC please stand up. Blood, 1994; 84:3991–3994.
2. Ogawa M. Differentiation and proliferation of hematopoietic stem cells. Blood 1995; 81:2844–2853.
3. Morrison S, Uchida N, Weissman I. The biology of hematopoietic stem cells. Annu Rev Cell Dev Biol 1995; 11: 35–71.
4. Sutherland HJ, Hogge DE, Eaves CJ. Characterization, quantitation and mobilization of early hematopoietic progenitors: implications for transplantation. Bone Marrow Transplant 1996; (suppl 1):S1–4.
5. Thomas ED, Storb R, Clift RA, Fefer A, Johnson FL, Neiman PE, Lerner KG, Glucksberg H, Buckner CD. Bone marrow transplantation (first of two parts). N Engl J Med 1975; 292:832–843.
6. Thomas ED, Storb R, Clift RA, Fefer A, Johnson FL, Neiman PE, Lerner KG, Glucksberg H, Buckner CD. Bone marrow transplantation (second of two parts). N Engl J Med 1975; 292:895–902.
7. Anderson WF. Prospects for human gene therapy. Science 1984; 226:401–409.
8. Dunbar CE. Gene transfer to hematopoietic stem cells: implications for gene therapy of human disease. Annu Rev Med 1996; 47:11–20.
9. Kohn DB. Gene therapy for haematopoietic and lymphoid disorders. Clin Exp Immunol 1997; 107(suppl 1):54–7.
10. Harrison DE, Astle CM. Population of lymphoid tissues in cured W-anemic mice by donor cells. Transplantation 1976; 22:42–46.
11. Nakano T, Waki N, Asai H, Kitamura Y. Lymphoid differentiation of the hematopoietic stem cell that reconstitutes total erythropoiesis of a genetically anemic W/Wv mouse. Blood 1989; 73:1175–1179.
12. Harrison DE, Astle CM, Lerner C. Number and continuous proliferative pattern of transplanted primitive immunohematopoietic stem cells. Proc Natl Acad Sci USA 1988; 85:822–826.
13. Dzierzak EA, Papayannopoulou T, Mulligan RC. Lineage specific expression of a human b-globin gene in murine bone marrow transplant recipients reconstituted with retrovirus-transduced stem cells. Nature 1988; 331:35–41.
14. Spangrude GJ., Heimfeld S, Weissman IL. Purification and characterization of mouse hematopoietic stem cells. Science 1988; 241:58–62.
15. Micklem HS, Ford CE, Evans EP, Ogden DA, Papworth DS. Competitive in vivo proliferation of foetal and adult

haematopoietic cells in lethally irradiated mice. J Cell Physiol 1972; 79:293–298.
16. Harrison DE. Competitive repopulation: a new assay for long-term stem cell capacity. Blood 1980; 55:77–86.
17. Russell ES. Hereditary anemias of the mouse: a review for geneticists. Advances Genetics 1979; 20:357–459.
18. Boggs DR, Boggs SS, Saxe DF, Gress LA, Canfield DR. Hematopoietic stem cells with high proliferative potential. Assay of their concentration in marrow by the frequency and duration of cure of W/Wv mice. J Clin Invest 1982; 70:242–253.
19. Till JE, McCulloch EA. A direct measurement of the radiation sensitivity of normal mouse bone-marrow cells. Rad Res 1961; 14:213–222.
20. Spangrude GJ, Brooks DM. Phenotypic analysis of mouse hematopoietic stem cells shows a Thy-1-negative subset. Blood 1992; 80:1957–1964.
21. Spangrude GJ, Brooks DM. Mouse strain variability in the expression of the hematopoietic stem cell antigen Ly-6A/E by bone marrow cells. Blood 1993; 82:3327–3332.
22. Orlie D, Fischer R, Nishikawa SI, Nienhuis AW, Bodine DM. Purification and characterization of heterogeneous pluripotent hematopoietic stem cell populations expressing high levels of c-kit receptor. Blood 1993; 82:762–770.
23. Okada S, Nakauchi H, Nagayoshi K, Nishikawa S, Miura Y, Suda T. Enrichment and characterization of murine hematopoietic stem cells that express c-kit molecule. Blood 1991; 78:1706–1712.
24. Okada S, Nakauchi H, Nagayoshi K, Nishikawa S, Miura Y, Suda T. In vivo and in vitro stem cell function of c-kit- and Sca-1-positive murine hematopoietic cells. Blood 1992; 80:3044–3050.
25. Ikuta K, Weissman IL. Evidence that hematopoietic stem cells express mouse c-kit but do not depend on steel factor for their generation. Proc Natl Acad Sci USA 1992; 89:1502–1506.
26. Orlie D, Anderson SA, Bodine DM. Biological properties of subpopulations of pluripotent hematopoietic stem cells enriched by elutriation and flow cytometry. Blood Cells 1994; 20:107–120.
27. Wolf NS, Kone A, Priestley GV, Bartelmez SH. In vivo and in vitro characterization of long-term repopulating primitive hematopoietic cells isolated by sequential Hoechst 33342-rhodamine 123 FACS selection. Exp Hematol 1993; 21:614–622.
28. Visser JVM, Bauman JGJ, Mulder AH, Eliason JF, de Leeux AM. Isolation of murine pluripotent hematopoietic stem cells. J Exp Med 1984; 59:1576–1590.
29. Spangrude GJ, Johnson GR. Resting and activated subsets of mouse multipotent hematopoietic stem cells. Proc Natl Acad Sci USA 1990; 87:7433–7437.
30. Goodell MA, Brose K, Paradis G, Conner AS, Mulligan RC. Isolation and functional properties of murine hematopoietic stem cells that are replicating in vivo. J Exp Med 1996; 183:1797–806.
31. Jones RJ, Collector MI, Barber JP, Vala MS, Fackler MJ, May WS, Griffin CA, Hawkins AL, Zehnbauer BA, Hilton J, Colvin OM, Sharkis SJ. Characterization of mouse lymphohematopoietic stem cells lacking spleen colony-forming activity. Blood 1996; 88:487–491.
32. McGrath ME, Palis J. Expression of homeobox genes, including an insulin promoting factor, in the murine yolk sac at the time of hematopoietic initiation. Mol Reprod Dev 1997; 48:145–153.
33. Silver L, Palis J. Initiation of murine embryonic erythropoiesis: a spatial analysis. Blood 1997; 89:1154–1164.
34. Yoder MC, Hiatt K, Mukherjee P. In vivo repopulating hematopoietic stem cells are present in the murine yolk sac at day 9.0 postcoitus. Proc Natl Acad Sci USA 1997; 94:6776–6780.
35. Yoder MC, Hiatt K, Dutt P, Mukherjee P, Bodine DM, Orlic D. Characterization of definitive lymphohematopoietic stem cells in the day 9 murine yolk sac. Immunity 1997; 7:335–344.
36. Medvinsky A, Dzierzak E. Definitive hematopoiesis is autonomously initiated by the AGM region. Cell 1996; 86:897–906.
37. Matthews W, Jordan CT, Wiegand GW, Pardoll D, Lemischka IR. A receptor tyrosine kinase specific to hematopoietic stem and progenitor cell-enriched populations. Cell 1991; 65:1143–1152.
38. Micklem HS, Anderson N, Ross E. Limited potential of circulating haemopoietic stem cells. Nature 1975; 256:41–43.
39. Bodine DM, Seidel NE, Zsebo KM, Orlic D. In vivo administration of stem cell factor to mice increases the absolute number of pluripotent hematopoietic stem cells. Blood 1993; 82:445–455.
40. Eaves CJ. Peripheral blood stem cells reach new heights. Blood 1993; 82:1957–1959.
41. Bodine DM, Orlie D, Birkett NC, Seidel NE, Zsebo KM. Stem cell factor increases colony-forming unit-spleen number in vitro in synergy with interleukin-6, and in vivo in S 1/S1d mice as a single factor. Blood 1992; 79:913–919.
42. Bodine DM, Seidel NE, Gale MS, Nienhuis AW, Orlie D. Efficient retrovirus transduction of mouse pluripotent hematopoietic stem cells mobilized into the peripheral blood by treatment with granulocyte colony-stimulating factor and stem cell factor. Blood 1994; 84:1482–1491.
43. Bodine DM, Seidel NE, Gale MS, Orlic D. In vivo administration of stem cell factor alone or in combination with granulocyte colony stimulating factor to mice mobilizes pluripotent hematopoietic stem cells into the peripheral blood which can be efficiently transduced by retroviral vectors. In: Stamatoyannopoulos G, ed. Biology of Hematopoiesis and Stem Cell Gene Transfer.
44. Neipp M, Zorina T, Domenick MA, Exner BG, Ildstad ST. Effect of FLT3 ligant and granulocyte colony-stimulating factor on expansion and mobilization of facilitating cells and hematopoietic stem cells in mice: kinetics and repopulating potential. Blood 1998; 92:3177–3188.
45. Molineux G, McCrea C, Yan XQ, Kerzik P, McNiece I. Flt-3 ligand synergizes with granulocyte colony-stimulat-

ing factor to increase neutrophil numbers and to mobilize peripheral blood stem cells with long-term repopulating potential. Blood 1997; 89:3998–4004.
46. Brasel K, McKenna HJ, Charrier K, Morrissey PJ, Williams DE, Lyman SD. Flt3 ligand synergizes with granulocyte-macrophage colony-stimulating factor or granulocyte colony-stimulating factor to mobilize hematopoietic progenitor cells into the peripheral blood of mice. Blood 1997; 90:3781–3788.
47. Neben S, Marcus K, Mauch P. Mobilization of hematopoietic stem and progenitor cell subpopulations from the marrow to the blood of mice following cyclophosphamide and/or granulocyte colony-stimulating factor. Blood 1993; 81:1960–1967.
48. Bodine DM, Seidel NE, Orlie D. Bone marrow collected 14 days after in vivo administration of granulocyte colony-stimulating factor and stem cell factor to mice has 10-fold more repopulating ability than untreated bone marrow. Blood 1996; 88:89–97.
49. Davenport C, Ildstad ST. Bone marrow transplantation: a natural form of gene therapy. Transplant Proc 1998; 30: 3484–3485.
50. Turhan AG, Humphries RK, Phillips GL, Eaves AC, Eaves CJ. Clonal hematopoiesis demonstrated by X-linked DNA polymorphisms after allogeneic bone marrow transplantation. N Engl J Med 1989; 320:1655–1661.
51. Amos TA, Gordon MY. Sources of human hematopoietic stem cells for transplantation-a review. Cell Transplant 1995; 4:547–569.
52. Broxmeyer HE. Questions to be answered regarding umbilical cord blood hematopoietic stem and progenitor cells and their use in-transplantation. Transfusion 1995; 35: 694–702.
53. Russell NH, Gratwohl A, Schmitz N. Developments in allogeneic peripheral blood progenitor cell transplantation. Br J Haematol 1998; 103:594–600.
54. Dexter TM, Lajtha LG. Proliferation of hematopoietic stem cells in vitro. Br J Hematol 1974; 28:25–30.
55. Sutherland HJ, Lansdorp PM, Henkleman DH, et al. Functional characterization of individual human hematopoietic stem cells cultured at limiting dilution on supportive marrow stromal cells. Proc Natl Acad Sci 1990; 87: 3584–3588.
56. Hao QL, Thiemann FT, Petersen D, Smogorzewska EM, Crooks GM. Extended long-term culture reveals a highly quiescent and primitive human hematopoietic progenitor population. Blood 1996; 88:3306–3313.
57. Eaves CJ, Sutherland HJ, Cashman JD, Otsuka T, Lansdorp PM, Humphries RK, Eaves AC, Hogge DE. Regulation of primitive human hematopoietic cells in long-term marrow culture. Semin Hematol 1991; 28:126–131.
58. Johnson A, Dorshkind K. Stromal cells in myeloid and lymphoid long-term bone marrow cultures can support multiple hemopoietic lineages and modulate their production of hemopoietic growth factors. Blood 1986; 68: 1348–1354.
59. Szilvassy SJ, Humpries RK, Lansdorp PM, Eaves AC. Quantitative assay for totipotent reconstituting hematopoietic stem cells by a competitive repopulation strategy. Proc Natl Acad Sci USA 1990; 87:8736–8740.
60. Zanjani ED, Almeida-Porada G, Flake AW. The human/sheep xenograft model: a large animal model of human hematopoiesis. Int J Hematol 1996; 63:179–192.
61. Mosier DE, ed. Humanizing the mouse. Semin Immunol 1996; 8:185–268.
62. Binns R. Bone marrow and lymphoid cell injection of the pig fetus resulting in transplantation tolerance or immunity, and immunoglobulin production. Nature 1969; 214: 179–181.
63. Flake AW, Harrison MR, Adzick NS, Zanjani ED. Transplantation of fetal hematopoietic cells in utero: the creation of hematopoietic chimeras. Science 1986; 233:776–778.
64. Zanjani ED, Pallavicini MG, Ascensao JL, et al. Engraftment and long term expression of human fetal hematopoietic stem cells in sheep following transplantation in utero. J Clin Invest 1992; 89:1178–1188.
65. Zanjani ED, Ascensao JL, Tavassoli M. Liver-derived fetal hemopoietic stem cells selectively and preferentially home to the fetal bone marrow. Blood 1993; 81:399–404.
66. Zanjani ED, Flake AW, Rice HE, Hedrick MH, Tavassoli M. Long term repopulation ability of xenogeneic transplanted human fetal liver hematopoietic stem cells (HSC) in sheep. J Clin Invest 1994; 93:1051–1055.
67. Zanjani ED, Ascensao JL, Harrison MR, Tavassoli M. Ex vivo incubation with growth factors enhances the engraftment of fetal hemopoietic stem cells transplanted in sheep fetuses. Blood 1992; 79:3045–3049.
68. Flake AW, Hendrick MH, Rice HE, Tavassoli M, Zanjani ED. Enhancement of human hematopoiesis by mast cell growth factor in human-sheep chimeras created by the in utero transplantation of human fetal hematopoietic cells. Exp Hematol 1995; 23:252–255.
69. Srour ED, Zanjani ED, Brandt JE, et al. Sustained human hematopoiesis in sheep transplanted in utero during early gestation with fractioned adult human bone marrow cells. Blood 1997; 79:1410–1412.
70. Srour EF, Zanjani ED, Cornetta K, et al. Persistance of human multilineage, self renewing lymphohematopoietic stem cells in chimeric sheep. Blood 1993; 82:3333–3342.
71. Zanjani ED, Srour EF, Hoffman R. Retention of long-term repopulating ability of xenogeneic transplanted purified adult human bone marrow hematopoietic stem cells in sheep. J Lab Clin Med 1995; 126:24–28.
72. Crombleholme TM, Harrison MR, Zanjani ED. In utero transplantation of hematopoietic cells in sheep: the role of T cells in engraftment and graft-vs-host disease. J Pediatr Surg 1990; 25:885–892.
73. Shultz LD. Hematopoiesis and models of immunodeficiency in the mouse. Semin Immunol 1991; 3:397–408.
74. Shultz LD. Immunological mutants of the mouse. Am J Anat 1991; 191:303–113.
75. Dick JE. Normal and leukemic human stem cells assayed in SCID mice. Semin Immunol 1996; 8:197–206.

76. Kamel-Reid S, Dick JE. Engraftment of immune-deficient mice with human hematopoietic stem cells. Science 1988; 242:1706–1709.
77. Nolta JA, Hanley MB, Kohn DB. Sustained human hematopoiesis in immunodeficient mice by cotransplantation of marrow stroma expressing human interleukin-3: analysis of gene transduction of long-lived progenitors. Blood 1994; 83:3041–3051.
78. Nolta JA, Dao M, Wells S, Smogorzewska E, Kohn D. Transduction of pluripotent human hematopoietic stem cells demonstrated by clonal analysis after engraftment in immune deficient mice. Proc Natl Acad Sci USA 1996; 93:2414–2419.
79. Triglia T, Peterson MG, Kemp DJ. A procedure for in vitro amplification of DNA segments that lie outside the boundries of known sequences. Nucl Acid Res 1988; 16: 8186.
80. Blunt T, Finnie NJ, Taccioli GE, Smith GCM, Demengeot J, Gottlieb TM, Mizuta R, Varghese AJ, Alt FW, Jeggo PA, Jackson SP. Defective DNA-dependent protein kinase activity is linked to V(D)J recombination and DNA repair defects associated with the murine scid mutation. Cell 1995; 80:813–823.
81. Lapidot T, Pflumino F, Doedens M, Murdoch B, Williams DE, Dick JE. Cytokine stimulation of multilineage hematopoiesis from immature human cells engrafted in scid mice. Science 1992; 255:1137–1141.
82. Bock TA, Orlic D, Dunbar CE, Broxmeyer HE, Bodine DM. Improved engraftment of human hematopoietic cells in severe combined immunodeficient (SCID) mice carrying human cytokine transgenes. J Exp Med 1995; 182: 2037–2043.
83. Shultz LD, Schweitzer PA, Christianson SW, Gott B, Schweitzer IB, Tennent B, McKenna S, Mobraaten L, Rajan TV, Greiner DL, Leiter EH. Multiple defects in inate and adaptive immunological function in NOD/LtSz-scid mice. J Immunol 1995; 154:180–191.
84. Namikawa R, Weilbaecher KN, Kaneshima H, Yee EJ, McCune JM. Long-term human hematopoiesis in the SCID-hu mouse. J Exp Med 1990; 172:1055–1063.
85. Krowka J, Sarin S, Namikawa R, McCune JM, Kaneshima H. The human T cells of the SCID-hu mouse are phenotypically normal and functionally competent. J Immunol 1991; 145:3751–3756.
86. Fraser C, Kaneshima H, Hansteen G, Kilpatrick M, Hoffman R, Chen BP. Human allogeneic stem cell maintenance and differentiation in a long-term multilineage SCID-hu graft. Blood 1995; 86:1680–1693.
87. Baum CM, Weissman IL, Tsukamoto AS, Buckle AM, Peault B. Isolation of a candidate human hematopoietic stem-cell population. Proc Natl Acad Sci USA 1992; 89: 2804–2808.
88. Terstappen LW, Huang S, Safford M, Lansdorp PM, Loken MR. Sequential generations of hematopoietic colonies derived from single nonlineage-committed CD34+CS38- progenitor cells. Blood 1991; 77: 1218–1227.
89. Kyoizumi S, Baum C, Kaneshima H, McCune JM, Yee EJ, Namikawa R. Implantation and maintenance of functional human bone marrow into SCID-hu mice. Blood 1992; 79: 1704–1711.
90. Vormoor J, Lapidot T, Pflumio F, Risdon G, Patterson B, Broxmeyer HE, Dick JE. Immature human cord blood progenitors engraft and proliferate to high levels in immune-deficient SCID mice. Blood 1994; 83:2489–2497.
91. Sutherland DR, Yeo EL, Stewart K, et al. Identification of CD34+ subsets following glycoprotease selection: engraftment of CD34+/Thyl+/Lin stem cells in fetal sheep. Exp Hematol 1996; 24:795–806.
92. Kawashima I, Zanjani FD, Alamaida-Porada G, Flake AW, Zeng H, Ogawa M. CD34+ human marrow cells that express low levels of Kit protein are enriched for long-term marrow engrafting cells. Blood 1996; 87:4136–4142.
93. Goodell MA, Rosenzweig M, Kim H, Marks DF, DeMaria M, Paradis G, Grupp SA, Sieff CA, Mulligan RC, Johnson RP. Dye efflux studies suggest that hematopoietic stem cells expressing low or undetectable levels of CD34 antigen exist in multiple species. Nat Med 1997; 3:1337–1345.
94. Zanjani ED, Almeida-Porada G, Livingston AG, Flake AW, Ogawa M. Human bone marrow CD34- cells engraft in vivo and undergo multilineage expression that includes giving rise to CD34+ cells. Exp Hematol 1998; 26: 353–360.
95. Bhatia M, Bonnet D, Murdoch B, Gan OI, Dick JE. A newly discovered class of human hematopoietic cells with SCID-repopulating activity. Nat Med 1998; 4:1038–1045.
96. Ponnazhagan S, Yoder MC, Srivastava A. Adeno-associated virus type 2-mediated transduction of murine hematopoietic cells with long-term repopulating ability and sustained expression of a human globin gene in vivo. J Virol 1997; 71:3098–3104.
97. Goodman S, Xiao X, Donahue RE, Moulton A, Miller J, Walsh C, Young NS, Samulski RJ, Nienhuis AW. Recombinant adeno-associated virus-mediated gene transfer into hematopoietic progenitor cells. Blood 1994; 94: 1492–1500.
98. Miller JL, Donahue RE, Sellers SE, Samulski RJ, Young NS, Nienhuis AW. Recombinant adeno-associated virus (rAAV)-mediated expression of a human gamma-globin gene in human progenitor-derived erythroid cells. Proc Natl Acad Sci USA 1994; 91:10183–10187.
99. Nienhuis AW, Bertran J, Hargrove P, Vanin E, Yang Y. Gene transfer into hematopoietic cells. Stem Cells 1997; (suppl 1):123–134.
100. Kohn DB, Hershfield MS, Carbonaro D, Shigeoka A, Brooks J, Smogorzewska EM, Barsky LW, Chan R, Burotto F, Annett G, Nolta JA, Crooks G, Kapoor N, Elder M, Wara D, Bowen T, Madsen E, Snyder FF, Bastian J, Muul L, Blaese RM, Weinberg K, Parkman R. T lymphocytes with a normal ADA gene accumulate after transplantation of transduced autologous umbilical cord blood CD34+ cells in ADA- deficient SCID neonates. Nat Med 1998; 4:775–780.

101. Aronow BJ, Silbiger RN, Dusing MR, Stock JL, Yager KL, Potter SS, Hutton JI, Wiginton DA. Functional analysis of the human adenosine deaminase gene thymic regulatory region and its ability to generate position-independent transgene expression. Mol Cell Biol 1992; 12:4170–4185.
102. Puck JM. Molecular and genetic basis of X-linked immunodeficiency disorders. J Clin Immunol 1994; 14:81–89.
103. Orlic D, Girard LJ, Lee D, Anderson SM, Puck JM, Bodine DM. Interleukin-7R alpha mRNA expression increases as stem cells differentiate into T and B lymphocyte progenitors. Exp Hematol 1997; 35:217–222.
104. Nienhuis AW, Walsh CE, Liu J. Viruses as therapeutic gene transfer vectors. In Viruses and Bone Marrow New York: Marcel Dekker, 1993:353–414.
105. Mulligan RC. The basic science of gene therapy. Science 1993; 260:926–932.
106. Varmus HE. Form and function of retroviral proviruses. Science 1982; 216:812–820.
107. Varmus H. Retroviruses. Science 1988; 240:1427–1435.
108. Miller AD. Retroviral vectors. Curr Top Microbiol Immunol 1992; 158:1–24.
109. Hunter E, and Swanstrom R. Retrovirus envelope glycoproteins. Curr Top Microbiol Immunol 1990; 157: 187–253.
110. Miller AD. Cell-surface receptors for retroviruses and implications for gene transfer. Proc Natl Acad Sci USA 1996; 93:11407–11413.
111. Albritton LM, Tseng L, Scadden D, Cunningham JM. A putative murine ecotropic retrovirus receptor gene encodes a multiple membrane-spanning protein and confers susceptibility to virus infection. Cell 1989; 57:659–666.
112. Kim JW, Closs EI, Albritton LM, Cunningham JM. Transport of cationic amino acids by the mouse ecotropic retrovirus receptor. Nature 1991; 352:725–728.
113. Albritton LM, Kim JW, Tseng L, Cunningham JM. Envelope-binding domain in the cationic amino acid transporter determines the host range of ecotropic murine retroviruses. J Virol 1993; 67:2091–2096.
114. Davey RA, Hamson CA, Healey JJ, Cunningham JM. In vitro binding of purified murine ectropic retrovirus envelope surface protein to its receptor, MCAT-1. J Virol 1997; 71:8096–8102.
115. Fass D, Davey RA, Hamson CA, Kim PS, Cunningham JM, Berger JM. Structure of a murine leukemia virus receptor-binding glycoprotein at 2.0 angstrom resolution. Science 1997; 277:1662–1666.
116. Miller DG, Edwards RH, Miller AD. Cloning of the cellular receptor for amphotropic murine retroviruses reveals homology to that for gibbon ape leukemia virus. Proc Natl Acad Sci USA 1994; 91:78–82.
117. van Zeijl M, Johann SV, Closs E, Cunningham J, Eddy R, Shows TB, O'Hara B. A human amphotropic retrovirus receptor is a second member of the gibbon ape leukemia virus receptor family. Proc Natl Acad Sci USA 1994; 92: 1168–1172.
118. Kavannaugh MP, Miller DG, Zhang W, Law W, Kozak SL, Kabat D, Miller AD. Cell-surface receptors for gibbon ape leukemia virus and amphotropic murine retrovirus are inducible sodium-dependent phosphate symporters. Proc Natl Acad Sci USA 1994; 91:7071–7075.
119. O'Hara B, Johann SV, Klinger HP, Blair DG, Rubinson H, Dunn KJ, Sass P, Vitek SM, Robins T. Characterization of a human gene conferring sensitivity to infection by gibbon ape leukemia virus. Cell Growth Differ 1990; 1: 119–127.
120. Johann SV, Gibbons JJ, O'Hara B. GLVR1, a receptor for gibbon ape leukemia virus, is homologous to a phosphate permease of Neurospora crassa and is expressed at high levels in the brain and thymus. J Virol 1992; 66: 1635–1640.
121. Miller AD, Garcia JV, von Suhr N, Lynch CM, Wilson C, Eiden MV. Construction and properties of retrovirus packaging cells based on gibbon ape leukemia virus. J Virol 1991; 65:2220–2224.
122. Bunnell BA, Metzger M, Byrne E, Morgan RA, Donahue RE. Efficient in vivo marking of primary CD4+ T lymphocytes in nonhuman primates using a gibbon ape leukemia virus-derived retroviral vector. Blood 1997; 89: 1987–1995.
123. Bunnell BA, Muul LM, Donahue RE, Blaese RM, Morgan RA. High-efficiency retroviral-mediated gene transfer into human and nonhuman primate peripheral blood lymphocytes. Proc Natl Acad Sci USA 1995; 92:7739–7743.
124. Miller AD, Chen F. Retrovirus packaging cells based on 10A1 murine leukemia virus for production of vectors that use multiple receptors for cell entry. J Virol 1996; 70: 5564–5571.
125. Burns JC, Friedmann T, Driever W, Burrascano M, Yee JK. Vesicular stomatitis virus G glycoprotein pseudotyped retroviral vectors: concentration to very high titer and efficient gene transfer into mammalian and nonmammalian cells. Proc Natl Acad Sci USA 1993; 90:8033–8037.
126. Yee JK, Miyanohara A, LaPorte P, Bouic K, Burns JC, Friedmann T. A general method for the generation of high-titer, pantropic retroviral vectors: highly efficient infection of primary hepatocytes. Proc Natl Acad Sci USA 1994; 91:9564–9568.
127. Schlegel R, Tralka TS, Willingham MC, Pastan I. Inhibition of VSV binding and infectivity by phosphatidylserine: is phosphatidylserine a VSV-binding site? Cell 1983; 32: 639–646.
128. Yang Y, Vanin EF, Whitt MA, Fornerod M, Zwart R, Schneiderman RD, Grosveld G, Neinhuis AW. Inducible, high-level production of infectious murine leukemia retroviral vector particles pseudotyped with vesicular stomatitis virus G envelope protein. Hum Gene Ther 1995; 6: 1203–1213.
129. Ory DS, Neugeboren BA, Mulligan RC. A stable human-derived packaging cell line for production of high titer retrovirus/vesicular stomatitis virus G pseudotypes. Proc Natl Acad Sci USA 1996; 93:11400–11406.
130. Chen ST, Iida A, Guo L, Friedmann T, Yee JK. Generation of packaging cell lines for pseudotyped retroviral vectors

of the G protein of vesicular stomatitis virus by using a modified tetracycline inducible system. Proc Natl Acad Sci USA 1996; 93:10057–10062.
131. Williams DA. Expression of introduced genetic sequences in hematopoietic cells following retroviral mediated gene transfer. Hum Gene Ther 1990; 1:229–239.
132. Sorrentino BP, McDonagh KT, Woods D, Orlic D. Expression of retroviral vectors containing the human multidrug resistance 1 cDNA in hematopoietic cells of transplanted mice. Blood 1995; 86:491–501.
133. Beck-Engeser G, Stocking C, Just U, Albritton L, Dexter M, Spooncer E, Ostertag W. Retroviral vectors related to the myeloproliferative sarcoma virus allow efficient expression in hematopoietic stem and precursor cell lines, but retroviral infection is reduced in more primitive cells. Hum Gene Ther 1991; 2:61–70.
134. Pawliuk R, Eaves CJ, Humphries RK. Sustained high-level reconstitution of the hematopoietic system by preselected hematopoietic cells expressing a transduced cell-surface antigen. Hum Gene Ther 1997; 8:1595–1604.
135. Onodera M, Nelson DM, Yachie A, Jagadeesh GJ, Bunnell BA, Morgan RA, Blaese RM. Development of improved adenosine deaminase retroviral vectors. J Virol 1998; 72: 1769–1774.
136. Chalita PM, Kohn DB. Lack of expression from a retroviral vector after transduction of murine hematopoietic stem cells is associated with methylation in vivo. Proc Natl Acad Sci USA 1994; 91:2567–2571.
137. Chalita PM, Skelton D, el-Khoueiry A, Yu XJ, Weinberg K, Kohn DB. Multiple modifications in cis elements of the long terminal repeat of retroviral vectors lead to increased expression and decreased DNA methylation in embryonic carcinoma cells. J Virol 1995; 69:748–755.
138. Robbins PB, Yu XJ, Skelton DM, Pepper KA, Wasserman RM, Zhu L, Kohn DB. Increased probability of expression from modified retroviral vectors in embryonal stem cells and embryonal carcinoma cells. J Virol 1997; 71: 9466–9474.
139. Cheng L, Du C, Lavau C, Chen S, Tong I, Chen BP, Scollay R, Hawley RG, Hill B. Sustained gene expression in retrovirally transduced, engrafting human hematopoietic stem cells and their lympho-myeloid progeny. Blood 1998; 92:83–92.
140. Harrison DE, Lerner CP. Most primitive hematopoietic stem cells are stimulated to cycle rapidly after treatment with 5-fluorouracil. Blood 1991; 78:1237–1240.
141. Reddy GP, Tiarks CY, Pang L, Wuu J, Hsieh CC, Quesenberry PJ. Cell cycle analysis and synchronization of pluripotent hematopoietic progenitor stem cells. Blood 1997; 90:2293–2299.
142. Habibian HK, Peters SO, Hsieh CC, Wuu J, Vergilis K, Grimaldi CI, Reilly J, Carlson JE, Frimberger AE, Stewart FM, Quesenberry PJ. The fluctuating phenotype of the lymphohematopoietic stem cell with cell cycle transit. J Exp Med 1998; 188:393–398.
143. Lewis P, Hensel M, Emerman M. Human immunodeficiency virus infection of cells arrested in the cell cycle. EMBO J 1992; 11:3053–3058.
144. Bukrinsky MI, Haggerty S, Dempsey MP, Sharova N, Adzhubel A, Spitz L, Lewis P, Goldfarb D, Emerman M, Stevenson M. A nuclear localization signal within HIV-1 matrix protein that governs infection of non-dividing cells. Nature 1993; 365:666–669.
145. Gallay P, Swingler S, Song J, Bushman F, Trono D. HIV nuclear import is governed by the phosphotyrosine-mediated binding of matrix to the core domain of integrase. Cell 1995; 83:569–576.
146. Naldini L, Blomer U, Gallay P, Ory D, Mulligan R, Gage FH, Verma IM, Trono D. In vivo gene delivery and stable transduction of nondividing cells by a lentiviral vector. Science 1996; 272:263–267.
147. Poeschla E, Gilbert J, Li X, Huang S, Ho A, Wong-Staal F. Identification of a human immunodeficiency virus type 2 (HIV-2) encapsidation determinant and transduction of nondividing human cells by HIV-2-based lentivirus vectors. J Virol 1998; 72:6527–6536.
148. Poeschla EM, Wong-Staal F, Looney DJ. Efficient transduction of nondividing human cells by feline immunodeficiency virus lentiviral vectors. Nat Med 1998; 4:354–357.
149. Sutton RE, Wu HT, Rigg R, Bohnlein E, Brown PO. Human immunodeficiency virus type 1 vectors efficiently transduce human hematopoietic stem cells. J Virol 1998; 72:5781–5788.
150. Williams DA, Lemischka IR, Nathan DG, Mulligan RC. Introduction of new genetic material into pluripotent haematopoietic stem cells of the mouse. Nature 1984; 310: 476–480.
151. Dick JE, Magli MC, Huszar D, Phillips RA, Bernstein A. Introduction of a selectable gene into primitive stem cells capable of reconstitution of the hemopoietic system of W/Wv mice. Cell 1985; 42:71–79.
152. Eglitis MA, Kantoff P, Gilboa E, Anderson WF. Gene expression in mice after high efficiency retroviral-mediated gene transfer. Science 1985; 230:1395–1398.
153. Lemischka IR, Raulet DH, Mulligan RC. Developmental potential and dynamic behavior of hematopoietic stem cells. Cell 1986; 45:917–927.
154. Jordan CT, Lemischka IR. Clonal and systemic analysis of long-term hematopoiesis in the mouse. Genes Dev 1990; 4:220–232.
155. Bodine DM, Karlsson S, Nienhuis AW. Combination of interleukins 3 and 6 preserves stem cell function in culture and enhances retrovirus-mediated gene transfer into hematopoietic stem cells. Proc Natl Acad Sci USA 1989; 86: 8897–8901.
156. Bodine DM, McDonagh KT, Seidel NE, Nienhuis AW. Survival and retrovirus infection of murine hematopoietic stem cells in vitro: Effects of 5-FU and method of infection. Exp Hematol 1991; 19:206–212.
157. Hodgson GS, Bradley TR. Properties of haematopoietic stem cells surviving 5-fluorouracil treatment: evidence for a pre CFU-S cell? Nature 1979; 281:381–382.
158. Bodine DM, Crozier PS, Clark SC. Effects of hematopoietic growth factors on the survival of primitive stem cells in liquid suspension culture. Blood 1991; 78:914–920.

159. Lusky BD, Rosenblatt M, Zsebo K, Williams DA. Stem cell factor, interleukin-3, and interleukin-6 promote retroviral-mediated gene transfer into murine hematopoietic stem cells. Blood 1992; 80:396–402.
160. Petzer AL, Zandstra PW, Piret JM, Eaves CJ. Differential cytokine effects on primitive (CD34+CD38−) human hematopoietic cells: novel responses to Flt3-ligand and thrombopoietin. J Exp Med 1996; 183:2551–2558.
161. Conneally E, Eaves CJ, Humphries RK. Efficient retroviral-mediated gene transfer to human cord blood stem cells with in vivo repopulating potential. Blood 1998; 91: 3487–3493.
162. Lim B, Apperly JF, Orkin SH, Williams DA. Long-term expression of human adenosine deaminase in mice transplanted with retrovirus infected hematopoietic stem cells. Proc Natl Acad Sci USA 1989; 86:8892–8896.
163. Belmont JW, MacGregor GR, Wagner-Smith K, Fletcher FA, Moore KA, Hawkins D, Villalon D, Chang SMW, Caskey CT. Expression of adenosine deaminase in murine hematopoietic cells. Mol Cell Biol 1988; 8:5116–5125.
164. Wilson JM, Danos O, Grossman M, Raulet DH, Mulligan RC. Expression of human adenosine deaminase in mice reconstituted with retrovirus-transduced hematopoietic stem cells. Proc Natl Acad Sci USA 1990; 87:439–443.
165. Correll PH, Kew Y, Perry LK, Brady RO, Fink JK, Karlsson S. Expression of human glucocerbrosidase in long-term reconstituted mice following retroviral-mediated gene transfer into hematopoietic stem cells. Hum Gene Ther 1990; 1:277–283.
166. Bender MA, Miller AD, Gelinas RE. Expression of the human b-globin gene after retroviral transfer into murine erythroleukemia cells and human BFU-E cells. Mol Cell Biol 1988; 8:1725–1735.
167. Wolfe JH, Sands MS, Barker JE, Gwynn B, Rowe LB, Vogler CA, Birkenmeier EH. Reversal of pathology in murine mucopolysaccharidosis type VII by somatic cell gene transfer. Nature 1992; 360:749–753.
168. Bjorgvinsdottir H, Ding C, Pech N, Gifford MA, Li LL, Dinauer MC. Retroviral-mediated gene transfer of gp91phox into bone marrow cells rescues defect in host defense against *Aspergillus fumigatus* in murine X-linked chronic granulomatous disease. Blood 1997; 89:41–48.
169. Mardiney M 3rd, Jackson SH, Spratt SK, Li F, Holland SM, Malech HL. Enhanced host defense after gene transfer in the murine p47 phoxdeficient model of chronic granulomatous disease. Blood 1997; 89:2268–2275.
170. Bunting KD, Sangster MY, Ihle JN, Sorrentino BP. Restoration of lymphocyte function in Janus kinase 3-deficient mice by retroviral-mediated gene transfer. Nat Med 1998; 4:58–64.
171. Bodine DM, McDonagh KT, Brandt SI, Ney PA, Agricola B, Byrne E, Nienhuis AW. Development of a high-titer retrovirus producer cell line capable of gene transfer into rhesus monkey hematopoietic stem cells. Proc Natl Acad Sci USA 87:3738–3742.
172. van Beusechem VW, Kukler A, Heidt PJ, Valerio D. Long-term expression of human adenosine deaminase in rhesus monkeys transplanted with retrovirus-infected bone marrow cells. Proc Natl Acad Sci USA 1992; 89:7640–7646.
173. Donahue RE, Kessler SW, Bodine D, McDonagh K, Dunbar C, Goodman S, Agricola B, Byrne E, Raffeld M, Moen R, Bacher J, Zsebo KM, Nienhuis AW. Helper virus induced T-cell lymphoma in nonhuman primates after retroviral mediated gene transfer. J Exp Med 1992; 176: 1125–1135.
174. Sykes M, Sachs DH, Nienhuis AW, Pearson DA, Moulton AD, Bodine DM. Specific prolongation of skin graft survival following retroviral transduction of bone marrow with an allogeneic major histocompatibility complex gene. Transplantation 1993; 55:197–202.
175. Moritz T, Dutt P, Xiao X, Carstanjen D, Vik T, Hanenberg H, Williams DA. Fibronectin improves transduction of reconstitution hematopoietic stem cells by retroviral vectors: evidence of direct viral binding to chymotryptic carboxy-terminal fragments. Blood 1996; 88:855–862.
176. Bodine DM, Moritz T, Donahue RE, Luskey B, Kessler S, Martin DIK, Orkin SH, Neinhuis AW, Williams DA. Long-term in vivo expression of a murine adenosine deaminase gene in Rhesus monkey hematopoietic cells of multiple lineages after retroviral mediated gene transfer into CD34+ bone marrow cells. Blood 1993; 82:1975–1980.
177. Sellers S, Tisdale JF, Bodine DM, Williams DA, Karlsson S, Meztger M, Donahue RE, Dunbar CE. No discrepancy between in vivo gene marking efficiency assessed in peripheral blood populations compared to bone marrow progenitors or CD34+ cells. Hum Gene Ther. In press.
178. Schuening FG, Kawahara K, Miller AD, To R, Goehle S, Steward D, Mullally K, Fisher L, Graham TC, Appelbaum FR, et al. Retrovirus-mediated gene transduction into long-term repopulating marrow cells of dogs. Blood 1991; 78: 2568–2576.
179. Schuening FG, Storb R, Stead RB, Goehle S, Nash R, Miller AD. Improved retroviral transfer of genes into canine hematopoietic progenitor cells kept in long term marrow culture. Blood 1989; 74:152–155.
180. Carter RF, Abrams-Ogg ACG, Dick JE, Kruth SA, Valli VE, Kamel-Reid S, Dube ID. Autologous transplantation of canine long-term marrow culture cells genetically marked by retroviral vectors. Blood 1992; 79:356–362.
181. Kiem HP, Darovsky B, Von Kalle C, Goehle S, Graham T, Miller AD, Storb R, Schuening FG. Long-term persistence of canine hematopoietic cells genetically marked by retrovirus vectors. Hum Gene Ther 1996; 7:89–96.
182. Brenner MK, et al. Gene marking to determine whether autologous marrow infusion restores long-term haemopoiesis in cancer patients. Lancet 1993; 342:1134–1137.
183. Dunbar CE, Cottler-Fox M, O'Shaughnessy JA, Doren S, Carter C, Berenson R, Brown S, Moen RC, Greenblatt J, Stewart FM, et al. Retrovirally marked CD34-enriched peripheral blood and bone marrow cells contribute to long-term engraftment after autologous transplantation. Blood 1995; 85:3048–3057.
184. Kohn DB, Weinberg KI, Nolta JA, Heiss LN, Lenarsky C, Crooks GM, Hanley ME, Annett G, Brooks JS, el-

Khoureiy A, et al. Engraftment of gene-modified umbilical cord blood cells in neonates with adenosine deaminase deficiency. Nat Med 1995; 1:1017–1023.

185. Malech HL, Maples PB, Whiting-Theobald N, Linton GF, Sekhsaria S, Vowells SJ, Li F, Miller JA, DeCarlo E, Holland SM, Leitman SF, Carter CS, Butz RE, Read EJ, Fleisher TA, Schneiderman RD, Van Epps DE, Spratt SK, Maack CA, Rokovich JA, Cohen LK, Gallin JI. Prolonged production of NADPH oxidase-corrected granulocytes after gene therapy of chronic granulomatous disease. Proc Natl Acad Sci USA 1997; 94:12133–12138.
186. Bordignon C, Notarangelo LD, Nobili N, Ferrari G, Casorati G, Panina P, Mazzolari E, Maggioni D, Rossi C, Servida P, et al. Gene therapy in peripheral blood lymphocytes and bone marrow for ADA-immunodeficient patients. Science 1995; 270:470–45.
187. Chuck AS, Clarke MF, Palsson BO. Retroviral infection is limited by Brownian motion. Hum Gene Ther 1996; 7: 1527–1534.
188. Bahnson AB, Dunigan JT, Baysal BE, Mohney T, Atchison RW, Nimgaonkar MT, Ball ED, Barranger JA. Centrifugal enhancement of retroviral mediated gene transfer. J Virol Methods 1995; 54:131–143.
189. Chuck AS, Palsson BO. Consistent and high rates of gene transfer can be obtained using flow-through transduction over a wide range of retroviral titers. Hum Gene Ther 1996; 7:743–750.
190. Hutchings M, Moriwaki K, Dilloo D, Hoffmann T, Kimbrough S, Johnsen HE, Brenner MK, Heslop HE. Increased transduction efficiency of primary hematopoietic cells by physical colocalization of retrovirus and target cells. J Hematother 1998; 7:217–224.
191. Hanenberg H, Xiao XL, Dilloo D, Hashino K, Kato I, Williams DA. Colocalization of retrovirus and target cells on specific fibronectin fragments increases genetic transduction of mammalian cells. Nat Med 1996; 2:876–882.
192. Sorrentino BP, Brandt SJ, Bodine D, Gottesman M, Pastan I, Cline A, Nienhuis AW. Selection of drug-resistant bone marrow cells in vivo after retroviral transfer of human MDR1. Science 1992; 257:99–103.
193. Podda S, Ward M, Himelstein A, Richardson C, de la Flor-Weiss E, Smith L, Gottesman M, Pastan I, and Bank A. Transfer and expression of the human multiple drug resistance gene into live mice. Proc Natl Acad Sci USA 1992; 89:9676–9680.
194. Rahman Z, Kavanagh J, Champlin R, Giles R, Hanania E, Fu S, Zu Z, Mehra R, Holmes F, Kudelka A, Claxton D, Verschraegen C, Gajewski J, Andreef M, Heimfeld S, Berenson R, Ellerson D, Calvert L, Mechetner E, Holzmayer T, Dayne A, Hamer J, Bachier C, Ostrove J, Deisseroth A, et al. Chemotherapy immediately following autologous stem-cell transplantation in patients with advanced breast cancer. Clin Cancer Res 1998; 4:2717–2721.
195. Hesdorffer C, Ayello J, Ward M, Kaubisch A, Vahdat L, Balmaceda C, Garrett T, Fetell M, Reiss R, Bank A, Antman K. Phase I trial of retroviral-mediated transfer of the human MDR 1 gene as marrow chemoprotection in patients undergoing high-dose chemotherapy and autologous stem-cell transplantation. J Clin Oncol 1998; 16:165–172.
196. Uchida N, Combs J, Chen S, Zanjani E, Hoffman R, Tsukamoto A. Primitive human hematopoietic cells displaying differential efflux of the rhodamine 123 dye have distinct biological activities. Blood 1996; 88:1297–1305.
197. Bunting KD, Galipeau J, Topham D, Benaim E, Sorrentino BP. Transduction of murine bone marrow cells with an MDR1 vector enables ex vivo stem cell expansion, but these expanded grafts cause a myeloproliferative syndrome in transplanted mice. Blood 1998; 92:2269–2279.
198. Corey CA, DeSilva AD, Holland CA, Williams DA. Serial transplantation of methotrexate-resistant bone marrow; protection of murine recipients from drug toxicity by progeny of transduced stem cells. Blood 75:337–343.
199. Allay JA, Persons DA, Galipeau J, Riberdy JM, Ashmun RA, Blakley RL, Sorrentino BP. In vivo selection of retrovirally transduced hematopoietic stem cells. Nat Med 1998; 4:1136–1143.
200. Osborne WR, Hock RA, Kaleko M, Miller AD. Long-term expression of human adenosine deaminase in mice after transplantation of bone marrow infected with amphotropic retroviral vectors. Hum Gene Ther 1990; 1:31–41.
201. Orlic D, Girard LJ, Jordan CT, Anderson SM, Cline AP, Bodine DM. The level of mRNA encoding the amphotropic retrovirus receptor in mouse and human hematopoietic stem cells is low and correlates with the efficiency of retrovirus transduction. Proc Natl Acad Sci USA 1996; 93:11097–11102.
202. Orlic D, Girard LJ, Anderson SM, Pyle LC, Yoder MC, Broxmeyer HE, Bodine DM, Identification of human and mouse hematopoietic stem cell populations expressing high levels of mRNA encoding retrovirus receptors. Blood 1998; 91:3247–3254.
203. Dunbar CE, Seidel NE, Doren S, Sellers S, Cline AP, Metzger ME, Agricola BA, Donahue RE, Bodine DM. Improved retroviral gene transfer into murine and rhesus peripheral blood or bone marrow repopulating cells primed in vivo with stem cell factor and granulocyte colony-stimulating factor. Proc Natl Acad Sci USA 1996; 93: 11871–11876.
204. Kiem HP, Andrews RG, Morris J, Peterson L, Heyward S, Allen JM, Rasko JE, Potter J, Miller AD. Improved gene transfer into baboon marrow repopulating cells using recombinant human fibronectin fragment CH-296 in combination with interleukin-6, stem cell factor, FLT-3 ligand, and megakaryocyte growth and development factor. Blood 1998; 92:1878–1886.
205. Tisdale JF, Hanazono Y, Sellers SE, Agricola BA, Metzger ME, Donahue RE, Dunbar CE. Ex vivo expansion of genetically marked rhesus peripheral blood progenitor cells results in diminished long-term repopulating ability. Blood 1998; 92:1131–1141.
206. Whitwam T, Haskins ME, Henthorn PS, Kraszewski JN, Kleiman SE, Seidel NE, Bodine DM, Puck JM. Retroviral

marking of canine bone marrow: long-term, high-level expression of human interleukin-2 receptor common gamma chain in canine lymphocytes. Blood 1998; 92: 1565–1575.

207. Dao MA, Taylor N, Nolta JA. Reduction in levels of the cyclin-dependent kinase inhibitor p27(kip-1) coupled with transforming growth factor beta neutralization induces cell-cycle entry and increases retroviral transduction of primitive human hematopoietic cells. Proc Natl Acad Sci USA 1998; 95:13006–13011.

208. Uchida N, Sutton RE, Friera AM, He D, Reitsma MJ, Chang WC, Veres G, Scollay R, Weissman IL. HIV, but not murine leukemia virus, vectors mediate high efficiency gene tranfer into freshly isolated G0/G1 human hematopoietic stem cells. Proc Natl Acad Sci USA 1998; 95: 11939–11944.

20

Gene Therapy for Hematopoietic Disorders

Mitchell E. Horwitz and Harry L. Malech
National Institute of Allergy and Infectious Diseases, National Institutes of Health, Bethesda, Maryland

I. INTRODUCTION

Clinical gene transfer to hematopoietic cells began on May 22, 1989, when autologous T lymphocytes of a cancer patient were gene marked and transplanted back into the patient (1). Gene-marking studies such as this have played an important role in the evolution of the field. Since 1989, over 150 patients have been enrolled in hematopoietic cell gene-marking or gene-therapy protocols. This chapter will review the practical issues involved in the conduct of a clinical gene-therapy trial, as well as the published trials to date.

There are two general strategies for clinical gene-transfer protocols for hematopoietic cells. The first strategy is to target the pleuripotential hematopoietic stem cell (HSC), which results in permanent gene transfer to all three hematopoietic cell lineages. Clinical HSC trials to date have involved transfer of both marker genes as well as therapeutic genes. The second strategy involves gene transfer into a single, terminally differentiated hematopoietic cell lineage. With this strategy, persistence of gene-corrected cells is dependent on the life span of the target cell. At present, this approach has been applied clinically only to lymphocytes.

Three broad categories of genes have been used in clinical trials: marker genes, suicide genes, and therapeutic genes. Marker genes provide a mechanism for detection of the transduced cells by introducing a gene product easily detectable by flow cytometry, by enzymatic activity, or by conferring a resistance phenotype. Antibiotic resistance genes such as the bacterial neomycin phosphotransferase gene are most commonly used as markers. Suicide genes allow for in vivo elimination of transduced cells. The herpes thymidine kinase, for example, confers sensitivity of the transduced cell to the drug gancyclovir. Of course, the ultimate goal of most gene-therapy studies is to transfer a therapeutic gene into the target cell. Table 1 summarizes the published clinical gene-transfer trials involving hematopoietic cells.

II. GENE TRANSFER VECTORS

A. Murine-Based Retroviral Vectors

All clinical gene-therapy trials to date targeting hematopoietic cells have utilized murine-based retroviral vectors from the oncovirinae subfamily. The simplicity of the murine retroviral genome has facilitated the development of a class of replication-incompetent vectors which can be produced by specially engineered producer cell lines (see Chapter 1). However, murine retroviral vectors can efficiently transfer genes only to actively replicating target cells (2). Relatively quiescent target cells such as HSCs, which reside predominantly in the G_0/G_1 phase of the cell cycle, are inefficiently transduced by murine retroviruses.

Most retroviral vectors that have been used clinically for hematopoietic gene transfer are based on the oncovirus called Moloney murine leukemia virus (MoMLV) (3). Some clinical vectors are derived from the Harvey Murine sarcoma virus (HaMSV), and more recently vectors derived from the murine stem cell virus (MSCV) have been employed in clinical trials. HaMSV and MSCV are similar to MoMLV in overall structure and function, as are the modifications incorporated to make them replication incompetent and safe to use in humans. The HaMSV and

Table 1 Published Clinical Trials of Hematopoietic Cell Gene Transfer

Transgene	Vector	Target cell	Ref.
Neomycin resistance[a]	Retroviral	Hematopoietic stem cell	36, 61, 62, 64, 67, 114
p47^{phox} (chronic granulomatous disease)	Retroviral	Hematopoietic stem cell	60
Adenosine deaminase (severe combined immunodeficiency)	Retroviral	Hematopoietic stem cell	37, 93, 95, 96
Multidrug resistance 1	Retroviral	Hematopoietic stem cell	87
Glucocerebrosidase (Gaucher's disease)	Retroviral	Hematopoietic stem cell	41
Neomycin resistance[a]	Retroviral	Lymphocyte	1, 109, 110
Adenosine deaminase (severe combined immunodeficiency)	Retroviral	Lymphocyte	56, 93, 111
Herpes simplex virus-thymidine kinase[b]	Retroviral	Lymphocyte	112, 113
Transdominant Rev protein (AIDS)	Retroviral	Lymphocyte	115

[a] Marker gene studies.
[b] Suicide gene studies.

MSCV long terminal repeats (LTRs) may function better in hematopoietic stem cells and may be less subject to silencing, but this has not been proven in humans or nonhuman primates. Modifications to the MoMLV LTR have been made by some investigators to achieve a similar goal of preventing silencing related to methylation by altering methylation-sensitive sites (4). The general description below of MoMLV also applies to the other related oncovirinae.

The MoMLV is composed of two copies of RNA ranging in size from 2 to 9 kb. In order to render these vectors replication incompetent, the *gag* (core proteins), *pol* (reverse transcriptase and integrase), and *env* (envelope protein determining the host cell range or tropism of the retrovirus) genes are deleted from the genome. What remains are the 5′ and 3′ LTR sequences on each end of the construct along with the packaging (Ψ) site. The 5′ LTR functions as the promoter and enhancer region, and the 3′ LTR contains the poly-A signal. The Ψ region serves as a binding site for the *gag* polyprotein, which packages the RNA into a viral core. The transgene is cloned into a site downstream of the Ψ region. In some vectors, splice donor and acceptor sites are retained or deliberately engineered into the Ψ region to generate, from a portion of the full-length mRNA, a subgenomic mRNA that more efficiently translates the downstream-inserted cDNA open reading frame.

Replication incompetent viral particles are produced in specifically engineered ''packaging cells.'' Packaging cell lines such as PA317 (5) (NIH3T3-derived murine fibroblasts), AM12 (6), Ψcrip (7), or 293SPA (8) (293 derived human embryonal kidney cells) constitutively express the *gag, pol,* and *env* proteins and therefore secrete empty virions into the culture media. When plasmid DNA of the retroviral vector is transfected into the packaging cells, clones of producer cells can be selected that secrete into the culture media replication-incompetent but infectious virions containing the transgene. The culture media, known as ''viral supernatant,'' can then be collected and used ex vivo to infect the desired target cells.

An important issue regarding retrovirus vector transduction of hematopoietic cells is that stem cells and lymphocytes express relatively low levels of the surface receptor required for binding of the most widely used amphotropic envelope packaging element (9). Some studies have suggested that packaging lines that use the gibbon ape leukemia virus (GALV) envelope may be advantageous for targeting both stem cells and T lymphocytes because these cells have higher levels of receptor for this envelope (10). However, recent advances in methods that enhance amphotropic retrovirus binding to stem cells, such as the coating of culture vessels with human fibronectin C-terminal fragment, may reduce these distinctions (11) (see below).

B. Non–Murine-Based Gene-Transfer Vectors

1. Lentiviral Vectors

Inefficient transduction by murine retroviral vectors of predominantly quiescent HSCs has prompted a search for vectors better suited for this target. Lentiviruses such as the human immunodeficiency virus (HIV) (see Chapter 1) have been shown to infect quiescent cells (reviewed in (12)). In its wild-type form, HIV causes the acquired immunodeficiency syndrome (AIDS). Construction of a replication-incompetent form packaged with alternate envelope genes such as the vesicular stomatitis virus-G (VSV-G) gene has resulted in a potentially safe and effective alternative to murine-based retroviral vectors. The VSV-G envelope confers upon the lentivirus vector both efficient cell binding and efficient entry of the contents of the virion into the cell. Furthermore, the VSV-G envelope also confers stability to the virus particle, allowing the use of physical processes such as ultracentrifugation for purification and concentration of virus particles without loss of activity. However, the ability of VSV-G to induce fusion of cell membranes that is so useful in the context of enhancing virion infectivity is toxic to the packaging cells that produce the virus particles, in part by facilitating syncytia formation. This toxicity limits production of VSV-G packaged lentivirus virions to a transient period after transfection of the packaging cells, with DNA vectors supplying the packaging elements. Thus, issues that still need to be resolved include the development of a stable packaging cell system and a better understanding of the possible interaction of HIV with other endogenous viruses that may be present in the host.

2. Spumavirus Vectors

Significantly less is known about another potential retroviral vector from the spumavirus genus called human foamy virus (HFV) (see Chapter 1). The advantage of HFV over HIV is that there is no evidence to date suggesting that HFV is pathogenic to humans. Furthermore, because HFV has the largest reported genome of any retrovirus, it may be able to accommodate larger transgenes (13). Although human cells are freely infected with HFV, its prevalence among humans appears to be quite low.

3. Adeno-Associated Virus Vectors

The adeno-associated virus (AAV) is a replication-defective single-stranded DNA parvovirus with significant potential as a gene-transfer vector. Integration into target cell genomic DNA occurs with the help of factors produced in *trans* from adenovirus or herpes virus superinfection. Like lentiviruses, AAV is able to infect nondividing cells, though the extent to which this is the case with purified nonreplicative AAV vectors in a variety of cells types is unclear (14–16). While transient episomal infection occurs in a large percentage of primitive hematopoietic precursors, transduction rates of 12% have been reported in AAV-transduced $CD34^{+}CD38^{-}$ cells cultured for 8 weeks (17). Large animal and human studies are needed to further evaluate the potential of AAV vectors in hematopoietic cell gene transfer. This topic is discussed in further detail in Chapter 3.

III. PRACTICAL CONSIDERATIONS OF HEMATOPOIETIC CELL GENE THERAPY

The following section outlines the three phases of a retroviral-based HSC and lymphocyte gene-transfer protocol: hematopoietic cell procurement, ex vivo gene transfer, and reinfusion of the corrected cells (Fig. 1).

A. Gene Transfer to Hematopoietic Stem Cells

1. Hematopoietic Stem Cell Procurement

Collection of large numbers of autologous hematopoietic stem cells is the first step in a HSC gene-therapy protocol. The three sites from which HSC can be harvested are bone marrow, cytokine or chemotherapy/cytokine-mobilized peripheral blood, and umbilical cord blood. Although the precise phenotype of a true HSC is unknown, large numbers of HSCs are contained in a population of cells expressing the CD34 antigen (18). $CD34^{+}$ cells make up 0.5–5% of nucleated cells in the bone marrow, and only a fraction of these are HSCs. HSCs be safely aspirated from bone marrow of the posterior superior iliac crest in a minor operative procedure. The major side effects of this procedure include mild discomfort at the aspiration site and an occasional hematoma. For smaller individuals, symptomatic anemia may require a blood transfusion, which, if anticipated in advance, can be an autologous unit. The major disadvantage of large-volume bone marrow aspiration is that it must be done under general anesthesia, which adds some risk to the procedure. Because of these issues repeated large-scale marrow harvests are not desirable.

In most individuals, administration of granulocyte colony-stimulating factor (G-CSF) at 10 μg/kg per day subcutaneously for 5 or 6 days results in a transient 20- to 100-fold increase in the frequency of $CD34^{+}$ stem cells in the circulation (a phenomenon termed mobilization). Other growth such as Flt-3-ligand (Flt3-L) (19–21), granulocyte-macrophage colony-stimulating factor (GM-CSF) (22–25), and stem cell factor (SCF) (26,27), which are used alone or in combination, are also effective for stem cell mobilization. Large numbers of HSC ($2–5 \times 10^{6}$ $CD34^{+}$ cells/kg patient weight) may be obtained from a single apheresis procedure following mobilization with growth factors. Often, apheresis procedures may be performed on two or three successive days at the peak of mobilization to maximize HSC collection. Furthermore, the mobilization process may be safely repeated at 4- to 8-week intervals. Unlike the procurement of bone marrow, no operative procedure is needed and the entire process can be done without a hospital admission.

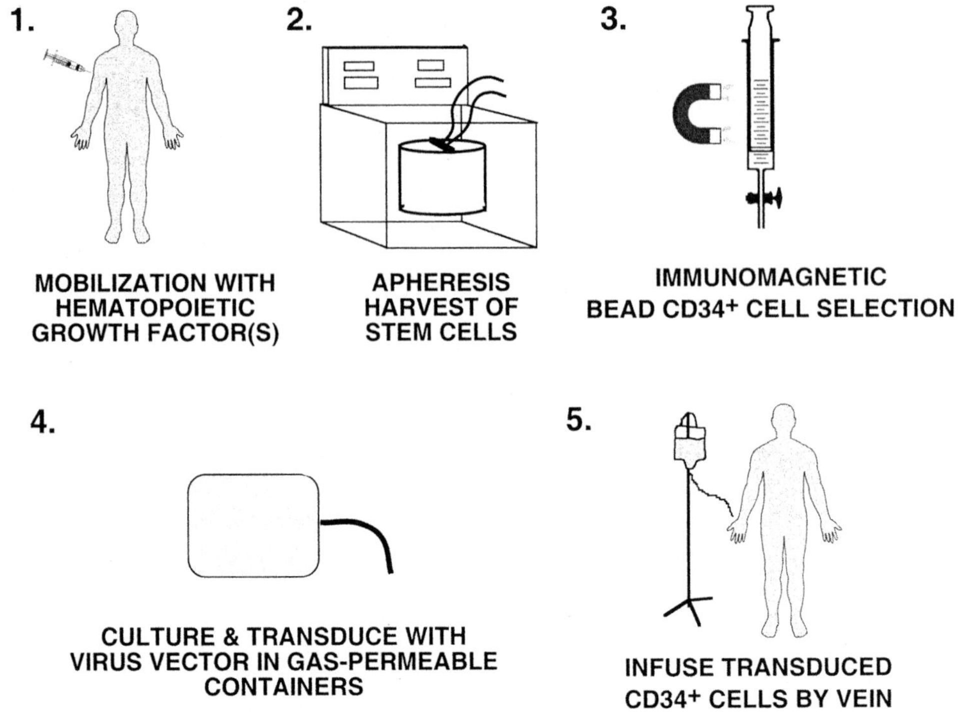

Figure 1 Hematopoietic stem cell gene therapy scheme.

Dunbar et al. (28) have shown improved gene marking in nonhuman primates when peripheral blood HSCs mobilized with G-CSF and SCF are compared to bone marrow HSCs. Furthermore, high-resolution cell-cycle analysis of cytokine-mobilized peripheral blood HSCs has revealed that these cells are more likely to have entered cell cycle and express higher levels of the amphotropic receptor mRNA (29–31). While certainly easier to collect, human gene-marking studies have yet to demonstrate unequivocally that cytokine-mobilized peripheral blood HSCs are better targets for retroviral transduction than bone marrow HSCs. However, the logistical advantages to obtaining peripheral blood HSCs dictate these as the preferred source for gene therapy and other transplant purposes except in settings where there is poor mobilization.

Umbilical cord blood contains a higher concentration of primitive hematopoietic progenitors than bone marrow (32). Recent data suggest that the HSCs from umbilical cord blood may also express higher levels of the amphotropic retrovirus receptor (33), which may result in more efficient transduction with amphotropic retroviral vectors. On average, 20×10^6 $CD34^+$ cells can be collected from the placenta at the time of delivery, which is approximately 10-fold less than can be collected from mobilized peripheral blood of an adult. Because of the low efficiency of HSC transduction with current techniques, clinical application for gene-corrected umbilical cord blood stem cells may be practical only in neonates.

2. Ex Vivo Gene Transfer

Optimization of ex vivo retroviral transduction conditions for HSCs has proven to be a formidable task. It appears that 48–72 hours of ex vivo culture in growth factors is required for quiescent lineage negative $CD34^+$ cells to enter the cell cycle (34). However, studies have shown that prolonged ex vivo culture of HSCs results in loss of long-term repopulating ability (35). This loss of repopulating potential with ex vivo culture may be gradual during culture. Thus, it may be possible to delineate optimum growth factor combinations and time in culture to allow entry into the cell cycle and subsequent retroviral transduction of some primitive cells that retain the ability to achieve long-term engraftment.

Measurable gene transfer into HSC in the clinical setting has been reported with ex vivo transduction periods ranging from 6 to 72 hours (36,37). While the report using a 6-hour regimen appeared to succeed in achieving measurable gene transfer without use of growth factors (36) most investigators have found that growth factors and an ex vivo culture period of 48–96 hours are required for optimum transduction. Growth factors are also essential to prevent apoptosis of HSC during prolonged ex vivo culture.

Some investigators have used autologous bone marrow stromal cell layers in an attempt to enhance transduction with retrovirus vectors while preserving reconstitutive potential (38–41). Despite encouraging results in small animal models, there is no evidence that use of bone marrow stromal layers produced better results in human clinical studies. Not only does the establishment of autologous stromal culture require a bone marrow aspiration, but this approach greatly increases the complexity and handling involved during clinical scale-up. Moreover, to achieve the highest level of transduction efficiency of HCSs grown on stromal layers, it is still essential to add growth factors to the culture.

Much current investigation is focused on the determination of growth factor combinations used without stromal layers that can achieve the highest transduction while maintaining reconstitutive potential of the transduced HSC. Flt3-L (42) and possibly also thrombopoietin (TPO) (42,43) have emerged as important agents to add to the ex vivo culture in relatively high concentrations (100–300 ng/mL) to achieve these dual goals. These growth factors work optimally in synergy with other growth factors. SCF at more modest doses of 50–100 ng/mL appears to be important as well. Interleukins 3 (IL-3) and 6 (IL-6) have also been widely used ex vivo in clinical trials to enhance cycling and may help to prevent apoptosis of HSC. However, use of concentrations of IL-3 higher than 30–50 ng/mL may be detrimental to preservation of cells with long-term engraftment potential. Other factors essential for maintenance and development of lymphoid progenitors from stem cells, such as IL-7, have not been used clinically but may in the future prove to be growth factors for the transduction of lymphocytes (44,45).

A number of techniques have been devised to encourage the interaction of hematopoietic progenitors with viral particles during the ex vivo transduction period. Most investigators have opted to transduce a cell population enriched for CD34 expression. $CD34^+$ cell enrichment enables an improved stem cell:viral particle ratio while using less of the valuable clinical grade retroviral supernatant. A variety of stem cell selection devices that use monoclonal antibodies specific for the CD34 antigen have been employed in experimental clinical protocols, (reviewed in Refs. 46,47). These devices are able to select large numbers of $CD34^+$ cells from bone marrow or an apheresis product at 50–70% efficiency, yielding a product consisting of 60–90% $CD34^+$ cells.

For reasons that are not well defined, centrifugation of target cells during incubation in a retrovirus vector supernatant increases transduction efficiency, a technique that has been termed ''spinocculation'' (48). The *g*-forces employed to achieve the effect are as low as $1200 \times g$ for 20 minutes, making it unlikely that the effect is due to sedimentation of individual virus particles. Co-cultivation of the target cells on a confluent layer of retrovirus producer cells has also been shown to enhance transduction. However, regulatory issues related to the safety of co-cultivation of HSCs with producer lines make this approach impractical for clinical application.

One of the more exciting new techniques to be described is the finding that a specific proteolytic fragment of fibronectin facilitates stem cell–retroviral particle interaction when this peptide is used to coat the surface of the culture vessel (11). Fibronectin, a prominent component of the extracellular matrix of bone marrow stromal cells, has numerous hematopoietic cell binding domains. Moritz et al. (49) demonstrated binding of both viral particles and hematopoietic target cells to a proteolytic fragment of fibronectin that contains the CS1-binding site. The CS1-binding site of fibronectin interacts with the VLA4 adhesion molecule found on hematopoietic stem cells (50). Thus, when HSC are incubated with retroviral particles in the presence of this specific fibronectin fragment, transduction efficiency is improved.

The availability of a clinical-grade recombinant human C-terminal fibronectin fragment (CH-296) has facilitated its use in several ongoing clinical gene-therapy trials targeting HSC. Even with retrovirus vectors of modest titer, acceptable transduction of $CD34^+$ cells can be achieved. Of note is that with retrovirus vectors at titers $> 5 \times 10^6$ infective particles per mL, the use of CH-296 fibronectin fragment–coated culture vessels can achieve transduction of 50–70% of $CD34^+$ cells routinely at clinical scale. It is also possible that use of fibronectin fragment coatings may help to preserve the long-term engraftment potential of cultured HSCs (51).

3. Transplantation of Transduced HSCs

Following transduction, the HSCs are infused into a peripheral vein of the patient. The role of bone marrow cytoreduction prior to infusion of transduced HSCs has yet to be defined. Experience with stem cell transplantation for treatment of hematological malignancies has shown that the bone marrow can be completely reconstituted by transplanted HSC (autologous or allogeneic) following myeloablative doses of chemotherapy and/or radiation. Because loss of long-term repopulating ability may occur during ex vivo transduction of HSCs, it would be unsafe to rescue hematopoiesis in a myeloablated patient with transduced HSCs only. Syngeneic transplant studies in mice have shown that engraftment of transplanted cells at levels that may be clinically relevant can occur without marrow conditioning when a large dose of donor HSCs is used (52–54). The stem cell dose in these studies may exceed that feasible for human gene-therapy studies unless the gene-corrected stem cells possess a survival advantage. In a murine model, partial engraftment of syngeneic HSC was facilitated by low doses of radiation (20–200 cGy) (55). Further studies are needed to determine whether a mild, nonmyeloablative regimen of bone marrow conditioning can aid in engraftment of transduced HSCs in humans.

B. Gene Transfer to Lymphocytes

1. Lymphocyte Procurement

With a few exceptions, large numbers of lymphocytes circulate in the peripheral blood and are therefore easily collected from gene-therapy candidates using apheresis. Lymphocytes may also be harvested from special sites such as tumors and are of particular interest because they may possess unique antitumor properties.

2. Ex Vivo Gene Transfer and Reinfusion

Compared to HSCs, fewer hurdles exist in the quest to optimize retroviral gene transfer of lymphocytes. Since these cells are terminally differentiated, loss of phenotype during ex vivo manipulation is not a concern. T lymphocytes, which are the most common target for lymphocyte-based gene therapy, are expanded in culture with agents such as IL-2 and/or monoclonal antibodies to CD3. While being cultured, many of the cells are stimulated into the active phase of the cell cycle and become more susceptible to permanent retroviral integration. It has been observed that with long-term culture of T lymphocytes, enrichment of CD8 T lymphocytes relative to CD4 T lymphocytes develops. This issue may be addressed by altering the ratio of cells added to the initial culture mixture (56).

Techniques that have been shown to improve lymphocyte transduction efficiency include (1) the use of retroviral vectors pseudotyped with the GALV envelope protein, (2) upregulation of amphotropic or GALV retroviral receptor expression by growth in phosphate depleted media, and (3) transduction in a culture vessel coated with the CS1 fibronectin fragment (57,58). Incorporation of these techniques together in the same protocol can yield transduction efficiency of 50–60%.

Reinfusion of the gene-corrected lymphocytes takes place as would any routine infusion of cell products. Cytoreductive conditioning of the recipient appears not to be necessary to achieve persistence of the transplanted lymphocytes, particularly where the therapeutic gene may provide a survival advantage (i.e., correction of adenosine deaminase severe combined immunodeficiency).

C. Clinical Scale-up

The transition from a laboratory-based gene-transfer assay to one that is ready for inclusion in a clinical protocol can be quite challenging. The most obvious differences relate to the number of hematopoietic progenitors that must be transduced at one time. Large volumes of retroviral supernatant must be produced in a facility licensed to provide clinical grade material. It is common to find a decrement in the viral titer of the clinical material compared to what is obtained in the laboratory. Besides the requisite sterility and endotoxin testing, the product must always be tested for the presence of replication-competent retrovirus. Regulatory and proprietary issues regarding use of reagents or devices often hinder the ability to replicate in the clinical setting what is done with case in the laboratory. Performing retroviral transduction in a clinically approved facility may require modifications of a laboratory optimized assay (59). Use of closed-system gas-permeable culture containers compatible with the standard sterile transfer techniques used by blood banks is one method that has been adapted for this purpose (60).

D. Regulatory Issues (United States)

All experimental clinical protocols are initially reviewed by an institutional human investigational review board. In addition, clinical use of retrovirus vectors generally requires review by an institutional biosafety committee. Human somatic gene-transfer proposals supported by NIH funding, including hematopoietic cell protocols, must be submitted for review by both the NIH Office of Recombinant DNA Activities (ORDA) and the U.S. Food and Drug Administration (FDA). Simultaneous submission to both agencies is currently allowed. These two agencies have consolidated their review process such that ORDA may recommend sole review by FDA for protocols that involve technologies that have already been reviewed and approved for previous protocols. A full review by ORDA's Recombinant DNA Advisory Committee (RAC) is usually required when novel approaches to gene delivery are utilized or new diseases are targeted. At the present time, germline gene-transfer studies will not be considered by the RAC. Further detail of the regulatory issues surrounding gene transfer protocols is discussed in Chapter 18.

IV. HUMAN GENE-TRANSFER TRIALS

A. Hematopoietic Stem Cell Gene-Transfer Studies

1. Marker Gene Studies

The insertion of marker genes into hematopoietic stem cells has been useful in the evolution of gene-transfer technology and has led to a better understanding of autologous stem cell transplantation. The first, and arguably the most successful, of these studies was reported by Brenner et al. in 1993 (36). This study enrolled 20 patients under the age of 20 who were candidates for autologous bone marrow transplantation for acute myelogenous leukemia or neuroblastoma. Bone marrow was harvested as the patient recovered from a cycle of cytotoxic chemotherapy. Two thirds of the harvest was immediately frozen, and the remaining one third was transduced with a retroviral vector containing the neomycin resistance gene. In vitro transduction efficiency was measured as percentage of hematopoietic colonies resistant to G418 (neomycin analog), and ranged from 2 to 14%. The transduced and unmanipulated bone marrow cells were infused after the administration of high-dose chemotherapy. Using PCR analysis, the marker gene was detected in approximately 5% of bone marrow mononuclear cells one month posttransplant. G418 resistance was observed in 5–20% of bone marrow colony-forming units (CFU) in 5 of 5 evaluable patients at 1 year, and in 2 patients at 18 months. Three important principals emerged from this study. First, the study proved that long-term repopulating cells could be successfully gene marked ex vivo. Second, the study demonstrated that autologous marrow infusion following high-dose chemotherapy participates in the marrow recovery. Finally, the authors also reported that tumor cells obtained from patients who relapsed after the gene-marked autologous BMT contained the neomycin resistance gene, suggesting tumor cell contamination of the autologous stem cell graft (61). Deisseroth et al. (62) performed a similar gene-marked autologous BMT study in patients with chronic myelogenous leukemia where gene marking of normal bone marrow CFU was demonstrated 6 months postinfusion. The investigators also demonstrated gene-marked tumor cells at relapse, suggesting tumor contamination of the autograft, (62). Two other studies were unsuccessful at demonstrating tumor contamination of autografts, which may be a consequence of much lower rates of ex vivo gene transfer (63,64).

Dunbar et al. employed HSC transduction conditions optimized by others with animal models (39,65,66) in an attempt to improve the low ex vivo transduction efficiency reported by Brenner et al. (36,61). This gene-marking study also set out to compare the engraftment capabilities of bone marrow and peripheral blood stem cells (PBSCs) and their suitability as targets for retroviral transduction (67). Bone marrow and chemotherapy/cytokine mobilized peripheral blood mononuclear cells were procured from breast cancer and multiple myeloma patients who were candidates for autologous stem cell transplantation. Two thirds of each product was cryopreserved without manipulation. $CD34^+$ cells were purified from the remaining one third of the mobilized peripheral blood and bone marrow product, and retroviral transduction of each product using one of two molecularly distinct retroviral vectors containing the neomycin resistance gene was performed. Since the bone marrow and peripheral blood $CD34^+$ cells were not transduced with the same vector, the contribution of each to engraftment following autologous stem cell transplantation could be tracked using PCR. Ex vivo transduction conditions consisted of a 72-hour culture of the target cells with retroviral supernatant supplemented with the hematopoietic cytokines IL-3, SCF, and IL-6 (IL-6 omitted from the culture of $CD34^+$ cells from multiple myeloma patients). All transduced and unmanipulated cells were pooled and reinfused following high-dose chemotherapy administration. The ex vivo transduction efficiency as measured by a clonogenic assay was 18–24%. Following transplantation, gene-marked bone marrow and peripheral blood cells were detected in 10 of 10 evaluable patients at a frequency of 0.1–1% using a semi-quantitative PCR technique. At 600 days postinfusion, only 1 patient had detectable levels of gene-marked cells. The authors did not identify any significant difference between bone marrow or peripheral blood stem cells as targets for retroviral gene transduction.

2. Chronic Granulomatous Disease

Chronic granulomatous disease (CGD) is an inherited immune deficiency caused by genetic mutations in any of the four subunits of the phagocyte NADPH oxidase ($p47^{phox}$, $p67^{phox}$ $gp91^{phox}$, $p22^{phox}$) resulting in the inability of phagocytes to produce microbicidal superoxide and hydrogen peroxide. CGD patients are prone to recurrent bacterial and fungal infections as well as granuloma formation (68). Stem cell transplantation can cure CGD (69–71), indicating that stem cells are the appropriate target for gene therapy. Preclinical work demonstrated that normal oxidase-positive neutrophils differentiate from CGD stem cells transduced with retroviral vectors encoding the corrective normal oxidase subunit cDNA (72–74). Based on this work, investigators at the National Institutes of Health have undertaken two clinical gene-transfer studies to treat CGD.

The first study targeted CGD patients with deficiency of the $p47^{phox}$ subunit (60). The $p47^{phox}$ cDNA was cloned into the MoMLV-based MFGS retrovirus vector, and this vector was packaged by the murine Ψ-crip amphotropic packaging cell line. Mobilized PBSC were apheresed from patients after treatment with G-CSF followed by $CD34^+$ enrichment using an immuno-paramagnetic bead-selection device (Nexell Isolex®). Retroviral transduction of the PBSCs was performed in serum-free media over a 6-hour period in the presence of hematopoietic cytokines (PIXY321, G-CSF) for 3 consecutive days. The transduced PBSC were then transfused into the patient without marrow conditioning. Ex vivo transduction efficiency was determined by several methods, including quantitative assessment of oxidase-positive (nitroblue tetrazolium dye test) myeloid colonies as well as determination of vector copy number using Southern blot hybridization. The percent of oxidase-positive colonies ranged from 9 to 29%. This was closely correlated with the vector copy number of 5–18% found in transduced and cultured PBSCs. Following intravenous infusion of transduced autologous $CD34^+$ cells into patients, the appearance of oxidase-normal neutrophils in the peripheral blood was assessed using a highly sensitive flow cytometry assay based on the increased fluorescence of oxidized dihydrorhodamine 123 (DHR) (75). Oxidase-normal neutrophils first appeared 2 weeks after transplantation, and peak correction occurred after 3–6 weeks. The frequency of corrected neutrophils ranged from 0.004 to 0.05%.

Preliminary results are available from a follow-up study that targeted CGD patients with the X-linked form of CGD caused by mutations in the transmembrane $gp91^{phox}$ subunit (personal communication, Ref. 76). All four of the patients enrolled in this trial had the $gp91^{phox}$ null form of X-linked CGD and had previously received allogeneic normal granulocytes as treatment for severe infection. A high-titer MFGS-$gp91^{phox}$ retroviral vector was prepared using the human-derived 293 (8) amphotropic envelope packaging cell line. In this study, GM-CSF combined with Flt-3 ligand (Immunex Corp.) was used to mobilize $CD34^+$ cells for apheresis. This novel cytokine combination was used to improve mobilization because previous studies had shown that CGD patients have a moderate defect in the mobilization response to G-CSF (77). Immune selected $CD34^+$ cells (Isolex 300I®) were exposed to retroviral supernatant in experimental gas-permeable containers, which were coated with a clinical-grade preparation of the CS-1 fibronectin fragment, Retronectin™ (Takara Shuzo). Transduction occurred on four consecutive days in serum-free media supplemented with Flt-3 ligand, Pixykine 321(Immunex Corp.), and stem cell factor. As in the first trial, cells were infused into the patient without marrow conditioning. Two or three cycles of gene therapy were administered at approximately 50-day intervals. Ex vivo transduction efficiency was assessed by flow cytometry using an anti-gp91 monoclonal antibody as well as by nitroblue tetrazolium dye testing for oxidase-positive colonies. Seventy-five to 85% of $CD34^+$ $CD38^-$, Lin^-, HLA DR^- cells were positive for the gp91 protein as detected by flow cytometry after 7 days of in vitro culture. Fifty percent of the myeloid CFU were found to be oxidase positive. Gene-corrected neutrophils were detected in two of the four patients treated beginning 2–3 weeks following the infusion of cells and remain detectable after 8 months of follow-up. One patient peaked at over 0.2% oxidase-positive neutrophils, and the other peaked at over 0.1%. Similar peaks of corrected neutrophils were seen after each cycle. While it is difficult to say definitively that the gene therapy resulted in clinical benefit to these patients, corrected neutrophils were recovered from the pus of a liver abscess in one patient who had a liver infection at the time of enrollment in the study. The inability to detect corrected neutrophils in two of the four patients may be a result of immune-mediated elimination of gene-corrected cells in this protein null inherited disorder.

3. Multidrug Resistance Gene Transfer

The multidrug resistance (MDR1) gene encodes a drug efflux pump called P-glycoprotein (reviewed in Refs. 78–80). This pump confers resistance to a variety of anticancer agents including doxorubicin, mitoxantrone, vincristine, etoposide, and taxol. MDR1 can be used as both a therapeutic and a selectable marker for other therapeutic genes (81).

In most cases, myelosuppression is the dose-limiting toxicity of chemotherapeutic agents. Therefore, if the transfer of MDR1 into HSCs is able to attenuate myelosuppression, higher and potentially more effective doses of chemotherapy could be delivered to the cancer patient. The proof of this principal was provided in transgenic mice engineered to constitutively express MDR1 (82). These mice could tolerate severalfold higher doses of taxol and daunomycin (83,84). A similar effect has been demonstrated using retroviral gene transfer of MDR1 into HSC (85–87).

Human clinical trials in MDR1 gene transfer have met with limited success. Hesdorffer et al. published the first study of MDR1 gene transfer in humans (88). In this phase 1 study, hematopoietic progenitor cells were collected from either bone marrow or mobilized peripheral blood. $CD34^+$ cells were enriched from the product, and two thirds of the cells were cryopreserved without manipulation. One third of the cells were incubated for 48 hours in the presence of cytokines on fibronectin-coated plates with a Harvey murine sarcoma virus–based retroviral vector containing the MDR1 cDNA. Ex vivo transduction efficiency as measured by a clonogenic assay ranged from 20 to 70%. Transduced and unmanipulated cells were infused after the administration of high-dose chemotherapy. PCR analysis of bone marrow samples posttransplant detected exogenous MDR1 cDNA in two of five patients treated at 3 and 10 weeks. The copy number of MDR1 in these two patients was estimated at less than 0.1%. PCR positivity from individual BFU-E and CFU-GM was not demonstrated. No toxicity was attributed to the gene-transfer component of this study, but both of the patients who had detectable gene transfer died from disease related complications. As a result, selection for transduced stem cells by subsequent chemotherapy administration could not be evaluated. Ongoing clinical trials in MDR1 gene transfer may help to answer the question of whether clinical benefit can be derived from this technique (89,90).

If selection of MDR1-transduced HSCs can be demonstrated in humans, the gene can then theoretically be used as an in vivo selectable marker. Sugimoto et al. (91) have developed a bicistronic Harvey sarcoma virus vector, which utilizes a viral-derived internal ribosome entry site (IRES) facilitating transcription of two transgenes. Fusion vectors containing cDNA for MDR1 and the Gaucher's disease gene glucocerebrosidase as well as the CGD gene $p47^{phox}$ have been developed and await clinical trail.

Safety issues regarding the use of MDR1 as a selectable marker have been brought into question by a recent study that demonstrates the development of a myeloproliferative syndrome in mice transplanted with MDR1-transduced cells. Of note is that the transplanted cells had been subjected to prolonged ex vivo culture (92). Further studies in large animal models are needed to confirm this possible toxicity. Use of MDR1 and other promising selectable markers such as mutant dihydrofolate reductase is discussed in further detail in Chapter 16.

4. Adenosine Deaminase Deficiency

The inherited deficiency of adenosine deaminase (ADA) is responsible for approximately one quarter of the cases of severe combined immunodeficiency (SCID). In the absence of ADA, lymphocytes accumulate high levels of 2′-deoxyadenosine, which is converted to the toxic compound deoxyadenosine triphosphate. The result is a patient with profound T- and B-lymphocyte dysfunction, who is therefore susceptible to infections with opportunistic pathogens. ADA deficiency is an attractive target for gene therapy because corrected lymphocytes have a survival advantage over noncorrected ADA-negative lymphocytes. Multiple gene-therapy trials for ADA SCID targeting HSCs as well as lymphocytes have been performed. Discussion in this section will focus on HSCs as the target for gene therapy of ADA SCID. It has been difficult to determine the clinical impact of HSC ADA gene-therapy trials because the current standard of care involves treatment of ADA-deficient SCID patients with polyethylene glycol–conjugated ADA (PEG-ADA) (93). However, there is compelling evidence suggesting that gene-corrected lymphocytes detected in these patients are responsible for improvement in a number of immunological laboratory parameters (94).

Van Beusechem et al. (95) laid the groundwork for HSC-based ADA gene transfer by demonstrating in nonhuman primates that prolonged low-level expression of human ADA from peripheral blood cells was possible after bone marrow cells were transduced with retrovirus containing the ADA cDNA. In perhaps the most successful clinical gene therapy trial to date, Bordignon et al. (94) transduced both peripheral blood lymphocytes and HSCs with two molecularly distinct retroviral vectors carrying the ADA gene. The two patients treated were transplanted with both gene-corrected lymphocytes and HSCs. One patient received nine injections of gene-corrected cells over a 2-year period. The other patient received five injections over 10 months. Prolonged detection of the transgene was observed in both the bone marrow and the peripheral blood for the entire 36-month period of follow-up. Until the 35-month time point, the vector used for HSC correction was detected only in circulating granulocytes and bone marrow cells. Gene-marked lymphocytes contained only the lymphocyte vector. At 35 months, however, lymphocytes derived from the gene-corrected HSCs were first detected and subsequently became more prevalent than those that carried the lymphocyte-specific vector.

Hoogerbrugge et al. performed a similar study, transducing bone marrow $CD34^+$ cells with a retroviral vector carrying the ADA cDNA (96). The transgene was detected transiently in the peripheral blood for 3 months following the infusion and was then lost. This disappointing result was attributed to low ex vivo HSC transduction.

Kohn et al. (37) transduced $CD34^+$ cells isolated from umbilical cord blood of three ADA-deficient neonates with a MoML V-based retroviral vector containing human ADA cDNA as well as the cDNA encoding the bacterial neomycin resistance gene (37). Cells were returned to the unconditioned recipient on the fourth day of life. Ex vivo transduction efficiency as measured by percent G418-resistant CFU ranged from 12 to 19%. Clonogenic myeloid precursors from the bone marrow were assayed at 1 year and found to be G418 resistant at a frequency of 4–6%. Concurrent with the infusion of gene-corrected HSCs, the patients began ADA replacement therapy with PEG-ADA. As a result, the selective advantage of ADA-positive clones was partially blunted. After 4 years of follow-up, the levels of gene-corrected cells in the peripheral blood mononuclear cell fraction has increased 50- to 100-fold in all three patients (97). The frequency of gene-corrected T lymphocytes increased to 1–10%. This rate of increase was far greater than observed in the granulocyte series (0.01–0.03%). In an attempt to assess clinical efficacy of gene transfer, PEG-ADA administration was discontinued in the patient with the highest level of gene-corrected T lymphocytes. This resulted in a fall in S-adenosylhomocysteine hydrolase activity and a loss of antigen-specific T-lymphocyte reactivity suggesting inadequate ADA production by the transduced cells. After 2 months, PEG-ADA replacement was restarted when oral monilia, sinusitis, and an upper respiratory tract infection developed. Despite the inability to demonstrate clinical benefit, the persistence of the transgene for over 4 years in both the lymphoid and the myeloid cell lines suggests that gene transfer into true long-term repopulating HSCs is possible from cells collected from umbilical cord blood.

5. Fanconi's Anemia

Fanconi's anemia (FA) is an autosomal recessive disorder manifested by aplastic anemia, physical malformations, and cancer susceptibility (98). Eight separate genotypic groups of FA have been described (FA-A through FA-H) (99). Cells carrying the FA mutation are hypersensitive to DNA-damaging agents such as mitomycin C (100). Since stem cell transplantation successfully treats the hematological manifestations of FA (101,102), it is a logical candidate for stem cell gene therapy. In addition, there is evidence to suggest that normal stem cells may have a selective growth advantage over HSCs with the mutated FA gene (103).

After demonstrating in vitro that HSCs from patients with the FA group C (FAC) gene mutation could be functionally corrected by retroviral gene transfer of the normal FAC gene, Liu et al. (104) initiated a clinical trial. Three children with the FAC mutation were treated with sequential cycles of autologous, G-CSF–mobilized CD34-selected progenitor cells, which were transduced with a MoMLV-based retroviral vector containing the cDNA for FAC and neomycin resistance. The cells were transduced in the presence of hematopoietic cytokines IL-3, IL-6, and SCF for 72 hours and infused into the patient without preceding marrow conditioning. FAC vector sequence was detected by PCR in the peripheral blood and bone marrow of all three patients at levels ranging from 0.01 to 3%. Multilineage peripheral blood marking was detected in one patient for a 16-month period during which the patient received four cycles of gene transfer. The other two patients had only transient bone marrow and peripheral blood positivity despite repeated cycles of gene therapy. Bone marrow sampling of each patient following the infusion of gene-corrected cells revealed an increase in the number of colonies resistant to the DNA-damaging effects of mitomycin C. No adverse effects were documented during the conduct of the trial (105).

6. Gaucher's Disease

Gaucher's disease is an autosomal recessive disorder that results in a deficiency of the lysosomal enzyme glucocerebrosidase (106). This leads to the accumulation of glucosylcerebroside in macrophages throughout the reticular endothelial system. Although the clinical course is quite variable, most patients develop hepatosplenomegaly and painful lytic bone lesions. Conventional treatment includes stem cell transplantation or glucocerebrosidase supplementation.

Dunbar et al. (41) published the first clinical gene therapy trial for Gaucher's disease. Three patients received CD34-selected (Cellpro Ceprate) bone marrow or mobilized PB transduced on autologous stroma $\pm$ cytokines with a retroviral vector containing the human glucocerebrosidase cDNA. Transduction efficiencies were low, ranging from 1 to 10% using a semi-quantitative PCR assay. Transgene was detected in peripheral blood mononuclear cells ($<0.02\%$) for 3 months in the patient whose cells were transduced with the highest efficiency.

7. Human Immunodeficiency Virus

HSCs and mature T lymphocytes are targets for anti-HIV gene therapy. Strategies include transfer of genes encoding ribozyme, which target the viral RNA genome, RNA decoys, and mutant transactivator genes that interfere with viral gene expression (107–109). These approaches, along with a review of the clinical trials, are discussed in Chapter 26.

8. Summary

Sustained engraftment of transduced HSCs whose progeny do not have a selective advantage is best demonstrated in the gene-marking studies (36,61,67). These studies all utilized cytotoxic marrow conditioning prior to infusion of transduced cells. Besides reducing the number of resident naive stem cells, marrow conditioning also results in a bone marrow microenvironment that is more conducive for engraftment of transduced HSCs. Sustained engraftment of transduced HSCs, (>6 months) has yet to be demonstrated without marrow conditioning. Improvement in retroviral transduction conditions that utilize cytokines such as FLT-3 ligand and thrombopoietin has resulted in impressive rates of HSC gene transfer in myeloablated nonhuman primates (35,110). It remains to be seen whether this can be translated to human gene-therapy trials.

B. Lymphocyte Gene-Transfer Studies

1. Gene-Marking Studies

The first clinical gene-therapy trial involved gene transfer into lymphocytes and was undertaken in the late 1980s as a means of characterizing tumor-infiltrating lymphocytes (TILs) (1). TILs were isolated from tumors of patients with metastatic melanoma. These cells were expanded and then transduced with a retroviral vector containing the neomycin resistance gene. Following reinfusion, the marker gene was used to track the migration of the marked lymphocytes. TILs were consistently found in the peripheral blood as well as tumor deposits for up to 2 months. A similar approach was employed to study the persistence of Epstein-Barr virus (EBV)–specific cytotoxic T lymphocytes (CTL) generated ex vivo and infused as treatment of post–bone marrow transplant EBV-related lymphoproliferation (111,112). EBV-specific CTLs marked with a neomycin resistance vector were detectable in the peripheral circulation for 10 weeks postinfusion.

2. Adenosine Deaminase Deficiency

Blaese et al. (56) were the first to use a therapeutic gene in a retroviral gene-transfer trial for ADA-deficient SCID patients. Two patients with an incomplete response to Peg-ADA therapy were infused with T lymphocytes transduced with a MoMLV-based retroviral vector containing the cDNA coding for ADA. The transduction efficiency of lymphocytes prior to infusion ranged from 0.1 to 10%. Patients were treated with multiple cycles of transduced T cells over a period of 1–2 years. Gene-corrected cells were detected in circulation for 2 years following the final cycle of gene therapy demonstrating a T-lymphocyte lifespan much longer than was predicted. There was clear-cut evidence of improved cellular and humoral immune response following gene therapy in one of the two patients treated. This discrepancy in patient response was attributed to superior ex vivo transduction efficiency obtained in the responding patient. No toxicity was attributed to the conduct of the protocol.

Using the identical experimental design and retroviral vector, Onodera et al. (113) accomplished similar results in one patient treated in Japan. These studies, in conjunction with the previously described Bordignon study (94), demonstrate the potential of lymphocyte-based gene therapy to provide prolonged clinical benefit.

3. Suicide Gene Transfer

The use of the herpes simplex virus thymidine kinase (HSV-TK) gene and other ''suicide'' genes for gene therapy is discussed in Chapter 17. Introduction of the HSV-TK gene into a cell allows for the phosphorylation of nucleoside analogs such as ganciclovir. Once phosphorylated, gancyclovir becomes toxic to the cell as it is incorporated into DNA. There are two published hematopoietic cell gene-therapy trials utilizing the HSV-TK. Lymphocytes were the target cells in both studies (114,115). In an attempt to make HIV therapy with autologous cytotoxic T cells safer, Riddell et al. (114) transduced HIV-specific cytotoxic T cells with the HSV-TK gene. The transduced cells could then be eliminated with gancyclovir treatment if toxicity were to arise from their presence. The vector used to transduce the lymphocytes also carried the hygromycin phosphotransferase gene. Unexpectedly, the transduced lymphocytes were rejected by a brisk host cytotoxic T-lymphocyte response against the transduced cells.

In allogeneic bone marrow transplantation, lymphocytes taken from the bone marrow donor are often infused into the recipient to treat tumor relapse or to aid in immune reconstitution. Significant toxicity may arise if transplanted lymphocytes mount an immunological attack against the recipient (graft-versus-host disease). As in the Riddell study, Bonini et al. (115) studied HSV-TK–transduced donor lymphocyte infusions as a method of protecting against graft-vs. host (GVHD) disease. The vector used for transduction also carried the marker gene that coded for a truncated form of the human low-affinity receptor for nerve growth factor (NGFR) as well as the neomycin resistance gene. Gene-marked lymphocytes were detected in seven of eight patients available for analysis with a range of 0.01–13.4% of the total circulating lymphocytes. Three of the patients developed GVHD and were treated with gancyclovir. The percent of genetically modified lymphocytes decreased dramatically with complete resolution of GVHD in two of three patients. Partial resolution of GVHD occurred in the other. While there was no evidence of an immune-mediated elimination of the transduced cells, these bone marrow transplant patients were likely immunocompromised even more profoundly than the HIV-positive patients studied by Riddell et al. (114).

V. CONCLUSION

To date, all clinical trials involving transduction of hematopoietic cells have utilized murine-based retroviral vectors. When lymphocytes are the target cell, modest clinical benefit was observed in both the ADA trials and the HSV-TK trial. This is attributable to the relatively high level of transduction efficiency using the latest techniques. Though clinical applicability of HSC gene transfer is much broader than for lymphocytes, long-term repopulating HSCs are less receptive to retroviral-based gene transfer. While alternate vectors such as lentivirus and adeno-associated viral vectors are promising, a number of studies have proven that the retroviral vector can successfully target the long-term repopulating cell, albeit with an extremely low efficiency. To improve the ability to transduce HSC, further knowledge of stem cell biology such as their cell cycle characteristics, their trigger for self-replication versus lineage commitment, and the optimal ex vivo growth conditions will aid in the ability to transduce these cells. The production of a high-titer, replication-defective retroviral supernatant is another technique that must be perfected. It is unclear to what extent host immune rejection of cells expressing the transgene will hinder progress of gene therapy for protein-null disorders or disorders where a heterologous gene product is produced. And finally, it is becoming clear that some degree of cytoreductive bone marrow conditioning will be necessary to achieve clinically significant levels of HSC gene transfer.

REFERENCES

1. Rosenberg SA, Aebersold P, Cornetta K, et al. Gene transfer into humans—immunotherapy of patients with advanced melanoma, using tumor-infiltrating lymphocytes modified by retroviral gene transduction [see comments]. N Engl J Med 1990; 323:570–578.
2. Roe T, Reynolds TC, Yu G, Brown PO. Integration of murine leukemia virus DNA depends on mitosis. Embo J 1993; 12:2099–2108.
3. Karlsson S. Treatment of genetic defects in hematopoietic cell function by gene transfer. Blood 1991; 78:2481–2492.
4. Challita PM, Skelton D, el-Khoueiry A, Yu XJ, Weinberg K, Kohn DB. Multiple modifications in cis elements of the long terminal repeat of retroviral vectors lead to increased expression and decreased DNA methylation in embryonic carcinoma cells. J Virol 1995; 69:748–755.
5. Miller AD, Buttimore C. Redesign of retrovirus packaging cell lines to avoid recombination leading to helper virus production. Mol Cell Biol 1986; 6:2895–2902.
6. Markowitz DG, Goff SP, Bank A. Safe and efficient ecotropic and amphotropic packaging lines for use in gene transfer experiments. Trans Assoc Am Physicians 1988; 101:212–218.
7. Danos O, Mulligan RC. Safe and efficient generation of recombinant retroviruses with amphotropic and ecotropic host ranges. Proc Natl Acad Sci USA 1988; 85: 6460–6464.
8. Davis JL, Witt RM, Gross PR, et al. Retroviral particles produced from a stable human-derived packaging cell line transduce target cells with very high efficiencies. Hum Gene Ther 1997; 8:1459–1467.
9. Orlic D, Girard LJ, Jordan CT, Anderson SM, Cline AP, Bodine DM. The level of mRNA encoding the amphotropic retrovirus receptor in mouse and human hematopoietic stem cells is low and correlates with the efficiency of retrovirus transduction. Proc Natl Acad Sci USA 1996; 93:11097–11102.
10. Kiem HP, Heyward S, Winkler A, et al. Gene transfer into marrow repopulating cells: comparison between amphotropic and gibbon ape leukemia virus pseudotyped retroviral vectors in a competitive repopulation assay in baboons. Blood 1997; 90:4638–4645.
11. Hanenberg H, Xiao XL, Dilloo D, Hashino K, Kato I, Williams DA. Colocalization of retrovirus and target cells on specific fibronectin fragments increases genetic transduction of mammalian cells. Nat Med 1996; 2:876–882.
12. Subbramanian RA, Cohen EA. Molecular biology of the human immunodeficiency virus accessory proteins. J Virol 1994; 68:6831–6835.
13. Yu SF, Baldwin DN, Gwynn SR, Yendapalli S, Linial ML. Human foamy virus replication: a pathway distinct from that of retroviruses and hepadnaviruses. Science 1996; 271:1579–1582.
14. Russell DW, Miller AD, Alexander IE. Adeno-associated virus vectors preferentially transduce cells in S phase. Proc Natl Acad Sci USA 1994; 91:8915–8919.
15. Podsakoff G, Wong KK, Jr., Chatterjee S. Efficient gene transfer into nondividing cells by adeno-associated virus-based vectors. J Virol 1994; 68:5656–5666.
16. Fisher-Adams G, Wong KK, Jr., Podsakoff G, Forman SJ, Chatterjee S. Integration of adeno-associated virus vectors in CD34+ human hematopoietic progenitor cells after transduction. Blood 1996; 88:492–504.
17. Chatterjee S, Li W, Wong CA, et al. Transduction of primitive human marrow and cord blood-derived hematopoietic progenitor cells with adeno-associated virus vectors. Blood 1999; 93:1882–1894.
18. Andrews RG, Singer JW, Bernstein ID. Precursors of colony-forming cells in humans can be distinguished from colony-forming cells by expression of the CD33 and CD34 antigens and light scatter properties. J Exp Med 1989; 169: 1721–1731.
19. Rusten LS, Lyman SD, Veiby OP, Jacobsen SE. The FLT3 ligand is a direct and potent stimulator of the growth of primitive and committed human CD34+ bone marrow progenitor cells in vitro. Blood 1996; 87:1317–1325.
20. Sudo Y, Shimazaki C, Ashihara E, et al. Synergistic effect of FLT-3 ligand on the granulocyte colony-stimulating factor-induced mobilization of hematopoietic stem cells and progenitor cells into blood in mice. Blood 1997; 89: 3186–3191.
21. Gabbianelli M, Pelosi E, Montesoro E, et al. Multi-level effects of flt3 ligand on human hematopoiesis: expansion of putative stem cells and proliferation of granulomonocytic progenitors/monocytic precursors. Blood 1995; 86: 1661–1670.
22. Lane TA, Law P, Maruyama M, et al. Harvesting and enrichment of hematopoietic progenitor cells mobilized into the peripheral blood of normal donors by granulocyte-macrophage colony-stimulating factor (GM-CSF) or G-CSF: potential role in allogeneic marrow transplantation. Blood 1995; 85:275–282.
23. Brugger W, Bross K, Frisch J, et al. Mobilization of peripheral blood progenitor cells by sequential administration of interleukin-3 and granulocyte-macrophage colony-stimulating factor following polychemotherapy with etoposide, ifosfamide, and cisplatin [see comments]. Blood 1992; 79: 1193–1200.
24. Socinski MA, Cannistra SA, Elias A, Antman KH, Schnipper L, Griffin JD. Granulocyte-macrophage colony stimulating factor expands the circulating haemopoietic progenitor cell compartment in man. Lancet 1988; 1:1194–1198.
25. Haas R, Ho AD, Bredthauer U, et al. Successful autologous transplantation of blood stem cells mobilized with recombinant human granulocyte-macrophage colony-stimulating factor. Exp Hematol 1990; 18:94–98.

26. Moskowitz CH, Stiff P, Gordon MS, et al. Recombinant methionyl human stem cell factor and filgrastim for peripheral blood progenitor cell mobilization and transplantation in non-Hodgkin's lymphoma patients—results of a phase I/II trial. Blood 1997; 89:3136–3147.
27. Andrews RG, Briddell RA, Knitter GH, et al. In vivo synergy between recombinant human stem cell factor and recombinant human granulocyte colony-stimulating factor in baboons enhanced circulation of progenitor cells. Blood 1994; 84:800–810.
28. Dunbar CE, Seidel NE, Doren S, et al. Improved retroviral gene transfer into murine and Rhesus peripheral blood or bone marrow repopulating cells primed in vivo with stem cell factor and granulocyte colony-stimulating factor. Proc Natl Acad Sci USA 1996; 93:11871–11876.
29. Lemoli RM, Tafuri A, Fortuna A, et al. Biological characterization of CD34+ cells mobilized into peripheral blood. Bone Marrow Transplant 1998; 22(suppl 5):S47–50.
30. Bregni M, Di Nicola M, Siena S, et al. Mobilized peripheral blood CD34+ cells express more amphotropic retrovirus receptor than bone marrow CD34+ cells. Haematologica 1998; 83:204–208.
31. Horwitz ME, Malech HL, Anderson SM, Girard LJ, Bodine DM, Orlic D. G-CSF Mobilized peripheral blood stem cells enter into G1 of the cell cycle and express higher levels of amphotropic retrovirus receptor mRNA. Exp Hematol 1999;27:1160–1167.
32. Broxmeyer HE, Hangoc G, Cooper S, et al. Growth characteristics and expansion of human umbilical cord blood and estimation of its potential for transplantation in adults. Proc Natl Acad Sci USA 1992; 89:4109–4113.
33. Orlic D, Girard LJ, Anderson SM, et al. Identification of human and mouse hematopoietic stem cell populations expressing high levels of mRNA encoding retrovirus receptors. Blood 1998; 91:3247–3254.
34. Jordan CT, Yamasaki G, Minamoto D. High-resolution cell cycle analysis of defined phenotypic subsets within primitive human hematopoietic cell population. Exp Hematol 1996; 24:1347–1355.
35. Tisdale JF, Hanazono Y, Sellers SE, et al. Ex vivo expansion of genetically marked rhesus peripheral blood progenitor cells results in diminished long-term repopulating ability. Blood 1998; 92:1131–1141.
36. Brenner MK, Rill DR, Holladay MS, et al. Gene marking to determine whether autologous marrow infusion restores long-term haemopoiesis in cancer patients. Lancet 1993; 342:1134–1137.
37. Kohn DB, Weinberg KI, Nolta JA, et al. Engraftment of gene-modified umbilical cord blood cells in neonates with adenosine deaminase deficiency. Nat Med 1995; 1: 1017–1023.
38. Nolta JA, Smogorzewska EM, Kohn DB. Analysis of optimal conditions for retroviral-mediated transduction of primitive human hematopoietic cells. Blood 1995; 86: 101–110.
39. Moore KA, Deisseroth AB, Reading CL, Williams DE, Belmont JW. Stromal support enhances cell-free retroviral vector transduction of human bone marrow long-term culture-initiating cells. Blood 1992; 79:1393–1399.
40. Wells S, Malik P, Pensiero M, Kohn DB, Nolta JA. The presence of an autologous marrow stromal cell layer increases glucocerebrosidase gene transduction of long-term culture initiating cells (LTCICs) from the bone marrow of a patient with Gaucher disease. Gene Ther 1995; 2: 512–520.
41. Dunbar CE, Kohn DB, Schiffman R, et al. Retroviral transfer of the glucocerebrosidase gene into CD34+ cells from patients with Gaucher disease: in vivo detection of transduced cells without myeloablation. Hum Gene Ther 1998; 9:2629–2640.
42. Luens KM, Travis MA, Chen BP, Hill BL, Scollay R, Murray LJ. Thrombopoietin, kit ligand, and flk2/flt3 ligand together induce increased numbers of primitive hematopoietic progenitors from human CD34+Thy-1+Lin- cells with preserved ability to engraft SCID-hu bone. Blood 1998; 91:1206–1215.
43. Borge OJ, Ramsfjell V, Cui L, Jacobsen SE. Ability of early acting cytokines to directly promote survival and suppress apoptosis of human primitive CD34+CD38- bone marrow cells with multilineage potential at the single-cell level: key role of thrombopoietin. Blood 1997; 90: 2282–2292.
44. Plum J, De Smedt M, Leclercq G, Verhasselt B, Vandekerckhove B. Interleukin-7 is a critical growth factor in early human T-cell development. Blood 1996; 88:4239–4245.
45. Peschon JJ, Morrissey PJ, Grabstein KH, et al. Early lymphocyte expansion is severely impaired in interleukin 7 receptor-deficient mice. J Exp Med 1994; 180:1955–1960.
46. Shpall EJ, et al. Peripheral blood stem cell harvesting and CD34-positive cell selection. Cancer Treat Res 1997; 77: 143–157.
47. Cagnoni PJ, et al. Mobilization and selection of CD34-positive hematopoietic progenitors. Blood Rev 1996; 10: 1–7.
48. Kotani H, et al. Improved methods of retroviral vector transduction and production for gene therapy. Hum Gene Ther 1994; 5:19–28.
49. Moritz T, Dutt P, Xiao X, et al. Fibronectin improves transduction of reconstituting hematopoietic stem cells by retroviral vectors: evidence of direct viral binding to chymotryptic carboxy-terminal fragments. Blood 1996; 88: 855–862.
50. Hurley RW, McCarthy JB, Verfaillie CM. Direct adhesion to bone marrow stroma via fibronectin receptors inhibits hematopoietic progenitor proliferation. J Clin Invest 1995; 96:511–519.
51. Dao MA, Hashino K, Kato I, Nolta JA. Adhesion to fibronectin maintains regenerative capacity during ex vivo culture and transduction of human hematopoietic stem and progenitor cells. Blood 1998; 92:4612–4621.
52. Nilsson SK, et al. Potential and distribution of transplanted hematopoietic stem cells in a nonablated mouse model. Blood 1997; 89:4013–4020.

53. Stewart FM, Crittenden RB, Lowry PA, Pearson-White S, Quesenberry PJ. Long-term engraftment of normal and post-5-fluorouracil murine marrow into normal nonmycloablated mice [see comments]. Blood 1993; 81: 2566–2571.
54. Rao SS, Peters SO, Crittenden RB, Stewart FM, Ramshaw HS, Quesenberry PJ. Stem cell transplantation in the normal nonmyeloablated host: relationship between cell dose, schedule, and engraftment. Exp Hematol 1997; 25: 114–121.
55. Mardiney M, 3rd, Malech HL. Enhanced engraftment of hematopoietic progenitor cells in mice treated with granulocyte colony-stimulating factor before low-dose irradiation: implications for gene therapy. Blood 1996; 87: 4049–4056.
56. Blaese RM, Culver KW, Miller AD, et al. T lymphocyte-directed gene therapy for ADA-SCID: initial trial results after 4 years. Science 1995; 270:475–480.
57. Lam JS, Reeves ME, Cowherd R, Rosenberg SA, Hwu P. Improved gene transfer into human lymphocytes using retroviruses with the gibbon ape leukemia virus envelope. Hum Gene Ther 1996; 7:1415–1422.
58. Bunnell BA, Muul LM, Donahue RE, Blaese RM, Morgan RA. High-efficiency retroviral-mediated gene transfer into human and nonhuman primate peripheral blood lymphocytes. Proc Natl Acad Sci USA 1995; 92:7739–7743.
59. Bosse R, Singhofer-Wowra M, Rosenthal F, Schulz G. Good manufacturing practice production of human stem cells for somatic cell and gene therapy. Stem Cells 1997; 15:275–280.
60. Malech HL, Maples PB, Whiting-Theobald N, et al. Prolonged production of NADPH oxidase-corrected granulocytes after gene therapy of chronic granulomatous disease. Proc Natl Acad Sci USA 1997; 94:12133–12138.
61. Brenner MK, Rill DR, Moen RC, et al. Gene-marking to trace origin of relapse after autologous bone-marrow transplantation. Lancet 1993; 341:85–86.
62. Deisseroth AB, Zu Z, Claxton D, et al. Genetic marking shows that Ph + cells present in autologous transplants of chronic myelogenous leukemia (CML) contribute to relapse after autologous bone marrow in CML. Blood 1994; 83:3068–3076.
63. Cornetta K, Srour EF, Moore A, et al. Retroviral gene transfer in autologous bone marrow transplantation for adult acute leukemia. Hum Gene Ther 1996; 7:1323–1329.
64. Bachier CR, Giles RE, Ellerson D, et al. Hematopoietic retroviral gene marking in patients with follicular non-Hodgkin's lymphoma. Leuk Lymphoma 1999; 32: 279–288.
65. Hughes PF, Thacker JD, Hogge D, et al. Retroviral gene transfer to primitive normal and leukemic hematopoietic cells using clinically applicable procedures. J Clin Invest 1992; 89:1817–1824.
66. Nolta JA, Kohn DB. Comparison of the effects of growth factors on retroviral vector-mediated gene transfer and the proliferative status of human hematopoietic progenitor cells. Hum Gene Ther 1990; 1:257–268.
67. Dunbar CE, Cottler-Fox M, O'Shaughnessy JA, et al. Retrovirally marked CD34-enriched peripheral blood and bone marrow cells contribute to long-term engraftment after autologous transplantation. Blood 1995; 85: 3048–3057.
68. Klempner MS, Malech, HL. Phagocytes: normal and abnormal neutrophil host defenses. In: Gorbach SL, Bartlett JG, Blacklow NR, eds. Infectious Diseases. Philadelphia: W.B. Saunders Co., 1997:41–46.
69. Ozsahin H, von Planta M, Muller I, et al. Successful treatment of invasive aspergillosis in chronic granulomatous disease by bone marrow transplantation, granulocyte colony-stimulating factor-mobilized granulocytes, and liposomal amphotericin-B. Blood 1998; 92:2719–2724.
70. Ho CM, Vowels MR, Lockwood L, Ziegler JB. Successful bone marrow transplantation in a child with X-linked chronic granulomatous disease. Bone Marrow Transplant 1996; 18:213–215.
71. Calvino MC, Maldonado MS, Otheo E, Munoz A, Couselo JM, Burgaleta C. Bone marrow transplantation in chronic granulomatous disease. Eur J Pediatr 1996; 155:877–879.
72. Sekhsaria S, Gallin JI, Linton GF, Mallory RM, Mulligan RC, Malech HL. Peripheral blood progenitors as a target for genetic correction of p47phox-deficient chronic granulomatous disease. Proc Natl Acad Sci USA 1993; 90: 7446–7450.
73. Li F, Linton GF, Sekhsaria S, et al. CD34+ peripheral blood progenitors as a target for genetic correction of the two flavocytochrome b558 defective forms of chronic granulomatous disease. Blood 1994; 84:53–58.
74. Weil WM, Linton GF, Whiting-Theobald N, et al. Genetic correction of p67phox deficient chronic granulomatous disease using peripheral blood progenitor cells as a target for retrovirus mediated gene transfer. Blood 1997; 89: 1754–1761.
75. Vowells SJ, Sekhsaria S, Malech HL, Shalit M, Fleisher TA. Flow cytometric analysis of the granulocyte respiratory burst: a comparison study of fluorescent probes. J Immunol Methods 1995; 178:89–97.
76. Malech HL, Horwitz ME, Linton GF, Theobold-Whiting N, Brown MR, Farrell CJ, Butz RE, Carter CS, Decarlo E, Miller JA, Von Epps DE, Read EJ, Fleisher TA. Extended production of oxidase normal neutrophils in x-linked chronic granulomatous disease following gene therapy with $gp91^{phox}$ transduced $CD34^{+}$ cells. Blood 1998;92:(sup)690a.
77. Sekhsaria S, Fleisher TA, Vowells S, et al. Granulocyte colony-stimulating factor recruitment of CD34+ progenitors to peripheral blood: impaired mobilization in chronic granulomatous disease and adenosine deaminase–deficient severe combined immunodeficiency disease patients. Blood 1996; 88:1104–1112.
78. Endicott JA, Ling V. The biochemistry of P-glycoprotein-mediated multidrug resistance. Annu Rev Biochem 1989; 58:137–171.

79. Gottesman MM, Pastan I. Biochemistry of multidrug resistance mediated by the multidrug transporter. Annu Rev Biochem 1993; 62:385–427.
80. Pastan I, Gottesman M. Multiple-drug resistance in human cancer. N Engl J Med 1987; 316:1388–1393.
81. Licht T, Gottesman MM, Pastan I. Transfer of the MDRI (multidrug resistance) gene: protection of hematopoietic cells from cytotoxic chemotherapy, and selection of transduced cells in vivo. Cytokines Mol Ther 1995; 1:11–20.
82. Galski H, Sullivan M, Willingham MC, et al. Expression of a human multidrug resistance cDNA (MDR1) in the bone marrow of transgenic mice: resistance to daunomycin-induced leukopenia. Mol Cell Biol 1989; 9: 4357–4363.
83. Mickisch GH, Licht T, Merlino GT, Gottesman MM, Pastan I. Chemotherapy and chemosensitization of transgenic mice which express the human multidrug resistance gene in bone marrow: efficacy, potency, and toxicity. Cancer Res 1991; 51:5417–5424.
84. Mickisch GH, Merlino GT, Galski H, Gottesman MM, Pastan T. Transgenic mice that express the human multidrug-resistance gene in bone marrow enable a rapid identification of agents that reverse drug resistance. Proc Natl Acad Sci USA 1991; 88:547–551.
85. Podda S, Ward M, Himelstein A, et al. Transfer and expression of the human multiple drug resistance gene into live mice. Proc Natl Acad Sci USA 1992; 89:9676–9680.
86. Sorrentino BP, Brandt SJ, Bodine D, et al. Selection of drug-resistant bone marrow cells in vivo after retroviral transfer of human MDR1. Science 1992; 257:99–103.
87. Hanania EG, Deisseroth AB. Serial transplantation shows that early hematopoietic precursor cells are transduced by MDR-1 retroviral vector in a mouse gene therapy model. Cancer Gene Ther 1994; 1:21–25.
88. Hesdorffer C, Ayello J, Ward M, et al. Phase I trial of retroviral-mediated transfer of the human MDR1 gene as marrow chemoprotection in patients undergoing high-dose chemotherapy and autologous stem-cell transplantation. J Clin Oncol 1998; 16:165–172.
89. O'Shaughnessy JA, Cowan KH, Nienhuis AW, et al. Retroviral mediated transfer of the human multidrug resistance gene (MDR-1) into hematopoietic stem cells during autologous transplantation after intensive chemotherapy for metastatic breast cancer. Hum Gene Ther 1994; 5: 891–911.
90. Deisseroth AB, Kavanagh J, Champlin R. Use of safety-modified retroviruses to introduce chemotherapy resistance sequences into normal hematopoietic cells for chemoprotection during the therapy of ovarian cancer: a pilot trial. Hum Gene Ther 1994; 5:1507–1522.
91. Sugimoto Y, Aksentijevich I, Murray GJ, Brady RO, Pastan I, Gottesman MM. Retroviral coexpression of a multidrug resistance gene (MDR1) and human alpha-galactosidase A for gene therapy of Fabry disease. Hum Gene Ther 1995; 6:905–915.
92. Bunting KD, Galipeau J, Topham D, Benaim E, Sorrentino BP. Transduction of murine bone marrow cells with an MDR1 vector enables ex vivo stem cell expansion, but these expanded grafts cause a myeloproliferative syndrome in transplanted mice. Blood 1998; 92:2269–2279.
93. Hershfield MS, Buckley RH, Greenberg ML, et al. Treatment of adenosine deaminase deficiency with polyethylene glycol-modified adenosine deaminase. N Engl J Med 1987; 316:589–596.
94. Bordignon C, Notarangelo LD, Nobili N, et al. Gene therapy in peripheral blood lymphocytes and bone marrow for ADA-immunodeficient patients. Science 1995; 270: 470–475.
95. van Beusechem VW, Kukler A, Heidt PJ, Valerio D. Long-term expression of human adenosine deaminase in rhesus monkeys transplanted with retrovirus-infected bone-marrow cells. Proc Natl Acad Sci USA 1992; 89:7640–7644.
96. Hoogerbrugge PM, van Beusechem VW, Fischer A, et al. Bone marrow gene transfer in three patients with adenosine deaminase deficiency. Gene Ther 1996; 3:179–183.
97. Kohn DB, Hershfield MS, Carbonaro D, et al. T lymphocytes with a normal ADA gene accumulate after transplantation of transduced autologous umbilical cord blood CD34+ cells in ADA-deficient SCID neonates. Nat Med 1998; 4:775–780.
98. Fanconi G. Familial constitutional panmyelocytopathy, Fanconi's anemia (F.A.). I. Clinical aspects. Semin Hematol 1967; 4:233–240.
99. Joenje H, Oostra AB, Wijker M, et al. Evidence for at least eight Fanconi anemia genes. Am J Hum Genet 1997; 61:940–944.
100. Liu JM, Buchwald M, Walsh CE, Young NS. Fanconi anemia and novel strategies for therapy. Blood 1994; 84: 3995–4007.
101. Gluckman E, Broxmeyer HA, Auerbach AD, et al. Hematopoietic reconstitution in a patient with Fanconi's anemia by means of umbilical-cord blood from an HLA-identical sibling. N Engl J Med 1989; 321:1174–1178.
102. Gluckman E, Auerbach AD, Horowitz MM, et al. Bone marrow transplantation for Fanconi anemia. Blood 1995; 86:2856–2862.
103. Lo Ten Foe JR, Kwee ML, Rooimans MA, et al. Somatic mosaicism in Fanconi anemia: molecular basis and clinical significance. Eur J Hum Genet 1997; 5:137–148.
104. Liu JM, Young NS, Walsh CE, et al. Retroviral mediated gene transfer of the Fanconi anemia complementation group C gene to hematopoietic progenitors of group C patients. Hum Gene Ther 1997; 8:1715–1730.
105. Lin JM, Kim S, Read EJ, Futaki M, Dokal I, Carter CS, Leitman SF, Pensiero M, Young NS, Walsh CE. Engraftment of hematopoietic progenitor cells transduced with Fanconi anemia group C gene (FANCC). Hum Gene Ther 1999;10:2337–2346.

106. Beutler E. Gaucher's disease. N Engl J Med 1991; 325: 1354–1360.
107. Sullenger BA, Gallardo HF, Ungers GE, Gilboa E. Overexpression of TAR sequences renders cells resistant to human immunodeficiency virus replication. Cell 1990; 63: 601–608.
108. Malim MH, Freimuth WW, Liu J, et al. Stable expression of transdominant Rev protein in human T cells inhibits human immunodeficiency virus replication. J Exp Med 1992; 176:1197–201.
109. Leavitt MC, Yu M, Yamada O, et al. Transfer of an anti-HIV-1 ribozyme gene into primary human lymphocytes. Hum Gene Ther 1994; 5:1115–1120.
110. Kiem HP, Andrews RG, Morris J, et al. Improved gene transfer into baboon marrow repopulating cells using recombinant human fibronectin fragment CH-296 in combination with interleukin-6, stem cell factor, FLT-3 ligand, and megakaryocyte growth and development factor. Blood 1998; 92:1878–1886.
111. Rooney CM, Smith CA, Ng CY, et al. Use of gene-modified virus-specific T lymphocytes to control Epstein-Barr-virus-related lymphoproliferation. Lancet 1995; 345:9–13.
112. Rooney CM, Smith CA, Ng CY, et al. Infusion of cytotoxic T cells for the prevention and treatment of Epstein-Barr virus-induced lymphoma in allogeneic transplant recipients. Blood 1998; 92:1549–1555.
113. Onodera M, Ariga T, Kawamura N, et al. Successful peripheral T-lymphocyte-directed gene transfer for a patient with severe combined immune deficiency caused by adenosine deaminase deficiency. Blood 1998; 91:30–36.
114. Riddell SR, Elliott M, Lewinsohn DA, et al. T-cell mediated rejection of gene-modified HIV-specific cytotoxic T lymphocytes in HIV-infected patients [see comments]. Nat Med 1996; 2:216–223.
115. Bonini C, Ferrari G, Verzeletti S, et al. HSV-TK gene transfer into donor lymphocytes for control of allogeneic graft-versus-leukemia [see comments]. Science 1997; 276: 1719–1724.

21

Gene Therapy for Cardiovascular Disease and Vascular Grafts

Afshin Ehsan, Michael J. Mann, and Victor J. Dzau
Brigham and Women's Hospital, and Harvard Medical School, Boston, Massachusetts

The earliest, and perhaps most obvious, clinical embodiments of gene-transfer technology have involved the treatment of rare genetic disorders. The development of effective methods of manipulating gene expression in vivo, however, coupled with an explosive growth in the understanding of changes in gene expression associated with the onset and progression of acquired diseases has created a prospect for revolutionizing the clinician's approach to common disorders. As researchers learn more about the genetic blueprints of disease, they gain the potential to alter, or even reverse, pathobiology at its roots. Nowhere are these possibilities more avidly sought, or more likely to impact a significant population of patients, than in the arena of cardiovascular disease.

Gene therapy has come to embrace both the introduction of functional genetic material into living cells as well as the sequence-specific blockade of certain active genes. These systems have included recombinant viral vectors that allow relatively efficient insertion of genetic information and oligonucleotides that can be used to alternative gene expression (1,2). This increased breadth of gene-manipulation technology has accompanied the identification of genes that are either activated or repressed during disease. Recent discoveries have uncovered therapeutic targets (2,3) both for the improvement of conventional cardiovascular therapies, such as balloon angioplasty or bypass grafting, and for the development of entirely novel approaches, such as the induction of angiogenesis in ischemic tissues. As enthusiasm grows for these new experimental strategies, it is important for clinicians to be aware of their limitations as well as their strengths and for careful processes of evaluation to pave the possible integration of these therapies into routine practice. This chapter will explore general principles of gene manipulation in the cardiovascular system and review a number of prominent examples of experimental reduction to practice. It is intended as a source to assist in the consideration of future developments in this exciting field.

I. GENETIC MANIPULATION OF CARDIOVASCULAR TISSUE

A. Gene Therapy Strategies

Gene therapy can be defined as any manipulation of gene activity, or gene "expression," that influences disease. This manipulation is generally achieved via the introduction of foreign DNA into cells in a process known as transduction or transfection. Gene therapy can involve either the delivery of whole, active genes (gene transfer) or the blockade of native gene expression by the transfection of cells with short chains of nucleic acids known as oligonucleotides.

The gene-transfer approach allows for replacement of a missing gene product or for the "overexpression" of a native or foreign protein that can prevent or reverse a disease process. The transfer of a gene into a target cell leading to subsequent gene expression is known as transduction, and the new gene can be referred to as the transgene. Gene replacement or augmentation involves the transfer of a gene that is either missing from a cell, present in a defective form, or simply underexpressed relative to the level of protein expression desired by the clinician. The protein expressed may be active only intracellularly, in which case a very high gene-transfer efficiency may be necessary to alter the overall function of an organ or tissue. Alternatively, proteins secreted by target cells may act on other cells in a paracrine or endocrine manner, in which case delivery to a small subpopulation may yield a sufficient therapeutic result.

Gene blockade can be accomplished by transfection of cells with short chains of DNA known as antisense oligodeoxynucleotides (ODN) (4). This approach attempts to alter cellular function by the inhibition of specific gene expression. Genes are defined by a specific sequence of bases that make up the DNA chain. Antisense ODN are designed to have a base sequence that is complementary in terms of Watson-Crick binding to a segment of the target gene. They are generally 15–20 bases in length, which confers specificity to a single site within the genome. This complementary sequence allows the ODN to bind specifically to the corresponding segment of messenger RNA (mRNA) that is transcribed from the gene during expression. This binding of ODN to mRNA prevents the translation of RNA into the protein product of the gene (4).

Another form of gene blockade is the use of ''ribozymes,'' segments of RNA that can act like enzymes to destroy specific sequences of target mRNA (5). Ribozymes contain both a catalytic region that can cleave other RNA molecules in sequence-specific manner and an adjacent sequence that confers the specificity of the target. Because the sequence-recognition portion of the ribozymes is generally limited to approximately six bases, these gene-inhibitory agents are generally more susceptible to nonspecific interactions than their antisense counterparts.

A third type of gene inhibition involves the blockade of gene-regulatory proteins known as transcription factors. Transcription factors regulate gene expression by binding to chromosomal DNA at specific promoter regions, and this binding turns on, or ''activates,'' an adjacent gene. Double-stranded ODN can therefore be designed to mimic the chromosome binding sites of these transcription factors and act as ''decoys,'' binding up the available transcription factor and preventing the subsequent activation of target genes (6).

The transfer of genetic sequences exogenous to the human genome have been envisioned, such as the gene encoding thymidine kinase (TK) from the herpes simplex virus. This has been used to enhance metabolic activation of the cytotoxic prodrug gancyclovir, which may be useful in treating vascular proliferative disorders such as restenosis (7). Scientists studying gene-transfer technology have often relied on a class of genes known as reporter or marker genes. These genes encode proteins, such as a form of β-galactosidase found in *Escherichia coli* (known as lacZ or β-gal) or a small fluorescent molecule known as green fluorescent protein (GFP), which can be detected easily via histochemistry, fluorescent microscopy, or other techniques that allow rapid identification and quantification of successful gene transfer.

B. Vectors for In Vivo Cardiovascular DNA Delivery

For the purpose of cardiovascular gene therapy, the ''ideal'' DNA-delivery vector would be capable of safe and highly efficient delivery to all cell types, both proliferating and quiescent, with the opportunity to select either short-term or indefinite gene expression. This ideal vector would also have the flexibility to accommodate genes of all sizes, incorporate control of the temporal pattern and degree of gene expression, and recognize specific cell types for tailored delivery or expression. While progress is being made on each of these fronts individually, researchers remain far from possessing a single vector with all of these characteristics. Instead, a spectrum of vectors has evolved, each of which may find a niche in different early clinical gene therapy strategies.

Viral vectors may represent nature's solution to the problem of efficient gene transfer, however, man's attempt to harness these resources has also been confounded by the biological barriers that have evolved to protect cells and organisms from viral infection. Immunologic responses not only limit the efficacy of viral gene transfer, particularly when repeat administrations are considered, but the inflammatory response to viral antigens, even those associated with replication-deficient vectors, may impede or negate the benefits of expression of the transferred gene (8). Furthermore, engineering of viral genomes does not always preclude residual cytotoxicity in infected cells and the possibility for regression to replication proficiency.

Scientists have therefore continued to explore nonviral avenues for achieving efficient DNA delivery. One advantage of nonviral delivery systems is that they can be used not only for gene transfer but also for the delivery of oligonucleotides and protein–nucleic acid complexes that can be used for alternative forms of genetic manipulation. Whereas *transduction* refers generally to the delivery of an intact gene to a target cell and *infection* is used to describe the process of viral gene delivery, *transfection* is a term used to describe nonviral (i.e., physical/chemical) delivery of genes or oligonucleotides. Below is a brief description of DNA-delivery vectors that have been exploited in the cardiovascular system (Table 1).

Table 1 Comparison of Vectors Used for Cardiovascular Gene Transfer

	Efficiency (in vivo)	DNA integration	Duration of gene expression	Level of expression (max.)	Ease of preparation	Host response	Risks
Viral							
Retrovirus	+	Yes	Life-long	+ +	+ + +	+	Oncogenesis; viral mutation
Adenovirus	+ + + +	No	1–2 weeks	+ + + +	+ +	+ + + +	Cytotoxicity; viral mutation
AAV	+	Sometimes	Life-long	+	+	+	Oncogenesis; viral mutation; viral contamination
Nonviral							
Liposomes	+	No	Limited	+	+ + + +	+	Cytotoxic at high concentrations
Fusigenic liposomes	+ +	No	Limited	+	+	+	Cytotoxic at high concentrations
Naked plasmid	+	No	Limited	+	+ + +	+	Cytotoxic at high concentrations

+ = Lowest; + + + + = highest; AAV = adenoassociated virus.

1. Retroviral Vectors

Recombinant, replication-deficient retroviral vectors have been used extensively for gene transfer in cultured cardiovascular cells in vitro, where cell proliferation can be manipulated easily. Their use in vivo has been more limited due to low transduction efficiencies, particularly in the cardiovascular system where most cells remain quiescent. Nabel et al. (9) first demonstrated the feasibility of transducing blood vessels with foreign DNA in vivo by infecting porcine iliofemoral arteries with a recombinant retroviral vector containing the β-galactosidase gene. Several cell types in the vessel wall were transduced, including endothelial and vascular smooth muscle cells (VSMC). Using a β-galactosidase retroviral vector to genetically modify endothelial cells in vitro, Wilson et al. (10) demonstrated expression up to 5 weeks after implantation of a prosthetic vascular graft seeded with genetically transformed cells. The random integration of traditional retroviral vectors such as MMLV (Malony murine leukemia virus) into chromosomal DNA involves the potential hazard of oncogene activation and neoplastic cell growth. While the risk may be exceedingly low, safety monitoring will be an important aspect of clinical trials using viral vectors. Recent improvements in packaging systems (particularly the development of ''pseudotyped'' retroviral vectors incorporating vesicular stomatitis virus G-protein) have improved the stability of retroviral particles and facilitated their use in a wider spectrum of target cells.

2. Adenoviral Vectors

Recombinant adenoviruses have become the most widely used viral vectors for experimental in vivo gene transfer and have been used extensively in animal models of cardiovascular disease (11). Adenoviruses can infect nondividing cells and generally do not integrate into the host genome. These vectors can therefore achieve relatively efficient gene transfer in quiescent vascular tissue, but transgenes are generally lost when cells are stimulated into rounds of cell division. Expression of DNA in a nonchromosomal or episomal state also appears to be less stable, and adenoviral transduction has proven to be transient in cells even in the absence of replication.

Many scientists have concluded that the immune response to adenoviral antigens represents the greatest limitation to their use in gene therapy. Conventional vectors have generally achieved gene expression for only 1–2 weeks after infection. It is not certain to what extent the destruction of infected cells contributes to the termination of transgene expression given that the suppression of episomal transgene promoters appears to occur as well. However, longer expression has been documented after injection of tissues in immune-deficient mice. Even in the context of such reactions, the adenoviral vector has been postulated to provide an adjuvant effect that amplifies the immune response. In the vasculature, physical barriers such as the internal elastic lamina apparently limits infection to the endothelium, with gene transfer to the media and adventitia only occurring after injury has disrupted the vessel architecture. Although gene delivery to 30–60% of cells after balloon injury has been reported with adenoviral vectors carrying reporter genes, the fact that atherosclerotic disease has also been found to limit the efficiency of adenoviral transduction may pose a significant problem for the treatment of human disease.

3. Adeno-Associated Viral Vectors

Adeno-associated virus (AAV) is a dependent human parvovirus that has not been linked to human disease (12). It can infect a wide range of target cells and can establish a latent infection by integration into the genome of the cell, thereby yielding stable gene transfer as in the case of retroviral vectors. Although AAV vectors transduce replicating cells at a more rapid rate, they possess the ability to infect nonreplicating cells both in vitro and in vivo. AAV is limited by its small size (transgenes cannot be longer than about 4 kb) and the need to eliminate helper viruses from viral preparations. The efficiency of AAV-mediated gene transfer to vascular cells and the potential use of AAV vectors for in vivo vascular gene therapy remains to be determined. However, a number of groups have reported successful transduction of myocardial cells after direct injection of AAV suspensions into heart tissue, and these infections have yielded relatively stable expression for greater than 60 days (13). It has not yet been clearly established whether long-term recombinant AAV transgenic expression is associated with genomic integration as is wild-type AAV infection. In general, AAV transgene expression does not occur at significant levels during the first 2–4 weeks after infection, although the reason for this delay remains unclear.

4. Lipid-Mediated Gene Transfer

Numerous nonviral methods are available for the delivery of DNA into cells in vitro, including calcium phosphate, electroporation, and particle bombardment. The development of similarly effective methods of in vivo transfection, however, has posed a significant challenge to cardiovascular and other clinical researchers who hope to avoid cumbersome and invasive steps of harvesting and culturing tissues or cells from the patient. The encapsulation of DNA in artificial lipid membranes (liposomes) can facilitate its uptake and cellular transport. The primary advantages of lipid-based gene-transfer methods are ease of preparation and flexibility in substituting different transgene constructs in comparison with the relatively complex process of producing recombinant viral vectors. Cationic liposomes have been used extensively for cellular delivery of plasmid DNA and antisense oligonucleotides (14). A wide variety of cationic lipid preparations is currently available for DNA transfer both in vitro and in vivo. In addition to cationic lipids, other substances, such as lipopolyamines and cationic polypeptides, are now being investigated as potential vehicles for enhanced DNA delivery both for gene transfer and gene blockade strategies (15).

5. Fusigenic Liposome–Mediated Gene Transfer (HVJ Liposomes)

This method utilizes a combination of fusigenic proteins of the Sendai virus (hemagglutinating virus of Japan, or HVJ) in conjunction with neutral liposomes. HVJ is an RNA virus and belongs to the paramyxovirus family, which has HN and F glycoproteins on its envelope (16). HN binds with glycol-type sialic acid groups, which act as receptors on the cell surface, and F protein can interact directly with a cellular lipid bilayer and induce fusion. HVJ liposomes consist of neutral liposomes complexed with UV light–inactivated HVJ virus. Fusion of HVJ liposome complexes with the cell membrane may result in the release of DNA directly into the cytosol and facilitating nuclear uptake. HVJ liposome methods have been successfully employed for gene transfer in vivo to many tissues including liver, kidney, and the vascular wall. A major limitation to current HVJ liposome techniques is the need to undertake a multistep liposome preparation procedure immediately prior to use and the poor long-term stability of the complexes.

6. Other In Vivo Gene Transfer Methods

Plasmids are circular chains of DNA that were originally discovered as a natural means of gene transfer between bacteria. Naked plasmids can also be used to transfer DNA into mammalian cells. The direct injection of plasmid DNA into tissues in vivo can result in transgene expression. Plasmid uptake and expression, however, has generally been achieved at reasonable levels only in skeletal and myocardial muscle (17). The uptake of naked oligonucleotides is also inefficient after either intravascular administration or direct injection. Various catheters that have been designed to enhance local drug delivery to isolated segments of target vessels have been proposed as vehicles for local vascular gene therapy. The controlled application of a pressurized environment to vascular tissue in a nondistended manner has recently been found to enhance oligonucleotide uptake and nuclear localization. This method may be particularly useful for ex vivo applications such as vein grafting or transplantation and may represent a means of enhancing plasmid gene delivery as well (18).

7. Regulatable Transgene Expression

In addition to effective gene delivery, many therapeutic settings will demand some degree of control over the duration, location, and degree of transgene expression. To this end, researchers have developed early gene promoter systems that allow the clinician to regulate the spatial or temporal pattern of gene expression. These systems include tissue-specific promoters that have been isolated from genetic sequences encoding proteins with natural restriction to the target tissue, such as the von Willebrand factor promoter in endothelial cells and the a-myosin heavy chain promoter in myocarium (19). Promoters have also been isolated from nonmammalian systems that can either promote or inhibit downstream gene expression in the presence of a pharmacological agent such as tetracycline, zinc, or steroids (20). In addition, regulation of transgene expression may even be relegated to the physiological conditions, with the incorporation of promoters or enhancers that respond to specific conditions such as hypoxia or increased oxidative stress (21).

II. GENE THERAPY FOR HYPERLIPIDEMIA AND SYSTEMIC DISEASES

Hyperlipidemia, in both its acquired and inherited forms, has been clearly shown to be an independent risk factor for the development of atherosclerotic vascular disease, myocardial infarction, and stroke. The use of drug therapies in the treatment of acquired forms of this disease, through either 3-hydroxy-3-methylglutaryl-coenzyme A (HMG CoA) reductase inhibitors or bile acid–binding resins, has proven effective in decreasing the morbidity and mortality associated with hyperlipidemia. However, these same regimens have had their limitations in the treatment of inherited disorders such as familial hypercholesterolemia (FH) and apo E deficiency. The shortcomings of conventional pharmacological therapy has therefore stimulated an interest in the genetic replacement of these missing proteins in hepatocytes as a potential means of reducing cholesterol levels in patients with these rare disorders.

A. Ex Vivo Approach

Familial hypercholesterolemia, caused by mutations in the low-density lipoprotein (LDL) receptor, is the most common genetically linked source of hypercholesterolemia, and the heterozygous form is the most common inherited cardiovascular disease (22). The receptor functions to facilitate the uptake of LDL in the liver and is essential for maintaining normal cholesterol levels. In a rabbit model of LDL receptor deficiency, Chowdhury et al. (23) surgically harvested autologous hepatocytes, and stably transferred the gene for the LDL receptor into those cells in culture using a replication-deficient retrovirus. The cells were then infused back into the animal's liver via the portal circulation, and ingraftment of the genetically engineered cells into the liver succeeded in lowering plasma cholesterol levels (23). These encouraging results spawned several clinical trials, the results of which were not as dramatic (24,25). Despite a 30% reduction in serum LDL levels for up to 6 months in the rabbit model, therapeutic reductions in LDL in the clinical trials ranged from 0 to 15%, with a significantly shorter duration. These differences likely reflect the need for a much higher number of genetically modified autologous cells in the human subject to produce significant therapeutic changes. The immunological response to these infected cells cultured in media containing nonhuman proteins may have also played a role in reducing the duration of clinical efficacy.

B. In Vivo Approach

Researchers have shown that after intravenous injection of adenovirus, more than 90% of transgene expression occurs in the liver. This finding led to the investigation of an in vivo approach to the genetic treatment of this FH. Several groups have reported complete correction of elevated LDL levels in mouse and rabbit models of FH after injection of a replication-deficient adenovirus containing the LDL receptor gene (26–29). However, these effects were found to be transient, once again likely due to the immune responses directed both to adenoviral proteins as well as to the transgene product. Additionally, Kozarsky et al. (30) reported effective adenoviral-mediated gene transfer of the VLDL receptor in a mouse model for FH with transient correction of hypercholesterolemia. Apo E deficiency has been shown to lead to marked hypercholesterolemia, hypertriglyceridemia, and increased levels of cholesterol-rich VLDL and chylomicron remnants. Apo E–deficient mice treated by adenovirus-mediated gene transfer of the human apoE3 gene resulted in a shift in the plasma lipoprotein distribution from primarily VLDL and LDL in the control mice to predominantly HDL in transfected mice (31). Furthermore, in normal mice, adenovirus-mediated transfer of a gene encoding apo A-I produced transient, physiologically relevant elevations of HDL cholesterol that were comparable to elevations observed in transgenic animals that overexpressed the apo A-I gene (32).

The progress achieved in the treatment of experimental FH through the in vivo genetic manipulation of hepatocytes has brought researchers a step closer towards the permanent correction of this devastating disease. With the development and/or improvement of gene-delivery vector systems that can produce long-term, stable integration and that do not lead to a significant inflammatory or immune response, one can also foresee a time where other systemic diseases like diabetes and coagulopathies such as hemophilia can be cured.

III. GENE THERAPY FOR VASCULAR DISEASES

A. Gene and Oligonucleotide Therapy of Restenosis

Recurrent narrowing of arteries following percutaneous angioplasty, atherectomy, or other disobliterative techniques is a common clinical problem that severely limits the durability of these procedures for patients with atherosclerotic occlusive diseases. In the case of balloon angioplasty, restenosis occurs in approximately 30–40% of treated coronary lesions and 30–50% of superficial femoral artery lesions within the first year. Intravascular stents reduce the restenosis rates in some settings, but the incidence remains significant and long-term data are limited. Despite impressive technological advances in the development of minimally invasive and endovascular approaches to treat arterial occlusions, the full benefit of these gains awaits the resolution of this fundamental biological problem.

Restenosis is an attractive target for gene therapy not only because of its frequency (and its associated costs incurred by the health-care system) but moreso because it is a local tissue reaction that develops precisely at a site of intervention to which access has already been accomplished. A potential advantage of the genetic approach over more conventional pharmacotherapies is that a single dose of a gene-therapy agent may have a protracted biological effect. It has been reasoned that the appropriate genetic modification, performed locally at the time of angioplasty, could induce a long-term benefit in patency by altering the healing response. The potential role for gene therapy in the prevention of restenosis will depend on the identification of an appropriate molecular target, a suitable vector system for efficiently targeting vessel wall cells, and methods of achieving local delivery without producing undue damage or distal tissue ischemia. Presently, considerable hurdles remain despite significant progress in each of these areas.

The pathophysiology of restenosis reflects a paradigm of the healing response of arteries that are injured by reconstructive techniques. It is comprised of a contraction and fibrosis of the vessel wall known as remodeling and an active growth of a fibrocellular lesion composed primarily of VSMC and extracellular matrix. The latter process, known as neointimal hyperplasia, involves the stimulation of the normally ''quiescent'' VSMC in the arterial media into the ''activated'' state characterized by rapid proliferation and migration. A number of growth factors are believed to play a role in the stimulation of VSMC during neointimal hyperplasia, including platelet-derived growth factor (PDGF), basic fibroblast growth factor (bFGF), transforming growth factor beta (TGF-β), and angiotensin II (33). Activated VSMC have also been found to produce a variety of enzymes, cytokines, adhesion molecules, and other proteins that not only enhance the inflammatory response within the vessel wall but also stimulate further vascular cell abnormality (34–37).

Although it is now thought that remodeling may account for the majority of late lumen loss after balloon dilation of atherosclerotic vessels, proliferation has been the predominant target of experimental genetic interventions. There have been two general approaches: cytostatic, in which cells are prevented from progressing through the cell cycle to mitosis, and cytotoxic, in which cell death is induced. A group of molecules known as cell cycle regulatory proteins act at different points along the cell cycle, mediating progression toward division. It has been hypothesized that by blocking expression of the genes for one or more of these proteins, one could prevent the progression of VSMC through the cell cycle and inhibit neointimal hyperplasia. Morishita et al. demonstrated near-complete inhibition of neointimal hyperplasia after carotid balloon injury via HVJ liposome–mediated transfection of the vessel wall with a combination of antisense ODN against cell cycle–regulatory genes (38,39). Arrest of the cell cycle via antisense blockade of either of two proto-oncogenes, c-myb or c-myc, has been found to inhibit neointimal hyperplasia in models of arterial balloon injury (40,41), although the specific antisense mechanism of the ODN used in these studies has subsequently been questioned (42,43).

In addition to transfection of cells with antisense ODN, cell cycle arrest can also be achieved through manipulation of transcription factor activity. The activity of a number of cell cycle–regulatory genes is influenced by a single transcription factor known as E2F (44). In quiescent cells, E2F is bound to a complex of other proteins, including a protein known as the retinoblastoma gene product (Rb), which prevents its interaction with chromosomal DNA and its stimulation of gene activity. In proliferating cells, E2F is released, resulting in cell cycle gene activation. A transcription factor decoy bearing the consensus binding sequence recognized by E2F can be employed as a means to inhibit cellular proliferation (Fig. 1). Morishita et al. demonstrated the use of this strategy to prevent VSMC proliferation and neointimal hyperplasia after rat carotid balloon injury (45). Alternatively, Chang et al. showed that localized arterial infection with a replication-defective adenovirus encoding a nonphosphorylatable, constitutively active form of Rb at the time of balloon angioplasty significantly reduced smooth muscle cell proliferation and neointima formation in both the rat carotid and porcine

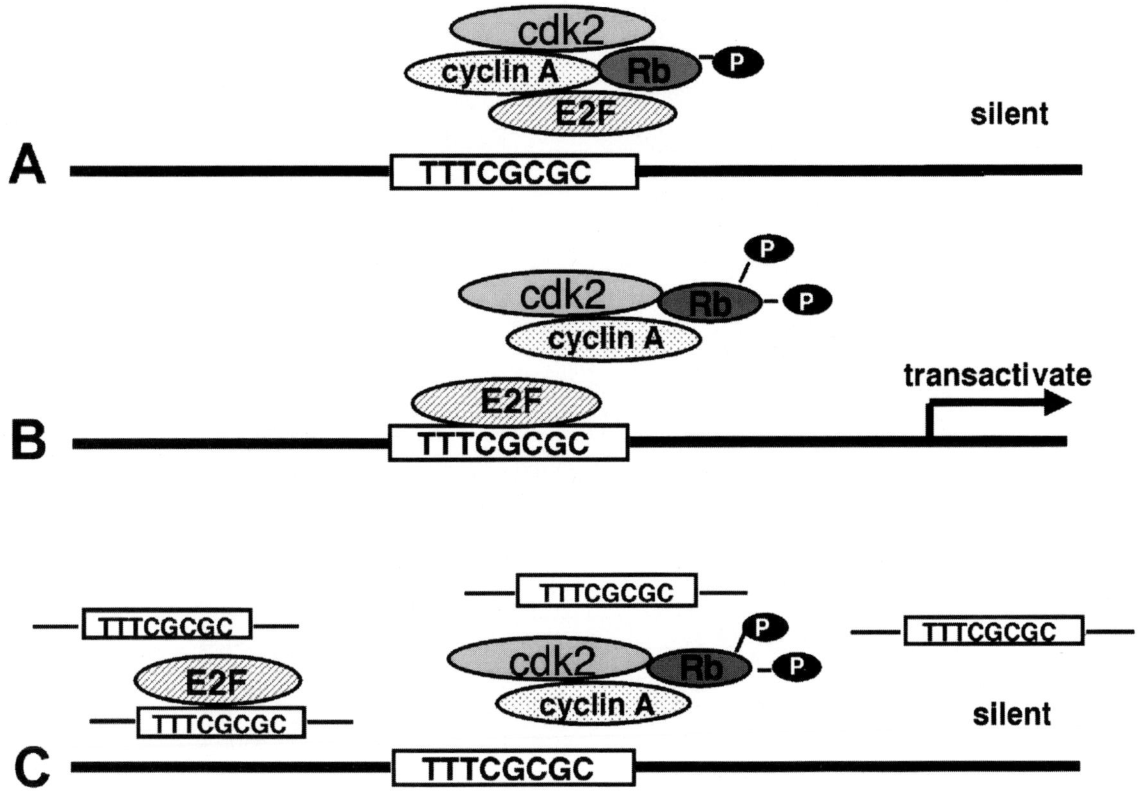

Figure 1 Principle of E2F ''decoy'' strategy. TTTCGCGC, consensus sequence for the E2F-binding site. (A) In quiescent cell state, the transcription factor E2F is complexed Rb (retinoblastoma gene product), cyclin A, and cyclin-dependent kinase cdK2. (B) Phosphorylation of releases free E2F, which binds to *cis* elements of the cell cycle–regulatory genes, resulting in the transactivation of these genes. (C) The E2F decoy *cis*-element double-stranded oligonucleotide binds to free E2F, preventing E2F-mediated transactivation of cell cycle–regulatory genes.

femoral artery models of restenosis (46). Similar results were also obtained by adenovirus-mediated overexpression of a ''natural'' inhibitor of cell cycle progression, the cyclin-dependent kinase inhibitor, p21, that likely prevents hyperphosphorylation of Rb in vivo (47). In addition to blockade of cell cycle gene expression, interruption of mitogenic signal transduction has been achieved in experimental models as well. For example, *Ras* proteins are key transducers of mitogenic signals from membrane to nucleus in many cell types. The local delivery of DNA vectors expressing *Ras* dominant negative mutants, which interfere with *Ras* function, reduced neointimal lesion formation in a rat carotid artery balloon injury model (48).

Nitric oxide mediates a number of biological processes that are thought to mitigate neointima formation in the vessel wall, such as inhibition of VSMC proliferation, reduction of platelet adherence, vasorelaxation, promotion of endothelial cell survival, and possible reduction of oxidative stress. In vivo transfer of plasmid DNA coding for endothelial cell nitric oxide synthase (ecNOS) has been investigated as a potential paracrine strategy to block neointimal disease. EcNOS cDNA driven by a β-actin promoter and CMV enhancer was transfected into the VSMC of rat carotid arteries after balloon injury. This model is known to have no significant regrowth of endothelial cells within 2–3 weeks after injury and therefore is capable of loss of endogenous ecNOS expression. Results revealed expression of the transgene in the vessel wall, along with improved vasomotor reactivity and a 70% inhibition of neointima formation (Fig. 2) (49).

An example of a direct cytotoxic approach to the prevention of neointima formation is the transfer of a ''suicide gene'' such as the herpes simplex virus-TK (HSV-TK) gene into VSMC. Using an adenoviral vector, HSV-TK was introduced into the VSMC of porcine arteries rendering the smooth muscle cells sensitive to the nucleoside

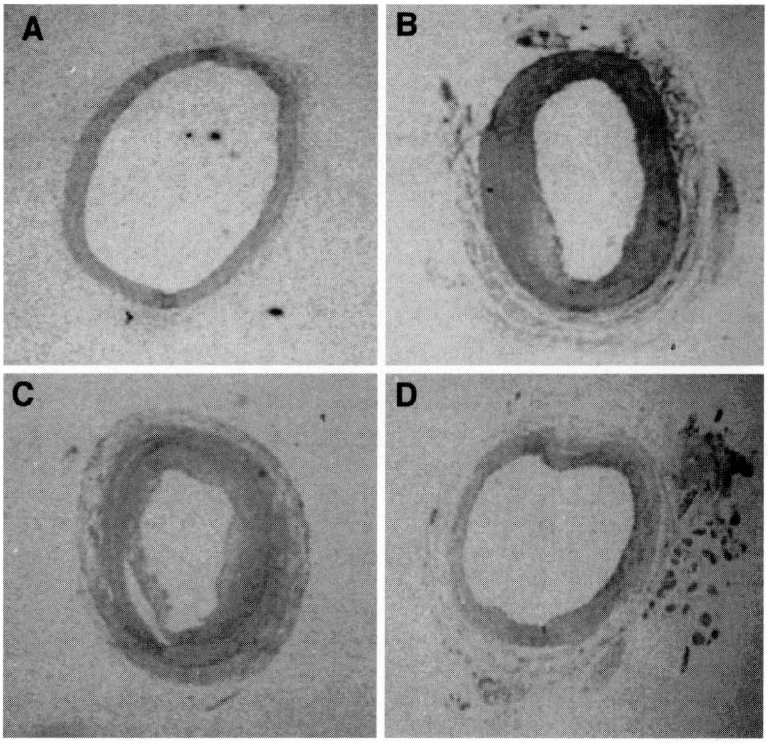

Figure 2 Inhibition of neointimal hyperplasia by in vivo gene transfer of endothelial cell–nitric oxide synthase (ecNOS) in balloon-injured rat carotid arteries. (A) Uninjured control artery (CTRL); (B) injured, untransfected artery (INJ); (C) injured, control vector-transfected artery (INJ + CV); (D) injured, ecNOS-transfected artery (INJ + NOS).

analog gancyclovir given immediately after balloon injury. After one course of gancyclovir treatment, neointimal hyperplasia decreased by about 50% (7). More recently, Pollman and associates (50) induced endogenous machinery for VSMC ''suicide'' in a strategy designed to inhibit the growth or achieve regression of neointimal lesions. This strategy involved antisense ODN blockade of a ''survival'' gene known as Bcl-x, which helps protect cells from activation of programmed cell death or apoptosis.

Another potentially relevant biological target for treatment of restenosis is reendothelialization, which might be accelerated by local delivery of a pro-angiogenic factor (e.g., vascular endothelial cell growth factor, VEGF) at the angioplasty site. This is the basis for the only current U.S. clinical trial of gene therapy for the prevention of restenosis in the peripheral circulation, in which the human VEGF gene is administered as a ''naked'' circular DNA plasmid directly to the injured arterial wall on the surface of the angioplasty balloon (51). The investigators hypothesize that the low efficiency of this delivery method is balanced by the high biological potency of this secreted angiogenic cytokine, enabling a significant local biological effect despite poor gene transfer.

Successful and efficient gene transfer to the injured, atherosclerotic arterial wall presents unique mechanical and kinetic challenges. For strategies designed to attenuate or prevent VSMC proliferation, the target cell mass lies within the media of the vessel wall. Following balloon angioplasty, mechanical disruption and dissection of plaque may facilitate particle delivery to deeper layers of the vessel wall, but uniform gene delivery to the bulk of target VSMC has been difficult to achieve despite the development of a number of specialized local delivery catheters. Experimental models of neointima formation in animals may not be clinically relevant given their high, uniform cellular content and absence of the more predominant noncellular components of complex atherosclerotic plaque in humans.

An ex vivo gene-transfer approach, involving implantation of genetically modified endothelial cells or VSMC at sites of arterial injury, is also being investigated. Conte et al. successfully demonstrated efficient repopulation of denuded rabbit arteries with genetically modified autologous endothelial cells (52). The need to harvest autologous donor tissue for target cells, coupled with the increased costs and complexity of tissue culture, have greatly dampened the enthusiasm for this strategy in favor of more direct methods. Nonetheless, it remains clinically feasible, and, in the case of endothelial cells, the implanted cells alone may confer beneficial properties to the healing arterial wall. Application of these cell transplantation approaches would be greatly facilitated by the development of ''universal donor'' cell lines in which major histocompatibility antigens have been ''knocked out.'' Such a development, while clearly years or decades away, may no longer be merely science fiction fantasy.

In summary, it would appear that the application of gene therapy for postangioplasty restenosis may be somewhat premature (53). In addition to major obstacles in delivering gene-transfer agents to the atherosclerotic vessel wall, the fundamental biological process remains incompletely understood. Nonetheless, continued progress on each of these fronts warrants an optimistic view for genetic approaches to control the arterial injury response. These developments will undoubtedly yield important corollaries for the surgical treatment of arterial occlusive diseases as well.

B. Gene Therapy Versus Molecular Therapy for Angiogenesis

The vascularization observed in neoplastic tissue led researchers such as Judah Folkman in the 1970s to investigate the role of molecular factors in the induction of new blood vessel growth (54). The subsequent identification and characterization of ''angiogenic'' growth factors created an opportunity not only to target the growth of solid tumors but also to attempt the therapeutic ''neovascularization'' of tissue rendered ischemic by occlusive disease in the native arterial bed. Angiogenesis has come to refer more strictly to the sprouting of new capillary networks from preexisting vascular structures, whereas vasculogenesis is the de novo development of both simple and complex vessels during embryonic development. Although it has been clearly established in a number of animal models that angiogenic factors can, in fact, stimulate the growth of capillary networks in vivo, it is less certain that these molecules can induce the development of larger, more complex vessels in adult tissues that would be capable of carrying significantly increased bulk blood flow. Nevertheless, the possibility of an improvement even of just the microvascular collateralization as a ''biological'' approach to the treatment of tissue ischemia has sparked the beginning of human clinical trials in neovascularization therapy.

After the first description of the angiogenic effect of fibroblast growth factors (FGFs), an abundance of ''pro-angiogenic'' factors were discovered to stimulate either endothelial cell proliferation, enhanced endothelial cell migration, or both. Many of these factors possess heparin-binding domains, which not only increase their retention in heparin-rich extracellular matrix but also play critical roles in mediating the interaction of the factors with cell surface receptors. Although the list of angiogenic factors includes such diverse molecules as insulin-like growth factor, hepatocyte growth factor, angiopocitin, and platelet-derived endothelial growth factor, the molecules that have received the most attention as potential therapeutic agents for neovascularization are vascular endothelial growth factor (VEGF) and two members of the FGF family, acidic FGF (FGF-1) and basic FGF (FGF-2).

Whereas all angiogenic factors share some ability to stimulate capillary growth in classical models such as the chick allantoic membrane, much debate persists regarding the optimum agent and the optimum route of delivery for angiogenic therapy in the ischemic human myocardium or lower extremity. VEGF may be the most selective agent for stimulating endothelial cell proliferation, although VEGF receptors are also expressed on a number of inflammatory cells including members of the monocyte-macrophage lineage (55). This selectivity has been viewed as an advantage, since the unwanted stimulation of fibroblasts and VSMC in native arteries might exacerbate the growth of neointimal or atherosclerotic lesions. Despite this theoretical selectivity, however, the experimental use of VEGF in animal models has been associated with not only capillary growth, but also the development of more complex vessels involving these other cell types (56). The FGFs are believed to be even more potent stimulators of endothelial cell proliferation, but, as their name implies, they are much less selective in their pro-proliferative action (57).

Optimizing the route of drug delivery depends heavily on the pharmacokinetic properties of the agent. Angiogenesis, however, is a very complex biological process involving multiple cell types engaged in multiple activities, including extracellular tissue dissolution and remodeling, cell proliferation, cell migration, cell recruitment, and programmed cell death. The role of any single agent must be understood within the complicated orchestration of multiple signaling agents and effectors. Despite the large amount of data that has become available in the past two decades, details of the cellular and molecular mechanisms of angiogenesis remain poorly understood. Still, it is believed that many of the known angiogenic factors, including VEGF and the FGFs, are exquisitely potent and would not, therefore, require large or prolonged dosing regimens. These conclusions are partly based on the results of in vivo experiments in which a broad range of dosing strategies, ranging from implantation of sustained release formulations to single intra-arterial boluses, have been reported to induce similarly successful increases in tissue perfusion (55).

The contribution of gene therapy to the potential development of therapeutic neovascularization is primarily one of drug delivery. The availability of the genetic sequences encoding these paracrine peptide agents provides an opportunity for the establishment of local tissue factories for drug production. Both intravascular as well as extravascular modes of gene product delivery are feasible, as gene transfer can be attempted either in the walls of vessels feeding the ischemic tissue or in the target myocardial or skeletal tissue itself. In fact, muscle tissue of both myocardial and skeletal origin is among the most receptive for gene transfer with the simplest of agents, pure plasmid DNA (58). Adenoviral vectors are also effective at achieving transgene expression in these muscle cells. A number of reports have suggested that plasmid injections can result in long-term gene expression in these muscle tissues, whereas the higher levels of expression associated with adenoviral vectors are likely limited to 1 or 2 weeks (18,59).

Preclinical studies of angiogenic gene therapy have utilized a number of models of chronic ischemia. An increase in capillary density was reported in an ischemic rabbit hind limb model after VEGF administration, and these results did not differ significantly regardless of whether VEGF was delivered as a single intra-arterial bolus of protein, plasmid DNA applied to surface of an upstream arterial wall or direct injection of the plasmid into the ischemic limb (55). Direct injection of an adenoviral vector encoding VEGF also succeeded in improving regional myocardial perfusion and ventricular fractional wall thickening at stress in a model of chronic myocardial ischemia induced via placement of a slowly occluding Ameroid constrictor around the circumflex coronary artery in pigs (60).

Unlike VEGF, FGF-1 and -2 do not possess signal sequences that facilitate secretion of the protein, so that transfer of these genetic sequences is less likely to yield an adequate supply of growth factor to target endothelial cells. To overcome this limitation, Tabata and associates constructed a plasmid encoding a modified FGF-1 molecule onto which a hydrophobic leader sequence had been added to enhance secretion (61). Delivery of this plasmid to the femoral artery wall, even at very low transfection efficiencies, was found to improve capillary density and reduce vascular resistance in the ischemic rabbit hind limb. Applying a similar strategy, Giordano et al. employed intracoronary infusion of 10^{11} viral particles of an adenoviral vector encoding human FGF-5, which does contain a secretory signal sequence at its amino terminus, to achieve enhanced wall thickening with stress and a higher number of capillary structures per myocardial muscle fiber 2 weeks after gene transfer (62).

Another novel approach to molecular neovascularization has been the combination of growth factor gene transfer with a potentially synergistic method of angiogenic stimulation: transmyocardial laser therapy. The formation of transmural laser channels, though not yet fully established as an effective means of generating increased collateral flow, has had documented clinical success in reducing angina scores and improving myocardial perfusion in otherwise untreatable patients. In a porcine Ameroid model, Sayced-shah et al. found that direct injection of plasmid DNA encoding VEGF in the region surrounding laser channel formation yielded better normalization of myocardial function than either therapy alone (63), and this therapeutic strategy can now be delivered either through minimally invasive thoracotomy or a percutaneous catheter-based approach (Fig. 3).

A number of phase I safety studies have been reported in which angiogenic factors or the genes encoding these factors have been administered to patients in small numbers (64,65). These studies have involved either the use of angiogenic factors in patients with peripheral vascular or coronary artery disease who were not candidates for conventional revascularization therapies, or the application of pro-angiogenic factors as an adjunct to conventional revascularization. The modest doses of either protein factors or genetic material delivered in these studies were not associated with any acute toxicities. Concerns remain, however, regarding the safety of potential systemic exposure to molecules known to enhance the growth of possible occult neoplasms or that can enhance diabetic retinopathy and potentially even occlusive arterial disease itself. Despite early enthusiasm, there is also little experience with the administration of live viral vectors in extremely large numbers to a large number of patients, and it is uncertain whether potential biological hazards of reversion to replication competent states or mutation and recombination will eventually become manifest.

In addition to issues of safety, it is also unclear whether the clinical success of conventional revascularization, which has involved the resumption of lost bulk blood flow through larger conduits, will be reproduced via biological strategies that primarily involve increase microscopic collateral networks. It must also be remembered that neovascularization is itself a naturally occurring process and that the addition of a single factor may not overcome conditions that have resulted in an inadequate endogenous neovascularization response in patients suffering from myocardial and lower limb ischemia. Despite these limitations, angiogenic gene therapy may provide an alternative not currently available to a significant number of patients suffering from untreatable disease and may offer an adjunct to

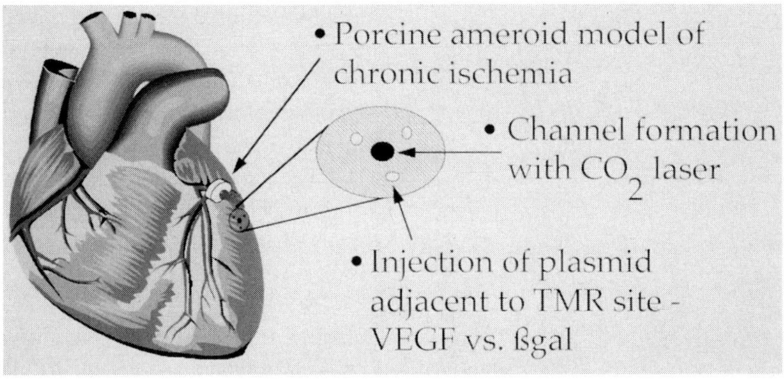

Figure 3 Combined gene transfer and transmyocardial laser revascularization (TMR). Schematic representation of chronic ischemia induced by placement of Ameroid constrictor around the circumflex coronary artery in pigs. Ischemic hearts that underwent TMR followed by injection of plasmid encoding VEGF demonstrated better normalization of myocardial function than either therapy alone.

traditional therapies that improves their long-term outcomes.

IV. GENE THERAPY FOR VASCULAR GRAFTS

A. Vein Graft Engineering with E2F Decoy ODN

The long-term success of surgical revascularization in the lower extremity and coronary circulations has been limited by significant rates of autologous vein graft failure. No pharmacological approach has been successful at preventing long-term graft diseases such as neointimal hyperplasia or graft atherosclerosis. Gene therapy offers a new avenue for the modification of vein graft biology that might lead to a reduction in clinical morbidity from graft failures. Intraoperative transfection of the vein graft also offers an opportunity to combine intact tissue DNA-transfer techniques with the increased safety of ex vivo transfection, and a number of studies have documented the feasibility of ex vivo gene transfer into vein grafts using viral vectors.

Neointimal disease is a significant part of graft remodeling and has been linked to the vast majority of vein graft failures (66). Although neointimal hyperplasia contributes to the reduction of wall stress in vein grafts after bypass, this process can also lead to luminal narrowing of the graft conduit during the first years after operation (67). Furthermore, the abnormal neointimal layer, with its production of pro-inflammatory proteins, is believed to form the basis for an accelerated form of atherosclerosis that causes late graft failure (68).

Similar to observations made in the arterial balloon injury model, it was found that a combination of antisense ODN that inhibit expression of at least two cell cycle–regulatory genes could significantly block neointimal hyperplasia in vein grafts (69). Additionally, E2F decoy ODN yielded similar efficacy in the vein graft when compared to the arterial injury model (70). In contrast to arterial balloon injury, however, vein grafts are not only subjected to a single injury at the time of operation, but are also exposed to chronic hemodynamic stimuli for remodeling. Despite these chronic stimuli, a single, intraoperative ODN treatment of vein grafts resulted in a resistance to neointimal hyperplasia that lasted at least 6 months in the rabbit model (69). During that time period, the grafts treated with antisense ODN were able to adapt to arterial conditions via hypertrophy of the medial layer. Furthermore, these genetically engineered conduits proved resistant to dict-induced graft atherosclerosis (Fig. 4) and were associated with preserved endothelial function (71).

A large-scale, prospective, randomized double-blind trial of human vein graft treatment with E2F decoy ODN has been initiated (18). Efficient delivery of the ODN is accomplished within 15 minutes during the operation by placement of the graft after harvest in a device that exposes the vessel to ODN in physiological solution and creates a nondistending pressurized environment of 300 mmHg. Preclinical findings indicated ODN delivery to greater than 80% of graft cells and effective blockade of target gene expression. This study will measure the effect of cell cycle gene blockade on primary graft failure rates and represents one of the first attempts to definitively determine the feasibility of clinical genetic manipulation in the treatment of a common cardiovascular disorder.

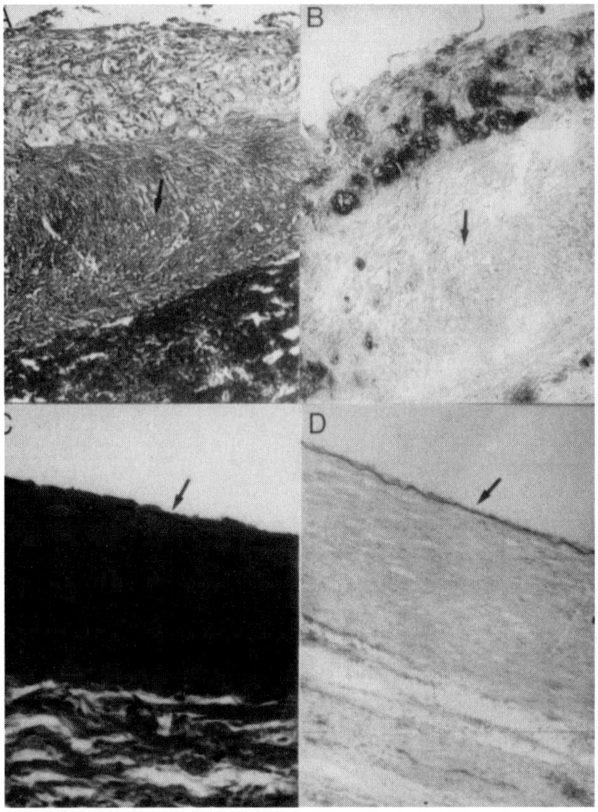

Figure 4 Control oligonucleotide-treated (A and B) and antisense oligonucleotide (against cdc2 kinase/PCNA)–treated vein grafts (C and D) in hypercholesterolemic rabbits, 6 weeks after surgery (70×). Sections were stained with hematoxylin/van Gieson (A and C) and a monoclonal antibody against rabbit macrophages (B and D). Arrows indicate the location of the internal elastic lamina.

B. Vein Graft Gene Transfer

With the development of viral-mediated gene-delivery methods, some investigators have begun to explore the possibility of using these systems ex vivo in autologous vein grafts. Chen et al. (72) demonstrated the expression of the marker gene b-galactosidase along the luminal surface and in the adventitia of 3-day porcine vein grafts infected with a replication-deficient adenoviral vector at the time of surgery. The vein segments were incubated in a high viral titer suspension for approximately 2 hours prior to implantation. Although these researchers documented expression of a soluble vascular cell adhesion molecule-1 (sVCAM-1) isomer on the luminal and abluminal surfaces of 3-day grafts infected with an adenoviral vector encoding this protein, no long-term expression or functional effect of this gene was reported. In a study previously alluded to, Kupfer et al. (73) explored the use of a novel adenovirus-based transduction system, in which adenoviral particles were linked to plasmid DNA via biotin/streptavidin-transferrin/polylysine complexes. β-Galactosidase expression was documented 3 and 7 days after surgery in rabbit vein grafts that had been incubated for 1 hour with complexes prior to grafting. Expression was again greatest on the luminal surfaces of the grafts, although presence of transfected cells in the medial and adventitial layers was also reported.

The feasibility of gene transfer in vein grafts has subsequently lead to the investigation of potential therapeutic endpoints such as neointima formation. George et al. (74), using a replication-deficient adenovirus expressing tissue inhibitor of mettaloproteinasee-2 (TIMP-2), was able to demonstrate a dramatic decrease in neointimal formation in a saphenous vein organ culture model. In vivo gene transfer has also been shown to effectively reduce neointima formation in experimental vein grafts. Bai et al. (75) performed intraoperative transfection of the senescent cell-derived inhibitor (sdi-1) gene, a downstream mediator of the tumor suppresser gene p53, using the HVJ liposome system, and was once again able to demonstrate a significant reduction in neointima formation. The use of gene transfer in vein grafts may reach beyond the treatment of the graft itself. The expression of therapeutic proteins by transduced grafts can lead to the treatment of diseases in tissues downstream to the location of graft implantation, further expanding the versatility of this bypass conduit.

C. Bioprosthetic Grafts

Prosthetic materials, such as PTFE or Dacron, often used as small-caliber arterial substitutes or in the construction of arteriovenous grafts, have been limited in their long-term use due to their thrombogenic surfaces. A bioengineering, cell-based strategy for decreasing or eliminating this thrombogenicity may therefore yield a prosthetic graft capable of maintaining normal flow. Successful isolation of autologous endothelial cells and their seeding onto prosthetic grafts in animal models has been well characterized (76). Furthermore, it has been hypothesized that one can enhance the function of these endothelial cells via the transfer of genes prior to seeding of the cells on the graft surface. Such a bioprosthesis could be useful for delivering genetically engineered factors that would enhance graft function and survival or even provide an avenue for intravascular drug delivery. First indication for the possible use of this strategy was presented by Wilson et al. (10), who demonstrated successful endothelialization of a prosthetic vascular graft with autologous endothelial cells transduced with a recombinant retrovirus encoding the lacZ gene. Additionally, seeding of transduced vascular smooth muscle cells into the interstices of a PTFE graft then luminally seeded with untreated endothelial cells revealed stable expression of the reporter gene after 3–5 weeks (77).

Successful clinical applications of these concepts, however, have not been reported. In an attempt to decrease graft thrombogenicity, Dunn et al. (78) seeded 4 mm Dacron grafts with retrovirally transduced endothelial cells encoding the gene for human tissue plasminogen activator (TPA) and implanted them into the femoral and carotid circulation of sheep. The proteolytic action of TPA resulted in a decrease in seeded endothelial cell adherence, with no improvement in surface thrombogenicity. The use of VEGF in this context also has potentially significant clinical applications. VEGF, a potent endothelial cell mitogen, when transduced into a limited number of endothelial cells and placed on the graft surface, may promote endothelial survival and replication and yield improved and more rapid graft coverage with a nonthrombogenic endothelial layer. Additionally, secretion of VEGF could lead to angiogenesis distal to the grafted area in what is likely to be an ischemic tissue bed. Yamamoto et al. (79) demonstrated successful seeding of PTFE grafts with VEGF-transduced adipose-derived endothelial cells and expression of the transgene after several weeks. Further studies are needed to determine the local effect of VEGF secretion on endothelial cell proliferation along with distant angiogenic stimuli.

V. GENE THERAPY FOR THE HEART

Failure of the myocardium due to insults such as ischemia, infection, metabolic disorders, or substance abuse afflicts millions of Americans annually. Traditional pharmacotherapy and surgical intervention has succeeded in ameliorating these problems, but the advent of gene-transfer technology has brought a heightened interest to either correcting, preventing, or limiting the functional deficits sustained by the myocardium. The myocardium has been shown to be receptive to the introduction of foreign genes. As seen in noncardiac muscle (80), measurable levels of gene activity have been found after direct injection of plasmids into myocardial tissue in vivo (81). Although limited to a few millimeters surrounding the injection site, these observations have laid the basis for consideration of gene transfer as a therapeutic approach to cardiac disease. The distribution of myocardial expression of genes after direct injection in rats has been enhanced via incorporation of the gene into an adenoviral vector (59). Additionally, both adenoviral and adeno-associated viral vectors can be delivered to the myocardial and coronary vascular cells via intracoronary infusion of highly concentrated preparations in rabbits and porcine models, respectively (82,83). Gene transfer into the myocardium has also been achieved via either direct injection or intracoronary infusion of myoblast cells that have been genetically engineered in cell culture (84).

A. Gene Therapy to Enhance Contractility

The β-adrenergic receptor (β-AR) is known to be a critical player in mediating the ionotropic state of the heart and has received significant attention as a target for genetic therapeutic intervention in congestive heart failure. Milano et al. (85), using transgenic mice expressing the β_2-AR under the control of the cardiac α-MHC promoter, demonstrated an approximately 200-fold increase in the level of β_2-AR along with highly enhanced contractility and increased heart rates in the absence of exogenous β-agonists. This genetic manipulation of the myocardium has generated considerable interest in the use of gene transfer of the β-AR gene into the ailing myocardium as a means of therapeutic intervention. To date, attempts at exploring this exciting possibility have been primarily limited to cell culture systems. Akhter et al. (86) successfully demonstrated improved contractility in rabbit ventricular myocytes, which have been chronically paced to produce hemodynamic failure after adenoviral-mediated gene transfer of the human β_2-AR. An enhanced chronotropic effect resulting from the injection of a β_2-AR plasmid construct into the right atrium of mice has been demonstrated by Edelberg et al. (87), but no evaluation of enhanced contractility by transfer of this gene into the ventricle has been reported. These results demonstrate the feasibility of using the β-adrenergic pathway and its regulators as a means by which to treat the endpoint effect of the variety of cardiac insults that exist.

There has also been recent interest in the enhancement of contractility through the manipulation of intracellular calcium levels. Sarcoplasmic reticulum Ca^{2+}-ATPase (SERCA2a) transporting enzyme, which regulates Ca^{2+} sequestration into the sarcoplasmic reticulum (SR), has been shown to be decreased in a variety of human and experimental cardomyopathies. Using adenoviral-mediated gene transfer, Hajjar et al. (88) were able to overexpress the SERCA2a protein in neonatal rat cardiomyocytes. This led to an increase in the peak $[Ca^{2+}]_i$ release, a decrease in resting $[Ca^{2+}]_i$ levels, and more importantly to enhanced contraction of the myocardial cells as detected by shortening measurements. The success of this approach to improving myocardial contractility has yet to be documented in vivo, but once again it provides a novel and potentially exciting means by which to treat the failed heart.

B. Gene Therapy for Myocardial Infarction

Coronary artery atherosclerosis and resulting myocardial ischemia is a leading cause of death in developed countries.

Reperfusion injury has been linked to significant cellular damage and progression of the ischemic insult. In addition to stimulating therapeutic neovascularization, genetic manipulation may be used as a means to limit the degree of injury sustained by the myocardium after ischemia and reperfusion.

The process of tissue damage resulting from ischemia and reperfusion has been well characterized. Briefly, the period of ischemia leads to an accumulation of adenosine monophosphate, which then leads to increased levels of hypoxanthine within and around cells in the affected area. Additionally, increased conversion of xanthine dehydrogenase into xanthine oxidase takes place, which upon exposure to oxygen during the period of reperfusion converts hypoxanthine to xanthine, leaving behind the cytotoxic oxygen radical, superoxide anion (O_2^-). O_2^- can then go on to form hydrogen peroxide (H_2O_2), another oxygen radical species. Ferrous iron (Fe^{2+}), which accumulates during ischemia, reacts with H_2O_2, which leads to the formation of the most potent oxygen radical, hydroxyl anion (OH^-) (89). These oxygen radicals result in cellular injury via lipid peroxidation of the plasma membrane, oxidation of sulfhydryl groups of intracellular and membrane proteins, nucleic acid injury, and breakdown of components of the extracellular matrix, such as collagen and hyaluronic acid (90). Natural oxygen radical scavengers, such as superoxide dismutase (SOD), catalase, glutathione peroxidase, and hemoxygenase (HO), function through various mechanisms to remove oxygen radicals produced in normal and injured tissues.

The degree of oxygen radical formation produced after ischemia-reperfusion in the heart can overwhelm the natural scavenger systems. Overexpression of either extracellular SOD (ecSOD) or manganese SOD (MnSOD) in transgenic mice has revealed improved postischemic cardiac function and decreased cardiomyocyte mitochondrial injury in adriamycin-treated mice, respectively (91,92). These findings suggest a role for gene transfer of these natural scavengers as a means by which to protect the myocardium in the event of an ischemia-reperfusion event. Li et al. (93) demonstrated substantial protection against myocardial stunning using intra-arterial injection of an adenovirus containing the gene for Cu/ZnSOD (the cytoplasmic isoform) into rabbits, although no studies have investigated the direct antioxidant effect and ensuing improvement in myocardial function of this treatment after ischemia and reperfusion. This application of gene therapy technology may offer a novel and exciting approach for prophylaxis against myocardial ischemic injury if incorporated into a system of long-term, regulatable transgene expression. In addition to the overexpression of antioxidant genes, some researchers have proposed intervening in the program of gene expression within the myocardium that leads to the downstream deleterious effects of ischemia reperfusion. For example, the transfection of rat myocardium with decoy oligonucleotides that block activity of the oxidation-sensitive transcription factor NFκ-B, linked to expression of a number of pro-inflammatory genes, succeeded in reducing infarct size after coronary artery ligation (94).

At the cellular level, myocardial infarction results in the formation of scar, which is composed of cardiac fibroblasts. Given the terminal differentiation of cardiomyocytes, loss of cell mass due to infarction does not result in the regeneration of myocytes to repopulate the wound. Researchers have therefore pursued the possibility of genetically converting cardiac fibroblasts into functional cardiomyocytes. The feasibility of this notion gained support from the work of Tam et al. (95), who demonstrated the in vitro conversion of cardiac fibroblasts into cells resembling skeletal myocytes via the forced expression of a skeletal muscle lineage–determining gene, *MyoD,* using retroviral-mediated gene transfer. Fibroblasts expressing the *MyoD* gene were observed to develop multinucleated myotubes similar to those seen in striated muscle which expressed MHC and myocyte-specific enhancer factor-2. Additionally, Murry et al. (96) also showed expression of myogenin and embryonic skeletal MHC after transfection of rat hearts injured by freeze-thaw with an adenovirus containing the *MyoD* gene. At this time, however, functional cardiomyocytes have not yet been identified in regions of myocardial scarring treated with in vivo gene transfer.

C. Gene Therapy for Immunomodulation

Genetic manipulation of donor tissues offers the opportunity to design organ-specific immunosuppression during cardiac transplantation. Although transgenic animals are being explored as potential sources for immunologically protected xenografts (97), the delivery of genes for immunosuppressive proteins, or the blockade of certain genes in human donor grafts, may allow site-specific, localized immunosuppression and a reduction or elimination of the need for toxic systemic immunosuppressive regimens. Gene activity has been documented in transplanted mouse hearts for at least 2 weeks after intraoperative injection of the tissue with either plasmid DNA, retroviral, or adenoviral vectors (98). The transfer of a gene for either TGF-β or IL-10 in a small area of the heart via direct injection in this model succeded in inhibiting cell-mediated immunity and delaying acute rejection (99,100). In another study, the systemic administration of antisense ODN directed against intercellular adhesion molecule-1 (ICAM-1) also prolonged graft survival and induced long-term graft tolerance when combined with a monoclonal antibody against the ligand for ICAM-1, leukocyte function antigen (101,102).

VI. SUMMARY

Gene therapy has begun a gradual ascent from the realm of pure theory and has entered a period of intense research into practical clinical applications. Although the first documentation of clinical success remains eagerly sought, gene manipulation strategies appear now to provide a meaningful addition to the tools available in the design of novel approaches to cardiovascular disease. Further refinement of both current gene therapy methodologies as well as the cardiovascular biologist's understanding of the molecular basis of complex disease processes will enhance the likelihood of such success and may prove essential to its realization. Nevertheless, ''proof of principle'' has been clearly established; a thoughtful and thorough scientific approach has therefore become warranted as these exciting new possibilities continue to expand.

REFERENCES

1. Danos O, Mulligan RO. Safe and efficient generation of recombinant retroviruses and amphotrophic and ecotrophic host ranges. Proc Natl Acad Sci USA 1988; 85: 6460–6464.
2. Dzau VJ, Gibbons GH, Cooke JP, et al. Vascular biology and medicine in the 1990s: Scope, concepts, potentials, and perspectives. Circulation 1993; 87:705–719.
3. Berg P, Singer MF. The recombinant DNA controversy twenty years later. Proc Natl Acad Sci USA 1995; 92: 9011–9013.
4. Colman A. Antisense strategies in cell and developmental biology. J Cell Sci 1990; 97:399–409.
5. Zaug A, Been M, Cech T. The Tetrahymena ribozyme acts like an RNA restriction endonuclease. Nature 1986; 324: 429–433.
6. Bielinska A, Schivdasani RA, Zhang L, et al. Regulation of gene expression with double-stranded phosphothioate oligonucleotides. Science 1990; 250:997–1000.
7. Ohno T, Gordon D, San H, Pompili VJ, et al. Gene therapy for vascular smooth muscle cell proliferation after arterial injury. Science 1994; 265:781–784.
8. Newman KD, Dunn PF, Owens JW, et al. Adenovirus-mediated gene transfer into normal rabbit arteries results in prolonged vascular cell activation, inflammation, and neointimal hyperplasia. J Clin Invest 1995; 96:2955–2965.
9. Nabel EG, Plautz G, Nabel GJ. Site-specific gene expression in vivo by direct gene transfer into the arterial wall. Science 1990; 249:1285–1288.
10. Wilson JM, Birinyi LK, Salomon RN, et al. Implantation of vascular grafts lined with genetically modified endothelial cells. Science 1989; 244:1344–1346.
11. Brody SL, Crystal RG. Adenovirus-mediated in vivo gene transfer. Ann NY Acad Sci 1994; 716:90–101.
12. Muzyczka N. Use of adeno-associated virus as a general transduction vector for mammalian cells. Curr Top Microbiol Immunol 1992; 158:97–129.
13. Svensson EC, Marshall DJ, Woodard K, et al. Efficient and stable transduction of cardiomyocytes after intramyocardial injection or intracoronary perfusion with recombinant adeno-associated virus vectors. Circulation 1999; 99: 201–205.
14. Felgner PL, Gader TR, Holm M, et al. Lipofectin: a highly efficient, lipid mediated DNA-transfection procedure. Proc Natl Acad Sci USA 1987; 84:7413–7417.
15. Qin L, Pahud DR, Ding Y, et al. Efficient transfer of genes into murine cardiac grafts by starburst polyamidoamone dendrimers. Hum Gene Ther 1998; 9:553–560.
16. Dzau VJ, Mann MJ, Morishita R, et al. Fusigenic viral liposome for gene therapy in cardiovascular diseases. Proc Natl Acad Sci USA 1996; 93:11421–11425.
17. Lin H, Parmacek MS, Morle G, et al. Expression of recombinant gene in myocardium in vivo after direct injection of DNA. Circulation 1990; 82:2217–2221.
18. Mann MJ, Whittemore AD, Donaldson MC, et al. Preliminary clinical experience with genetic engineering of human vein grafts: Evidence for target gene inhibition. Circulation 1997; 96:I4.
19. Kadambi VJ, Ponniah S, Harrer JM, et al. Cardiac-specific overexpression of phospholamban alters calcium kinetics and resultant cardiomyocyte mechanics in transgenic mice. J Clin Invest 1996; 97:533–539.
20. Yu Z, Redfern CS, Fishman GI. Conditional transgene expression in the heart. Circ Res 1996; 79:691–697.
21. Prentice H, Bishopric NH, Hicks MN, et al. Regulated expression of a foreign gene targeted to the ischemic myocardium. Cardiovasc Res 1997; 35:567–574.
22. Grundy SM, Vega GL. Causes of high blood cholesterol. Circulation 1990; 81:412–427.
23. Chowdhury JR, Grossman M, Gupta S, et al. Long term improvement of hypercholesterolemia after ex vivo gene therapy in LDLR-deficient rabbits. Science 1991; 254: 1802–1805.
24. Randall T. First gene therapy for inherited hypercholesterolemia a partial success. JAMA 1993; 269:837–838.
25. Grossman M, Raper SE, Kozarsky KF, et al. Successful ex vivo gene therapy directed to liver in patient with familial hypercholesterolemia. Nat Genet 1994; 6:335–341.
26. Kobayashi K, Oka K, Forte T, et al. Reversal of hypercholesterolemia in low density lipoprotein receptor knockout mice by adenovirus-mediated gene transfer of the very low density lipoprotein receptor. J Biol Chem 1996; 274: 6852–6860.
27. Kozarsky KF, McKinley DR, Austin LL, et al. In vivo correction of low density lipoprotein receptor deficiency in the Watanabe heritable hyperlipidemic rabbit with recombinant adenovirus. J Biol Chem 1994; 269: 13695–13702.

28. Ishibashi S, Brown MS, Goldstein JL, et al. Hypercholesterolemia in low density lipoprotein receptor knockout mice and its reversal by adenovirus-mediated gene delivery. J Clin Invest 1993; 92:883–893.
29. Li J, Fang B, Eisensmith RC, et al. In vivo gene therapy for hyperlipidemia: phenotypic correction in Watanabe rabbits by hepatic delivery of the rabbit LDL receptor gene. J Clin Invest 1995; 95:768–773.
30. Kozarsky KF, Jooss K, Donahee MJF, et al. Effective treatment of familial hypercholesterolemia in the mouse model using adenovirus-mediated transfer of the VLDL receptor gene. Nat Genet 1996; 3:54–62.
31. Stevenson SC, Marshall-Neff J, Teng B, et al. Phenotypic correction of hypercholesterolemia in apoE-deficient mice by adenovirus-mediated in vivo gene transfer. Arterioscler Thromb Vasc Biol 1995; 15:479–484.
32. Kopfler WP, Willard M, Betz T, et al. Adenovirus-mediated transfer of a gene encoding human apolipoprotein A-I into normal mice increases circulating high-density lipoprotein cholesterol. Circulation 1994; 90:1319–1327.
33. Gibbons GH, Dzau VJ. The emerging concept of vascular remodeling. N Engl J Med 1994; 330:1431–1438.
34. Tanaka H, Sukhova GK, Swanson SJ, et al. Sustained activation of vascular cells and leukocytes in the rabbit aorta after balloon injury. Circulation 1993; 88:1788–1803.
35. Bendeck MP, Irvin C, Reidy MA. Inhibition of matrix metaloproteinase activity inhibits smooth muscle cell migration but not neointimal thickening after arterial injury. Circ Res 1996; 78:38–42.
36. Loppnow H, Libby P. Proliferating or interleukin 1-activated human vascular smooth muscle cells secrete copious interleukin 6. J Clin Invest 1990; 85:731–738.
37. Wenzel VO, Fouqueray B, Grandaliano G, et al. Thrombin regulates expression of monocyte chemoattractant protein-1 in vascular smooth muscle cells. Cir Res 1995; 77: 503–509.
38. Morishita R, Gibbons GH, Ellison KE, et al. Single intraluminal delivery of antisense cdc2 kinase and proliferating-cell nuclear antigen oligonucleotides results in chronic inhibition of neointimal hyperplasia. Proc Natl Acad Sci USA 1993; 90:8474–8478.
39. Morishita R, Gibbons GH, Kaneda Y, et al. Pharmacokinetics of antisense oligodeoxynucleotides (cyclin B1 and cdc2 kinase) in the vessel wall in vivo: enhanced therapeutic utility for restenosis by HVJ-liposome delivery. Gene 1994; 149:13–19.
40. Simons M, Edelman ER, DeKeyser JL, et al. Antisense c-myb oligonucleotides inhibit intimal arterial smooth muscle cell accumulation in vivo. Nature 1992; 359:67–70.
41. Shi Y, Fard A, Galeo A, et al. Transcatheter delivery of c-myc antisense oligomers reduce neointimal formation in a porcine model of coronary artery balloon injury. Circulation 1994; 90:944–951.
42. Villa AE, Guzman LA, Poptic EJ, et al. Effects of antisense c-myb oligonucleotides on vascular smooth muscle cell proliferation and response to vessel wall injury. Circ Res 1995; 76:505–513.
43. Burgess TL, Fisher EF, Ross SL, et al. The antiproliferative activity of c-myb and c-myc antisense oligonucleotides in smooth muscle cells is caused by nonantisense mechanism. Proc Natl Acad Sci USA 1995; 92: 4051–4055.
44. Hiebert SW, Lipp M, Nevins JR, et al. E1A-dependent trans-activation of the human MYC promoter is mediated by the E2F factor. Proc Natl Acad Sci USA 1989; 89: 3594–3598.
45. Morishita R, Gibbons GH, Horiuchi M, et al. A novel molecular strategy using cis element ''decoy'' of E2F binding site inhibits smooth muscle proliferation in vivo. Proc Natl Acad Sci USA 1995; 92:5855–5859.
46. Chang MW, Barr E, Seltzer J, et al. Cytostatic gene therapy for vascular proliferative disorders with a constitutively active form of the retinoblastoma gene product. Science 1995; 267:518–522.
47. Chang MW, Barr E, Lu MM, et al. Adenovirus-mediated over-expression of the cyclin/cyclin dependent kinase inhibitor, p21 inhibits vascular smooth muscle cell proliferation and neointima formation in the rat carotid artery model of balloon angioplasty. J Clin Invest 1995; 96:2260–2268.
48. Indolfi C, Avvedimento EV, Rapacciuolo A, et al. Inhibition of cellular ras prevents smooth muscle cell proliferation after vascular injury in vivo. Nature Med 1995; 1: 541–545.
49. von der Leyen HE, Gibbons GH, Morishita R, et al. Gene therapy inhibiting neointimal vascular lesion: in vivo gene transfer of endothelial-cell nitric oxide synthase gene. Proc Natl Acad Sci USA 1995; 92:1137–1141.
50. Pollman MJ, Hall JL, Mann MJ, et al. Inhibition of neointimal cell bcl-x expression induces apoptosis and regression of vascular disease. Nat Med 1998; 4:222–227.
51. Isner JM, Walsh K, Rosenfield K, et al. Clinical protocol: arterial gene therapy for restenosis. Hum Gene Ther 1996; 7:989–1011.
52. Conte, MS, Birinyi LK, Miyata T, et al. Efficient repopulation of denuded rabbit arteries with autologous genetically modified endothelial cells. Circulation 1994; 89: 2161–2169.
53. DeYoung MB, Dichek DA. Gene therapy for restenosis. Are we ready? Circ Res 1998; 82:306–313.
54. Folkman J, Merler E, Abernathy C, et al. Isolation of a tumor factor responsible or angiogenesis. J Exp Med 1971; 133:275–288.
55. Ware JA, Simons M. Angiogenesis in ischemic heart disease. Nat Med 1997; 8:158–164.
56. Banai S, Jaklitsch MT, Shou M, et al. Angiogenic-induced enhancement of collateral blood flow to ischemic myocardium by vascular endothelial growth factor in dogs. Circulation 1994; 89:2183–2189.
57. Folkman J, Klagsburn M. Angiogenic factors. Science 1987; 235:442–447.
58. Buttrick PM, Kass A, Kitsis RN, et al. Behavior of genes directly injected into the rat heart in vivo. Circ Res 1992; 70:193–198.

59. Guzman RJ, Lemarchand P, Crystal RG, et al. Efficient gene transfer into myocardium by direct injection of adenovirus vectors. Circ Res 1993; 73:1202–1207.
60. Mack CA, Patel SR, Schwarz EA, et al. Biologic bypass with the use of adenovirus-mediated gene transfer of the complementary deoxyribonucleic acid for vascular endothelial growth factor 121 improves myocardial perfusion and function in the ischemic porcine heart. J Thorac Cardiovasc Surg 1998; 115:168–176.
61. Tabata H, Silver M, Isner JM. Arterial gene transfer of acidic fibroblast growth factor for therapeutic angiogenesis in vivo: critical role of secretion signal in use of naked DNA. Cardiovasc Res 1997; 35:470–479.
62. Giordano FJ, Ping P, McKirnan MD, et al. Intracoronary gene transfer of fibroblast growth factor-5 increases blood flow and contractile function in an ischemic region of the heart. Nat Med 1996; 2:534–539.
63. Sayeed-Shah U, Mann MJ, Martin J, et al. Complete reversal of ischemic wall motion abnormalities by combined use of gene therapy with transmyocardial laser revascularization. J Thorac Cardiovasc Surg 1998; 116:763–769.
64. Schumacher B, Pecher P, von Specht BU, et al: Induction of neoangiogenesis in ischemic myocardium by human growth factors: first clinical results of a new treatment of coronary heart disease. Circulation. 1998; 97:645–50.
65. Losordo DW, Vale PR, Symes JF, et al. Gene therapy for myocardial angiogenesis: initial clinical results with direct myocardial injection of phVEGF165 as sole therapy for myocardial ischemia. Circulation 1998; 98:2800–2804.
66. Bryan AJ, Angelini GD. The biology of saphenous vein graft occlusion: etiology and strategies for prevention. Curr Opin Cardiol 1994; 9:641–649.
67. Zwolak RM, Adams MC, Clowes AW. Kinetics of vein graft hyperplasia: association with tangential stress. J Vasc Surg 1987; 5:126–136.
68. Cox JL, Chiasson DA, Gotlieg AI. Stranger in a strange land: the pathogenesis of saphenous vein graft stenosis with emphasis on structural and functional differences between veins and arteries. Prog Cardiovasc Dis 1991; 84: 45–68.
69. Mann MJ, Gibbons GH, Kernoff RS, et al. Genetic engineering of vein grafts resistant to atherosclerosis. Proc Natl Acad Sci USA 1995; 92:4502–4506.
70. Mann MJ, Dzau VJ. Vein graft gene therapy using E2F-decoy oligonucleotides: target gene inhibition in human veins and long-term resistence to atherosclerosis in rabbits. Surg Forum 1997; 48:242–244.
71. Mann MJ, Gibbons GH, Tsao PS, et al. Cell cycle inhibition preserves endothelial function in genetically engineered rabbit vein grafts. J Clin Invest 1997; 99: 1295–1301.
72. Chen S-J, Wilson JM, Muller DWM. Adenovirus-mediated gene transfer of soluble vascular cell adhesion molecule to porcine interposition vein grafts. Circulation 1994; 89:1922–1928.
73. Kupfer JM, Ruan XM, Liu G, et al. High efficiency gene transfer to autologous rabbit jugular vein grafts using adenovirus-transferrin/polylysine-DNA complexes. Hum Gene Ther 1994; 5:1437–1443.
74. George SJ, Baker AH, Angelini GD, et al. Gene transfer of tissue inhibitor of metalloproteinase-2 inhibits metalloproteinase activity and neointima formation in human saphenous veins. Gene Ther 1998; 5:1552–1560.
75. Bai H, Morishita R, Kida I, et al. Inhibition of intimal hyperplasia after vein grafting by in vivo transfer of human senescent cell-derived inhibitor-1 gene. Gene Ther 1998; 5:761–769.
76. Herring MB. Endothelial cel seeding. J Vasc Surg 1991; 13:731–732.
77. Geary RL, Clowes AW, Lau S, et al. Gene transfer in baboons using prosthetic vascular grafts seeded with retrovirally transduced smooth muscle cells: a model for local and systemic gene therapy. Hum Gene Ther 1994; 5: 1211–1216.
78. Dunn PF, Newman KD, Jones M, et al. Seeding of vascular grafts with genetically modified endothelial cells. Secretion of recombinant TPA results in decreased seeded cell retention in vitro and in vivo. Circulation 1996; 93: 1439–1446.
79. Yamamoto K, Takahashi K, Dzau VJ, et al. Human VEGF gene transfer into vascular prosthesis. Circulation 1996; 94(suppl I):I–637.
80. Wolff JA, Malone RW, Williams P. Direct gene transfer into mouse muscle in vivo. Science 1990; 247:1465–1468.
81. Lin H, Parmacek MS, Leiden JM. Expression of recombinant genes in myocardium in vivo after direct injection of DNA. Circulation 1990; 82:2217–2221.
82. Barr E, Carroll J, Kalynych AM, et al. Efficient catheter-mediated gene transfer into the heart using replication-defective adenovirus. Gene Ther 1994; 1:51–58.
83. Kaplitt MG, Xiao X, Samulski RJ, et al. Long-term gene transfer in porcine myocardium after coronary infusion of an adeno-associated virus vector. Ann Thorac Surg 1996; 62:1669–1676.
84. Blau HM, Springer ML. Muscle-mediated gene therapy. N Engl J Med 1995; 333:1554–1556.
85. Milano CA, Allen LF, Rockman HA, et al. Enhanced myocardial function in transgenic mice overexpressing the beta 2-adrenergic receptor. Science 1994; 265:582–586.
86. Akhter SA, Skaer CA, Kypson AP, et al. Restoration of beta-adrenergic signaling in failing cardiac ventricular myocytes via adenoviral-mediated gene transfer. Proc Natl Acad Sci USA 1997; 94:12100–12105.
87. Edelberg JM, Aird WC, Rosenberg RD. Enhancement of murine cardiac chronotropy by the molecular transfer of human beta2 adrenergic receptor DNA. J Clin Invest 1998; 101:337–343.
88. Hajjar RJ, Kang JX, Gwathmey JK. Physiological effects of adenoviral gene transfer of sarcoplasmic reticulum calcium ATPase in isolated rat myocytes. Circulation 1997; 95:423–429.
89. Flaherty JT. Myocardial injury mediated by oxygen free radicals. Am J Med 1991; 91(suppl 3C):79S–85S.

90. Grace PA. Ischaemia-reperfusion injury. Br J Surg 1994; 81:637–647.
91. Chen EP, Bittner HB, Davis D, et al. Extracellular superoxide dismutase transgene overexpression preserves postischemic myocardial function in isolated murine hearts. Circulation 1996; 94[suppl II]:II412–II417.
92. Yen H-C, Oberley TD, Vichitbandha S, et al. The protective role of manganese superoxide dismutase against adriamycin-induced acute cardiac toxicity in transgenic mice. J Clin Invest 1996; 98:1253–1260.
93. Li Q, Bolli R, Qiu Y, et al. Gene therapy with extracellular superoxide dismutase attenuates myocardial stunning in conscious rabbits. Circulation 1998; 98:1438–1448.
94. Morishita R, Sugimoto T, Aoki M, et al. In vivo transfection of cis element ''decoy'' against nuclear factor-kappaB binding site prevents myocardial infarction. Nat Med 1997; 3:894–899.
95. Tam SK, Gu W, Nadal-Ginard B. Molecular cardiomyoplasty: potential cardiac gene therapy for chronic heart failure. J Thorac Cardiovasc Surg 1995; 109:918–924.
96. Murry CE, Kay MA, Bartosek T, et al. Muscle differentiation during repair of myocardial necrosis in rats via gene transfer with MyoD. J Clin Invest 1996; 98:2209–2217.
97. McCurry KR, Diamond LE, Kooyman DL, et al. Human complement regulatory proteins expressed in transgenic swine protect swine xenografts from humoral injury. Transplant Proc 1996; 28:758.
98. Qin L, Chavin KD, Ding Y, et al. Multiple vectors effectively achieve gene transfer in a murine cardiac transplantation model. Immunosuppression with TGF-beta 1 or vIL-10. Transplantation 1995; 59:809–816.
99. Qin L, Ding Y, Bromberg, JS. Gene transfer of transforming growth factor-beta 1 prolongs murine cardiac allograft survival by inhibiting cell-mediated immunity. Hum Gene Ther 1996; 7:1981–1988.
100. Qin L, Chavin KD, Ding Y, et al. Retrovirus-mediated transfer of viral IL-10 gene prolongs murine cardiac allograft survival. J Immunol 1996; 156:2316–2323.
101. Stepkowski SM, Tu Y, Condon TP, et al. Blocking of heart allograft rejection by intracellular adhesion molecule-1 antisense oligonucleotides alone or in combination with other immunosuppressive modalities. J Immunol 1994; 153: 5336–5346.
102. Poston RS, Mann MJ, Rode S, et al: Ex vivo gene therapy and LFA-1 monoclonal antibody combine to yield long-term tolerance to cardiac allografts. J Heart Lung Transplant 1997; 16:41.

22

Gene Therapy for Cancer

Karsten Brand
Humboldt-University Berlin, Berlin-Buch, Germany

Gerhard Wolff
Theragen AG, Biomedical Research Campus, Berlin-Buch, Germany

Michael Strauss†
Humboldt-University Berlin, Berlin-Buch, Germany

I. INTRODUCTION

Gene therapy for cancer is one of the most advanced applications of gene transfer technology in medicine. The field has experienced great interest for nearly a decade and intensive experimental and clinical investigations are underway. In general, it comprises different technologies to deliver a cDNA of choice to cancer cells or normal tissue for a variety of diagnostic and therapeutic applications. Based on the complex nature of cancer, these technologies are very heterogeneous, as demonstrated by different concepts such as immunomodulation, the ''suicide strategy'' (i.e., transfer of the cDNA of a prodrug converting enzyme), gene-replacement strategies like transfer of a tumor suppressor and/or an oncogene, viral oncolysis, antiangiogenic gene therapy, or the delivery of drug-resistance genes into hematopoietic precursor cells. Thus, gene therapy for cancer has multiple goals, including cancer cell death, prevention of metastasis, and protection of hematopoietic precursor cells.

II. THERAPEUTIC PRINCIPLES

A. Immunomodulation

It has been long recognized that tumors exhibit to a certain extent immunogenicity (1). As demonstrated by several studies, the human immune system seems to respond to this immunogenicity by recognizing specific tumor antigens and, consequently, by mounting humoral and cellular responses. However, during cancer development, this response is of limited intensity and time of duration (2,3). As the mechanisms by which cancer cells manage to escape detection by the immune system are being elucidated, more and more strategies are developed to reconstitute an effective antitumor immune response. The tremendous increase in knowledge about the immunobiology of cancer has made immunological approaches (e.g., immunomodulation) the most dominant strategy in gene therapy for cancer during recent years (4). In general, immunomodulation studies can be categorized according to (a) the target cells (tumor cells, host cells, T cells, or antigen presenting cells such as dendritic cells or other cells), (b) the mode of gene delivery (which vector, in vitro, ex vivo, or in vivo), or (c) the transferred transgenes (cytokines, costimulatory molecules, tumor-associated antigens). To illustrate the variety of these approaches, four examples will be described in more detail.

One of the most attractive target cell types to be genetically modified are T lymphocytes. The application of cytokine-transduced tumor-infiltrating T lymphocytes (TILs) (5–8) was among the earliest clinical protocols for gene therapy. More recently, T lymphocytes have been the target for ex vivo genetic modification by cytokine gene transfer

† Deceased.

and redirection by chimeric receptor genes (one side against tumor antigen, one side against, e.g., CD3 or GM-CSF) or have been isolated from genetically modified tumors or their draining lymph nodes (9–11). More recent developments enhance T-cell reactivity with antibodies targeted directly at the respective receptors on T cells (12,13). These approaches are completed in different ways to enhance antigen recognition on the surface of tumor cells.

Another immunological approach to generate a local inflammatory response is the use of short-range communications between immune and nonimmune cells by transferring cytokine-transfected tumor cells or fibroblasts, which are then supposed to directly activate specific as well as nonspecific immune cells. In this context, the continuous local release of cytokines has been shown to increase the therapeutic index. Additionally or alternatively, costimulatory molecules can be transferred. In tumor cells where major histocompatibility complex (MHC) molecules or costimulatory molecules such as B7 are downregulated, the transfer of the corresponding wild-type cDNA can reactivate antigen recognition on the surface of the transduced tumor cells.

During the last decade, more and more tumor-derived antigens have been defined, providing an interesting target for gene-transfer approaches (14). Besides application of the respective peptides, some of these antigens were transferred by viral vectors or as naked DNA either directly to the tumors or via dendritic cells, and an immune response against the tumor was evoked. Detection of new tumor antigens with powerful new methods such as SEREX [serological analysis of tumor antigens by recombinant expression cloning (2,15)] holds great promise for the future. Finally, antibody-based immunotherapy should be mentioned in this context (16). The underlying concept of this strategy is to raise monoclonal antibodies against soluble tumor antigens or against antigens that are expressed on the surface of the malignant cells or on the tumor stroma.

B. Prodrug-Converting Enzymes ("Suicide Strategy")

The "suicide strategy" in oncology combines classical cytotoxic chemotherapy with gene transfer technology. The underlying concept is to limit the action of a known cytotoxic drug to the local area of the tumor lesion. To this end, the cDNA of a prodrug-converting enzyme is delivered into the tumor by a vector system of choice. This is followed by regional or systemic application of the corresponding nontoxic prodrug. Once the prodrug reaches the tumor and is taken up by the tumor cells that express the prodrug-converting enzyme, it is converted into the cytotoxic drug. In conventional chemotherapy, toxic and myeloablative side effects can be dose limiting. In contrast, when using the suicide gene concept, cytotoxic effects of the converted drug are mainly restricted to the area of tumor infiltration and the time of action is limited to the presence of the cancer cells expressing the prodrug converting enzyme. In addition, the suicide strategy takes advantage of the "bystander effect." This molecular mechanism allows the killing of even uninfected tumor cells in the neighborhood of infected cells due to intercellular communication mediated, e.g., by gap junctions. However, this mechanism is still not fully understood. There are different prodrug-converting enzymes in experimental or clinical investigation, and the number of systems developed has increased rapidly (17). (For a more detailed overview of the application of the suicide strategy in gene therapy for cancer, (see Chapter 17.)

The most often used prodrug-converting enzyme for clinical approaches is the herpes simplex virus thymidine kinase gene (HSV-tk). The enzyme thymidine kinase (tk) phosphorylates the prodrug ganciclovir (GCV) to GCV monophosphate, which is then further phosphorylated to toxic GCV triphosphate. Inhibition of the DNA polymerase by GCV triphosphate finally leads to cell death. As demonstrated by different reports, tumor eradication has been achieved even if only 10% of the tumor mass is transduced (18). This effect is probably due to a very potent bystander effect. In preclinical animal experiments, a vector carrying the HSV-tk gene is usually applied intratumorally. In several reports using immunocompromised animals, a reduction of tumor volume of more than 50% of the controls was achieved in various experimental settings, and even complete remissions were frequently observed. In addition to these experimental studies in immunocompromised animals, reports in immunocompetent animals suggest that the immune system may play a supportive role in the efficacy of this approach (19). Promising results of tumor growth inhibition are not without side effects induced by the HSV-tk system. Using an in vivo model of adenovirus-mediated gene transfer to the liver of mice and rats, there was liver toxicity due to unwanted transduction of normal tissue, which can be eliminated either by targeted vectors or tissue-specific gene expression (20,21). However, promising preclinical studies of glioblastoma treatment by the HSV-tk system resulted in the first multicenter clinical trial for patients with glioblastoma (22).

As in other gene therapy strategies, the ability of the suicide strategy to kill cancer cells in experimental and clinical studies is limited by overall low efficacy of gene transfer in vivo. Independent of the vector system used, there is only a partial transduction with a nonhomogeneous intratumoral vector distribution. This more general problem was approached by the use of retroviral vector producer cells (VPCs). These cells, which were engineered to continuously produce HSV-tk–positive retroviruses, were proven to be more effective than direct vector application in experimental animal studies. In several ongoing clinical multicenter trials for the treatment of patients with glioblastoma, VPCs are being used. Another alternative to improve the efficacy of suicide approaches is the regional application of the vector into the normal tissue surrounding the tumor. By adenovirus-mediated gene transfer of cytosine deaminase (CD), which converts 5-fluorocytosine into the cytotoxic drug 5-fluorouracil, this approach was demonstrated to be a strategy to treat liver metastasis of colorectal cancer (23). Together with others, these preclinical studies led to the first clinical trial to treat patients with colorectal cancer metastatic to the liver (24).

C. Tumor Suppressor Genes and Antioncogenes

During the last decade, a number of genes has been identified that become dysregulated during carcinogenesis. During this complex and multifactorial process, leading finally to the macroscopic presence of cancer, genes become dysregulated by different molecular mechanisms, including gene deletion and mutation or promotor silencing. At the end of these processes of genetic alteration resulting in activation or inactivation of multiple genes, the cancer cell proliferates in an uncontrolled fashion. Genes promoting cellular proliferation, such as oncogenes, become activated, whereas genes suppressing cellular proliferation, such as tumor suppressor genes, become inactivated. Although classifying oncogene versus tumor suppressor genes is a very strong simplification of the underlying mechanisms of the regulation of signal transduction, it helps to characterize the variety of different therapeutic approaches.

The approach presents an opportunity for treatment strategies that can specifically target cancer cells. Current approaches include the inactivation of overexpressed oncogenes by antisense molecules or dominant negative mutants or alternatively the reconstitution of cells with tumor suppressor genes that have been lost or were mutated. The rationale is not so much the reversion of tumor cells back into normal cells. This task would be difficult to solve because usually more than one mutation is acquired by the tumor cell during the transformation process. The aim is rather to define the weak point in the cell's regulatory balance and consequently the gene or combination of genes that would have the greatest impact in the exertion of cell cycle arrest or better apoptosis. To this end, it is of crucial importance to acquire a sufficient understanding of the cell's balance with respect to signal transduction, cell cycle regulation, and finally susceptibility to apoptosis. The targeting of the genes known to be dysfunctional in the respective tumor is usually the most efficient procedure. This does, however, not always hold true. It is, for example, still a matter of controversy whether retransfer of p53 into p53-negative tumor cells does generally result in efficient apoptosis induction, because, for example, the presence of often highly overexpressed mutant p53 can compete with the transferred intact gene. In other cases, a combination of several genes could increase specificity and efficacy. The main obstacle to this therapeutic approach is the need for a particularly high efficacy of gene transfer.

Although a mild bystander effect has been reported in the context of p53 gene transfer (25), a transfer efficacy close to 100% is usually necessary for eradication of tumors if the immune system as an adjuvant is excluded. Such high transfer efficacies are the exception with current vectors, such that the breakthrough of this highly tumor-specific approach will particularly depend on future vector development. Gene therapy directed against oncogenes has targeted several types of cancer and several clinical trials are underway (see Section IV). Among the tumor suppressor genes, only p53 has made it into the clinic. Besides proapoptotic bax (26) and, bcl-x_s (27) genes, genes involved in the regulation of the G1 phase of the cell cycle have been evaluated in animal experiments. Tumor growth was inhibited by transfer of wild-type and truncated pRb (28,29), which in its active form binds E2F-1 and prevents entry into the S phase, as well as by the cdk/cyclin inhibitors p16 (30,31) and p21 (32), which keep pRb in its hypophosphorylated, active state. It remains to be shown whether cell cycle arrest is sufficient for therapy of established tumors or whether apoptosis induction is required. Undoubtedly, restoration of tumor cells with p53 or p21 can increase the cells sensitivity to radiation (33–35) and chemotherapy (36–39). Also, combinations of tumor suppressor genes could prove to have more than additive tumoricidal effects, as shown for the combination of p53 and p16 (30).

D. Tumor Lysis by Recombinant Viruses

Since the early beginnings, cancer therapy by viral oncolysis has been one of the most challenging strategies to treat human malignancies (40). The idea that viruses may be used as selective anticancer agents dates back almost a century (41). In 1957, four years after their discovery, replicating adenoviruses were used in cancer therapy. Of patients with advanced cervical carcinoma receiving intratumoral or intra-arterial injections of wild-type human adenoviruses, 65% had a marked to moderate local tumor response, and only 3 patients out of 30 patients on steroids had a viral syndrome of short duration (42). The underlying concept of this strategy is to inject the virus directly into the tumor, leading to the transduction of a certain number of cells in which viral replication takes place. Consequently, the infected cells are finally disrupted and viral progeny are released, allowing the spread of the infection and an increase in transfer efficacy. Interest and research in the area of molecular biology has exploded, and the available virus-production techniques and purification techniques have been markedly improved. Thus, much larger amounts of adenovirus can now been applied. However, one major concern has been how to limit the viral replication to the site of the tumor. One strategy to confer tumor-specific replication has been created by utilizing the dependence of the replicating adenovirus on the genetic status of p53 in the infected host cell. Like many DNA viruses, adenoviruses have also developed specific gene products that seem to counteract apoptosis-inducing molecules like p53. Among the adenoviral genes, the E1B 55 kDa gene blocks p53, the best known inducer of cell cycle arrest and potent inducer of apoptosis. In this intriguing approach, (43) the E1B gene was deleted from the adenoviral genome allowing viral replication only in p53-negative tumor cells but creating apoptosis upon viral infection in p53-positive normal cells (43,44). Since more than 50% of the common solid tumors lack functional p53, this approach was thought to be widely applicable. In the meantime, both the lack of replication in p53-positive cells as well as potent replication in p53-negative cells (45) have been questioned. A further understanding of how exactly E1B 55 kDa interacts with p53 is certainly needed. Independent of the outcome of this debate, this concept has already stimulated virologists and cancer biologists to develop the next generation of conditionally replication-dependent adenoviruses.

Another way to achieve cancer-specific replication uses tissue-specific gene expression. The adenoviral E1A region, which is responsible for viral replication, was placed under the control of a tissue-specific promoter instead of the E1A promoter. This approach has allowed specific replication in prostate cancer cells if the PSA promoter was used (46). However, as mentioned for tissue-specific expression of transgenes in a viral context, a loss of tissue specificity can also occur, as we observed after insertion of the CEA promoter to express the E1A gene (author's unpublished observations). A reason for this loss of specificity may be the influence of the adenoviral E1A enhancer. Appropriate engineering of the adenoviral genome will probably solve this problem. Besides adenoviruses, other oncolytic viruses have been tested in animal models. Like adenoviruses, herpes simplex virus (HSV), a neurotrophic DNA virus, directly lyses cells during viral shedding. First-generation HSV contains a 360 bp deletion in the thymidine kinase gene, which seems to prevent replication in quiescent cells but allows replication in rapidly proliferating cells (47,48). Second-generation viruses with additional mutations have been generated to further reduce neurovirulence (49). Newcastle disease virus (NDV) is a chicken paramyxovirus associated with minimal disease in humans. Cytotoxicity for numerous human tumor cell lines and resistance of several human fibroblast lines have been reported (50). The mechanism that causes tumor selectivity remains unclear. Tumor cell killing may involve virus replication and direct cell lysis and/or induction of tumor necrosis factor (TNF) secretion and increased sensitivity of tumor cells to TNF-mediated killing (51,52).

Autonomous parvoviruses are DNA viruses with small genomes, which depend on helper viruses or specific cellular functions for replication. The cytopathic effect seems to be dependent on DNA replication as well as on the expression of nonstructural gene products and enhanced sensitivity to their effects (49).

In the future, the tremendous increase in knowledge in the field of tumor and virus biology can be used to create appropriate vectors. Several factors that potentially influence clinical efficacy have been defined. Among these are (a) characteristics of the viruses such as the size, the time between infection and lysis, the number of virions produced, or the induction of a humoral or cellular immune response and (b) characteristics of the tumor such as distribution of the vasculature or physical barriers to virus spread such as fibrosis. An example of surmounting such a natural barrier is the recent demonstration that inactivation of particular adenoviral serotypes by preformed antibodies can be circumvented if other serotypes are used (53).

E. Antiangiogenic Gene Therapy

This therapy targets the endothelial cells of blood vessels. Several naturally produced or synthetic angiogenesis inhibitors have been shown to inhibit proliferation of intratumoral endothelial cells and consequently tumor growth (54,55). Recently, two antiangiogenic gene therapeutic approaches have been discussed (56). In both cases, the genes for the soluble form of endothelial cell receptor proteins (Tie2 and FLT-1) that interact with angiogenetic factors were transfered in vivo or ex vivo and resulted in significant inhibition of tumor growth (57,58). Antiangiogenic therapy itself is only in its infancy, and the future development of this treatment modality will obviously have a great impact on the corresponding gene therapeutic approach. Both approaches can be used after surgery or after radiotherapy to prevent recurrence of distant metastases or in combination with conventional chemotherapy or immunotherapy and, of course, with other types of gene therapy. There are several advantages of molecular therapy over direct application of the effector substance. First, the use of targeted vectors allows increased intratumoral concentrations of antiangiogenic factors without the risk of potential negative side effects on wound healing, endometrial maturation, or embryo growth (59). Another advantage of antiangiogenetic gene therapy may be reduced expense as compared to prolonged protein therapy with angiogenesis inhibitors such as angiostatin and endostatin. Moreover, experimental data suggest that effective antiangiogenic therapy requires the continuous presence of the inhibitor in the blood, which may be more efficiently achieved by gene therapy than by bolus protein therapy.

F. Drug-Resistance Genes

Instead of killing tumor cells, this strategy is aimed at preventing toxic side effects of modern chemotherapy, e.g., by making normal cells resistant to chemotherapeutic toxicity. This approach is based on the fact that the cytotoxicity of chemotherapy cannot discriminate between normal and cancer cells. Proliferating normal cells like hematopoietic precursor cells are especially affected, as evidenced by the fact that bone marrow suppression is still dose-limiting in most chemotherapeutic courses. To overcome this limitation, different experimental approaches were developed. One strategy to make hematopoietic precursor cells resistant to chemotherapy is the direct gene transfer of drug-resistance genes like MDR1. The MDR1 gene encodes for the P-glycoprotein, a cell membrane multidrug transporter that effluxes a broad spectrum of hydrophobic and amphipathic compounds, including several chemotherapeutic drugs currently used in clinical studies (60). Transfer and expression of the MDR1 gene in hematopoietic progenitor cells has been shown to increase the resistance of hematopoietic precursor cells to chemotherapy (61–65). Therefore, several clinical trials have been initiated. As in other gene therapy strategies, one of the limitations that needs to be eliminated before using such strategies for clinical application is the specificity of gene transfer into the target cells.

III. VECTORS FOR GENE THERAPY FOR CANCER

A. Virus-Based Gene-Transfer Vectors

In this chapter, the different gene-transfer vectors (e.g., adenovirus- and retrovirus-based vectors) will be discussed with respect to their specific relevance for efficacy and toxicity in cancer gene therapy. For general biology, development, and design of the vectors, the reader is referred to the corresponding chapters in this book that focus on the particular vectors.

One of the most widely used vectors for in vivo application in gene therapy for cancer is the replication-deficient recombinant adenovirus. First-generation adenoviral vectors (Ad vector) can be generated to the highest titers (up to 10^{12}/mL) among viral vectors (66). Moreover, they easily infect cells of epithelial origin, including cancer cells, because these cells express the appropriate receptors (67) and integrins (68) for binding and internalization, respectively (CAR, integrins). Since Ad vectors infect dividing and nondividing cells, dormant tumor cells that can make up a considerable fraction of the tumor mass can also be killed. These properties have made first-generation adenoviruses one of the vectors of choice for clinical studies. Ad vector–mediated gene transfer can be accompanied by toxic side effects towards normal tissue, mainly due to residual adenoviral gene expression in occasionally transduced normal cells (69–74). This toxicity can be reduced using second-generation Ad vectors where adenoviral genes such as the E4 region or the E2a gene are deleted (66,75–79) or minimal or gutless adenoviral vectors, which are completely devoid of all viral genes (80–82). The side effects of first-generation Ad vectors such as toxicity and immunity can be turned into an adjuvant situation for cancer therapy as demonstrated by the group of Rosenberg et al. (83). However, in gene therapy for cancer where vector toxicity to the tumor cells at the first glance may even be desirable, this may also be a disadvantage. For instance, leakage of intratumorally injected vectors carrying a prodrug-converting enzyme (''suicide gene strategy'') into the host organ has been shown to produce severe side effects (20). Even more dangerous, regional and systemic application of vectors will transduce normal tissue, and finally anticancer strategies based on transduction of normal tissue (e.g., some immunological approaches) will depend on safer vectors such as helper-dependent (HD) vectors for in vivo gene transfer. Moreover, HD-Ad vectors have an extremely high packaging capacity, which allows an increased level of adaptation to the tumor cells' particularities. At this time titers of 10^{10} infectious particles/mL (from 10^{8} cells) are about one to two magnitudes below what can be achieved with first-generation vectors (84; author's unpublished observations) but already comparable to adeno-associated virus (AAV) titers obtained with modern techniques. Significant advantages in vector design and isolation procedures keep the contamination with helper Ads below 1%. With further improvement in vector technology preventing the frequent recombinatorial events, HD-Ad vectors will find their application in gene therapy for cancer.

Another very popular vehicle for gene transfer are retrovirus-based vectors derived from murine leukemia virus (MLV). These were the first vectors where all the viral genes were provided by vector producer cells (VPCs) and the retroviruses themselves contained only the LTRs, the packaging signal, and the transgene. Due to the initially low achievable titers of 10^6/mL in the retroviral supernatant, the VPCs themselves were directly applied to the tumors with the rationale that these VPCs would deliver retroviruses until they were eliminated by the immune system (85). As for adenoviral vectors, many animal studies including in vivo gene transfer into established tumors were carried out, and complete remissions of microscopic tumors have been reported (85). Current packaging lines give titers of $>10^7$ infectious particles per mL (86). Moreover, the use of different envelope proteins, such as the G protein from vesicular-stomatitis virus, has improved titers following concentration to greater than 10^9/mL (86). Although these titers are still far away from what is achievable with adenoviruses, direct application of retroviruses may have its particular application in gene therapy for cancer. The fact that they only infect dividing cells may prevent toxicity to nondividing normal tissue. On the other hand, these vectors also leave out dormant cancer cells, which may decrease their efficacy. Other than MLV-based vectors, lentiviral retroviruses are able to infect certain nondividing cells (87) and may therefore be of interest for gene therapy for cancer (88–90). Based on their tropism for neuronal tissues, HSVs are the preferred gene-transfer vectors for neurological cancer therapy. In general, they can infect dividing and nondividing cells. Similar to adenoviruses, cytotoxic genes have to be deleted from the viral genome and are to be provided by helper viruses or cell lines in order to prevent toxicity, which is even higher than that of first-generation adenoviruses. Successful attempts in this direction have been made (91–96).

Other vectors that have become very interesting for gene therapy of cancer are AAV-based vectors. These helper virus (e.g., adenovirus)–dependent vectors do not induce a cellular immune response and have the potential to integrate into the host genome. Therefore, they are very promising candidate vectors when long-term expression is required, as in the protection of hematopoietic precursor cells during high-dose chemotherapy. (For the general biology of AAV-based gene-transfer vectors, see Chapter 3.)

Fowlpox viruses and vaccinia viruses infect a wide variety of cells types. In addition, they are safe and have a high packaging capacity (97). Due to their high intrinsic immunogenicity, they have been used as adjuvant and transfer vehicles for immunogene therapy of cancer, and two clinical studies have already been initiated [Genetic Medicine Clinical Trials Database online (www.wiley.co.uk/genetherapy/DATABASE)]. In the context of tumor vaccination, poliovirus-based gene transfer would also be a suitable approach (98). In addition, several other viruses have been used for the transfer of genes into cancer cells; they usually have some interesting features but also certain disadvantages, which have so far prevented widespread use. Epstein-Barr Viruses (EBV) have a natural tropism for B cells, but the potential development of wild-type transforming viruses by homologous recombination raises a safety concern. Baculoviruses are insect viruses and cannot replicate in human cells but have been shown to efficiently infect a variety of human cell lines (99,100). However, the human complement system rapidly inactivates these vectors such that extensive modifications of the cell surface are required (100,101). Alphaviruses like Sindbis virus (102) and Semliki Forest virus (103) can efficiently multiply their RNA genome in target cells, which allows a very high transgene expression. Further improvements in their packaging systems could make these vectors very interesting for the future. Autonomous parvoviral vectors (104) such as H1, MVM, and LIII can only replicate during the S phase of the host cell. These small viruses could become excellent tumor-specific tools if appropriate packaging cell lines can be generated.

Solutions for most of the problems of the current state of technology to construct viral vectors for cancer gene therapy are imaginable. However, some natural limitations such as packaging capacity, site-specific integration, or preexisting antibodies will require some effort to overcome. Chimeric vectors, which are constructed by the use of two or more viruses, may have some advantages. To date, attempts have mainly been made to combine the high transfer efficacy of adenoviruses with the long duration of gene expression of AAVs or retroviruses (105), but specific applications for gene therapy of cancer will certainly evolve in the future.

B. Non–Virus-Based Gene-Transfer Vectors

In general, nonviral vector systems exhibit much lower efficacy of gene transfer into tumor cells than viral vector systems. This problem has been approached using different methods like repeated injections or continuous application through pump systems. These applications are easier to perform with nonviral vectors than with many viral vectors, but the rate of gene transfer is still limited (106). A physical method of gene transfer that is applicable in vivo is particle bombardment (107–109). Small (1–3 μm) gold or tungsten particles are covered with plasmid DNA accelerated in an electrical field and fired onto the target tissue. Due to a depth of penetration of up to 50 cell layers, this approach may be applicable to superficial lymphoma of the skin.

Another very commonly used medium for gene transfer are cationic liposomes. This technique is based on the overall positive charge of the liposomes and the overall negative charge of the cell surface. Liposomes have been used in several clinical studies for tumor vaccination and were injected intratumorally in these cases.

Several approaches have attempted to combine viral and nonviral elements. Successful gene transfer was achieved with a combination of the cationic polypeptide polylysin, a covalently bound asialoglycoprotein receptor, and the negatively charged DNA complexed to the polylysin (110). An up to 1000-fold increase of the expression of transferred genes was seen by additional integration of inactivated adenovirus into the complex, which prevents lysosomal digestion (111–113).

C. Cancer-Specific Expression Cassette

Expression cassettes are the cDNA of a transgene and its control elements, for instance, promotors or enhancers packed for the transfer into the target organ or target cell. For a variety of applications, simple expression cassettes can be used containing the wild-type cDNA of the gene to be transferred under the control of a constitutive promotor. However, the complex molecular biology of cancer sometimes requires the expression of more specific therapeutic genes. For instance, as demonstrated by the interaction between mutated and wild-type (wt) p53, transgenes can be inactivated by their intratumoral defective version (114). In this case the wt version of p53 would not be the best choice. On the other hand, genes are regulated differently in tumors and in normal cells, as demonstrated by drug-resistance genes (115,116). Therefore, the field of vectorology focuses on the construction of specific expression cassettes for gene therapy of cancer by modifying the cDNA of the transgene or applying cancer-specific promotors or enhancer elements.

As in other fields of gene therapy, the packaging size of the vector to be used for gene transfer is one of the most important limitations for the construction of cancer-specific expression cassettes. So far, vectorologists have mainly worked with the intron-free cDNA coding for the transgene. Recently, the availability of vectors with substantially increased packaging capacity such as HD adenoviruses has allowed the inclusion of whole mini-genes into a viral vector (81,117–119). These approaches are aimed at an optimal and physiological regulation of the transgene, a property that may be of future relevance in gene therapy of cancer. Gene therapy of cancer needs to be evaluated according to its efficacy to kill cancer cells without side effects. To meet these criteria, strong viral promoters with usually ubiquitous and constitutive activity have been the preferred expression control elements used so far. However, these promoters can lead to toxicity, because they allow undesired high-level expression of potentially toxic transgenes in normal cells once they are transduced (20,21,120). To avoid such side effects, the use of tissue-specific promoters may allow an increase in the therapeutic index. Their use is particularly interesting in the situation of metastatic cancer, where the tissue-specific promotor allows transgene expression in the metastatic tumor cell but not in the surrounding normal tissue, even if it is transduced by the vector. For instance, the carcinoembryonic antigen (CEA), which is physiologically expressed predominantly on colon tissue but not in liver tissue, allows a transgene expression predominantly in colon cancer cells metastatic to the liver. Other examples for such a promoter strategy are the AFP (alpha-fetoprotein) promoter for hepatocellular carcinoma (HCC), the promoters of erbB2, an oncogene often found in breast tumors, or the promoter of the tyrosinase gene, which has specificity for melanoma.

However, the maintenance of tissue specificity can be a problem. For adenoviral vectors, loss as well as maintenance of tissue specificity has been reported (21,121–126). In this context, the orientation of the expression cassette can play an important role. For instance, the transcriptional activity of the E1A enhancer, which is not deleted in E1-deficient first-generation adenoviruses, can induce loss of tissue specificity. This can even occur if the expression cassette is inserted in the reverse orientation to the adenoviral reading frame (author's unpublished observations). In contrast, insertion of expression cassettes in reverse orientation into retroviral vectors normally maintains tissue specificity, whereas orientation in frame puts the transgene under the influence of the strong retroviral LTR with subsequent loss of specificity (127). Alternatively, SIN vectors, which lose their own LTR upon integration into the host cell genome (128), can be used or the LTR can be replaced by the tissue-specific promoter. The problems of tissue-specific expression seen in adenovirus or retrovirus vectors do not seem to occur in AAV vectors (129,130), probably because the flanking ITRs possess no regulative activity.

In contrast to constitutive promotors, tumor specificity in patients resistant to chemotherapy could be mediated by therapy-inducible promoters. In this respect, the examination of gene regulation in cancer cells, like the multidrug resistance gene (MDR1), the x-irradiation–induced tissue-type plasminogen activator (t-PA), the early growth-response gene (Egr-1), the human heat-shock protein HSP 70, or the glucose-regulated protein (GRP78), led to the discovery of a class of promoter sequences that are involved in such stress responses. These promoters carry responsive elements that are inducible by either radiotherapy, cytostatic drugs, or hyperthermia, which are conventional treatment modalities. It has already been shown that the expression of therapeutic genes, if placed under the control of therapy-inducible promoters, could be enhanced and the efficacy increased (131). The combination of therapeutic genes under the control of therapy-inducible promoters with conventional cancer treatment methods could enhance the overall treatment efficacy and also retain specificity.

D. Targeted Vectors

The currently used viral vectors for gene transfer can infect a broad variety of target cells and tissues. Whereas this is of interest for cell type–independent gene expression, it is a disadvantage when tissue-specific gene expression is required as in gene therapy for cancer. Therefore the surface of the vector needs to be modified such that the cancer cell is infected in a more specific manner (retargeting). Based on the increasing knowledge about the molecular biology of viral vectors, the most advanced systems are retrovirus- or adenovirus-based chimeric vectors.

The efficacy of binding to the surface of a given target cell by an adenovirus depends on the presence of specific receptors like the coxsackie and adenovirus receptor (CAR) and the alpha$_2$ domain of MHC class I, which interact with the adenoviral fiber coat protein (67,68,132,133). Consequently, several approaches have been developed to redirect the tropism of adenoviral vectors in favor of cancer cells. Among these were replacement of the Ad5 fiber knob by a fiber knob from another adenovirus (134,135) or the insertion of polylysin or an RGD motive as ligand for widely expressed heparan or alpha v integrin receptors, respectively, into the fiber knob leading to an increase in gene-transfer efficiency of up to two logs (136,137). Another way to optimize adenovirus-mediated gene transfer into cancer cells can be accomplished by bridging of virus and cellular receptors through bispecific antibodies (138–140). Here, a true retargeting was achieved by blocking of the native adenoviral fiber knob (138).

Retargeting of retroviral vectors is usually based on murine leukemia viruses (MoMLV). The Pit-2 receptor of the amphotropic MoMLV vectors is widely distributed on human tissues (141), which could lead to an undesirable transduction of many cell types following in vivo administration of the vector. In addition, several cell types are inefficiently transduced by these vectors. Several modification of the viral envelope that broadened the host cell spectrum in vitro have been reported. This genetic pseudotyping by other envelope proteins includes vesicular stomatitis virus G (VSV-G) glycoprotein [(142), generation of high titers], gibbon ape leukemia virus (GaLV) (143), human foamy virus (HFV) (144), simian immunodeficiency virus (145), HIV-1 envelope protein (146), and N-terminus of murine stem cell factor (147). However, no in vivo gene transfer has yet been reported.

IV. CLINICAL TARGETS FOR GENE THERAPY FOR CANCER

A. Breast Cancer

One of the most important target malignancies for cancer gene therapy is breast cancer. Breast cancer will affect one in every nine women in the United States, and a similar incidence is seen in Europe (148). Conventional treatment like surgery, radiotherapy, and adjuvant systemic therapy allows disease-free survival for many years. However, the loco regional recurrence rate and the rate of disseminated disease is high, and even 10–40% of patients without obvious axillary lymph node involvement at the time of surgery relapse (149). In these cases, a curability by conventional methods is very unlikely.

Based on the unsatisfying outcome of classical strategies to improve cancer treatment, different gene-transfer approaches are under experimental and clinical investigation. These include immunological approaches or the transfer of tumor suppressor genes or prodrug-activating enzymes. Several immunological strategies are based on the use of tumor-specific antigens to improve recognition of breast cancer cells by the effector cells of the immune system. In this respect, different tumor-specific antigens are under experimental investigation to set up a specific vaccination strategy for patients with breast cancer. Candidate antigens are mucin 1 (MUC-1), MAGE-1, carcinoembryonal antigen (CEA) and members of the erbB gene family of cell surface receptors (150). Among the first immunological approaches for breast cancer patients is an ongoing phase I study of immunotherapy of cutaneous metastasis using allogenic (A2, HLA-B13) and xenogenic [HLA-H-2K(k)] MHC–DNA liposome complexes (151).

Gene-transfer strategies for patients with breast cancer can also be used to improve classical strategies in therapy of breast cancer like chemotherapy. In this respect, purging techniques in high-dose chemotherapy are under intensive experimental investigation. Before high-dose chemotherapy to treat woman with breast cancer, autologous stem cell transplants are collected from the patient and are given back after finishing the therapeutic protocol. Because these preparations can still be contaminated by tumor cells, it is the goal of different strategies to purge these stem cell transplants from contamination. However, magnetic purging techniques are expensive and not very efficient, and pharmacological purging is very effective but not restricted to the tumor (152). Therefore, to limit the toxicity of pharmacological purging of contaminating cancer cells, either hematopoietic precursor cells of the autologous stem cell transplants need to be made resistant to chemotherapy or contaminating tumor cells need to be made more sensitive to chemotherapy. Thus, one genetic approach attempts to infect only hematopoietic cells, making them resistant to chemotherapy by transfer of a multidrug-resistant gene (153). The other strategy, making contaminating tumor cells more sensitive to chemotherapy, is demonstrated by adenovirus-mediated gene transfer of a prodrug-activating enzyme like HSV-tk or CD (121,154,155). This approach uses the fact that breast cancer cells contaminating autologous steam cell transplants express more adenovirus-internalizing integrins than hematopoietic precursor cells (156–158). That the concept of adenovirus-mediated gene transfer into contaminating breast cancer cells of autologous stem cells is a real alternative strategy for a direct clinical application is demonstrated by a preclinical study (159).

Another strategy that has been adapted for gene therapy of breast cancer is the use of antioncogene and tumor suppressor genes. Adenovirus-mediated transfer of the cDNA of the pro-apoptotic bcl-x_S into breast cancer cells demonstrated a significant reduction of tumor growth after the transduced cells were transplanted into immunodeficient mice (27,160). As described for colorectal cancer, breast cancer also develops by a succession of genetic alterations (161–165). Although the degree of genetic heterogeneity is particularly high in breast cancer, these multiple genetic changes may interfere with just a few critical cell cycle–regulatory pathways and therefore represent suitable targets for corrective gene therapy (166). Successful in vitro approaches include oligonucleoutide-mediated transfer of antisense myc (167,168), ErbB-2 (169,170), cyclin D1 (171), and TGF-α (172) and the transfer of genes for intracellular antibodies, which prevent growth factor receptors to reach the cell surface as reported for ErbB-2 (173). Inhibition of breast tumor growth in vivo was shown by retroviral transfer of antisense C-FOS (174). However, whether these approaches meet the criteria for clinical applications needs to be demonstrated. The best in vivo data exist so far for adenoviral transfer of the tumor suppressor p53, which argues for the fruitfulness of combining a highly efficient gene-transfer vehicle with a nearly universal apoptosis inducer (175). In addition, good efficacy of tumor growth reduction was achieved using liposomes for the transfer of a p53 cDNA (176,177). The importance of the p53 status for the efficacy of chemotherapeutic drugs is a matter of intensive debate. Whereas in the majority of studies the loss of p53 has been associated with decreased sensitivity to chemotherapy, the opposite was reported for the chemotherapeutic drug taxol (178).

B. Colorectal Cancer

Colorectal cancer is the third most frequent cancer in the United States (179). Surgical removal of the primary tumor is the established first-line therapy allowing this strategy to be a curative approach if all cancer cells are eliminated. However, already at a very early stage of tumor development, colorectal cancer metastasizes to the liver, making this organ in 60% of all cases the only manifestation of distant metastasis (180). Consequently, liver metastasis of colorectal cancer is one of the very few indications where treatment of metastasis can lead to a significant improvement of the prognosis of the disease.

Single liver metastasis of colorectal cancer represents a promising target for intratumoral and/or regional gene therapy. Studies in experimental animals demonstrated significant tumor reduction by gene transfer of the tumor suppressor gene p53 or by the suicide approach using gene transfer of prodrug-activating enzymes like cytosine deaminase or HSV-tk followed by systemic application of corresponding prodrug 5-fluorocytosine or ganciclovir (GCV) (23,181). Single dose of adenovirus transferring the HSV-tk gene followed by a 10-day intraperitoneal GCV treatment led to a reduced tumor growth of more than 90% and a significant reduction of the tumor volume (182). This experimental approach was extended by the combination of adenovirus vectors carrying the transgene of different cytokines with the adenovirus encoding for HSV-tk. The results so far suggest that the HSV-tk/GCV effect can be increased by simultaneous cytokine gene expression (182). However, in an orthotopic model of colon carcinoma metastatic to the liver, the HSV-tk strategy was compromised by severe hepatic toxicity and the death of several animals (20). Similar toxicity was seen if the vector was applied intraportally for the treatment of HCC in mice or rats (120). In contrast, no toxicity was observed with retroviral vectors (183). The liver toxicity observed using adenovirus vectors could be abrogated if the CMV promoter was replaced by the colon-specific CEA promoter in these vectors (21). Another alternative to generate tumor cell–specific transgene expression in colorectal liver metastases by adenovirus vectors can be accomplished by modification of the adenoviral fiber protein by inclusion of the CEA receptor (112). These approaches are now in the phase of preclinical testing.

Multiple liver metastases are also targets for immunological gene therapy strategies. In this respect, CEA is one of the most promising candidates under investigation. An immunization study using a plasmid containing the cDNA of the CEA gene is already in the stage of a clinical phase I trial. So far, after treatment of 12 patients with deltoid injections of up to 10 μg plasmid, no acute toxicities have been noted (184). In addition, significant tumor growth inhibition of xenografts from colon tumor cells in established animal models has also been accomplished by different approaches including vaccinia virus–mediated transfer of B7-1 and IL-12 (185), adenovirus-mediated transfer of IL-12 (183), liposomal transfer of MHC class I molecules (186), or the transfer of fibroblasts that had been transduced in vitro with IL-2 (187). The results of these experimental studies indicate that the dormant or suppressed immunogenicity of colon tumor cells can be evoked by several immunomodulatory mechanisms. Moreover, the good antitumor efficacy achieved even with vector systems that traditionally suffer from low gene-transfer efficacy suggests that a certain level of gene transfer may be sufficient to induce an immune response.

C. Glioblastoma

Glioblastoma is the most common primary brain tumor. Despite advances in diagnosis and treatment, the median survival time is still only one year from the time of diagnosis (188). This tumor rarely metastasizes to distant organs, suggesting that improvements in local treatment could be of great benefit. Therefore, glioblastoma has been one of the model diseases for gene therapy with suicide genes. The first preclinical studies for gene therapy for cancer were performed using retrovirus-mediated transfer of the HSV-tk gene into established intracranial glioblastomas in Fisher rats (85). Based on the early promising results, other vector systems have been tested for the HSV-tk/GCV approach including adenoviruses, liposomes AAV, or HSV. All of these vectors have been successfully used in animal studies where complete remissions with long-term survival could be frequently observed (Table 1). Consequently, different clinical phase I, II, and III trials were initiated making the gene therapy of glioblastoma by the HSV-tk/GSV approach the most advanced system for gene therapy for cancer. As demonstrated by results from a multicenter phase II trial in Germany, there is no ''clear-cut'' clinical outcome so far. A one-year follow-up study reports of 10 patients with recurrent glioblastoma multiforme where retroviral vector packaging cells were administered into the tumor followed by application of GCV. Of the 10 patients, 4 died because of tumor progression. Of the other 6 patients, one presented a complete remission at 12 months and 5 had progressive disease but with a significant increase in quality of life (189). Other reports demonstrated responses in the CT scan where a clear enhancement was visible in the areas where the retroviral VPCs carrying the transgene had been injected. Clinical responses, however, were rare and not marked. Some responders were also observed in trials using adenoviral vectors, but therapy was accompanied by severe neurological symptoms (190,191). As discussed in the context of colorectal liver metastases, toxicity can in principle be abrogated by tissue-specific expression of the transgene or targeted vectors. The suicide gene approach has been combined with surgery by first removing as much malignant tissue as possible and leaving the local infiltrating parts for multiple vector injections. This strategy leaves out the large isles of healthy tissue within the tumor network, which is a characteristic of this tumor and is the reason why complete resections can be rarely performed.

Besides the strategy of using prodrug-converting enzymes, gene transfer of the tumor suppressor gene p53 has also been tested in experimental models with success (192). The cell cycle inhibitor p16 is very often inactivated in glioblastoma. Therefore, adenovirus-mediated gene transfer of p16 generated significant tumor growth reduction in glioblastoma tumors that were negative for p16 (193). For the transcription factor E2F-1, it could be demonstrated that adenovirus-mediated overexpression resulted in a tumor growth reduction in p53 wild-type expressing glioblastoma cells (194). In addition to the use of molecules regulating cell cycle and apoptosis, several immunomodulatory genes have been tested to treat experimental glioblastoma tumors either alone and in combination. Growth inhibition was seen in most cases, which indicates that although the brain is an ''immunoprivileged'' site, this barrier could effectively be surmounted, at least in some tumors.

D. Head and Neck Cancer

Each year in the United States, approximately 40,000 individuals will be diagnosed with carcinoma of the head and neck (SCCHN) and upper aerodigestive tract (195). More than two thirds of the individuals with SCCHN present with stages III or IV of the disease (196), and 50–60% of these patients will ultimately develop local recurrence despite optimal local therapy. They therefore represent an ideal target for local or regional gene therapeutic approaches. Based on the good infectability of cancer cells of the head and neck, this tumor is one of the targets for adenovirus vector–mediated approaches. Because a high percentage of these tumors are negative for p53, different clinical phase I studies with p53 as the transferred transgene are underway. To evaluate toxicity and efficacy of intratumoral adenovirus-mediated gene transfer of p53 (Ad p53), patients with squamous head and neck cancer were injected intratumorally with Ad p53 (197). Whereas individual promising results have been reported, only evaluation of the results at the end of the studies will give a clear picture.

Table 1 Gene Therapy for Cancer, In Vivo Gene Transfer: Preclinical Studies

Strategy	Transgene	Vector	Route	Dose	Efficacy	Animal model, organ, cell line, site, pretreatment size	Ref.*
Anti-oncogenes	c-fos	Retro	i.p.	5×10^5	80% (weight)[a]	Nude[e], breast cancer (MCF-7), s.c., 1–4 μm^{3f}	Arteaga and Holt, 1996
	anti Erbβ-2 antibody	Ad	i.p.	500 pfu/cell	12-fold decreased risk of death	SCID, ovarian cancer (SKOV-3), i.p.	Deshane et al., 1995
	anti-K-RAS	Lip		100 μg^c, $3\times^g$	83% (cures)[d]	Nude, pancreatic cancer (AsPC-1), i.p.	Aoki et al., 1995
	anti-Cyclin G1	Retro	i.tu.	1×10^7, 10×	79% (vol)[a]	Nude, osteosarcoma (MNNG/HOS), s.c., 50–60 mm^3	Chen et al., 1997
	bcl-x_5	Ad	i.tu.	7×10^7	50% (vol)	Nude, breast cancer (MCF-7), s.c.	Ealovega et al., 1996
Tumor suppressor genes	p53	Ad	i.tu.	2.2×10^8, 10×	231: 86% (vol) 468: 74% (vol) 435: n.s. (vol)	Nude, breast cancer (MDA-MB-231, −468, −435, s.c. or ortho[h]	Nielsen et al., 1997
	p53	Lip	i.v.	1 × 16 μg, 1 × 12 μg	MDA-435: 75% (vol) MCF-7: 40% (vol)	Nude, breast cancer (MDA-MB-435: 17.6 mm^3, MCF-7: 12.8 mm^3), ortho	Xu et al., 1997
	p53	Lip	i.v.	35 μg, 6×	60% (vol) 97% (metastasis)	Nude, breast cancer (MDA-MB-435) ortho	Lesoon-Wood et al., 1995
	p53	Ad	i.tu.		45% (cures)	SCID, ovarian cancer (SK-OV-3), s.c., 5–6 mm	Gallardo et al., 1996
	p53	Ad	i.tu.	1–2 × 10^8, 6–8×	>65% (cures)	Nude, prostate cancer (C4-2), s.c.	Ko et al., 1996
	p53	Ad	i.tu.	5×10^9	p53: 21% (vol)	129/SV mice, prostate cancer (148-1PA, s.c., 24–40 mm^3	Eastham et al., 1995
	p53	Ad	i.tu.	5×10^9, 6× CDDP, i.p.	83% (vol) 91% (vol)	Nude, lung cancer (II1299), s.c., 250 mm^3	Nguyen et al., 1996
	p53	Ad	i.tu.	2×10^9, 8×	97% (vol)	Nude, lung cancer (SCLC, NIH-H69), s.c., 40 mm^3	Wills et al., 1994
	p53	Ad	i.tra.	5×10^7, 2×	73% (vol)	Lung cancer (NSCLC, H226Br)	Zhang et al., 1994
	p53	Ad, cisplatin	i.tu.	2×10^7	74% (vol)	Nude, lung cancer (NSCLC, H358), s.c., 5–6 mm	Fujiwara et al., 1994b
	p53	Retro	i.tru.	100 μL, 3×	64–100% (vol)	Nude, lung cancer (NSCLc, H226Br)	Fujiwara et al., 1994a
	p53	Ad	i.tu.	10^8	100% (cures) MDA 886: 33% (cures)	Nude, head and neck cancer (Tu-138, Tu-177, MDA 686-LN, MDA 886), s.c., microscopic	Clayman et al., 1995
	p53	Ad	i.tu.	10^8	98% (vol)	Nude, head and neck cancer (Tu-138, Tu-177), s.c., 6 mm	Liu et al., 1994
	p53	Ad	i.tu.	1×10^7	Tumor growth suppression	Nude, head and neck cancer, SCCHN (MDA686LN), s.c.	Liu et al., 1995

Table 1 (Continued)

Strategy	Transgene	Vector	Route	Dose	Efficacy	Animal model, organ, cell line, site, pretreatment size	Ref.*
	p53	Ad	i.tu.	10^4	40% (vol)	Wistar ral. glioma (9L), ortho	Badie et al., 1995
	p53	Ad	i.tu.	10^9, 5×	68% (vol)	Nude, colon cancer (DLD-1), s.c.	Harris et al., 1996
	p53	Ad	i.tu.	3.3 × 10^9, 3×	SW620: 62% (vol) KM12L4: 69% (vol)	Nude, colorectal cancer (SW620, KM12L4), s.c., 200 mm^3	Spitz et al., 1996
	p53	Ad	i.tu.	2 × 10^9	B16: 38% (vol) SK: 24% (vol)	Nude, melanoma (B16-G3.26, s.c., 1200 mm^3, SK-MEL-24, s.c., 300 mm^3)	Cirielli et al., 1995
	p53	Ad	i.a. (hepatic artery)	4 × 10^9, 4×	>64% (tu nodules)	Buffalo rat, HCC (McA-RH7777), ortho	Anderson et al., 1998
	E1A	Lip	i.p.	15 μg DNA, weekly	400% (surv)[b]	Nude, ovarian cancer (SKOV-3), i.p.	Yu et al., 1995
	E1A	Ad	i.v.	10^8, 6×	71% (vol)	Nude, lung cancer (NCl H820), ortho	Chang et al., 1996
	Mutant SV40 T Ag	AgLip	i.p.	15 μg DNA 30×	Incr. survival [40% >1 year vs. 0% >3 months, (control)]	Nude, ovarian cancer (SKOV-3), i.p.	Xing et al., 1996
	p21	Ad	i.tu.	5 × 10^9	p21: 68% (vol)	129/Sv, prostate cancer (148-1PA), s.c., 25–40 mm^3	Eastham et al., 1995
	p21	Retro-VPCs	i.tu.	1 × 10^6, 3×	58% (vol)	Nude, squamous carcinoma (HN8), s.c., 3 mm^3	Cardinali et al., 1998
	Rb	Ad	i.tu.	5 × 10^7 particles	125% (surv)	$Rh^{+/-}$ mice, pituitary cancer, ortho	Riley et al., 1996
	Truncated Rb	Ad	i.tu.	5 × 10^8, pfu, 6×	95% (vol)	Nude, bladder cancer (5637) s.c.	Xu et al., 1996
	BRCA-1	Retro	i.p.	Titer: 10^7/mL	300% (surv)	Nude, breast cancer (MCF-7), i.p., 3–5 mm	Holt et al., 1996
	bcl-x_x	Ad	i.tu.	7 × 10^7 pfu, 4×	50% (vol)	Nude, breast cancer (MCF-7), s.c.	Ealovega et al., 1996
Prodrug-activating genes	HSV-tk	AAV	i.tu.	9.6 × 10^9, 3×	>80% (cures)	Nude, glioma (U251-SP) ortho, 2 mm	Mizuno et al., 1998
	HSV-tk	Ad	i.tu.	10^8 pfu	83% (vol)	C57BL6, pancreatic cancer (PANC02), to liver, 4.5 mm	Block et al., 1997
	HSV-tk	Ad	i.port.	2 × 10^{10}	63% (cures)	Wistar/Ico rats, HCC (DENA induced), multiple 1–7 mm	Qian et al., 1997
	HSV-tk	Ad	i.tu.		84% (vol)	SCID, colon cancer (LS 174), s.c.	Brand et al., 1998
	HSV-tk	Ad	i.tu.	3 × 10^8	>75% (vol)	C3H/He, bladder cancer (MBT-2), s.c., 40 mm^3	Sutton et al., 1997
	HSV-tk	Ad	i.tu.	5 × 10^8	66% (weight), 112% (surv)	C57/BL6, prostate cancer (RM-1), ortho	Hall et al., 1997
	HSV-tk	Ad	i.tu.	5 × 10^8	84% (vol), 150% (surv)	C57/BL6, prostate cancer (RM-1), s.c., 50 mm^3	Eastham et al., 1996

Table 1 (Continued)

Strategy	Transgene	Vector	Route	Dose	Efficacy	Animal model, organ, cell line, site, pretreatment size	Ref.*
	HSV-tk	Ad	i.p.	2×10^9, 3×	>300% (surv)	Nude, ovarian cancer (Ov-ca-2774), i.p.	Tong et al., 1996
	HSV-tk	Ad	i.p.	10^9, 2×	91% (weight)	Nude, breast cancer (MCF-7), i.p.	Chen et al., 1995
	HSV-tk	Ad	i.tu.	10^9, 2×	HuH7: (cures), SK-Hep-1: (red vol)	Nude, HCC (Huh7: 83.2 mm^3, SK-Hep-1: 10.9 mm^3), s.c.	Kaneko et al., 1995
	HSV-tk	Ad	i.tu.	10^{10}	40–50% (vol)	Nude, melanoma (B16), s.c., 6–8 mm	Bonnekoh et al., 1995
	HSV-tk	Ad	i.tu.	1.2×10^9	100% (cures)	Fisher rats, glioma (9L), ortho, 1.7 mm^2	Perez-Cruet et al., 1994
	HSV-tk	Ad	i.tu.	3×10^8	99.8% (vol)	Nude, glioma (C_6), ortho, 4 mm	Chen et al., 1994b
	HSV-tk	Ad	i.thecal	2×10^9	126% (symptom-free latency)	Fisher rat, glioma (9L), ortho	Vincent et al., 1996a
	HSV-tk	Ad	i.p.	6.5×10^8	340% (surv) 28% (weight)	Nude, breast cancer (MDA-MB-435A), i.p.	Yee et al., 1996
	HSV-tk	HSV	i.thecal	10^8	90% (cures)	Fisher rats, glioma (9L), ortho	Kramm et al., 1996
	HSV-tk	HSV-tk-positive tumor cells	i.tu.	1×10^5	Retardation of tumor growth	Fisher rat, glioma (9L)	Namba et al., 1998
	HSV-tk	Lip	i.tu.	3 μg, 14×	69% (vol)	Nude, colon cancer (Colo201), s.c.	Takakuwa et al., 1997
	HSV-tk	Lip	i.tu.	3 μg DNA, 10×	Colo 320DM0: 57%, A-431: 75%, Nakajima, KF: not sig (vol)	Nude, colon cancer (Colo 320 DM), vulva (A 431), ovarian cancer (Nakajima, KF), s.c., 40–60 mm^3	Sugaya et al., 1996
	HSV-tk	Plasmid	i.tu.		40–50% (weight)	C57B1/6, melanoma (B16F1) s.c.	Soubrane et al., 1996
	HSV-tk	Retro	i.tu.	10^8	29% (cures)	Fisher rat, glioma (9L), ortho	Kruse et al., 1997
	HSV-tk	Retro-VPC	i.tu.	3×10^6	79% (cures)	Fisher rat, glioma (9L), ortho, micro	Culver et al., 1992
	HSV-tk	Retro-VPC	i.tu.	5×10^5	140% (surv)	Fisher rat, glioma (9L), ortho	Rainov et al., 1996
	HSV-tk	Retro-VPC	i.tu.	2×10^7	95% (vol)	Nude, head and neck cancer (UMSCC 29), s.c., 5 mm	Wilson et al., 1996
	HSV-tk	Ad, retro-VPC	i.tu.	Ad: 5×10^8 pfu, retro VPC: 5×10^6	Ad > retro-VPC (surv)	Fisher rat, glioma (9L), ortho	Vincent et al., 1996b
	CD	Ad	i.v.	10^9	97% (vol)	BALB/c, colon cancer (CT26) to liver, ortho, microscopic	Topf et al., 1998
	CD	Ad	i.p.	1×10^9	64–85% (weight)	Nude, i.p. gastric cancer (MKN45)	Lan et al., 1997
	CD	Ad	i.tu.	10^9	70% (vol)	C57BL/6, pancreatic cancer (PAN02), s.c.	Evoy et al., 1997
	CD	Ad	i.tu.	1×10^9	81% (vol)	Nude, breast cancer (MDA-MB-231), s.c.	Li et al., 1997
	CD	Ad	i.tu.	10^9	70–85% (vol)	Nude, HCC (PLC/PRF/5), s.c., >100 mm^3	Kanai et al., 1997

Table 1 (Continued)

Strategy	Transgene	Vector	Route	Dose	Efficacy	Animal model, organ, cell line, site, pretreatment size	Ref.*
	CD	Ad	peri.tu.		Growth suppression	Nude, colon cancer (HT29) to liver, ortho	Ohwada et al., 1996
	CD	Lip	i.tu.	10 μg or 50 μg, 10×	Incr (surv)	C57/BL6, melanoma (B16(F10), s.c.	Szala et al., 1996
Immunotherapeutic genes	MHC II	Tumor cells			60% (cures) (2–5 mm) 40% (cures) (4–7 mm)	A/J, sarcoma (Sal), s.c., 2–5 mm, 4–7 mm	Baskar et al., 1994
	MHCI H-2Ks	Lip	i.tu.	1 μg, several times	9/12 tu. growth retardation	BALB/c, colon cancer (CT-26), s.c.	Plautz et al., 1993
	IL-2	Tumor cells		2×10^6, 5×	70% (vol)	C57BL/6, pancreatic cancer (Panc 02), s.c.	Clary et al., 1997
	IL-2	Tumor cells	s.c.	2×10^6	64% (vol)	Nude, melanoma (DM92), s.c.	Abdel-Wahab et al., 1994
	IL-2	Tumor cells	s.c., i.p., i.pleu.	5×10^6, 3×	No effect (s.c.) 80% (cures, i.pleu.) 100% (cures, i.p.)	C57BL/6, lung cancer, (Lewis lung carcinoma), i.p., i.pleu, s.c.	Heike et al., 1997
	IL-2	Fibroblasts	s.c., i.cr.		Incr surv., i.cr.>i.s.	C57BL/6, glioma (GL261), ortho	Glick et al., 1997
	IL-2	Ad	i.tu.	2×10^9, 3×	65% (diameter)	C3H, fibrosarcoma (FSA), breast cancer (MCA-K), s.c., 3–5 mm	Toloza et al., 1996
	IL-2	Ad	i.tu.	2×10^9, 3×	95.2% tumor growth delay	SCID, HCC (HepG2, Hep3B), 4–6 mm	Bui et al., 1997
	IL-2	Fibroblasts	s.c.	2×10^6, 4×	44% (cures)	Nude, colon cancer (CT-26), s.c.	Fakhrai et al., 1995
	IL-4 + systemic IL-2	Fibroblasts	s.c.	10^6	100% (tumor growth delay)	C57BL/6, fibrosarcoma (MCA105)	Pippin et al., 1994
	IL-4	Tumor cells	s.c.	4×10^6	180% (surv)	C57BL/6, melanoma (B16), s.c.	Dranoff et al., 1993
	IL-4		s.c.	1×10^6, weekly 3×	70% (cures)	BALB/c, renal cancer (Renca), s.c.	Golumbek et al., 1991
	IL-4	Lip	i.tu.	10 μg	89% (vol)	C57BL/6, melanoma (B16(F10)), s.c.	Missol et al., 1995
	IL-12	Tumor cells	s.c.	5×10^6	100% (cures)	BALB/c, fibrosarcoma (CMS5a), s.c.	Schmitt et al., 1997
	IL-12	Tumor cells	s.c.		d1: 30% (cures), d7: 10% (cures)	BALB/c breast cancer (TSA), microscopic (d1), 2.4 mm (d7)	Cavallo et al., 1997
	IL-12	Ad	i.tu.	5×10^8	77% (vol)	BALB/c, colon cancer (MCA-26), to liver, ortho, 16–25 mm^2	Caruso et al., 1996
	IL-12	Gene gun	i.d.	5 μg, 2×	94% (diameter)	BALB/c, sarcoma (Meth A), i.d.	Rakhmilevich et al., 1997
	IL-12	Gene gun	i.d.	5 μg, 2–4×	P815: 28% (vol), B16: 47% (vol) (cures): Renca, L5178Y: 87.5%, MethA: 57%, SA-1: 37.5%	BALB/c: renal cancer (Renca), sarcoma (MethA), i.d., Sarcoma (SA-1), DBA 2 mice: lymphoma (L5178Y), mastocytoma (P815), i.d., AJ/C57BL/6: sarcoma (SA-1), melanoma, (B16), 5–8 mm	Rakhmilevich et al., 1996

Table 1 (Continued)

Strategy	Transgene	Vector	Route	Dose	Efficacy	Animal model, organ, cell line, site, pretreatment size	Ref.*
	IL-12	Plasmid	i.d.		78% (vol)	BALB/c, renal cancer (Renca), s.c.	Tan et al., 1996
	IL-12	HSV	i.tu.	7×10^5, 2× (helper)	94% (vol) 145% (surv)	BALB/c, colon cancer (CT-26), s.c., 5 mm	Toda et al., 1998
	B7-1	Tumor cells	MTX chemo	10^6, 2–4×	87% (red met) 200% (surv)	F344 rats, osteosarcoma (MSK-8G), ortho	Hayakawa et al., 1997
	B7-1	Ad	i.tu.	10^9	No regression	C3H mice melanoma (K 1735), s.c., 27 mm^3	Boxhorn et al., 1998
	B7	Tumor cells	i.p.		60% (cures)	C57/BL6, lymphoma (EL4), s.c.	Chen et al., 1994a
	B7-1	Tumor cells	s.c.	5×10^6	13% (cures n.s. (surv)	A/J, neuroblastoma (N-2a), s.c., 3–7 mm	Heuer et al., 1996
	Tumor peptides	Dendritic cells	i.v.	$3–5 \times 10^5$, several times	MCA205 82% (vol) TS/A >50% (vol) C3 100% (cures)	C57BL/6, fibrosarcoma (MCA205), C3, i.d. BALB/c, breast cancer (TS/A), i.d.	Zitvogel et al., 1996a
	gp100	VV-generated T cells	i.v., rhIL-2 i.p.	1×10^7	96% (number of metastases)	C57BL/6, melanoma (B16), i.v.	Overwijk et al., 1998
Combinations	p16 + p53	Ad	i.tu.	6×10^9, 2×	84% (vol)	Nude, HCC, (HuH7) s.c.	Sandig et al., 1997
	p21 + MHC class 1, H-2Kb	Ad	i.tu.	2×10^8, 7×	62.5% (cures)	BALB/c, renal cancer (Renca), s.c., 4 mm^2	Ohno et al., 1997
	HSV-tk + IL-2	Ad	i.tu.	2.5×10^8	87% (area)	Lewis lung cancer (LL2) in liver, 4–5 mm	Kwong et al., 1997
	CD + GM-CSF	Ad		10^9, 2×	79% (vol)	C57BL/6, melanoma (B16F10), s.c.	Cao et al., 1998
	IL-2 + TNF	Plasmid	s.c.	5×10^6, 6×	Growth retardation	C57/BL6, lung cancer (Lewis lung cancer carcinoma), s.c.	Ohira et al., 1994
	IL-2, IFN-γ, GM-CSF	Tumor cells	i.d.	10^6, 3×	60% (cures) (s.c.) no (cures), surv benefit (orth)	Copenhagen rats, prostate cancer, (R3327-MatLylu), s.c., ortho	Vieweg et al., 1994
	IL-2, IFN-γ	Tumor cells	i.p.	1×10^6, 4×	IL-2 53% (number of metastases) γIFN 81% (number of metastases) no add, effect	C57/BL6, melanoma (B16), i.v.	Abdel-Wahab et al., 1997
	B7-1, MHC class II	Tumor cells	i.p.	10^6, 1×	60% (cures)	A/J mice, sarcoma (Sal/N), s.c., 2–5 mm	Baskar et al., 1995
	B7-1, GM-CSF, IL-12	Tumor cells	i.d.	1×10^6, 3×	IL-12 30% (cures), 70% (vol) B7-1, GM-CSF no eff.	C57BL/6, lung cancer (LLC), i.d.	Sumimoto et al., 1998
	B7-1, IL-12	Fibroblasts	peri.tu.	$1–2 \times 10^6$, 2/3×	55% (vol)	BALB/c, breast cancer (TS/A), i.d., 25–36 mm^2	Zitvogel et al., 1996b
	B7-1, IL-12		s.c.	5×10^6, weekly	IL-2 80% (cures) B7-1 no impact	DBA/2, mastocytoma (P1. HTR.C), s.c.	Fallarino et al., 1997

Table 1 (Continued)

Strategy	Transgene	Vector	Route	Dose	Efficacy	Animal model, organ, cell line, site, pretreatment size	Ref.*
	B7-1, B7-2	Tumor cells	s.c.	10^6, 6×	RMA: 40% (cures) TS/A (B7-2): 22% (cures), TS/A (B7-1): no (cures) B16 no response	BALB/c, C57BL/6, lymphaoma (RMA T), breast cancer (TS/A), melanoma (B16 F10) s.c.	Martin-Fontecha et al., 1996
	GM-CSF, IL-4	Tumor cells	s.c.	3 × 10^6, d5	GM-CSF: 90 IL-4: 170% (surv)	BALB/c, lymphoma (A20), i.v.	Levitsky et al., 1996
	GM-CSF + IFN-γ	Tumor cells	s.c.	10^6	145% (surv)	A/J, neuroblastoma (neuro 2a), ortho	Bausero et al., 1996
	IFN-γ, IL-4	Monocyte macrophage cell line (J774A.1)	i.tu.	2–4 × 10^6	IL-4 or IFN-gamma: 50% IL-4 + IFN-gamma: 25% (vol)	C57BL/6, melanoma (B16), s.c.	Nishihara et al., 1995

* Table references follow text references on page 468.

i.p.: Intraperitoneal; tu.: intratumoral; i.pleu.: intrapleural; i.port.: intraportal; i.a.: intraarterial; s.c.: subcutaneous; i.cr.: intracranial; i.d.: intradermal; ortho: orthotopic (typical site of primary tumor); HCC: hepatocellular carcinoma; Ad: adenovirus; Retro: retrovirus; Retro-VPC: retrovirus vector producer cells; VV: vaccinia virus; Lip: liposomes; vol: volume; surv: survival.

[a] Reduction of tumor weight or volume in percent of untreated control.

[b] Increase in survival in percent of the control.

[c] The amount of DNA is indicated.

[d] Cures: tumor-free animals and long-term survivers.

[e] Mice if not stated otherwise.

[f] Calcilated volumes or diameters.

[g] Number of repetitions.

[h] Orthotopic, usually the organ where the cell line originates from.

Based on the bulky mass of head and neck cancer, it is unlikely that the large tumor burdens that remain even after radical surgery can be sufficiently transduced even by the highly efficacious replication-deficient adenoviral vectors. Therefore, and because of the good accessibility, head and neck cancer has become the model disease for therapy with selectively replication-competent adenoviruses. The underlying concept of the use of replication-competent recombinant adenoviruses is based on the capability of adenovirus to induce cell lysis by its progeny inside of an infected target cell (198,199). To limit the cytotoxicity only to tumor cells and not to normal cells, the fact was used that about 50% of tumors carry a mutation in the tumor suppressor gene p53. A recombinant replication-competent adenovirus was constructed that should specifically replicate only in p53-negative tumor cells (43). This was achieved by deletion of the adenoviral E1B gene coding for a 55 kDa protein, which inactivates the apoptosis promoting effect of p53. Consequently, this adenovirus replicates in p53-negative tumor cells leading to cell lysis and the spread of the virus to neighboring tumor cells. Once these cells are infected, the lytic cycle starts again. However, when such viruses reach a p53-positive cell, e.g., normal tissue, the missing E1B 55 kDa gene product cannot block p53 and, therefore, replication is terminated by apoptosis. This replication-competent recombinant adenovirus can be used without and in combination with classical chemotherapy (44). However, this intriguing concept has recently been seriously questioned by the observation that the presence of p53 was necessary for viral replication, indicating that only p53-negative tumor cells are resistant to viral replication (45). Further experiments are needed to study the underlying molecular mechanism in more detail. Despite the incomplete understanding of the underlying concept of the mode of action of the vector, the first clinical trials are underway and preliminary data are encouraging. So far, over 90 patients with head and neck cancer have been treated with direct intratumoral vector injections. In this study, replication of ONYX-015 with associated cytopathic effects in p53-negative tumors was demonstrated (200).

E. Hematological and Lymphatic Malignancies

These malignancies are the domain of chemotherapy. Due to the development of advanced protocols, the initial rate of remission and the rate of long-term survivors has dramatically increased. In all stages, the primary therapeutic intention is curative. The usual treatment regime consists of several cycles of intensive or high-dose chemotherapy up to a full eradication of the patient's bone marrow followed by autologous or allogeneic bone marrow transplantation. Due to the good susceptibility of leukemic and lymphatic cells to chemotherapy, conventional treatment usually leaves minimal residual disease, which then could be the target of gene therapeutic intervention to prevent relapses, which usually have a bad prognosis and occur in 80% of patients with leukemia (201). Several immunological approaches have been conducted: among several cytokines, IL-4 and GM-CSF protected best against tumor challenge and GM-CSF–transduced cells also inhibited further progression of preestablished lymphatic tumors (202). Transfer of IL-2 into lymphomas is already the subject of a clinical phase I study (203). TNF-α was used for T-cell lymphoma (204) and myeloma (205), B7 for several lymphomas (206,207), and GM-CSF for T-cell leukemia (208).

The generation of chimeric T-cell receptors (TCRs) has been another strategy to generate antitumor immunity for B-cell lymphoma. T cells are directed against target cells by grafting an antibody V region of desired specificity onto the TCR and the constant regions. Specificity of this approach in vitro has been shown (209). Vaccinations with the DNA of tumor antigens have also been carried out. Gene therapy provides here an advantage over the use of the respective protein when this is difficult to obtain in the required amount or in the correctly glycosylated form.

A successful approach to the treatment of B-cell lymphoma has been the transfer of donor leukocytes (210) or EBV-specific cytotoxic T lymphocytes (211). A potential problem of this strategy, however, could be graft-versus-host disease (GvHD). An ingenious way to circumvent this problem is the transduction of the donor T cells with a suicide gene like HSV-tk to be able to kill the donor T cells by GCV if signs of GvHD appear (212).

Lymphomas and leukemias have also been targeted with oligonucleotides against myc (167,213,214), bcl-2 (215), myb (216), bcr-abl (213,214), and bcr-abl ribozymes (217). Transfer efficacy of antisense oligonucleotides in vitro and in vivo is highly controversial, and time will show whether this remarkably simple technique will play a role in gene therapy for cancer.

Therapy-associated side effects like infections and hemorrhages account for 70% of the deaths of adult patients with acute leukemia (218). The transfer of MDR genes into hematopoietic stem cells for chemoprotection holds promise, and clinical studies of the transduction of the MDR gene in patients with relapsed and resistant lymphomas are already underway. This approach, however, bears the danger that tumor cells are transduced, making them resistant to chemotherapy, and only the future will show whether this problem can be circumvented, e.g., by targeted vectors.

F. Hepatocellular Carcinoma

Whereas hepatocellular carcinoma (HCC) is of moderate epidemiological relevance in the western world, it is the most common cancer in large areas in Asia. HCC often remains localized to the liver, but only a minority of patients is amenable to local therapy, such as surgery, liver transplantation or cryo-ablation, and standard chemotherapy is largely ineffective. Therefore, HCC is a good target for intratumoral application of therapeutic genes. As demonstrated, adenovirus vectors can easily infect and express different types of genes in tumor cells of HCC (30,69). In addition, in the α-fetoprotein (AFP) promoter, an extremely HCC-specific promoter is available (219). Using adenovirus-mediated gene transfer, different experimental approaches were studied demonstrating significant tumor volume reductions by IL-12 (220), HSV-tk/GCV (221), or combinatorial expression of p53 and p16 (30). A pilot study to assess the therapeutic potential of percutaneous injection of wild-type p53 (wt-p53) in five patients with primary HCC was initiated in 1996. Five patients with primary HCC received percutaneous injections of a wild-type p53 DNA-liposome complex. Three out of five patients showed reduction of tumor volume, as reported by computer tomographic scans. The serum levels of AFP also diminished significantly (222).

G. Melanoma

Malignant melanoma is a tumor of average incidence worldwide but with extremely high incidence in certain areas, such as Australia. Worldwide, a yearly increase in its incidence of 6–7% was reported (223). Melanoma is probably the tumor with the highest resistance to treatment. Treatment schedules including radiation, chemotherapy, and combinations of both have no significant impact on the overall survival of patients (224,225). Although the primary tumor can usually easily be excised, distant metastases cause death in nearly all patients. This is one reason why this disease is an important target for immunological approaches from which a systemic antitumor efficacy can be expected. The other reason is the naturally high immunogenicity of melanomas, which facilitates the recognition of the tumor by the immune system. Basically, all principles of immuno-modulation described above have been applied to melanoma. This is also reflected by the number of clinical gene therapy studies—30—for melanoma at the time of writing, which make this tumor the predominant target for clinical gene therapy. The earliest trials were based on the transfer of TNF-transduced TILs (6). Phase I trials are now closed, but due to minor success no further trials entirely focusing on TILs have been initiated. However, in a more recent trial, TILs obtained from a patients tumor nodules were injected with the B7 molecule, expanded, and reinfused, and direct immunological effects were demonstrated (226).

Costimulatory molecules have also been transferred in vitro to tumor cells, which were then applied or their DNA directly injected into tumors in preclinical or clinical trials

(227). More than 50 patients in five different studies have received intratumoral injections of B7 DNA using cationic liposomes (203,228). DNA or protein was detected in the great majority of the patients. Toxicity not attributable to the mechanical irritations was the exception, and local or even general responses were seen in one third of the cases. For malignant melanoma, there exist an abundance of preclinical data about the transfer of irradiated autologous tumor cells transfected with cytokines. The initial trials used IL-2–transfected and later IL-4– and IL-7–transfected tumor cells. Sometimes, also autologous fibroblasts, which are easier to generate than autologous tumor cells or heterologous tumor cells, were used. More recently, a preclinical study and a first clinical phase I trial were performed using vaccination with IL-12 gene-modified autologous melanoma cells where the genes coding for the p35 and p40 chain of interleukin-12 (IL-12) were inserted in two independent eukaryotic expression vectors. In the phase I trial, six patients with terminal metastatic melanoma were treated. In vitro, biologically active IL-12 was secreted. High levels were obtained by magnetic enrichment of transduced cells prior to irradiation. Transduced irradiated autologous cells were reinjected subcutaneously five or six times during the 6-week treatment course. In two of the six patients, an increase in tumor-reactive CTLs and proliferative cells was detected after vaccination. Although three patients showed disease stabilization and one patient had a mixed clinical response for several months, no complete or partial response was achieved (229).

Expectations have newly been laid regarding cytokine gene transfer into dendritic cells, which are easy to transfect with adenoviral vectors and which are the most effective antigen-presenting cells known to date. Recently, in vivo transfer of specific tumor antigens using dendritic cells has been reported. Especially MART-1 antigen–transfected dendritic cells generated MART-1–specific immunity and arrested the growth of established tumors (230,231).

Besides the illustrated immunological approaches that clearly dominate gene therapy of melanoma, preclinical suicide gene (Table 1) and tumor suppressor gene (p53) (Table 1) therapies have also been performed. Combinatorial approaches, e.g., cotransfer of suicide genes and cytokines, have resulted in additive tumor growth inhibition (205,232).

H. Lung Cancer

In the western world, lung cancer has become the most frequent tumor in males (218). The main reason for this is smoking, as more than 90% of the patients are or were smokers. The prognosis for this cancer is bad. Due to regional or systemic metastases, tumors can be resected in only 25% of the patients. Of these patients, only one fourth survive 5 years such that only 6% of the patients are curable. Because of the tendency for early metastasis, gene therapeutic approaches aiming at a systemic response such as immuno gene therapy are needed. Only recently has a potent evocation of an immune response been reported in animal experiments (233).

The combination of early metastasis of lung cancer and the low intrinsic immunogenicity make this tumor a very difficult target for gene therapy. On the contrary, the high epidemiological relevance of lung cancer creates an urgent need to develop alternative strategies to the standard therapeutic approaches. This is especially true for non–small-cell lung cancer (NSCLC). Because NSCLC is in most cases highly resistant to any kind of chemotherapy and well-documented studies about genetic defects in NSCLC exist, this tumor was from the beginning an attractive target for the use of tumor suppressor genes, e.g., p53. Impressive results have been obtained in preclinical studies demonstrating significant tumor growth inhibition in subcutaneous and orthotopic animal models (234,235). Therefore, the first clinical trial to treat NSCLC by gene transfer of p53 was initiated. A retroviral vector containing the wild-type p53 gene under control of a β-actin promoter was used. Nine patients whose conventional treatments had failed received direct injections into the tumor. Despite a low efficacy of gene transfer and lacking evidence for involvement of T-cell–mediated immunity, partial tumor regression was noted in three patients and tumor growth was stabilized in three other patients (236). To improve the in vivo gene-transfer efficacy, in the next step an adenovirus vector was used for p53 gene transfer (237). In a clinical phase 1 protocol that is still ongoing, this vector was combined with cisplatin chemotherapy to induce programmed cell death (apoptosis) in NSCLC (238).

Lung cancer has also been a model disease for antioncogene therapy. The K-ras oncogene is frequently overexpressed in lung cancer. Intratracheal transfer of retroviruses carrying an antisense K-ras construct markedly reduced tumor size and number of lung tumors in nude mice (239). Another candidate for antisense therapy is the ErbB2 transmembrane protein kinase receptor, whose abberant expression has been shown to contribute to malignant transformation and progression. The promoter of the ErbB2 gene could be used for expression of toxic transgenes. Also promoters that are activated by ionizing radiation (240) have been used for this purpose. It is hoped that in the future sufficient specificity for tumor deposits will be achieved such that even metastases can be efficiently transduced without toxicity for the surrounding normal tissue. Under these circumstances, combinations of gene therapy with conventional therapy could be a particularly attractive strategy, as discussed above for p53 and cisplatin.

I. Osteosarcoma

Osteosarcoma primarily afflicts young people within the first decades of life and accounts for 5% of all childhood malignancies (241). The overall 2-year metastasis-free survival rate approaches 66% (242,243). Metastases, mainly to the lung, are the predominant cause of mortality. Therefore, immunological approaches, e.g., the in vivo transfer of the B7 gene (244), may be particularly fruitful. However, with the osteocalcin promoter a tissue-specific promoter is available, which potentially allows systemic or regional treatment with cytotoxic genes and which has already been proven to be efficient in vivo in an adenoviral context (245).

J. Ovarian Cancer

Like the other two gynecological malignancies, namely cancer of the cervix and breast, ovarian cancer is also a relevant target for gene therapeutic approaches. Ovarian cancer is the leading cause of death from gynecological malignancies in women (246). Due to improvements in surgical, radiation, and chemotherapeutic techniques, the 5-year survival rate has improved over the last 20 years. However, over two thirds of the patients have advanced stage disease at presentation, and despite transient responses, the long-term survival of these patients rarely exceeds 15–30%. Although even patients with advanced stages often have their disease confined to their abdomen for extended periods of time, intraperitoneal chemotherapies have only moderate success basically because they do not provide the reduced toxicity profiles initially hoped for. Therefore, ovarian cancer has become one of the model diseases for gene therapeutic approaches with intracavital vector applications. Clinical studies have been initiated with HSV-tk as transgene and either retroviral VPCs (247) or adenoviruses (248) as vectors. In both cases, in preclinical experiments, intraperitoneal vector application and consecutive GCV treatment significantly prolonged the survival of mice with established tumors. The superiority of either vector will be seen when the studies are closed. Phase I trials have also been initiated for adenoviral delivery of an anti-erbB-2 single-chain antibody gene (248,249). This "intrabody" approach could become a potent alternative to antisense strategies. A fourth study where HSV-tk–positive tumor cells are delivered into the peritoneal cavity relies on the bystander effect and additionally aims at a potent induction of an immunological response (250). Lastly, adenoviral transfer of p53 (34) and liposomal transfer of E1A (251) or mutant SV 40T antigen (252) also resulted in significant growth retardation in animal experiments.

K. Pancreatic Cancer

This disease has a low incidence but a very bad prognosis, mainly because the primary tumors are usually not resectable at the time of discovery. Moreover, the tumors are highly chemoresistant, and only very recently have partial remissions of up to 15% of the cases been seen with the new drug gemcitabine (218).

More than 80% of pancreatic tumors contain a mutation of the ras oncogene in position 12 (253). Since this mutation as well as others are recognized by the immune system, peptide-based immunotherapy has been successful in mice and clinical studies are already underway (254,255). The fact that the local disease is often life limiting in pancreatic cancer makes the disease attractive for cytotoxic gene therapy approaches (256–258). An interesting target gene may also be the DPC-4 (deleted in pancreatic cancer) gene, which is homozygously deleted or mutated in more than 50% of the pancreatic carcinomas (259).

L. Prostate Carcinoma

Prostate cancer is the most frequently diagnosed cancer in men in the United States and the second leading cause of death from malignancy (246,260). Locally restricted tumors can be treated by surgical resection or radiotherapy. Androgen ablative therapy often induces dramatic responses, but virtually all patients progress to an androgen refractory state with a median survival of 12–18 months. The prostate is a unique accessory organ and expresses several hundred unique gene products as potential targets for gene therapy. Prostate cancer can therefore serve as a model disease for tumor-specific gene therapy. Among the already initiated clinical trials are three using common immunological approaches (two for GM-CSF, IL-2 + IFN-γ) and three that use the prostate-specific PSA antigen for immunization. A current trial for HSV-tk gene transfer uses the universal RSV promoter for tk gene expression. The efficacy and specificity of the PSA promoter has already been proven in animal experiments (261) such that the use of this regulatory element can be expected in the future. This promoter has also been used to confer prostate-specific replication of conditionally replication-competent adenoviruses (46). Others report the transfer of the anti-IGF-1 receptor (262), p53 (263,264), p21 (264), and anti-sense myc (265). The future use of prostate-specific regulatory elements and target genes holds the promise that treatment of disseminated disease, which is the major cause of death in prostate cancer patients, will eventually be possible if systemic application of the vectors harboring cytotoxic genes can be done without major toxicity.

V. CONCLUSIONS

The use of a vehicle to transfer a gene into the human body is less direct and usually more complicated than conventional methods for cancer therapy. However, the interposition of several steps between application of an active substance and the generation of an observable effect allows an unusually great amount of freedom of regulation and at the same time requires that this freedom be used intelligently. On the one hand, one can comply with the biology and especially the weak spots of the cancer cells to a degree never seen before, but on the other hand, the gene therapeutic approach suffers from low specificity and sometimes discouraging efficacy if these requirements are not exactly met. Since we are still far from a tight adaptation of our vectors to the specificities of the cancer cells and these specificities themselves are not yet fully known, it comes as no surprise that clinical efficacy needs to be improved. We would, however, like to stress that the potential fruitfulness of a new method cannot be judged by its initial success, but rather by the general limitations of the whole concept. Since in the area of gene therapy for cancer such limitations are not yet evident, a breakthrough in therapeutic efficacy will most likely be a matter of time. Therefore, optimism about the development of a successful treatment of cancer with gene therapeutic approaches is probably justified.

ACKNOWLEDGMENTS

We thank Martin Schmidt for excellent technical assistance and Axel Schumacher and Zhihai Qin for critical reading of the manuscript.

TEXT REFERENCES

1. Ottgen HF, Old LJ. The history of cancer immunotherapy. In: DeVita VT, Hellmann S, Rosenberg SA, eds. Biological Therapy of Cancer: Principles and Practice. JB Lippincott, 1991:87–111.
2. Sahin U, Tureci O, Schmitt H, Cochlovirus B, Johannes T, Schmits R, Stenner F, Luo G, Schobert I, Pfreundschuh M. Human neoplasms elicit multiple specific immune responses in the autologous host. Proc Natl Acad Sci USA 92:11810–11813.
3. Pardoll DM. Tumour antigens. A new look for the 1990s [news; comment]. Nature 1994; 369:357–358.
4. Blankenstein T, Cayeux S, Qin Z. Genetic approaches to cancer immunotherapy. Rev Physiol Biochem Pharmacol 1996; 129:1–49.
5. Riddell SR, Greenberg PD. Principles for adoptive T cell therapy of human viral diseases. Annu Rev Immunol 1995; 13:545–586.
6. Rosenberg SA, Aebersold P, Cornetta K, Kasid A, Morgan RA, Moen R, Karson EM, Lotze MT, Yang JC, Topalian SL, et al. Gene transfer into humans—immunotherapy of patients with advanced melanoma, using tumor-infiltrating lymphocytes modified by retroviral gene transduction [see comments]. N Engl J Med 1990; 323:570–578.
7. Merrouche Y, Negrier S, Bain C, Combaret V, Mercatello A, Coronel B, Moskovtchenko JF, Tolstoshev P, Moen R, Philip T, et al. Clinical application of retroviral gene transfer in oncology: results of a French study with tumor-infiltrating lymphocytes transduced with the gene of resistance to neomycin. J Clin Oncol 1995; 13:410–418.
8. Friedmann T. Genetically modified tumor-infiltrating lymphocytes for cancer therapy. Cancer Cells 1991; 3: 271–274.
9. Greenberg PD. Adoptive T cell therapy of tumors: mechanisms operative in the recognition and elimination of tumor cells. Adv Immunol 1991; 49:281–355.
10. Rosenberg SA. Cancer vaccines based on the identification of genes encoding cancer regression antigens. Immunol Today 1997; 18:175–182.
11. Yee C, Gilbert MJ, Riddell SR, Brichard VG, Fefer A, Thompson JA, Boon T, Greenberg PD. Isolation of tyrosinase-specific CD8+ and CD4+ T cell clones from the peripheral blood of melanoma patients following in vitro stimulation with recombinant vaccinia virus. J Immunol 1996; 157:4079–4086.
12. Leach DR, Krummel MF, Allison JP. Enhancement of antitumor immunity by CTLA-4 blockade [see comments]. Science 1996; 271:1734–1736.
13. Melero I, Shuford WW, Newby SA, Aruffo A, Ledbetter JA, Hellstrom KE, Mittler RS, Chen L. Monoclonal antibodies against the 4-1BB T-cell activation molecule eradicate established tumors. Nat Med 1997; 3:682–685.
14. van der Bruggen P, Traversari C, Chomez P, Lurquin C, De PE, Van d EB, Knuth A, Boon T. A gene encoding an antigen recognized by cytolytic T lymphocytes on a human melanoma. Science 1991; 254:1643–1647.
15. Sahin U, Tureci O, Pfreundschuh M. Serological identification of human tumor antigens. Curr Opin Immunol 1997; 9:709–716.
16. Riethmuller G, Schneider GE, Schlimok G, Schmiegel W, Raab R, Hoffken K, Gruber R, Pichlmaier H, Hirche H, Pichlmayr R, et al. Randomised trial of monoclonal antibody for adjuvant therapy of resected Dukes' C colorectal carcinoma. German Cancer Aid 17-1A Study Group [see comments]. Lancet 1994; 343:1177–1183.
17. Connors TA. The choice of prodrugs for gene directed enzyme prodrug therapy of cancer. Gene Ther 1995; 2: 702–709.
18. Moolten FL, Wells JM, Heyman RA, Evans RM. Lymphoma regression induced by ganciclovir in mice bearing a herpes thymidine kinase transgene. Hum Gene Ther 1990; 1:125–134.

19. Barba D, Hardin J, Sadelain M, Gage FH. Development of anti-tumor immunity following thymidine kinase-mediated killing of experimental brain tumors. Proc Natl Acad Sci USA 1994; 91:4348–4352.
20. Brand K, Arnold W, Bartels T, Lieber A, Kay MA, Strauss M, Dorken B. Liver-associated toxicity of the HSV-tk/GCV approach and adenoviral vectors, Cancer Gene Ther 1997; 4:9–16.
21. Brand K, Löser P, Arnold W, Bartels T, Strauss M. Tumor cell-specific transgene expression prevents liver toxicity of adeno-HSVtk/GCV approach. Gene Ther 1998; 5: 1363–1371.
22. Eck SL, Alavi JB, Alavi A, Davis A, Hackney D, Judy K, Mollman J, Phillips PC, Wheeldon EB, Wilson JM. Treatment of advanced CNS malignancies with the recombinant adenovirus H5.010RSVTK: a phase I trial. Hum Gene Ther 1996; 7:1465–1482.
23. Ohwada A, Hirschowitz EA, Crystal RG. Regional delivery of an adenovirus vector containing the *Escherichia coli* cytosine deaminase gene to provide local activation of 5-fluorocytosine to suppress the growth of colon carcinoma metastatic to liver. Hum Gene Ther 1996; 7:1567–1576.
24. Crystal RG, Hirschowitz E, Lieberman M, Daly J, Kazam E, Henschke C, Yankelevitz D, Kemeny N, Silverstein R, Ohwada A, Russi T, Mastrangeli A, Sanders A, Cooke J, Harvey BG. Phase I study of direct administration of a replication deficient adenovirus vector containing the *E. coli* cytosine deaminase gene to metastatic colon carcinoma of the liver in association with the oral administration of the pro-drug 5-fluorocytosine. Hum Gene Ther 1997; 8:985–1001.
25. Bouvet M, Ellis LM, Nishizaki M, Fujiwara T, Liu W, Bucana CD, Fang B, Lee JJ, Roth JA. Adenovirus-mediated wild-type p53 gene transfer down-regulates vascular endothelial growth factor expression and inhibits angiogenesis in human colon cancer. Cancer Res 1998; 58: 2288–2292.
26. Bargou RC, Wagener C, Bommert K, Mapara MY, Daniel PT, Arnold W, Dietel M, Guski H, Feller A, Royer HD, Dorken B. Overexpression of the death-promoting gene bax-alpha which is downregulated in breast cancer restores sensitivity to different apoptotic stimuli and reduces tumor growth in SCID mice [see comments]. J Clin Invest 1996; 97:2651–2659.
27. Ealovega MW, McGinnis PK, Sumantran VN, Clarke MF, Wicha MS. bcl-xs gene therapy induces apoptosis of human mammary tumors in nude mice. Cancer Res 1996; 56:1965–1969.
28. Riley DJ, Nikitin AY, Lee WH. Adenovirus-mediated retinoblastoma gene therapy suppresses spontaneous pituitary melanotroph tumors in Rb+/− mice. Nat Med 1996; 2: 1316–1321.
29. Xu HJ, Zhou Y, Seigne J, Perng GS, Mixon M, Zhang C, Li J, Benedict WF, Hu SX. Enhanced tumor suppressor gene therapy via replication-deficient adenovirus vectors expressing an N-terminal truncated retinoblastoma protein. Cancer Res 1996; 56:2245–2249.
30. Sandig V, Brand K, Herwig S, Lukas J, Bartek J, Strauss M. Adenovirally transferred p16INK4/CDKN2 and p53 genes cooperate to induce apoptotic tumor cell death. Nat Med 1997; 3:313–319.
31. Jin X, Nguyen D, Zhang WW, Kyritsis AP, Roth JA. Cell cycle arrest and inhibition of tumor cell proliferation by the p16INK4 gene mediated by an adenovirus vector. Cancer Res 1995; 55:3250–3253.
32. Yang ZY, Perkins ND, Ohno T, Nabel EG, Nabel GJ. The p21 cyclin-dependent kinase inhibitor suppresses tumorigenicity in vivo [see comments]. Nat Med 1995; 1: 1052–1056.
33. Chang EH, Jang YJ, Hao Z, Murphy G, Rait A, Fee WJ, Sussman HH, Ryan P, Chiang Y, Pirollo KF. Restoration of the G1 checkpoint and the apoptotic pathway mediated by wild-type p53 sensitizes squamous cell carcinoma of the head and neck to radiotherapy. Arch Otolaryngol Head Neck Surg 1997; 123:507–512.
34. Gallardo D, Drazan KE, McBride WH. Adenovirus-based transfer of wild-type p53 gene increases ovarian tumor radiosensitivity. Cancer Res 1996; 56:4891–4893.
35. Spitz FR, Nguyen D, Skibber JM, Meyn RE, Cristiano RJ, Roth JA. Adenovirus-mediated wild-type p53 gene expression sensitizes colorectal cancer cells to ionizing radiation. Clin Cancer Res 1996; 2:1665–1671.
36. Blagosklonny MV, El DW. Acute overexpression of wt p53 facilitates anticancer drug-induced death of cancer and normal cells. Int J Cancer 1998; 75:933–940.
37. Fujiwara T, Grimm EA, Mukhopadhyay T, Zhang WW, Owen SL, Roth JA. Induction of chemosensitivity in human lung cancer cells in vivo by adenovirus-mediated transfer of the wild-type p53 gene. Cancer Res 1994; 54: 2287–2291.
38. Skladanowski A, Larsen AK. Expression of wild-type p53 increases etoposide cytotoxicity in M1 myeloid leukemia cells by facilitated G2 to M transition: implications for gene therapy. Cancer Res 1997; 57:818–823.
39. Li WW, Fan J, Hochhauser D, Bertino JR. Overexpression of p21waf1 leads to increased inhibition of E2F-1 phosphorylation and sensitivity to anticancer drugs in retinoblastoma-negative human sarcoma cells. Cancer Res 1997; 57:2193–2199.
40. Kovesdi I, Brough DE, Bruder JT, Wickham TJ. Adenoviral vectors for gene transfer. Curr Opin Biotechnol 1997; 8:583–589.
41. Dock G. Am J Med Sci 1904; 127:563.
42. Smith R, et al. Studies on the use of viruses in the treatment of carcinoma of the cervix. Cancer 1956; 9:1211–1218.
43. Bischoff JR, Kirn DH, Williams A, Heise C, Horn S, Muna M, Ng L, Nye JA, Sampson JA, Fattaey A, McCormick F. An adenovirus mutant that replicates selectively in p53-deficient human tumor cells [see comments], Science 1996; 274:373–376.
44. Heise C, Sampson JA, Williams A, McCormick F, Von HD, Kirn DH. ONYX-015, an E1B gene-attenuated adenovirus, causes tumor-specific cytolysis and antitumoral effi-

cacy that can be augmented by standard chemotherapeutic agents [see comments]. Nat Med 1997; 3:639–645.
45. Hall AR, Dix BR, O'Carroll SJ, Braithwaite AW. p53-dependent cell death/apoptosis is required for a productive adenovirus infection [see comments]. Nat Med 1998; 4: 1068–1072.
46. Rodriguez R, Schuur ER, Lim HY, Henderson GA, Simons JW, Henderson DR. Prostate attenuated replication competent adenovirus (ARCA) CN706: a selective cytotoxic for prostate-specific antigen-positive prostate cancer cells. Cancer Res 1997; 57:2559–2563.
47. Martuza RL, Malick A, Markert JM, Ruffner KL, Coen DM. Experimental therapy of human glioma by means of a genetically engineered virus mutant. Science 1991; 252: 854–856.
48. Jia WW, McDermott M, Goldie J, Cynader M, Tan J, Tufaro F. Selective destruction of gliomas in immunocompetent rats by thymidine kinase-defective herpes simplex virus type 1 [see comments]. J Natl Cancer Inst 1994; 86: 1209–1215.
49. Kirn D. Selectively replicating viruses as therapeutic agents against cancer. In: Lattime EC, Gerson SL, eds. Gene Therapy of Cancer. New York: Academic Press, 1999:235–247.
50. Reichard KW, Lorence RM, Cascino CJ, Peeples ME, Walter RJ, Fernando MB, Reyes HM, Greager JA. Newcastle disease virus selectively kills human tumor cells. J Surg Res 1992; 52:448–453.
51. Cassel WA, Garrett RE. Newcastle disease virus as an antineoplastic agent. Cancer 1965; 18:863–868.
52. Lorence RM, Rood PA, Kelley KW. Newcastle disease virus as an antineoplastic agent: induction of tumor necrosis factor-alpha and augmentation of its cytotoxicity. J Natl Cancer Inst 1988; 80:1305–1312.
53. Kass-Eisler A, Leinwand L, Gall J, Bloom B, Falck PE. Circumventing the immune response to adenovirus-mediated gene therapy. Gene Ther 1996; 3:154–162.
54. O'Reilly MS, Boehm T, Shing Y, Fukai N, Vasios G, Lane WS, Flynn E, Birkhead JR, Olsen BR, Folkman J. Endostatin: an endogenous inhibitor of angiogenesis and tumor growth. Cell 1997; 88:277–285.
55. Brem H, Goto F, Budson A, Saunders L, Folkman J. Minimal drug resistance after prolonged anti-angiogenic therapy with AGM-1470. Surg Forum 1994; XLV:674–677.
56. Folkman J. Antiangiogenic gene therapy. Proc Natl Acad Sci USA 1998; 95:9064–9066.
57. Lin P, Buxton JA, Acheson A, Radziejewski C, Maisonpierre PC, Yancopoulos GD, Channon KM, Hale LP, Dewhirst MW, George SE, Peters KG. Antiangiogenic gene therapy targeting the endothelium-specific receptor tyrosine kinase Tie2. Proc Natl Acad Sci USA 1998; 95: 8829–8834.
58. Goldman CK, Kendall RL, Cabrera G, Soroceanu L, Heike Y, Gillespie GY, Siegal GP, Mao X, Bett AJ, Huckle WR, Thomas KA, Curiel DT. Paracrine expression of a native soluble vascular endothelial growth factor receptor inhibits tumor growth, metastasis, and mortality rate. Proc Natl Acad Sci USA 1998; 95:8795–8800.
59. Klauber N, Rohan RM, Flynn E, D'Amato RJ. Critical components of the female reproductive pathway are suppressed by the angiogenesis inhibitor AGM-1470. Nat Med 3: 1997; 3:443–446.
60. Gottesman MM, Hrycyna CA, Schoenlein PV, Germann UA, Pastan I. Genetic analysis of the multidrug transporter. Annu Rev Genet 1995; 29:607–649.
61. Mickisch GH, Aksentijevich I, Schoenlein PV, Goldstein LJ, Galski H, Stahle C, Sachs DH, Pastan I, Gottesman MM. Transplantation of bone marrow cells from transgenic mice expressing the human MDR1 gene results in long-term protection against the myelosuppressive effect of chemotherapy in mice. Blood 1992; 79:1087–1093.
62. Podda S, Ward M, Himelstein A, Richardson C, De IFWE, Smith L, Gottesman M, Pastan I, Bank A. Transfer and expression of the human multiple drug resistance gene into live mice. Proc Natl Acad Sci USA 1992; 89:9676–9680.
63. Sorrentino BP, Brandt SJ, Bodine D, Gottesman M, Pastan I, Cline A, Nienhuis AW. Selection of drug-resistant bone marrow cells in vivo after retroviral transfer of human MDR1. Science 1992; 257:99–103.
64. Sorrentino BP, McDonagh KT, Woods D, Orlic D. Expression of retroviral vectors containing the human multidrug resistance 1 cDNA in hematopoietic cells of transplanted mice. Blood 1995; 86:491–501.
65. Licht T, Aksentijevich I, Gottesman MM, Pastan I. Efficient expression of functional human MDR1 gene in murine bone marrow after retroviral transduction of purified hematopoietic stem cells. Blood 1995; 86:111–121.
66. Wilson JM. Adenoviruses as gene-delivery vehicles. N Engl J Med 1996; 334:1185–1187.
67. Bergelson JM, Cunningham JA, Droguett G, Kurt JE, Krithivas A, Hong JS, Horwitz MS, Crowell RL, Finberg RW. Isolation of a common receptor for coxsackie B viruses and adenoviruses 2 and 5. Science 1997; 275: 1320–1323.
68. Wickham TJ, Mathias P, Cheresh DA, Nemerow GR. Integrins alpha v beta 3 and alpha v beta 5 promote adenovirus internalization but not virus attachment. Cell 1993; 73: 300–319.
69. Brand K, Klocke R, Poßling A, Paul D, Strauss M. Induction of apoptosis and G2/M arrest by infection with replication deficient adenovirus at high multiplicity of infection. Gene Ther 1999; 6:1054–1063.
70. Amalfitano A, Hauser MA, Hu H, Serra D, Begy CR, Chamberlain JS. Production and characterization of improved adenovirus vectors with the E1, E2b, and E3 genes deleted. J Virol 1998; 72:926–933.
71. Nevins JR. Mechanism of activation of early viral transcription by the adenovirus E1A gene product. Cell 1981; 26:213–220.
72. Yang Y, Nunes FA, Berencsi K, Gonczol E, Engelhardt JF, Wilson JM. Inactivation of E2a in recombinant adenoviruses improves the prospect for gene therapy in cystic fibrosis. Nat Genet 1994; 7:362–369.

73. Lieber A, He CY, Meuse L, Schowalter D, Kirillova I, Winther B, Kay MA. The role of Kupffer cell activation and viral gene expression in early liver toxicity after infusion of recombinant adenovirus vectors. J Virol 1997; 71: 8798–8807.
74. Spergel JM, Chen KS. Interleukin 6 enhances a cellular activity that functionally substitutes for E1A protein in transactivation. Proc Natl Acad Sci USA 1991; 88: 6472–6476.
75. Bramson J, Hitt M, Gallichan WS, Rosenthal KL, Gauldie J, Graham FL. Construction of a double recombinant adenovirus vector expressing a heterodimeric cytokine: in vitro and in vivo production of biologically active interleukin-12. Hum Gene Ther 1996; 7:333–342.
76. Gao GP, Yang Y, Wilson JM. Biology of adenovirus vectors with E1 and E4 deletions for liver-directed gene therapy. J Virol 1996; 70:8934–8943.
77. Wang Q, Finer MH. Second-generation adenovirus vectors. Nat Med 1996; 2:714–716.
78. Wang Q, Jia XC, Finer MH. A packaging cell line for propagation of recombinant adenovirus vectors containing two lethal gene-region deletions. Gene Ther 1995; 2: 775–783.
79. Yeh P, Dedieu JF, Orsini C, Vigne E, Denefle P, Perricaudet M. Efficient dual transcomplementation of adenovirus E1 and E4 regions from a 293-derived cell line expressing a minimal E4 functional unit. J Virol 1996; 70: 559–565.
80. Haecker SE, Stedman HH, Balice GR, Smith DB, Greelish JP, Mitchell MA, Wells A, Sweeney HL, Wilson JM. In vivo expression of full-length human dystrophin from adenoviral vectors deleted of all viral genes. Hum Gene Ther 1996; 7:1907–1914.
81. Parks RJ, Chen L, Anton M, Sankar U, Rudnicki MA, Graham FL. A helper-dependent adenovirus vector system: removal of helper virus by Cre-mediated excision of the viral packaging signal. Proc Natl Acad Sci USA 1996; 93:13565–13570.
82. Parks RJ, Graham FL. A helper-dependent system for adenovirus vector production helps define a lower limit for efficient DNA packaging. J Virol 1997; 71:3293–3298.
83. Chen PW, Wang M, Bronte V, Zhai Y, Rosenberg SA, Restifo NP. Therapeutic antitumor response after immunization with a recombinant adenovirus encoding a model tumor-associated antigen. J Immunol 1996; 156:224–231.
84. Morsy MA, Gu M, Motzel S, Zhao J, Lin J, Su Q, Allen H, Franlin L, Parks RJ, Graham FL, Kochanek S, Bett AJ, Caskey CT. An adenoviral vector deleted for all viral coding sequences results in enhanced safety and extended expression of a leptin transgene. Proc Natl Acad Sci USA 1998; 95:7866–7871.
85. Culver KW, Ram Z, Wallbridge S, Ishii H, Oldfield EH, Blaese RM. In vivo gene transfer with retroviral vector-producer cells for treatment of experimental brain tumors [see comments]. Science 1992; 256:1550–1552.
86. Cosset FL, Takeuchi Y, Battini JL, Weiss RA, Collins MK. High-titer packaging cells producing recombinant retroviruses resistant to human serum. J Virol 1995; 69: 7430–7436.
87. Robbins PD, Tahara H, Ghivizzani SC. Viral vectors for gene therapy. Trends Biotechnol 1998; 16:35–40.
88. Blomer U, Naldini L, Verma IM, Trono D, Gage FH. Applications of gene therapy to the CNS. Hum Mol Genet 1996; 5 Spec No:1397–1404.
89. Naldini L, Blomer U, Gage FH, Trono D, Verma IM. Efficient transfer, integration, and sustained long-term expression of the transgene in adult rat brains injected with a lentiviral vector. Proc Natl Acad Sci USA 1996; 93: 11382–11388.
90. Naldini L, Blomer U, Gallay P, Ory D, Mulligan R, Gage FH, Verma IM, Trono D. In vivo gene delivery and stable transduction of nondividing cells by a lentiviral vector [see comments]. Science 1996; 272:263–267.
91. Fink DJ, Ramakrishnan R, Marconi P, Goins WF, Holland TC, Glorioso JC. Advances in the development of herpes simplex virus-based gene transfer vectors for the nervous system. Clin Neurosci 1995; 3:284–291.
92. Marconi P, Krisky D, Oligino T, Poliani PL, Ramakrishnan R, Goins WF, Fink DJ, Glorioso JC. Replication-defective herpes simplex virus vectors for gene transfer in vivo. Proc Natl Acad Sci USA 1996; 93:11319–11320.
93. Fink DJ, Glorioso JC. Herpes simplex virus-based vectors: problems and some solutions. Adv Neurol 1997; 72: 149–156.
94. Fink DJ, Glorioso JC. Engineering herpes simplex virus vectors for gene transfer to neurons. Nat Med 1997; 3: 357–359.
95. Wu N, Watkins SC, Schaffer PA, DeLuca NA. Prolonged gene expression and cell survival after infection by a herpes simplex virus mutant defective in the immediate-early genes encoding ICP4, ICP27, and ICP22. J Virol 1996; 70:6358–6369.
96. Zhu Z, DeLuca NA, Schaffer PA. Overexpression of the herpes simplex virus type 1 immediate-early regulatory protein, ICP27, is responsible for the aberrant localization of ICPO and mutant forms of ICP4 in ICP4 mutant virus-infected cells. J Virol 1996; 70:5346–5356.
97. Scheiflinger F, Dorner F, Falkner FG. Construction of chimeric vaccinia viruses by molecular cloning and packaging. Proc Natl Acad Sci USA 1992; 89:9977–9981.
98. Ansardi DC, Moldoveanu Z, Porter DC, Walker DE, Conry RM, LoBuglio AF, McPherson S, Morrow CD. Characterization of poliovirus replicons encoding carcinoembryonic antigen. Cancer Res 1994; 54:6359–6364.
99. Hofmann C, Sandig V, Jennings G, Rudolph M, Schlag P, Strauss M. Efficient gene transfer into human hepatocytes by baculovirus vectors. Proc Natl Acad Sci USA 1995; 92:10099–10103.
100. Sandig V, Hofmann C, Steinert S, Jennings G, Schlag P, Strauss M. Gene transfer into hepatocytes and human liver tissue by baculovirus vectors. Hum Gene Ther 1996; 7: 1937–1945.
101. Hofmann C, Strauss M. Baculovirus-mediated gene transfer in the presence of human serum or blood facilitated by

inhibition of the complement system, Gene Ther 1998; 5: 531–536.
102. Xiong C, Levis R, Shen P, Schlesinger S, Rice CM, Huang HV. Sindbis virus: an efficient, broad host range vector for gene expression in animal cells. Science 1989; 243: 1188–1191.
103. Berglund P, Sjoberg M, Garoff H, Atkins GJ, Sheahan BJ, Liljestrom P. Semliki forest virus expression system: production of conditionally infectious recombinant particles. Biotechnol NY 1993; 11:916–920.
104. Maxwell IH, Spitzer AL, Long CJ, Maxwell F. Autonomous parvovirus transduction of a gene under control of tissue-specific or inducible promoters. Gene Ther 1996; 3:28–36.
105. Recchia A, Parks RJ, Lamartina S, Toniatti C, Pieroni L, Palombo F, Ciliberto G, Graham FL, Cortese R, La-Monica N, Colloca S. Site-specific integration mediated by a *hybrid adenovirus*/adeno-associated virus vector. Proc Natl Acad Sci USA. 1999; 96:2615–2620.
106. Ledley FD. Nonviral gene therapy: the promise of genes as pharmaceutical products. Hum Gene Ther 1995; 6: 1129–1144.
107. Burkholder JK, Decker J, Yang NS. Rapid transgene expression in lymphocyte and macrophage primary cultures after particle bombardment-mediated gene transfer. J Immunol Methods 1993; 165:149–156.
108. Cheng L, Ziegelhoffer PR, Yang NS. In vivo promoter activity and transgene expression in mammalian somatic tissues evaluated by using particle bombardment. Proc Natl Acad Sci USA 1993; 90:4455–44.
109. Yang NS, Burkholder J, Roberts B, Martinell B, McCabe D. In vivo and in vitro gene transfer to mammalian somatic cells by particle bombardment, Proc Natl Acad Sci USA 1990; 87:9568–9572.
110. Wilson JM, Grossman M, Wu CH, Chowdhury NR, Wu GY, Chowdhury JR. Hepatocyte-directed gene transfer in vivo leads to transient improvement of hypercholesterolemia in low density lipoprotein receptor-deficient rabbits. J Biol Chem 1992; 26:963–967.
111. Cristiano RJ, Smith LC, Kay MA, Brinkley BR, Woo SL. Hepatic gene therapy: efficient gene delivery and expression in primary hepatocytes utilizing a conjugated adenovirus-DNA complex. Proc Natl Acad Sci USA 1993; 90: 11548–11552.
112. Curiel DT, Wagner E, Cotten M, Birnstiel ML, Agarwal S, Li CM, Loechel S, Hu PC. High-efficiency gene transfer mediated by adenovirus coupled to DNA-polylysine complexes. Hum Gene Ther 1992; 3:147–154.
113. Wagner E, Plank C, Zatloukal K, Cotten M, Birnstiel ML. Influenza virus hemagglutinin HA-2 N-terminal fusogenic peptides augment gene transfer by transferrin-polylysine-DNA complexes: toward a synthetic virus-like gene-transfer vehicle. Proc Natl Acad Sci USA 1992; 89:7934–7938.
114. Vogelstein B, Kinzler KW. p53 function and dysfunction. Cell 1992; 70:523–526.
115. Bargou RC, Jurchott K, Wagener C, Bergmann S, Metzner S, Bommert K, Mapara MY, Winzer KJ, Dietel M, Dorken B, Royer HD. Nuclear localization and increased levels of transcription factor YB-1 in primary human breast cancers are associated with intrinsic MDR1 gene expression [see comments]. Nat Med 1997; 3:447–450.
116. Baldini N. Multidrug resistance—a multiplex phenomenon [news; comment]. Nat Med. 1997; 3:378–380.
117. Fisher KJ, Choi H, Burda J, Chen SJ, Wilson JM. Recombinant adenovirus deleted of all viral genes for gene therapy of cystic fibrosis. Virology 1996; 217:11–22.
118. Kochanek S, Clemens PR, Mitani K, Chen HH, Chan S, Caskey CT. A new adenoviral vector: replacement of all viral coding sequences with 28 kb of DNA independently expressing both full-length dystrophin and beta-galactosidase, Proc Natl Acad Sci USA 1996; 93:5731–5736.
119. Mitani K, Graham FL, Caskey CT, Kochanek S. Rescue, propagation, and partial purification of a helper virus-dependent adenovirus vector. Proc Natl Acad Sci USA 1995; 92:3854–3858.
120. van der Eb MM, Cramer SJ, Vergouwe Y, Schagen FH, van KJ, van, dEA, Rinkes IH, van dVC, Hoeben RC. Severe hepatic dysfunction after adenovirus-mediated transfer of the herpes simplex virus thymidine kinase gene and ganciclovir administration. Gene Ther 1998; 5:451–458.
121. Chen L, Chen D, Manome Y, Dong Y, Fine HA, Kufe DW. Breast cancer selective gene expression and therapy mediated by recombinant adenoviruses containing the DF3/MUC1 promoter. J Clin Invest 1995; 96:2775–2782.
122. Connelly S, Gardner JM, McClelland A, Kaleko M. High-level tissue-specific expression of functional human factor VIII in mice. Hum Gene Ther 1996; 7:183–195.
123. Imler JL, Dupuit F, Chartier C, Accart N, Dieterle A, Schultz H, Puchelle E, Pavirani A. Targeting cell-specific gene expression with an adenovirus vector containing the lacZ gene under the control of the CFTR promoter. Gene Ther 1996; 3:49–58.
124. Sandig V, Loser P, Lieber A, Kay MA, Strauss M. HBV-derived promoters direct liver-specific expression of an adenovirally transduced LDL receptor gene. Gene Ther 1996; 3:1002–1009.
125. Siders WM, Halloran PJ, Fenton RG. Transcriptional targeting of recombinant adenoviruses to human and murine melanoma cells. Cancer Res 1996; 56:5638–5646.
126. Tanaka T, Kanai F, Lan KH, Ohashi M, Shiratori Y, Yoshida Y, Hamada H, Omata M. Adenovirus-mediated gene therapy of gastric carcinoma using cancer-specific gene expression in vivo. Biochem Biophys Res Commun 1997; 231:775–779.
127. Wu X, Holschen J, Kennedy SC, Ponder KP. Retroviral vector sequences may interact with some internal promoters and influence expression. Hum Gene Ther 1996; 7:159–171.
128. Yu SF, von Rüden T, Kantoff PW, Garber C, Seiberg M, Ruther U, Anderson WF, Wagner EF, Gilboa E. Self-inactivating retroviral vectors designed for transfer of whole genes into mammalian cells. Proc Natl Acad Sci USA 1986; 83:3194–3198.

129. Su H, Chang JC, Xu SM, Kan YW. Selective killing of AFP-positive hepatocellular carcinoma cells by adeno-associated virus transfer of the herpes simplex virus thymidine kinase gene. Hum Gene Ther 1996; 7:463–470.
130. Zhou SZ, Li Q, Stamatoyannopoulos G, Srivastava A. Adeno-associated virus 2-mediated transduction and erythroid cell-specific expression of a human beta-globin gene. Gene Ther 1996; 3:223–229.
131. Joki T, Nakamura M, Ohno T. Activation of the radiosensitive EGR-1 promoter induces expression of the herpes simplex virus thymidine kinase gene and sensitivity of human glioma cells to ganciclovir. Hum Gene Ther 1995; 6: 1507–1513.
132. Tomko RP, Xu R, Philipson L. HCAR and MCAR: the human and mouse cellular receptors for subgroup C adenoviruses and group B coxsackieviruses. Proc Natl Acad Sci USA 1997; 94:3352–3356.
133. Hong SS, Karayan L, Toumier J, Curiel DT, Boulanger PA. Adenovirus type 5 fiber knob binds to MHC class I alpha2 domain at the surface of human epithelial and B lymphoblastoid cells. Embo J 1997; 16:2294–2306.
134. Stevenson SC, Rollence M, White B, Weaver L, McClelland A. Human adenovirus serotypes 3 and 5 bind to two different cellular receptors via the fiber head domain. J Virol 1995; 69:2850–2857.
135. Roelvink PW, Kovesdi I, Wickham TJ. Comparative analysis of adenovirus fiber-cell interaction: adenovirus type 2 (Ad2) and Ad9 utilize the same cellular fiber receptor but use different binding strategies for attachment. J Virol 1996; 70:7614–7621.
136. Wickham TJ, Roelvink PW, Brough DE, Kovesdi I. Adenovirus targeted to heparan-containing receptors increases its gene delivery efficiency to multiple cell types. Nat Biotechnol 1996; 14:1570–1573.
137. Brooks PC, Montgomery AM, Rosenfeld M, Reisfeld RA, Hu T, Klier G, Cheresh DA. Integrin alpha v beta 3 antagonists promote tumor regression by inducing apoptosis of angiogenic blood vessels. Cell 1994; 79:1157–1164.
138. Douglas JT, Rogers BE, Rosenfeld ME, Michael SI, Feng M, Curiel DT. Targeted gene delivery by tropism-modified adenoviral vectors. Nat Biotechnol 1996; 14:1574–1578.
139. Wickham TJ, Segal DM, Roelvink PW, Carrion ME, Lizonova A, Lee GM, Kovesdi I. Targeted adenovirus gene transfer to endothelial and smooth muscle cells by using bispecific antibodies. J Virol 1996; 70:6831–6838.
140. Goldman CK, Rogers BE, Douglas JT, Sosnowski BA, Ying W, Siegal GP, Baird A, Campain JA, Curiel DT. Targeted gene delivery to Kaposi's sarcoma cells via the fibroblast growth factor receptor. Cancer Res 1997; 57: 1447–1451.
141. Chien ML, Foster JL, Douglas JL, Garcia JV. The amphotropic murine leukemia virus receptor gene encodes a 71-kilodalton protein that is induced by phosphate depletion. J Virol 1997; 71:4564–4570.
142. Yee JK, Miyanohara A, LaPorte P, Bouic K, Burns JC, Friedmann T. A general method for the generation of high-titer, pantropic retroviral vectors: highly efficient infection of primary hepatocytes. Proc Natl Acad Sci USA 1998; 91:9564–9568.
143. von Kalle C, Kiem HP, Goehle S, Darovsky B, Heimfeld S, Torok SB, Storb R, Schuening FG. Increased gene transfer into human hematopoietic progenitor cells by extended in vitro exposure to a pseudotyped retroviral vector. Blood 1994; 84:2890–2897.
144. Lindermann D, Bock M, Schweizer M, Rethwilm A. Efficient pseudotyping of murine leukemia virus particles with chimeric human foamy virus envelope proteins. J Virol 1997; 71:4815–4820.
145. Indraccolo S, Minuzzo S, Feroli F, Mammano F, Calderazzo F, Chieco BL, Amadori A. Pseudotyping of Moloney leukemia virus-based retroviral vectors with simian immunodeficiency virus envelope leads to targeted infection of human CD4+ lymphoid cells. Gene Ther 1998; 5: 209–217.
146. Mammano F, Salvatori F, Indraccolo S, De RA, Chieco BL, Gottlinger HG. Truncation of the human immunodeficiency virus type 1 envelope glycoprotein allows efficient pseudotyping of Moloney murine leukemia virus particles and gene transfer into CD4+ cells. J Virol 1997;
147. Yajima T, Kanda T, Yoshiike K, Kitamura Y. Retroviral vector targeting human cells via c-Kit-stem cell factor interaction. Hum Gene Ther 1998; 9:779–787.
148. Harris JR, Morrow M, Bonadonng EA. Cancer of the breast. In: DeVita, Hellman S, Rosenberg SA, eds. Cancer: Principles and Practice of Oncology. 4th ed. Philadelphia: JB Lippincott, 1993:1264–1332.
149. Miller BA, Feuer EJ, Hankey BF. Recent incidence trends for breast cancer in women and the relevance of early detection: an update [see comments]. Ca Cancer J Clin 1993; 43:27–41.
150. Ruppert JM, Wright M, Rosenfeld M, Grushcow J, Bilbao G, Curiel DT, Strong TV. Gene therapy strategies for carcinoma of the breast, Breast Cancer Res Treat 1997; 44: 93–114.
151. Hui KM, Ang PT, Huang L, Tay SK. Phase I study of immunotherapy of cutaneous metastases of human carcinoma using allogeneic and xenogeneic MHC DNA-liposome complexes. Gene Ther 1997; 4:783–790.
152. Hildebrandt M, Mapara MY, Korner IJ, Bargou RC, Moldenhauer G, Dorken B. Reverse transcriptase-polymerase chain reaction (RT-PCR)-controlled immunomagnetic purging of breast cancer cells using the magnetic cell separation (MACS) system: a sensitive method for monitoring purging efficiency, Exp Hematol 1997; 25:57–65.
153. Frey BM, Hackett NR, Bergelson JM, Finberg R, Crystal RG, Moore MA, Rafii S. High-efficiency gene transfer into ex vivo expanded human hematopoietic progenitors and precursor cells by adenovirus vectors. Blood 1998; 91:2781–2792.
154. Yee D, McGuire SE, Brunner N, Kozelsky TW, Allred DC, Chen SH, Woo SL. Adenovirus-mediated gene transfer of herpes simplex virus thymidine kinase in an ascites model

of human breast cancer. Hum Gene Ther 1996; 7: 1251–1257.

155. Garcia Sanchez F, Pizzorno G, Fu SQ, Nanakorn T, Krause DS, Liang J, Adams E, Leffert JJ, Yin LH, Cooperberg MR, Hanania E, Wang WL, Won JH, Peng XY, Cote R, Brown R, Burtness B, Giles R, Crystal R, Deisseroth AB. Cytosine deaminase adenoviral vector and 5-fluorocytosine selectively reduce breast cancer cells 1 million-fold when they contaminate hematopoietic cells: a potential purging method for autologous transplantation. Blood 1998; 92:672–682.

156. Seth P, Brinkmann U, Schwartz GN, Katayose D, Gress R, Pastan I, Cowan K. Adenovirus-mediated gene transfer to human breast tumor cells: an approach for cancer gene therapy and bone marrow purging. Cancer Res 1996; 56: 1346–1351.

157. Wroblewski JM, Lay LT, Van ZG, Phillips G, Seth P, Curiel D, Meeker TC. Selective elimination (purging) of contaminating malignant cells from hematopoietic stem cell autografts using recombinant adenovirus. Cancer Gene Ther 1996; 3:257–264.

158. Li Z, Shanmugam N, Katayose D, Huber B, Srivastava S, Cowan K, Seth P. Enzyme/prodrug gene therapy approach for breast cancer using a recombinant adenovirus expressing *Escherichia coli* cytosine deaminase. Cancer Gene Ther 1997; 4:113–117.

159. Wolff G, Korner IJ, Schumacher A, Arnold W, Dorken B, Mapara MY. Ex vivo breast cancer cell purging by adenovirus-mediated cytosine deaminase gene transfer and short-term incubation with 5-fluorocytosine completely prevents tumor growth after transplantation. Hum Gene Ther 1998; 9:2277–2284.

160. Clarke MF, Apel IJ, Benedict MA, Eipers PG, Sumantran V, Gonzalez GM, Doedens M, Fukunaga N, Davidson B, Dick JE, et al. A recombinant bcl-x s adenovirus selectively induces apoptosis in cancer cells but not in normal bone marrow cells. Proc Natl Acad Sci USA 1995; 92: 11024–11028.

161. Mars WM, Saunders GF. Chromosomal abnormalities in human breast cancer. Cancer Metastasis Rev. 1990; 9: 35–43.

162. Cox LA, Chen G, Lee EY. Tumor suppressor genes and their roles in breast cancer. Breast Cancer Res Treat 1994; 32:19–38.

163. Devilee P, Cornelisse CJ. Somatic genetic changes in human breast cancer. Biochim Biophys Acta 1994; 1198: 113–130.

164. Parsons R, Li GM, Longley MJ, Fang WH, Papadopoulos N, Jen J, De ICA, Kinzler KW, Vogelstein B, Modrich P. Hypermutability and mismatch repair deficiency in RER+ tumor cells. Cell 1993; 75:1227–1236.

165. Cho KR, Vogelstein B. Suppressor gene alterations in the colorectal adenoma-carcinoma sequence. J Cell Biochem Suppl. 1992; 16G:137–141.

166. Lukas J, Aagaard L, Strauss M, Bartek J. Oncogenic aberrations of p16INK4/CDKN2 and cyclin D1 cooperate to deregulate G1 control. Cancer Res 1995; 55:4818–4823.

167. McManaway ME, Neckers LM, Loke SL, al NA, Redner RL, Shiramizu BT, Goldschmidts WL, Huber BE, Bhatia K, Magrath IT. Tumour-specific inhibition of lymphoma growth by an antisense oligodeoxynucleotide. Lancet 1990; 335:808–811.

168. Watson PH, Pon RT, Shiu RP. Inhibition of c-myc expression by phosphorothioate antisense oligonucleotide identifies a critical role for c-myc in the growth of human breast cancer. Cancer Res 1991; 51:3996–4000.

169. Bertram J, Killian M, Brysch W, Schlingensiepen KH, Kneba M. Reduction of erbB2 gene product in mamma carcinoma cell lines by erbB2 mRNA-specific and tyrosine kinase consensus phosphorothioate antisense oligonucleotides. Biochem Biophys Res Commun 1994; 200: 661–667.

170. Casalini P, Menard S, Malandrin SM, Rigo CM, Coinaghi MI, Cultraro CM, Segal S. Inhibition of tumorigenicity in lung adenocarcinoma cells by c-erbB-2 antisense expression. Int J Cancer 1997; 72:631–636.

171. Zhou P, Jiang W, Zhang YJ, Kahn SM, Schieren I, Santella RM, Weinstein IB. Antisense to cyclin D1 inhibits growth and reverses the transformed phenotype of human esophageal cancer cells. Oncogene 1995; 11:571–580.

172. Kenney NJ, Saeki T, Gottardis M, Kim N, Garcia MP, Martin MB, Normanno N, Ciardiello F, Day A, Cutler ML, et al. Expression of transforming growth factor alpha antisense mRNA inhibits the estrogen-induced production of TGF alpha and estrogen-induced proliferation of estrogen-responsive human breast cancer cells. J Cell Physiol 1993; 156:497–514.

173. Wright M, Grim J, Deshane J, Kim M, Strong TV, Slegal GP, Curiel DT. An intracellular anti-erbB-2 single-chain antibody is specifically cytotoxic to human breast carcinoma cells overexpressing erbB-2. Gene Ther 1997; 4: 317–322.

174. Arteaga CL, Holt JT. Tissue-targeted antisense c-fos retroviral vector inhibits established breast cancer xenografts in nude mice. Cancer Res 1996; 56:1098–1103.

175. Nielsen LL, Dell J, Maxwell E, Armstrong L, Maneval D, Catino JJ. Efficacy of p53 adenovirus-mediated gene therapy against human breast cancer xenografts. Cancer Gene Ther 1997; 4:129–138.

176. Xu M, Kumar D, Srinivas S, Detolla LJ, Yu SF, Stass SA, Mixson AJ. Parenteral gene therapy with p53 inhibits human breast tumors in vivo through a bystander mechanism without evidence of toxicity. Hum Gene Ther 1997; 8:177–185.

177. Lesoon Wood LA, Kim WH, Kleinman HK, Weintraub BD, Mixson AJ. Systemic gene therapy with p53 reduces growth and metastases of a malignant human breast cancer in nude mice. Hum Gene Ther 1995; 6:395–405.

178. Wahl AF, Donaldson RL, Fairchild C, Lee FY, Foster SA, Demers GW, Galloway DA. Loss of normal p53 function confers sensitization to taxol by increasing G2/M arrest and apoptosis [see comments]. Nat Med 1996; 2:72–79.

179. Parker SL, Tong T, Bolden S, Wingo PA. Cancer statistics, 1997 [published erratum appears in CA Cancer J Clin 1997; 47(2):68]. Ca Cancer J Clin 1997; 47:5–27.

180. Kemeny N, Seiter K. Treatment option for patients with metastatic colorectal cancer. In: Niederhuber J, ed. Current Therapy in Oncology. St. Louis: Mosby Year Book, 1993: 447–457.
181. Hirschowitz EA, Ohwada A, Pascal WR, Russi TJ, Crystal RG. In vivo adenovirus-mediated gene transfer of the *Escherichia coli* cytosine deaminase gene to human colon carcinoma-derived tumors induces chemosensitivity to 5-fluorocytosine. Hum Gene Ther 1995; 6:1055–1063.
182. O'Malley BJ, Sewell DA, Li D, Kosai K, Chen SH, Woo SL, Duan L. The role of interleukin-2 in combination adenovirus gene therapy for head and neck cancer. Mol Endocrinol 1997; 11:667–673.
183. Caruso M, Pham NK, Kwong YL, Xu B, Kosai KI, Finegold M, Woo SL, Chen SH. Adenovirus-mediated interleukin-12 gene therapy for metastatic colon carcinoma. Proc Natl Acad Sci USA 1996; 93.
184. White SA, Conry RM, Strong TV, Curiel DT, LoBuglio AF. Polynucleotide-mediated immunization of cancer. In: Lattime EC, Gerson SL, eds. Gene Therapy of Cancer, New York: Academic Press, 1992:271–283.
185. Rao JB, Chamberlain RS, Bronte V, Carroll MW, Irvine KR, Moss B, Rosenberg SA, Restifo NP. IL-12 is an effective adjuvant to recombinant vaccinia virus-based tumor vaccines: enhancement by simultaneous B7-1 expression, J Immunol 1996; 156:3357–3365.
186. Plautz GE, Yang ZY, Wu BY, Gao X, Huang L, Nabel GJ. Immunotherapy of malignancy by in vivo gene transfer into tumors [see comments]. Proc Natl Acad Sci USA 1993; 90:4645–4649.
187. Fakhrai H, Shawler DL, Gjerset R, Naviaux RK, Koziol J, Royston L, Sobol RE. Cytokine gene therapy with interleukin-2-transduced fibroblasts: effects of IL-2 dose on anti-tumor immunity. Hum Gene Ther 1995; 6:591–601.
188. Mahaley MJ, Mettlin C, Natarajan N, Laws EJ, Peace BB. National survey of patterns of care for brain-tumor patients. J Neurosurg 1989; 71:826–836.
189. Weber F, Bojar H, Priesack HB, Floeth F, Lenartz D, Kiwit J, Bock W. Gene therapy of glioblastoma—one year clinical experience with ten patients. J Mol Med 1997; 75:B40.
190. Alavi JB, Judy K, Alavi A, Hackney D, Phillips P, Smith J, Recio A, Wilson J, Eck S. Phase I trial of gene therapy in primary brain tumors. In: American Society of Gene Therapy 1st Annual Meeting, Seattle, 1998.
191. Trask TW, Aguilar-Cordova E, Goodman JC, Guevara R, Wyde P, Shine HD, Grossman RG. A phase I study of adenoviral vector delivery of the HSV-TK gene and the intravenous administration of ganciclovir in adults with malignant tumors of the central nervous system. In: American Society of Gene Therapy 1st Annual Meeting, Seattle, 1998.
192. Badie B, Drazan KE, Kramar MH, Shaked A, Black KL. Adenovirus-mediated p53 gene delivery inhibits 9L glioma growth in rats. Neurol Res 1995; 17:209–216.
193. Fueyo J, Gomez MC, Yung WK, Clayman GL, Liu TJ, Bruner J, Levin VA, Kyritsis AP. Adenovirus-mediated p16/CDKN2 gene transfer induces growth arrest and modifies the transformed phenotype of glioma cells. Oncogene 1996; 12:103–10.
194. Fueyo J, Gomez MC, Yung WK, Liu TJ, Alemany R, McDonnell TJ, Shi X, Rao JS, Levin VA, Kyritsis AP. Overexpression of E2F-1 in glioma triggers apoptosis and suppresses tumor growth in vitro and in vivo. Nat Med 1998; 4:685–690.
195. American Cancer Society. American Cancer Society Facts and Figures. Publ. No. 93–400. Washington, DC: American Cancer Society, 1993.
196. Dimery IW, Hong WK. Overview of combined modality therapies for head and neck cancer. J Natl Cancer Inst 1993; 85:95–111.
197. Burt K, Chema D, Timmons T. Tracing the dissemination of adenoviral vectors in patient body fluids. J Mol Med 1997; 75:B28.
198. Horwitz MS. Adenoviruses. In: Fields BN et al., eds. Fields Virology. 3d ed. Philadelphia: Lippincott-Raven, 1996: 2149–2171.
199. Shenk T. Adenoviridae: the viruses and their replication. In: Fields BN et al., eds. Fields Virology. 3d ed. Philadelphia: Lippincott-Raven, 1996:2111–2148.
200. Kirn D, Nemunaitis J, Ganly I, Posner M, Vokes E, Kuhn J, Heise C, Maac C, Kaye S. A phase II trial of intratumoral injection with an E1b-deleted adenovirus, Onyx-015, in patients with recurrent, refractory head and neck cancer. In: Proceedings American Society of Clinical Oncology Thirty-Fourth Annual Meeting, Los Angeles, 1998, p. 391a.
201. Braun SE, Chen K, Battiwalla M, Cornetta K. Gene therapy strategies for leukemia. Mol Med Today 1997; 3: 39–46.
202. Levitsky HI, Montgomery J, Ahmadzadeh M, Staveley OCK, Guarnieri F, Longo DL, Kwak LW. Immunization with granulocyte-macrophage colony-stimulating factor-transduced, but not B7-1-transduced, lymphoma cells primes idiotype-specific T cells and generates potent systemic antitumor immunity. J Immunol 1996; 156: 3858–65.
203. Hersh EM, Nabel G, Silver H, et al. Intratumoral injection of plasmid DNA in cationic lipid vectors for cancer gene therapy. Cancer Gene Ther 1996; 3:511.
204. Gillio TA, Cignetti A, Rovera G, Foa R. Retroviral vector-mediated transfer of the tumor necrosis factor alpha gene into human cancer cells restores an apoptotic cell death program and induces a bystander-killing effect. Blood 1996; 87:2486–2495.
205. Cao X, Ju DW, Tao Q, Wang J, Wan T, Wang BM, Zhang W, Hamada H. Adenovirus-mediated GM-CSF gene and cytosine deaminase gene transfer followed by 5-fluorocytosine administration elicit more potent antitumor response in tumor-bearing mice. Gene Ther 1998; 5:1130–1136.
206. Chen L, McGowan P, Ashe S, Johnston J, Li Y, Hellstrom I, Hellstrom KE. Tumor immunogenicity determines the effect of B7 costimulation on T cell-mediated tumor immunity. J Exp Med 1994; 179:523–532.

207. Martin Fontecha A, Cavallo F, Bellone M, Heltai S, Iezzi G, Tornaghi P, Nabavi N, Forni G, Dellabona P, Casorati G. Heterogeneous effects of B7-1 and B7-2 in the induction of both protective and therapeutic anti-tumor immunity against different mouse tumors. Eur J Immunol 1996; 26:1851–1859.
208. Hsieh CL, Pang VF, Chen DS, Hwang LH. Regression of established mouse leukemia by GM-CSF-transduced tumor vaccine: implications for cytotoxic T lymphocyte responses and tumor burdens. Hum Gene Ther 1997; 8: 1843–1854.
209. Gross G, Levy S, Levy R, Waks T, Eshhar Z. Chimaeric T-cell receptors specific to a B-lymphoma idiotype: a model for tumour immunotherapy. Biochem Soc Trans 1995; 23:1079–11082.
210. Mackinnon S, Papadopoulos EB, Carabasi MH, Reich L, Collins NH, O'Reilly RJ. Adoptive immunotherapy using donor leukocytes following bone marrow transplantation for chronic myeloid leukemia: Is T cell dose important in determining biological response? Bone Marrow Transplant 1995; 15:591–594.
211. Rooney CM, Smith CA, Ng CY, Loftin S, Li C, Krance RA, Brenner MK, Heslop HE. Use of gene-modified virus-specific T lymphocytes to control Epstein-Barr-virus-related lymphoproliferation. Lancet 1995; 345:9–13.
212. Verzeletti S, Bonini C, Marktel S, Nobili N, Ciceri F, Traversari C, Bordignon C. Herpes simplex virus thymidine kinase gene transfer for controlled graft-versus-host disease and graft-versus-leukemia: clinical follow-up and improved new vectors. Hum Gene Ther 1998; 9:2243–2251.
213. Skorski T, Nieborowska SM, Campbell K, lozzo RV, Zon G, Darzynklewicz Z, Calabretta B. Leukemia treatment in severe combined immunodeficiency mice by antisense oligodeoxynucleotides targeting cooperating oncogenes. J Exp Med 1995; 182:1645–1653.
214. Skorski T, Nieborowska SM, Wlodarski P, Zon G, lozzo RV, Calabretta B. Antisense oligodeoxynucleotide combination therapy of primary chronic myelogenous leukemia blast crisis in SCID mice. Blood 1996; 88:1005–1012.
215. Madrigal M, Janicek MF, Sevin BU, Perras J, Estape R, Penalver M, Averette HE. In vitro antigene therapy targeting HPV-16 E6 and E7 in cervical carcinoma. Gynecol Oncol 1997; 64:18–25.
216. Ratajczak MZ, Kant JA, Luger SM, Hijiya N, Zhang J, Zon G, Gewirtz AM. In vivo treatment of human leukemia in a scid mouse model with c-myb antisense oligodeoxynucleotides. Proc Natl Acad Sci USA 1992; 89: 11823–11827.
217. Lange W, Cantin EM, Finke J, Dolken G. In vitro and in vivo effects of synthetic ribozymes targeted against BCR/ABL mRNA. Leukemia 1993; 7:1786–1794.
218. Mertelsmann R. Blutbildendes und Lymphatisches Systen. In: Weihrauch TR, ed. Internistische Therapie 98/99. Urban und Schwarzenberg München 1998, 689–737.
219. Ido A, Nakata K, Kato Y, Nakao K, Murata K, Fujita M, Ishii N, Tamaoki T, Shiku H, Nagataki S. Gene therapy for hepatoma cells using a retrovirus vector carrying herpes simplex virus thymidine kinase gene under the control of human alpha-fetoprotein gene promoter. Cancer Res 1995; 55:3105–3109.
220. Bui LA, Butterfield LH, Kim JY, Ribas A, Seu P, Lau R, Glaspy JA, McBride WH, Economou JS. In vivo therapy of hepatocellular carcinoma with a tumor-specific adenoviral vector expressing interleukin-2 [see comments]. Hum Gene Ther 1997; 8:2173–2182.
221. Qian C, Idoate M, Bilbao R, Sangro B, Bruna O, Vazquez J, Prieto J. Gene transfer and therapy with adenoviral vector in rats with diethylnitrosamine-induced hepatocellular carcinoma. Hum Gene Ther 1997; 8:349–358.
222. Habib NA, Ding SF, el-Masry R, Mitry RR, Honda K, Michail NE, Dalla SG, Izzi G, Greco L, Bassyouni M, el TM, Abdel GY. Preliminary report: the short-term effects of direct p53 DNA injection in primary hepatocellular carcinomas. Cancer Detect Prev 1996; 20:103–107.
223. Monson JR. Malignant melanoma: a plague of our times. Br J Surg 1989; 76:997–998.
224. Ho VC, Sober AJ. Therapy for cutaneous melanoma: an update. J Am Acad Dermatol 1990; 22(2 Pt 1):159–176.
225. Ahmann DL, et al. Complete responses and long-term survivals after systemic chemotherapy for patients with advanced malignant melanoma. Cancer 1989; 63:224–227.
226. DeBruyne LA, Chang AE, Cameron MJ, Yang Z, Gordon D, Nabel EG, Nabel GJ, Bishop DK. Direct transfer of a foreign MHC gene into human melanoma alters T cell receptor V beta usage by tumor-infiltrating lymphocytes. Cancer Immunol Immunother 1996; 43:49–58.
227. Nabel GJ, Nabel EG, Yang ZY, Fox BA, Plautz GE, Gao X, Huang L, Shu S, Gordon D, Chang AE. Direct gene transfer with DNA-liposome complexes in melanoma: expression, biologic activity, and lack of toxicity in humans. Proc Natl Acad Sci USA 1993; 90:11307–11311.
228. Vogelzang NJ, Sudakoff G, Hersh EM, et al. Clinical experience in phase I and phase II testing of direct intratumoral administration with Allovectin-7: a gene-based immunotherapeutic agent. Proc Am Soc Clin Oncol 1996; 15:235.
229. Sun Y, Jurgovsky K, Moller P, Alijagic S, Dorbic T, Georgieva J, Wittig B, Schadendorf D. Vaccination with IL-12 gene-modified autologous melanoma cells: preclinical results and a first clinical phase I study. Gene Ther 1998; 5:481–490.
230. Butterfield LH, Ribas A, Economou JS. DNA and dendritic cell-based genetic immunization against cancer. In: Lattime EL, Gerson SL, eds. Gene Therapy of Cancer. New York: Academic Press, 1999:285–298.
231. Ribas A, Butterfield LH, McBride WH, Jilani SM, Bui LA, Vollmer CM, Lau R, Dissette VB, Hu B, Chen AY, Glaspy JA, Economou JS. Genetic immunization for the melanoma antigen MART-1/Melan-A using recombinant adenovirus-transduced murine dendritic cells. Cancer Res 1997; 57:2865–2869.
232. Bonnekoh B, Greenhalgh DA, Bundman DS, Eckhardt JN, Longley MA, Chen SH, Woo SL, Roop DR. Inhibition of

melanoma growth by adenoviral-mediated HSV thymidine kinase gene transfer in vivo. J Invest Dermatol 1995; 104: 313–317.
233. Esandi MC, Van SG, Bout A, Mulder AH, Van BD, Valerio D, Noteboom JL. IL-1/IL-3 gene therapy of non-small cell lung cancer (NSCLC) in rats using 'cracked' adenoproducer cells. Gene Ther 1998; 5:778–788.
234. Zhang WW, Fang X, Mazur W, French BA, Georges RN, Roth JA. High-efficiency gene transfer and high-level expression of wild-type p53 in human lung cancer cells mediated by recombinant adenovirus. Cancer Gene Ther 1994; 1:5–13.
235. Fujiwara T, Cai DW, Georges RN, Mukhopadhyay T, Grimm EA, Roth JA. Therapeutic effect of a retroviral wild-type p53 expression vector in an orthotopic lung cancer model [see comments]. J Natl Cancer Inst 1994; 86: 1458–1462.
236. Roth JA, Nguyen D, Lawrence DD, Kemp BL, Carrasco CH, Ferson DZ, Hong WK, Komaki R, Lee JJ, Nesbitt JC, Pisters KM, Putnam JB, Schea R, Shin DM, Walsh GL, Dolormente MM, Han CT, Martin FD, Yen N, Xu K, Stephens LC, McDonnell TJ, Mukhopadhyay T, Cai D. Retrovirus-mediated wild-type p53 gene transfer to tumors of patients with lung cancer [see comments]. Nat Med 1996; 2:985–991.
237. Zhang WW, Alemany R, Wang J, Koch PE, Ordonez NG, Roth JA. Safety evaluation of Ad5CMV-p53 in vitro and in vivo. Hum Gene Ther 1995; 6:155–164.
238. Roth JA. Modification of tumor suppressor gene expression and induction of apoptosis in non-small cell lung cancer (NSCLC) with an adenovirus vector expressing wild-type p53 and cisplatin, Hum Gene Ther 1996; 7: 1013–1030.
239. Georges RN, Mukhopadhyay T, Zhang Y, Yen N, Roth JA. Prevention of orthotopic human lung cancer growth by intratracheal instillation of a retroviral antisense K-ras construct. Cancer Res 1993; 53:1743–1746.
240. Weichselbaum RR, Hallahan DE, Beckett MA, Mauceri HJ, Lee H, Sukhatme VP, Kufe DW. Gene therapy targeted by radiation preferentially radiosensitizes tumor cells. Cancer Res 1994; 54:4266–4269.
241. Hudson M, Jaffe MR, Jaffe N, Ayala A, Raymond AK, Carrasco H, Wallace S, Murray J, Robertson R. Pediatric osteosarcoma: therapeutic strategies, results, and prognostic factors derived from a 10-year experience. J Clin Oncol 1990; 8:1988–1997.
242. Link MP, Goorin AM, Miser AW, Green AA, Pratt CB, Belasco JB, Pritchard J, Malpas JS, Baker AR, Kirkpatrick JA, et al. The effect of adjuvant chemotherapy on relapse-free survival in patients with osteosarcoma of the extremity. N Engl J Med 1986; 314:1600–1606.
243. Goorin AM, Perez AA, Gebhardt M, Andersen JW, Wilkinson RH, Delorey MJ, Watts H, Link M, Jaffe N, Frei ED, et al. Weekly high-dose methotrexate and doxorubicin for osteosarcoma: the Dana-Farber Cancer Institute/the Children's Hospital—study III. J Clin Oncol 1987; 5: 1178–1184.
244. Hayakawa M, Kawaguchi S, Ishii S, Murakami M, Uede T. B7-1-transfected tumor vaccine counteracts chemotherapy-induced immunosuppression and prolongs the survival of rats bearing highly metastatic osteosarcoma cells. Int J Cancer 1997; 71:1091–1102.
245. Ko SC, Cheon J, Kao C, Gotoh A, Shirakawa T, Sikes RA, Karsenty G, Chung LW. Osteocalcin promoter-based toxic gene therapy for the treatment of osteosarcoma in experimental models. Cancer Res 1996; 56:4614–4619.
246. Boring CC, Squires TS, Tong T, Montgomery S. Cancer statistics, 1994. Ca Cancer J Clin 1994; 44:7–26.
247. Link CJ, Moorman D, Seregina T, Levy JP, Schabold KJ. A phase I trial of in vivo gene therapy with the herpes simplex thymidine kinase/ganciclovir system for the treatment of refractory or recurrent ovarian cancer. Hum Gene Ther 1996; 7:1161–1179.
248. Alvarez RD, Curiel DT. A phase I study of recombinant adenovirus vector-mediated intraperitoneal delivery of herpes simplex virus thymidine kinase (HSV-TK) gene and intravenous ganciclovir for previously treated ovarian and extraovarian cancer patients. Hum Gene Ther 1997; 8:597–613.
249. Deshane J, Siegal GP, Alvarez RD, Wang MH, Feng M, Cabrera G, Liu T, Kay M, Curiel DT. Targeted tumor killing via an intracellular antibody against erbB-2. J Clin Invest 1995; 96:2980–2989.
250. Freeman SM, McCune C, Robinson W, Abboud CN, Abraham GN, Angel C, Marrogi A. The treatment of ovarian cancer with a gene modified cancer vaccine: a phase I study. Hum Gene Ther 1995; 6:927–939.
251. Yu D, Matin A, Xia W, Sorgi F, Huang L, Hung MC. Liposome-mediated in vivo E1A gene transfer suppressed dissemination of ovarian cancer cells that overexpress HER-2/neu. Oncogene 1995; 11:1383–1388.
252. Xing X, Matin A, Yu D, Xia W, Sorgi F, Huang L, Hung MC. Mutant SV40 large T antigen as a therapeutic agent for HER-2/neu-overexpressing ovarian cancer. Cancer Gene Ther 1996; 3:168–174.
253. Abrams SI, Hand PH, Tsang KY, Schlom J. Mutant ras epitopes as targets for cancer vaccines. Semin Oncol 1996; 23:118–134.
254. Gjertsen MK, Bakka A, Breivik J, Saeterdal I, Gedde DTR, Stokke KT, Solheim BG, Egge TS, Soreide O, Thorsby E, Gaudernack G. Ex vivo ras peptide vaccination in patients with advanced pancreatic cancer: results of a phase I/II study. Int J Cancer 1996; 65:450–453.
255. Abrams SI, Khleif SN, Bergmann-Leitner ES, Kantor JA, Chung Y, Hamilton JM, Schlom J. Generation of stable CD4+ and CD8+ T cell lines from patients immunized with ras oncogene-derived peptides reflecting codon 12 mutations. Cell Immunol 1997; 182:137–151.
256. Block A, Chen SH, Kosai K, Finegold M, Woo SL. Adenoviral-mediated herpes simplex virus thymidine kinase gene transfer: regression of hepatic metastasis of pancreatic tumors. Pancreas 1997; 15:25–34.
257. Aoki K, Yoshida T, Sugimura T, Terada M. Liposome-mediated in vivo gene transfer of antisense K-ras construct

inhibits pancreatic tumor dissemination in the murine peritoneal cavity. Cancer Res 1995; 55:3810–3816.

258. Evoy D, Hirschowitz EA, Naama HA, Li XK, Crystal RG, Daly JM, Lieberman MD. In vivo adenoviral-mediated gene transfer in the treatment of pancreatic cancer. J Surg Res 1997; 69:226–231.
259. Hahn SA, Schutte M, Hoque AT, Moskaluk CA, Da CL, Rozenblum E, Weinstein CL, Fischer A, Yeo CJ, Hruban RH, Kern SE. DPC4, a candidate tumor suppressor gene at human chromosome 18q21.1 [see comments]. Science 1996; 271:350–353.
260. Carter HB, Coffey DS. The prostate: an increasing medical problem. Prostate 1990; 16:39–48.
261. Gotoh A, Ko SC, Shirakawa T, Cheon J, Kao C, Miyamoto T, Gardner TA, Ho LJ, Cleutjens CB, Trapman J, Graham FL, Chung LW. Development of prostate-specific antigen promoter-based gene therapy for androgen-independent human prostate cancer. J Urol 1998; 160:220–229.
262. Burfeind P, Chernicky CL, Rininsland F, Ilan J, Ilan J. Antisense RNA to the type I insulin-like growth factor receptor suppresses tumor growth and prevents invasion by rat prostate cancer cells in vivo. Proc Natl Acad Sci USA 1996; 93:7263–7268.
263. Ko SC, Gotoh A, Thalmann GN, Zhau HE, Johnston DA, Zhang WW, Kao C, Chung LW. Molecular therapy with recombinant p53 adenovirus in an androgen-independent, metastatic human prostate cancer model. Hum Gene Ther 1996; 7:1683–1691.
264. Eastham JA, Hall SJ, Sehgal I, Wang J, Timme TL, Yang G, Connell CL, Elledge SJ, Zhang WW, Harper JW, et al. In vivo gene therapy with p53 or p21 adenovirus for prostate cancer. Cancer Res 1995; 55:5151–5155.
265. Steiner MS, Anthony CT, Lu Y, Holt JT. Antisense c-myc retroviral vector suppresses established human prostate cancer. Hum Gene Ther 1998; 9:747–755.

TABLE REFERENCES

Abdel Wahab Z, Dar M, Osanto S, Fong T, Vervaert CE, Hester D, Jolly D, Seigler HF. Eradication of melanoma pulmonary metastases by immunotherapy with tumor cells engineered to secrete interleukin-2 or gamma interferon. Cancer Gene Ther 1997; 4:33–41.

Abdel Wahab Z, Li WP, Osanto S, Darrow TL, Hessling J, Vervaert CE, Burrascano M, Barber J, Seigler HF. Transduction of human melanoma cells with interleukin-2 gene reduces tumorigenicity and enhances host antitumor immunity: a nude mouse model. Cell Immunol 1994; 159:26–39.

Anderson SC, Johnson DE, Harris MP, Engler H, Hancock W, Huang WM, Wills KN, Gregory RJ, Sutjipto S, Wen SF, Lofgren S, Shepard HM, and Maneval DC. p53 gene therapy in a rat model of hepatocellular carcinoma: intra-arterial delivery of a recombinant adenovirus. Clin Cancer Res 1998; 4: 1649–1659.

Aoki K, Yoshida T, Sugimura T, Terada M. Liposome-mediated in vivo gene transfer of antisense K-ras construct inhibits pancreatic tumor dissemination in the murine peritoneal cavity. Cancer Res 1995; 55:3810–3816.

Arteaga CL, Holt JT. Tissue-targeted antisense c-fos retroviral vector inhibits established breast cancer xenografts in nude mice. Cancer Res 1996; 56:1098–1103.

Badie B, Drazan KE, Kramar MH, Shaked A, Black KL. Adenovirus-mediated p53 gene delivery inhibits 9L glioma growth in rats. Neurol Res 1995; 17:209–216.

Baskar S, Glimcher L, Nabavi N, Jones RT, Ostrand Rosenberg S. Major histocompatibility complex class II + B7 − 1 + tumor cells are potent vaccines for stimulating tumor rejection in tumor-bearing mice. J Exp Med 1995; 181:619–629.

Baskar S, Azarenko V, Garcia Marshall E, Hughes E, Ostrand Rosenberg S. MHC class II-transfected tumor cells induce long-term tumor-specific immunity in autologous mice. Cell Immunol 1994; 155:123–133.

Bausero MA, Panoskaltsis Mortari A, Blazar BR, Katsanis E. Effective immunization against neuroblastoma using double-transduced tumor cells secreting GM-CSF and interferon-gamma. J Immunother Emphasis Tumor Immunol 1996; 19: 113–124.

Block A, Chen SH, Kosai K, Finegold M, Woo SL. Adenoviral-mediated herpes simplex virus thymidine kinase gene transfer: regression of hepatic metastasis of pancreatic tumors. Pancreas 1997; 15:25–34.

Bonnekoh B, Greenhalgh DA, Bundman DS, Eckhardt JN, Longley MA, Chen SH, Woo SL, Roop DR. Inhibition of melanoma growth by adenoviral-mediated HSV thymidine kinase gene transfer in vivo. J. Invest. Dermatol. 1995; 104:313–317.

Boxhorn HKE, Smith JG, Chang YJ, Guerry D, Lee WMF, Rodeck U, Turka LA, Eck SL. Adenoviral transduction of melanoma cells with B7-1: antitumor immunity and immunosuppressive factors. Cancer Immunol Immunother 1998; 46: 283–292.

Brand K, Löser P, Arnold W, Bartels T, Strauss M. Tumor cell-specific transgene expression prevents liver toxicity of the adeno-HSVtk/GCV approach. Gene Ther 1998; 5:1363–1371.

Bui LA, Butterfield LH, Kim JY, Ribas A, Seu P, Lau R, Glaspy JA, McBride WH, Economou JS. In vivo therapy of hepatocellular carcinoma with a tumor-specific adenoviral vector expressing interleukin-2 [see comments]. Hum Gene Ther 1997; 8:2173–2182.

Cao X, Ju DW, Tao Q, Wang J, Wan T, Wang BM, Zhang W, Hamada H. Adenovirus-mediated GM-CSF gene and cytosine deaminase gene transfer followed by 5-fluorocytosine administration elicit more potent antitumor response in tumor-bearing mice. Gene Therapy 1998; 5:1130–1136.

Cardinali M, Jakus J, Shah S, Ensley JF, Robbins KC, Yeudall WA. p21(WAF1/Cip1) retards the growth of human squamous cell carcinomas in vivo. Oral Oncology 1998; 34:211–218.

Caruso M, Pham Nguyen K, Kwong YL, Xu B, Kosai KI, Finegold M, Woo SL, Chen SR. Adenovirus-mediated interleukin-12 gene therapy for metastatic colon carcinoma. Proc Natl Acad Sci USA 1996; 93:11302–11306.

Cavallo F, Signorelli P, Giovarelli M, Musiani P, Modesti A, Brunda MJ, Colombo MP, Eorni G. Antitumor efficacy of adenocarcinoma cells engineered to produce interleukin 12 (IL-12) or other cytokines compared with exogenous IL-12. J Natl Cancer Inst 1997; 89:1049–1058.

Chang JY, Xia W, Shao R, Hung MC. Inhibition of intratracheal lung cancer development by systemic delivery of E1A. Oncogene 1996; 13:1405–1412.

Chen DS, Zhu NL, Hung G, Skotzko MJ, Hinton DR, Tolo V, Hall FL, Anderson WF, Gordon EM. Retroviral vector-mediated transfer of an antisense cyclin G1 construct inhibits osteosarcoma tumor growth in nude mice. Hum Gene Ther 1997; 8: 1667–1674.

Chen L, Chen D, Manome Y, Dong Y, Fine HA, Kufe DW. Breast cancer selective gene expression and therapy mediated by recombinant adenoviruses containing the DF3/MUC1 promoter. J Clin Invest 1995; 96:2775–2782.

Chen L, McGowan P, Ashe S, Johnston J, Li Y, Hellstrom I, Hellstrom KE. Tumor immunogenicity determines the effect of B7 costimulation on T cell-mediated tumor immunity. J Exp Med 1994a; 179:523–532.

Chen SH, Shine HD, Goodman JC, Grossman RG, Woo SL. Gene therapy for brain tumors: regression of experimental gliomas by adenovirus-mediated gene transfer in vivo. Proc Natl Acad Sci USA 1994b; 91:3054–3057.

Cirielli C, Riccioni T, Yang C, Pili R, Gloe T, Chang J, Inyaku K, Passaniti A, Capogrossi MC. Adenovirus-mediated gene transfer of wild-type p53 results in melanoma cell apoptosis in vitro and in vivo. Int J Cancer 1995; 63:673–679.

Clary BM, Coveney EC, Philip R, Blazer DG-3, Morse M, Gilboa E, Lyerly HK. Inhibition of established pancreatic cancers following specific active immunotherapy with interleukin-2 gene-transduced tumor cells. Cancer Gene Ther 1997; 4: 97–104.

Clayman GL, el Naggar AK, Roth JA, Zhang WW, Goepfert H, Taylor DL, Liu TJ. In vivo molecular therapy with p53 adenovirus for microscopic residual head and neck squamous carcinoma. Cancer Res 1995; 55:1–6.

Culver KW, Ram Z, Wallbridge S, Ishii H, Oldfield EH, Blaese RM. In vivo gene transfer with retroviral vector-producer cells for treatment of experimental brain tumors [see comments]. Science 1992; 256:1550–1552.

Deshane J, Siegal GP, Alvarez RD, Wang MH, Feng M, Cabrera G, Liu T, Kay M, Curiel DT. Targeted tumor killing via an intracellular antibody against erbB-2. J Clin Invest 1995; 96: 2980–2989.

Dranoff G, Jaffee E, Lazenby A, Golumbek P, Levitsky H, Brose K, Jackson V, Hamada H, Pardoll D, Mulligan RC. Vaccination with irradiated tumor cells engineered to secrete murine granulocyte-macrophage colony-stimulating factor stimulates potent, specific, and long-lasting anti-tumor immunity. Proc Natl Acad Sci USA 1993; 90:3539–3543.

Ealovega MW, McGinnis PK, Sumantran VN, Clarke MF, Wicha MS. bcl-xs gene therapy induces apoptosis of human mammary tumors in nude mice. Cancer Res 1996; 56:1965–1969.

Eastham JA, Chen SH, Sehgal I, Yang G, Timme TL, Hall SJ, Woo SL, Thompson TC. Prostate cancer gene therapy: herpes simplex virus thymidine kinase gene transduction followed by ganciclovir in mouse and human prostate cancer models. Hum Gene Ther 1996; 7:515–523.

Eastham JA, Hall SJ, Sehgal I, Wang J, Timme TL, Yang G, Connell Crowley L, Elledge SJ, Zhang WW, Harper JW, et al. In vivo gene therapy with p53 or p21 adenovirus for prostate cancer. Cancer Res 1995; 55:5151–5155.

Evoy D, Hirschowitz EA, Naama HA, Li XK, Crystal RG, Daly JM, Lieberman MD. In vivo adenoviral-mediated gene transfer in the treatment of pancreatic cancer. J Surg Res 1997; 69:226–231.

Fakhrai H, Shawler DL, Gjerset R, Naviaux RK, Koziol J, Royston I, Sobol RE. Cytokine gene therapy with interleukin-2-transduced fibroblasts: effects of IL-2 dose on anti-tumor immunity. Hum Gene Ther 1995; 6:591–601.

Fallarino F, Ashikari A, Boon T, Gajewski TF. Antigen-specific regression of established tumors induced by active immunization with irradiated IL-12- but not B7-1-transfected tumor cells. Int Immunol 1997; 9:1259–1269.

Fujiwara T, Cai DW, Georges RN, Mukhopadhyay T, Grimm EA, Roth JA. Therapeutic effect of a retroviral wild-type p53 expression vector in an orthotopic lung cancer model [see comments]. J Natl Cancer Inst 1994a; 86:1458–1462.

Fujiwara T, Grimm EA, Mukhopadhyay T, Zhang WW, Owen Schaub LB, Roth JA. Induction of chemosensitivity in human lung cancer cells in vivo by adenovirus-mediated transfer of the wild-type p53 gene. Cancer Res 1994b; 54:2287–2291.

Gallardo D, Drazan KE, McBride WH. Adenovirus-based transfer of wild-type p53 gene increases ovarian tumor radiosensitivity. Cancer Res 1996; 56:4891–4893.

Glick RP, Lichtor T, Mogharbel A, Taylor CA, Cohen EP. Intracerebral versus subcutaneous immunization with allogeneic fibroblasts genetically engineered to secrete interleukin-2 in the treatment of central nervous system glioma and melanoma. Neurosurgery 1997; 41:898–906.

Golumbek PT, Lazenby AJ, Levitsky HI, Jaffee LM, Karasuyama H, Baker M, Pardoll DM. Treatment of established renal cancer by tumor cells engineered to secrete interleukin-4. Science 1991; 254:713–716.

Hall SJ, Mutchnik SE, Chen SH, Woo SL, Thompson TC. Adenovirus-mediated herpes simplex virus thymidine kinase gene and ganciclovir therapy leads to systemic activity against spontaneous and induced metastasis in an orthotopic mouse model of prostate cancer. Int J Cancer 1997; 70:183–187.

Harris MP, Sutjipto S, Wills KN, Hancock W, Cornell D, Johnson DE, Gregory RJ, Shepard HM, Maneval DC. Adenovirus-mediated p53 gene transfer inhibits growth of human tumor cells expressing mutant p53 protein. Cancer Gene Ther 1996; 3:121–130.

Hayakawa M, Kawaguchi S, Ishii S, Murakami M, Uede T. B7-1-transfected tumor vaccine counteracts chemotherapy-induced immunosuppression and prolongs the survival of rats bearing highly metastatic osteosarcoma cells. Int J Cancer 1997; 71: 1091–1102.

Heike Y, Takahashi M, Ohira T, Naruse I, Hama S, Ohe Y, Kasai T, Fukumoto H, Olsen KJ, Podack EE, Saijo N. Genetic immunotherapy by intrapleural, intraperitoneal and subcutaneous injection of IL-2 gene-modified Lewis lung carcinoma cells. Int J Cancer 1997; 73:844–849.

Heuer JG, Tucker McClung C, Gonin R, Hock RA. Retrovirus-mediated gene transfer of B7-1 and MHC class II converts a poorly immunogenic neuroblastoma into a highly immunogenic one. Hum Gene Ther 1996; 7:2059–2068.

Holt JT, Thompson ME, Szabo C, Robinson Benion C, Arteaga CL, King MC, Jensen RA. Growth retardation and tumour inhibition by BRCA1 [see comments]. Nat Genet 1996; 12: 298–302.

Kanai F, Lan KH, Shiratori Y, Tanaka T, Ohashi M, Okudaira T, Yoshida Y, Wakimoto H, Hamada H, Nakabayashi H, Tamaoki T, Omata M. In vivo gene therapy for alpha-fetoprotein-producing hepatocellular carcinoma by adenovirus-mediated transfer of cytosine deaminase gene. Cancer Res 1997; 57: 461–465.

Kaneko S, Hallenbeck P, Kotani T, Nakabayashi H, McGarrity G, Tamaoki T, Anderson WF, Chiang YL. Adenovirus-mediated gene therapy of hepatocellular carcinoma using cancer-specific gene expression. Cancer Res 1995; 55:5283–5287.

Ko SC, Gotoh A, Thalmann GN, Zhau HE, Johnston DA, Zhang WW, Kao C, Chung LW. Molecular therapy with recombinant p53 adenovirus in an androgen-independent, metastatic human prostate cancer model. Hum Gene Ther 1996; 7:1683–1691.

Kramm CM, Rainov NG, Sena Esteves M, Barnett FH, Chase M, Herrlinger U, Pechan PA, Chiocca EA, Breakefield XO. Long-term survival in a rodent model of disseminated brain tumors by combined intrathecal delivery of herpes vectors and ganciclovir treatment. Hum Gene Ther 1996; 7:1989–1994.

Kruse CA, Roper MD, Kleinschmidt DeMasters BK, Banuelos SJ, Smiley WR, Robbins JM, Burrows FJ. Purified herpes simplex thymidine kinase Retrovector particles. I. In vitro characterization, in situ transduction efficiency, and histopathological analyses of gene therapy-treated brain tumors. Cancer Gene Ther 1997; 4:118–128.

Kwong YL, Chen SH, Kosai K, Finegold M, Woo SL. Combination therapy with suicide and cytokine genes for hepatic metastases of lung cancer. Chest 1997; 112:1332–1337.

Lan KH, Kanai F, Shiratori Y, Ohashi M, Tanaka T, Okudaira T, Yoshida Y, Hamada H, Omata M. In vivo selective gene expression and therapy mediated by adenoviral vectors for human carcinoembryonic antigen-producing gastric carcinoma. Cancer Res 1997; 57:4279–4284.

Lesoon-Wood LA, Kim WH, Kleinman HK, Weintraub BD, Mixson AJ. Systemic gene therapy with p53 reduces growth and metastases of a malignant human breast cancer in nude mice. Hum Gene Ther 1995; 6:395–405.

Levitsky HI, Montgomery J, Ahmadzadeh M, Staveley O-K, Guarnieri F, Longo DL, Kwak LW. Immunization with granulocyte-macrophage colony-stimulating factor-transduced, but not B7-1-transduced, lymphoma cells primes idiotype-specific T cells and generates potent systemic antitumor immunity. J Immunol 1996; 156:3858–3865.

Li Z, Shanmugam N, Katayose D, Huber B, Srivastava S, Cowan K, Seth P. Enzyme/prodrug gene therapy approach for breast cancer using a recombinant adenovirus expressing Escherichia coli cytosine deaminase. Cancer Gene Ther 1997; 4:113–117.

Liu TJ, el Naggar AK, McDonnell TJ, Steck KD, Wang M, Taylor DL, Clayman GL. Apoptosis induction mediated by wild-type p53 adenoviral gene transfer in squamous cell carcinoma of the head and neck. Cancer Res 1995; 55:3117–3122.

Liu TJ, Zhang WW, Taylor DL, Roth JA, Goepfert H, Clayman GL. Growth suppression of human head and neck cancer cells by the introduction of a wild-type p53 gene via a recombinant adenovirus. Cancer Res 1994; 54:3662–3667.

Martin Fontecha A, Cavallo F, Bellone M, Heltai S, Iezzi G, Tornaghi P, Nabavi N, Forni G, Dellabona P, Casorati G. Heterogeneous effects of B7-1 and B7-2 in the induction of both protective and therapeutic anti-tumor immunity against different mouse tumors. Eur J Immunol 1996; 26:1851–1859.

Missol E, Sochanik A, Szala S. Introduction of murine Il-4 gene into B16(F10) melanoma tumors by direct gene transfer with DNA-liposome complexes. Cancer Lett 1995; 97:189–193.

Mizuno M, Yoshida J, Colosi P, Kurtzman G. Adeno-associated virus vector containing the herpes simplex virus thymidine kinase gene causes complete regression of intracerebrally implanted human gliomas in mice, in conjunction with ganciclovir administration. Jpn J Cancer Res 1998; 89:76–80.

Namba H, Tagawa M, Iwadate Y, Kimura M, Sueyoshi K, Sakiyama S. Bystander effect-mediated therapy of experimental brain tumor by genetically engineered tumor cells [see comments]. Hum. Gene Ther 1998; 9:5–11.

Nguyen DM, Spitz FR, Yen N, Cristiano RJ, Roth JA. Gene therapy for lung cancer: enhancement of tumor suppression by a combination of sequential systemic cisplatin and adenovirus-mediated p53 gene transfer. J Thorac Cardiovasc Surg 1996; 112:1372–1376.

Nielsen LL, Dell J, Maxwell E, Armstrong L, Maneval D, Catino JJ. Efficacy of p53 adenovirus-mediated gene therapy against human breast cancer xenografts. Cancer Gene Ther 1997; 4: 129–138.

Nishihara K, Barth RF, Wilkie N, Lang JC, Oda Y, Kikuchi H, Everson MP, Lotze MT. Increased in vitro and in vivo tumoricidal activity of a macrophage cell line genetically engineered to express IFN-gamma, IL-4, IL-6, or TNF-alpha. Cancer Gene Ther 1995; 2:113–124.

Ohira T, Ohe Y, Heike Y, Podack ER, Olsen KJ, Nishio K, Nishio M, Miyahara Y, Funayama Y, Ogasawara H, et al. Gene therapy for Lewis lung carcinoma with tumor necrosis factor and interleukin 2 cDNAs co-transfected subline. Gene Ther 1994; 1:269–275.

Ohno T, Yang Z, Ling X, Jaffe M, Nabel EG, Normolle D, Nabel GJ. Combination gene transfer to potentiate tumor regression. Gene Ther 1997; 4:361–366.

Ohwada A, Hirschowitz EA, Crystal RG. Regional delivery of an adenovirus vector containing the Escherichia coli cytosine deaminase gene to provide local activation of 5-fluorocytosine to suppress the growth of colon carcinoma metastatic to liver. Hum Gene Ther 1996; 7:1567–1576.

Overwijk WW, Tsung A, Irvine KR, Parkhurst MR, Goletz TJ, Tsung K, Carroll MW, Liu C, Moss B, Rosenberg SA, Restifo NP. gp100/pmel 17 is a murine tumor rejection antigen: induction of ''self''-reactive, tumoricidal T cells using high-affinity, altered peptide ligand. J Exp Med 1998; 188:277–286.

Perez Cruet MJ, Trask TW, Chen SH, Goodman JC, Woo SL, Grossman RG, Shine HD. Adenovirus-mediated gene therapy of experimental gliomas. J Neurosci Res 1994; 39:506–511.

Pippin BA, Rosenstein M, Jacob WF, Chiang Y, Lotze MT. Local IL-4 delivery enhances immune reactivity to murine tumors: gene therapy in combination with IL-2. Cancer Gene Ther 1994; 1:35–42.

Plautz GE, Yang ZY, Wu BY, Gao X, Huang L, Nabel GJ. Immunotherapy of malignancy by in vivo gene transfer into tumors [see comments]. Proc Natl Acad Sci USA 1993; 90: 4645–4649.

Qian C, Idoate M, Bilbao R, Sangro B, Bruna O, Vazquez J, Prieto J. Gene transfer and therapy with adenoviral vector in rats with diethylnitrosamine-induced hepatocellular carcinoma. Hum Gene Ther 1997; 8:349–358.

Rainov NG, Kramm CM, Aboody Guterman K, Chase M, Ueki K, Louis DN, Harsh GR, Chiocca A, Breakefield XO. Retrovirus-mediated gene therapy of experimental brain neoplasms using the herpes simplex virus-thymidine kinase/ganciclovir paradigm. Cancer Gene Ther 1996; 3:99–106.

Rakhmilevich AL, Janssen K, Turner J, Culp J, Yang NS. Cytokine gene therapy of cancer using gene gun technology: superior antitumor activity of interleukin-12. Hum Gene Ther 1997; 8:1303–1311.

Rakhmilevich AL, Turner J, Ford MJ, McCabe D, Sun WH, Sondel PM, Grota K, Yang NS. Gene gun-mediated skin transfection with interleukin 12 gene results in regression of established primary and metastatic murine tumors. Proc Natl Acad Sci USA 1996; 93:6291–6296.

Riley DJ, Nikitin AY, Lee WH. Adenovirus-mediated retinoblastoma gene therapy suppresses spontaneous pituitary melanotroph tumors in Rb+/− mice. Nat Med 1996; 2:1316–1321.

Sandig V, Brand K, Herwig S, Lukas J, Bartek J, Strauss M. Adenovirally transferred p16INK4/CDKN2 and p53 genes cooperate to induce apoptotic tumor cell death. Nat Med 1997; 3:313–319.

Schmitt M, Ikeda H, Nagata Y, Gu X, Wang L, Kuribayashi K, Shiku H. Involvement of T-cell subsets and natural killer (NK) cells in the growth suppression of murine fibrosarcoma cells transfected with interleukin-12 (IL-12) genes. Int J Cancer 1997; 72:505–511.

Soubrane C, Mouawad R, Rixe O, Calvez V, Ghoumari A, Verola O, Weil M, Khayat D. Direct gene transfer of a plasmid carrying the herpes simplex virus-thymidine kinase gene (HSV-TK) in transplanted murine melanoma: in vivo study. Eur J Cancer 1996; 32A:691–695.

Spitz FR, Nguyen D, Skibber JM, Cusack J, Roth JA, Cristiano RJ. In vivo adenovirus-mediated p53 tumor suppressor gene therapy for colorectal cancer. Anticancer Res 1996; 16: 3415–3422.

Sugaya S, Fujita K, Kikuchi A, Ueda H, Takakuwa K, Kodama S, Tanaka K. Inhibition of tumor growth by direct intratumoral gene transfer of herpes simplex virus thymidine kinase gene with DNA-liposome complexes. Hum. Gene Ther 1996; 7: 223–230.

Sumimoto H, Tani K, Nakazaki Y, Tanabe T, Hibino H, Wu MS, Izawa K, Hamada H, Asano S. Superiority of interleukin-12-transduced murine lung cancer cells to GM-CSF or B7-1 (CD80) transfectants for therapeutic antitumor immunity in syngeneic immunocompetent mice. Cancer Gene Ther 1998; 5:29–37.

Sutton MA, Berkman SA, Chen SH, Block A, Dang TD, Kattan MW, Wheeler TM, Rowley DR, Woo SL, and Lerner SP. Adenovirus-mediated suicide gene therapy for experimental bladder cancer. Urology. 49:173–180, 1997.

Szala S, Missol E, Sochanik A, Strozyk M. The use of cationic liposomes DC-CHOL/DOPE and DDAB/DOPE for direct transfer of *Escherichia coli* cytosine deaminase gene into growing melanoma tumors. Gene Ther 1996; 3:1026–1031.

Takakuwa K, Fujita K, Kikuchi A, Sugaya S, Yahata T, Aida H, Kurabayashi T, Hasegawa I, Tanaka K. Direct intratumoral gene transfer of the herpes simplex virus thymidine kinase gene with DNA-liposome complexes: growth inhibition of tumors and lack of localization in normal tissues. Jpn J Cancer Res 1997; 88:166–175.

Tan J, Newton CA, Djeu JY, Gutsch DE, Chang AE, Yang NS, Klein TW, Hua Y. Injection of complementary DNA encoding interleukin-12 inhibits tumor establishment at a distant site in a murine renal carcinoma model. Cancer Res 1996; 56: 3399–3403.

Toda M, Martuza RL, Kojima H, Rabkin SD. In situ cancer vaccination: an IL-12 defective vector/replication-competent herpes simplex virus combination induces local and systemic antitumor activity. J Immunol 1998; 160:4457–4464.

Toloza EM, Hunt K, Swisher S, McBride W, Lau R, Pang S, Rhoades K, Drake T, Belldegrun A, Glaspy J, Economou JS. In vivo cancer gene therapy with a recombinant interleukin-2 adenovirus vector. Cancer Gene Ther 1996; 3:11–17.

Tong XW, Block A, Chen SH, Contant CF, Agoulnik I, Blankenburg K, Kaufman RH, Woo SL, Kieback DG. In vivo gene therapy of ovarian cancer by adenovirus-mediated thymidine kinase gene transduction and ganciclovir administration. Gynecol Oncol 1996; 61:175–179.

Topf N, Worgall S, Hackett NR, Crystal RG. Regional 'pro-drug' gene therapy: intravenous administration of an adenoviral vector expressing the *E. coli* cytosine deaminase gene and systemic administration of 5-fluorocytosine suppresses growth of hepatic metastasis of colon carcinoma. Gene Ther 1998; 5: 507–513.

Vieweg J, Rosenthal FM, Bannerji R, Heston WD, Fair WR, Gansbacher B, Gilboa E. Immunotherapy of prostate cancer in the Dunning rat model: use of cytokine gene modified tumor vaccines. Cancer Res 1994; 54:1760–1765.

Vincent AJ, Esandi MD, van Someren G, Noteboom JL, Avezaat CJ, Vecht C, Smitt PA, van Bekkum DW, Valerio D, Hoogerbrugge PM, Bout A. Treatment of leptomeningeal metastases in a rat model using a recombinant adenovirus containing the HSV-tk gene. J Neurosurg 1996a; 85:648–654.

Vincent AJ, Vogels R, Someren GV, Esandi MC, Noteboom JL, Avezaat CJ, Vecht C, Bekkum DW, Valerio D, Bout A, Hoogerbrugge PM. Herpes simplex virus thymidine kinase gene therapy for rat malignant brain tumors. Hum Gene Ther 1996b; 7:197–205.

Wills KN, Maneval DC, Menzel P, Harris MP, Sutjipto S, Vaillancourt MT, Huang WM, Johnson DE, Anderson SC, Wen SF, et al. Development and characterization of recombinant adenoviruses encoding human p53 for gene therapy of cancer. Hum Gene Ther 1994; 5:1079–1088.

Wilson KM, Stambrook PJ, Bi WL, Pavelic ZP, Pavelic L, Gluckman JL. HSV-tk gene therapy in head and neck squamous cell carcinoma. Enhancement by the local and distant bystander effect. Arch Otolaryngol Head Neck Surg 1996; 122:746–749.

Xing X, Matin A, Yu D, Xia W, Sorgi F, Huang L, Huang MC. Mutant SV40 large T antigen as a therapeutic agent for HER-2/neu-overexpressing ovarian cancer. Cancer Gene Ther 1996; 3:168–174.

Xu HJ, Zhou Y, Seigne J, Perng GS, Mixon M, Zhang C, Li J, Benedict WF, Hu SX. Enhanced tumor suppressor gene therapy via replication-deficient adenovirus vectors expressing an N-terminal truncated retinoblastoma protein. Cancer Res 1996; 56:2245–2249.

Xu M, Kumar D, Srinivas S, Detolla LJ, Yu SF, Stass SA, Mixson AJ. Parenteral gene therapy with p53 inhibits human breast tumors in vivo through a bystander mechanism without evidence of toxicity. Hum Gene Ther 1997; 8:177–185.

Yee D, McGuire SE, Brunner N, Kozelsky TW, Allred DC, Chen SH, Woo SL. Adenovirus-mediated gene transfer of herpes simplex virus thymidine kinase in an ascites model of human breast cancer. Hum Gene Ther 1996; 7:1251–1257.

Yu D, Matin A, Xia W, Sorgi F, Huang L, Hung MC. Liposome-mediated in vivo E1A gene transfer suppressed dissemination of ovarian cancer cells that overexpress HER-2/neu. Oncogene 1995; 11:1383–1388.

Zhang WW, Fang X, Mazur W, French BA, Georges RN, Roth JA. High-efficiency gene transfer and high-level expression of wild-type p53 in human lung cancer cells mediated by recombinant adenovirus. Cancer Gene Ther 1994; 7:5–13.

Zitvogel L, Mayordomo JI, Tjandrawan T, DeLeo AB, Clarke MR, Lotze MT, Storkus WJ. Therapy of murine tumors with tumor peptide-pulsed dendritic cells: dependence on T cells, B7 costimulation, and T helper cell 1-associated cytokines [see comments]. J Exp Med 1996a; 183:87–97.

Zitvogel L, Robbins PD, Storkus WJ, Clarke MR, Maeurer MJ, Campbell RL, Davis CG, Tahara H, Schreiber RD, Lotze MT. Interleukin-12 and B7.1 co-stimulation cooperate in the induction of effective antitumor immunity and therapy of established tumors. Eur J Immunol 1996b; 26:1335–1341.

23

Barriers to Efficient Airway Epithelial Gene Transfer: Lessons from Cystic Fibrosis

Larry G. Johnson and Richard C. Boucher
University of North Carolina at Chapel Hill, Chapel Hill, North Carolina

I. INTRODUCTION

The identification of human genes linked to clinical disease from human genome research has raised hopes for the development of specific genetic therapies for many inherited and acquired diseases. Cystic fibrosis (CF) is a common inherited disorder with a high morbidity and mortality that makes it an attractive target for gene therapy. The autosomal inheritance pattern of this monogenic disorder in which heterozygotes are phenotypically normal, combined with the relatively large numbers of patients available for clinical studies, has led to the establishment of CF as the prototypical disease for investigation of gene therapy in the lung.

The normal phenotype of CF heterozygotes suggests that introduction of a single wild-type (normal) copy of the gene into defective CF epithelial cells should restore the normal phenotype. Restoration of CFTR-mediated Cl^- transport function following introduction of wild-type *CFTR* into CF airway epithelial cells in vitro using retrovirus, vaccinia virus, liposomes, and adenoviral vectors is consistent with this concept (1–6). These studies established the feasibility of gene therapy for CF and promoted the intense investigation necessary to develop it for clinical application.

An important factor in the development of gene therapy for CF is the identification of the appropriate cellular targets in human airways. The site where CF lung disease begins is still debated, with both the superficial columnar epithelial cells lining the lumen of the small airways and the serous cells of submucosal glands having been identified as rational targets. Clinical data tend to support the theory that the disease begins in the small airways (7,8). Where the disease begins is relevant since luminal (airway) delivery of gene-transfer vectors targets the superficial columnar airway epithelium, while intravenous (blood) delivery will be required to target the submucosal glands.

Following initial in vitro complementation studies, investigators rapidly moved to clinical safety and efficacy trials of gene-transfer vectors delivered by luminal application to the airways of CF patients. While some evidence for gene transfer was detected, the efficiency and efficacy of gene transfer failed to meet expectations and did not fully correct the known biochemical defects ascribed to this disorder. This failure has forced investigators in the field to carefully explore the barriers to gene transfer in airways and has stimulated efforts to develop strategies to overcome these barriers. In this chapter, we review data from published clinical gene-transfer safety and efficacy studies, discuss the barriers that have become apparent as a result of these trials and ongoing laboratory investigation, and explore new ideas or strategies to overcome the limitations of airway gene transfer.

II. CLINICAL TRIALS IN CYSTIC FIBROSIS PATIENTS

The characteristic features, advantages, and disadvantages of adenoviral (Ad), adeno-associated viral (AAV), and cationic liposomal vectors have been extensively reviewed elsewhere (9–14). Clinical gene-transfer safety and efficacy trials of each of these vectors have been initiated in airway epithelia of CF patients. Initial phase I trials evaluated single administration of Ad-*CFTR* vectors to the nasal and/or lower airway epithelia of CF patients. Subsequent trials of Ad vectors have evaluated the feasibility of repetitive dosing and the safety and efficacy of aerosolized adenovirus vector administration. Trials of cationic liposomes complexed to CFTR plasmid DNA (lipoplexes) have increased rapidly in number, and two trials of AAV-mediated gene transfer to CF airways have been initiated. Data have been published from a number of these trials and are reviewed below.

A. Adenoviral Vector Trials

The results of several trials (Table 1) evaluating single, aerosolized, or repetitive administration of Ad-*CFTR* vectors have been published (15–20). In an initial uncontrolled study, Ad-mediated correction of the Cl^- transport defect in the nasal epithelium of three CF subjects (MOIs of 1, 3, and 25) and expression of CFTR by RNA-specific (RS)-PCR in two of the three subjects studied (MOIs of 3 and 25) was detected (15). A major criticism of this study has been the failure of the investigators to include the low Cl^- maneuver in the nasal potential difference (PD) technique used to measure Cl^- secretion in their study. The low Cl^- maneuver is a very sensitive discriminator of CF airway from non-CF airway Cl^- secretory responses when performed in the presence of isoproterenol (21).

Expression of mRNA by RT-PCR and immunohistochemical detection of CFTR from bronchial brushings in one of four (not the same patient) patients was reported by Crystal and colleagues (16) in their study of Ad-mediated gene transfer to nasal airway epithelia followed 24 hours later by delivery to the bronchial epithelium. A systemic inflammatory syndrome occurred in one subject that was characterized by headache, fatigue, fever, tachycardia, hypotension, pulmonary infiltrates, and a decrease in lung function 12–24 hours after Ad-*CFTR* administration (2×10^9 pfu) to the right lower lobe bronchus. Increased interleukin-6 (IL-6) levels relative to the levels of the other study subjects were detected in association with the onset of symptoms. Clinical signs and symptoms resolved by 14 days with broad-spectrum antibiotics, antipyretics, nasal

Table 1 Clinical Gene-Transfer Safety and Efficacy Trials of Adenoviral Vectors in Cystic Fibrosis

Principal investigator(s)	Description of trial
Ronald Crystal	A phase I study, in cystic fibrosis patients, of the safety, toxicity, and biological efficacy of a single administration of a replication-deficient, recombinant adenovirus carrying the cDNA of the normal human cystic fibrosis transmembrane conductance regulator gene in the lung
Ronald Crystal	Evaluation of repeat administration of a replication-deficient, recombinant adenovirus containing the normal cystic fibrosis transmembrane conductance regulator cDNA to the airways of individuals with cystic fibrosis
Michael Welsh, Alan E. Smith	Cystic fibrosis gene therapy using an adenovirus vector: in vivo safety and efficacy in nasal epithelium
Michael Welsh, Joseph Zabner	Adenovirus-mediated gene transfer of CFTR to the nasal epithelium and maxillary sinus of patients with cystic fibrosis
James M. Wilson	Gene therapy of cystic fibrosis lung disease using E1-deleted adenoviruses: a phase I trial/intrapulmonary administration of a third-generation adenoviral vector in adults with cystic fibrosis
Richard C. Boucher, Michael R. Knowles	Gene therapy for cystic fibrosis using E1-deleted adenovirus: a phase I trial in the nasal cavity
Robert W. Wilmott, Jeffrey Whitsett	A phase I study of gene therapy of cystic fibrosis utilizing a replication-deficient recombinant adenovirus vector to deliver the human cystic fibrosis transmembrane conductance regulator cDNA to the airways
Henry L. Dorkin	Adenovirus-mediated gene transfer for cystic fibrosis: safety of single administration in the lung (lobar instillation)
Henry L. Dorkin	Adenovirus-mediated gene transfer for cystic fibrosis: safety of single administration in the lung (aerosol administration)
G. Bellon	Aerosol administration of recombinant adenovirus expressing CFTR to cystic fibrosis patients: a phase I trial

oxygen, and IV fluids, but chest radiographic abnormalities persisted for up to 25 days and lung function did not return to baseline for 30 days. Subsequently, the functional data from administration of Ad-*CFTR* (2×10^5–$2 \times 10^{8.5}$ pfu) to the nasal epithelium of nine CF patients, including data from the first four patients discussed above, was reported (17). Partial correction of both Na^+ hyperabsorption and Cl^- secretion (33% of that measured in non-CF individuals) was detected using the nasal PD technique when averaged over 14 days. A dose-dependent relationship between vector and function was not apparent in this particular study.

Knowles and colleagues (18) detected transduced CFTR-mRNA by RT-PCR and/or in situ hybridization in five of the six patients at the highest doses (MOI 100 and 1000) and in one of six patients at lower MOIs (MOI = 10) in a double-blinded, vehicle-controlled, dose-escalation study in the nasal epithelium of CF subjects. No correction of defective CFTR-mediated Cl^- transport or normalization of raised Na^+ transport was measured using the nasal potential difference technique. In situ hybridization studies of mucosal biopsies from these subjects demonstrated transduction of less than 1% of the cells consistent with the functional assessment. Mucosal inflammation was detected in the Ad5-CB*CFTR* dosed nostril in two of three patients at MOI 1000. Subsequent in vivo studies in rats suggested that the mucosal inflammation arose from vector-induced neurogenic inflammation (22). A 15-fold increase in neutralizing antibody titer was detected in one of the high-dose patients.

The results of a trial evaluating aerosol administration of recombinant Ad-*CFTR* has been published (19). In a dose-escalation study with cohorts of two patients each, six CF patients were dosed with Ad-*CFTR* via nasal instillation followed 24 hours later by aerosol administration. The doses of vector for nasal instillation were 1×10^5, 1×10^7, and 4×10^8 pfu in a volume of 400 μL and 1×10^7, 1×10^8, and 5.4×10^8 pfu for aerosol administration with a volume of 1.6 mL in a breath-activated jet nebulizer (OPTINEB, Air Liquide, Paris, France). The estimated dose of vector delivered to the airways was 25% of the dose in the nebulizer or 2.6×10^6, 2.5×10^7, and 1.35×10^8 pfu, respectively, for each cohort. Transduced CFTR mRNA was detected by RT-PCR in nasal brush specimens obtained from all six patients and in bronchial brush specimens from one of six subjects 1–15 days post–Ad-*CFTR* administration, but was not detected in either nasal or bronchial specimens obtained from subjects at baseline (prior to vector administration). CFTR expression by immunohistochemistry was also detected in nasal brush specimens from all six subjects post–nasal instillation and in bronchial brush specimens obtained from two of six subjects post–aerosolized vector administration. The fraction of cells transduced by immunohistochemistry from nasal brush specimens ranged from 1.5 to 14.6% (mean 5.2%) post–vector administration. However, functional correlates of Ad-mediated CFTR gene transfer were not measured. No safety concerns were raised in this particular study.

Zabner et al. have reported their results from the repeat administration of a second-generation Ad2-*CFTR* vector to the nasal epithelia of six CF patients (20). The study was double-blinded in the last four subjects. Vector (200–600 μL) was delivered over 30 minutes to the inferior turbinate of one nostril with an equal volume of placebo (saline) delivered to the contralateral nostril in each subject. Five doses of vector were administered with an average of 44 days between doses. The doses of vector delivered were as follows: 2×10^7, 2×10^8, 2×10^9, 6.6×10^9, and 1×10^{10} IU. No adverse clinical effects were detected. However, a fourfold increase in IgG antibody titer in three subjects at doses greater than or equal to 2×10^9 IU and a fourfold increase in neutralizing antibody in three subjects at a dose of 6.6×10^9 IU were detected. No increase in levels of IgA antibody in nasal lavage fluid could be detected postdosing. Importantly, no correction of sodium transport was measured, and only a partial correction of Cl^- transport was present at 2–6×10^9 IU (primarily in two of six subjects).

These trials demonstrated that the efficiency of Ad-mediated transduction of CFTR in the airway epithelium of CF patients was low and stimulated a more thorough investigation of the barriers to Ad gene transfer. Moreover, safety concerns were raised in humans with this vector system. Further improvements in Ad-mediated gene-transfer efficiency and safety will be required to safely achieve sufficient efficacy.

B. Adeno-Associated Virus Vectors

Two clinical safety and efficacy trials of AAV vectors for CF gene therapy have been initiated (Table 2): one exam-

Table 2 Clinical Gene-Transfer Safety and Efficacy Trials of Adeno-Associated Viral Vectors in Cystic Fibrosis

Principal investigator	Description of trial
Terence R. Flotte	A phase I study of an adeno-associated virus–CFTR gene vector in adult CF patients with mild lung disease
Phyllis Gardner	A phase I/II study of tgAAV-CF for the treatment of chronic sinusitis in patients with cystic fibrosis

ines the utility of AAV-*CFTR* vectors in the nasal and lower airway epithelium, while the other investigates potential utility in the maxillary sinus, which is also lined by respiratory (airway) epithelium. Wagner et al. recently reported the initial results from an unblinded study of 10 CF patients—patients received a single dose to one sinus and 5 subjects received a low dose to one sinus with the next highest dose vector to contralateral sinus (23). Doses of AAV-*CFTR* used in this study were as follows: 10^2, 10^3, 10^4, 5×10^4, and 10^5 replicating units (RU). However, the specifics of repetitive dosing are not described in detail. DNA was detectable by PCR in all patients receiving 10^4 RU or greater at 14 days, but RT-PCR was negative for mRNA. A hyperpolarization of maxillary PD with low $C1^-$/isoproterenol perfusion was reported at doses of $\geq 10^4$ RU, but no controls were described, the data were not shown, and the ion transport physiology of sinus epithelium in normal individuals has not been studied. The results from studies of AAV-*CFTR* in the nasal and lower airway epithelia of CF patients have not been published. Thus it is difficult to assess the efficacy of AAV from these trials.

C. Cationic Liposomes

Several trials of cationic liposome-mediated CFTR gene transfer to the nasal epithelium of CF patients have been initiated (Table 3). Caplen et al. reported a double-blinded, placebo-controlled trial in which nine cystic fibrosis subjects received CFTR plasmid DNA (pSV-CFTR) complexed with DC-Chol/DOPE liposomes in a 1:5 (w/w) DNA-to-lipid ratio (24). Six CF subjects received only DC-Chol/DOPE liposomes to the nasal epithelia. The doses of DNA utilized were 10, 100, and 300 μg plasmid DNA per nostril delivered by nasal spray. The highest dose was delivered in 200 μL aliquots to each nostril every 10 minutes, requiring a total time of 7.5 hours. A mean hyperpolarization of the nasal PD (more negative PD) following low $C1^-$ perfusion in patients receiving the CFTR plasmid DNA-liposome complex (lipoplexes) equal to ~20% of that measured in normals was reported. No differences in nasal PDs between CF controls dosed with liposomes only and CF patients dosed with CFTR lipoplexes were detected following treatment with isoprenaline, a cAMP-mediated agonist. RT-PCR detected vector-derived CFTR mRNA in nasal biopsies of five of eight patients who received the DNA liposome complex, but was also positive in one of five patients who received placebo (liposomes only). Importantly, no toxicity was observed and DC-Chol/DOPE liposomes without plasmid DNA delivered to the nasal epithelium in six normal and three CF subjects did not alter nasal ion transport parameters, lung function, or alter antibiotic sensitivities of CF sputum bacterial isolates (25).

Gill and coworkers have reported data from a double-blinded placebo-controlled trial of DC-Chol/DOPE liposomes complexed to CFTR plasmid under the transcriptional control of an RSV 3′LTR promoter (26). A unique feature of this trial was the use of an empty plasmid vector complexed to liposomes in two of the four placebo patients (the other two received buffer). The 12 patients in this study received either placebo (4 patients), lipoplexes with 40 μg CFTR plasmid DNA (4 patients), or lipoplexes with

Table 3 Clinical Gene-Transfer Safety and Efficacy Trials of Cationic Liposomes in Cystic Fibrosis

Principal investigator(s)	Lipid	Description of trial
Eric W. F. W. Alton, Duncan M. Geddes	DC-Chol/DOPE	Liposome-mediated CFTR gene transfer to the nasal epithelium of patients with cystic fibrosis
Stephen Hyde	DC-Chol/DOPE	A placebo-controlled study of liposome-mediated gene transfer to the nasal epithelium of patients with cystic fibrosis
Michael J. Welsh, Joseph Zabner	GL-67	Cationic lipid-mediated gene transfer of CFTR: safety of a single administration to the nasal epithelia
Eric W. F. W. Alton, Duncan M. Geddes	GL-67	Safety and efficacy of lipid #67 in the airway epithelium of CF patients
Eric J. Sorscher, James L. Logan	DMRIE/DOPE	Gene therapy for cystic fibrosis using cationic liposome-mediated gene transfer; a phase I trial of safety and efficacy in the nasal airway
Eric J. Sorscher	GL-67	Phase I study of liposome gene transfer therapy
David Porteus, J.A. Innes	DOTAP	DOTAP liposome delivery of gene therapy for cystic fibrosis; a phase I trial in the human nose
Michael R. Knowles, Peadar Noone	EDMPC	A double-blind, placebo-controlled, dose-ranging study to evaluate the safety and biological efficacy of the lipid-DNA complex GR213487B in the nasal epithelium of adult patients with cystic fibrosis

400 μg CFTR plasmid DNA (4 patients) to each nostril delivered via direct instillation over 2 days. Hyperpolarization of the nasal PD into the range of non-CF individuals with superfusion of a low $C1^-$ solution plus amiloride was reported in two of eight subjects dosed with vector (one from each cohort receiving CFTR lipoplexes), but not in placebo-treated subjects. Functional gene transfer was detectable at the single-cell level in five of eight patients by SPQ analysis. However, a positive SPQ signal did not predict a parallel response in the nasal PD maneuver that tests the bioelectric function of the epithelium. No evidence for correction of the raised basal PD (a measure of Na^+ transport) was detected, and immunohistochemical and molecular analysis were not performed. Interestingly, one high-dose (400 μg) patient developed a transient earache on the evening of initial dosing with an associated injected tympanic membrane for 15 days. Because rhinovirus was cultured from nasal lavage fluid on day 14, delineation of infection versus neurogenic inflammation (22) as the etiology of the earache and inflamed tympanic membrane was not feasible.

Single administration of 400 μg pCMV-CFTR/2.4 mg DOTAP lipoplexes has been reported (27) in a double-blinded placebo-controlled trial in the nasal epithelium of 16 CF patients (8 placebo and 8 CFTR lipoplex). Vector-specific CFTR mRNA was detectable by RT-PCR in 2 of 8 patients receiving CFTR lipoplexes, but no significant CFTR-related functional changes were detectable by either the nasal PD technique or SPQ analysis of cells obtained by nasal brushing.

A randomized, double-blinded study of single administration of CFTR plasmid DNA (pCF1-CFTR) GL-67 lipoplexes versus CFTR plasmid (pCF1-CFTR) alone (naked DNA) the nasal epithelium has been completed (28). Eighteen subjects were evaluated: 6 non-CF subjects received lipid alone for safety testing, 9 CF subjects received pCF1-CFTR (1.25 mg) naked DNA to one nostril vs CFTR lipoplex (1.25:2 w/w DNA:lipid ratio) in the contralateral nostril, and 3 CF subjects received pCF1-CFTR vs pNull naked DNA (1.25 mg each). Vector-specific DNA was detected in 8 of 9 CFTR lipoplex nostrils and 9 of 9 pCF1-CFTR naked DNA nostrils. Vector-specific mRNA was detected by RT-PCR in one of three lipoplex nostrils and 2 of 3 naked CFTR DNA nostrils in which GAPDH was also detected. The other 6 nasal samples were negative for both CFTR and GAPDH. No correction of basal PD was measured. However, a small hyperpolarization with low chloride/tertabuline superfusion in CFTR lipoplex (~2.5 mV) and naked CFTR DNA-treated nostrils (~3.5 mV) was detected consistent with a partial correction of chloride secretion. The surprise was that the relative magnitude of partial corrections by lipoplexes and naked DNA were similar. No significant toxicity was measured.

These data would suggest that CFTR lipoplex–mediated gene transfer to CF airways in vivo is also inefficient. Similar barriers to gene transfer as those affecting Ad vectors may be present.

D. Lessons from Gene-Transfer Safety and Efficacy Trials

The data from the trials above are summarized in Table 4. Several lessons may be discerned from the data: (1) in vivo gene-transfer efficacy to CF airways is low; (2) because this conclusion relates to all vectors tested, common barriers to gene transfer may exist in addition to vector specific barriers; and (3) immune or inflammatory reactions may also limit gene transfer particularly with regard to Ad vectors and some lipoplexes. In the next section, we will focus on barriers at the cellular level that limit binding, entry, and expression. Immune barriers, e.g., neutralizing antibodies and immune/inflammatory responses to the administered vector that limit transgene expression, will not be discussed.

III. BARRIERS TO AIRWAY GENE TRANSFER

The markedly inflammed CF lung has barriers to airway gene transfer at virtually all levels, including nonspecific barriers and vector specific barriers. Nonspecific barriers include CF airway mucus, glycoconjugates, and the inflammatory milieu, while vector specific barriers (see Table 5) include factors affecting binding and entry, e.g., receptor localization and endocytic capacity, nuclear translocation, and factors limiting transgene expression post–nuclear entry. These barriers combine to make in vivo gene transfer to human CF airways inefficient.

A. Nonspecific Barriers to Gene Transfer

In cystic fibrosis, the manifestation of mutant CFTR as defective ion transport leads to abnormal secretions, ineffective mucociliary clearance, bacterial proliferation with multiresistant organisms, bronchiectasis, and ultimately death (29). Expression of mutant CFTR in airway epithelia is also associated with an inflammatory response characterized by a massive influx of neutrophils, which act as a source of oxidants and proteolytic enzymes promoting tissue injury and bronchiectasis. This influx of neutrophils increases the load of DNA and actin in the airway secretions of the CF lung, leading to a markedly increased sputum viscosity and with markedly elevated levels of proinflammatory cytokines, including TNFα, IL-1β, IL-6, and

Table 4 Summary Data from Published Gene-Transfer Safety and Efficacy Trials in CF Patients

Principal investigator(s) [Ref.]	Vector	No. of subjects	Vector DNA	Vector-specific RNA	Immunohistochemistry	Functional correction	
						Cl	Na
Welsh/Smith [15]	Adenovirus	3	NR	2/3	No	Partial	No
Crystal [16]	Adenovirus	4	Yes	1/4	1/4	NR	NR
Crystal/Hay [17]	Adenovirus	9	NR	NR	NR	Partial	Partial
Knowles/Boucher [18]	Adenovirus	12	Yes	6/12	NR	No	No
Bellon [19]	Adenovirus	6	Yes	6/6	6/6	NR	NR
Welsh/Zabner [20]	Adenovirus	6	Yes	NR	NR	Partial	No
Wagner/Gardner [23]	AAV	10	Yes	NR	No	Yes[a]	NR
Alton/Geddes [24]	Cationic liposomes	9	Yes	5/8	NR	Partial	No
Gill/Hyde [26]	Cationic liposomes	12	NR	NR	NR	Partial	No
Porteus/Innes [27]	Cationic liposomes	16	Yes	2/8	NR	No	No
Zabner/Welsh [28]	Cationic liposomes	18[a]	Yes	1/9	NR	Partial	No

[a] Includes six non-CF subjects.
NR = Not reported.

IL-8, that perpetuate the inflammatory response (30). Furthermore, inflammation with abnormal secretions and *Pseudomonas* colonization is established early, often in the first year of life (31–33). Given the inability of current therapies to eradicate the chronic pulmonary infection and inflammation of the CF lung, vectors directed at gene transfer to the superficial epithelium will likely have to overcome the inflammatory response to gain access to the epithelium.

Stern et al. investigated the effect of fresh sputum obtained from CF patients on gene transfer to primary airway cells and to CF cell lines in vitro (34). A dose-dependent inhibition of gene transfer to COS-7, 16HBE14o, and 2-CFSMEO cells mediated by the cationic liposome DC-Chol/DOPE and an Ad-lacZ vector was detected in the presence of ultraviolet light–sterilized CF sputum. The effects of CF sputum on liposomal gene transfer were partially reversible using rDNAse pretreatment and completely reversible when rDNAse pretreatment preceded Ad gene transfer. However, pretreatment with other mucolytic agents including nacystelyn, lysine, *n*-acetylysteine, and rAlginase failed to increase liposomal or adenoviral gene-transfer efficiency. This effect could be simulated by application of genomic DNA to cultures prior to transduction with DC-Chol/DOPE or an Ad-*lacZ* vector. These data would suggest that noninfectious sputum components can inhibit gene transfer mediated by cationic liposomes and adenoviruses and that excessive DNA is a major contributor to this inhibitory response.

Van Heeckeren et al. investigated the effect of bronchopulmonary inflammation induced by *Pseudomonas aeruginosa* on Ad-mediated gene transfer to airway epithelial cells in vivo (35). These investigators used an animal model of chronic bronchopulmonary infection in which mice inoculated with *P. aeruginosa*–laden agarose beads develop bronchitis, bronchopneumonia, bronchiectasis, mucus plugging, and alveolar exudate with acute and chronic inflammatory cells. Their studies demonstrated a

Table 5 Barriers to Efficient In Vivo Airway Gene Transfer

Vector	Binding	Entry	Nuclear transport	Second strand synthesis
Adenovirus	Yes	Yes	No	N/A
Adeno-associated virus	Yes	Yes	No	Yes
Retrovirus				
MuLV	Yes	Yes	Yes	N/A
Lentivirus	Yes	Yes	No	N/A
Cationic liposomes	Yes	Yes	Yes	N/A

N/A = Not applicable.

greater than twofold reduction in gene-transfer efficiency mediated by nasal instillation of an Ad-*lacZ* vector in mice in which the *Pseudomonas*-laden beads were instilled compared to mice that had sterile beads or Ad vector alone instilled. In a subsequent study, Parsons et al. demonstrated that Ad-*lacZ* gene transfer to nasal airways of *Pseudomonas* (PA01 strain)–infected mice was reduced 10-fold relative to noninfected nasal airways (36). Thus, the inflammatory milieu induced by *Pseudomonas* is a formidable barrier to transduction.

Innate immunity has been suggested as a potential barrier to lung gene transfer by several investigators. Components of the innate immune system serving as potential barriers include alveolar macrophages and airway surface fluid. Using Ad-specific probes and Southern analysis, Worgall et al. demonstrated a 70% loss of Ad-*lacZ* genomes in both immunocompetent and immunodeficient mice 24 hours following transtracheal administration of an Ad-*lacZ* vector (37). Elimination of macrophages by administration of liposomes containing dichloromethylene biphosphonate with subsequent administration of the Ad-*lacZ* vector resulted in a significant (100%) increase in lung DNA and subsequent βgal expression. In contrast to the persistence of Ad vector DNA in epithelial cell lines in vitro studies in cultured human alveolar macrophages demonstrate rapid loss of Ad vector genomes. These data suggest that alveolar macrophages may play a significant role in reducing the efficiency of Ad gene transfer in the lung parenchyma.

Alveolar macrophages have also been shown to inhibit retrovirus mediated gene transfer to airway epithelia in vitro (38). McCray et al. demonstrated that transduction of human airway epithelial cells by an amphotropic enveloped retroviral vector was inhibited 40% in the presence of alveolar macrophages and more than 60% in the presence of LPS activated alveolar macrophages (38). Incubation of macrophages with dexamethasone (1 μM) partially reversed this inhibition of retroviral transduction. Furthermore, rapid uptake of labeled vector into vesicles of macrophages was associated with loss of DNA within 24 hours, consistent with rapid degradation, rather than rapid transduction, of alveolar macrophages. These data suggest that macrophages can play a significant role in inhibiting in vivo gene transfer to lung epithelia.

Airway surface liquid may also have potential inhibitory effects on airway gene transfer. Batra and colleagues demonstrated that high concentrations of proteoglycans and glycosaminoglycans in pleural fluid from patients with malignant pleural effusion can have inhibitory effects on amphotropic and other pseudotyped retroviral vectors in vitro (39). Because human airways are lined by a glycocalyx, which may contain proteoglycans and glycosaminoglycans, molecules shed from this glycocalyx into the airway surface liquid may potentially inhibit gene transfer. In a study by McCray and coworkers, airway surface liquid from well-differentiated human epithelial cell cultures harvested in a small volume of distilled water failed to inhibit retroviral transduction to naïve airway cells in vitro (38). Johnson and coworkers also reported that freshly isolated murine bronchoalveolar lavage fluid had no effect on transduction of airway epithelial cells by VSV-G pseudotyped retroviral vectors (40). Similar findings documenting no effect of airway surface fluid obtained by washing the surfaces of well-differentiated airway cell cultures and bronchial xenografts on transduction mediated by AAV vectors have also been reported (41). Although the samples of the airway surface fluid used in these studies were dilute, these data would suggest that insignificant levels of vector-inhibitory substances are present within the soluble components of airway surface fluid.

B. Vector-Specific Barriers to Luminal Airway Gene Transfer

Coincident with the initiation of clinical gene-transfer efficacy and safety trials, in vitro and in vivo preclinical studies began to show evidence for inefficient transduction of airway epithelial cells when vector was delivered to the luminal surface. In this section, we review data identifying the barriers to gene transfer for vectors that are either currently used in clinical trials or exhibit potential for use in clinical trials.

1. Ad Vectors

Despite reports of efficient Ad gene transfer to primary human airway epithelia in vitro and to cotton rat airway epithelial in vivo (42–46), preclinical studies in airway epithelia of nonhuman primates revealed inefficient airway gene transfer (47). One explanation offered for this difference in transduction was that Ad-mediated transduction of different cell types in vivo occurred with different efficiencies (48). Grubb et al., using a model of mechanical injury, demonstrated that luminal application of an Ad-*lacZ* vector efficiently transduced basal cells, the predominant cell type at the site of mechanical injury in human and mouse tracheal explants, whereas lumen facing columnar cells in uninjured areas were resistant to gene transfer (48). This observation has been confirmed in model systems of well-differentiated rat and human airway epithelia and extended to human intrapulmonary (bronchial) airways (49). Parallel experiments in excised human airway specimens have demonstrated preferential transduction of undifferentiated regenerating or wound repairing cells by Ad vectors, but not well-differentiated pseudostratified columnar epithelia (50).

More recent studies have explored the reason for the inefficiency of Ad gene transfer to well-differentiated epithelial cells following luminal application. An early observation was that $\alpha_v\beta_{3/5}$ integrins, which were generally believed to mediate uptake of Ad vectors (51) after initial binding to a high-affinity receptor, were not expressed on the apical surface of well-differentiated columnar cells, potentially limiting cellular entry and hence efficient gene transfer (52). In a subsequent series of studies using radio and fluorescent labeled Ad vectors, decreased binding to the target cell surface and a low rate of vector internalization were demonstrated as the barriers to efficient gene transfer in well-differentiated columnar airway epithelial cells (53,54). Zabner et al. demonstrated that the apical membrane of well-differentiated airway cells lacked functional high-affinity fiber receptors necessary for binding of Ad vectors and subsequent efficient transduction (53). Furthermore, application of exogenous penton base protein and/or RGD peptides failed to inhibit transduction, suggesting that interactions of penton base with $\alpha_v\beta_{3/5}$ integrins were not essential for transduction. Pickles et al. used immunohistochemical techniques and confocal microscopy to demonstrate that decreased binding and markedly decreased uptake of labeled Ad vectors out of proportion to the reduction in Ad binding as compared to poorly differentiated cells was responsible for inefficient Ad gene transfer across the apical membrane of well-differentiated cells (54). Decreased Ad vector binding resulted from lack of expression of the high-affinity coxsackie-adenoviral receptor (CAR) on the apical membrane of well-differentiated airway epithelial cells (54). Instead, CAR was localized to the basolateral membrane of these cells. Functional studies demonstrating preferential transduction of well-differentiated airway epithelia by application of vector to the basolateral membrane as compared to the apical membrane confirmed the immunohistochemical localization of CAR in well-differentiated airway epithelia (54). These investigators also demonstrated that $\alpha_v\beta_{3/5}$ integrins were expressed at low levels in the apical membrane of well-differentiated airway cells, which correlated with low levels of Ad-mediated transduction in well-differentiated airways. Thus, a low level of integrin expression appears to correlate with low levels of Ad-mediated transduction in well-differentiated airways. Studies with RGD peptides, however, suggested that integrin expression may not be crucial for gene transfer (53,54). Some reports have suggested that the resistance of the epithelium to Ad-mediated gene transfer may be partially overcome by increasing the duration of Ad vector incubation with well-differentiated epithelia, presumably by nonspecific mechanisms (55,56). However, direct measurements of nonspecific (fluid-phase) endocytosis using radiolabeled markers detected a markedly reduced rate of endocytic uptake in well-differentiated airway epithelia as compared to poorly differentiated airway epithelia (54). Thus, minimal enhancement of gene transfer would be generated by increases in nonspecific binding of Ad vectors to well-differentiated airway epithelia.

The aforementioned studies confirm that vector-specific barriers to Ad-mediated gene transfer are present in the apical membrane of well-differentiated airways, including lack of receptors and integrins leading to decreased uptake and decreased entry of gene-transfer vectors. Strategies to improve vector access with luminal application must address these considerations.

2. AAV Vectors

Evidence is evolving that transduction of well-differentiated airway epithelia by luminal application of AAV vectors may also be inefficient. Summerford et al. have identified a membrane-associated heparan sulfate proteoglycan as a receptor for adeno-associated virus serotype 2 (AAV-2), the most common serotype used in AAV vectors (57). Immunohistochemical studies using anti-heparan sulfate proteoglycans monoclonal antibodies have localized the receptor to the basal surface, but not the apical membrane of well-differentiated airway epithelial cultures (41). This receptor localization correlates with preferential transduction of these cells when vector is applied to the basolateral membrane relative to the apical membrane. In this particular study, binding and uptake of radiolabeled AAV vector was also reduced on the apical membrane relative to the basal membrane. A postentry barrier to transduction identified in undifferentiated primary cells is the persistence of AAV genomes as single-stranded episomes, which are inefficiently converted to double-stranded DNA, a requirement for transgene expression (58–62). Similar observations have been made in well-differentiated airway epithelia in bronchial xenografts (59). Fortunately, the latter limitation may be overcome by DNA-damaging agents, topoisomerase inhibitors, and Ad early gene products (62–64). Thus, barriers to AAV transduction include decreased binding and uptake of vector due to decreased receptor expression on the apical membrane and inefficient single strand–to–double strand conversion of AAV genomes.

3. Cationic Liposomes

Although efficient cationic liposome-mediated gene transfer has been reported in vitro in a variety of cell types (65–69), several undifferentiated cell lines or cell types are resistant to transfection by cationic liposomes (70). In these nontransfectable undifferentiated cells, nuclear entry has been identified as the rate-limiting factor for efficient liposome-mediated gene transfer (70). In contrast, gene transfer to well-differentiated airway epithelial cells is limited by failure of DNA-liposome complexes to enter the cell (71). Matsui et al. used rat and human airway cells grown as islands on permeable collagen substrates in which poorly differentiated cells form on the edges of the islands and polarized (well-differentiated) cells form in the central portions to investigate the relative efficiency of liposome-mediated gene transfer (71). Using fluorescent probes, physiological blockers, and confocal microscopy, Matsui et al. demonstrated loss of phagocytic entry mechanisms, decreased cell surface binding, and decreased uptake in differentiated airway epithelial cells (central cells) as compared to poorly differentiated cells (edge cells) as the reason for inefficient transduction. In a subsequent study, Fasbender and colleagues confirmed the observations of Matsui by demonstrating decreased amounts of cell-associated lipoplexes in differentiated airway epithelia as compared to poorly differentiated epithelia (72). These investigators also documented enhanced gene transfer in proliferating cells relative to quiescent cells by lipoplexes, raising the possibility of enhanced nuclear transport of DNA during mitosis due to breakdown of the nuclear envelope. The choice of lipid used in these two studies did not affect the low efficiency of gene transfer to differentiated epithelia. Thus, barriers to efficient transduction of well-differentiated airway cells by lipoplexes include decreased binding and uptake of lipoplexes and poor nuclear translocation of DNA.

4. Retroviral Vectors

Retroviral vectors have not been used in clinical gene-transfer safety and efficacy studies in cystic fibrosis patients. However, they remain attractive for CF and other genetic diseases due to their potential for long-term expression as a result of integration into the host cell genome. The lack of cell proliferation in well-differentiated airway epithelia in vivo (73) and low titers have served as major barriers to the use of retroviral vectors derived from Moloney murine leukemia virus (MuLV) for in vivo airway gene transfer. The development of lentiviral vectors derived from human immunodeficiency virus (HIV) (74) and equine infectious anemia virus (EIAV) (75), which can transduce nondividing airway cells, may soon overcome the requirement for cell proliferation (76). Advances in retroviral technology including production techniques and pseudotyping of vectors to permit concentration of vector stocks may also soon overcome the limitations of titer (77,78).

However, other barriers to efficient transduction of well-differentiated airway cells by retroviruses clearly exist. Wang et al. have demonstrated efficient transduction of polarized well-differentiated airway cells stimulated to proliferate with keratinocyte growth factor (KGF) when amphotropic enveloped MuLV vectors were applied to basolateral surface as compared to minimal to no gene transfer when vector was applied to the apical surface (79). These data are consistent with localization of the amphotropic receptor, RAM-1, to the basolateral surface of cultured well-differentiated airway cells. Western blot data from this study suggested that receptor levels were extremely low in the absence of KGF (79).

Similar finding may occur with other enveloped retroviral vectors. Wild-type vesicular stomatitis virus (VSV) has been shown to preferentially infect polarized MDCK cells, a model for polarized airway epithelia, across the basolateral membrane (80). Since the envelope glycoprotein of vesicular stomatitis virus has been used to pseudotype MuLV and lentiviral vectors derived form HIV and EIAV, VSV-G pseudotyped retroviral and lentiviral vectors would also be expected to preferentially transduce polarized MDCK cells from the basolateral surface. Preliminary studies of transduction have confirmed this notion in MDCK cells and in well-differentiated airway cells (81,82).

In summary, a variety of barriers to efficient transduction of airways in vivo by luminal application of vector exist (see Table 5). Decreased binding and uptake of vector due to lack of apical membrane receptors and internalization pathways appears to be a common barrier to all vectors. Other barriers such as second-strand synthesis and nuclear entry are more vector specific. Thus strategies that permit better apical membrane entry or that allow access of vector to the basolateral surface are likely to be generally useful.

IV. STRATEGIES TO OVERCOME APICAL MEMBRANE BARRIERS TO EFFICIENT TRANSDUCTION

Since the apical membrane of well-differentiated cells is a major barrier to efficient transduction by all the current gene transfer vectors, strategies to overcome apical membrane barriers are crucial. Although intravenous approaches have been considered (83), the multiple barriers that must be crossed, e.g., endothelium, endothelial basement membrane, interstitium, and epithelial basement membrane, have made luminal delivery of vectors attractive. Two strategies for improving gene-transfer efficiency using luminal application of vector have been proposed. One strategy focuses on modification of the host by increasing the paracellular permeability of airway epithelia to allow access of vector to the receptors on the basolateral membrane of the airway cells and the other strategy modifies vectors to target receptors expressed on the apical membrane of airways in vivo that have the capacity to internalize.

A. Host Modification

A number of agents have been used in the literature to modify paracellular permeability (36,40,84,85) and are listed in Table 6. These agents can generally be grouped into those agents that have relatively nonspecific effects and those that target specific components of the intercellular junction. In vitro and in vivo studies have recently begun to appear in the literature establishing the feasibility of such approaches. Inhalation of the oxidant gas sulfur dioxide promotes denuding of the surface epithelium in a dose-dependent manner while also increasing paracellular permeability in less severely injured regions (40,86). In a recent study, Johnson and colleagues demonstrated that this oxidant model could be used to stimulate epithelial cell proliferation and enable relatively efficient gene transfer to the airways of mice using a VSV-G pseudotyped retroviral vector (40). In a subsequent study, Parsons and colleagues demonstrated that low doses of the surface-active detergent or enhancer polidocanol increased airway permeability (measured by lanthanum permeation into the intercellular junctions) of polidocanol-treated murine airways, but not that of control animals without inducing frank morphological injury (36). Pretreatment of nasal airways with this surface-active agent enhanced gene transfer mediated by an Ad-*lacZ* vector and facilitated partial correction of the Cl transport defect in the nasal epithelium of CF mice following a single dose of vector. The single dose of Ad-CFTR vector used following pretreatment with the surface agent polidocanol generated the same degree of CFTR correction previously reported by Grubb in which four doses of an Ad vector were required to generate a 40–50% correction of Cl^- transport (48).

Recently, investigators have begun to target the adherens junction of the intercellular junctional complex. Wang et al. demonstrated enhanced retroviral gene transfer mediated by an amphotropic enveloped vector applied to the apical membrane of well-differentiated airway epithelia following pretreatment with the calcium chelator, EGTA, and hypotonic solutions (79). Increasing paracellular permeability using the EGTA/hypotonic solution maneuver enabled the investigators to correct the Cl^- transport defect in well-differentiated human CF airway epithelial cell cultures stimulated to proliferate with KGF when vector was applied to the luminal surface. Because the effects of EGTA and hypotonic solution are reversible, these data suggest that transient modification of the host by permeabilization of the paracellular path is a feasible approach to transduction of well-differentiated airway epithelia in vivo using luminal application of gene-transfer vectors. In parallel studies, Duan et al. reported a 7- to 10-fold increase in AAV-mediated transduction of well-differentiated primary airway cell cultures using an AAV GFP vector and transient permeabilization with EGTA/hypotonic solution (41). Thus, these studies establish the feasibility of using the transient modification of the host by permeabilization of the paracellular path to enhance airway gene transfer in vivo mediated by vectors whose receptors are located on the basolateral membrane. A key concern of using this approach is the relative safety of these reagents in vivo. Such studies have not been performed to date.

Table 6 Modulators of Paracellular Permeability

Nonspecific	Specific
Oxidant gases	Calcium chelators
Surfactant enhancers	Cytoskeletal agents
Bile acid conjugates	Tyrosine phosphatase inhibitors
	Protein kinase inhibitors
	Small peptides
	Antisense oligonucleotides
	Toxins

B. Vector Modification

An alternative strategy is to modify the vector. This strategy focuses on targeting the vector to receptors that are specifically expressed on the apical membrane of well-differentiated human airway epithelial cells. The concept of targeting gene-transfer vectors to alternative (non–wild-type) receptors is well established in the literature for adenoviral, retroviral, and nonviral vectors (87–99). Three general strategies have been used for Ad vectors (Fig. 1): (1) genetic engineering of peptide ligand sequences or single chain antibody fragments (scFv) into the fiber knob domain of Ad (89,91); (2) the use of scFv-fusion proteins with specificities for an Ad epitope while bearing a ligand-binding domain for a specific cell surface receptor—the adenobody approach (88); and (3) the use of bispecific antibodies composed of two antibodies—one directed against the Ad vector and the other against the specific cell surface receptor—that have been crosslinked (90). Similar strategies have been employed with retroviral vectors with the creation of chimeric envelopes bearing a ligand or single chain antibody specific for a cell surface receptor in the N-terminal domain of envelope protein (93–96) or, as has recently been reported, fused directly to transmembrane domain of envelope with the use of a spacer (97). Incorporation of ligand molecules into the lipid bilayers of

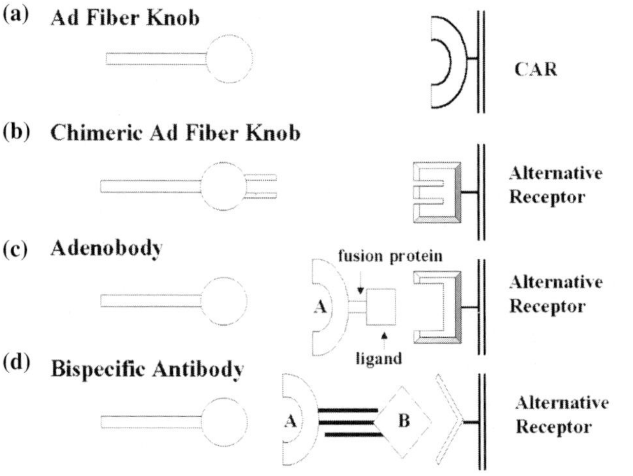

Figure 1 Strategies for retargeting of Ad vectors to alternative receptors. Depicted is a schematic representation of the binding domain (Ad fiber knob) with modifications to permit binding to alternative receptors. (a) The wild-type Ad2/5 fiber knob–binding domain and its natural receptor, the coxsackie-adenoviral receptor (CAR). (b) A genetically engineered chimeric Ad fiber knob domain, which can now bind to an alternative receptor. (c) An adenobody in which antibody fragment A binds to the adenovirus while a ligand connected to the antibody via a fusion protein targets the adenovirus to an alternative receptor on the cell membrane. (d) A bispecific antibody in which antibody A, which binds to the ad fiber knob domain, is fused to antibody B, which targets the adenoviral-antibody complex to an alternative receptor.

liposomes is well described, and biotinylation of ligands for use with streptavidin-labeled DNA polymers has also been reported (98,99).

While each of these methods has been successful at increasing binding, successful vector-specific transduction has been more difficult. Genetic incorporation of ligands is limited by the size of the peptide sequence and the ability to incorporate the chimeras into viral particles, while bispecific antibodies and adenobodies must fold properly to bind specifically and enter with the target receptor (94,95). Furthermore, a membrane or endosomolytic fusion event must occur for the vector to gain access to the cytoplasm and, henceforth, the nucleus. Nevertheless, the aforementioned approaches have been successfully used in vitro to target a variety of receptors including α_v integrins (89), the epidermal growth factor receptor (88), stem cell factor receptor (96,98), and T-cell receptors such as CD3 (90).

Since most growth receptors are expressed on the basolateral membrane of well-differentiated cells, major concerns are which receptors are expressed on the apical membrane and whether the levels of expression are sufficient to promote successful gene transfer. Seven transmembrane receptors, a class of receptors that normally mediates acute airway epithelial cell responses to the luminal environment, have been proposed as an attractive target on the apical membrane. A member of the purinergic class of seven transmembrane receptors, $P2Y_2$-R, is expressed on the apical membrane of the airways (100,101). This receptor internalizes extracellular ATP and UTP into coated pits in response to agonist stimulation. Targeting this receptor with an Ad-ligand (UTP) complex would allow apical entry into the endosomal compartment via $P2Y_2$-R while the penton base of Ad should promote endosomolysis (endosomal escape) and subsequent nuclear transport and expression. Preliminary studies in nonpolarized cells have documented that bispecific monoclonal antibody Ad vector complexes directed toward epitope-tagged external domains of $P2Y_2$-R can produce efficient gene transfer via this pathway (102). Furthermore, transduction can be achieved via epitope-tagged $P2Y_2$-R when it is expressed in the apical membrane of polarized cells (102). Targeted transduction of wild-type $P2Y_2$-R–expressing cell lines mediated by vector conjugates composed of Ad complexed to chemically modified ligands, such as biotin-UTP, has also been demonstrated in preliminary studies (103). The experience with targeting or modification of the vector to date suggests that such a strategy will be applicable to a variety of vectors, including adenoviral, AAV, retroviral, lentiviral, and nonviral vectors. Thus, it may be possible to overcome the lack of naturally occurring apical membrane receptors for efficient airway gene transfer by current vector systems and subsequent inefficient gene transfer by retargeting vectors to seven transmembrane receptors known to be expressed in airways.

V. SUMMARY

Data from published clinical gene-transfer safety and efficacy trials have suggested that the efficiency and efficacy of gene transfer is too low to offer a clinical benefit. Extensive laboratory investigation has elucidated a variety of barriers that limit gene transfer to airway epithelia. Of these, the major barrier has been localized to the apical membrane where minimal binding and entry have been documented for all current gene-transfer vectors. Strategies to modify the host and to modify the vector offer hope for overcoming these barriers. Hopefully, the lessons we have learned from our investigation of barriers will help us to further refine the strategies outlined to make CF gene therapy a clinical reality.

ACKNOWLEDGMENTS

The authors thank Ms. Elizabeth Godwin for clerical assistance in the preparation of this manuscript. The authors also thank Ms. Miriam Kelly and Ms. Hong Ni for their assistance with the preparation of the figure and tables in this manuscript.

REFERENCES

1. Drumm ML, Pope HA, Cliff WH, Rommens JM, Marvin SA, et al. Correction of the cystic fibrosis defect in vitro by retrovirus-mediated gene transfer. Cell 1990; 62: 1227–1223.
2. Rich DP, Anderson MP, Gregory RJ, Cheng SH, Paul S, et al. Expression of the cystic fibrosis transmembrane conductance regulator corrects defective chloride channel regulation in cystic fibrosis airway epithelial cells. Nature 1990; 347:358–363.
3. Olsen JC, Johnson LG, Stutts MJ, Sarkadi B, Yankaskas JR, Swanstrom R, Boucher RC. Correction of the apical membrane chloride permeability defect in polarized cystic fibrosis airway epithelia following retroviral-mediated gene transfer. Hum Gene Ther 1992; 3:253–266.
4. Zabner J, Couture LA, Smith AE, Welsh MJ. Correction of cAMP-stimulated fluid secretion in cystic fibrosis airway epithelia: efficiency of Ad-mediated gene transfer in vitro. Hum Gene Ther 1994; 5:585–593.
5. Egan M, Flotte T, Afione S, Solow R, Zeitlin PL, Carater BJ, Guggino WB. Defective regulation of outwardly rectifying $C1^-$ channels by protein kinase A corrected by the insertion of CFTR. Nature 1992; 358:581–584.
6. Lee ER, Marshall J, Siegel CS, Jiang C, Yew NS, et al. Detailed analysis of structures and formulations of cationic lipids for efficient gene transfer to the lung. Hum Gene Ther 1996; 7:1701–1717.
7. Brasfield D, Hicks G, Soong SJ, Peters J, Tiller RE. Evaluation of a scoring system of the chest radiograph in cystic fibrosis: a collaborative study. Am J Roentgen 1980; 134: 1195–1198.
8. Tepper RS, Montgomery GL, Ackerman V, Eigen H. Longitudinal evaluation of pulmonary function in infants and very young children with cystic fibrosis. Pediatr Pulmonol 1993; 16:96–100.
9. Curiel DT, Garver Jr. RI. Adenoviral vectors for gene therapy of inherited and acquired disorders of the lung. In: Brigham K, ed. Lung Biology in Health and Disease: Gene Therapy for Diseases of the Lung. New York: Marcel Dekker, 1997:29–52.
10. Chiocca S, Cotten M. Cellular responses to adenovirus entry. In: Brigham K, ed. Lung Biology in Health and Disease: Gene Therapy for Diseases of the Lung. New York: Marcel Dekker, 1997:83–97.
11. Zeitlin PL. Adeno-associated virus-based delivery systems. In: Brigham K, ed. Lung Biology in Health and Disease: Gene Therapy for Diseases of the Lung. New York: Marcel Dekker, 1997:53–81.
12. Rabinowitz JE, Samulski J. Adeno-associated virus expression systems for gene transfer. Curr Opin Biotechnol 1998; 9:470–475.
13. Gao X. Cationic lipid-based gene delivery: an update. In: Brigham K, ed. Lung Biology in Health and Disease: Gene Therapy for Diseases of the Lung. New York: Marcel Dekker, 1997:99–112.
14. Stecenko AA. Liposome/viral hybrid gene delivery systems. In: Brigham K, ed. Lung Biology in Health and Disease: Gene Therapy for Diseases of the Lung. New York: Marcel Dekker, 1997:113–131.
15. Zabner J, Couture LA, Gregory RJ, Graham SM, Smith AE, Welsh MJ. Ad-mediated gene transfer transiently corrects the chloride transport defect in nasal epithelia of patients with cystic fibrosis. Cell 1993; 75:207–216.
16. Crystal RG, McElvaney NG, Rosenfeld MA, Chu C-S, Mastrangeli A, Hay JG, Brody SL, Jaffe HA, Eissa NT, Danel C. Administration of an adenovirus containing the human CFTR cDNA to the respiratory tract of individuals with cystic fibrosis. Nat Genet 1994; 8:42–51.
17. Hay JG, McElvaney NG, Herena J, Crystal RG. Modification of nasal epithelial potential differences of individuals with cystic fibrosis consequent to local administration of a normal CFTR cDNA adenovirus gene transfer vector. Hum Gene Ther 1995; 6:1487–1496.
18. Knowles MR, Hohneker K, Zhou Z-Q, Olsen JC, Noah TL, et al. A controlled study of adenoviral vector mediated gene transfer in the nasal epithelium of patients with cystic fibrosis. N Engl J Med 1995; 333:823–831.
19. Bellon G, Michel-Calemard L, Thouvenot D, Jagneaux V, Poitevin F, et al. Aerosol administration of a recombinant adenovirus expressing CFTR to cystic fibrosis patients: a phase I clinical trial. Hum Gene Ther 1997; 8:15–25.
20. Zabner J, Ramsey BW, Meeker DP, et al. Repeat administration of an adenovirus vector encoding cystic fibrosis transmembrane conductance regulator to the nasal epithelium of patients with cystic fibrosis. J Clin Invest 1996; 97:1504–1511.
21. Knowles MR, Paradiso AM, Boucher RC. In vivo nasal potential difference: techniques and protocols for assessing efficacy of gene transfer in cystic fibrosis. Hum Gene Ther 1995; 6:445–457.
22. Piedimonte G, Pickles RJ, Lehmann JR, McCarty D, Costa DL, Boucher RC. Replication-deficient adenoviral vector for gene transfer potentiates airway neurogenic inflammation. Am J Respir Cell Mol Biol 1997; 16:250–258.
23. Wagner JA, Reynolds T, Moran ML, Moss RB, Wine JJ, Flotte TR, Gardner P. Efficient and persistent gene transfer of AAV-CFTR in maxillary sinus. Lancet 1998; 351: 1702–1703.
24. Caplen NJ, Alton EWFW, Middleton PG, Dorin JR, Stevenson BJ, et al. Liposome-mediated CFTR gene transfer to the nasal epithelium of patients with cystic fibrosis. Nat Med 1995; 1:39–46.
25. Middleton PG, Caplen NJ, Gao X, Huang L, Gaya H, Geddes DM, Alton EWFW. Nasal application of the cationic liposome DC-Chol:DOPE does not alter ion transport, lung function or bacterial growth. Eur Respir J 1994; 7: 442–445.

26. Gill DR, Southern KW, Mofford KA, Seddon T, Huang L, et al. A placebo-controlled study of liposome-mediated gene transfer to the nasal epithelium of patients with cystic fibrosis. Gene Ther 1997; 4:199–207.
27. Porteous DJ, Dorin JR, McLachlan G, Davidson-Smith H, Davidson H, Stevenson BJ, et al. Evidence for safety and efficacy of DOTAP cationic liposome mediated CFTR gene transfer to the nasal epithelium of patients with cystic fibrosis. Gene Ther 1997; 4:210–218.
28. Zabner J, Cheng SH, Meeker D, Launspach J, Balfour R, Perricone MA, Morris JE, Marshall J, Fasbender A, Smith AE, Welsh MJ. Comparison of DNA-lipid complexes and DNA alone for gene transfer to cystic fibrosis airway epithelia in vivo. J Clin Invest 1997; 100:1529–1537.
29. Davis PB. Clinical pathophysiology and manifestations of lung disease. In: Yankaskas, JR, Knowles MR, eds. Cystic Fibrosis in Adults. Philadelphia: Lippincott-Raven, 1999: 45–67.
30. Bonfil TL. Inflammatory cytokines in cystic fibrosis lungs. Am J Respir Crit Care Med 1995; 152:2111–21118.
31. Khan TZ, Wagener JS, Bost T, Martinez J, Accurso FJ, Riches DW. Early pulmonary inflammation in infants with cystic fibrosis. Am J Respir Crit Care Med 1995; 151(4): 1075–1082.
32. Kirchner KK, Wagener JS, Copenhaver SC, Accurso FJ. Increased DNA levels in bronchoalveolar lavage fluid obtained from infants with cystic fibrosis. Am J Respir Crit Care Med 1996; 154:1426–1429.
33. Noah TL, Black HR, Cheng PW, Wood RE, Leigh MW. Nasal and bronchoalveolar lavage fluid cytokines in early cystic fibrosis. J Infect Dis 1997; 175:638–647.
34. Stern M, Caplen NJ, Browning JE, Griesenbach U, Sorgi F, Huang L, Gruenert DC. The effect of mucolytic agents on gene transfer across a CF sputum barrier in vitro. Gene Ther 1998; 5:91–98.
35. Van Heeckeren A, Ferkol T, Tosi M. Effects of bronchopulmonary inflammation induced by pseudomonas aeruginosa on adenovirus-mediated gene transfer to airway epithelial cells in mice. Gene Ther 1998; 5:345–351.
36. Parsons DW, Grubb B, Johnson LG, Boucher RC. Enhancement of in vivo adenoviral gene transfer via modification of host barrier properties with a surface active agent. Hum Gene Ther 1998; 9:2661–2672.
37. Worgall S, Leopold PL, Wolfe G, Ferris B, Van Roijen N, Crystal RG. Role of alveolar macrophages in rapid elimination of adenovirus vectors administered to the epithelial surface of the respiratory tract. Hum Gene Ther 1997; 8:1675–1684.
38. McCray Jr PB, Wang G, Kline JN, Zabner J, Chada S, Jolly DJ, Chang SMW, Davidson BL. Alveolar macrophages inhibit retrovirus-mediated gene transfer to airway epithelia. Hum Gene Ther 1997; 8:1087–1093.
39. Batra RJ, Olsen JC, Hoganson DK, Caterson B, Boucher RC. Retroviral gene transfer is inhibited by chondroitin sulfate proteoglycans/glycosaminoglycans in malignant pleural effusions. J Biol Chem 1997; 272:11736–11743.
40. Johnson LG, Mewshaw JP, Ni H, Friedmann T, Boucher RC, Olsen JC. Effect of host modification and age on airway epithelial gene transfer mediated by a murine leukemia virus-derived vector. J Virol 1998; 72:8861–8872.
41. Duan D-S, Yue Y-P, Yan Z, McCray Jr PB, Engelhardt JF. Polarity influences the efficiency of recombinant adeno-associated virus infection in differentiated airway epithelia. Hum Gene Ther 1998; 9:2761–2776.
42. Engelhardt JF, Yang Y, Stratford-Perricaudet LD, Allen ED, Kozarsky K, Perricaudet M, Yankaskas JR, Wilson JM. Direct gene transfer of human CFTR into human bronchial epithelia of xenografts with El-deleted adenoviruses. Nat Genet 1993; 4:27–34.
43. Rich DP, Couture LA, Cardoza LM, Guiggio VM, Armentano D, Espino PC, Hehir K, Welsh MJ, Smith AE, Gregory RJ. Development and analysis of recombinant adenoviruses for gene therapy of cystic fibrosis. Hum Gene Ther 1993; 4:461–476.
44. Zabner J, Wadsworth SC, Smith AE, Welsh MJ. Adenovirus-mediated generation of cAMP-stimulated $C1^-$ transport in cystic fibrosis airway epithelia in vitro: effect of promoter and administration method. Gene Ther 1996; 3: 458–465.
45. Rosenfeld MA, Siegfried W, Yoshimura K, Yoneyama K, Fukayama M, Stier LE, Paakko PK, Gilardi P, Stratford-Perricaudet LD, Perricaudet M, Jallat S, Pavirani A, Lecocq J-P, Crystal RG. Ad-mediated transfer of a recombinant α_1-antitrypsin gene to the lung epithelium in vivo. Science 1991; 252:431–434.
46. Rosenfeld MA, Yoshimura K, Trapnell BC, Yoneyama K, Rosenthal ER, Dalemans W, Fukayama M, Bargon J, Stier LE, Stratford-Perricaudet L, Perricaudet M, Guggino WB, Pavirani A, Lecocq J-P, Crystal RG. In vivo transfer of the human cystic fibrosis transmembrane conductance regulator gene to the airway epithelium. Cell 1992; 68: 143–155.
47. Engelhardt JF, Simon RH, Yang Y, Zepeda M, Pendleton SW, Doranz B, Grossman M, Wilson JM. Ad-mediated transfer of the CFTR gene to lung of non-human primates: biological efficacy study. Hum Gene Ther 1993; 4: 759–769.
48. Grubb BR, Pickles RJ, Ye H, Yankaskas JR, Vick RN, Engelhardt JF, Wilson JM, Johnson LG, Boucher RC. Inefficient gene transfer by adenovirus vector to cystic fibrosis airway epithelia of mice and humans. Nature 1994; 371: 802–806.
49. Pickles RJ, Barker PM, Ye H, Boucher RC. Efficient Ad-mediated gene transfer to basal but not columnar cells of cartilaginous airway epithelia. Hum Gene Ther 1996; 7: 921–931.
50. Dupuit F, Zahm JH-M, Pierrot D, Brezillon S, Bonnet N, Imler J-L, Pavirani A, Puchelle E. Regenerating cells in human airway surface epithelium represent preferential targets for recombinant adenovirus. Hum Gene Ther 1995; 6:1185–1193.
51. Wickham TJ, Mathias P, Cheresh DA, Nemerow GR. Integrins $\alpha_v\beta_3$ and $\alpha_v\beta_5$ promote adenovirus internalization but not virus attachment. Cell 1993; 73:309–319.

52. Goldman MJ, Wilson JM. Expression of $\alpha_v\beta_5$ integrin is necessary for efficient Ad-mediated gene transfer in the human airway. J Virol 1995; 69:5951–5958.
53. Zabner J, Freimuth P, Puga A, Fabrega A, Welsh MJ. Lack of high affinity fiber receptor activity explains the resistance of ciliated airway epithelia to adenovirus infection. J Clin Invest 1997; 100:1144–1149.
54. Pickles RJ, McCarty D, Matsui H, Hart PJ, Randell SH, Boucher RC. Limited entry of adenovirus vectors into well-differentiated airway epithelium is responsible for inefficient gene transfer. J Virol 1998; 72:6014–6023.
55. Zabner J, Zeiher BG, Friedman E, Welsh MJ. Adenovirus-mediated gene transfer to ciliated airway epithelia requires prolonged incubation time. J Virol 1996; 70:6994.
56. Jiang C, Akita GY, Colledge WH, Ratcliff RA, Evans MJ, Hehir KM, St. George JA, Wadsworth SC, Cheng SH. Increased contact time improves adenovirus-mediated CFTR gene transfer to nasal epithelium of CF mice. Hum Gene Ther 1997; 8:671–680.
57. Summerford C, Samulski RJ. Membrane-associated heparan sulfate proteoglycan is a receptor for adeno-associated virus type 2 virions. J Virol 1998; 72:1438–1445.
58. Halbert CL, Alexander IE, Wolgamot GM, Miller AD. Adeno-associated virus vectors transduce primary cells much less efficiently than immortalized cells. J Virol 1995; 69:1473–1479.
59. Goldman MJ, Weitzman MD, Fisher KJ, et al. Recombinant adeno-associated virus enters but does not transduce lung epithelium in a human bronchial xenograft model. Ped Pulmonol 1996; 13(suppl):256.
60. Ferrari FK, Samulski T, Shenk T, Samulski RJ. Second-strand synthesis is a rate-limiting step for efficient transduction by recombinant adeno-associated virus vectors. Virol 1996; 70:3227–3234.
61. Fisher KJ, Gao GP, Weitzman MD, DeMatteo R, Burda JF, Wilson JM. Transduction with recombinant adeno-associated virus for gene therapy is limited by leading-strand synthesis. J Virol 1996; 70:520–532.
62. Teramoto S, Bartlett JS, McCarty D, Xiao X, Samulski RJ, Boucher RC. Factors influencing adeno-associated virus-mediated gene transfer to human cystic fibrosis airway epithelial cells: comparison to adenovirus vectors. J Virol 1998; 72:8904–8912.
63. Alexander IE, Russell DW, Miller AD. DNA-damaging agents greatly increase the transduction of nondividing cells by adenoassociated virus vectors. J Virol 1994; 68: 8282–8287.
64. Russell DW, Alexander IE, Miller AD. DNA synthesis and topoisomerase inhibitors increase transduction by adeno-associated virus vectors. Proc Natl Acad Sci USA 1995; 92:5719–5723.
65. Zhou X, Huang L. DNA transfection mediated by cationic liposomes containing lipopolylysine: characterization and mechanism of action. Biochim Biophys Acta 1994; 1189: 195–203.
66. Debs R, Pian M, Gaensler K, Clements J, Friend DS, Dobbs L. Prolonged transgene expression in rodent lung cells. Am J Respir Cell Mol Biol 1992; 7:406–413.
67. Jarnagin WR, Debs RJ, Wang S-S, Bissell DM. Cationic lipid-mediated transfection of liver cells in primary culture. Nucleic Acids Res 1992; 20:4205–4211.
68. Felgner PL, Gadek TR, Holm M, Roman R, Chan HW, Wenz M, Northrop JP, Ringold GM, Danielsen M. Lipofection: a highly efficient, lipid-mediated DNA transfection procedure. Proc Natl Acad Sci 1987; 84:7413–7417.
69. Lu L, Zeitlin PL, Guggino WB, Craig RW. Gene transfer by lipofection in rabbit and human secretory epithelial cells. Pflugers Arch 1989; 415:198–203.
70. Zabner J, Fasbender AJ, Moninger T, Poellinger KA, Welsh MJ. Cellular and molecular barriers to gene transfer by a cationic lipid. J Biol Chem 1995; 270:18997–19007.
71. Matsui H, Johnson LG, Randell SH, Boucher RC. Loss of binding and entry of liposome-DNA complexes decreases transfection efficiency in differentiated rat tracheal epithelial cells. J Biol Chem 1997; 272:1117–1126.
72. Fasbender A, Zabner J, Zeiher BG, Welsh MJ. A low rate of cell proliferation and reduced DNA uptake limit cationic lipid-mediated gene transfer to primary cultures of ciliated human airway epithelia. Gene Ther 1997; 4:1173–1180.
73. Leigh MW, Kylander JE, Yankaskas JR, Boucher RC. Cell proliferation in bronchial epithelium and submucosal glands of cystic fibrosis patients. Am J Respir Cell Mol Biol 1995; 12:605–612.
74. Naldini L, Blomer U, Gallay P, Ory D, Mulligan R, Gage FH, Verma IM, Trono D. In vivo gene delivery and stable transduction of nondividing cells by a lentiviral vector. Science 1996; 272:263–267.
75. Olsen JC. Gene transfer vectors derived from equine infectious anemia virus. Gene Ther 1998; 5:1481–1487.
76. Miller DG, Adam MA, Miller AD. Gene transfer by retrovirus vectors occurs only in cells that are actively replicating at the time of infection. Mol Cell Biol 1990; 10:4329.
77. Burns JC, Friedmann T, Driever W, Burrascano M, Yee J-K. Vesicular stomatitis virus G glycoprotein pseudotyped retroviral vectors: concentration to very high titer and efficient gene transfer into mammalian and nonmammalian cells. Proc Natl Acad Sci USA 1993; 90:8033–8037.
78. Kitten O, Cosset FL, Ferry N. Highly efficient retrovirus-mediated gene transfer into rat hepatocytes in vivo. Hum Gene Ther 1997; 8:1491–1494.
79. Wang G, Davidson BL, Melchert P, Slepushkin VA, Van Es HHG, Bodner M, Jolly DJ, McCray Jr. PB. Influence of cell polarity on retrovirus-mediated gene transfer to differentiated human airway epithelia. J Virol 1998; 72: 9818–9826.
80. Fuller S, Von Bonsdorff CH, Simons K. Vesicular stomatitis virus infects and matures only through the basolateral surface of the polarized epithelial cell line, MDCK. Cell 1984; 38:65–77.
81. Johnson LG, Mewshaw JP, Boucher RC, Olsen JC. In vivo airway gene transfer using pseudotyped retroviral vectors. Am J Respir Crit Care Med 1998; 157:A480.
82. Olsen JC, Fu J, Patel M. Lentiviral vector-mediated gene transfer to polarized epithelia. Pediatr Pulmonol 1998; 17(suppl):268.

83. Ferkol T, Perales JC, Eckman E, Kaetzel CS, Hanson RW, Davis PB. Gene transfer into the airway epithelium of animals by targeting the polymeric immunoglobulin receptor. J Clin Invest 1995; 95:493–502.
84. Lutz KL, Siahaan TJ. Molecular structure of the apical junction complex and its contribution to the paracellular barrier. Pharmaceut Sci 1997; 86:977–984.
85. Anderson JM, Van Itallie CM. Tight junctions and the molecular basis for regulation of paracellular permeability. Am J Physiol 1995; 269:G467–G475.
86. Hulbert WC, Man SF, Rosychuk MK, Braybrook G, Mehta JG. The response phase—the first six hours after acute airway injury by SO_2 inhalation: an in vivo and in vitro study. Scanning Microscopy 1989; 3:369–378.
87. Douglas JT, Rogers BE, Rosenfeld ME, Michael SI, Feng M, Curiel DT. Targeted gene delivery by tropism modified adenoviral vectors. Nat Biotechnol 1996; 14:1574–1578.
88. Watkins SJ, Mesyanzhinov VV, Kurochkina LP, Hawkins RE. The adenobody approach to viral targeting: specific and enhanced adenoviral gene delivery. Gene Ther 1997; 4:1004–1012.
89. Wickham TJ, Tzeng E, Shears II LL, Roelvink PW, Li Y, Lee GM, Brough DF, Lizonova A, Kovesdi I. Increased in vitro and in vivo gene transfer by adenovirus vectors containing chimeric fiber proteins. J Virol 1997; 71: 8221–8229.
90. Wickham TJ, Lee GM, Titus JA, Sconocchia G, Bakacs T, Kovesdi L, Segal DM. Targeted adenovirus-mediated gene delivery to T cells via CD3. J Virol 1997; 71: 7663–7669.
91. Dmitriev I, Krasnykh V, Miller CR, Wang M, Kashentseva E, Mikheeva G, Belousova N, Curiel DT. An adenovirus vector with genetically modified fibers demonstrates expanded tropism via utilization of a coxsackie virus and adenovirus receptor-independent cell entry mechanism. J Virol 1998; 72:9706–9713.
92. Paillard F. Commentary: cell-specific targeting with retroviral vectors. Hum Gene Ther 1998; 9:767–768.
93. Kasahara N, Dozy AM, Kan YW. Tissue-specific targeting of retroviral vectors through ligand-receptor interactions. Science 1994; 266:1373–1376.
94. Cosset FL, Morling FJ, Takeuchi Y, Weiss RA, Collins MKL, Russel SJ. Retroviral retargeting by envelopes expressing an N-terminal binding domain. J Virol 1995; 69: 6314–6322.
95. Schierle BS, Moritz D, Jeschke M, Groner B. Expression of chimeric envelope proteins in helper cell lines and integration into moloney murine leukemia virus particles. Gene Ther 1996; 3:334–342.
96. Yajima T, Kanda T, Yoshiike K, Kitamura Y. Retroviral vector targeting human cells via c-kit-stem cell factor interaction. Hum Gene Ther 1998; 9:779–788.
97. Jiang A, Chu T-HT, Nocken F, Cichutek K, Dornburg R. Cell-type specific gene transfer into human cells with retroviral vectors that display single-chain antibodies. J Virol 1998; 72:10148–10156.
98. Schwarzenberger P, Spence SE, Gooya JM, Michiel D, Curiel DT, Ruscetti FW, Keller JR. Targeted gene transfer to human hematopoietic progenitor cell lines through the c-kit receptor. Blood 1996; 87:472–478.
99. Schreier H, Moran P, Caras IW. Targeting of liposomes to cells expressing CD4 using glycosylphosphatidylinositol-anchored gp120. J Biol Chem 1994; 12:9090–9098.
100. Mason SJ, Paradiso AM, Boucher RC. Regulation of transepithelial ion transport and intracellular calcium by extracellular ATP in human normal and cystic fibrosis airway epithelium. Br J Pharmacol 1991; 103:1649–1656.
101. Hwang TH, Schwiebert EM, Guggino WB. Apical and basolateral ATP stimulates tracheal epithelial chloride secretion via multiple purinergic receptors. Am J Physiol 1996; 270:C1611–C1623.
102. Pickles RJ, Kreda S, Olsen J, Johnson L, Gerard R, Segal D, Boucher RC. High efficiency gene transfer to polarised epithelial cells by re-targeting adenoviral vectors to $P2Y_2$ purinoceptors with bi-specific antibodies. Pediatr Pulmonol 1998; 17(suppl):261.
103. Kreda SM, Pickles R, Lazarowski E, Boucher RC. $P2Y_2$ receptor agonists to produce conjugates for gene transfer. Pediatr Pulmonol 1998; 17(suppl):258.

24

Gene Transfer to the Central Nervous System

Ulrike Blömer
Medical School Hannover, Hannover, Germany

I. M. Verma and F. H. Gage
The Salk Institute for Biological Studies, La Jolla, California

I. INTRODUCTION

A. Background

Inherited and acquired neurological disease still has numerous unidentified causes, but a large number of gene defects or deletions have been identified. Transplantation and gene transfer to correct the dysfunctional gene or to apply gene products that may reduce cellular dysfunction have developed as strategies toward therapy in the future.

Restoration of neuronal pathways in the central nervous system (CNS) is a major scientific challenge, which has become obtainable following the development of powerful tools and techniques applicable to cellular and molecular aspects in neurobiology. Over the past two decades a significant scientific effort has been directed towards the evaluation of novel strategies for anatomical and functional regeneration in the CNS. One of the major breakthroughs in this area is the concept that neurotrophic and inhibitory proteins governing the processes involved in brain and spinal cord repair. Cell replacement and gene therapies have added valuable tools to overcome the intrinsic limitations in regeneration observed in the CNS.

The CNS, with its unique complex structures consisting of a variety of cell types and tracts kept in a privileged environment separated from the blood system by the blood-brain barrier (BBB), represents a barrier to gene therapy. However, this protection may also provide an immunologically privileged status for the CNS that may be useful in mitigating the immunologically mediated elimination of genetically modified or implanted cells. Since mechanisms of the CNS repair often involve specific targeting and only limited amounts of gene products are necessary, gene transfer in the CNS is potentially amenable to current gene-transfer protocols. Since the majority of neurons are terminally differentiated in the adult CNS, direct gene transfer into these cells is still limited to only a few vector systems. The delivery of transgene products or even a viral vector may also be performed by retrograde transport from peripheral organ systems. Neuronal processes, particularly axons, terminate at a significant distance from their perikarya, which are the site of their transcriptional and translational centers. Protein products can diffuse or can be transported anterogradely or retrogradely into the CNS and even viral vectors can be taken up by either endocytosis, receptor-mediated transport, or membrane-to-membrane fusion. On the other hand, CNS cells build contacts with each other, providing a conduit for the transfer of the introduced transgenes or their products. Neuronal-glial or interneuronal contacts are routed for potential transport of transgene products.

Currently there are two main approaches for performing somatic gene therapy: the ex vivo and in vivo strategies. In the ex vivo approach, gene transfer is performed in cell culture (in vitro) and the cell is transplanted into the organism. In the in vivo approach, the gene is directly delivered within an organism for in situ gene transfer into the cells (Fig. 1). Increasing knowledge about the host and donor

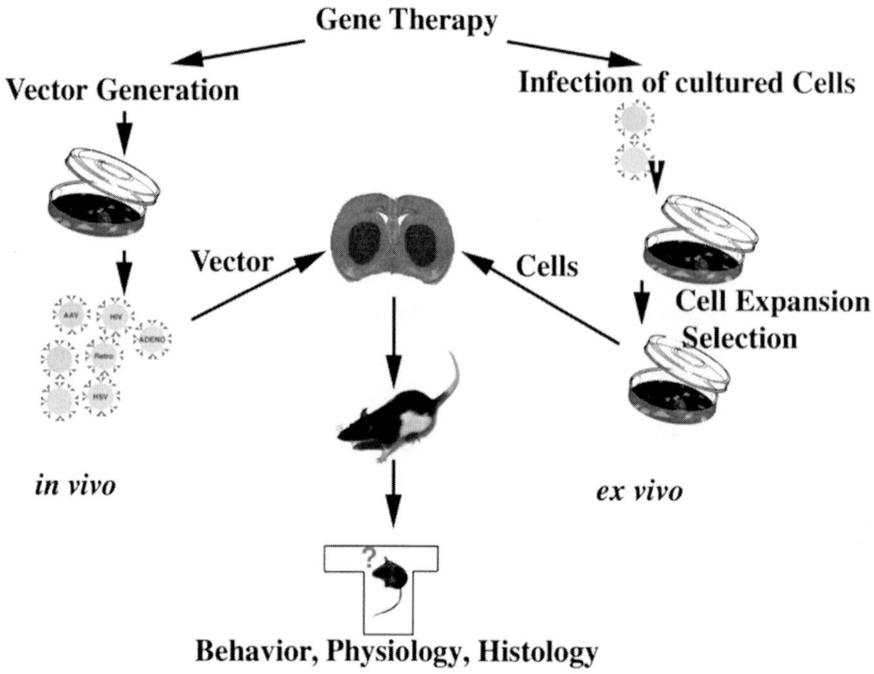

Figure 1 Different approaches to gene therapy. Ex vivo the gene transfer is performed in cell culture and cells are transplanted into the organism. In vivo the gene is directly delivered into the organism for in situ gene transfer into the cells.

cells, conditions for their maintenance in culture, and transplantation techniques has led to the realization that gene therapy applies not only to genetic diseases, but also to many acquired disorders or trauma in the central nervous system. Somatic gene transfer can be applied at different points in the disease, since there are molecules that can be used prophylactically and other molecules that can be applied after the damage has occurred in order to replace the lacking gene product. Neuronal damage caused by toxic compounds, like free radicals or excessive excitatory compounds, can be reduced by implanting cells that produce free radical scavengers or express amino acid receptors. Cells dying due to a lack of supporting neurotrophic factors can be rescued by implanted cells genetically engineered to supply trophic support. Direct gene transfer into in vivo models has been shown to genetically modify the target cell without interrupting the cell circuit. A limited number of studies have shown in several systems that viral vector–based gene transfer is able to attain stable transgene expression with biological effect (1,2).

B. History

Following Thompson's first reports a century ago (3) of transplantation of the cortex of adult cats and dogs into the neocortical cavities of other adult cats and dogs, with presumably limited survival of neuronal cells, the first successful CNS tissue transplantation was performed by E. Dunn in 1917 (4). Results from her study revealed important information about graft survival close to the ventricle in pups rather than adults. Meanwhile Cajal, supposing that everything in the CNS may die but nothing regenerates, transplanted ganglia and pieces of peripheral nerves successfully and revealed important connections between trophism and tropism and glial-neuronal interaction (5). Studies by Clark (6) and Glees (7) investigated the transplantation of developing CNS tissue into the mammalian brain and demonstrated the survival of differentiating cells. The improvement in microscopy, especially the electron microscope, and of transplantation techniques allowed for more detailed studies on graft survival and interaction between graft and host cells. The first real functional studies were performed by Knigge and Halasz, showing the endocrinological effect of transplanted pituitary tissue in different locations, restoring hypophysis function in hypophysectomized rats (8,9). In the 1970s the experimental approaches of transplantation in the parkinsonian model showed significant effects (10,11).

Recent isolation and identification of an increasing number of trophic factors has led to a broad series of studies of these factors in the CNS. The first factor identified, the nerve growth factor (12,13), has been shown to influence both differentiated and developing neurons, and the discovery of a growing number of neurotrophins with different effects has encouraged their application in a variety of in vitro and in vivo models.

Increasing knowledge of interactions demands more sophisticated methods to deliver genes, not only via transplanted cells but also especially into the cells already available in the CNS. Neurobiology has focused on methods to deliver reagents rapidly in the organism, in particular to cell populations. Evolution taught us that viruses were able to transfer genes into host cells to survive by employing either RNA or DNA as their genetic material that encodes for a limited set of virus-specific functions and infects either stable or transiently. The development of viral-based vectors as gene-transfer vehicles has proven to be possible; however, it is still limited in many ways.

II. EX VIVO GENE TRANSFER

A. Donor Cells

Many studies have explored somatic gene therapy focusing on the ex vivo approach (Fig. 1). In spite of the complexity of the majority of human neurological disorders and the relative difficulty in accessing dysfunctional areas of the brain, intracerebral grafts of fetal- and/or adult-derived cells are useful in somatic gene therapy. Cells of diverse origins survive transplantation into the brain and can replace or supplement deficient molecules. Behavioral abnormalities in animal models of CNS damage and those seen in neurological diseases can be successfully reversed using cell transplantation (4,15). Although fetal tissue grafts have been a cell-replacement source, genetically modified cells for intracerebral transplantation promise far greater benefits. For example, engineered cells can be autologous and therefore minimize the problems of cellular rejection. In addition, molecular biological methods allow the genetic modification of cells to produce a more controlled and broader range of desired factors than can be obtained with nonengineered cells. Following neuronal trauma, toxic compounds can be reduced or eliminated by cells engineered to produce free radical scavengers (16). In neurodegenerative disorders, cells that lose their vital source of trophic factors, e.g., nerve growth factor (NGF), brain-derived neurotrophic factor (BDNF), or neurotrophins (NT-3 and NT4-5), can be supported by transplantation of cells modified to produce these factors (17,18). The application of neurotransmitters and neuromodulators in models of neuronal degeneration has been found to restore neuronal function, although grafted cells are not able to mimic the normal dynamic functions of intercellular contact (19).

Engineered cells may also serve as a drug-delivery system in cancer therapy, delivering suicide genes or toxic compounds to rapidly dividing tumor cells. Preferential incorporation of drug-sensitive genes into tumor cells enables the cells to produce enzymes metabolizing drugs into toxic derivatives. These toxic derivatives result in the destruction of tumor cells following systematic administration of the appropriate drug, whereas the majority of healthy brain cells remain immune because they are quiescent (20).

In choosing a target cell, the potential for the cell to survive the gene-transfer process, the ability of transgene synthesis at biologically relevant levels, and cell survival after transplantation need to be considered. Immortalized neuronal and nonneuronal cell lines (C6, neuroblastoma, AT20) have been used for gene therapy; however, the persistence of growth leads to tumor formation and limits therapeutic applications (21,22).

1. Nonneuronal Cells

Nonneuronal primary fibroblasts have been studied extensively because they are readily available, easily maintained in cell culture for weeks, and can be genetically modified by various methods. Contact inhibition in high-density cultures leads to decreased cell division and also prevents tumor-like growth (17,23) in the CNS as well as in peripheral tissue (24). The morphology of these grafts is similar to fibroblasts normally found in the skin, and viability has been demonstrated by collagen staining and abundant fibronectin production within the graft border (25,26). Transplanted genetically engineered fibroblasts producing neurotrophic factors have been successful in various rodent models diminishing the neuronal loss following surgical and toxic lesion (27). Also, primary myoblasts have been shown to survive well in the brain after transplantation (28–30).

Astrocytes and oliogodendrocytes are very attractive cells for grafting studies, due to their intrinsic supportive role in the CNS (31). However, their use has been limited to fetal or neonatal tissue and has been slow because of insufficient growth in vitro and the related low transduction rates with retroviral vectors (32). In addition, Schwann cells have been used in vitro, producing tyrosine hydroxylase (23).

2. Chromaffin Cells

Chromaffin cells from adrenal medulla have been used as graft donor cells and revealed only poor survival, and constitutional production of catecholamines without any genetic modification was low (14,34). Survival of these cells transplanted together with peripheral nerve fragments is the result of NGF supplementation. In vitro studies demonstrated that chromaffin cells convert to sympathetic neurons when NGF is included in the medium (34,35). Cografting of NGF-producing fibroblasts with chromaffin cells has shown not only enhanced survival but also transdifferentiation (36,37).

Obtaining autologous grafts includes major surgical procedures involving patients already compromised by the primary disease. This may be the limiting factor in the transplantation of autologous materials into the CNS; however, no functional recovery was observed (38).

3. Neuronal Progenitor Cells

Immature neuronal progenitor cells isolated from the adult and fetal brain have been successfully cultured and characterized (39–43). These cells are found early in development and can survive in vitro in growth factor enriched media over many passages, expressing glial and neuronal markers (40,44). Immortalized rodent progenitor cell lines have been successfully transplanted in various regions of the brain, with subsequent migration and integration into the host system. These cells are accessible to ex vivo gene therapy because they grow fast ex vivo and allow retroviral vector modification. Also, their pluripotentiality allows them to assume different cell phenotypes in different regions of the brain, depending on the local cues (45,46). The culturing and manipulation of neuronal cells, integration into the host system without uncontrolled proliferation and potential to differentiate into mature neurons make these cells a promising tool for ex vivo gene therapy (47). However, in order to achieve an unlimited supply of well-characterized uniform cells, the biological properties of immortalized progenitors and stem-like cells need further research.

4. Immortalized and Regulatable Neuronal Cells

Oncogenes (e.g., v-myc, r-ras) have been used for the immortalization of slow-dividing cells. These genes maintain cells in a highly mitotic, undifferentiated state and expression for as long as 22 months in vivo (39). Transplantation of oncogene-expressing cells has revealed chromosomal damage and varied cell morphologies and survival potential (48,49). Oncogene-expressing cells can also exhibit uncontrolled growth, with resulting tumor formation (50,51).

To obtain regulatable expression of transgenes, the temperature-sensitive mutant of SV40 large T antigen (TsA58) has been used (52). SV40 regulates the expression of oncogenes at 25°C and leaves cells in an undifferentiated rapidly dividing state (53). Down regulation of oncogene expression and differentiation of these cells into neurons occurs at 37°C. However, this has been obtained only incompletely. To externally regulate transgene expression a regulatable retroviral vector in which the oncogene v-myc is driven by a tetracycline-controlled transactivator has also been used for conditional immortalization of adult progenitor cells (54). The suppression of the v-myc oncogene expression was sufficient to make proliferating cells exit from the cell cycles and induce terminal differentiation.

B. Vector Systems

Viruses can be thought of as cell parasites that require the function of the host cell in order to live and duplicate. Depending on the viral family, DNA or RNA encode a limited set of viral proteins encased in a capsid and surrounded by a lipid coat. Viral proteins embedded in the outer coat layer interact with cellular receptors. The tropism of different viruses for specific target cells is due to differences in viral protein coatings. Viruses transfer their genes into host cells and use the cell machinery for replication and generation of progeny virus.

Viral vectors are modified viruses engineered to contain a gene of interest that is typically flanked by viral sequences, encoding signals for coating, reverse transcription, and packaging. Typically viral vectors are replication defective and capable of a single round of host cell infection without viral spread. The gene transfer can be either transient, with the transgene staying episomal, or permanent, with integration of the viral genome into the host cell DNA. Adeno and herpes simplex viral vectors, for example, transiently infect cells, but the transgene is lost over time by dilution during cell division.

Wild-type retroviral and adeno-associated viral (AAV) vectors, however, are able to stably insert the viral gene and the gene of interest into the host chromosome. The stable integration of foreign genes yields permanent alteration of the genome in the transduced cell and their progeny (Fig. 2). To obtain integration into the host cell genome, simple retroviral vectors like Moloney murine leukemia virus–derived vectors require the breakdown of the nuclear membrane that occurs during cell division. Although long-lasting transduction is achieved by retroviral vectors, the major limitation lies in the exclusion of quiescent, terminally differentiated cells like neurons and liver and muscle cells. The AAV vector, although integrating into the host cell genome of dividing and nondividing cells, depends on helper viral function, either the adeno or herpes simplex virus, to be efficient in transduction. However, lentiviruses, for example, the human immunodeficiency virus (HIV), a subclass of retroviruses, allow the stable transduction of nondividing cells.

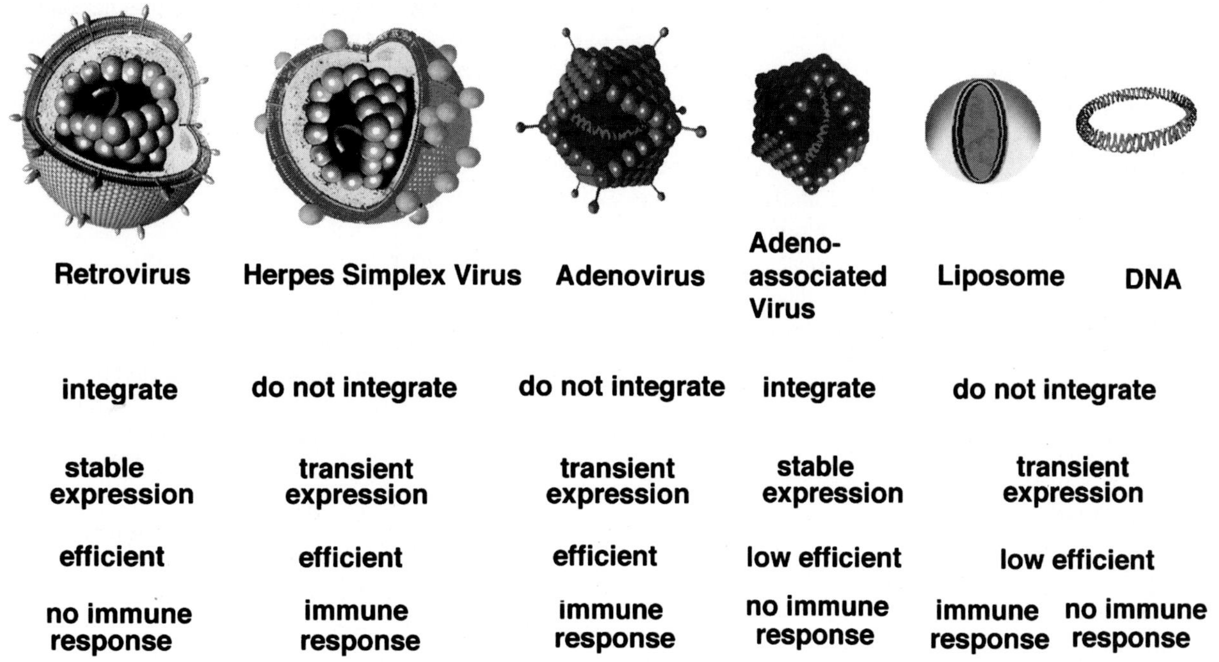

Figure 2 Viral vectors are derived from different viruses. The advantages and disadvantages are mostly depending upon integration, efficacy and immunogenicity of the parent virus.

Transgene expression efficiency and persistency of viral vectors in general depend on the promoter driving the transgene and also on the host immune response. The immune response, directly related to the amount of viral proteins made by the transduced cell, can be avoided by reducing viral vector proteins to the minimal set of coding viral sequences.

C. Functional Genes

1. Neurotrophic and Inhibitory Factors

Neurotrophins are a large family consisting of NGF, BDNF, glial cell-line–derived neurotrophic factor (GDNF), and neurotrophin-3, -4, -5, and -6 (55). Neurotrophins affect a large number of neuronal cells in developing and adult neuronal populations of the peripheral (PNS) and central nervous systems (CNS). Furthermore, neurotrophins can provide neuroprotection to neurons axotomized by traumatic injury or by neurotoxins.

GDNF was characterized as a trophic factor for midbrain dopaminergic neurons (56) and has been found to play an important role in survival and development of a broad number of neuronal and nonneuronal cells. The progressive loss of dopaminergic neurons of the substantia nigra, with resulting reduction of dopamine (DA) in the target area (striatum), causes Parkinson's disease. A large number of studies have tried to increase the DA production of the remaining dopaminergic cells by delivering GDNF to provide more dopamine in the target region.

Neurotrophins exert their activity by binding to tyrosine kinase receptors. Neurotrophin-3 (NT-3) binds primarily to trkC (57). Most dorsal root ganglions (DRG) express the mRNA for trk receptors, and trkC mRNA is expressed by 17% of the neurons that project to the muscle (58). Importantly during embryogenesis trkC is expressed by many neurons of the dorsal root ganglion but is downregulated except in a very few large neurons (59). In vivo data suggest that NT-3 is required for survival of dorsal root ganglions already at the time of formation in the chick, since the application of antibodies leads to complete elimination of neurons (60). Maturation and proliferation of DRG neurons in vitro by applications of NT-3 suggest that NT-3 may also play a role in the differentiation of precursor cells in the early sensory ganglion (61,62).

2. Antiapoptotic Factors

Traumatic axotomy, toxins, and trophic factor withdrawal are some of the death-inducing insults to neurons, in that they require active participation of the neuronal metabolism for their demise, which is reflected by metabolic changes, the induction of a stress response, and the requirement for ongoing macromolecular synthesis. During early lesions neurons maintain many of their functional properties, including the ability to respond to trophic factors with survival, until Bcl-2 and caspases become critical for the induction of apoptosis. This suggests that, in degenerative diseases or after injury in which Bcl-2 and caspases are required for effecting neuronal survival, inhibitors of these two control mechanisms should be able to stabilize degenerating neurons prior to the onset of irreversible damage. The Bcl-2 family of proteins includes apoptosis-promoting (Bax, Bak, Bcl-xS) and survival-maintaining (Bcl-2, Bcl-xL) members that function at least in part through competing homo- and heterodimer formation (63).

III. IN VIVO GENE TRANSFER

A. Herpes Simplex Virus

Because the herpes simplex virus (HSV) is a neurotropic virus, the HSV system is a useful tool to deliver foreign genes to the nervous system. Neurons and glial cells can be transduced, but HSV clearly has greater efficiency in transducing neurons (1,52). HSV is a large, 150-kb DNA virus containing approximately 70 genes, which are not all required for growth in cell culture. Many of the HSV vectors used are recombination-competent and basically concentrated units of the original plasmid, allowing a single insert of the gene of interest. In contrast defective amplicon HSV vectors have multiple copies of the gene of interest, which are packaged into HSV virions. Once an HSV vector infects the host cell, the capsid is released into the cytoplasm and transported to the nucleus, where the viral DNA enters through the nuclear pore. Progeny viral particles are produced and released by the infected cell and infect other cells, resulting in cell lysis or latency in the host cell (1,64).

HSV vector constructs have been used with viral and nonviral promoters and foreign gene inserts in mouse brain (65) and rat hippocampus (66). Transient expression peaks after inoculation and loss of expression after 2 weeks have been reported (52,67,68). The loss of transgene expression is either due to the promoter shut-off or to the host's immune response. Current brain tumor strategies utilize HSV vector mutants that are attenuated for growth in nondividing cells but replicate within growing tumor cells. This allows the virus to enter one tumor cell, make multiple copies, kill the cell, and spread to additional tumor cells. The surrounding brain tissue contains nondividing cells and therefore is unable to support the replication (69). These studies in immune-compromised animals have shown promising results, but the treatment has to be reevaluated in the context of a competent immune system. Although HSV has a broad host range and gene transfer in many types of culture cells is possible, widespread use of this transfer approach will be restricted until problems concerning the spread of the vector in vivo are solved. In addition it will be necessary to remove viral-induced cytotoxic functions, including those required for the lytic replication (70).

B. Adenovirus

Adenoviruses, which are linear double-stranded DNA viruses, contain approximately 36,000 base pairs encapsulated in a protein coat. Adenoviruses transiently transduce nondividing cells with high expression of viral proteins, causing a pathogenic response by cytotoxic T lymphocytes (71–73). Several reports have documented the expression of a transgene for up to 8 weeks after injection into the brain, for over 6 months in fetal and in immune-compromised animals (74–76). Adenoviral vectors are available in two different forms that are replication deficient and reduced in their oncogenic potential. The first vector lacks two early viral genes (E1A, E1B), which are involved in the host cell cycle progression. In some adenoviral constructs the E3 region, which inhibits the cytolysis of the infected cell by cytotoxic T lymphocytes (CTL), and tumor necrosis factor (TNF) were deleted (77–80). Despite these manipulations an increasing number of adenoviral vector experiments in the brain has revealed a significant immune response due to the remaining expression of viral proteins (81,82). The second generation of adenoviral vectors differs from the first generation in that the E3 region is only partially deleted. The vector retains the expression of the E3 19 kDa protein responsible for the immune suppression ability of adenoviruses and subsequently reduces the immune response (83,84). Still, this vector continues to express viral genes at low levels and often leads to an inflammatory response (85), death of infected cells, and rapid loss of transgene expression. In order to develop a third generation of adenoviral vectors, the removal of the E4 region, which can probably cause oncogenic transformation in the host cell, is desired (86). However, elimination of E4 causes drastic reduction of gene expression (87). Recently, ''gutless'' vectors have been developed showing improved expression and decreased toxicity in vivo.

C. AAV

Adeno-associated viruses, which are single-stranded DNA parvoviruses, are nonpathogenic for mammals. In adeno-associated viral vectors all viral coding sequences can be deleted, reducing the deleterious effects of viral protein expression, except for the minimum AAV sequences required for transduction. AAV vectors allow integration into the host cell genome, but the efficiency may be very low. Studies of immortalized and primary cell cultures have shown that the vast majority of AAV vector genomes remain episomal and nonintegrated (88). Helper viruses, either adeno or HSV, provide proteins that are necessary for translation and transcription of the AAV and perform a similar role during the transcription of the helper virus itself (88). Recently it has been shown that the adenoviral E4 region is the limiting step in the AAV life cycle, specifically in the second strand synthesis (89). For efficient transduction, however, the role of the helper viruses needs to be further elucidated. Helper viruses may have important implications for the use of AAV vectors in gene therapy protocols, because patients treated with recombinant viruses may subsequently be infected with wild-type helper viruses and the interaction of recombinant viruses is only poorly understood (90,91). Low vector titers, low transduction efficiency, and the dependency on helper viruses seem to limit the use of AAV.

D. Retrovirus

Retroviruses were discovered as oncogenic agents, although the vast majority of retroviruses do not cause any pathology. These oncogenic viruses transform cells by expression of viral oncogenic sequences originally transduced from host cell genomes or by integration near cellular oncogenes with subsequent activation of the host oncogene. Their wide host range and their ability to carry foreign genes and stably integrate into the host cell genome make them ideal vectors for gene transfer (92). Retroviral vector constructs, based on the Moloney murine leukemia virus (MLV), are significantly reduced in their viral genome, lowering viral protein expression and subsequently the host immune response. The gene of interest is flanked by minimal viral gene signals for packaging and retroviral transcription. The lacking viral proteins like gag, pol, and env can be supplied by helper viruses in packaging cell lines to generate retroviral vectors. The host cell specificity of retroviral vectors can be increased by replacing the ecotropic envelope gene with amphotropic envelope genes (93). Although retroviruses provide an efficient method for stable gene delivery, there are difficulties in obtaining high titers of vector without the risk of recombination and production of replication-competent virus particles (94).

In contrast to other viral vectors, which may have been attenuated but retain some ability to infect other cells, replication-deficient retroviral vectors infect only once and do not spread in vivo. Retroviral vectors have a broad host cell range, but their use is limited to dividing cells (95,96). As cell division is limited in the CNS, the application of this system is restricted mostly to ex vivo experiments.

To target nondividing terminally differentiated cells, especially neurons of the CNS, a new vector system has been developed based on HIV. Like other lentiviruses, HIV is able to infect dividing as well as quiescent cells, such as monocyte-derived macrophages and growth-arrested cell (97). Hijacking the nuclear import machinery, the lentiviral genome and its gene of interest are actively transported through the nuclear pore (98–101). The HIV-derived vector does not express the HIV virus envelope but uses the vesicular stomatits virus protein envelope (VSV.G), which increases stability and allows high titers during the vector preparation. Gene delivery using this vector has been tested by intracerebral injection of highly concentrated vector (10^8 TU/mL) into the striatum and the hippocampus of adult rats. Four weeks after injection the reporter gene (β-galactosidase) was still detectable in every injection site and terminally differentiated neurons were transduced (102) (Fig. 3). Obvious pathological changes or signs of immune response were not detected in the rat brain tissue. In comparison, control animals injected with a MLV-based retroviral vector did not express the β-galactosidase reporter gene after 6 weeks. Long-term transgene expression, stable integration, and lack of expression of viral proteins associated with immune responses make this vector an attractive tool in CNS gene therapy.

E. Synthetic Vectors

Similar to viral vector systems, nonviral systems need efficient gene-delivery systems and effective gene expression in the target cell. Essentially challenging is the fact that plasmids encoding for the transgene product are negatively charged and have hydrodynamic diameters of more than 100–200 nm. A variety of nonviral gene-delivery systems have been developed using liposomes, cationic lipids, polymers, and endosomal lysis peptides.

In vitro gene transfer by calcium phosphate ($CaPO_4$) precipitation is frequently used to transfect single cell layers (103). It is thought that the Ca-DNA complex forms a particle that precipitates onto the surface of the cell, leading to nonspecific uptake by the cell (104). The efficacy depends on the quality of the precipitation reaction and the precipitate size. In ideal situations a rate of 10–50% uptake of DNA is achieved. However, many cells are resistant to this type of transfection, and the cells that are transduced are only transiently infected since the DNA remains episomal or as an extrachromosomal element in the nucleus. Stable infection is as low as 10% in vitro. Integration is random and multiple integrations are frequent, depending on the DNA concentration (105). Calcium precipitation is limited to the in vitro application similar to microinjection

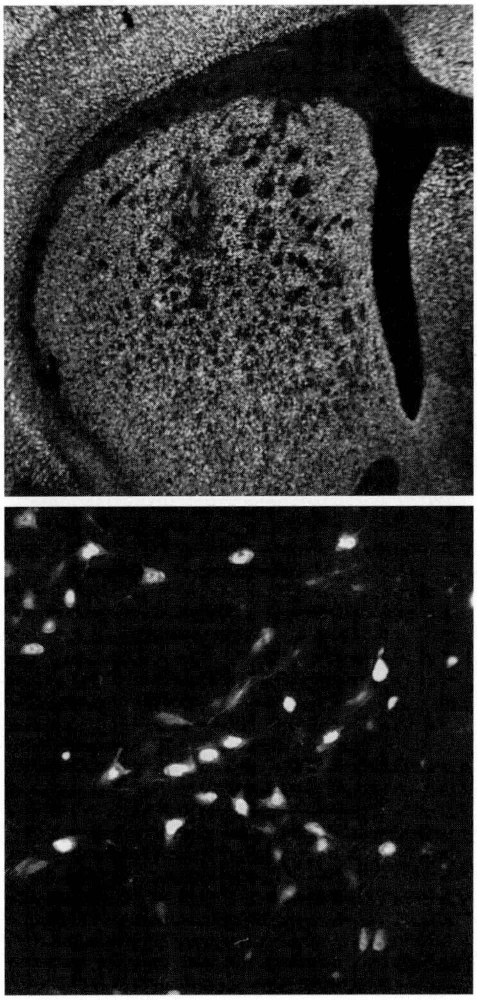

Figure 3 (A) Coronal section through the striatum of an adult rat injected 2 years before with lentiviral vector expressing the reporter gene (β-gal). Large numbers of cells stably express the transgene, without immune response. (B) Higher magnification of cells expressing the transgene (GFP). The cell body and processes are filled with the transgene product.

of DNA into the target cell, which results in occasional integration (106).

Studies using direct injection of purified DNA into various tissues have shown uptake and expression of the injected gene in various species like rats, mice, rabbits, and baboons (30). Efficiency is very low around the injection tract, but it was used to inject the gene for muscle dystrophy in models for Duchenne muscular dystrophy (107,108). Cationic lipids have been used successfully to deliver genes to the lung in the animals for cystic fibrosis (109) and into tumors for anticancer therapy (110,111).

F. Model Systems

Identification of the mutant genes and mechanisms responsible for neurological disorders provides an opportunity to consider new approaches to their treatment. The identification of gene products and delineation of the cellular dysfunction and cell death in animal models may suggest new therapeutic options. In this review we will focus on neurodegenerative diseases; therefore, a number of intriguing topics, like Huntington's disease, Lesch-Nyhan's disease, and lysosomal storage disorders must unfortunately be excluded and are reviewed elsewhere.

1. Parkinson's Disease

Parkinson's disease (PD), with 0.1–1% prevalence, is one of the most widespread neurodegenerative disorders. The biological cause is generally unknown but may be related to oxidative stress, lack of neurotrophic support, or exposure to toxins. The disease is characterized by a loss of dopamine-producing neurons, specifically dopaminergic neurons of the substantia nigra that project to the striatum. Tremor, rigidity, and movement disorder result from the loss of inhibitory input on the extrapyramidal system. The current treatment, oral L-dopa therapy, becomes less effective with progression of the disease and the number of side effects increases.

The effect of oral L-dopa indicates that the restoration of the neuronal circuitry is not necessary for improvement, but local delivery of L-dopa is an alternative therapy. The enzyme tyrosine hydroxylase (TH) is responsible for the biosynthesis of L-dopa from tyrosine. Therefore, a single gene introducing TH to cells in regions of terminal loss can increase the local supply of L-dopa (112,113).

An established animal model in rodents allows testing of the efficiency of gene therapy in Parkinson's disease. The injection of a neurotoxin, 6-hydroxydopamine, destroys nigro-striatal dopaminergic neurons and results in elimination of nigral dopaminergic input and upregulation of dopamine receptors in the lesioned striatum, while the striatal dopamine receptor density in the unlesioned side remains unchanged. The asymmetry caused by the resulting differential postsynaptic receptor sensitivities between denervated and intact striatum results in rotational behavior after application of apomorphine.

Direct gene delivery of the TH gene into the denervated striatum has been obtained with several viral vectors. During and colleagues (1) used defective HSV vector encoding TH and Kaplitt et al. (114) showed long-term expression in vivo in lesioned animals using the AAV vector. Previous reports mostly using adenoviral vectors were not able to retain long-term transgene expression (82,115,116).

While fetal tissue has been effective in experimental models and partially in applications in humans, access to tissue and characterization prior to transplantation are problematic. Adrenal chromaffin cells, on the other hand, have proven to be unsuccessful in preclinical and clinical trials (117,118). As a result genetic modification of cells producing TH has become one of the major interests in gene therapy. Fibroblasts, retrovirally transfected with the TH gene and implanted into the striatum, are able to reduce the circling frequency (119). Although grafted cells were found more than 2 months after injection, the number of expressing cells decreased with increasing time (120). These data also have shown that a small number of TH-producing graft cells are able to result in behavior improvement. The hypothesis that oxidative stress causes the loss of transplanted cells was tested in transplantation studies with transgenic mice overexpressing Cu/Zn superoxide dismutase (Cu/Zn-SOD). This enzyme is crucial in the detoxification of free radicals. Transgenic mice producing Cu/Zn-SOD have been shown to be more resistant to neuronal damage induced by oxidative stress. The transplantation of neurons of Cu/Zn-SOD mice into immune-suppressed animals showed a four times higher cell survival of genetically engineered neurons with concomitant functional recovery after 6-dihydroxydopamine lesion (16).

2. Alzheimer's Disease

Alzheimer's disease (AD) is a common dementia (0.02–5% prevalence) of older patients and belongs in a large group of degenerative brain disorders. Only a small number of cases are inherited compared to the large number of acquired cases. The neuropathology is characterized by progressive dementia caused by cortical atrophy, neuronal loss, neurofibrillary tangles, senile plaques, and vascular deposits of β-amyloid in various regions of the cerebral cortex and the hippocampus. β-Amyloid and its precursor play a crucial role in the pathogenesis of AD (121,122). The degeneration of forebrain cholinergic neurons responsible for memory acquisition and retention is well known, but the cause of the cell loss is not known. A well-established model for degeneration of cholinergic neurons in rodents is created by the fimbria fornix lesion. This lesion disconnects the cholinergic neurons of the medial septum to their NGF supply. Exogenous replacement of NGF in this model can prevent cholinergic neurons from degeneration and ameliorates some form of memory deficit (123,124). Direct intraventricular infusion of NGF into adult rats from the time of fimbria fornix lesion onward prevents the death of most of the axotomized cholinergic neurons. Furthermore, even noncholinergic septal neurons are destined to die and are likely not to be saved by NGF administration (123,125). Based on this observation, NGF infusions into aged, cognitively impaired rats demonstrated that rats with intact pumps showed improvement in learning tasks compared to noninfused, cognitively impaired rats (126–128). Additional studies extended the findings showing the age range and magnitude of the deficits that can be ameliorated by NGF infusions and that performance on the learning task is improved even if NGF is dosage dependent (119,126). Based on these results, primary fibroblasts, genetically modified to produce NGF, were implanted in the nucleus basalis Meynert (NBM) of aged impaired rats (129). Amerlioration of learning and memory associated with significant increase in size and number of NGF receptor–positive neurons in the basal forebrain was observed.

Therapeutic strategies for AD have also targeted the replacement or replenishment of deficient neurotransmitters, for example, acetylcholine (ACh). In one assessment of graft effect on cognitive impairments, cholinergic-rich tissue from the septum was implanted into the hippocampus of aged impaired rats (130,131). When compared to nongrafted impaired rats, the septal grafted rats showed significant improvement in spatial tasks. Fibroblasts retrovirally transduced to produce ACh survived within the brain and released ACh at least 10 days postimplantation (15,132). ACh-producing fibroblasts implanted into the frontal and parietal cortices of rats with bilateral lesions of the NBM could ameliorate cognitive dysfunction in a rat model of AD (133). The entorhinal cortex (EC) is also one of the first regions affected by neuropathological changes associated with AD. Lesions of the perforant pathway, which connects the EC with the hippocampus, resulted in selective loss of glutaminergic neurons (134). Transplants of fibroblast growth factor–producing fibroblasts prevented cell death of glutaminergic neurons of the endorhinal cortex.

3. Huntington's Disease

Huntington's disease (HD) is a movement disorder with disruption of the major input-output circuits of the basal ganglia. Major emotional and cognitive dysfunctions with involuntary movements (chorea) develop over 10–20 years of the disease in average. The cognitive disturbance may be due to degeneration of the striatal projecting neurons. γ-Aminobutyric acid (GABA) is the main transmitter of these neurons, and it has been shown by direct injection of GABA antagonists into the lateral part of the globus pallidus that choreitic movements can be induced (135). GABA receptor active substances injected in various regions in the striatum also had effects on motor behavior (136–138).

Neuronal transplantation in the HD model is based on the idea of restitution of striatum-like structures at the striatal lesion and replacement of functions lost by the destruction of striatal projecting neurons. The ibotenic acid lesion or kainic acidic lesion of the caudate putamen is chosen by causing significant loss of up to 90% in the injected area accompanied by degeneration loss of transmitters (139). Reduction of volume of the lesion site of up to 50% results after 3 months under building of a glial scar (140–142).

In addition dopaminergic structures of the lesioned site are reduced significantly (143). Until now studies investigating the effect of fetal transplants have been shown to reconstitute the volume of the lesioned striatum up to 80% (143). Interestingly, local cues seem to influence the graft development, showing that graft size is larger in denervated striata than in other regions of the brain or unlesioned globus pallidus (145). Studies investigating the transmitter status of grafts revealed the reconstitution of transmitter of both Chat and GAD up to normal activity levels (143,145). Positron emission studies of glucose consumption showed that striatal grafts have functional influence on reduction of motoric imbalance, supporting the idea that transplanted neurons establish functional connections with the host brain.

Early studies in nonhuman primates with cross-species grafts of fetal rat striatum under immunosuppression showed reduced apomorphine-induced dyskenisia. However, HD is a progressive disease, and transplanted neurons may undergo degeneration as well, destroying the transplant.

4. Peripheral Nerve Lesions

In humans, acoustic nerve injury may occur mainly by trauma or tumor affection, e.g., by vestibular (acoustic) schwannomas. Spontaneous regeneration of severed human acoustic nerve has not yet been described, although the acoustic nerve of lower vertebrates can spontaneously regenerate after injury (146–152). Lesions of the acoustic nerve in adult mammals do not normally result in regeneration (153,154).

Recently, the monoclonal antibody IN-1, which neutralizes the myelin-associated inhibitors of neurite growth, has been shown to enable injured CNS axons to regenerate in vivo (155–158). Behavioral studies showed that regenerating fibers in the spinal cord may form connections that lead to functional recovery (159).

All neurotrophins have more recently been shown to promote the survival of spinal and cranial sensory neurons in varying degrees in culture (59,160–168), while BDNF and NT-3 also have been shown to be crucial in vivo for development of chicken neurons (60) Mice carrying a deletion of NT-3 develop with severe sensory deficits, including a reduction of 60% of the lumbar root ganglion neurons (59,169,170). NT-3 supports neurons mediating limb proprioception in culture (171,172) and in vivo (173,174), as well as mechanoreceptive neurons supplying Meckel sensory organ innervation (Arvidsson, personal communication).

After cochlea nerve injury and treatment with the recombinant Fab fragment of the IN-1 antibody, the number of regenerating axons was low. Cochlear nerve axotomy resulted in a marked degeneration of proximal parent neurons in the spiral ganglion. Nissl staining of the axotomized spiral ganglion revealed a significant decrease in the number of neurons (90%). Retrograde degeneration of adult mammalian primary auditory neurons has been described following cochlear nerve axotomy (154,175).

The number of surviving primary auditory neurons may play a very important role in the number of regenerating axons after treatment with IN-1 Fab fragment. Therefore, efforts were made to treat the axotomized spiral ganglion neurons with NT-3. NT-3 has been shown to play a major role as a survival factor in developing spinal ganglion neurons (176). Lack of NT-3 resulted in the loss of 87% of spiral ganglion neurons in gene-ablated mice (59). Tatagiba et al. have shown that application of NT-3 to the lesion site results in an approximate five-fold increase in the number of surviving spiral ganglion neurons compared to nontreated animals (177).

5. Brain Tumors

Brain tumors have become a major target of novel gene transfer during the last decade, probably presenting the best model of an acquired genetic disease. The growth rate of malignant tumor cells is different from mature brain cells, which are mostly quiescent. Rapidly dividing cells are theoretically an ideal target for gene-transfer methods, without transfection of the surrounding brain tissue. Current therapeutic strategies include the direct killing of tumor cells, the production of new tumor antigens on the cell surface to induce tumor rejection, and the transfer of drug-sensitivity genes to tumor cells.

A large number of animal models and lately even clinical trials have taken advantage of the thymidine kinase (TK) model (102,178–180). The transfection of cells with the TK gene enables the transfected cell to metabolize the antiviral drug ganciclivir (GCV) into ganciclovir-triphosphate, which is cytotoxic and causes cell death. Only cells transduced with the TK gene are sensitive to GCV treatment. The poor efficiency in early studies by direct injection of viral vectors carrying the TK gene into the tumor bed was overcome by implantation of producer cells, continuously supplying the vector, which has only a short half-life time (2–4 h) (103). Culver et al. demonstrated this approach by injecting inoculated 9L glioma tumors with fibroblasts producing HSV thymidine kinase recombinant retroviruses (181). Using retroviral vectors, only rapidly dividing cells (e.g., tumor cells) are infected and killed because the majority of quiescent cells of the brain do not adopt the foreign gene. To achieve a cure, it was originally thought that 100% of tumor cells had to be transfected with TK and subsequently killed by GCV. In rodent studies several groups have seen tumor regression even with rates of 70% and less, due to the bystander effect (182). The bystander effect is based on the observation that HSV-TK–containing tumor cells in the presence of GCV are directly toxic to unmodified adjacent tumor cells.

To stimulate the immune response and increase tumor rejection, the delivery of interleukins and granulocytes–macrophage stimulating factors has been investigated (183,184). In addition, several studies successfully used the increasing immune response against tumors after vaccination strategies with irradiated tumor cells. In clinical trials, patients with primary or metastatic brain tumors have been treated in pilot studies with HSV-TK–producing cells and ganciclovir, but solid conclusions are not yet available.

IV. HURDLES TO APPLICATIONS

A. Toxicity and Safety of Viral Vectors in the CNS

Retroviral vectors have found broad application because they have small toxicity in vitro and in vivo. The lack of viral protein synthesis avoids any immune response, humoral as well as cellular (185–189). The advantage of retroviral as well as lentiviral vectors includes efficiency of gene transfer and stable integration of provirus into the host cell genome as described above.

They have undergone a variety of modifications through several generations to increase their safety. The disadvantage of retroviral vectors is the limited size of the insert (8–10 kbp). The insertion of the provirus into the host cell genome is stable, but the location is random and therefore the expression levels vary and the disruption of a normal gene may cause mutagenesis (90–93). Recent development of packaging cell lines has been shown to minimize the possibility of homologous recombination (187–189). The main disadvantage of the MLV-based retroviruses that require active replication and synthesis of DNA for provirus integration to occur has been overcome by lentiviral vectors, which have been shown to be able to efficiently infect nondividing cells in vivo and in vitro without decreasing expression and immune response (102,185,186,194,195).

Adeno-associated viral vectors have also been shown to have advantages like stable integration into the host cell, lack of any human-related disease, and the ability to infect nondividing cells, although integration here is still discussed. The efficiency and need for adenovirus to produce AAV vectors are still the most disappointing aspects and limit the in vivo approach significantly.

Herpes simplex viral vectors have been developed over the years, and changes have reduced the cytopathic effect of lytic infection; however, direct applications still cause local tissue damage and severe cell damage, mostly due to persistent expression of viral proteins. The advantage of HSV is its long-term persistence in a latent nonintegrated state in neuronal cell nuclei, as well as the large packaging size, allowing for large inserts of ≥15 kbp. During latency the lytic viral genes are silent.

Adenoviral vectors have found broad application, but the immune response based on the remaining expression of viral proteins is still the major problem and limits long-term expression. New generations provide more promising adenoviral vectors and efficiency and persistency, although nonintegration of the transgene has reported expression up to 6 months (2,196–198).

B. Regulatable Expression

Genetic engineering of cells in vivo or in vitro for transplantation purposes demands stable long-term expression of the transgene. Next to transcriptional efficacy, stability of the RNA and protein, the main regulation system is the promoter system driving the transgene. The choice now is viral promoters, because they have high levels of transgene expression in dividing cells (199). In posttransplantation systems, however, these promoters may be deactivated, resulting in the transgene shut-off (24). The other group of promoters uses the tissue-specific promoters, allowing for transgene expression in selected subgroups of cells like neuron-specific enolase and glial-fibrillary acidic promoters (200). The addition of enhancer elements was shown to increase the expression level in a variety of cell types.

In many biological systems the regulation of transgene expression is also required. Therefore, different strategies have been used to construct regulatable promoters containing bacterial as well as eukaryotic regulatory elements and to allow for the regulation of transgene expression, at least in vitro. The tetracycline repressor system, developed by Gossen (201–203), is currently under investigation in many in vitro (54) and in vivo models (204).

V. CONCLUSIONS

Technical problems of cell transplantation models in vitro as well as for direct in vivo gene transfer via viral vectors present the future challenge in order to develop methods for therapeutic gene transfer into the CNS. Improved knowledge about transplantation of cells, trophic factors, and the role of local cues will allow for more successful transplant survival and even functional effects of cells. The discovery of mechanisms involved in gene expression will lead to more efficient viral vectors, reduction of toxicity, and, in the long run, regulation of transgene expression. Stable producer cell lines will enable us to obtain viral vectors in quantities allowing for application in larger organisms. Recent developments of stable expression in terminally differentiated cells like neurons bring the goal of direct gene transfer in the CNS within reach. In addition, the increasing knowledge of cell cycle and antiapoptotic factors broadens the range of factors available to rescue cells, prevent cell death, or even allow cell regeneration in the CNS.

REFERENCES

1. During MJ, Naegele JR, O'Malley KL, et al. Long-term behavioral recovery in parkinsonian rats by an HSV vector expressing tyrosine hydroxylase [see comments]. Science 1994; 266:1399–1403.
2. Mallet J, et al. Adenovirus mediated gene transfer to the central nervous system. Gene Ther 1994; 1(suppl 1):552.
3. Thompson EG. Successful brain grafting. NY Med J 1890; 51:701–702.
4. Dunn EH. Primary and secundary findings in a series of attempts to transplant cerebral cortex into the albino rat. J Comp Neurol 1917; 27:565–582.
5. Cajal SR. Degeneration and Regeneration in the Central Nervous System. Oxford: Oxford University Press, 1928.
6. Clark WEL. Neuronal differentiation in implanted foetal cortical tissue. J Neurol Psychiatry 1940; 14:376–384.
7. Glees B. Studies of cortical regeneration with special reference to cerebral transplants. In: Windle WE, ed. Regeneration in the Central Nervous System. Springfield, IL: Charles C Thomas, 1955:94–111.
8. Halasz L, Pupp L, Uhlarik S, Timak L. Further studies on the hormon secretion of the anterior pituitary gland transplanted into the hypophysiotrophic areas of rat hypothalamus. Endocrinology 1965; 77:343–355.
9. Knigge KM. Gonadotrophic action of neonatal pituitary glands implanted in the rat brain. Am J Physiol 1962; 202: 387–391.
10. Perlow M, Freed WJ, Hoffer BJ, Seiger A, Olson L, Wyatt RJ. Brain grafts reduce motor abnormalities produced by distraction of nigrostriatal dopamine system. Science 1979; 204:643–647.
11. Björklund A, Stenevi U. Reconstruction of the nigrostriatal dopamine pathway by intracerebral transplants. Brain Res 1979; 177:555–560.
12. Mobley WC, et al. Nerve growth factor increases choline acetyltransferase activity in developing basal forebrain neurons. Brain Res 1986; 387:53–62.
13. Martinez HJ, Dreyfus CF, Jonakait GM, Black IB. Nerve growth factor promotes cholinergic development in brain striatal cultures. Proc Natl Acad Sci USA 1985; 82: 7777–7781.
14. Freed WJ. Neural transplantation: a special issue [editorial]. Exp Neurol 1993; 122:1–4.
15. Fisher LJ, Raymon HK, Gage FH. Cells engineered to produce acetylcholine: therapeutic potential for Alzheimer's disease. Ann NY Acad Sci 1993; 695:278–284.
16. Nakao N, et al. Overexpressing Cu/Zn superoxide dismutase enhances survival of transplanted neurons in a rat model of Parkinson's disease [see comments]. Nat Med 1995; 1:226–231.
17. Kawaja MD, Rosenberg MB, Yoshida K, Gage FH. Somatic gene transfer of nerve growth factor promotes the survival of axotomized septal neurons and the regeneration of their axons in adult rats. J Neurosci 1992; 12: 2849–2864.
18. Rosenberg MB et al. Grafting genetically modified cells to the damaged brain: restorative effects of NGF expression. Science 1988; 242:1575–1578.
19. Fisher LJ, Gage FH. Intracerebral transplantation: basic and clinical applications to the neostriatum. FASEB J 1994; 8:489–496.
20. Barba D, Hardin J, Sadelain M, Gage FH. Development of anti-tumor immunity following thymidine kinase-mediated killing of experimental brain tumors. Proc Natl Acad Sci USA 1994; 91:4348–4352.
21. Brautigam M, Dreesen R, Flosbach CW, Herken H. Mouse neuroblastoma clone N1E-115: a suitable model for studying the action of dopamine agonists of tyrosine hydroxylase activity. Biochem Pharmacol 1982; 31:1279–1282.
22. Brautigam M, Dreesen R, Herken H. Dopa-release from mouse neuroblastoma clone N 1 E-115 into the culture medium. A test for tyrosine hydroxylase activity. Naunyn Schmiedebergs Arch Pharmacol 1981; 320:85–89.
23. Kawaja M, Gage FH. Reactive astrocytes are substrates for the growth of adult CNS nerve oxons in the presence of elevated levels of nerve growth factor. Neuron 1991; 7:1019–1030.
24. Palmer TD, Rosman GJ, Osborne WR, Miller AD. Genetically modified skin fibroblasts persist long term after transplantation but gradually inactivate introduced genes. Proc Natl Acad Sci 1991; 88:1330–1334.
25. Lucidi-Phillipi CA, et al. Brain-derived neurotrophic factor-transduced fibroblasts: production of BDNF and effects of grafting to the adult rat brain. J Comp Neurol 1995; 354:361–376.
26. Kawaja MD, Gage FH. Morphological and neurochemical features of cultured primary skin fibroblasts of Fischer 344 rats following striatal implantation. J Comp Neurol 1992; 317:102–116.
27. Frim DM, et al. Implanted fibroblasts genetically engineered to produce brain-derived neurotrophic factor pre-

vent 1-methyl-4-phenylpyridinium toxicity to dopaminergic neurons in the rat. Proc Natl Acad Sci USA 1994; 91:5104–5108.

28. Dai Y, Roman M, Naviaux RK, Verma IM. Gene therapy via primary myoblasts: long-term expression of factor IX protein following transplantation in vivo. Proc Natl Acad Sci USA 1992; 89:10892–10895.
29. Jiao S, et al. Direct gene transfer into nonhuman primate myofibers in vivo. Hum Gene Ther 1992; 3:21–33.
30. Jiao S, Wolff JA. Long-term survival of autologous muscle grafts in rat brain. Neurosci Lett 1992; 137:207–210.
31. Cunningham LA, Short MP, Breakefield XO, Bohn MC. Nerve growth factor released by transgenic astrocytes enhances the function of adrenal chromaffin cell grafts in a rat model of Parkinson's disease. Brain Res 1994; 658: 219–231.
32. Ridoux V, et al. The use of adenovirus vectors for intracerebral grafting of transfected nervous cells. Neuroreport 1994; 5:801–804.
33. Owens GC, Johnson R, Bunge RP, O'Malley KL. L-3,4-dihydroxyphenylalanine synthesis by genetically modified Schwann cells. J Neurochem 1991; 56:1030–1036.
34. Kordower JH, Cochran E, Penn RD, Goetz CG. Putative chromaffin cell survival and enhanced host-derived TH-fiber innervation following a functional adrenal medulla autograft for Parkinson's disease. Ann Neurol 1991; 29: 405–412.
35. Strömberg I, et al. Rescue of basal forebrain cholinergic neurons after implantation of genetically midified cells producing recombinant NGF. The Journal of Neuroscience Research 1990; 25:405–411.
36. Niijima K, et al. Enhanced survival and neuronal differentiation of adrenal chromaffin cells cografted into the striatum with NGF-producing fibroblasts. J Neurosci 1995; 15: 1180–1194.
37. Culliton BJ. Gene therapy on the move [news]. Nature 1991; 354:429.
38. Chalmers GR, Fisher LJ, Niijima K, Patterson PH, Gage FH. Adrenal chromaffin cells transdifferentiate in response to basic fibroblast growth factor and show directed outgrowth to a nerve growth factor source in vivo. Exp Neurol 1995; 133:32–42.
39. Snyder EY, et al. Multipotent neural cell lines can engraft and participate in development of mouse cerebellum. Cell 1992; 68:33–51.
40. Gage FH, et al. Survival and differentiation of adult neuronal progenitor cells transplanted to the adult brain. Proc Natl Acad Sci USA 1995; 92:11879–11883.
41. Gage FH, Ray J, Fisher LJ. Isolation, characterization, and use of stem cells from the CNS. Annu Rev Neurosci 1995; 18:159–192.
42. Bjorklund A, Stenevi U, Dunnett SB, Gage FH. Cross-species neural grafting in a rat model of Parkinson's disease. Nature 1982; 298:652–654.
43. Bjorklund A. Neurobiology. Better cells for brain repair [news; comment]. Nature 1993; 362:414–415.
44. Gage FH, Thompson RG. Differential distribution of norepinephrine and serotonin along the dorsal-ventral axis of the hippocampal formation. Brain Res Bull 1980; 5: 771–773.
45. Suhonen JO, Peterson DA, Ray J, Gage FH. Differentiation of adult hippocampus-derived progenitors into olfactory. Nature 1996; 383:624–627.
46. Ray J, Palmer T, Takahashi J, Gage, FH. Neurogenesis in the adult brain: Lessons learned from the studies of progenitor cells from the embryonic and adult central nervous systems. In: YC, ed. Isolation, Characterization and Utilization of CNS Stem Cells. Paris: Springer, 1996: 129–150.
47. Lacorazza HD, Flax JD, Snyder EY, Jendoubi M. Expression of human beta-hexosaminidase alpha-subunit gene (the gene defect of Tay-Sachs disease) in mouse brains upon engraftment of transduced progenitor cells. Nat Med 1996; 2:424–429.
48. Cepko CL. Immortalization of neural cells via retrovirus-mediated oncogene transduction. Annu Rev Neurosci 1989; 12:47–65.
49. Cepko CL, Ryder EF, Austin CP, Walsh C, Fekete DM. Lineage analysis using retrovirus vectors. Methods Enzymol 1993; 225:933–960.
50. Aguzzi A, Kleihues P, Heckl K, Wiestler OD. Cell type-specific tumor induction in neural transplants by retrovirus. Oncogene 1991; 6:113–118.
51. Kleihues P, Aguzzi A, Wiestler OD. Cellular and molecular aspects of neurocarcinogenesis. Toxicol Pathol 1990; 18:193–203.
52. Andersen JK, Frim DM, Isacson O, Breakefield XO. Herpesvirus-mediated gene delivery into the rat brain: specificity and efficiency of the neuron-specific enolase promoter. Cell Mol Neurobiol 1993; 13:503–515.
53. Frederiksen K, McKay RD. Proliferation and differentiation of rat neuroepithelial precursor. J Neurosci 1988; 8: 1144–1151.
54. Hoshimaru M, Ray J, Sah DW, Gage FH. Differentiation of the immortalized adult neuronal progenitor cell line HC2S2 into neurons by regulatable suppression of the v-myc oncogene. Proc Natl Acad Sci USA 1996; 93: 1518–1523.
55. Bothwell M. Functional interactions of neurotrophins and neurotrophin receptors. Annu Rev Neurosci 1995; 18: 223–253.
56. Lin LF, Doherty DH, Lile JD, Bektesh S, Collins F. GDNF: a glial cell line-derived neurotrophic factor for midbrain dopaminergic neurons [see comments]. Science 1993; 260: 1130–1132.
57. Lamballe F, Klein R, Barbacid M. trkC, a new member of the trk family of tyrosine protein kinases, is a receptor for neurotrophin-3. Cell 1991; 66:967–979.
58. McMahon SB, Priestley JV. Peripheral neuropathies and neurotrophic factors: animal models and clinical perspectives. Curr Opin Neurobiol 1995; 5:616–624.
59. Ernfors P, Lee KF, Kucera J, Jaenisch R. Lack of neurotrophin-3 leads to deficiencies in the peripheral nervous sys-

tem and loss of limb proprioceptive afferents. Cell 1994; 77:503–512.
60. Gaese F, Kolbeck R, Barde YA. Sensory ganglia require neurotrophin-3 early in development. Development 1994; 120:1613–1619.
61. Kalcheim C, Carmeli C, Rosenthal A. Neurotrophin 3 is a mitogen for cultured neural crest cells. Proc Natl Acad Sci USA 1992; 89:1661–1665.
62. Kalcheim C. The role of neurotrophins in development of neural-crest cells that become sensory ganglia. Phil Trans R Soc Lond B Biol Sci 1996; 351:375–381.
63. Korsmeyer SJ, Yin XM, Oltvai ZN, Veis-Novack DJ, Linette GP. Reactive oxygen species and the regulation of cell death by the Bcl-2 gene family. Biochim Biophys Acta 1995; 1271:63–66.
64. Mellerick DM, Fraser NW. Physical state of the latent herpes simplex virus genome in a mouse. Virology 1987; 158:265–275.
65. Palella TD, Silverman LJ, Homa FL, Levine M, Kelley WN. Transfer of human HPRT gene sequences into neuronal cells by a herpes simplex virus derived vector. Adv Exp Med Biol 1989; 253A:549–554.
66. Fink DJ, et al. In vivo expression of beta-galactosidase in hippocampal neurons by HSV-mediated gene transfer. Hum Gene Ther 1992; 3:11–19.
67. Andersen JK, Garber DA, Meaney CA, Breakefield XO. Gene transfer into mammalian central nervous system using herpes virus vectors: extended expression of bacterial lacZ in neurons using the neuron-specific enolase promoter. Hum Gene Ther 1992; 3:487–499.
68. Chiocca EA, et al. Transfer and expression of the lacZ gene in rat brain neurons mediated by herpes simplex virus mutants. New Biol 1990; 2:739–746.
69. Martuza RL, Malick A, Markert JM, Ruffner KL, Coen DM. Experimental therapy of human glioma by means of a genetically engineered virus mutant. Science 1991; 252: 854–856.
70. Johnson PA, Miyanohara A, Levine F, Cahill T, Friedmann T. Cytotoxicity of a replication-defective mutant of herpes simplex virus type 1. J Virol 1992; 66:2952–2965.
71. Brody SL, Jaffe HA, Han SK, Wersto RP, Crystal RG. Direct in vivo gene transfer and expression in malignant cells using adenovirus vectors. Hum Gene Ther 1994; 5: 437–447.
72. Brody SL, Crystal RG. Adenovirus-mediated in vivo gene transfer. Ann NY Acad Sci 1994; 716:90–101.
73. Brody SL, Metzger M, Danel C, Rosenfeld MA, Crystal RG. Acute responses of non-human primates to airway delivery of an adenovirus vector containing the human cystic fibrosis transmembrane conductance regulator cDNA. Hum Gene Ther 1994; 5:821–836.
74. Haase G, et al. Gene therapy of murine motor neuron disease using adenoviral vectors for neurotrophic factors [see comments]. Nat Med 1997; 3:429–436.
75. Akli S, et al. Restoration of hexosaminidase A activity in human Tay-Sachs fibroblasts via adenoviral vector-mediated gene transfer. Gene Ther 1996; 3:769–774.
76. Caillaud C, et al. Adenoviral vector as a gene delivery system into cultured rat neuronal and glial cells. Eur J Neurosci 1993; 5:1287–1291.
77. Gooding LR. Virus proteins that counteract host immune defenses. Cell 1992; 71:5–7.
78. Gooding LR. Regulation of TNF-mediated cell death and inflammation by human adenoviruses. Infect Agents Dis 1994; 3:106–115.
79. Kaplan JM, et al. Characterization of factors involved in modulating persistence of transgene expression from recombinant adenovirus in the mouse lung. Hum Gene Ther 1997; 8:45–56.
80. Sparer TE, et al. Generation of cytotoxic T lymphocytes against immunorecessive epitopes after multiple immunizations with adenovirus vectors is dependent on haplotype. J Virol 1997; 71:2277–2284.
81. Davidson BL, et al. Expression of Escherichia coli beta-galactosidase and rat HPRT in the CNS of Macaca mulatta following adenoviral mediated gene transfer. Exp Neurol 1994; 125:258–267.
82. Davidson BL, Bohn MC. Recombinant adenovirus: a gene transfer vector for study and treatment of CNS diseases. Exp Neurol 1997; 144:125–130.
83. Engelhardt JF, Ye S, Doranz B, Wilson JM. Ablation of E2A in recombinant adenoviruses improves transgene persistence and decreases inflammatory response in mouse liver. Proc Natl Acad Sci USA 1994; 91:6196–6200.
84. Engelhardt JF, Litzky L, Wilson JM. Prolonged transgene expression in cotton rat lung with recombinant adenoviruses defective in E2a. Hum Gene Ther 1994; 5: 1217–1229.
85. Byrnes AP, Rusby JE, Wood MJ, Charlton HM. Adenovirus gene transfer causes inflammation in the brain. Neuroscience 1995; 66:1015–1024.
86. Javier RT. Adenovirus type 9 E4 open reading frame 1 encodes a transforming protein required for the production of mammary tumors in rats. J Virol 1994; 68:3917–3924.
87. Halbert DN, Cutt JR, Shenk T. Adenovirus early region 4 encodes functions required for efficient DNA replication, late gene expression, and host cell shutoff. J Virol 1985; 56:250–257.
88. Muzyczka N. Use of adeno-associated virus as a general transduction vector for mammalian cells. Curr Top Microbiol Immunol 1992; 158:97–129.
89. Ferrari FK, Samulski T, Shenk T, Samulski RJ. Second-strand synthesis is a rate-limiting step for efficient transduction by recombinant adeno-associated virus vectors. J Virol 1996; 70:3227–3234.
90. Afione SA, et al. In vivo model of adeno-associated virus vector persistence and rescue. J Virol 1996; 70: 3235–3241.
91. Afione SA, Conrad CK, Flott TR. Gene therapy vectors as drug delivery systems. Clin Pharmacokinet 1995; 28: 181–189.
92. Bishop JM, Varmus H. Functions and Origins of Retroviral Transforming Genes: RNA Tumor Viruses. Cold Spring Harbor, NY: Cold Spring Harbor Laboratories, 1984.

93. Miller AD, Rosman GJ. Improved retroviral vectors for gene transfer and expression. Biotechniques 1989; 7: 980–982, 984–986, 989–990.
94. Pear WS, Nolan GP, Scott ML, Baltimore D. Production of high-titer helper-free retroviruses by transient transfection. Proc Natl Acad Sci USA 1993; 90:8392–8396.
95. Varmus HE, Padgett T, Heasley S, Simon G, Bishop JM. Cellular functions are required for the synthesis and integration of avian sarcoma virus-specific DNA. Cell 1977; 11:307–319.
96. Humphries EH, Glover C, Reichmann ME. Rous sarcoma virus infection of synchronized cells establishes provirus integration during S-phase DNA synthesis prior to cellular division. Proc Natl Acad Sci USA 1981; 78:2601–2605.
97. Lewis P, Henselj M, Emerman M. Human immunodeficiency virus infection of cells arrested in the cell cycle. EMBO J 1992; 11:3053–3058.
98. von Schwedler U, Kornbluth RS, Trono D. The nuclear localization signal of the matrix protein of human immunodeficiency virus type 1 allows the establishment of infection in macrophages and quiescent T lymphocytes. Proc Natl Acad Sci USA 1994; 91:6992–6996.
99. Gallay P, Stitt V, Mundy C, Oettinger M, Trono D. Role of the karyopherin pathway in human immunodeficiency virus type 1 nuclear import. J Virol 1996; 70:1027–1032.
100. Gallay P, Swingler S, Song J, Bushman F, Trono D. HIV nuclear import is governed by the phosphotyrosine-mediated binding of matrix to the core domain of integrase. Cell 1995; 83:569–576.
101. Gallay P, Swingler S, Aiken C, Trono D. HIV-1 infection of nondividing cells: C-terminal tyrosine phosphorylation of the viral matrix protein is a key regulator. Cell 1995; 80:379–388.
102. Naldini L, et al. In vivo gene delivery and stable transduction of nondividing cells by a lentiviral vector. Science 1996; 272:263–267.
103. Loyter A, Scangos G, Juricek D, Keene D, Ruddle FH. Mechanisms of DNA entry into mammalian cells. II. Phagocytosis of calcium phosphate DNA co-precipitate visualized by electron microscopy. Exp Cell Res 1982; 139:223–234.
104. Loyter A, Scangos GA, Ruddle FH. Mechanisms of DNA uptake by mammalian cells: fate of exogenously added DNA monitored by the use of fluorescent dyes. Proc Natl Acad Sci USA 1982; 79:422–426.
105. Ruddle FH. A new era in mammalian gene mapping: somatic cell genetics and recombinant DNA methodologies. Nature 1981; 294:115–120.
106. Capecchi MR. High efficiency transformation by direct microinjection of DNA into cultured mammalian cells. Cell 1980; 22:479–488.
107. Danko I, Wolff JA. Direct gene transfer into muscle. Vaccine 1994; 12:1499–1502.
108. Danko I, et al. High expression of naked plasmid DNA in muscles of young rodents. Hum Mol Genet 1997; 6: 1435–1443.
109. Yoshimura K, et al. Expression of the human cystic fibrosis transmembrane conductance regulator gene in the mouse lung after in vivo intratracheal plasmid-mediated gene transfer. Nucleic Acids Res 1992; 20:3233–3240.
110. Plautz GE, et al. Immunotherapy of malignancy by in vivo gene transfer into tumors [see comments]. Proc Natl Acad Sci USA 1993; 90:4645–4649.
111. Plautz GE, et al. Direct gene transfer for the understanding and treatment of human disease. Ann NY Acad Sci 1994; 716:144–153.
112. Jiao S, Gurevich V, Wolff JA. Long-term correction of rat model of Parkinson's disease by gene therapy. Nature 1996; 380:734.
113. Jiao S, Gurevich V, Wolff JA. Long-term correction of rat model of Parkinson's disease by gene therapy. Nature 1996; 362:450–453.
114. Kaplitt MG, et al. Long-term gene expression and phenotypic correction using adeno-associated virus vectors in the mammalian brain. Nat Genet 1994; 8:148–154.
115. Le Gal La Salle G, et al. An adenovirus vector for gene transfer into neurons and glia in the brain. Science 1993; 259:988–990.
116. Horellou P, et al. Exogenous expression of L-dopa and dopamine in various cell lines following transfer of rat and human tyrosine hydroxylase cDNA: grafting in an animal model of Parkinson's disease. Prog Brain Res 1990; 82: 23–32.
117. Lindvall O. Cell transplantation: a future therapy for Parkinson's disease? Neurologia 1994; 9:101–107.
118. Kopin IJ, Bankiewicz KS, Plunkett RJ, Jacobowitz DM, Oldfield EH. Tissue implants in treatment of parkinsonian syndromes in animals and implications for use of tissue implants in humans. Adv Neurol 1993; 60:707–714.
119. Fisher LJ, Jinnah HA, Kale LC, Higgins GA, Gage FH. Survival and function of intrastriatally grafted primary fibroblasts genetically modified to produce L-dopa. Neuron 1991; 6:371–380.
120. Kawaja M, Gage FH. Nerve growth factor receptor immonreactivity in the rat septo-hippocampal pathway; a light and electronmicroscopical investigation. J Comp Neurol 1991; 307:512–530.
121. Games D, et al. Alzheimer-type neuropathology in transgenic mice overexpressing V717F beta-amyloid precursor protein [see comments]. Nature 1995; 373: 523–527.
122. Selkoe DJ. The molecular pathology of Alzheimer's disease. Neuron 1991; 6:487–498.
123. Williams LR, et al. Continuous infusion of nerve growth factor prevents basal forebrain neuronal death after fimbria fornix transection. Proc Natl Acad Sci USA 1986; 83: 9231–9235.
124. Hefti F, et al. Promotion of neuronal survival in vitro by thermal proteins and poly(dicarboxylic)amino acids. Brain Res 1991; 541:273–283.
125. Gage FH, Bjorklund A. Trophic and growth-regulating mechanisms in the central nervous system monitored by

intracerebral neural transplants. Ciba Found Symp 1987; 126:143–159.
126. Koliatsos VE, et al. Highly selective effects of nerve growth factor, brain-derived neurotrophic factor, and neurotrophin-3 on intact and injured basal forebrain magnocellular neurons. J Comp Neurol 1994; 343:247–262.
127. Koliatsos VE, et al. Recombinant human nerve growth factor prevents retrograde degeneration of axotomized basal forebrain cholinergic neurons in the rat. Exp Neurol 1991; 112:161–173.
128. Fischer A, Schatz C. Gene therapy. Therapie 1995; 50: 369–374.
129. Chen KS, Gage FH. Somatic gene transfer of NGF to the aged brain: behavioral and morphological amelioration. J Neurosci 1995; 15:2819–2825.
130. Gage FH, Bjorklund A, Stenevi U, Dunnett SB, Kelly PA. Intrahippocampal septal grafts ameliorate learning impairments in aged rats. Science 1984; 225:533–536.
131. Gage FH, Dunnett SB, Bjorklund A. Spatial learning and motor deficits in aged rats. Neurobiol Aging 1984; 5: 43–48.
132. Fisher LJ, et al. In vivo production and release of acetylcholine from primary fibroblasts genetically modified to express choline acetyltransferase. J Neurochem 1993; 61: 1323–1332.
133. Winkler J, Suhr ST, Gage FH, Thal LJ, Fisher LJ. Essential role of neocortical acetylcholine in spatial memory [see comments]. Nature 1995; 375:484–487.
134. Peterson DA, Lucidi-Phillipi CA, Eagle KL, Gage FH. Perforant path damage results in progressive neuronal death and somal atrophy in layer II of entorhinal cortex and functional impairment with increasing postdamage age. J Neurosci 1994; 14:6872–6885.
135. Crossman AR, Mitchell IJ, Sambrook MA, Jackson A. Chorea and myoclonus in the monkey induced by gamma-aminobutyric acid antagonism in the lentiform complex. The site of drug action and a hypothesis for the neural mechanisms of chorea. Brain 1988; 111:1211–1233.
136. Gale K, Casu M. Dynamic utilization of GABA in substantia nigra: regulation by dopamine and GABAin the striatum, and its clinical and behavioral implications. Mol Cell Biochem 1981; 39:369–405.
137. Scheel-Kruger J. Dopamine-GABA interactions: evidence that GABA transmits, modulates and mediates dopaminergic functions in the basal ganglia and the limbic system. Acta Neurol Scand Suppl 1986; 107:1–54.
138. Scheel-Kruger J, Arnt J. New aspects on the role of dopamine, acetylcholine, and GABA in the development of tardive dyskinesia. Psychopharmacology Suppl 1985; 2: 46–57.
139. Isacson O, Brundin P, Kelly PA, Gage FH, Bjorklund A. Functional neuronal replacement by grafted striatal neurones in the ibotenic acid-lesioned rat striatum. Nature 1984; 311:458–460.
140. Dusart I, Isacson O, Nothias F, Gumpel M, Peschanski M. Presence of Schwann cells in neurodegenerative lesions of the central nervous system. Neurosci Lett 1989; 105: 246–250.
141. Dusart I, Nothias F, Roudier F, Besson JM, Peschanski M. Vascularization of fetal cell suspension grafts in the excitotoxically lesioned adult rat thalamus. Brain Res Dev Brain Res 1989; 48:215–228.
142. Dusart I, Marty S, Peschanski M. Glial changes following an excitotoxic lesion in the CNS—II. Astrocytes. Neuroscience 1991; 45:541–549.
143. Isacson O, Brundin P, Gage FH, Bjorklund A. Neural grafting in a rat model of Huntington's disease: progressive neurochemical changes after neostriatal ibotenate lesions and striatal tissue grafting. Neuroscience 1985; 16: 799–817.
144. Labandeira-Garcia JL, et al. Intrathalamic striatal grafts survive and after circling behaviour in adult rats with excitotoxically lesioned striatum. Neuroscience 1995; 68: 737–749.
145. Schmidt RH, Bjorklund A, Stenevi U. Intracerebral grafting of dissociated CNS tissue suspensions: a new approach for neuronal transplantation to deep brain sites. Brain Res 1981; 218:347–356.
146. Davis RL. Specificity of VIIIth nerve regeneration in lower vertebrates. J Exp Zool 1992; 261:254–260.
147. Davis RL, Sewell WF. Neurite regeneration from single primary-auditory neurons in vitro. Hear Res 1992; 58: 107–121.
148. Newman A, Kuruvilla A, Pereda A, Honrubia V. Regeneration of the eight cranial nerve. I. Anatomic verification in the bullfrog. Laryngoscope 1986; 96:484–493.
149. Newman A, Honrubia V. Regeneration of the eight cranial nerve in the bullfrog, Rana catesbeiana. Exp Neurol 1992; 115:115–120.
150. Zakon H, Capranica RR. Reformation of organized connections in the auditory system after generation of the eighth nerve. Science 1981; 213:242–244.
151. Zakon H, Capranica RR. An anatomical and physiological study of regeneration of the eighth nerve in the leopard frog. Brain Res 1981; 209:325–338.
152. Zakon H. Reorganization of connectivity in amphibian central auditory system following VIIIth nerve regeneration: time course. J Neurophysiol 1983; 49:1410–1427.
153. Corwin JT. Regeneration in the auditory system. Exp Neurol 1992; 115:7–12.
154. Spoendlin H. Factors inducing retrograde degeneration of the cochlear nerve. Ann Otol Rhinol Laryngol Suppl 1984; 112:76–82.
155. Weibel D, Cadelli D, Schwab ME. Regeneration of lesioned rat optic nerve fibers is improved after neutralization of myelin-associated neurite growth inhibitors. Brain Res 1994; 642:259–266.
156. Schnell L, Schwab ME. Axonal regeneration in the rat spinal cord produced by an antibody against myelin-associated neurite growth inhibitors. Nature 1990; 343: 269–272.
157. Schnell L, Schwab ME. Sprouting and regeneration of lesioned corticospinal tract fibres in the adult rat spinal cord. Eur J Neurosci 1993; 5:1156–1171.

158. Schnell L, Schneider R, Kolbeck R, Barde YA, Schwab ME. Neurotrophin-3 enhances sprouting of corticospinal tract during development and after adult spinal cord lesion. Nature 1994; 367:170–173.
159. Bregman BS, et al. Recovery from spinal cord injury mediated by antibodies to neurite growth inhibitors [see comments]. Nature 1995; 378:498–501.
160. Hallbook F, Ibanez CF, Ebendal T, Perrson H. Cellular localization of brain-derived neurotrophic factor and neurotrophin-3 mRNA expression in the early chicken embryo. Eur J Neurosci 1993; 5:1–14.
161. Hallbook F, et al. Neurotrophins and their receptors in chicken neuronal development. Int J Dev Biol 1995; 39: 855–868.
162. Hallbook F, Backstrom A, Kullander K, Ebendal T, Carri NG. Expression of neurotrophins and trk receptors in the avian retina. J Comp Neurol 1996; 364:664–676.
163. Ernfors P, Kucera J, Lee KF, Loring J, Jaenisch R. Studies on the physiological role of brain-derived neurotrophic factor and neurotrophin-3 in knockout mice. Int J Dev Biol 1995; 39:799–807.
164. Ernfors P, Van De Water T, Loring J, Jaenisch R. Complementary roles of BDNF and NT-3 in vestibular and auditory development. Neuron 1995; 14:1153–1164.
165. Ernfors P, Duan ML, ElShamy WM, Canlon B. Protection of auditory neurons from aminoglycoside toxicity by neurotrophin-3. Nat Med 1996; 2:463–467.
166. Ibanez CF, et al. Neurotrophin-4 is a target-derived neurotrophic factor for neurons of the trigeminal ganglion. Development 1993; 117:1345–1353.
167. Ibanez CF, Ilag LL, Murray Rust J, Persson H. An extended surface of binding to Trk tyrosine kinase receptors in NGF and BDNF allows the engineering of a multifunctional pan-neurotrophin. EMBO J 1993; 12:2281–2293.
168. Ibanez CF. Neurotrophic factors: from structure-function studies to designing effective therapeutics [published erratum appears in Trends Biotechnol 1995; 13(8):310]. Trends Biotechnol 1995; 13:217–227.
169. Farinas I, Jones KR, Backus C, Wang XY, Reichardt LF. Severe sensory and sympathetic deficits in mice lacking neurotrophin-3. Nature 1994; 369:658–661.
170. Farinas I, Yoshida CK, Backus C, Reichardt LF. Lack of neurotrophin-3 results in death of spinal sensory neurons and premature differentiation of their precursors. Neuron 1996; 17:1065–1078.
171. Hory Lee F, Russell M, Lindsay RM, Frank E. Neurotrophin 3 supports the survival of developing muscle sensory neurons in culture. Proc Natl Acad Sci USA 1993; 90: 2613–2617.
172. Hohn A, Leibrock J, Bailey K, Barde YA. Identification and characterization of a novel member of the nerve growth factor/brain-derived neurotrophic factor family. Nature 1990; 344:339–341.
173. Oakley RA, Garner AS, Large TH, Frank E. Muscle sensory neurons require neurotrophin-3 from peripheral tissues during the period of normal cell death. Development 1995; 121:1341–1350.
174. Oakley RA, et al. Neurotrophin-3 promotes the differentiation of muscle spindle afferents in the absence of peripheral targets. J Neurosci 1997; 17:4262–4274.
175. Leake PA, Snyder RL, Merzenich MM. Topographic organization of the cochlear spiral ganglion demonstrated by restricted lesions of the anteroventral cochlear nucleus. J Comp Neurol 1992; 320:468–478.
176. Fritzsch B, Silos-Santiago I, Bianchi LM, Farinas I. The role of neurotrophic factors in regulating the development of inner ear innervation. Trends Neurosci 1977; 20: 159–164.
177. Tatagiba M, Brösamle C, Skerra A, Schwab ME. Regeneration of the axotomized auditory nerve in the adult rat promoted by intrathecal application of the IN-1 antibody [Abstract]. Clin Neuropathol 1996; 15:296.
178. Barba D, Hardin J, Ray J, Gage FH. Thymidine kinase-mediated killing of rat brain tumors. J Neurosurg 1993; 79:729–735.
179. Tuszynski MH, et al. Fibroblasts genetically modified to produce nerve growth factor induce robust neuritic ingrowth after grafting to the spinal cord. Exp Neurol 1994; 126:1–14.
180. Ram Z, et al. The effect of thymidine kinase transduction and ganciclovir therapy on tumor vasculature and growth of 9L gliomas in rats. J Neurosurg 1994; 81:256–260.
181. Culver KW, et al. In vivo gene transfer with retroviral vector-producer cells for treatment of experimental brain tumors. Science 1992; 256:1550–1552.
182. Marini FCR, Nelson JA, Lapeyre JN. Assessment of bystander effect potency produced by intratumoral implantation of HSVtk-expressing cells using surrogate marker secretion to monitor tumor growth kinetics. Gene Ther 1995; 2:655–659.
183. Berns AJ, et al. Phase I study of non-replicating autologous tumor cell injections using cells prepared with or without GM-CSF gene transduction in patients with metastatic renal cell carcinoma. Hum Gene Ther 1995; 6:347–368.
184. Dranoff G, et al. Involvement of granulocyte-macrophage colony-stimulating factor in pulmonary homeostasis. Science 1994; 264:713–716.
185. Kafri T, Blömer U, Gage F, Verma I. Highly efficient and sustained gene transfer in muscle and liver with lentiviral vector. Nat Genetics 1997; 17:314–317.
186. Blömer U, et al. Highly efficient and sustained gene transfer in adult neurons with a lentiviral vector. J Virol 1997; 71:6641–6649.
187. Miller AD, Chen F. Retrovirus packaging cells based on 10A1 murine leukemia virus for production of vectors that use multiple receptors for cell entry. J Virol 1996; 70: 5564–5571.
188. Miller AD. Cell-surface receptors for retroviruses and implications for gene transfer. Proc Natl Acad Sci USA 1996; 93:11407–11413.
189. Miller AD, Miller DG, Carcia JV, Lynch CM. Use of retroviral vectors for gene transfer and expression. Methods Enzymol 1993; 217:581–599.

190. Cosset FL, Takeuchi Y, Battini JL, Weiss RA, Collins MK. High-titer packaging cells producing recombinant retroviruses resistant to human serum. J Virol 1995; 69: 7430–7436.
191. Cosset FL, Russell SJ. Targeting retrovirus entry. Gene Ther 1996; 3:946–956.
192. Coffin JM. Virology 1990; 1437–1500.
193. Coffin J. Structure of the retroviral genome. In: Furmanski P, ed. RNA Tumor Viruses. Cold Spring Harbor, NY: Cold Spring Harbor Laboratory, 1984.
194. Blömer U, Naldini L, Verma IM, Trono D, Gage FH. Applications of gene therapy to the CNS. Hum Mol Genet 1996; 5:1397–1404.
195. Naldini L, Blömer U, Gage FH, Trono D, Verma IM. Efficient transfer, integration and sustained long-term expression of the transgene in adult rat brains injected with a lentiviral vector. Proc Natl Acad Sci USA 1996; 93: 11382–11387.
196. Ho DY, Sapolsky RM. Gene therapy for the nervous system. Sci Am 1997; 276:116–120.
197. Horellou P, et al. Direct intracerebral gene transfer of an adenoviral vector expressing tyrosine hydroxylase in a rat model of Parkinson's disease. Neuroreport 1994; 6:49–53.
198. Horellou P, et al. Behavioural effects of genetically engineered cells releasing dopa and dopamine after intracerebral grafting in a rat model of Parkinson's disease. J Physiol (Paris) 1991; 85:158–170.
199. Hock RA, Miller AD, Osborne WR. Expression of human adenosine deaminase from various strong promoters after gene transfer into human hematopoietic cell lines. Blood 1989; 74:876–881.
200. Kaplitt MG, et al. Preproenkephalin promoter yields region-specific and long-term expression in adult brain after direct in vivo gene transfer via a defective herpes simplex viral vector. Proc Natl Acad Sci USA 1994; 91: 8979–8983.
201. Gossen M, Bujard H. Tight control of gene expression in mammalian cells by tetracycline-responsive promoters. Proc Natl Acad Sci USA 1992; 89:5547–5551.
202. Gossen M, Bonin AL, Bujard H. Control of gene activity in higher eukaryotic cells by prokaryotic regulatory elements. Trends Biochem Sci 1993; 18:471–475.
203. Gossen M, Bujard H. Efficacy of tetracycline-controlled gene expression is influenced by cell type: commentary. Biotechniques 1995; 19:213–217.
204. Raymon HK, Thode, S, Palmer TD, Winkler J, Ray J, Fisher LJ, Kang UJ, Thal LJ, Gage FH. Exogenous regulation of human tyrosine hydroxylase transgene expression in genetically modified fibroblasts and neuronal progenitors. Symposium of ventral mesencephalic cell cultures sponsored by NINDS, 1996.

25

Principles of Gene Therapy for Inborn Errors of Metabolism

Jon A. Wolff and Cary O. Harding
University of Wisconsin–Madison, Madison, Wisconsin

I. INTRODUCTION

A. Historical Perspective on Inborn Errors of Metabolism

Inborn errors of metabolism (IEM) have played a central role in the formulation of modern genetics. The hallmark of IEM is the accumulation of a biochemical in a bodily tissue. With the development of chemical analytical techniques, it became possible to identify and measure these biochemicals and correlate them with specific diseases (Fig. 1). Knowledge of metabolic pathways enabled enzymatic defects to be identified, which eventually led to discovery of the cognate proteins and genes.

The appreciation that inborn susceptibilities play important roles in diseases was first promulgated at the beginning of the twentieth century by Alfred Garrod. He formulated the concept of an inherited metabolic disease on the basis of his studies of patients with alkaptonuria, albinism, cystinuria, and pentosuria. Cognizant of the laws of Mendel, he postulated that the relevant biochemical accumulates due to a metabolic block that is inherited in a recessive process.

The one gene–one enzyme principle developed by Beadle and Tatum provided the next conceptual framework for understanding IEM. This principle provides that metabolic processes are the result of specific enzymatic steps, which are under the control of a single gene. A mutation in a gene leads to deficiency of the enzyme that catalyzes the specific step. The molecular basis for a defective enzyme was provided by Pauling and Ingram's experiments on sickle cell anemia, while the molecular basis for a defective gene was provided by Watson and Crick and subsequent elaboration of the central dogma. This dogma defines the flow of information as proceeding from DNA to RNA to protein. The objective of gene therapy is to modulate the flow of genetic information so as to attenuate the disease state.

B. Historical Perspective on Gene Therapy of IEM

IEM have also played a central role in the formulation of gene therapy (1). In fact, many of the first human clinical trials in gene therapy were for IEM. In the late 1960s, S. Rogers attempted to treat three siblings with arginase deficiency by injecting them with the Shope virus on the basis of the incorrect assumption that the virus contained an arginase gene. While being ahead of his time in anticipating the development of viral vectors, the injections had no effect on the subjects' arginine levels. In the more modern era of gene therapy, the first human trials for treating a disease involved children with severe combined immunodeficiency (SCID) caused by a deficiency in adenosine deaminase (ADA).

In addition to human gene therapy trials, IEM have played an important role in the development of gene therapy tools (1). Cell lines deficient in hypoxanthine phosphoribosyl transferase (HPRT) and hypoxanthine/aminopterin/thymidine (HAT) selection media (developed by W. and E. Szybalski) enabled the selection for genetically modified cells that take up the HPRT gene in conjunc-

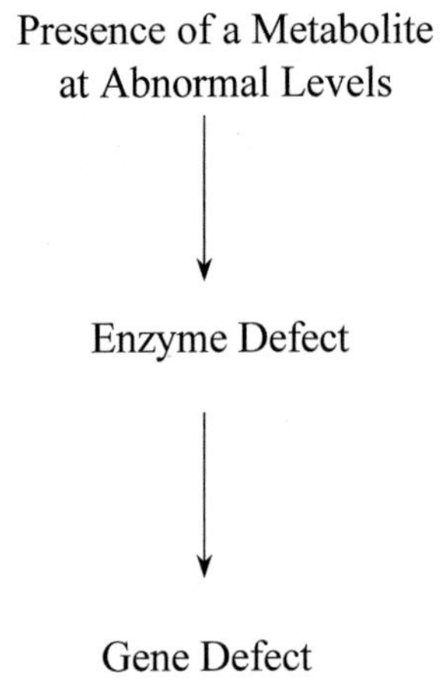

Figure 1 Flow of information in elucidating the genetic basis of metabolic disorders.

tion with other foreign genes. Similarly, cell lines deficient in thymidine kinase (TK) can be used for gene-transfer selection.

With the advent of positional cloning and the human genome project, disorders are being linked to defective genes without any understanding of how metabolism has been disrupted. The current challenge will be to identify how the defective gene leads to a disturbance in development or homeostasis. Gene transfer and expression in animals and humans will provide critical tests for hypotheses of pathogenesis.

II. BASIS FOR GENE THERAPY FOR IEM

A. Types of IEM

One common type of IEM is caused by deficiency of an enzyme that catalyzes the conversion of one chemical to another (Fig. 2a). Deficiency of a specific enzyme can cause disease through three separate mechanisms: (1) excessive accumulation of substrate to toxic levels, (2) deficiency of an essential product, or (3) metabolism of the substrate through alternative biochemical pathways leading to toxic secondary metabolites. Examples of such IEM include phenylketonuria and methylmalonic aciduria.

IEM can also be caused by deficiency of protein that is involved in the transport of metabolite (Fig. 2b). Examples include the cystine transporter in cystinosis and the LDL (low-density lipoprotein) receptor in familial hypercholesterolemia.

Other genes relevant to IEM are required for the proper formation of organelles (Fig. 2c). Neonatal adrenoleukodystrophy and Zellweger syndrome are caused by defects in genes that are required for the proper formation of peroxisomes.

B. Different Pathogenesis Models for IEM

The pathogenesis of IEM can be explained by several models (Fig. 3). One major category includes IEM in which organ dysfunction occurs by a circulating toxic metabolite (Fig. 3a). Another major category is organ dysfunction resulting from a cell autonomous process (Fig. 3b). While these concepts are useful in formulating gene therapy approaches, it should be appreciated that they are only models and that our understanding of the pathogenesis for many IEM is incomplete. In fact, gene therapy trials may provide decisive information concerning the mechanism by which the metabolic defect leads to the diseased state.

C. Circulating Toxic Metabolite

In this class of disorder, a metabolite accumulates in one tissue as result of an enzymatic deficiency (Fig. 3a). This leads to increased metabolite levels in the blood and toxicity in other tissues. The prototype for this type of disorder is phenylketonuria in which deficiency of hepatic phenylalanine hydroxylase leads to increased blood levels of phenylalanine and toxic effects to the developing brain. Familial hypercholesterolemia is another IEM that fits this model. Deficiency of the LDL receptor in the liver leads to increased levels of LDL and subsequent damage to the coronary arteries.

A corollary of this model is intraorgan toxicity from a metabolite that accumulates in an extracellular space within the affected tissue. It is particularly applicable to the central nervous system. Some IEM associated with neurological dysfunction may be caused by a toxic metabolite that accumulates within the brain and circulates in the cerebral spinal fluid (CSF). Gene therapy could then be predicated on providing gene expression in any cell within the brain as long as the expressed enzyme could lower levels of the toxic metabolite in the CNS. The cerebral spinal fluid could provide the conduit for such exchange.

A metabolic defect in one tissue could also harm another tissue by decreasing the circulating level of a metabolite. For example, a defect in gluconeogenesis that occurs in the liver and muscle (e.g., glycogen storage disorder) can cause hypoglycemia and damage to the brain.

D. Cell Autonomous Toxicity

In other IEM, the metabolic defect only leads to toxicity to the cell that has the metabolic deficiency (Fig. 3b). Cellular toxicity results from either increased or decreased levels of a metabolite within the affected cell. For these disorders, gene therapy would be effective only if the normal gene is targeted to the dysfunctional cell.

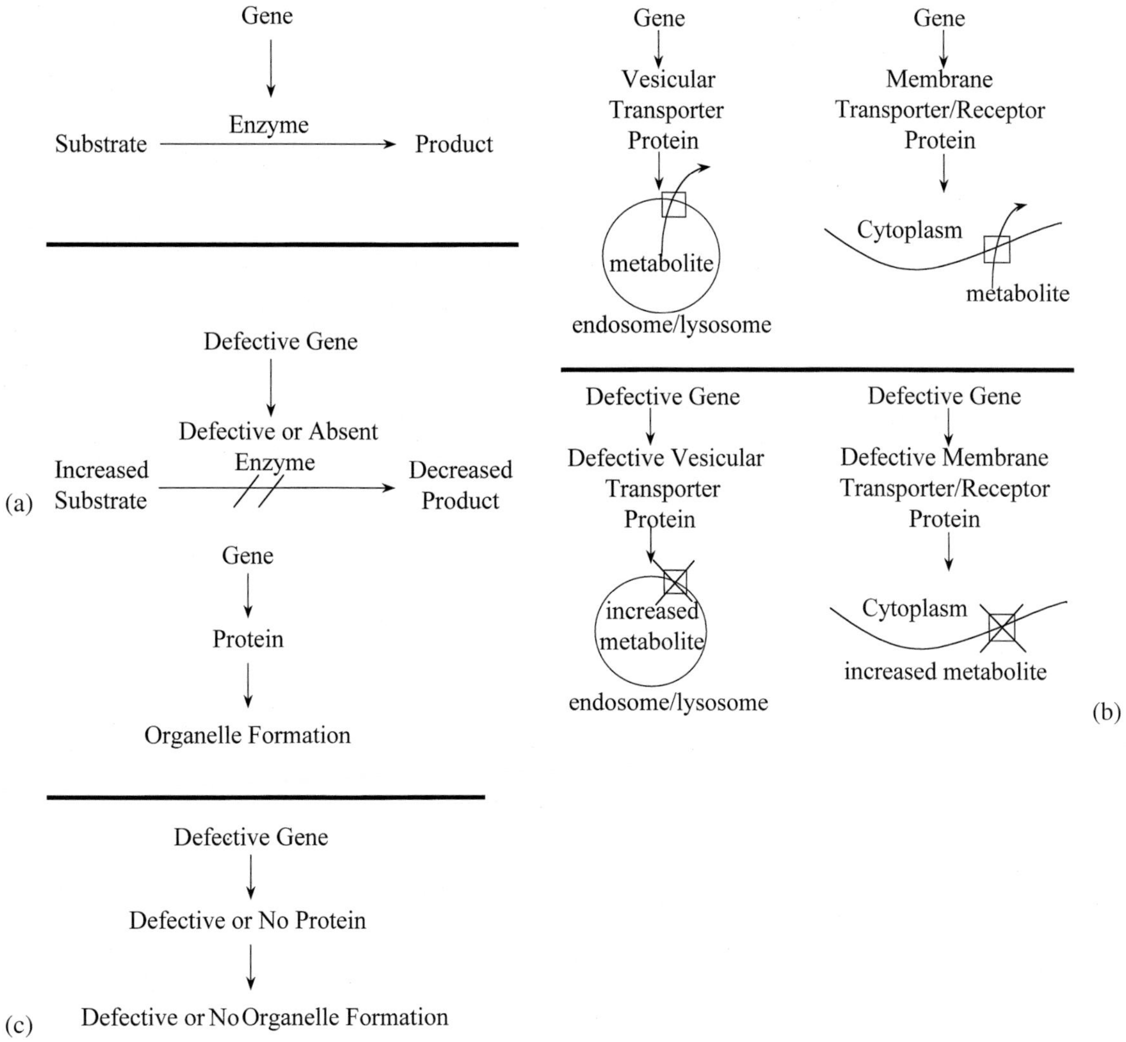

Figure 2 The types of normal functions that are disrupted in IEMs: (a) defects in enzymatic activity; (b) defects in the uptake or transport of metabolites; (c) defects in the formation of organelles.

E. Method of Gene Correction

A variety of parameters of expression are important determinants of the ability of gene therapy to treat specific disorders. Some generalizations can be made concerning the expression requirements for IEM (Table 1). Most IEM are recessive conditions, and addition of a single gene copy is sufficient to correct the disease phenotype. In effect, gene addition converts the patient to a biochemical state analogous to that of a carrier. For those patients with single point mutations, targeted gene correction using gene conversion or homologous recombination is a possible therapy, but gene correction is not necessary if a functional gene can be added. The obvious therapeutic gene to be added in IEM is the human gene that is defective in the disease state, but it is conceivable that a therapeutic effect could be achieved using another gene. For example, a gene from another species could metabolize a toxic metabolite by a different mechanism.

F. Requirements for Expression Persistence

For most IEM, gene expression does not have to be regulated and can be constant. Most genes involved in IEM are considered ''housekeeping'' genes. In contrast, in diabetes mellitus, insulin expression has to be regulated in response to blood glucose levels.

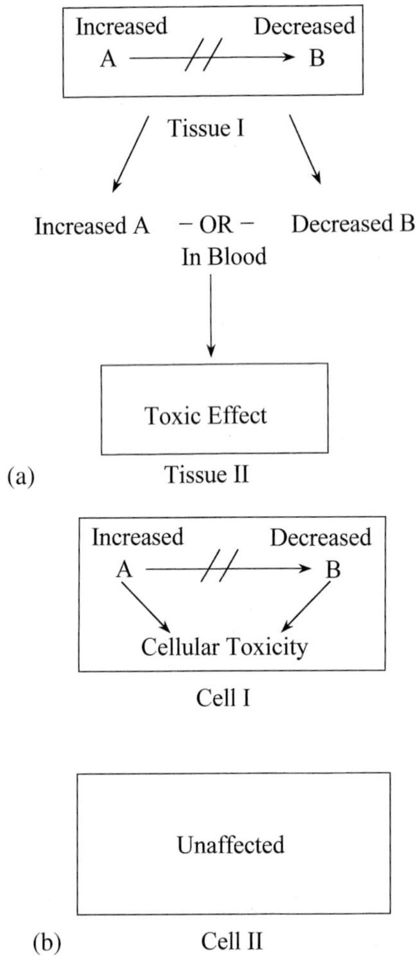

Figure 3 Two models by which IEM leads to cellular toxicity: (a) circulating toxic metabolite; (b) cell autonomous toxicity.

Table 1 Generalizations Concerning Expression Requirements for Gene Therapy of IEM

Expression parameter	Requirement
Method of modification	Gene addition is sufficient
Therapeutic gene	Normal gene that is defective in patient
Duration	Persistent
Regulation	Not needed
Levels	>5% of normal levels
Target tissues	Liver, CNS, blood cells, muscle, heterologous expression possible in some disorders

Given that IEM are chronic conditions, persistent expression is needed. It would be best if gene correction and therefore a ''cure'' could be done with one or few administrations. If expression cannot be persistent after one gene dose, then repetitive administrations are required. Repetitive administrations can be problematic for some vectors such as adenoviral vectors that induce neutralizing antibodies. Loss of expression from vectors can be a result of removal of the foreign DNA, promoter suppression, or rejection of the foreign gene product.

Immune effects can arise even if the gene product is intracellular since all parts of proteins are presented to the immune system via the MHC I complex. The important issue is whether, in the disease state, the patient expresses any residual native protein and is immunologically tolerant to the normal gene product. One measure of this is whether tissues from the patient exhibit cross-reactive material (CRM), protein that cross-reacts with antibodies against the native protein. This is best determined by performing immunoblot (Western blot) analysis. Even if protein is not present, native protein could have been produced but be unstable. Expression of the foreign gene in such a patient may not induce an immune effect since the protein is not recognized as foreign. Further experience is necessary to determine whether the immune system will prevent stable expression of the normal gene in patients with IEM.

G. Requirements for Expression Levels

The level of expression is a critical determinant for the success of a gene therapy. For most IEM, foreign gene expression only has to be greater than 5% of normal levels in order to attenuate the majority of the diseased state. This is based upon clinical experience in which the percent of residual enzyme activity is correlated with the phenotype. In many IEM, people with more than 5% of normal enzymatic activity are free of symptoms. If enzymatic activity is between 1 and 5%, their clinical course is less severe than patients with 0% of enzymatic activity.

While the total enzymatic activity is one measure, the percent of cells expressing the foreign gene may also be important. Overexpression in a few cells may not lead to a therapeutic effect if the expressed enzyme alone cannot completely produce the metabolic conversion. The protein deficient in the patient may be part of an enzymatic complex so that overexpression of one component would not necessarily lead to higher activity of the complete complex. Similarly, other enzymatic steps, cofactors, or transport of metabolites may limit the ability for the cell to perform the required metabolic conversion at a rate higher than the normal level. If so, the therapeutic gene has to be expressed in more than 5% of the target cells.

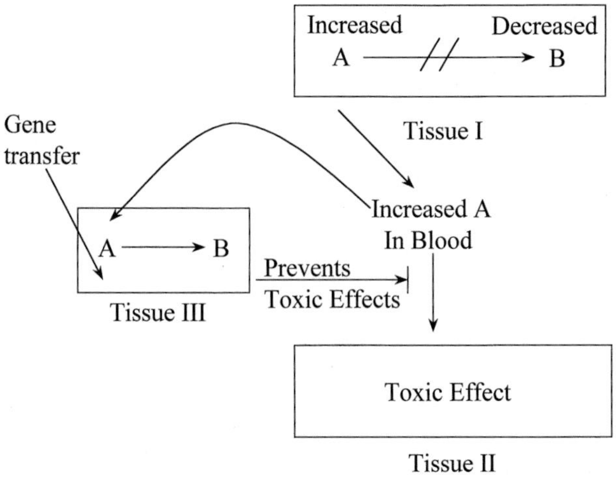

Figure 4 Heterologous tissue expression of a therapeutic gene to treat an IEM in which a circulating toxic metabolite causes the diseased state.

H. Target Tissues

Details of the pathogenesis for the IEM need to be understood, and the target tissue has to be tailored for each disorder. For IEM that fit the ''circulating toxic metabolite'' model, the therapeutic gene does not necessarily have to be targeted to the tissue that normally expresses the affected gene (Fig. 4). Although correction of the deficient enzymatic activity in the affected organ would be most straightforward, expression within a heterologous tissue (different from that that normally expresses the enzyme) could clear the circulating toxic metabolite and attenuate the disease state. In order for this approach to be effective, the enzyme must be functional within the heterologous tissue. Restrictions on enzymatic function can include requirements for protein subunits, cofactors, substrate, and clearance of product. Given the ability for several gene-transfer systems (e.g., plasmid DNA, adenoviral vectors, and AAV vectors) to express foreign genes stably in muscle, it will be a useful tissue for many heterologous gene therapy approaches. Blood cells derived from genetically modified stem cells are another candidate tissue for heterologous gene expression if the problems associated with stable foreign expression are solved.

For IEM that fit the ''cell autonomous'' model, expression within the affected cell is generally required. The exception is for the lysosomal storage disorders in which the enzyme can be transferred from one cell to another.

For IEM that affect the brain, ''global'' gene expression throughout the brain may be required. Alternatively, specific neurological symptoms could be treated by targeting specific regions of the brain. For example, in Lesch-Nyhan syndrome, choreathetoid movements could be treated by targeting the basal ganglia.

I. Mitochondrial Disorders of Oxidative Phosphorylation

Several IEM are caused by defective oxidative phosphorylation within the respiratory chain complex of mitochondria. An unique feature of mitochondria is that 13 of the more than 80 respiratory chain subunits are encoded within the mitochondrial genome. The mitochondria also contain 22 transfer RNA (tRNA) and two ribosomal RNA that enable protein synthesis within the mitochondria. The remaining 70 or so respiratory chain subunits are encoded within the nuclear genome. These proteins are produced within the cytoplasm and contain an amino terminus that target their entry into the mitochondria by interacting with a number of chaperone and transport proteins.

For disorders caused by mutations in the nuclear encoded respiratory chain genes, the gene therapy approaches described above are germane. However, disorders caused by mutations in the mitochondrial genome offer additional challenges for gene therapy. One approach would be to express the deficient subunit within the nucleus regardless of its native mitochondrial origin. The subunit could be modified to contain an amino leader sequence to enable entry into the mitochondria.

The other approach of genetically modifying the mitochondrial genome is at an early conceptual stage. Toward this end, a peptide mitochondria-targeting sequence has been covalently attached to oligonucleotide to enable mitochondrial entry. The oligonucleotide could correct a point mutation by some type of gene conversion or recombination process. Point mutations occur in mitochondrial disorders such as Leber hereditary optic atrophy (LHON), myoclonic epilepsy and ragged-red fiber disease (MERRF), and mitochondrial encephalomyopathy, lactic acidosis, and strokelike episodes (MELAS). An alternative treatment approach would be the addition of functional tRNA genes to patients with mitochondrial disorders such as MERRF or MELAS that are caused by tRNA mutations. The treatment of mitochondrial DNA deletion diseases would require the delivery of larger DNA sequences ($>$ 5 kb), which would be more challenging. Deletions occurs in disorders such as Kearns-Sayre syndrome. Another option would be to deliver normal mitochondria en toto.

Different mitochondria can proliferate in a tissue at different rates. This may explain why inborn and somatic (acquired) mitochondrial defects often present in later life. Any genetic modification of mitochondria must enable the corrected mitochondria to have a proliferation advantage over the abnormal mitochondria in order to achieve a permanent cure. A final challenge for mitochondrial disorders is that they often involve the nervous system, which is less accessible than other organs to therapeutic endeavors.

J. Newborn and Prenatal Screening

Gene therapy for IEM will have a significant impact on newborn screening programs and vice versa. Screening for IEM at birth enables gene therapy to be initiated prior to the onset of symptoms and any irreversible tissue damage and thereby increases the value of the gene therapy. Irreversible brain damage occurs in many IEM when a neonatal metabolic crisis is not prevented. For example, the extent of perinatal hyperammonemia in a urea cycle defect, ornithine transcarbomylase deficiency (OTC), has been directly correlated with intelligence in later life.

One criterion for the initiation of newborn screening for a particular disorder is whether an effective treatment exists. The development of effective gene therapy for a disorder could satisfy this criterion. Another criterion is the availability of a reliable, inexpensive laboratory method for disease detection.

Currently, most states in the United States and many other nations are screening for phenylketonuria and galactosemia. Screening for maple syrup urine disease or homocysteinemia is less common. Tandem mass spectroscopy procedures are being developed for analyzing in blood spots amino acids and organic acids conjugated to carnitine (acylcarnitines) in order to detect many of the disorders in amino acid and fat metabolism and organic acidurias. Such comprehensive newborn screening programs developed in conjunction with new gene therapies will have a major impact on the morbidity and mortality of IEM.

Many IEM can be reliably diagnosed in the prenatal period. As intrauterine gene therapy approaches are developed, IEM will be good candidates for such approaches. One potential advantage of prenatal approaches may be a decreased chance of an immune recognition of the therapeutic gene product.

III. GENE THERAPY OF SPECIFIC DISORDERS

A comprehensive review of the tremendous progress in the gene therapy for IEM is beyond the scope of this review. In fact, gene therapy studies have been conducted in almost every type of IEM. Instead, specific IEM were chosen either because they illustrate the above principles or for their important historical role.

A. Aminoacidopathies

The aminoacidopathies are a heterogeneous group of recessively inherited enzyme deficiencies that are associated with the accumulation of specific amino acids in blood and other tissues. The best known and most studied aminoacidopathy is phenylketonuria (PKU) (Table 2) caused by deficiency of the liver enzyme phenylalanine hydroxylase (PAH) (Fig. 5). PAH deficiency prevents the hydroxylation of phenylalanine to tyrosine and leads to excessive accumulation of phenylalanine in the body. If PKU is left untreated in an infant, poor brain and physical growth, seizures, and mental retardation will result from increased levels of the circulating toxic metabolite phenylalanine. Other examples of aminoacidopathies include tyrosinemia, maple syrup urine disease, homocystinuria, and ornithine transcarbamoylase (OTC) deficiency (Table 2). Each of these enzyme deficiencies leads to the accumulation of a different specific substrate and causes a different symptom complex.

Contemporary therapy for these diseases is based upon an understanding of the pathogenesis involved in each case, and the design of any gene therapy protocol must also be grounded upon a rational understanding of the specific disease pathophysiology. For example, high levels of phenylalanine in PKU are toxic to the developing brain, and reducing blood phenylalanine levels is critical to successful treatment of PKU. However, some symptoms of PKU may be caused by deficiencies of specific neurotransmitters, such as dopamine, that are synthesized from tyrosine. In tyrosinemia, elevated tyrosine levels do not appear to be directly toxic, but production of the toxic metabolite succinylacetone through an alternative biochemical pathway causes severe liver damage. So, for PKU, a successful therapy will both remove phenylalanine and restore tyrosine levels, while removal of tyrosine from individuals with tyrosinemia is less important than stopping the production of succinylacetone. These considerations must play a role in the design of any gene therapy protocol.

In many aminoacidopathies, the deficient enzyme is normally either exclusively or primarily expressed in liver; liver is the obvious target for gene transfer in these diseases (2). However, for select disorders, circulating toxic metabolites may be effectively removed from the body by enzyme expressed in a tissue other than liver. The concept of expressing in an alternative tissue a protein that is normally restricted to a specific organ is known as heterologous gene therapy. As an example, PAH expression in skeletal muscle, if supplied with the necessary cofactors, might effectively clear phenylalanine from the circulation of a person with PKU. Gene targeting to the liver may not be essential for some aminoacidopathies. For other diseases, specific pathophysiological features limit the effectiveness of a heterologous gene therapy approach. In OTC deficiency, the substrate for OTC, carbamyl phosphate, is produced only locally in the liver and does not appear in the circulation.

Table 2 Summary of Select Amino Acidopathies

Disease	Deficient enzyme	Elevated blood amino acids	Animal model?
Phenylketonuria	Phenylalanine hydroxylase (PAH)	Phenylalanine	*Pah*^{enu2} mouse
Tyrosinemia type I	Fumarylacetoacetate hydrolase (FAH)	Tyrosine	FAH knockout mouse
Ornithine transcarbamoylase deficiency	Ornithine transcarbamoylase (OTC)	Glutamine; elevated blood ammonia	Sparse fur (*spf*) mouse
Maple syrup urine disease (MSUD)	Branched-chain keto acid dehydrogenase	Leucine, valine, isoleucine	Hereford inbred calf maple syrup urine disease
Homocystinuria	Cystathionine β-synthase	Homocystine	None

In tyrosinemia, liver damage is mediated by local production of succinylacetone in hepatocytes; removal of succinylacetone from the circulation without preventing its production in the liver might not alter the course of tyrosinemia. If possible, disease-specific pathophysiological features and the effectiveness of any gene therapy approach should be demonstrated in an animal model of the disease, if one is available, prior to application of the method in humans. Table 2 lists animal models available for the study of some amino acidopathies.

Gene-transfer experiments to treat PKU illustrate the difficulties and complexities of gene therapy for aminoacidopathies and other liver diseases (2). The availability of a mouse model, the *Pah*^{enu2} mouse, that accurately portrays human PAH deficiency has allowed significant advances in PKU gene therapy research. Soon after cloning the PAH gene, Dr. Savio Woo and colleagues pioneered gene transfer into liver and demonstrated that PAH activity could be expressed in cultured fibroblasts or PAH-deficient hepatocytes from a PAH cDNA. This was accomplished using a variety of gene transfer vectors including recombinant retrovirus. Scaling up to perform retroviral-mediated liver-directed gene therapy in a whole animal proved more problematic. Integration of the retroviral DNA into the target genome requires mitotic division of the target cell; the mitotic rate of hepatocytes in vivo is estimated to be only about 1% per year in humans. So, retroviral-mediated liver-directed gene therapy requires an ex vivo approach in which part of the liver is surgically removed from an animal, the hepatocytes are cultured, allowed to divide, transfected with the recombinant retrovirus, and then the treated hepatocytes are infused back into the animal via the portal venous system. Using this approach and the β-galactosidase reporter gene, Woo and colleagues demonstrated that approximately 1% of the hepatocytes in the liver of a dog could be induced to permanently express the reporter gene. Unfortunately, successful treatment of PKU (and probably other aminoacidopathies) requires enzymatic reconstitution of at least 5–10% of the liver. Successful retroviral-mediated ex vivo gene therapy in the PKU mouse has not been reported. This approach has, however, been employed successfully in the treatment of murine tyrosinemia type I (3). In this mouse model, enzymatically corrected hepatocytes have a survival advantage over enzyme-deficient cells in the host; although they initially constitute only a very small fraction of the liver, retrovirus-treated enzyme-expressing hepatocytes gradually repopulate the entire liver. Recombinant retroviral-mediated gene therapy may be useful for disorders that require correction of only 1–2% of the liver to effect a phenotypic change or in situations where corrected cells have a competitive advantage over the native hepatocytes.

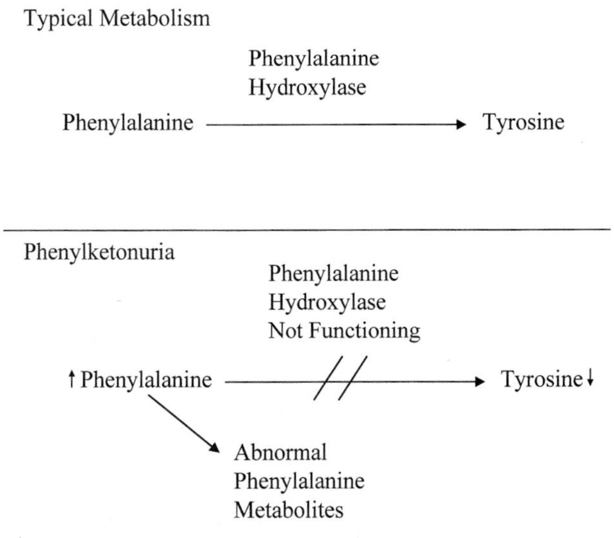

Figure 5 Pathogenesis of phenylketonuria.

Recombinant adenoviral vectors are another promising gene delivery vehicle for in vivo application. In contrast to retroviral vectors, recombinant adenovirus can be produced and purified to higher titers and are capable of efficiently infecting nondividing cells. A recombinant adenovirus containing the PAH cDNA has been infused into the portal circulation of PKU mice (4). In this experiment, hepatic PAH activity was reconstituted to 5–20% of control levels. Complete normalization of plasma phenylalanine levels occurred in animals with hepatic PAH activity equivalent to at least 10% of that in control animals. However, the effect had disappeared by 3 weeks following the treatment, and no hepatic PAH activity was detected following a second treatment with the adenoviral vector. The stability of expression from adenoviral vectors administered in vivo is limited by the immune response of the host against the vector or the reporter gene product. In experimental trials of adenovirus-mediated, liver-directed gene therapy employing a variety of different therapeutic genes to treat several different animal models, gene expression has been stable for 7–10 days and then has decreased to undetectable levels over the next few weeks.

Further alteration of the adenoviral genome has resulted in recombinant adenovirus that is less immunogenic than first-generation adenovirus vectors. Liver OTC deficiency in the sparse fur mouse was corrected for at least 2 months following infusion of a second-generation recombinant adenovirus containing the human OTC cDNA (15). This vector is currently being used in a human clinical trial involving adult females with partial OTC deficiency. Further efforts to develop even more effective adenoviral vectors continues.

The search for the ideal liver-directed gene-transfer vector continues. Along with further modification of recombinant adenovirus vectors, the development of new viral and nonviral vectors targeted to liver has expanded the therapeutic armamentarium of the gene therapist. Early animal trials with recombinant adeno-associated virus (AAV) and lentivirus vectors have shown substantially better persistence of gene expression than with recombinant adenovirus and much higher levels of gene product than with recombinant retrovirus. Nonviral methods such as infusion of naked plasmid DNA under physical and osmotic pressure directly into the venous circulation of liver or the bile duct aim to altogether avoid difficulties with immunogenic effects of a viral delivery system. Although much further research in animal models is needed before human clinical trials should be attempted, several new gene-delivery systems demonstrate the promise of physiologically significant stable gene expression in liver.

B. Organic Acidurias

Propionic aciduria and methylmalonic aciduria are two organic acidurias that have been well studied and are excellent candidates for gene therapy (Fig. 6). In severe cases, patients present in the neonatal period with coma, metabolic ketoacidosis, and hyperammonemia. With vigorous medical support, they can survive this initial metabolic crisis, but they then must adhere to a strict diet restricted in protein intake. Despite dietary therapy, they continue to have metabolic crises that can be life-threatening. Given the inadequacy of dietary therapy, a gene therapy approach is needed.

Both disorders are caused by enzyme deficiencies in the metabolism of three-carbon species that are generated from the catabolism of amino acids and other metabolites (Fig. 6). Methylmalonic aciduria is caused by a deficiency of methylmalonyl-CoA carboxylase activity that is a result of a defect either in the apoenzyme or in the active form of vitamin B_{12}. Patients with the latter defect often respond well to treatment with large amounts of vitamin B_{12} and are therefore in less need of gene therapy.

The prominent target tissue for both disorders is presumed to be the liver. Hepatorenal transplantation has been successfully employed in a patient with a severe form of methylmalonic aciduria. Nonetheless, the major pathology associated with these organic acidurias is due to circulating toxic metabolites. The associated enzymes are normally expressed in many tissues including leukocytes, muscle, and fibroblasts. Therefore, these heterologous tissues should be explored in gene therapy preclinical studies. Unfortunately, animal models for these disorders do not exist at the present time.

Five percent of normal enzymatic activity in either propionic aciduria or methylmalonic aciduria is associated with a benign clinical course, indicating that this level of expression in a gene therapy should be sufficient to realize a large clinical benefit. This level of expression may have to be distributed over approximately 5% of the cells because overexpression of the relevant genes may not lead to a proportional increase in metabolic flux through the three-carbon pathway. For example, in propionic aciduria, the propionyl-CoA carboxylase has two different subunits, α and β. In patients with a defect in the β subunit, overexpression would require gene transfer with both subunits. However, in patients with a defect in the α subunit, overexpression of the α subunit may be sufficient because the β subunit is produced in a fivefold excess over that of the α subunit.

C. Lysosomal Storage Diseases

The common feature of lysosomal storage diseases is the inappropriate accumulation of normal cellular components within lysosomes. This storage of material is visible in cells by light microscopy as very large lysosomes that displace

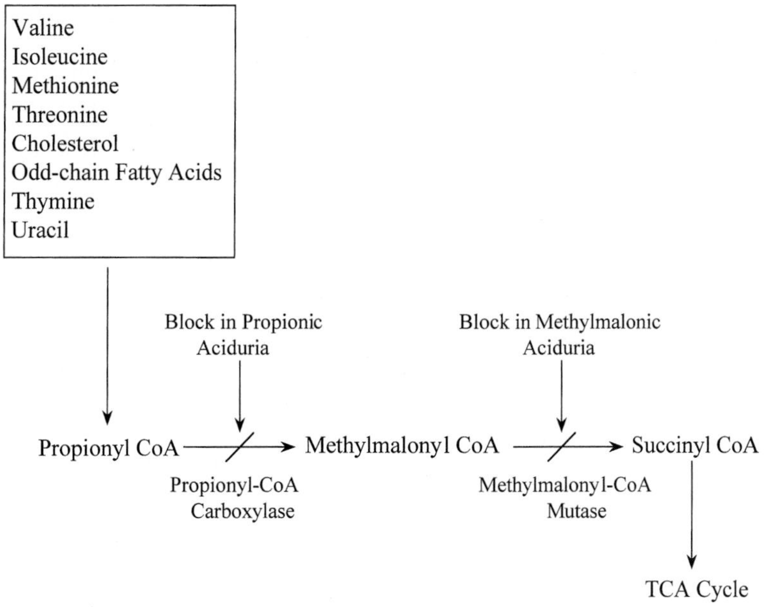

Figure 6 Enzymatic deficiencies in methylmalonic aciduria or propionic aciduria. TCA = Tricarboxylic acid cycle.

a large part of the cytoplasm. This class of disorders is caused by deficiency of specific lysosomal enzymes that are required for the degradation and recycling of glycoproteins and other cellular components. Without a specific degradative enzyme, the substrate for the reaction accumulates and cannot be removed from the lysosome. The clinical phenotype of each disease is dependent upon the tissue type most affected by storage and by the accumulation rate. Physical findings that are suggestive of lysosomal storage include enlargement of the liver and spleen, anemia and thrombocytopenia due to replacement of normal bone marrow by stored material, destruction of bone, and for those enzymatic deficiencies that cause lysosomal storage in neurons, severe developmental regression, seizures, and other neurological symptoms. Not all of these problems are present in all lysosomal storage diseases; each different enzymatic deficiency presents with a specific phenotypic complex.

The challenges of gene therapy for lysosomal storage diseases are illustrated by the results of contemporary treatment with enzyme-replacement therapy or bone marrow transplantation. A major challenge to treating a lysosomal storage disease with gene therapy (in contrast to treatment of a liver enzymopathy) is the necessity of reversing lysosomal storage in multiple separate tissues. No currently available gene-transfer technique is capable of delivering DNA to multiple target tissues efficiently. However, many lines of evidence demonstrate that lysosomal enzyme proteins can be produced in isolated tissues or even purified ex vivo and effectively delivered to most target tissues. For example, glucocerebrosidase, the enzyme deficient in Gaucher' disease can be produced in vitro using standard recombinant techniques, chemically modified to facilitate lysosomal targeting, and delivered to affected organs by simple intravenous infusion. This therapy if repeated periodically dramatically reduces liver and spleen size, corrects anemia and thrombocytopenia, and possibly prevents bone deterioration, all major debilitating features of Gaucher's disease. So, at least for gene therapy of Gaucher's disease, the enzyme would not need to be locally produced in all affected tissues. The enzyme could potentially be produced in a single target tissue, secreted into the circulation, and taken up by other diseased tissues. The major limitation of this approach is the difficulty of engineering a secreted form of the enzyme that would be efficiently taken up by other cells and incorporated into lysosomes.

Alternatively, the enzyme could be transferred from the site of production to diseased tissues via circulating blood cells. Seminal experiments demonstrated that functional lysosomal enzymes may be transferred directly from a normal cell to an enzyme-deficient cell in tissue culture. Bone marrow transplantation in the treatment of lysosomal storage diseases exploits this phenomenon. Replacement of enzyme-deficient host bone marrow with enzyme-sufficient donor bone marrow yields a population of circulating blood cells of the reticuloendothelial lineage that infiltrates tissues and transfers lysosomal enzyme to the native cells. Bone marrow transplantation has been employed successfully in Gaucher's disease and in select other storage diseases that do not exhibit brain involvement. Apparently either insufficient numbers of corrected cells penetrate the central nervous system or insufficient enzyme is transferred to neurons to successfully ameliorate the neurological phenotype of many lysosomal storage disorders. Presumably, difficulties with correcting enzyme deficiency in the brain will also be a major obstacle to successful gene therapy.

Gene therapy for lysosomal storage diseases has to date focused upon gene transfer into bone marrow stem cells for the purpose of supplying enzyme via circulating reticuloendothelial cells (6). Enzymatic correction of Gaucher bone marrow cells in culture has been accomplished with recombinant retroviral vectors. Similar experiments using other lysosomal enzymes in both cultured bone marrow and fibroblasts have been successful. Persistent production of enzyme in circulating blood cells has been demonstrated in rodents. Phenotypic improvement following retroviral-mediated gene transfer into bone marrow has been shown in gus^{mps}/gus^{mps} mice, a β-glucuronidase–deficient mouse model of human mucopolysaccharidosis type VII. As expected, enzymatic correction of bone marrow resulted in amelioration of the somatic symptoms but did not arrest progressive neurological deterioration in this model. However, lysosomal storage in the brain did decrease in mice that had received intracerebral β-glucuronidase–expressing fibroblast implants. Clinical trials of retroviral-mediated bone marrow stem cell–directed gene therapy are underway in humans with Gaucher's disease and in patients with Hunter's syndrome (mucopolysaccharidosis type II) who have little central nervous system involvement.

D. Lesch-Nyhan Syndrome

This X-linked syndrome is caused by a deficiency in hypoxanthine phosphoribosyl transferase (HPRT), an enzyme required for salvaging purines (Fig. 7). It is characterized clinically by increased blood and urine uric acid, mental retardation, choreoathetoid movements, and, most extraordinarily, self-mutilation. It is not understood how a deficiency in HPRT leads to these remarkable neurological sequelae. A genetic mouse model completely lacking HPRT activity does not exhibit any neurological dysfunction except when stressed with amphetamine administration or inhibition of adenine phosphoribosyl transferase (APRT) with 9-ethyladenine. The choreoathetoid movement disorder, however, is postulated to be due to dysfunction within the basal ganglion secondary to disturbed dopamine metabolism.

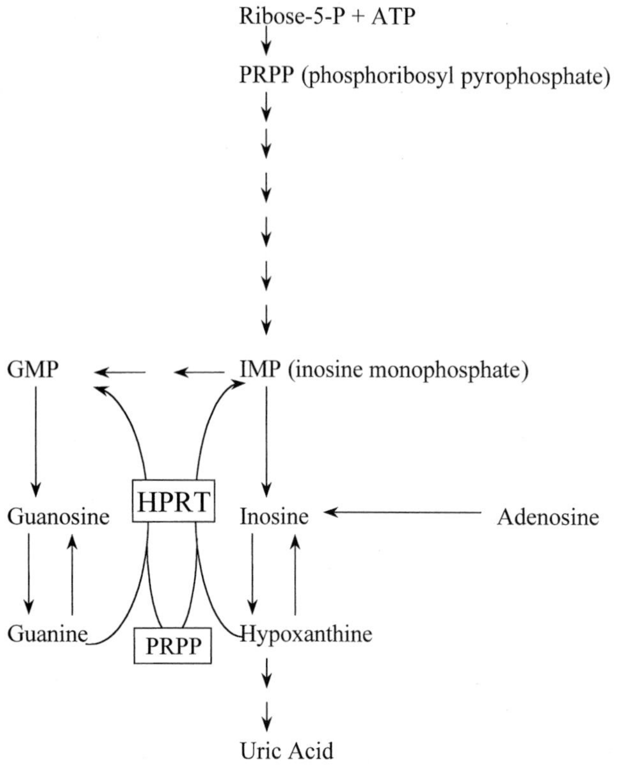

Figure 7 Enzymatic deficiency in Lesch-Nyhan syndrome.

While the hyperuric acidemia and its sequela can be controlled with allopurinol, the absence of treatment for the neurological symptoms has prompted the search for gene therapy approaches. Historically, Lesch-Nyhan syndrome has played an important role in the development of gene therapy. One of the first demonstrations of the ability of retroviral vectors to correct a genetic mutation was done using the human HPRT gene. The first animal experiment in which a foreign gene was expressed in the brain was done by intracerebrally transplanting fibroblasts genetically modified to express the human HPRT (7). Although HPRT is expressed in all cells, its high levels in the basal ganglia suggest that this area of the brain should be targeted for gene transfer. Prevention of the mental retardation may require more global expression within the brain.

The amount of normal gene expression required to effect relief can be extrapolated from clinical experience. While it was previously thought that the severity of the syndrome was not correlated with residual enzymatic activity, it is now realized that its severity does correlate with the amount of HPRT activity in whole cells. Patients with

1.6–8% of normal activity had choreoathetosis but not mental retardation or self-mutilation.

In summary, this syndrome is an example of a genetic disorder in which therapy is lacking even when so much is known about its genetic and molecular basis. The development of effective gene-transfer methods into the brain may not only provide a therapy but will be quite revealing about its pathogenesis.

E. Familial Hypercholesterolemia

Gene therapy has the potential to significantly improve the clinical status of patients with familial hypercholesterolemia (FH), which is caused by a defect in the LDL receptor (LDLR) (Fig. 8). Deficiency in this receptor leads to reduced clearance of LDL by the liver and higher blood levels of LDL. In addition, affected individuals synthesize more cholesterol since the inhibitory effect of LDL on cholesterol synthesis is lost. This inhibition results from decreased HMG CoA reductase activity, the rate-limiting step in cholesterol synthesis.

Heterozygotes with LDLR deficiency occur at a frequency of 1:500 (as common as insulin-dependent diabetes mellitus), making it one of the most common genetic disorders in the United States, Europe, and Japan. Such patients have a twofold elevation in plasma cholesterol levels (300–600 mg/dL) and may develop coronary artery disease by the fourth decade of life. Three to six percent of survivors of myocardial infarctions are heterozygotes for FH.

Homozygotes with LDLR deficiency occur much more infrequently (1 in a million), but have much higher cholesterol levels (600–1000 mg/dL) and invariably die from coronary artery disease in their twenties. The severity of the sequelae is attenuated in the homozygotes by a few percent residual LDLR activity. Deaths were much less frequent in those homozygotes who had at least 10% of normal LDLR activity. This indicates that clinical benefit could be achieved by a gene therapy in which only a small percentage of LDLR activity is restored. Furthermore, the severity of this disorder increases the benefit-to-risk ratio of clinical trials and thereby facilitates them. A gene therapy protocol can be first tested in the homozygotes (aided by Orphan Drug Status) and then extended to the more common heterozygotes.

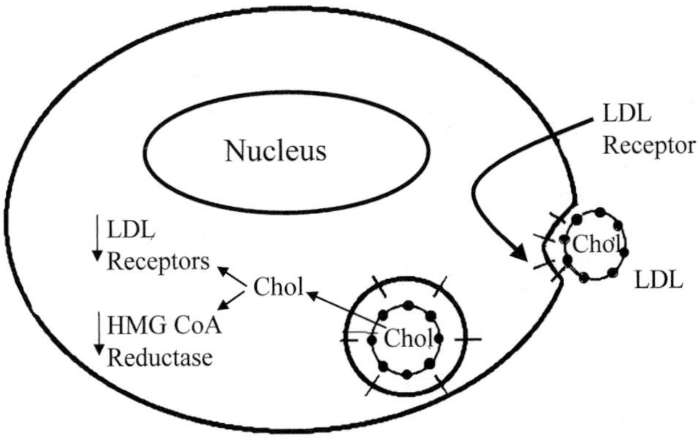

Figure 8 Pathogenesis of familial hypercholesterolemia. Chol = Cholesterol; HMG = 3-hydroxymethylglutaryl.

Liver transplantation in children has proven that correction of the LDL receptor defect in the liver can normalize cholesterol levels. For this reason, gene therapy techniques for FH have been directed at the hepatocyte. Based upon preclinical studies in mouse and rabbit LDLR-deficient models, ex vivo gene therapy in five homozygous FH patients using retrovirus-mediated LDL receptor gene transfer was performed. This technically challenging protocol yielded a highly variable metabolic response with some improvement in only one of the patients (8). This study indicates that important modifications must be made to the ex vivo gene-transfer method before gene therapy can be used as a general therapeutic procedure for such patients (9).

Given the borderline results of the human clinical trial, efforts were initiated with adenoviral vectors carrying the LDLR gene. In vivo adenovirus-mediated transfer of the LDL receptor was shown to be highly effective in reversing the hypercholesterolemia in LDL receptor knockout mice and WHHL rabbits (10). The important limitation of adenoviral-mediated gene transfer remains the transient expression in vivo after infection of somatic cells with recombinant adenovirus. Nonetheless, these studies demonstrate the proof of principle for the gene therapy of FH by the transfer of the normal LDLR gene and highlight the inadequacies of current gene-transfer methods.

Current therapy for hypercholesterolemia (not limited to homozygotic FH) includes the use of HMG-CoA reductase inhibitors, which work by secondarily inducing expression of the LDLR, thereby lowering plasma LDL levels. These agents not only lower serum cholesterol but also lower all-cause mortality by at least 30% in men and women who have coronary disease and total cholesterol levels of 215–300 mg/dL. However, 2% of patients suffer liver toxicity and 0.2% develop muscle disease requiring cessation of drug administration. These drugs have to be taken once or twice every day for extended periods of time, and compliance is often difficult. A gene therapeutic agent that is administered less than every month (even by intravenous injection) would offer substantial benefit to the patient.

At high efficiencies of liver gene transfer, LDLR gene transfer into the liver could be used to prevent coronary artery disease in the general population. Taking into account all types of hypercholesterolemias, the third National Health and Nutrition Examination Survey (NHANES III) concluded that lipid lowering therapy was required for 29% of Americans over 20 years of age (11). The Cholesterol and Recurrent Events study showed that patients with coronary artery disease but having "normal" LDL cholesterol levels benefited from treatment with a single statin therapy (12). The positive correlation between LDL levels and coronary artery disease is a continuum. In addition, overexpression of the normal LDL receptor in the liver of transgenic mice (four to five times that of the endogenous receptor) prevented diet-induced hypercholesterolemia, suggesting that unregulated overexpression of the LDLR by liver gene therapy would be therapeutic in humans with hypercholesterolemia of various causes (13).

Many individuals develop coronary artery disease from other causes not amenable to statin therapy but that are potentially treatable by gene therapy. Liver gene therapy using the apoB mRNA editing enzyme (Apobec 1) or the VLDL receptor genes could modify LDL cholesterol levels. Other lipoprotein factors besides LDL cholesterol levels influence the onset of coronary artery disease and are amenable to modulation by liver gene transfer. Additional expression of apoA-I in the liver by foreign gene transfer could raise high-density lipoprotein (HDL) levels and prevent atherosclerosis, as has been demonstrated in mouse and rabbit models. Hypertension, a predisposing factor for coronary artery disease, could be treated by delivering the kalikrein gene to the liver.

IV. SUMMARY

The foundation for treating many IEM by gene therapy has been established. It is clear that the expression of the cognate gene can correct the metabolic disturbance and the disease state in most IEM. As in other types of disorders, clinical success has been thwarted by inefficiencies in the gene-delivery and expression systems. As new vectors and expression systems are developed and improved over the next few years, it is anticipated that clinical efficacy will be demonstrated for an increasing number of IEM.

ACKNOWLEDGMENT

This work was supported by National Institutes of Health grants DK49117 and DK02405.

REFERENCES

1. Wolff JA, Lederberg J. An early history of gene transfer and therapy. Hum Gene Ther 1994; 5:469–480.
2. Eisensmith RC, Woo SL. Somatic gene therapy for phenylketonuria and other hepatic deficiencies. J Inherited Metab Dis 1996; 19:412–423.
3. Overturf K, Al-Dhalimy M, Manning K, Ou CN, Finegold M, Grompe M. Ex vivo hepatic gene therapy of a mouse model of Hereditary Tyrosinemia Type I. Hum Gene Ther 1998; 9:295–304.
4. Fang B, Eisensmith RC, Li XHC, Finegold MJ, Shedlovsky A, Dove W. Gene therapy for phenylketonuria: phenotypic correction in a genetically deficient mouse model by adenovirus-mediated hepatic gene therapy. Gene Ther 1994; 1: 247–254.
5. Ye X, Robinson MB, Batshaw ML, Furth EE, Smith I, Wilson JM. Prolonged metabolic correction in adult ornithine transcarbamylase-deficient mice with adenoviral vectors. J Biol Chem 1996; 271:3639–3646.
6. Salvetti A, Heard JM, Danos O. Gene therapy of lysosomal storage disorders. Br Med Bull 1995; 51:106–122.
7. Gage FH, Wolff JA, Rosenberg MB, Xu L, Yee J-K, Shultz C, Friedmann T. Grafting genetically modified cells to the brain. Neuroscience 1987; 23:795–807.
8. Grossman M, Rader DJ, Muller DW, Kolansky DM, Kozarsky K, Clark B Jr, Stein EA, Lupien PJ, Brewer HB Jr, Raper SE, et al. A pilot study of ex vivo gene therapy for homozygous familial hypercholesterolaemia. Nat Med 1995; 1:1148–1154.
9. Brown MS, Goldstein JL, Havel RJ, Steinberg D. Gene therapy for cholesterol. Nat Genetics 1994; 7:349–350.
10. Ishibashi S, Brown MS, Goldstein JL, Gerard RD, Hammer RE, Herz J. Hypercholesterolemia in low density lipoprotein receptor knockout mice and its reversal by adenovirus-mediated gene delivery. J Clin Invest 1993; 92:883–893.
11. Sempos CT, Cleeman JI, Carroll MD, et al. Prevalence of high blood cholesterol among US adults: an update based on guidelines from the second report of the National Cholesterol Education Program Adult Treatment Panel. JAMA 1993; 269:3009.
12. Sacks FM, Pfeffer MA, Moye LA, Rouleau JL, Rutherford JD, et al. The effect of pravastatin on coronary events after myocardial infarction in patients with average cholesterol levels. N Engl J Med 1996; 35:1001–1009.
13. Yokode M, Hammer RE, Ishibashi S, Brown MS, Goldstein JL. Diet-induced hypercholesterolemia in mice: prevention by overexpression of LDL receptors. Science 1990; 250: 1273–1275.

26

Gene Therapy and HIV-1 Infection

Ralph Dornburg and Roger J. Pomerantz
Thomas Jefferson University, Philadelphia, Pennsylvania

I. INTRODUCTION

Since the discovery that the acquired immunodeficiency syndrome (AIDS) is caused by a retrovirus, termed human immunodeficiency virus type I (HIV-1), enormous efforts have been undertaken to develop new pharmaceutical agents to control the spread of this epidemic disease. Such conventional drugs are specifically designed to block the action of HIV-1–specific enzymes, such as the reverse transcriptase or the protease. However, as a result of the high mutation rate of the virus, new virus variants continously emerge, which are resistant to such conventional therapies. Thus, great efforts are currently being made in many laboratories worldwide to develop alternative genetic approaches to inhibit the replication of this virus. With growing insight into the mechanism and regulation of HIV-1 replication, genetic antivirals have been developed that attack basically every step in the viral life cycle. Tissue culture cells have been transduced with genes encoding for such antivirals, and it has been shown that such transduced cells can become rather resistant to HIV-1 infection. However, although such antivirals have been proven to be very effective in vitro, their beneficiary effect in vivo is very difficult to evaluate and still remains to be shown. Furthermore, the delivery of genes encoding for such genetic antivirals still constitutes one of the main problems, since no efficient gene-delivery tools are available at this point that would enable the robust delivery to the actual target cell in vivo. This chapter summarizes the experimental approaches and current gene-delivery techniques to inhibit HIV-1 infection.

II. HIV-1 INFECTION AND CONVENTIONAL PHARMACEUTICAL AGENTS

The acquired immuno deficiency syndrome is caused by the human immunodeficiency virus type I. This retrovirus primarily infects and destroys cells of the human immune system, in particular $CD4^+$ T cells and macrophages. The destruction of such cells leads to a severe immunodeficiency, e.g., the inability to fight other infectious agents or tumor cells. Thus, AIDS patients usually die from secondary infections (e.g., tuberculosis, pneumonia) or cancer (e.g., Kaposi's sarcoma). Enormous efforts have been made to study the life cycle and pathogenesis of HIV-1 in order to find potential targets to block the replication of this virus. For a description of the life cycle of HIV-1, see Figure 1. Some viral proteins, such as the protease and reverse transcriptase, have been crystallized and their three-dimensional structures have been determined. These studies were performed to design specific compounds, which would irreversibly bind to the active sites of such enzymes and, therefore, inhibit their function. Indeed, specific chemical compounds that efficiently block the activity or function of these viral proteins are now commercially available and in use worldwide (1–5).

Recent studies have demonstrated that administration of a mixture of three such antiviral compounds (called combination chemotherapy or highly active retroviral therapy, HAART) can lead to significant reduction of viral load in vivo. Utilizing two reverse transcriptase and one protease inhibitor in treatment-naive patients, the serum HIV-1 RNA levels may be reduced to an undetectable level. How

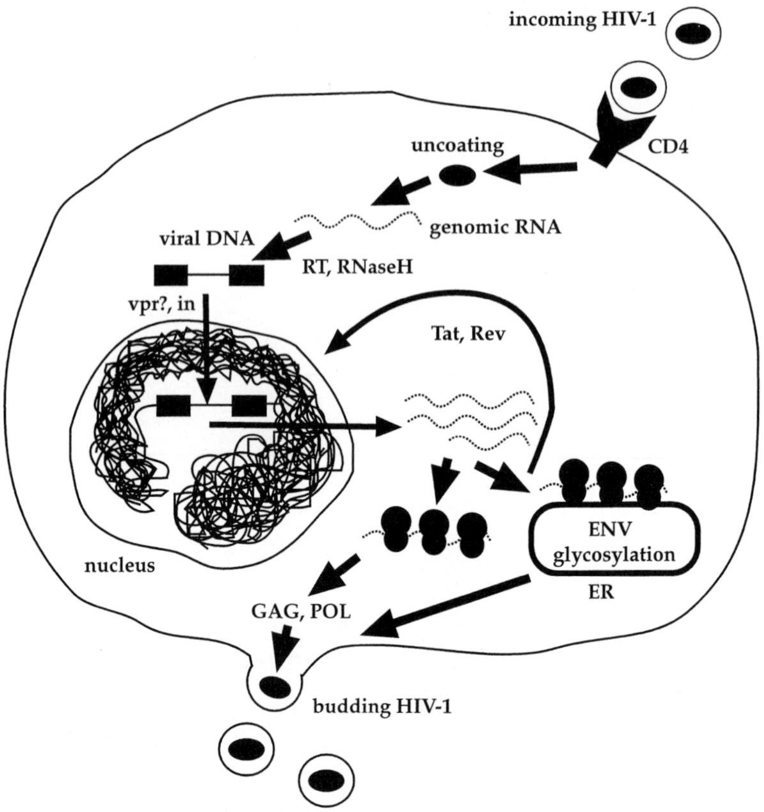

Figure 1 Life cycle of HIV-1. The life cycle of the human immunodeficiency virus type I is similar to that of all retroviruses studied. HIV-1 attaches to the target cell mainly by binding to the CD4 molecule. After fusion of the viral and cellular membranes, retroviral core particles are released into the cytoplasm. The RNA genome is converted into a double-stranded DNA by the viral reverse transcriptase (RT) and ribonuclease H (RNaseH) and actively transported into the nucleus, probably aided by the viral protein vpr. The viral DNA is integrated into the genome of the host cell by the viral integrase (in). The integrated DNA form of the virus is called the provirus. In contrast to other retroviruses, transcription and RNA splicing of the provirus is regulated by viral accessory proteins. For example, the viral protein Tat must bind to a specific sequence in the HIV genome (termed TAR) to enable highly efficient transcription of the provirus. Rev is required to control RNA splicing and the transport of RNAs into the cytoplasm. Finally, in the cytoplasm, virus core particles are assembled by encapsidating full-length geriomic viral RNAs (recognized by specific encapsidation sequences). At the cell membrane virus particle assembly is completed by the interaction of the core with the viral membrane proteins and new particles ''bud'' (are released) from the infected cell. For more details regarding regulatory proteins, see Figure 5. Env = Envelope; ER = endoplasmatic reticulum.

long this response will last in these patients remains an open issue. Reports of patients have emerged describing variant strains of HIV-1 that are resistant to this combination chemotherapy.

In particular, patients who have been treated with one antiviral inhibitor alone in the past appear to already carry a virus strain that is resistant to one of such compounds and, therefore, are partially resistant to combination therapy. Such virus strains have a higher chance to further mutate and escape the inhibitory effects of the other chemical compounds. In particular, the viral enzyme reverse transcriptase, which converts the viral RNA genome into a double-stranded DNA, does not have proofreading capabilities. On average, it inserts at least one incorrect nucleotide into the viral genome per replication cycle. This error rate is one million times higher than that of the cellular DNA polymerase I, which is the main enzyme for the replication of the eukaryotic genome. This high mutation rate explains why drug-resistant virus mutants emerge rapidly in HIV-1–infected patients (6). This high mutation rate also explains why new mutant viruses continuously arise that are ''new'' to and, therefore, not recognized and inactivated by the immune system. Consequently, in the clinically latent stage of HIV-1 infection, high virus loads persist, which consistently change their genetic outfit to escape drugs that inhibit virus replication and the immune system (7–9).

In summary, the clinical application of all drugs for the treatment of AIDS has not led to a cure for the disease, and even the new combination therapy may only halt the development of AIDS in infected people temporarily, as new drug-resistant variants of the HIV-1 virus start to emerge. Thus, efforts are underway in many laboratories to develop alternative therapeutics.

III. GENETIC "BULLETS" TO BLOCK HIV-1 REPLICATION

The primary target cells for HIV-1 are cells of the hematopoietic system, in particular $CD4^+$ T lymphocytes and macrophages. During HIV-1 infection these cells are destroyed by the virus, leading to immunodeficiency of the infected individual. In order to prevent the destruction of the cells of the immune system, many efforts are now underway to make such cells resistant to the HIV-1 virus. This approach has been termed "intracellular immunization" (10). In particular, the development of genetic agents that attack the virus at several points simultaneously inside the cell and/or are independent from viral mutations has gained great attention.

Such potential agents, also termed "genetic antivirals," should have four features to overcome the shortcomings of conventional treatments: First, they should be directed against a highly conserved moiety in HIV-1, which is absolutely essential for virus replication, eliminating the chance that new mutant variants arise that can escape this attack. Second, they have to be highly effective, greatly reducing or, ideally, completely blocking the production of progeny virus. Third, they have to be nontoxic. A fourth criteria that also should not be overlooked is that the antiviral agent has to be tolerated by the immune system. It would not make much sense to endow immune cells with an antiviral agent that elicits an immune response against itself leading to the destruction of the HIV-1–resistant cell after a short period of time.

In the past few years, many strategies have been developed and proposed for clinical application to block HIV-1 replication inside the cell (see also Fig. 2). Such strategies use either antiviral RNAs or proteins. They include antisense oligonucleotides, ribozymes, RNA decoys, transdominant mutant proteins, products of toxic genes, and single-chain antigen-binding proteins (for reviews, see Refs. 11–23). Antiviral strategies that employ RNAs have the advantage that they are less likely to be immunogenic than protein-based antiviral agents. However, protein-based systems have been engineered that use inducible promoters that only become active upon HIV-1 infection.

A. RNA-Based Inhibitors of HIV-1 Replication

1. Antisense RNAs and Ribozymes

It is very well known that prokaryotes and bacteriophages express antisense RNAs, which provide regulatory control over gene expression by hybridizing to specific RNA sequences (24). In animal cells, artificial antisense oligonucleotides (RNAs or single-stranded DNAs) have been successfully used to selectively prevent expression of various genes (e.g., oncogenes, differentiation genes, viral genes) (24,25). Furthermore, the presence of double-stranded RNA inside the cell can induce the production of interferon and/or other cytokines stimulating an immune response. Indeed, it has also been reported that the expression of RNAs capable of forming a double-stranded RNA molecule with the HIV-1 RNA (antisense RNAs) can significantly reduce the expression of HIV-1 proteins and consequently the efficiency of progeny virus production (24–29).

Ribozymes are very similar to antisense RNAs, e.g., they bind to specific RNA sequences, but they are also capable of cleaving their target at the binding site catalytically. Thus, they have the advantage that they may not need to be overexpressed in order to fulfill their function. Certain ribozymes (e.g., hairpin and hammerhead ribozymes) (Fig. 3) require only a GUC sequence. Thus, many sites in the HIV-1 genome can be targeted. However, several questions remain to be answered: for example, it is unclear, (1) whether efficient subcellular co-localization can be obtained, in particular in vivo, or (2) whether the target RNA will be efficiently recognized due to secondary and tertiary folding of the target RNA, or (3) whether RNA-binding proteins would prevent efficient binding. Thus, more experimentation will be necessary to address these problems (30–43).

2. RNA Decoys

In contrast to ribozymes and antisense RNAs, RNA decoys do not attack the viral RNAs directly. RNA decoys are mutant RNAs that resemble authentic viral RNAs that have crucial functions in the viral life cycle. They mimic such RNA structures and decoy viral and/or cellular factors required for the propagation of the virus (30,44–53). For example, HIV-1 replication largely depends on the two regulatory proteins—Tat and Rev. These proteins bind to specific regions in the viral RNA, the transactivation response (TAR) loop, and the Rev response element (RRE), respectively. Tat binding to TAR is crucial in the initiation of RNA transcription; Rev binding to RRE is essential in

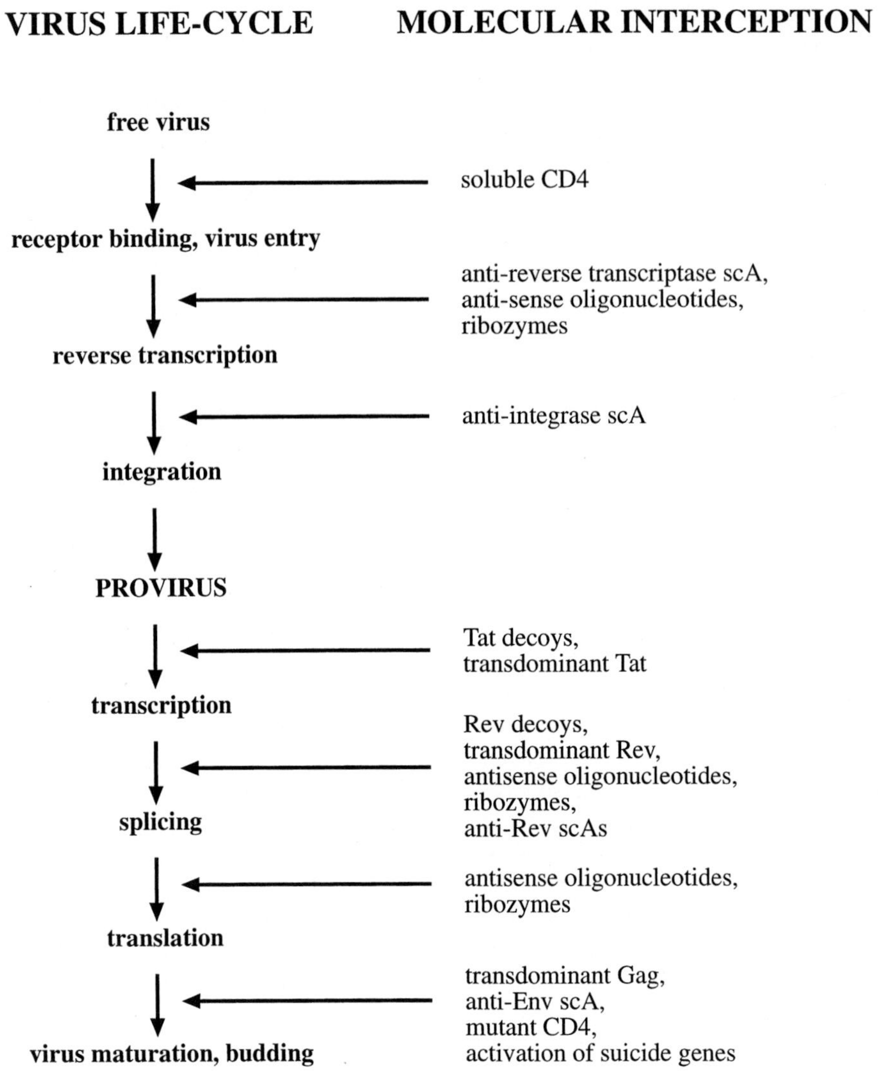

Figure 2 Overview of possible genetic targets to block HIV-1 replication. The different approaches are described in detail in the text.

controlling splicing, RNA stability, and the transport of the viral RNA from the nucleus to the cytoplasm. These two complex secondary RNA structures within the HIV-1 genome appear to be unique to the HIV-1 virus, and no cellular homologous structures have been identified. Thus, such structures appear to be valuable targets for attack with genetic antivirals.

The strategy here is to endow HIV-1 target cells with genes that overexpress short RNAs containing TAR or RRE sequences. The rationale for this is to have RNA molecules within the cells in abundance, which will capture Tat or Rev proteins, preventing the binding of such proteins to their actual targets. Consequently, HIV-1 replication is markedly impaired. This strategy has the advantage over antisense RNAs and ribozymes in that mutant Tat or Rev, which will not bind to the RNA decoys, will also not bind to their actual targets. Thus, the likelihood that mutant strains would arise that would bypass the RNA decoy trap is low. However, it still remains to be elucidated whether cellular factors also bind to Tat or Rev decoys and whether overexpression of decoy RNAs would lead to the sequestering of the resulting protein-RNA complexes in the cell.

B. Protein-Based Inhibitors of HIV-1 Replication

1. Transdominant Mutant Proteins

During HIV-1 replication, several regulatory proteins are essential for viral gene expression and gene regulation. Mu-

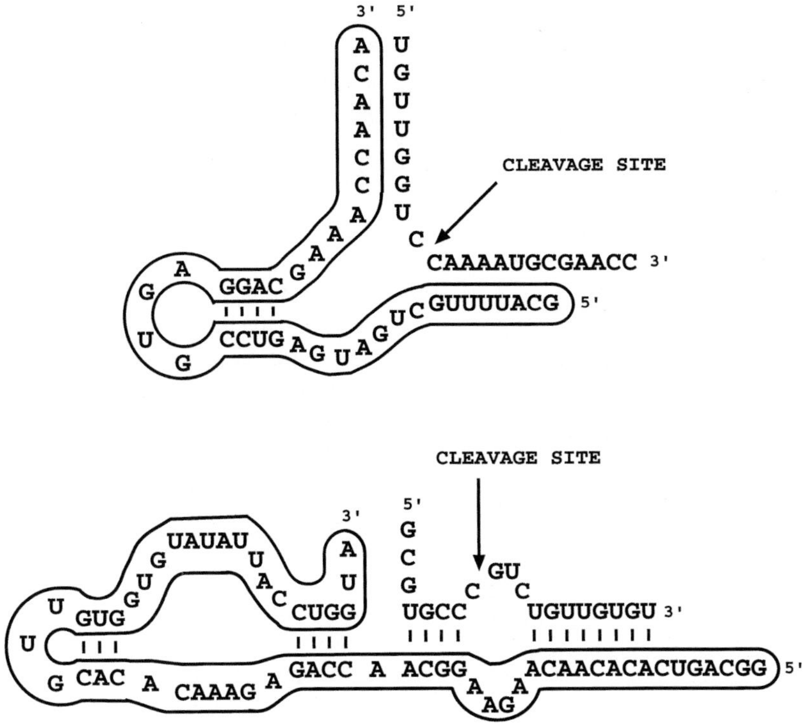

Figure 3 Schematic representation of two ribozymes to block HIV-1 replication. The structures shown are paired with actual HIV-1 target sequences. (Top) A hammerhead ribozyme pairs specifically with a sequence in the gag region of the HIV-1 genome. (Bottom) A hairpin ribozyme designed to bind to and cleave the 5′ end of the viral genome, abolishing the reverse transcription and integration of progeny virus.

tant forms of such proteins greatly reduce the efficiency of viral replication. Transdominant (TD) mutants are genetically modified viral proteins that still bind to their targets but are unable to perform their actual function. They compete with the corresponding native, wild-type protein inside the cell. The competition of several TD proteins with the wild-type counterpart has been shown to greatly reduce virus replication, especially when such TD mutants are expressed from strong promoters (e.g., the cytomegalovirus immediate early promoter, CMV-IE) (10,17,54–62).

For example, transcription from the HIV-1 long terminal repeat (LTR) promoter is dependent on the Tat protein. Mutant Tat proteins, which still bind to the nascent viral RNA, but which are unable to further trigger RNA elongation of transcription, greatly reduce the production of HIV-1 RNAs and consequently the production of progeny virus. In a similar way, mutant Rev proteins interfere with regulated posttranscriptional events and also greatly reduce the efficiency of virus replication in an infected cell.

Although TD mutants have been shown to be effective in vitro, it still remains unclear how long cells endowed with such proteins will survive in vivo. There is a significant possibility that peptides of such proteins will be displayed via HLA leading to the destruction of the HIV-1–resistant cell by the patient's own immune system. There is, however, the potential to express such proteins from the HIV-1 LTR promoter, which only becomes activated upon HIV-1 infection. However, this would rule out that a TD Tat can be used, because TD Tat may also abolish its own expression. Even if other TD proteins are expressed from inducible promoters, it still remains unclear whether such inducible promoters are really silent enough so that no protein is made (and no immune response) as long as there is no viral infection.

2. Toxic Genes

Another approach to reduce the production of progeny virus is to endow the target cells of HIV-1 with toxic genes, which become activated immediately after virus infection. The activation of the toxic gene leads to immediate cell death, and, therefore, no new progeny virus particles can be produced. Theoretically, this would lead to an overall reduction of the virus load in the patient. In vitro experiments have shown that the production of HIV-1 virus particles was indeed reduced if target cells were endowed with genes coding for the herpes simplex virus (HSV) thymidine kinase or a mutant form of the bacterial diphtheria toxin protein. Such genes were inserted downstream of the HIV-1 LTR promoter, which only becomes activated upon HIV-1 infection, when the viral Tat protein is expressed (63–68).

Besides the question regarding the ''silence'' of the HIV-1 LTR promoter without Tat (discussed above), the main problem with this approach is the actual number of cells that carry a toxic gene present in the patient. Since the HIV-1 virus will not only infect cells that carry the toxic gene, but also many other cells of its host, this approach may only ''slow down'' virus replication for a short period of time until all cells that carry the toxic genes undergo self-destruction upon infection.

3. CD4 as Decoy

The CD4 molecule is the major receptor for the HIV-1 virus for entry into T lymphocytes. Thus, in a similar way to RNA decoys, mutant CD4, which stays inside the endoplasmatic reticulum (ER), has been shown to inactivate HIV-1 envelope maturation, preventing formation of infectious particles. In another approach, soluble CD4 has been used to block the envelope of free extracellular virus particles and to prevent binding to fresh target cells. However, the question remains if soluble and/or mutant CD4 in the blood of the patient will also serve as a trap for natural CD4 ligands leading to the impairment of important physiological functions (69–71).

4. Single-Chain Antibodies

Single-chain antibodies (scA) were originally developed for *Escherichia coli* expression to bypass the costly production of monoclonal antibodies in tissue culture or mice (72,73). They comprise only the variable domains of both the heavy and light chains of an antibody. These domains are expressed from a single gene, in which the coding region for these domains are separated by a short spacer sequence coding for a peptide bridge, which connects the two variable domain peptides. The resulting scA (also termed single-chain variable fragment, scFv) can bind to its antigen with similar affinity as a Fab fragment of the authentic antibody molecule.

scFvs have been developed by our group and others to combat HIV-1 replication when expressed intracellularly (23,70,74–80). Both pre (e.g., integrase, reverse transcriptase, matrix protein– and post (e.g., Rev and Tat)–integration sites of the viral life cycle have been targeted, with varying success. Further studies using constructs combining multiple scFvs for potential synergistic antiviral potency are under development and should be of importance in developing robust anti-HIV-1 molecular therapeutics.

IV. GENETIC "GUNS" TO DELIVER GENETIC ANTIVIRALS

In all therapeutic approaches listed above, the therapeutical agent cannot be delivered directly to the cell. Instead, the corresponding genes have to be transduced to express the therapeutic agent of interest within the target cell. Genes can be delivered using a large variety of molecular tools. Such tools range from nonviral delivery agents (liposomes or even naked DNA) to viral vectors. Since HIV-1 remains and replicates in the body of an infected person for many years, it will be essential to stably introduce therapeutic genes into the genome of target cells for either continuous expression or for availability upon demand. Thus, gene-delivery tools such as naked DNA, liposomes, or adenoviruses (AV), which are highly effective for transient expression of therapeutic genes, may not be useful for gene therapy of HIV-1 infection.

Adeno-associated virus (AAV), a nonpathogenic single-stranded DNA virus of the parvovirus family, has recently gained a great deal of attention as a vector, because it is not only capable of inserting its genome specifically at one site at chromosome 19 in human cells, but it is also capable of infecting nondividing cells. However, vectors derived from AAV are much less efficient and lose their ability to target chromosome 19 (81,82). Another shortcoming of AAV is the need for it to be propagated with replication-competent AV, since AAV alone is replication defective. It also remains to be shown how efficiently AAV vectors transduce genes into human hematopoietic stem cells and/or mature T lymphocytes and macrophages. Because gene therapy of HIV-1 infection may also require multiple injections of the vector (in vivo gene therapy, see below) or of ex vivo manipulated cells, it also remains to be shown whether even small amounts of contaminating AV, which is used as a helper agent to grow AAV, will cause immune problems.

The most efficient tools for stable gene delivery are retroviral vectors (83–89), which stably integrate into the genome of the host cell, as this is a part of the retroviral life cycle (Fig. 1). This is why virus-based gene-delivery systems have been derived from this class of viruses. This is also why they are being used in almost all current human gene therapy trials, including ongoing clinical AIDS trials.

Retroviral vectors are basically retroviral particles that contain a genome in which all viral protein coding sequences have been replaced with the gene(s) of interest. As a result, such viruses cannot further replicate after one round of infection. Furthermore, infected cells do not express any retroviral proteins, which makes cells that carry a vector provirus (the integrated DNA form of a retrovirus) invisible to the immune system (83–89).

A. Retroviral Vectors Derived from C-Type Retroviruses

All current retroviral vectors used in clinical trials have been derived from murine leukemia virus (MLV), a C-type retrovirus with a rather simple genomic organization (Fig. 4). MLV contains only two gene units, which code for the inner core structure proteins and the envelope protein, respectively. It does not contain regulatory genes like HIV-1. Thus, the construction of safe gene-delivery systems is rather simple and straightforward. Such delivery systems consist of two components: (1) the retroviral vector, a genetically modified viral genome that contains the gene of interest replacing retroviral protein coding sequences, and (2) a helper cell that supplies the retroviral proteins for the encapsidation of the vector genome into retroviral particles (Fig. 4). Modern helper cells contain separate plasmid constructs, which express all retroviral proteins necessary for replication. After transfection of the vector genome into such helper cells, the vector genome is encapsidated into virus particles (due to the presence of specific encapsidation sequences). Virus particles are released from the helper cell carrying a genome containing only the gene(s) of interest (Fig. 4). Thus, once established, retrovirus helper cells can produce gene transfer particles for very long time periods (e.g., several years). In the last decade, several retroviral vector systems have also been derived from other C-type chicken retroviruses (83,85,89).

B. Retroviral Vectors Derived from HIV-1

Retroviral vectors derived from MLV have been shown to be very useful to transfer genes into a large variety of human cells. However, they poorly infect human hematopoietic cells because such cells lack the receptor that is recognized by the MLV envelope protein. Furthermore, retroviral vectors derived from C-type retroviruses are unable to infect quiescent cells: such viruses (and their vectors)

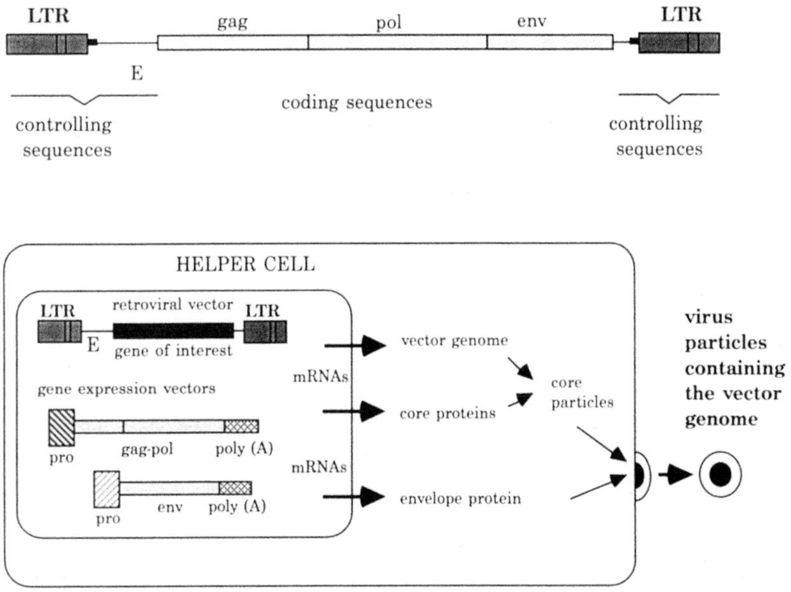

Figure 4 Retroviral helper cells derived from C-type retroviruses. A C-type retroviral provirus (the DNA intermediate of a retrovirus) is shown at the top. The protein coding genes (gag-pol and env) are flanked by *cis*-acting or controlling sequences, which play essential roles during replication. (Below) In a retroviral helper cell, the retroviral protein coding genes, which code for all virion proteins, are expressed (ideally) from heterologous promoters (pro) and polyadenylated via a heterologous polyadenylation signal sequence [poly(A)]. To minimize reconstitution of a full-length provirus by recombination, the gag-pol and env genes are split to different gene expression vectors. In the retroviral vector, the viral protein coding sequences are completely replaced by the gene(s) of interest. Since the vector contains specific encapsidation sequences (E), the vector genome is encapsidated into retroviral vector particles, which bud from the helper cell. The virion contains all proteins necessary to reverse transcribe and integrate the vector genome into that of a newly infected target cell. However, since there are no retroviral protein coding sequences in the target cell, vector replication is limited to one round of infection. LTR = Long terminal repeat.

can only establish a provirus after one cell division, during which the nuclear membrane is temporarily dissolved. Thus, efforts are underway in many laboratories to develop retroviral vectors from lentiviruses, e.g., HIV-1 or the simian immunodeficiency virus (SIV), which are able to establish a provirus in nondividing cells (although the mechanism by which these viruses penetrate the nucleus is not fully understood). However, the fact that lentiviruses contain several regulatory proteins, which are essential for virus replication, makes the construction of lentiviral packaging cells more complicated. Furthermore, the fact that the lentiviral envelope proteins (e.g., that of HIV-1) can cause syncytia and/or that some viral regulatory proteins are toxic to the cells further hampers the development of stable packaging lines.

The ''envelope problem'' has been solved by generating packaging cells that express the envelope protein of MLV or the envelope of vesicular stomatitis virus (VSV). Such envelope proteins are efficiently incorporated into lentiviral particles. The second and major problem for generating stable packaging lines is the toxicity of some retroviral regulatory proteins to the cell. Thus, retroviral vectors can only be generated in transient systems: 293T cells (human tissue culture cells highly susceptible for transfecting DNAs) are simultaneously transfected with all plasmid constructs to express the particle proteins and the vector genome. Fig. 5 shows plasmid constructs used to make HIV-1–derived packaging cells. Vector virus can be harvested from the transfected cells for a limited time period and used to infect fresh target cells. Although this gene-transfer system has been shown to be functional, it is not highly efficient and better packaging cells still need to be developed. In addition, may questions regarding the safety of such vectors still need to addressed. It is known that plasmid DNAs can recombine with each other very efficiently immediately after transfection. Thus, the question needs to be addressed whether there is a chance that replication-competent viruses arise by recombination, which may cause a disease in gene-transduced patients.

C. Cell-Type–Specific Retroviral Vectors

All retroviral vectors currently used in human gene therapy trials contain the envelope protein of amphotropic (ampho) MLV or VSV. Ampho-MLV as well as VSV have a very broad host range and can infect various tissues of many species, including humans. Thus, the use of vectors containing such envelope proteins enables the transduction into many different human tissues. However, due to this broad host range, gene transfer has to be performed ex vivo. If injected directly into the blood stream, the chances that the vector particles would infect their actual target cells are very low. Furthermore, such vector particles may infect germline cells (which are continuously dividing). Thus, the target cells have to be isolated, and the gene transfer is being performed in tissue culture. Gene-transduced cells are then selected and reintroduced into the patient.

However, this protocol has major shortcomings in regard (not only) to gene therapy of HIV-1 infection. First, it is very expensive and requires highly trained personal. Second, human cells kept in tissue culture change their physiological behavior and/or take up fetal bovine proteins (a component of the tissue culture medium) and display bovine peptides via HLA on the cell surface. Consequently, such cells become immunogenic and are eliminated by the immune system of the patient. To bypass such ex vivo protocols, efforts are now underway in many laboratories to develop cell-type–specific gene-delivery systems, which would involve injecting the gene-delivery vehicle directly into the patient's blood stream or tissue of interest. In the past few years, several attempts have been made to develop cell-type–specific gene-delivery tools, again with retrovirus-derived vectors leading the field.

The cell-type specificity of a virus particle is determined by the nature of the retroviral envelope protein that mediates the binding of the virus to a receptor of the target cell (90). Thus, experiments have been initiated in several laboratories to modify the envelope protein of retroviruses in order to alter the host range of the vector. One of the first attempts to specifically deliver genes into distinct target cells has been performed in the laboratory of Dr. H. Varmus. Using retroviral vectors derived from avian leukosis virus (ALV), these investigators incorporated the human CD4 molecule into virions to specifically transduce genes into HIV-1–infected cells (91). However, such particles were not infectious for unknown reasons. Recent reports indicate the MLV particles that carry CD4 can infect HIV-1–infected cells, although at very low efficiencies (92).

In another attempt to target retroviral particles to specific cells, Roux et al. were able to infect human cells with eco-MLV by adding two different antibodies to the virus particle solution. The antibodies were connected at their carboxy termini by streptavidine. One antibody was directed against a cell surface protein; the other antibody was directed against the retroviral envelope protein (93,94). Although this approach was not practical (infectivity was very inefficient and was performed at 4°C), these experiments showed that cells that do not have an appropriate receptor for a particular virus can be infected with that virus if binding to the cell surface is facilitated. These data also indi-

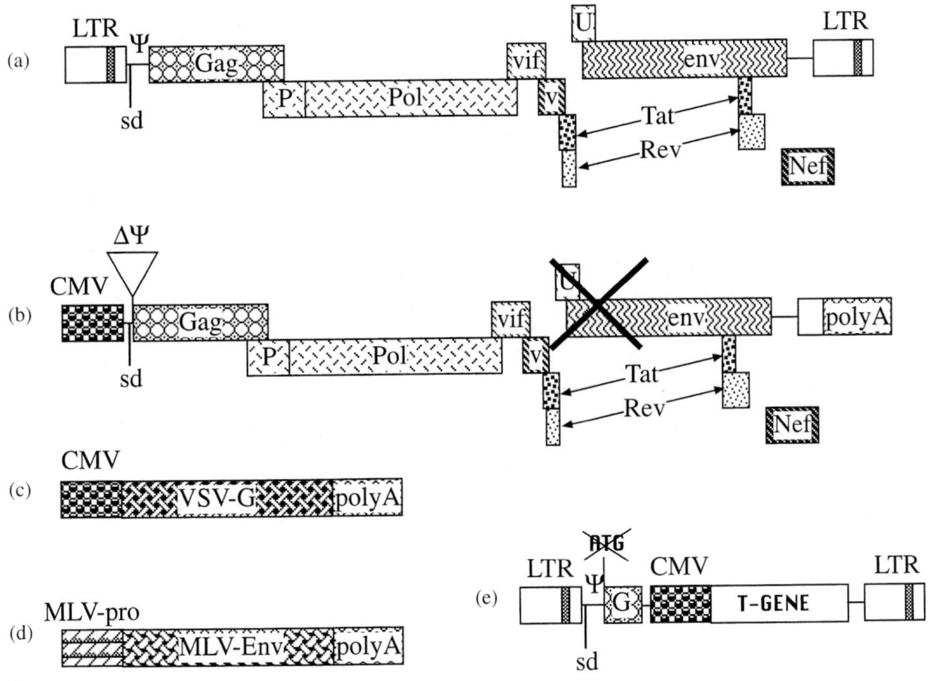

Figure 5 Retroviral packaging system derived from HIV-1: (a) a provirus of HIV-1; (b–d) plasmid constructs to express pseudotyped HIV-1 retroviral particles; (e) a plasmid construct to encapsidate and transduce genes with a HIV-1 vector (the plasmid sequences to propagate such constructs in bacteria are not shown). Besides the genes encoding for HIV-1 proteins, which form the core of the virus (e.g., Gag = structural core proteins, P = protease, Pol = reverse transcriptase and integrase) and the envelope (e.g., env = envelope protein), the HIV-1 genome also codes for several regulatory proteins (Vif, U = Vpu, V = Vpr, Tat, Rev, Nef), which are expressed from spliced mRNAs and which have important functions in the viral life cycle. The plasmid construct in (b) expresses the core and regulatory proteins. To avoid encapsidation and transduction of genes coding for such proteins, the following modifications have been made: the 5′ LTR promoter of the HIV-1 provirus has been replaced with the promoter of cytomegalovirus (CMV) to enable constitutive gene expression; the 3′ LTR has been partially replaced with the polyadenylation signal sequence of simian virus 40 (poly A); the encapsidation signal has been deleted ($\Delta\Psi$); the reading frames for the envelope and vpu genes have been blocked. The plasmid constructs in (c) and (d) express the envelope proteins of the vesicular stomatitis virus (VSV-G) or the envelope protein of murine leukemia virus (MLV), respectively. In the absence of HIV-1 envelope proteins, which are rather toxic to the cell, HIV-1 efficiently incorporates the envelope proteins of VSV or MLV into virions. The use of such envelopes also further reduces the risk of the reconstitution of a replication-competent HIV-1 by homologous recombination between the plasmid constructs. A retroviral vector (e) is used to package and transduce a gene of interest (T-gene) with HIV-1–derived vectors. Since the encapsidation sequence extends into the Gag region, part of the gag gene (G) has been conserved in the vector. However, the ATG start codon has been mutated. The gene of interest is expressed from an internal promoter, since the HIV-1 LTR promoter is silent without Tat. sd = Splice donor site.

cated that antibody-mediated cell targeting with retroviral vectors was possible.

To overcome the technical problems of creating an antibody bridge, it was logical to incorporate the antibody directly into the virus particle. However, complete antibodies are very bulky and are not suitable for this approach. The problem has been solved using single-chain antibody technology (95–98). Using hapten model systems, it has been shown that retroviral vectors that contained scAs fused to the envelope are competent for infection (96,97). Retroviral vector particles derived from spleen necrosis virus (SNV, an avian retrovirus) that display various scAs against human cell surface proteins are competent for infection on human cells that express the antigen recognized by the antibody (95,96,98).

Most recently it became possible to use scA-displaying SNV to introduce genes into human T cells with the same high efficiency obtained with vectors containing wild-type envelope. In all such experiments, the wild-type envelope of SNV had to be co-present in the virus particle to enable efficient infection of human cells. However, since SNV vector particles with wild-type SNV envelope do not infect human cells at all, this requirement is not a drawback for using such vector particles for human gene therapy (99,100).

Although successful gene transfer using scA-displaying MLV vector particles has been reported from one laboratory (101), further experimentation in the laboratories of several other investigators revealed that MLV-derived vector particles that display various scAs are not competent for infection in human cells (93,94,102–105). The difference between MLV and SNV cell-targeting vectors is certainly based on the different features of the wild-type envelope and the mode of virus entry (reviewed in Ref. 106). Moreover, wild-type ampho-MLV infects human hematopoietic cells extremely poorly, most likely due to the absence of an ampho-MLV receptor on such cells (107). Thus, MLV-derived vectors are certainly not the best candidates for human gene therapy of AIDS, and alternative vectors need to be developed.

D. Other New Potential Vector Systems

Most recently, other very interesting attempts have been made to combat HIV-1–infected cells. Recombinant VSV has been engineered, which lacks its own glycoprotein gene. Instead, genes coding for the HIV-1 receptor CD4 and a chemokine co-receptor, CXCR4, have been inserted. The corresponding virus was able to efficiently infect HIV-1–infected cells, which display the HIV-1 glycoprotein on the cell surface. Since VSV is a virus that normally kills infected cells, the engineered virus only infects and kills HIV-1–infected cells. It has been reported that this virus indeed reduced HIV-1 replication in tissue culture cells up to 10,000 fold (108). This novel approach to combat one virus with another will certainly gain a great deal of further attention. However, it remains to be shown how effective this approach will be in vivo. Will the ''antivirus'' succeed in eliminating a large load of HIV-infected cells before it will be cleared by the immune system? On the other hand, since HIV-1 preferentially kills activated immune cells, will it destroy the immune cells, which are attempting to clear the body from its own ''enemy''? How will the body tolerate a virus that does not look like one because it carries human cell surface proteins on the viral surface? The answers to these and other questions are eagerly awaited (109).

E. Other Potential Problems

Even if we find a gene-transfer system that can transduce enough cells within the body to inhibit virus replication significantly, many other questions remain to be answered. For example, it is not clear whether a cell that has been endowed with an HIV-1 resistance gene will be able to fulfil its normal biological function in vivo. It has to be considered that in order to become resistant against HIV-1, the cells usually have to overproduce the corresponding HIV-1 resistance gene. Does this overproduction result in a loss of other functions, e.g., because the cell has to supply a significant part of its energy supply to the production of the HIV-1 resistance gene? Will the body be able to eliminate all HIV-1–infected cells, or will the infected person become a life-long carrier of the virus, which is still replicating in his or her body although at levels that cause no clinical symptoms due to the presence of HIV-1 resistance genes? Will the patient be capable of infecting new individuals? Finally, as genetic therapies can all be overcome with in vitro challenges of very high MOIs of HIV-1, will there be a difference in antiviral effects in peripheral blood versus lymphoid tissues?

V. ANIMAL MODEL SYSTEMS

One of the major problems with any therapeutic agent against HIV-1 infection is the lack of an appropriate and inexpensive animal model system to test the efficiency of an antiviral agent. Since HIV-1 causes AIDS only in humans, it is very difficult to test and evaluate the therapeutic effect of novel antiviral agents in vivo. Furthermore, the evaluation of the efficacy of a new drug is further complicated by the very long latency period of the virus until the onset of AIDS (possibly 10 years or more). Although a virus similar to HIV-1 has been found in monkeys—the simian immunodeficiency virus (SIV)—results obtained with this virus do not necessarily reflect the onset of AIDS in humans caused by HIV-1. Furthermore, many antivirals that block HIV-1 are ineffective in blocking SIV. Thus, other animal model systems need to be developed to study the effect of anti-HIV-1 therapies.

In the past decade, many strains of laboratory mice have been bred that lack components of the immune system. Severe combined-immunodeficient (SCID) mice are deficient in functional B and T lymphocytes. Thus, they are unable to reject allogeneic organ grafts (110–115). SCID mice have been used extensively to study human leukemia and other malignancies and for modeling human retroviral pathogenesis including antiviral gene therapy. Furthermore, in the past few years, much progress has been made to transplant hematopoietic stem cells into SCID mice to mimic and study human hematopoiesis. It has been shown that transplantation of human hematopoietic cells into such mice can lead to the repopulation of the mouse's blood with human CD4- and CD8-positive cells. Thus, SCID mice appear also to be very good candidates to develop mouse model systems for HIV-1 infection.

At present, two different SCID mice model systems are used to study the effect of anti-HIV-1 antiviral agents. The two systems are somewhat different, because they represent different components of the human immune system. One is called the hu-PBL SCID model, and the other is termed the SCID-hu mouse.

In the hu-PBL SCID mouse system, human peripheral blood leukocytes are injected into the peritoneum of the animal. Thus, cells residing in such animals are mature $CD4^+$ and $CD8^+$ lymphocytes. The presence of activated and/or memory T cells ($CD45RO^+$ cells) has also been demonstrated. Such human cells can be recovered from various organs in the mouse, e.g., the spleen or lymph nodes. Since these animals contain human $CD4^+$ T cells, they can be infected easily with HIV-1. Furthermore, HIV-1 virus replicates in the animal leading to the depletion of $CD4^+$ T cells over a period of several weeks after infection. Thus, this experimental system is very valuable to test the effect of antiviral agents (116,117). For example, experiments have been performed to test the effect of monoclonal antibodies against the HIV-1 envelope protein (neutralizing the receptor binding V3 domain). It has been shown that this antibody indeed could block the replication of the viral strain for which the antibody was specific. This model system has also been used to test the efficiency of a vaccinia virus–derived vaccine.

In the SCID-hu mouse model system, various human fetal hematopoietic tissues (e.g., liver, lymph nodes, and/or thymus) are transplanted into the mouse. For example, human fetal thymus and liver tissues are engrafted under the murine kidney capsule. It has been shown that normal thymopoiesis takes place for up to one year after implantation, and human $CD4^+$ and $CD8^+$ T cells are found in the mouse blood at low levels. In contrast to the hu-PBL-SCID mouse, human cells are also found that express the CD45RA antigen, which is considered a marker for "naive" T lymphocytes. Such mice can also be infected with HIV-1, although the injection of a high virus dose directly into the implant is necessary to establish an infection. However, once an infection has been established, the pathological effects observed are very similar to those observed in the thymuses of infected human adults, children, and fetuses. Moreover, a depletion of $CD4^+/CD8^-$ T cells is observed.

Both SCID mice model systems are very useful to study pathogenesis and the effect of anti-HIV-1 drugs and to test the effect of anti-HIV antiviral genes. However, one has to keep in mind that such model systems only represent a portion of the human immune system, and HIV-1 also infects other cells in humans, such as dendritic cells, microvascular endothelial cells, and neurons in the brain. Thus, the pathogenesis observed in SCID mice certainly does not accurately reflect the pathogenesis in humans. Moreover, it is not clear whether SCID mice transplanted with human immune cells do have a functional immune system.

VI. CLINICAL TRIALS

Recently certain initial in vivo studies have been conducted for intracellular immunization against primate lentiviruses. A trans-dominant negative Rev protein (RevM10) has been studied in humans infected with HIV-1 by Dr. G. Nabel's group. In these initial studies, it was demonstrated that cells transduced with RevM10 had a significantly longer half-life than control cells when reinfused into patients in different stages of disease. These early initial phase I trials were performed using murine retroviral vectors (MLV), as well as microparticulate bombardment using a "gene gun" (118).

In addition, a very exciting study has recently been reported by R. Morgan's group in which an antisense construct to Tat and Rev genes in SIV was used to transduce T cells from rhesus macaques (119). The monkeys were then challenged with SIV intravenously. Of note, the animals with the transduced cells had significantly lower viral loads and higher CD4 counts compared to control monkeys. This suggests that, for the first time, gene therapy against lentiviruses may have significant efficacy in vivo. Clearly, these are both very preliminary studies in humans and in primates, which require more detailed evaluation. Other trials using a variety of different approaches are ongoing in initial phase I studies.

In summary, considering all facts and problems of current gene-transfer technologies and considering our lack of knowledge regarding many functions of the immune system, how should we move forward with more phase I gene therapy trials to combat HIV-1? In spite of the lack of knowledge of many aspects of this disease, we have to remain optimistic and can only hope that one approach or the other will lead to measurable progress towards a cure or will at least significantly prolong the life expectancy of the infected person. Clearly, in addition to further exploring novel molecular therapeutics in vivo, significant attention must be paid to answering critical basic science questions pertaining to "intracellular immunization."

REFERENCES

1. Johnston MI, Allaudeen HS, Sarver N. HIV proteinase as a target for drug action. Trends Pharmacol Sci 1989; 10: 305–307.

2. Erickson JW, Burt SK. Structural mechanisms of HIV drug resistance. Annu Rev Pharmacol Toxicol 1996; 36: 545–571.
3. de Clercq E. Non-nucleoside reverse transcriptase inhibitors (nnrtis) for the treatment of human immunodeficiency virus type 1 (HIV-1) infections: strategies to overcome drug resistance development. Med Res Rev 1996; 16: 125–157.
4. Sandstrom PA, Folks TM. New strategies for treating AIDS. Bioessays 1996; 18:343–346.
5. Fulcher D, Clezy K. Antiretroviral therapy. Med J Aust 1996; 164:607.
6. Richman D. HIV drug resistance. AIDS Res Hum Retroviruses 1992; 8:1065–1071.
7. Baltimore D. The enigma of HIV infection. Cell 1995; 82: 175–176.
8. Embretson JE, Zupanic M, Ribas JL, Burke A, Racz P, Tenner-Racz K, Haase AT. Massive covert infection of helper T lymphocytes and macrophages by HIV during incubation period of AIDS. Nature 1993; 362:359–362.
9. Pantaleo G, Graziosi C, Demarest JF, Butini L, Montroni M, Fox CH, Orenstein JM, Kotler DP, Fauci AS. HIV infection is active and progressive in lymphoid tissue during the clinically latent stage of disease. Nature 1993; 362: 355–358.
10. Baltimore D. Intracellular immunization. Nature 1988; 235:395–396.
11. Dropubic B, Jeang K-T. Gene therapy for human immunodeficiency virus infection: genetic antiviral strategies and targets for intervention. Hum Gene Ther 1994; 5:927–939.
12. Yu M, Poeschla E, Wong-Staal F. Progress towards gene therapy for HIV infection. Gene Ther 1994; 1:13–26.
13. Kaplan JC, Hirsch MS. Therapy other than reverse transcriptase inhibitors for HIV infection. Clin Lab Med 1994; 14:367–391.
14. Gilboa E, Smith C. Gene therapy for infectious diseases: the AIDS model. Trends Genet 1994; 10:139–144.
15. Anderson WF. Gene therapy for AIDS [editorial]. Hum Gene Ther 1994; 5:149–150.
16. Sarver N, Rossi J. Gene therapy: a bold direction for HIV-1 treatment. AIDS Res Hum Retroviruses 1993; 9:483–487.
17. Bahner I, Zhou C, Yu XJ, Hao QL, Guatelli JC, Kohn DB. Comparison of trans-dominant inhibitory mutant human immunodeficiency virus type 1 genes expressed by retroviral vectors in human T lymphocytes. J Virol 1993; 67: 3199–3207.
18. Blaese RM. Steps toward gene therapy: 2. Cancer and AIDS. Hosp Pract 1995; 30:37–45.
19. Bridges SH, Sarver N. Gene therapy and immune restoration for HIV disease. Lancet 1995; 345:427–432.
20. Bunnell BA, Morgan RA. Gene therapy for AIDS. Mol Cells 1996; 6:1–12.
21. Cohen J. Gene therapy—new role for HIV-a vehicle for moving genes into cells. Science 1996; 272:195.
22. Ho AD, Li XO, Lane TA, Yu M, Law P, Wongstaal F. Stem cells as vehicles for gene therapy—novel strategy for HIV infection. Stem Cells 1995; 13:100–105.
23. Pomerantz RJ, Trono D. Genetic therapies for HIV infections: promise for the future. AIDS 1995; 9:985–993.
24. Stein CA, Cheng YC. Antisense oligonucleotides as therapeutic agents: Is the bullet really magical? Science 1993; 261:1004–1012.
25. Agrawal S. Antisense oligonucleotides as antiviral agents. Trends Biotechnol 1992; 10:152–158.
26. Castanotto D, Rossi JJ, Sarver N. Antisense catalytic RNAs as therapeutic agents. Adv Pharmacol 1994; 25: 289–317.
27. Rossi JJ, Sarver N. Catalytic antisense RNA (ribozymes): their potential and use as anti-HIV-1 therapeutic agents. Adv Exp Med Biol 1992; 312:95–109.
28. Rothenberg M, Johnson G, Laughlin C, Green I, Cradock J, Sarver N, Cohen JS. Oligodeoxynucleotides as anti-sense inhibitors of gene expression: therapeutic implications. J Natl Cancer Inst 1989; 81:1539–1544.
29. Cohen JS. Antisense oilgonucleotides as antiviral agents. Antiviral Res 1991; 16:121–133.
30. Bahner I, Kearns K, Hao OL, Smogorzewska EM, Kohn DB. Transduction of human cd34+ hematopoietic progenitor cells by a retroviral vector expressing an rre decoy inhibits human immunodeficiency virus type 1 replication in myelomonocytic cells produced in long-term culture. J Virol 1996; 70:4352–4360.
31. Biasolo MA, Radaelli A, Del Pup L, Franchin E, De Giuli-Morghen C, Palu G. A new antisense tRNA construct for the genetic treatment of human immunodeficiency virus type 1 infection. J Virol 1996; 70:2154–2161.
32. Larsson S, Hotchkiss G, Su I, Kebede T, Andang M, Nyholm T, Johansson B, Sonnerborg A, Vahlne A, Britton S, Ahrlund-Richter L. A novel ribozyme target site located in the HIV-1 nef open reading frame. Virology 1996; 219: 161–169.
33. Heusch M, Kraus G, Johnson P, Wong-Staal F. Intracellular immunization against SIVmac utilizing a hairpin ribozyme. Virology 1996; 216:241–244.
34. Poeschla EM, Wong-Staal F. Gene therapy and HIV disease. AIDS Clin Rev 1995; 1–45.
35. Chuah MK, Vandendriessche T, Chang HK, Ensoli B, Morgan RA. Inhibition of human immunodeficiency virus type-1 by retroviral vectors expressing antisense-tar. Hum Gene Ther 1994; 5:1467–1475.
36. Yu M, Poeschla E, Yamada O, Degrandis P, Leavitt MC, Heusch M, Yees JK, Wong-Staal F, Hampel A. In vitro and in vivo characterization of a second functional hairpin ribozyme against HIV-1. Virology 1995; 206:381–386.
37. Leavitt MC, Yu M, Yamada O, Kraus G, Looney D, Poeschla E, Wong-Staal F. Transfer of an anti-HIV-1 ribozyme gene into primary human lymphocytes. Hum Gene Ther 1994; 5:1115–1120.
38. Poeschla E, Wong-Staal F. Antiviral and anticancer ribozymes. Curr Opin Oncol 1994; 6:601–606.
39. Sullivan SM. Development of ribozymes for gene therapy. J Invest Dermatol 1994; 103:85S–89S.
40. Yu M, Ojwang I, Yamada O, Hampel A, Rapapport I, Looney D, Wong-Staal F. A hairpin ribozyme inhibits

expression of diverse strains of human immunodeficiency virus type 1 [published erratum appears in Proc Natl Acad Sci USA 1993; 90(17):8303]. Proc Natl Acad Sci USA 1993; 90:6340–6344.

41. Weerasinghe M, Liem SE, Asad S, Read SE, Joshi S. Resistance to human immunodeficiency virus type 1 (HIV-1) infection in human CD4+ lymphocyte-derived cell lines conferred by using retroviral vectors expressing an HIV-1 RNA-specific ribozyme. J Virol 1991; 65:5531–5534.
42. Leavitt MC, Yu M, Wongstaal F, Looney DJ. Ex vivo transduction and expansion of CD4(+) lymphocytes from HIV + donors—prelude to a ribozyme gene therapy trial. Gene Ther 1996; 3:599–606.
43. Wongstaal F. Ribozyme gene therapy for HIV infection—intracellular immunization of lymphocytes and CD34+ cells with an anti-HIV-1 ribozyme gene. Adv Drug Del Rev 1995; 17:363–368.
44. Lisziewicz J, Sun D, Lisziewicz A, Gallo RC. Anti-tat gene therapy: a candidate for late-stage AIDS patients. Gene Ther 1995; 2:218–222.
45. Cesbron JY, Agut H, Gosselin B, Candotti D, Raphael M, Puech F, Grandadam M, Debre P, Capron A, Autran B. SCID-hu mouse as a model for human lung HIV-1 infection. CR Acad Sci III 1994; 317:669–674.
46. Bahner I, Kearns K, Hao QL, Smogorzewska EM, Kohn DB. Transduction of human CD34(+) hematopoietic progenitor cells by a retroviral vector expressing an rre decoy inhibits human immunodeficiency virus type 1 replication in myelomonocytic cells produced in long-term culture. J Virol 1996; 70:4352–4360.
47. Lee SW, Gallardo HF, Gilboa E, Smith C. Inhibition of human immunodeficiency virus type 1 in human t cells by a potent rev response element decoy consisting of the 13-nucleotide minimal rev-binding domain. J Virol 1994; 68: 8254–8264.
48. Smythe JA, Sun D, Thomson M, Markham PD, Reitz MS Jr, Gallo RC, Lisziewicz J. A rev-inducible mutant gag gene stably transferred into T lymphocytes: an approach to gene therapy against human immunodeficiency virus type 1 infection. Proc Natl Acad Sci USA 1994; 91: 3657–3661.
49. Matsuda Z, Yu X, Yu QC, Lee TH, Essex M. A virion-specific inhibitory molecule with therapeutic potential for human immunodeficiency virus type 1. Proc Natl Acad Sci USA 1993; 90:3544–3548.
50. Lisziewicz J, Sun D, Smythe J, Lusso P, Lori F, Louie A, Markham P, Rossi J, Reitz M, Gallo RC. Inhibition of human immunodeficiency virus type 1 replication by regulated expression of a polymeric tat activation response RNA decoy as a strategy for gene therapy in AIDS. Proc Natl Acad Sci USA 1993; 90:8000–8004.
51. Brother MB, Chang HK, Lisziewicz J, Su D, Murty LC, Ensoli B. Block of tat-mediated transactivation of tumor necrosis factor beta gene expression by polymeric-tar decoys. Virology 1996; 222:252–256.
52. Chang HK, Gendelman R, Lisziewicz J, Gallo RC, Ensoli B. Block of HIV-1 infection by a combination of antisense tat RNA and tar decoys: a strategy for control of HIV-1. Gene Ther 1994; 1:208–216.
53. Sullenger BA, Gallardo HF, Ungers GE, Gilboa E. Overexpression of TAR sequences renders cells resistant to HIV replication. Cell 1990; 63:601–608.
54. Trono D, Feinberg MB, Baltimore D. HIV-1 gag mutants can dominantly interfere with the replication of wild-type virus. Cell 1988; 59:113–120.
55. Buchschacher GL, Freed EO, Panganiban AT. Cells induced to express a human immunodeficiency virus type 1 envelope mutant inhibit the spread of the wild-type virus. Hum Gene Ther 1992; 3:391–397.
56. Freed EO, Delwart EL, Buchschacher GL, Panganiban AT. A mutation in the human immunodeficiency virus type 1 transmembrane glycosylation gp41 dominantly interferes with fusion and infectivity. Proc Natl Acad Sci USA 1992; 89:70–74.
57. Wu X, Liu H, Xiao H, Conway JA, Kappes JC. Inhibition of human and simian immunodeficiency virus protease function by targeting vpx-protease-mutant fusion protein into viral particles. J Virol 1996; 70:3378–3384.
58. Ragheb JA, Bressler P, Daucher M, Chiang L, Chuah MK, Vandendriessche T, Morgan RA. Analysis of trans-dominant mutants of the HIV type 1 rev protein for their ability to inhibit rev function, HIV type 1 replication, and their use as anti-HIV gene therapeutics. AIDS Res Hum Retroviruses 1995; 11:1343–1353.
59. Liu J, Woffendin C, Yang ZY, Nabel GJ. Regulated expression of a dominant negative form of rev improves resistance to HIV replication in T cells. Gene Ther 1994; 1:32–37.
60. Lori F, Lisziewicz J, Smythe J, Cara A, Bunnag TA, Curiel D, Gallo RC. Rapid protection against human immunodeficiency virus type 1 (HIV-1) replication mediated by high efficiency non-retroviral delivery of genes interfering with HIV-1 tat and gag. Gene Ther 1994; 1:27–31.
61. Liem SE, Ramezani A, Li X, Joshi S. The development and testing of retroviral vectors expressing trans-dominant mutants of HIV-1 proteins to confer anti-HIV-1 resistance. Hum Gene Ther 1993; 4:625–634.
62. Caputo A, Grossi MP, Bozzini R, Rossi C, Betti M, Marconi PC, Barbantibrodano G, Balboni PG. Inhibition of HIV-1 replication and reactivation from latency by tat transdominant negative mutants in the cysteine rich region. Gene Ther 1996; 3:235–245.
63. Dinges M-M, Cook DR, King J, Curiel TJ, Zhang XQ, Harrison GS. HIV-regulated diphtheria toxin a chain gene confers long-term protection against HIV type 1 infection in the human promonocytic cell line u937. Hum Gene Ther 1995; 6:1437–1445.
64. Curiel TJ, Cook DR, Wang Y, Hahn BH, Ghosh SK, Harrison GS. Long-term inhibition of clinical and laboratory human immunodeficiency virus strains in human T-cell lines containing an HIV-regulated diphtheria toxin a chain gene. Hum Gene Ther 1993; 4:741–747.
65. Caruso M, Klatzmann D. Selective killing of CD4+ cells harboring a human immunodeficiency virus-inducible sui-

cide gene prevents viral spread in an infected cell population. Proc Natl Acad Sci USA 1992; 89:182–186.
66. Caruso M. Gene therapy against cancer and HIV infection using the gene encoding herpes simplex virus thymidine kinase. Mol Med Today 1996; 2:212–217.
67. Dinges MM, Cook DR, King J, Curiel TJ, Zhang XQ, Harrison GS. HIV-regulated diphtheria toxin a chain gene confers long-term protection against HIV type 1 infection in the human promonocytic cell line u937. Hum Gene Ther 1995; 6:1437–1445.
68. Brady HJ, Miles CG, Pennington DJ, Dzierzak EA. Specific ablation of human immunodeficiency virus Tat-expressing cells by conditionally toxic retroviruses. Proc Natl Acad Sci USA 1994; 91:365–369.
69. Vandendriessche T, Chuah MK, Chiang L, Chang HK, Ensoli B, Morgan RA. Inhibition of clinical human immunodeficiency virus (HIV) type 1 isolates in primary CD4+ t lymphocytes by retroviral vectors expressing anti-HIV genes. J Virol 1995; 69:4045–4052.
70. Morgan RA, Baler-Bitterlich G, Ragheb JA, Wong-Staal F, Gallo RC, Anderson WF. Further evaluation of soluble CD4 as an anti-HIV type 1 gene therapy: demonstration of protection of primary human peripheral blood lymphocytes from infection by HIV type 1. AIDS Res Hum Retroviruses 1994; 10:1507–1515.
71. Morgan RA, Looney DJ, Muenchau DD, Wong-Staal F, Gallo RC, Anderson WF. Retroviral vectors expressing soluble CD4: a potential gene therapy for AIDS. AIDS Res Hum Retroviruses 1990; 6:183–191.
72. Bird RE, Hardman KD, Jacobson JW, Johnson S, Kaufmann BM, Lee S-M, Lee T, Pope SH, Riordan GS, Whitlow M. Single-chain antigen-binding proteins. Science 1988; 242:423–426.
73. Whitlow M, Filpula D. Single-chain Fv proteins and their fusion proteins. Methods Enzymol 1991; 2:1–9.
74. Duan L, Pomerantz RJ. Intracellular antibodies for HIV-1 gene therapy. Sci Med 1996; 3:24–36.
75. Chen SY, Bagley J, Marasco WA. Intracellular antibodies as a new class of therapeutic molecules for gene therapy. Hum Gene Ther 1994; 5:595–601.
76. Chen SY, Khouri Y, Bagley J, Marasco WA. Combined intra- and extracellular immunization against human immunodeficiency virus type 1 infection with a human anti-gp120 antibody. Proc Natl Acad Sci USA 1994; 91: 5932–5936.
77. Buonocore L, Rose JK. Blockade of human immunodeficiency virus type 1 production in CD4+ t cells by an intracellular CD4 expressed under control of the viral long terminal repeat. Proc Natl Acad Sci USA 1993; 90: 2695–2699.
78. Duan L, Zhang H, Oakes JW, Bagasra O, Pomerantz RJ. Molecular and virological effects of intracellular anti-rev single-chain variable fragments on the expression of various human immunodeficiency virus-1 strains. Hum Gene Ther 1994; 5:1315–1324.
79. Duan L, Bagasra O, Laughlin MA, Oakes JW, Pomerantz RJ. Potent inhibition of human immunodeficiency virus type 1 replication by an intracellular anti-rev single-chain antibody. Proc Natl Acad Sci USA 1994; 91:5075–5079.
80. Pomerantz RJ, Bagasra O, Baltimore D. Cellular latency of human immunodeficiency virus type 1. Curr Opin Immunol 1992; 4:475–480.
81. Muzyczka N. Use of adeno-associated virus as a general transduction vector for mammalian cells. Curr Top Microbiol Immunol 1992; 158:97–129.
82. Hallek M, Wendtner CM. Recombinant adeno-associated virus (RAAV) vectors for somatic gene therapy—recent advances and potential clinical applications. Cytokines Mol Ther 1996; 2:69–79.
83. Miller AD. Retrovirus packaging cells. Hum Gene Ther 1990; 1:5–14.
84. Morgan RA, Andserson WF. Human gene therapy. Annu Rev Biochem 1993; 62:191–217.
85. Dornburg R. Reticuloendotheliosis viruses and derived vectors. Gene Ther 1995; 2:301–310.
86. Temin HM. Retrovirus vectors for gene transfer: efficient integration into and expression of exogenous DNA in vertebrate cell genomes. In: Kucherlapati R, ed. Gene Transfer. New York: Plenum Press, 1986:144–187.
87. Gilboa E. Retroviral gene transfer: applications to human gene therapy. Prog Clin Biol Res 1990; 352:301–311.
88. Eglitis MA, Anderson WF. Retroviral vectors for introduction of genes into mammalian cells. Biotechniques 1988; 6:608–614.
89. Gunzburg WH, Salmons B. Development of retroviral vectors as safe, targeted gene delivery systems [review]. J Mol Med 1996; 74:171–182.
90. Hunter E, Swanstrom R. Retrovirus envelope glycoproteins. Curr Top Microbiol Immunol 1990; 157:187–253.
91. Young JAT, Bates P, Willert K, Varmus HE. Efficient incorporation of human CD4 protein into avian leukosis virus particles. Science 1990; 250:1421–1423.
92. Matano T, Odawara T, Iwamoto A, Yoshikura H. Targeted infection of a retrovirus bearing a CD4-env chimera into human cells expressing human immunodeficiency virus type 1. J Gen Virol 1995; 76:3165–3169.
93. Etienne-Julan M, Roux P, Carillo S, Jeanteur P, Piechaczyk M. The efficiency of cell targeting by recombinant retroviruses depends on the nature of the receptor and the composition of the artificial cell-virus linker. J Gen Virol 1992; 73:3251–3255.
94. Roux P, Jeanteur P, Piechaczyk M. A versatile and potentially general approach to the targeting of specific cell types by retroviruses: application to the infection of human by means of major histocompatibility complex class I and class II antigens by mouse ecotropic murine leukemia virus-derived viruses. Proc Natl Acad Sci USA 1989; 86: 9079–9083.
95. Chu T-H, Dornburg R. Retroviral vector particles displaying the antigen-binding site of an antibody enable cell-type-specific gene transfer. J Virol 1995; 69:2659–2663.
96. Chu T-H, Martinez I, Sheavy WC, Dornburg R. Cell targeting with retroviral vector particles containing antibody-envelope fusion proteins. Gene Ther 1994; 1:292–299.

97. Russell SJ, Hawkins RE, Winter G. Retroviral vectors displaying functional antibody fragments. Nucl Acid Res 1993; 21:1081–1085.
98. Chu T-H, Dornburg R. Towards highly-efficient cell-type-specific gene transfer with retroviral vectors that display a single chain antibody. J Virol 1997; 71:720–725.
99. Dougherty JP, Wisniewski R, Yang S, Rhode BW, Temin HM. New retrovirus helper cells with almost no nucleotide sequence homology to retrovirus vectors. J Virol 1989; 63:3209–3212.
100. Purchase HG, Witter RL. The reticuloendotheliosis viruses. Curr Top Microbiol Immunol 1975; 71:103–124.
101. Somia NV, Zoppe M, Verma IM. Generation of targeted retroviral vectors by using single-chain variable fragment: an approach to in vivo gene delivery. Proc Natl Acad Sci USA 1995; 92:7570–7574.
102. Marin M, Noel D, Valsesia-Wittman S, Brockly F, Etienne-Julan M, Russell S, Cosset F-L, Piechaczyk M. Targeted infection of human cells via major histocompatibility complex class I molecules by Moleney leukemia virus-derived viruses displaying single chain antibody fragment-envelope fusion proteins. J Virol 1996; 70: 2957–2962.
103. Valsesia-Wittmann S, Morling F, Nilson B, Takeuchi Y, Russell S, Cosset F-L. Improvement of retroviral retargeting by using acid spacers between an additional binding domain and the N terminus of Moloney leukemia virus SU. J Virol 1996; 70:2059–2064.
104. Nilson BHK, Morling FJ, Cosset F-L, Russell SJ. Targeting of retroviral vectors through protease-substrate interactions. Gene Ther 1996; 3:280–286.
105. Schnierle BS, Moritz D, Jeschke M, Groner B. Expression of chimeric envelope proteins in helper cell lines and integratyion into Moloney murine leukemia virus particles. Gene Ther 1996; 3:334–342.
106. Dornburg R. From the natural evolution to the genetic manipulation of the host range of retroviruses. Biol Chem 1997; 378:457–468.
107. Orlic D, Girard LJ, Jordan CT, Anderson SM, Cline AP, Bodine DM. The level of mRNA encoding the amphotropic retrovirus receptor in mouse and human hematopoietic stem cells is low and correlates with the efficiency of retrovirus transduction. Proc Natl Acad Sci USA 1996; 93:11097–11102.
108. Schnell MJ, Johnson IE, Buonocore L, Rose JK. Construction of a novel virus that targets HIV-1-infected cells and controls HIV-1 infection. Cell 1997; 90:849–857.
109. Nolan GP. Harnessing viral devices as pharmaceuticals: fighting HIV-1's fire with fire. Cell 1997; 90:821–824.
110. Uckun FM. Severe combined immunodeficient mouse models of human leukemia. Blood 1996; 88:1135–1146.
111. Dick JE. Future prospects for animal models created by transplanting human haematopoietic cells into immune-deficient mice. Res Immunol 1994; 145:380–384.
112. Dick JE, Sirard C, Pflumio F, Lapidot T. Murine models of normal and neoplastic human haematopoiesis. Cancer Surv 1992; 15:161–181.
113. Dick JE. Immune-deficient mice as models of normal and leukemic human hematopoiesis [review]. Cancer Cells 1991; 3:39–48.
114. Mueller BM, Reisfeld RA. Potential of the SCID mouse as a host for human tumors. Cancer Metastasis Rev 1991; 10:193–200.
115. Shen RN, Lu L, Broxmeyer HE. New therapeutic strategies in the treatment of murine diseases induced by virus and solid tumors: biology and implications for the potential treatment of human leukemia, AIDS, and solid tumors. Crit Rev Oncol Hematol 1990; 10:253–265.
116. Gauduin M-C, Parren PWHI, Weir R, Barbas CF, Burton DR, Koup RA. Passive immunization with a human monoclonal antibody protects hu-PBL-SCID mice against challenge by primary isolates of HIV-1. Nat Med 1997; 3: 1389–1393.
117. Gauduin M-C, Allaway GP, Olson WC, Weir R, Maddon PJ, Koup RA. CD4-immunoglobulin G2 protects hu-PBL-SCID mice against challenge by primary human immunodeficiency virus type 1 isolates. J Virol 1998; 72: 3475–3478.
118. Ranga U, Woffendin C, Verma S, Xu L, June CH, Bishop DK, Nabel GJ. Enhanced T cell engraftment after retroviral delivery of an antiviral gene in HIV-infected individuals. Proc Natl Acad Sci USA 1998; 95:1201–1205.
119. Donahue RE, Bunnell BA, Zink MC, Metzger ME, Westro RP, Kirby MR, Unangst T, Clements JE, Morgan RA. Reduction in SIV replication in rhesus macaques infused with autologous lymphozytes engineered with antiviral genes. Nat Med 1998; 4:181–186.

27

Gene Delivery to the Skin

Paul A. Khavari
VA Palo Alto Healthcare System, Palo Alto, and Stanford University School of Medicine, Stanford, California

I. INTRODUCTION

The skin is composed of two major compartments, the stratified squamous epithelium of the epidermis and the fibrous mesenchymal tissue of the dermis (Fig. 1) (1). The epidermis is a self-renewing tissue comprised of a multilayered array of keratinocytes expressing either of two mutually exclusive programs of gene expression. The basal program is devoted to proliferation of keratinocytes and adhesion of these cells to the underlying basement membrane, while the suprabasal program is directed at keratinocyte terminal differentiation and skin barrier formation (2–4). The dermis is a supporting collagenous stroma within which are embedded fibroblasts, blood vessels, epidermal appendages such as hair and sweat glands, and an array of diverse cell types (14). The skin is the site of a number of debilitating hereditary and acquired diseases, such as epidermolysis bullosa and cutaneous T-cell lymphoma, for which effective therapy is currently unavailable. However, the elucidation of the molecular basis for several skin disorders has focused attention on therapeutic gene delivery. The attractive features of the skin in this regard are considerable and include the ability to grow primary skin cells in culture and then to regenerate tissue elements in vivo, the ready accessibility of genetically engineered skin to clinical monitoring, the ability of skin to produce and deliver polypeptides to the systemic circulation, and the potential for topical regulation of inserted transgenes (5–9). However, as might be expected in a tissue representing an important frontier that blocks microbial invasion and therefore the insertion of foreign DNA, the obstacles to effective gene insertion into cells of skin tissue are not trivial.

II. CANDIDATE DISEASES

The skin represents a gene therapy target tissue for both cutaneous and systemic diseases. Because of its accessibility, the skin offers an attractive opportunity to refine gene-transfer capabilities relative to current efforts underway in visceral tissues (10–13).

A. Selected Candidate Skin Diseases

The genetic basis for a number of hereditary skin diseases has been elucidated (Table 1) with the remaining uncharacterized genodermatoses currently foci of intensive investigation. Human genetic lesions leading to skin blistering, abnormal cutaneous cornification, and cancer predisposition have been well characterized. In the epidermis, these mutations affect genes expressed selectively in either basal or suprabasal layers as well as those expressed in both compartments. The site of such genetic defects within the epidermis can produce characteristic corresponding phenotypic abnormalities. Mutations in important basal layer genes commonly lead to skin fragility and blistering, such as is seen with laminin 5 chain gene defects in a subset of junctional epidermolysis bullosa patients (14–17). Suprabasal defects lead to abnormal terminal epidermal differentiation manifested often as hyperkeratosis, as seen in the case of transglutaminase 1 gene mutations in lamellar ichthyosis (18–20). A number of these disorders, espe-

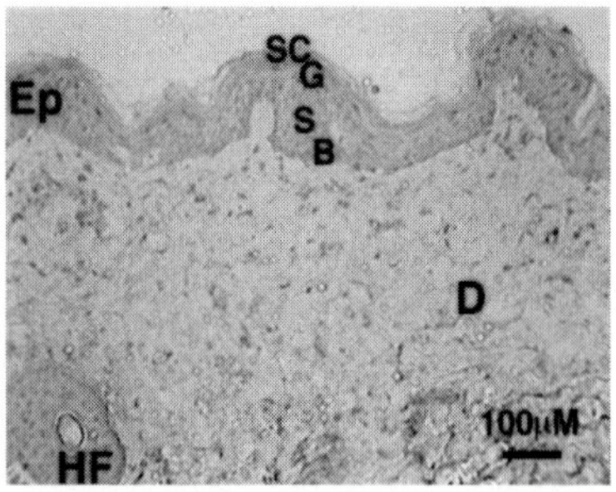

Figure 1 Tissue architecture of skin. Ep = Epidermis; D = dermis; HF = hair follicle; B = basal layer of the epidermis; S = squamous layer; G = granular layer; SC = stratum corneum. (Scale bar = 100 μM.)

cially those involving mutations in large structural proteins such as Type VII collagen in dystrophic epidermolysis bullosa (21–23), are likely to be intractable to small-molecule pharmacotherapy and may be only effectively approached by the return of normal protein expression.

Table 1 Selected Candidate Skin Diseases

Disorder	Selected gene(s)	Ref.
Lamellar ichthyosis subset	Transglutaminase 1	18,19
X-linked ichthyosis	Steroid sulfatase	73
EB simplex	Keratins 5 and 14	51,52
	Plectin	117
Pachyonychia congenita type 1/2	Keratins 6a and 16/17	81,82
Epidermolytic hyperkeratosis	Keratins 1 and 10	27,28
Epidermolytic PPK	Keratin 9	78,79
Nonepidermolytic PPK	Keratin 16	80
Vohwinkel's syndrome	Loricrin	113
Ichthyosis bullosa of Siemens	keratin 2e	114
Junctional EB	Laminin 5 $\alpha3$, $\beta3$, and $\gamma2$	14,15
	BPAG2 [BP180]	115
	$\beta4$ Integrin	116
Dystrophic EB	Type VII collagen	21,22
Xeroderma pigmentosum	XP group genes	94,95
Basal cell nevus syndrome	Patched	118,119

EB = epidermolysis bullosa; PPK = palmoplantar keratoderma; XP = xeroderma pigmentosum.

In addition to identification of disease genes, successful corrective gene delivery to the skin requires an understanding of disease pathogenesis, gene expression characteristics, stem cell biology, effective gene delivery, and immune modulation (5–9). Progress in cutaneous gene therapy for genetic disease, however, has lagged behind other tissues, and future advances depend on rigorous studies in well-defined skin disease model systems. An understanding of the molecular basis of disease pathogenesis in these disorders, however, represents the first step in the rational design of genetic therapies. Correction of recessive disorders, in principal, requires only reexpression of the normal protein product corresponding to the previously absent or defective genes. This has been recently achieved in model efforts, as noted below (24–26). A greater challenge exists in the dominant disorders due to dominant-negative mutant proteins that effectively ''poison'' any wild-type protein present, as in the case of keratin 1 and 10 mutants in epidermolytic hyperkeratosis (27,28). Effective genetic correction in these latter instances requires circumventing the negative effects of such mutants in an effort to restore function of the normal protein. Because of the considerable additional technical challenges associated with gene delivery to human somatic tissue, the recessive genetic skin disorders have been the focus of many current efforts to date.

B. Gene Therapy for Systemic Disease via the Skin

The skin has been used as a site of polypeptide production for delivery to the systemic circulation (29) via both keratinocytes and fibroblasts in models involving human skin xenografts onto mice as well as mouse skin grafts onto mice. Polypeptides that have been successfully delivered from the skin include such proteins as Factor IX (30), apolipoprotein E (31), transferrin (32), and growth hormone (33,34). In addition, skin fibroblasts that were implanted in a variety of noncutaneous visceral tissue sites have shown encouraging results in animal models of disorders such as mucopolysaccharidosis and anemia (35). This work was performed with a variety of grafting approaches using either normal or transformed cells as well as full-thickness transgenic murine skin tissue and indicates that genetically engineered epidermis and dermis can deliver a variety of polypeptides to the systemic circulation. Potential limitations due to protein size and charge, however, are still incompletely understood. While much progress has been recently made in the development of therapeutic cutaneous gene delivery in model systems, significant barriers must be addressed before widespread application in humans will be possible.

III. MAJOR APPROACHES TO CUTANEOUS GENE DELIVERY

Two rapidly developing approaches to therapeutic gene delivery to the skin in model systems utilize different strategies (Fig. 2). First, in the ex vivo approach, cells are harvested from the host by skin biopsy; this is followed by growth of the cells in vitro and gene transfer to the cells while they are growing in tissue culture. The cells are then grafted back onto the recipient. Gene transfer by this approach has been most successfully achieved with integrating retroviral vectors (24,25,36–38). Grafting efforts have benefited from a wide variety of experience obtained primarily in the treatment of burn and cutaneous ulcer patients (39,40). These include refinement of approaches ranging from the application of simple sheets of epithelium grown in vitro to the use of complex grafts composed of living cells seeded in natural or synthetic matrices. Ex vivo cutaneous gene delivery allows the application of selection criteria to specific engineered skin cell populations, such as drug selection, and the production of entirely engineered regions of grafted skin tissue in vivo (24,26,41). However, this approach is labor intensive in that it involves extensive tissue culture and grafting efforts, with the latter involving a potentially scarring surgical procedure.

The second major strategy for cutaneous gene transfer involves direct administration of genetic material to intact skin tissue using either viral or nonviral delivery vectors. Gene-delivery vectors contain and deliver therapeutic genes. Viral gene-delivery vectors (which include retrovirus, adenovirus, adeno-associated virus, herpes simplex virus, and others) incorporate therapeutic genes into a modified viral genome and use viral mechanisms for entering host cells. Nonviral vectors commonly use naked plasmid DNA, either alone or complexed to lipid and/or protein elements. The direct approach to administering vectors to skin includes the topical application of either naked plasmid DNA complexed with liposomes (42) or viral vectors such as adenovirus and modified herpes virus (43,44), direct injection of viral vectors (44) or naked plasmid DNA in buffered saline (45,46), and particle bombardment utilizing vector-coated microspheres (''gene gun'') (47). In addition, other emerging methods for direct gene transfer to intact skin, including ultrasound, electroporation, and high-frequency oscillating needle bundles, have recently been presented (48). Each of these new approaches uses physical methods to assist in delivering genes across the epidermal permeability barrier, however, substantial additional work is required to define their future potential utility over other current approaches. Direct in vivo gene transfer to the skin is less labor-intensive in general than ex vivo approaches and can produce biologically active levels of gene expression and protein production. Direct approaches have, however, been plagued by low levels of gene transfer that achieve transgene expression in only a minority of cells

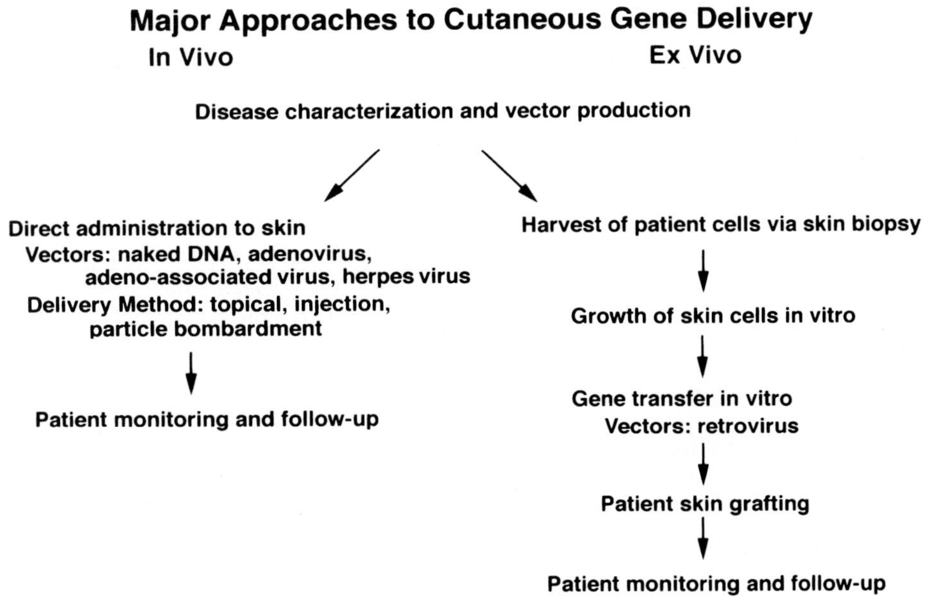

Figure 2 Major strategies for cutaneous gene delivery. Ex vivo and direct in vivo gene-delivery approaches along with selected vectors used for each approach are noted.

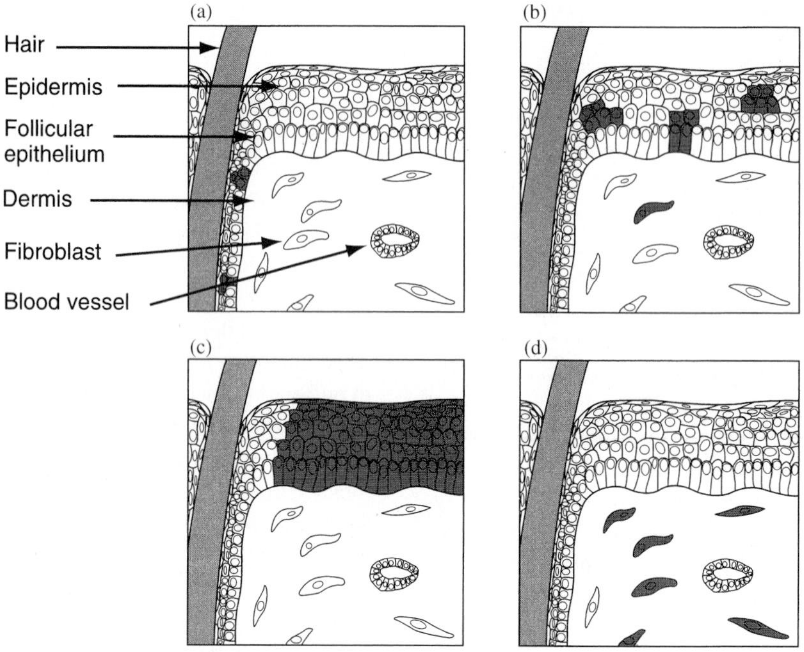

Figure 3 Gene expression patterns obtained in skin by differing gene-transfer approaches. Schematic representation of gene expression patterns obtained in epidermis following different delivery approaches (cells expressing delivered genes are shaded). (a) Topical application of nonviral vector in liposome complex shows focal expression in follicular epithelium. (b) Injected nonviral or viral vectors by direct superficial injection of the skin show localized expression primarily in the epidermis. (c) High-efficiency ex vivo gene transfer to keratinocytes followed by grafting show transgene expression in all epidermal cells with the exception of follicular epithelium (follicular structures are not regenerated by this approach so that hair follicle denotes the border of the grafted skin). (d) High-efficiency ex vivo gene transfer to fibroblasts is followed by grafting of cells embedded in dermal substrates (follicular structures are not regenerated by this approach so the follicle would denote the border of the grafted skin as above).

for periods as short as a few days (43,45). The patterns of gene expression obtained by different gene-delivery approaches can vary dramatically, from the patchy perifollicular pattern seen with topical application of lipid-complexed DNA to the more uniform interfollicular epidermal distribution seen with ex vivo delivery using retroviral gene transfer, as noted schematically in (Fig. 3).

IV. DIFFERING REQUIREMENTS FOR SPECIFIC APPLICATIONS IN CUTANEOUS GENE DELIVERY

A recurrent theme in gene therapy efforts in all tissues is the need to tailor gene transfer approaches to specific therapeutic applications (10). In addition to genetic skin diseases, the skin is a potential tissue site for a number of distinct therapeutic gene-transfer efforts, and these differ considerably in their gene-transfer requirements (Table 2). Such potential efforts include cutaneous gene transfer for immunization (49) and for production of polypeptides for delivery to the systemic circulation (31,50). Each of these three major applications has distinctive requirements regarding efficiency of gene transfer, durability, regulation of expression of the introduced gene (the "transgene"), and transgene immunogenicity.

High-efficiency gene transfer that restores normal gene expression to all cells of a diseased tissue has been among the most challenging goals in many tissues, but not all applications require it. Immunization via gene transfer to the skin does not require uniform transgene delivery to all cells in a given tissue compartment. This is also the case in systemic delivery of proteins expressed in skin, where the absolute magnitude of total transgene product delivered from the skin impacts the therapeutic outcome more that the percentage of cells in the skin that express it. Lasting correction of genetic skin disease, in contrast, may require high-efficiency gene transfer, as could be predicted in the case of cancer prevention in patients with xeroderma pigmentosum and in the correction of cell-intrinsic structural defects such as keratin 5 and 14 mutations in epidermolysis

Table 2 Cutaneous Gene-Transfer Properties by Therapeutic Goal

	Efficiency[a]	Durability[b]	Expression level	Immunogenicity
Genodermatosis	High	Sustained	Consistent	None
Immunization	Variable	Transient	Regulated	High
Systemic delivery	High	Sustained[c]	Regulated	None

[a] Percentage of cells in skin tissue that receive the therapeutic gene.
[b] Sustainability of capability for gene expression after gene transfer.
[c] certain applications (e.g., pulsed delivery of hematopoietic growth factors after bone marrow transplantation) may require transient periods of gene delivery.

bullosa simplex (51,52). In such cases, a focal lack of corrective gene expression may be sufficient to perpetuate major elements of disease pathology (i.e., neoplastic transformation in xeroderma pigmentosum and skin fragility in epidermolysis bullosa). High-efficiency genetic correction, therefore, may be of importance in gene therapy of genodermatoses.

Gene transfer efforts in human visceral tissues have been unsuccessful in reliably sustaining therapeutic gene expression (10–13), and the ability to sustain therapeutic gene delivery for prolonged periods is another capability important in gene therapy for genetic skin disease. While the need for such long-term gene delivery may be variable to nonexistent in both genetic immunization and protein delivery to the circulation from the skin (Table 2), curative efforts in genodermatoses depend on lasting restoration of normal gene expression. Because this requires durable gene-delivery vectors, gene targeting to long-lived skin stem cells, and avoidance of immune clearing, achieving such sustainability has proven to be a formidable challenge. While periodic administration of therapeutic genes in the form of grafting with genetically engineered cells or by direct transfer of vectors to intact human skin tissue may be envisioned in certain lethal genetic skin disorders, achievement of sustainable cutaneous gene delivery is a major requirement for ultimate success.

The skin, by virtue of its accessibility to target gene regulation by topically applied agents, is an attractive tissue for regulated therapeutic gene production. Such regulated delivery may be of importance in delivery of proteins to the systemic circulation, such as the hematopoietic growth factor erythropoeitin (53). Many of the genes affected in genetic skin disease, however, are expressed at constant levels within a given tissue compartment, as in the case of laminin 5 and keratin genes within the basal and suprabasal layers, respectively. Precise regulation of the magnitude of therapeutic gene expression in genetic skin disease, therefore, may be unneeded in most cases, provided gene expression may be restored to levels within a physiological range.

The ability of a therapeutic transgene to induce a specific immune response, while central for success of intradermal genetic immunization, represents a feared complication in gene-transfer efforts for monogenic skin disease. Surprisingly, such unwanted transgene-specific immune responses have not been widely reported in current gene therapy trials in other tissues, in stark contrast to inflammatory responses seen in humans with viral gene-delivery vectors such as adenovirus (54). Because current preclinical models of therapeutic cutaneous gene transfer lack an intact human immune system, the extent to which unwanted immune reactions will pose a challenge may only become clear in human clinical trials. Central requirements for successful genetic correction of genetic skin disease, then, may include high-efficiency genetic correction, durability, consistent transgene expression levels, and a lack of unwanted immune clearing of the therapeutic gene.

V. MODEL SYSTEMS FOR THERAPEUTIC GENE DELIVERY TO THE HUMAN SKIN

Preclinical efforts to deliver genes via the skin have used entirely animal models such as those in the mouse and pig (33,45) or human skin tissue grafted on immune-deficient mice (24,26). The latter approach is especially attractive in the case of cutaneous tissue because human skin can differ dramatically from that of animal models in such characteristics as epidermal thickness, turnover time, and degree of accessibility to direct gene transfer. In the case of human skin–immune-deficient mouse models, severe combined immunodeficiency (SCID) and nude mice have most commonly been used to accept either (1) composite grafts made of cells that have been seeded on a variety of natural and synthetic substrates (55–57), (2) epithelial sheets of engineered cells (50), or (3) full-thickness human skin (58). Immune-deficient mice are useful in models of gene delivery to the skin because they readily accept grafted human tissue without developing an immune response to the foreign transplanted tissue. Human epidermis, either regenerated from cells grown in culture or as full-thickness grafts from intact skin on immune-deficient mice, displays the histological features, gene-expression pattern, pigmentary characteristics, and functional properties of the skin of the individual human donor—whether that individual had normal or diseased skin (24,57,58). This retention of disease phenotype in living human tissue in vivo is of particular value in developing approaches to correct monogenic disorders, where the defect in gene expression is intrinsic to the skin and does not stem from abnormal circulating peptides or systemic immune elements.

VI. CURRENT PROGRESS IN MODEL SYSTEMS

A number of efforts using model systems as noted above have been made to achieve therapeutic gene delivery to the skin (Table 3). These efforts fall into two major categories: treatment of primary cutaneous disease, including wounds, and the use of the skin to deliver polypeptides to the systemic circulation. A major focus has been the direct treatment of primary cutaneous disease. These studies have included the recent corrective efforts with primary genetic skin diseases, including lamellar ichthyosis (24,25), X-linked ichthyosis (26), and epidermolysis bullos (59). In the case of the former two diseases, keratinocytes that had been freshly isolated from the skin of affected patients were genetically engineered in vitro using a retroviral vector, then used to regenerate skin in vivo on immune-deficient mice. This process led to phenotypic correction of central disease features at the levels of gene expression (transglutaminase 1 and steroid sulfatase gene expression was restored), tissue architecture (the stratum corneum was restored to normal thickness), clinical appearance, and barrier function (24,26). Gene-delivery efforts for the treatment of disorders localized to the skin have also included direct gene delivery to induce local production of growth factors or cytokines in models of wound healing (60,61) and cancer (62) (Table 3).

VII. PROGRESS IN GENETIC SKIN DISEASE

A. Recessive Ichthyoses

The ichthyotic disorders are a heterogeneous family of diseases characterized by abnormal epidermal cornification (63). Recently the genetic basis for several of these disorders has been characterized (64) and found to involve key enzymatic or structural proteins involved in epithelial maturation and cutaneous barrier function. Among the recessive ichthyoses are lamellar ichthyosis and X-linked recessive ichthyosis. Consistent with the nature of their gene defects in the suprabasal epidermal gene expression program, these disorders are characterized by clinical hyperkeratosis.

Lamellar ichthyosis has been associated with the *TGM1* gene (18–20) in a subset of patients by genetic linkage and mutation analysis and has proven to be a valuable prototype disorder for gene therapy (24,25) due to its dramatic clinical and biochemical phenotype. The *TGM1* gene encodes keratinocytes transglutaminase (TGase1) (65,66) a membrane-linked enzyme active in forming the cornified envelope in differentiating keratinocytes. TGase1 catalyzes the formation of isodipeptide crosslinks between cornified envelope precursor molecules (67,68) and is believed necessary for normal terminal differentiation and barrier formation in the outer epidermis. While not present in all lamellar ichthyosis patients (69,70), *TGM1* gene mutations in affected patients may produce enzymatically inactive TGase1 protein (18). Restoration of functional TGase1 en-

Table 3 Selected Cutaneous Gene-Delivery Models

Disease model	Delivered gene	Delivery method	Ref.
Atherosclerosis	Apolipoprotein E	Ex vivo	50
Hemophilia B	Factor IX	Ex vivo	30
Growth hormone deficiency	Growth hormone	Ex vivo	33,34
Transferrin deficiency	Transferrin	Ex vivo	32
Lamellar ichthyosis	Transglutaminase 1	Ex vivo	24
X-linked ichthyosis	Steroid sulfatase	Ex vivo	26
Junctional epidermolysis bullosa	Laminin 5 $\gamma 2$	Ex vivo	59
Wound healing	Epidermal growth factor,	In vivo	60,61
	transforming growth factor $\beta 1$	In vivo	
Neoplasia	Interleukin-12 and others	In vivo	62

zymatic activity to skin from TGase1-negative patients represents a possible means of correcting this disorder.

In order to achieve this, recent work developed an approach to achieving high-efficiency transfer of the normal TGase1 gene to skin from patients characterized as TGase1-negative (25). This approach relied on amphotropic retroviral gene-delivery vectors for the TGase1 gene (25). Following high-efficiency gene transfer into primary patient keratinocytes grown in vitro, restoration of full-length TGase1 protein expression and transglutaminase enzymatic activity was verified. These keratinocytes were then grafted to immune-deficient mice to regenerate human skin in vivo. Lamellar ichthyosis patient keratinocytes genetically engineered with the TGase1 vector regenerated skin displaying restored TGase1 protein expression in vivo and normalized histology, clinical surface appearance, and barrier function; patient cells that received a control vector produced skin with the hyperkeratosis and defective skin barrier function characteristic of the disease (24). These findings indicated that successful phenotypic correction of human genetic skin disease tissue can be achieved via this gene-transfer approach, but this correction failed to extend beyond the 1-month timepoint after which transgene expression is commonly lost in many cutaneous gene-transfer models (5,24,26,30,41,71). Such loss may be due to a number of potential factors; however, in this approach it appears to be due to silencing of vector promoter elements (41). Correction of lamellar ichthyosis patient skin tissue then could be achieved but not sustained.

X-linked ichthyosis is a genodermatosis that is generally much milder than lamellar ichthyosis (63,72). Due to a loss of functional arylsulfatase O (73–76), a steroid sulfatase believed necessary for a normal desquamation (77), X-linked ichthyosis constitutes another prototype recessive disorder for refinement of cutaneous gene transfer. High-efficiency retroviral gene transfer followed by grafting of genetically engineered cells has also recently been used to correct X-linked ichthyosis patient skin at the level of tissue architecture, gene expression, clinical appearance, and function (26). While also not sustained for periods significantly longer than 1 month, this corrective gene-transfer disease model offers another opportunity to address the challenge of durable therapeutic gene delivery to the skin.

Among the other inherited disorders of cornification are dominant disorders due to keratin mutations, such as epidermolytic hyperkeratosis (K1/K10) (27,28), palmoplantar keratoderma subtypes (epidermolytic:K9, nonepidermolytic:K16) (78–80), and pachyonychia congenita subtypes (K6a/16/17) (81,82). In principal, these diseases represent much greater challenges to even achieving short-term correction than the recessive disorders because of the presence of proposed dominant-negative mutant keratin molecules. Additional wild-type gene expression in this setting may be ineffective because such mutants can disrupt function of normal keratin subunits in forming the intermediate filaments that give structural integrity to the cell (3,83). A number of strategies to overcoming the challenge of dominant-negative mutants via genetic approaches are being studied, including in situ gene repair by oligonucleotide recombination and homologous gene recombination, but none have yet been shown successful in achieving functional correction in a genodermatosis model.

B. Epidermolysis Bullosa

The array of inherited blistering skin disorders known as epidermolysis bullosa represent prototypes of gene defects in affecting the basal epidermal program of gene expression (16,17,84–86). The recent characterization of the genes responsible for specific subtypes of this disease have revealed a corresponding heterogeneity in molecular defects (Table 1). A common theme emerging from these studies has been the appreciation that these defects affect structural proteins forming the vital link from the cytoplasm of basal keratinocytes through basement membrane zone components and on down into the uppermost dermis (17). Because of the structural nature of these proteins and the fact that many have multiple functional domains and can polymerize to form higher order structures, purely medicinal therapy has proven of little benefit. Especially in the case of more severe subtypes of epidermolysis bullosa, a key hope centers on correction of specific underlying genetic defects.

Molecular alterations in a number of specific genes responsible for epidermolysis bullosa have been increasingly well characterized over the past 5 years (17,84–87). Malfunction in any of their corresponding proteins mediating epidermal adhesion, which could be envisioned to function as a series of connected links in a chain, results in skin fragility and blistering. The association of these genes with specific clinical phenotypes has shed additional light on their pathogenesis as, for example, in the case of compound heterozygous mutations identified in the Type VII collagen gene in dystrophic epidermolysis bullosa (88) as well as BPAG2 (89) and laminin 5 chains (90,91) in junctional epidermolysis bullosa. The majority of genes implicated in epidermolysis bullosa are effectively produced within keratinocytes of the basal epidermal layer (92). This, combined with the fact that some of these genes are expressed in internal epithelia in addition to skin, underscore the fact that attempts at genetic correction in these disorders must be correctly targeted. In this regard, it is unknown whether restored expression of a basement membrane protein throughout the epidermis may result in disordered epithelial polarity, therefore, it is formally possible that proteins such as laminin 5 and BPAG2 require expression limited to the basal epidermal layer. This is in contrast to corrective efforts with TGase1 and steroid sulfatase where mRNA expression throughout the epidermis via vector promoters active in all layers failed to impair their corrective impact (24,25). The fact that genetically corrected epidermolysis bullosa patient keratinocytes may have a selective adhesive advantage over uncorrected cells, however, may mitigate against these and other unanticipated potential pitfalls.

While at an earlier stage than the ichthyoses, efforts at genetic correction epidermolysis bullosa in model systems have focused on laminin 5 (59) and BPAG2 in junctional disease and Type VII collagen in the dystrophic subtypes. Of interest, revertant mosaicism in the BPAG2 gene—where a defective gene reverts to normal in a mosaic pattern in the skin—has been described in generalized benign atrophic epidermolysis bullosa and has been noted to resemble a natural form of cutaneous gene therapy (93). In the case of laminin 5, defects in one of the three chains of the laminin 5 trimer ($\alpha3$, $\beta3$, or $\gamma2$) are associated with junctional epidermolysis bullosa of a severity that extends to include the severe Herlitz subtype (14,15,84). Laminin 5 $\gamma2$ chain gene transfer via both modified adenoviral- and retroviral-based approaches has been described in the immortalized L5V5 keratinocyte line (59). Such gene transfer led to restoration of normal features laminin 5 trimer expression in a basal-polarized fashion, and this finding was confirmed in cysts of immortalized cells formed in vivo after subcutaneous injection into nude mice (59). A next phase of work in genetic correction of epidermolysis bullosa will involve nontransformed tissue from patients in spatially intact epidermis.

C. Xeroderma Pigmentosum

Xeroderma pigmentosum has been associated with defects in a number of DNA repair genes and is characterized by specific inadequacies in DNA repair following ultraviolet injury (94,95). From the standpoint of gene targeting, xeroderma pigmentosum represents a pan-epidermal prototype disorder affecting both basal and suprabasal compartments, including melanocytes. The disease is characterized by photosensitivity with early onset of cutaneous neoplasias, including basal cell carcinoma, squamous cell carcinoma, and malignant melanoma (96). Much progress has been made in identifying the genes corresponding to the separate genetic complementation groups of xeroderma pigmentosum and its variants. This progress has been followed by attempts at genetic correction in xeroderma pigmentosum cells grown in tissue culture. The XPA and XPD genes have been among those best studied in this regard, and their restoration to cells lacking these genes has been shown to return parameters of DNA repair and cell survival after ultraviolet injury back toward normal (97,98). While corrective gene delivery to all layers of the epithelium is readily achieved to keratinocytes by regeneration of skin using genetically engineered cells (24,26), the need to target melanocytes represents an additional formidable challenge in xeroderma pigmentosum that has not yet been systematically approached. Xeroderma pigmentosum, then, represents another serious genetic disorder in which efforts in models of genetic correction have been initiated yet in which major technical challenges remain.

D. Challenges in Gene Delivery to Skin

Many of the current challenges facing gene therapy in the skin are shared with efforts in visceral tissues (10). Improvements are needed in the ability to target therapeutic genes to specific cells and tissues and in the capacity to regulate and sustain therapeutic gene production. Therapeutic gene targeting to specific tissue compartments in the skin is possible by selective ex vivo gene transfer to only keratinocytes or fibroblasts prior to grafting back to the host as well as by use of cell-type–specific promoters. In the case of the epidermis, different promoters exist to target gene expression to specific layers of the epithelium, such as the basal layer–specific keratin 14 promoter and the suprabasal layer–specific keratin 10 promoter (4,99,100). While ex vivo efforts allow controlled production of relatively homogeneous populations of genetically engineered cell types, an ability to accomplish precise and uniform vector targeting to only one cell type (i.e., keratinocytes and not melanocytes) via direct gene insertion to intact skin has not been clearly characterized. The challenge to achieve precise control over therapeutic molecule dosage that is so formidable in many tissues may be circumvented in the skin because of the potential use of topical regulation agents that can act on therapeutic gene promoters, including retinoid and corticosteroid ligands.

Although transient gene expression in the skin may be currently sufficient for short-term applications such as immunization, long-term gene delivery for efforts such as lasting correction of genetic diseases and supplementation of low levels of systemic polypeptides in the circulation is currently an area of significant challenge. Gene expression following the administration of nonviral vectors by direct-delivery approaches is lost within 2–7 days (45). In the case of gene transfer via retroviral and adenoviral vectors, the gene expression is also transient, with high levels of uniform epidermal gene expression usually ceasing within 1–4 weeks (24,30,41,43,71). The achievement of sustained transgene expression in skin hinges on meeting specific criteria, among which are (1) successful gene transfer to long-lived progenitor stem cells, (2) retention of genetic elements within such cells, (3) maintenance of retained gene expression via gene-delivery promoter elements, and (4) avoidance of immune responses against introduced genes that result in clearing of genetically engineered cells. Precise molecular markers identifying cutaneous stem cells (101) and effective approaches to engineer them by direct gene transfer in vivo have not been clearly defined in animals or humans. However, it appears that long-lived progenitors from both keratinocytes and fibroblasts can survive ex vivo gene transfer to regenerate skin elements for prolonged periods in vivo (32,41). Nonviral vector gene sequences appear to be rapidly lost from the skin after direct administration, but retroviral vector sequences that have been integrated in keratinocytes ex vivo before grafting the cells in vivo in mice have been shown to persist for multiple epidermal turnover cycles long after the loss of transgene expression (41). This latter finding suggests that there is a potential silencing phenomenon that contributes to a loss of gene expression by the retained vector sequences. Another important factor that may limit the durability of therapeutic gene delivery to the skin involves undesired immune responses. The skin is a tissue that is continuously exposed to microbial pathogens and therefore is a site of generation of potent immune responses (102). As in visceral tissues, vigorous immune responses to viral vector proteins, most notably to adenoviral proteins, may hinder attempts to achieve sustained gene delivery to the skin. Recent progress in immune modulation offers hope that this barrier may be surmounted. This progress includes the blockade of co-stimulatory molecules such as CD28 and CD40, an intervention recently shown capable of allowing successful skin xenotransplantation in immune-competent mice (103). In addition, oral tolerization to viral vector components (104), a process in which the feeding of viral proteins induces immune tolerance upon subsequent viral rechallenge, may comprise important future avenues to circumvent unwanted immune clearing of therapeutic genes expressed in the skin.

VIII. REQUIRED NEW CAPABILITIES AND ALTERNATIVE APPROACHES

Widespread successful application of cutaneous genetic therapies is dependent upon the advancement of our understanding of fundamental biological processes in the skin as well as the acquisition of new gene-delivery capabilities. Important biological questions in therapeutic gene transfer involve the characterization of cutaneous stem cells and an increased understanding of cutaneous gene expression. While impressive advances have recently been made in our understanding of the characteristics of epidermal stem cells (101,105–108), no markers solely specific for these cells have yet been identified. Furthermore, our understanding of the factors controlling stem cell division and the genetic programs unique to these tissue progenitors is still in the early stages. In addition to targeting genetic elements to stem cells, long-term corrective gene delivery requires sustained transgene expression. Such expression is dependent on the gene-regulatory milieu within a given tissue, and, as noted above, this has not supported achievement of long-term uniform gene expression throughout genetically engineered skin tissue by current approaches, even when vector sequences persist (5,24,26,30,41,71). The factors causing this loss of transgene expression may involve mechanisms fundamental to eukaryotic gene regulation, such as promoter methylation and heterochromatin formation (109,110). Recently, however, new vectors have been developed that show promise in achieving longer-term gene expression in human epidermis (112). An understanding of fundamental relevant biological processes will be important to future improvements in cutaneous gene transfer.

Parallel to these advances in fundamental skin biology, new technical capabilities in gene delivery are required for sustained genetic correction of the genodermatoses. Among these are development of highly efficient vectors that can be directly administered to intact skin without unwanted immune hypersensitivity reactions. Current viral and nonviral approaches for direct gene transfer fail to meet these criteria (43,45). An unsuccessful attempt to correct human lamellar ichthyosis patient skin tissue by direct TGasel expression plasmid injection highlights some of the current challenges facing this approach to gene therapy for genodermatoses (111). The development of new vectors and the use of immune downmodulation by blockade of co-stimulatory molecules such as CD28 and CD40 (103) show some promise in this regard. A lack of intrinsic vector stamina, however, must be addressed as well, and the characterization of genetic elements conferring durable expression on therapeutic vector sequences is an important effort in achieving lasting genetic correction (112).

Correction of abnormal gene expression in genodermatoses may be approached by avenues distinct from transfer of the normal gene. Among such methods are oligonucleotide-based repair of mutated genes by genetic recombination, direct application of recombinant proteins to affected skin, and heterologous cell therapy that circumvents immune rejection. These approaches, along with other emerging innovative strategies, may offer attractive future ways to avoid the traumatic and complicated process of grafting genetically engineered cells that represents a current focus of models of gene therapy of genetic disease.

A summary of some of the challenges facing efforts in widespread application of cutaneous gene therapy in humans includes the following:

1. Achievement of high-efficiency, targeted, and sustained gene delivery be achieved via direct gene transfer to intact skin.
2. Development of sustainable gene-delivery approaches that produce regions of stably genetically engineered skin without competitive repopulation by unengineered cells (i.e., from adjacent hair follicles).
3. Identification of the specific markers and gene-targeting requirements of cutaneous stem cells.
4. Characterization of the limits on polypeptide delivery to circulation from skin in terms of protein, size, charge, and transport kinetics.
5. Development of approaches for effective topical regulation of therapeutic gene expression in the skin.
6. Avoidance of unwanted immune reactions to delivered gene products.

IX. SUMMARY

The skin is a readily accessible tissue for gene therapy, with a diverse array of potential therapeutic gene-delivery vectors and strategies. Key barriers confronting therapeutic gene delivery include the problem of achieving sustained therapeutic gene production, the difficulty in targeting genes to long-lived stem cells and the challenge of achieving uniform transfer of therapeutic genes to specific skin tissue compartments. Because the skin is the primary tissue site affected by a widespread collection of human diseases, as well as being able to produce therapeutic polypeptides for delivery to the systemic circulation, it remains an attractive tissue for future development of new capabilities in therapeutic gene delivery.

REFERENCES

1. Lever WF, Schaumberg-Lever G. Histopathology of the skin. Philadelphia: Lippincott, 1990:622–634.
2. Leask A, Rosenberg M, Vassar R, Fuchs E. Regulation of a human epidermal keratin gene: sequences and nuclear factors involved in keratinocyte-specific transcription. Genes Dev 1990; 4:1985–98.
3. Freedberg IM. Keratin: a journey of three decades. J Dermatol 1993; 20:321–328.
4. Goldsmith LA. Physiology, Biochemistry, and Molecular Biology of the Skin. 2d ed. New York: Oxford University Press, 1991.
5. Taichman LB. Epithelial gene therapy. In: Leigh I, Lane B, Watt F, eds. The Keratinocyte Handbook. Cambridge University Press, 1994:543.
6. Greenhalgh DA, Rothnagel JA, Roop DR. Epidermis: an attractive target tissue for gene therapy. J Invest Dermatol 1994; 103:63S–69S.
7. Khavari PA, Krueger GG. Cutaneous gene therapy. Dermatol Clin 1997; 15:27–35.
8. Vogel JC. Keratinocyte gene therapy. Arch Dermatol, 1993; 129:1478–1483.
9. Krueger GG, Morgan JR, Jorgensen CM, Schmidt L, Li HL, Kwan MK, Boyce ST, Wiley HS, Kaplan J, Petersen MJ. Genetically modified skin to treat disease: potential and limitations. J Invest Dermatol, 1994; 103:76S–84S.
10. Blau HM, Khavari PA. Gene therapy: progress, problems and prospects. Nat Med 1997; 3:13–14.
11. Davis BM, Koc ON, Lee K, Gerson SL. Current progress in the gene therapy of cancer. Curr Opin Oncol 1996; 8: 499–508.
12. Hess P. Gene therapy: a brief review. Clin Lab Med 1996; 16:197–211.
13. Sokol DL, Gewirtz AM. Gene therapy: basic concepts and recent advances. Crit Rev Eukaryot Gene Expr 1996; 6: 29–57.
14. Aberdam D, Galliano MF, Vailly J, Pulkkinen L, Bonifas J, Christiano AM, Tryggvason K, Uitto J, Epstein EH, Jr., Ortonne JP, et al. Herlitz's junctional epidermolysis bullosa is linked to mutations in the gene (LAMC2) for the gamma 2 subunit of nicein/kalinin (LAMININ-5). Nat Genet 1994; 6:299–304.
15. Pulkkinen L, Christiano AM, Airenne T, Haakana H, Tryggvason K, Uitto J. Mutations in the gamma 2 chain gene (LAMC2) of kalinin/laminin 5 in the junctional forms of epidermolysis bullosa. Nat Genet 1994; 6:293–7.
16. Eady RA, Dunnill MG. Epidermolysis bullosa: hereditary skin fragility diseases as paradigms in cell biology. Arch Dermatol Res 1994; 287:2–9.
17. Uitto J, Pulkkinen L. Molecular complexity of the cutaneous basement membrane zone. Mol Biol Rep 1996; 23: 35–46.
18. Huber M, Rettler I, Bernasconi K, Frenk E, Lavrijsen SP, Ponec M, Bon A, Lautenschlager S, Schorderet DF, Hohl D. Mutations of keratinocyte transglutaminase in lamellar ichthyosis. Science 1995; 267:525–528.
19. Russell LJ, DiGiovanna JJ, Rogers GR, Steinert PM, Hashem N, Compton JG, Bale SJ. Mutations in the gene for transglutaminase 1 in autosomal recessive lamellar ichthyosis. Nat Genet 1995; 9:279–283.
20. Russell LJ, DiGiovanna JJ, Hashem N, Compton JG, Bale SJ. Linkage of autosomal recessive lamellar ichthyosis to chromosome 14q. Am J Hum Genet 1994; 55:1146–1152.
21. Hilal L, Rochat A, Duquesnoy P, Blanchet-Bardon C, Wechsler J, Martin N, Christiano AM, Barrandon Y, Uitto J, Goossens M, et al. A homozygous insertion-deletion in the type VII collagen gene (COL7A1) in Hallopeau-Siemens dystrophic epidermolysis bullosa. Nat Genet 1993; 5:287–293.
22. Christiano AM, Greenspan DS, Hoffman GG, Zhang X, Tamai Y, Lin AN, Dietz HC, Hovnanian A, Uitto J. A

missense mutation in type VII collagen in two affected siblings with recessive dystrophic epidermolysis bullosa. Nat Genet 1993; 4:62–66.
23. Christiano AM, Anhalt G, Gibbons S, Bauer EA, Uitto J. Premature termination codons in the type VII collagen gene (COL7A1) underlie severe, mutilating recessive dystrophic epidermolysis bullosa. Genomics 1994; 21: 160–168.
24. Choate KA, Medalie DA, Morgan JR, Khavari PA. Corrective gene transfer in the human skin disorder lamellar ichthyosis. Nat Med 1996; 2:1263–1267.
25. Choate KA, Kinsella TM, Williams ML, Nolan GP, Khavari PA. Transglutaminase 1 delivery to lamellar ichthyosis keratinocytes. Hum Gene Ther 1996; 7:2247–2253.
26. Freiberg RA, Choate KA, Deng H, Alperin ES, Shapiro LJ, Khavari PA. A model of corrective gene transfer in X-linked ichthyosis. Hum Mol Genet 1997; 6:937–933.
27. Rothnagel JA, Dominey AM, Dempsey LD, Longley MA, Greenhalgh DA, Gagne TA, Huber M, Frenk E, Hohl D, Roop DR. Mutations in the rod domains of keratins 1 and 10 in epidermolytic hyperkeratosis. Science 1992; 257: 1128–1130.
28. Cheng J, Syder AJ, Yu QC, Letai A, Paller AS, Fuchs E. The genetic basis of epidermolytic hyperkeratosis: a disorder of differentiation-specific epidermal keratin genes. Cell 1992; 70:811–819.
29. Boyce ST. Epidermis as a secretory tissue [editorial; comment]. J Invest Dermatol 1994; 102:8–10.
30. Gerrard AJ, Hudson DL, Brownlee GG, Watt FM. Towards gene therapy for haemophilia B using primary human keratinocytes. Nat Genet 1993; 8:180–183.
31. Fenjves ES, Gordon DA, Pershing LK, Williams DL, Taichman LB. Systemic distribution of apolipoprotein E secreted by grafts of epidermal keratinocytes: implications for epidermal function and gene therapy. Proc Natl Acad Sci USA 1989; 86:8803–8807.
32. Petersen MJ, Kaplan J, Jorgensen CM, Schmidt LA, Li L, Morgan JR, Kwan MK, Krueger GG. Sustained production of human transferrin by transduced fibroblasts implanted into athymic mice: a model for somatic gene therapy. J Invest Dermatol 1995; 104:171–176.
33. Wang X, Zinkel S, Polonsky K, Fuchs E. Transgenic studies with a keratin promoter-driven growth hormone transgene: prospects for gene therapy. Proc Natl Acad Sci USA 1997; 94:219–226.
34. Morgan JR, Barrandon Y, Green H, Mulligan RC. Expression of an exogenous growth hormone gene by transplantable human epidermal cells. Science 1987; 237:1476–1479.
35. Naffakh N, Henri A, Villeval JL, Rouyer-Fessard P, Moullier P, Blumenfeld N, Danos O, Vainchenker W, Heard JM, Beuzard Y. Sustained delivery of erythropoietin in mice by genetically modified skin fibroblasts. Proc Natl Acad Sci USA 1995; 92:3194–3198.
36. Garlick JA, Katz AB, Fenjves ES, Taichman LB. Retrovirus-mediated transduction of cultured epidermal keratinocytes. J Invest Dermatol 1991; 97:824–829.
37. Eming SA, Lee J, Snow RG, Tompkins RG, Yarmush ML, Morgan JR. Genetically modified human epidermis overexpressing PDGF-A directs the development of a cellular and vascular connective tissue stroma when transplanted to athymic mice—implications for the use of genetically modified keratinocytes to modulate dermal regeneration. J Invest Dermatol 1995; 105:756–763.
38. Fenjves ES. Approaches to gene transfer in keratinocytes. J Invest Dermatol 1994; 103:70S–75S.
39. Gallico GGd, O'Connor NE, Compton CC, Kehinde O, Green H. Permanent coverage of large burn wounds with autologous cultured human epithelium. N Engl J Med 1984; 311:448–451.
40. Limova M, Mauro T. Treatment of leg ulcers with cultured epithelial autografts: clinical study and case reports. Ostomy Wound Manage 1995; 41:48–50, 52, 54–60.
41. Choate KA, Khavari PA. Sustainability of keratinocyte gene transfer and cell survival in vivo. Hum Gene Ther 1997; 8:895–901.
42. Li L, Hoffman RM. The feasibility of targeted selective gene therapy of the hair follicle. Nat Med 1995; 1: 705–706.
43. Lu B, Federoff HJ, Wang Y, Goldsmith LA, Scott G. Topical application of viral vectors for epidermal gene transfer. J Invest Dermatol 1997; 108:803–808.
44. Setoguchi Y, Jaffe HA, Danel C, Crystal RG. Ex vivo and in vivo gene transfer to the skin using replication-deficient recombinant adenovirus vectors. J Invest Dermatol 1994; 102:415–421.
45. Hengge UR, Chan EF, Foster RA, Walker PS, Vogel JC. Cytokine gene expression in epidermis with biological effects following injection of naked DNA. Nat Genet 1995; 10:161–166.
46. Hengge UR, Walker PS, Vogel JC. Expression of naked DNA in human, pig, and mouse skin. J Clin Invest 1996; 97:2911–2916.
47. Cheng L, Ziegelhoffer PR, Yang NS. In vivo promoter activity and transgene expression in mammalian somatic tissues evaluated by using particle bombardment. Proc Natl Acad Sci USA 1993; 90:4455–4459.
48. Ciernik IF, Krayenbuhl BH, Carbone DP. Puncture-mediated gene transfer to the skin. Hum Gene Ther 1996; 7: 893–899.
49. Raz E, Carson DA, Parker SE, Parr TB, Abai AM, Aichinger G, Gromkowski SH, Singh M, Lew D, Yankauckas MA, et al. Intradermal gene immunization: the possible role of DNA uptake in the induction of cellular immunity to viruses. Proc Natl Acad Sci USA 1994; 91:9519–9523.
50. Fenjves ES, Smith J, Zaradic S, Taichman LB. Systemic delivery of secreted protein by grafts of epidermal keratinocytes: prospects for keratinocyte gene therapy. Hum Gene Ther 1994; 5:1241–1248.
51. Coulombe PA, Hutton ME, Letai A, Hebert A, Paller AS, Fuchs E. Point mutations in human keratin 14 genes of epidermolysis bullosa simplex patients: genetic and functional analyses. Cell 1991; 66:1301–1311.

52. Bonifas JM, Rothman AL, Epstein EH, Jr. Epidermolysis bullosa simplex: evidence in two families for keratin gene abnormalities [see comments]. Science 1991; 254: 1202–1205.
53. Bohl D, Naffakh N, Heard JM. Long-term control of erythropoietin secretion by doxycycline in mice transplanted with engineered primary myoblasts [see comments]. Nat Med 1997; 3:299–305.
54. Knowles MR, Hohneker KW, Zhou Z, Olsen JC, Noah TL, Hu PC, Leigh MW, Engelhardt JF, Edwards LJ, Jones KR, et al. A controlled study of adenoviral-vector-mediated gene transfer in the nasal epithelium of patients with cystic fibrosis [see comments]. N Engl J Med 1995; 833: 823–831.
55. Hansbrough JF, Morgan J, Greenleaf G, Parikh M, Nolte C, Wilkins L. Evaluation of Graftskin composite grafts on full-thickness wounds on athymic mice. J Burn Care Rehabil 1994; 15:346–353.
56. Cuono CB, Langdon R, Birchall N, Barttelbort S, McGuire J. Composite autologous-allogeneic skin replacement: development and clinical application. Plast Reconstr Surg 1987; 80:626–637.
57. Medalie DA, Eming SA, Tompkins RG, Yarmush ML, Krueger GG, Morgan JR. Evaluation of human skin reconstituted from composite grafts of cultured keratinocytes and human acellular dermis transplanted to athymic mice. J Invest Dermatol 1996; 107:121–127.
58. Kim YH, Woodley DT, Wynn KC, Giomi W, Bauer EA. Recessive dystrophic epidermolysis bullosa phenotype is preserved in xenografts using SCID mice: development of an experimental in vivo model. J Invest Dermatol 1992; 98:191–197.
59. Gagnoux-Palacios L, Vailly J, Durand-Clement M, Wagner E, Ortonne JP, Meneguzzi G. Functional Re-expression of laminin-5 in laminin-gamma2-deficient human keratinocytes modifies cell morphology, motility, and adhesion. J Biol Chem 1996; 271:18437–18444.
60. Andree C, Swain WF, Page CP, Macklin MD, Slama J, Hatzis D, Eriksson E. In vivo transfer and expression of a human epidermal growth factor gene accelerates wound repair. Proc Natl Acad Sci USA 1994; 91:12188–12192.
61. Benn SI, Whitsitt JS, Broadley KN, Nanney LB, Perkins D, He L, Patel M, Morgan JR, Swain WF, Davidson JM. Particle-mediated gene transfer with transforming growth factor-betal cDNAs enhances wound repair in rat skin. J Clin Invest 1996; 98:2894–2902.
62. Rakhmilevich AL, Turner J, Ford MJ, McCabe D, Sun WH, Sondel PM, Grota K, Yang NS. Gene gun-mediated skin transfection with interleukin 12 gene results in regression of established primary and metastatic murine tumors. Proc Natl Acad Sci USA 1996; 93:6291–6296.
63. Williams ML, Elias PM. Genetically transmitted, generalized disorders of cornification. The ichthyoses. Dermatol Clin 1987; 5:155–178.
64. Bale SJ, Doyle SZ. The genetics of ichthyosis: a primer for epidemiologists. J Invest Dermatol 1994; 102:49S–50S.
65. Thacher SM, Rice RH, Greenberg CS, Birckbichler PJ, Rice RH. Keratinocyte-specific transglutaminase of cultured human epidermal cells: relation to cross-linked envelope formation and terminal differentiation. Transglutaminases: multifunctional cross-linking enzymes that stabilize tissues. Cell 1985; 10:685–695.
66. Phillips MA, Stewart BE, Qin Q, Chakravarty R, Floyd EE, Jetten AM, Rice RH. Primary structure of keratinocyte transglutaminase. Proc Natl Acad Sci USA 1990; 87: 9333–9337.
67. Greenberg CS, Birckbichler PJ, Rice RH. Transglutaminases: multifunctional cross-linking enzymes that stabilize tissues. FASEB J 1991; 5:3071–3077.
68. Kim SY, Chung SI, Steinert PM. Highly active soluble processed forms of the transglutaminase 1 enzyme in epidermal keratinocytes. J Biol Chem 1995; 270: 18026–18035.
69. Huber M, Rettler I, Bernasconi K, Wyss M, Hohl D. Lamellar ichthyosis is genetically heterogeneous—cases with normal keratinocyte transglutaminase. J Invest Dermatol 1995; 105:653–654.
70. Bale SJ, Russell LJ, Lee ML, Compton JG, DiGiovanna JJ. Congenital recessive ichthyosis unlinked to loci for epidermal transglutaminases. J Invest Dermatol 1996; 107: 808–811.
71. Fenjves ES, Yao SN, Kurachi K, Taichman LB. Loss of expression of a retrovirus-transduced gene in human keratinocytes. J Invest Dermatol 1996; 106:576–578.
72. Paige DG, Emillion GG, Bouloux PM, Harper JI. A clinical and genetic study of X-linked recessive ichthyosis and contiguous gene defects. Br J Dermatol 1994; 131: 622–629.
73. Yen PH, Allen E, Marsh B, Mohandas T, Wang N, Taggart RT, Shapiro LJ. Cloning and expression of steroid sulfatase cDNA and the frequent occurrence of deletions in STS deficiency: implications for X-Y interchange. Cell 1987; 49:443–454.
74. Ballabio A, Shapiro LJ. Steroid sulfatase deficiency and X-linked ichthyosis. In: Scriver CR, Beaudet AL, Sly WS, Valle D, eds. The Metabolic and Molecular Bases of Inherited Disease. New York: McGraw-Hill, 1995:2999.
75. Alperin ES, Shapiro LJ. Characterization of point mutations in patients with X-linked ichthyosis. Am J Hum Genet 1994; 55:209.
76. Shapiro LJ, Yen P, Pomerantz D, Martin E, Rolewic L, Mohandas T. Molecular studies of deletions at the human steroid sulfatase locus. Proc Natl Acad Sci USA 1989; 86: 8477–8481.
77. Epstein EH Jr, Williams ML, Elias PM. Steroid sulfatase, X-linked ichthyosis, and stratum corneum cell cohesion. Arch Dermatol 1981; 117:761–763.
78. Reis A, Hennies HC, Langbein L, Digweed M, Mischke D, Drechsler M, Schrock E, Royer-Pokora B, Franke WW, Sperling K, et al. Keratin 9 gene mutations in epidermolytic palmoplantar keratoderma (EPPK). Nat Genet 1994; 6:174–179.

79. Torchard D, Blanchet-Bardon C, Serova O, Langbein L, Narod S, Janin N, Goguel AF, Bernheim A, Franke WW, Lenoir GM, et al. Epidermolytic palmoplantar keratoderma cosegregates with a keratin 9 mutation in a pedigree with breast and ovarian cancer. Nat Genet 1994; 6: 106–110.
80. Shamsher MK, Navsaria HA, Stevens HP, Ratnavel RC, Purkis PE, Kelsell DP, McLean WH, Cook LJ, Griffiths WA, Gschmeissmer S, et al. Novel mutations in keratin 16 gene underly focal non-epidermolytic palmoplantar keratoderma (NEPPK) in two families. Hum Mol Genet 1995; 4:1875–1881.
81. Bowden PE, Haley JL, Kansky A, Rothnagel JA, Jones DO, Turner RJ. Mutation of a type II keratin gene (K6a) in pachyonychia congenita. Nat Genet 1995; 10:363–365.
82. McLean WH, Rugg EL, Lunny DP, Morley SM, Lane EB, Swensson O, Dopping-Hepenstal PJ, Griffiths WA, Eady RA, Higgins C, et al. Keratin 16 and keratin 17 mutations cause pachyonychia congenita. Nat Genet 1995; 9: 273–278.
83. Fuchs E. Keratins and the skin. Ann Rev Cell Dev Biol 1995; 11:123–153.
84. Uitto J, Pulkkinen L, Christiano AM. Molecular basis of the dystrophic and junctional forms of epidermolysis bullosa: mutations in the type VII collagen and kalinin (laminin 5) genes. J Invest Dermatol 1994; 103:39S–46S.
85. Korge BP, Krieg T. The molecular basis for inherited bullous diseases. J Mol Med 1996; 74:59–70.
86. Paller AS. The genetic basis of hereditary blistering disorders. Curr Opin Pediatr 1996; 8:367–371.
87. Marinkovich MP. The molecular genetics of basement membrane diseases. Arch Dermatol 1993; 129: 1557–1565.
88. Tamai K, Ishida-Yamamoto A, Matsuo S, Iizuka H, Hashimoto I, Christiano AM, Uitto J, McGrath JA. Compound heterozygosity for a nonsense mutation and a splice site mutation in the type VII collagen gene (COL7A1) in recessive dystrophic epidermolysis bullosa. Lab Invest 1997; 76:209–217.
89. McGrath JA, Gatalica B, Li K, Dunnill MG, McMillan JR, Christiano AM, Eady RA, Uitto J. Compound heterozygosity for a dominant glycine substitution and a recessive internal duplication mutation in the type XVII collagen gene results in junctional epidermolysis bullosa and abnormal dentition [see comments]. Am J Pathol 1996; 148:1787–1796.
90. McGarth JA, Christiano AM, Pulkkinen L, Eady RA, Uitto J. Compound heterozygosity for nonsense ans missense mutations in the LAMB3 gene in nonlethal junctional epidermolysis bullosa. J Invest Dermatol 1996; 106: 1157–1159.
91. Christiano AM, Pulkkinen L, Eady RA, Uitto J. Compound heterozygosity for nonsense and missense mutations in the LAMB3 gene in nonlethal junctional epidermolysis bullosa. J Invest Dermatol 1996; 106:775–777.
92. Marinkovich MP, Keene DR, Rimberg CS, Burgeson RE. Cellular origin of the dermal-epidermal basement membrane. Dev Dyn 1993; 197:255–267.
93. Jonkman MF, Scheffer H, Stulp R, Pas HH, Nijenhuis M, Heeres K, Owaribe K, Pulkkinen L, Uitto J. Revertant mosaicism in epidermolysis bullosa caused by mitotic gene conversion. Cell 1997; 88:543–551.
94. Kraemer KH. Xeroderma pigmentosum knockouts. Lancet 1996; 347:278–279.
95. Li L, Bales ES, Peterson CA, Legerski RJ. Characterization of molecular defects in xeroderma pigmentosum group C. Nat Genet 1993; 5:413–417.
96. Kraemer KH, Seetharam S, Seidman MM, Bredberg A, Brash D, Waters HL, Protic-Sabljic M, Peck G, DiGiovanna J, Moshell A, et al. Defective DNA repair in humans: clinical and molecular studies of xeroderma pigmentosum. Basic Life Sci 1990; 53:95–104.
97. Marionnet C, Quilliet X, Benoit A, Armier J, Sarasin A, Stary A. Recovery of normal DNA repair and mutagenesis in trichothiodystrophy cells after transduction of the XPD human gene. Cancer Res 1996; 56:5450–5456.
98. Myrand SP, Topping RS, States JC. Stable transformation of xeroderma pigmentosum group A cells with an XPA minigene restores normal DNA repair and mutagenesis of UV-treated plasmids. Carcinogenesis 1996; 17: 1909–1917.
99. Byrne C, Fuchs E. Probing keratinocyte and differentiation specificity of the human K5 promoter in vitro and in transgenic mice. Mol Cell Biol 1993; 13:3176–3190.
100. Carroll JM, Albers KM, Garlick JA, Harrington R, Taichman LB. Tissue- and stratum-specific expression of the human involucrin promoter in transgenic mice. Proc Natl Acad Sci USA 1993; 90:10270–10274.
101. Jones PH, Harper S, Watt FM. Stem cell patterning and fate in human epidermis. Cell 1995; 80:83–93.
102. Williams IR, Kupper TS. Immunity at the surface: homeostatic mechanisms of the skin immune system. Life Sci 1996; 58:1485–1507.
103. Larsen CP, Elwood ET, Alexander DZ, Ritchie SC, Hendrix R, Tucker-Burden C, Cho HR, Aruffo A, Hollenbaugh D, Linsley PS, Winn KJ, Pearson TC. Long-term acceptance of skin and cardiac allografts after blocking CD40 and CD28 pathways. Nature 1996; 381:434–438.
104. Ilan Y, Prakash R, Davidson A, Jona, Droguett G, Horwitz MS, Chowdhury NR, Chowdhury JR. Oral tolerization to adenoviral antigens permits long-term gene expression using recombinant adenoviral vectors. J Clin Invest 1997; 99:1098–1106.
105. Jones PH, Watt FM. Separation of human epidermal stem cells from transit amplifying cells on the basis of differences in integrin function and expression. Cell 1993; 73: 713–724.
106. Mathor MB, Ferrari G, Dellambra E, Cilli M, Mavilio F, Cancedda R, De Luca M. Clonal analysis of stably transduced human epidermal stem cells in culture. Proc Natl Acad Sci USA 1996; 93:10371–10376.
107. Rochat A, Kobayashi K, Barrandon Y. Location of stem cells of human hair follicles by clonal analysis. Cell 1994; 76:1063–1073.

108. Bata-Csorgo Z, Hammerberg C, Voorhees JJ, Cooper KD. Kinetics and regulation of human keratinocyte stem cell growth in short-term primary ex vivo culture. Cooperative growth factors from psoriatic lesional T lymphocytes stimulate proliferation among psoriatic uninvolved, but not normal, stem keratinocytes. J Clin Invest 1995; 95: 317–327.
109. Hoeben RC, Migchielsen AA, van der Jagt RC, van Ormondt H, van der Eb AJ. Inactivation of the Moloney murine leukemia virus long terminal repeat in murine fibroblast cell lines is associated with methylation and dependent on its chromosomal position. J Virol 1991; 65: 904–912.
110. Wolffe AP. New insights into chromatin function in transcriptional control. FASEB J 1992; 6:3354–3361.
111. Choate KA, Khavari PA. Direct cutaneous gene delivery in a human genetic skin disease. Hum Gene Ther 1997; 8:1671–1677.
112. Deng H, Lin Q, Khavari PA. Sustainable cutaneous gene delivery. Nat Biotechnol 1997; 15:1388–1391.
113. Maestrini E, Monaco AP, McGrath JA, Ishida-Yamamoto A, Camisa C, Hovnanian A, Weeks DE, Lathrop M, Uitto J, Christiano AM. A molecular defect in loricrin, the major component of the cornified cell envelope, underlies Vohwinkel's syndrome. Nat Genet 1996; 13:70–77.
114. Rothnagel JA, Traupe H, Wojcik S, Huber M, Hohl D, Pittelkow MR, Saeki H, Ishibashi Y, Roop DR. Mutations in the rod domain of keratin 2e in patients with ichthyosis bullosa of Siemens. Nat Genet 1994; 7:485–490.
115. McGrath JA, Gatalica B, Christiano AM, Li K, Owaribe K, McMillan JR, Eady RA, Uitto J. Mutations in the 180-kD bullous pemphigoid antigen (BPAG2), a hemidesmosomal transmembrane collagen (COL17A1), in generalized atrophic benign epidermolysis bullosa. Nat Genet 1995; 11:83–86.
116. Vidal F, Aberdam D, Miquel C, Christiano AM, Pulkkinen L, Uitto J, Ortonne JP, Meneguzzi G. Integrin beta 4 mutations associated with junctional epidermolysis bullosa with pyloric atresia. Nat Genet 1995; 10:229–234.
117. Smith FJ, Eady RA, Leigh IM, McMillan JR, Rugg EL, Kelsell DP, Bryant SP, Spurr NK, Geddes JF, Kirtschig G, Milana G, de Bono AG, Owaribe K, Wiche G, Pulkkinen L, Uitto J, McLean WH, Lane EB. Plectin deficiency results in muscular dystrophy with epidermolysis bullosa. Nat Genet 1996; 13:450–457.
118. Johnson RL, Rothman AL, Xie J, Goodrich LV, Bare JW, Bonifas JM, Quinn AG, Myers RM, Cox DR, Epstein EH, Jr., Scott MP. Human homolog of patched, a candidate gene for the basal cell nevus syndrome. Science 1996; 272: 1668–1671.
119. Hahn H, Wicking C, Zaphiropoulous PG, Gailani MR, Shanley S, Chidambaram A, Vorechovsky I, Holmberg E, Unden AB, Gillies S, Negus K, Smyth I, Pressman C, Leffell DJ, Gerrard B, Goldstein AM, Dean M, Toftgard R, Chenevix-Trench G, Wainwright B, Bale AE. Mutations of the human homolog of Drosophila patched in the nevoid basal cell carcinoma syndrome. Cell 1996; 85:841–851.

28

DNA Vaccines

Jong J. Kim
Merck & Company, West Point, Pennsylvania

David B. Weiner
University of Pennsylvania, Philadelphia, Pennsylvania

I. IMPORTANCE OF VACCINES

A. Historical Importance of Vaccines

Vaccination is a deliberate introduction of materials into humans to protect against diseases (1). The history of vaccine use dates back to ancient times. In the seventh century, Indian Buddhists drank snake venom to protect themselves from snake bites (1). In ninth-century China, *The Correct Treatment of Small Pox* was written by a Buddhist nun. The manuscript recommended that a mixture of ground dried smallpox scabs and herbs be blown into the nostrils of children. Even with such a long history, immunization was not widely used until Edward Jenner deliberately injected cowpox virus was humans to protect them from the ravages of smallpox. Since that time the wide use of vaccines against pathogenic microorganisms has become the most important advance in the history of medicine. Vaccines have provided protection not only from smallpox, but also from poliomyelitis, measles, mumps, rubella, yellow fever, pertussis (whooping cough), hepatitis A, hepatitis B, and varicella, as well as others. These vaccines have dramatically reduced morbidity from infectious agents and have directly protected more human lives than all other avenues of modern medicine combined. Yet, as increased standards for effectiveness and safety and the increased costs of developing and manufacturing vaccines have become more restrictive, the development of new vaccines has slowed. Furthermore, as new pathogens continue to emerge, it is important that novel methods for vaccine production be developed and tested to meet more demanding requirements in the twenty-first century.

B. Vaccine Immunology

Traditional vaccines have relied on either live-replicating or nonliving preparations of microorganisms. The injected material functions as a vaccine by generating immunity against the inoculum, and the resulting immune responses function to prevent disease. This type of induced immunity is referred to as protective immunity and results from the vaccine activating specific B and T lymphocytes, which compose the lymphocyte subsets of the white blood cells of the immune system (2).

As the major components of humoral immune response, B cells are lymphocytes that develop in fetal liver and subsequently mature in the bone marrow. Mature B cells carry surface immunoglobulins, which act as their antigen receptor. They then move through the circulation to secondary lymphoid tissues, the lymph nodes and spleen, where they respond to antigenic stimuli by dividing and differentiating into plasma cells under direction of cytokines produced by T cells. When they are activated, B lymphocytes are terminally differentiated to become plasma cells, which are entirely devoted to the production of secreted antibody. Antibodies are large water-soluble serum proteins that are induced following contact with antigen. Antibodies bind to the specific antigens that induced their formation and either directly neutralize or inactivate them. Antibodies can also direct other cells of the immune system, such as macrophages and phagocytes, to dispose of the antigen. Furthermore, they can direct complements, highly toxic soluble immune mediators, to bind to and destroy an invading pathogen.

T cells are lymphocytes that develop in the thymus. T cells acquire their antigen receptors in the thymus and differentiate into a number of subpopulations that have separate functions and can be recognized by their different cell surface markers. T lymphocytes develop as one of two subsets of white blood cells termed T-helper cells and T cytotoxic or T-killer cells in the thymus. These cells become the basis of cell-mediated immune responses and function to eradicate pathogens in different ways. T-helper cells help and direct B cells to produce antibodies, which target mostly extracellular pathogens. T-helper cells also cooperate with cytotoxic T lymphocytes in the destruction of virally infected cells. Activated T-helper cells secrete small protein messengers termed cytokines or lymphokines, which activate and expand either or both humoral and cellular immune responses. On the other hand, activated T-cytotoxic cells seek out and destroy cells that have been infected with pathogens. These T-killer cells bind and destroy allogeneic and virally infected cells, which display recognizable antigen-MHC class I molecules. T-killer cells induce these pathogen-infected cells to die either through the release of toxic proteins such as granzyme B or through initiating apoptosis or programmed cell death in the target cells. In addition to defense against pathogens, cytotoxic T lymphocytes (CTL) are particularly important in eradicating misbehaving host cells such as cancer cells. Humoral or cellular immunity can act independently or in concert to destroy the pathogenic organism within a vaccinated host.

C. Traditional Vaccines

In the case of live vaccines, the infectious material has been manipulated to be weakened or attenuated so that it no longer induces disease. In the case of the nonlive preparations, the vaccine material has been manufactured to contain killed organisms that can no longer grow when inoculated into a host. In some instances, specific components can be purified away from other portions of the microorganism or artificially manufactured in the laboratory to function as a subunit vaccine. Both categories of vaccines are presently utilized throughout the world to protect individuals against specific pathogens. Each has its own general characteristics for generating immunity and exhibits properties that can be beneficial or deleterious to an individual.

Live attenuated vaccines, such as the polio and smallpox vaccines, stimulate protective immunity as they replicate in the body of an immunized host. These vaccines emulate the natural infection of pathogens and generate a broad spectrum of immune responses. Because they are a weakened form of the pathogen, no disease occurs. This category of vaccine induces broad protective immunity with induction of both antibodies and activated T cells. More specifically, because CTLs are only induced if an infectious agent or vaccine actually is produced within host cells, live attenuated vaccines are the most effective inducer of CTL. Attenuated vaccines have an additional benefit in that they provide life-long immunity. In contrast, nonliving inactivated vaccines (including subunit preparations), such as the vaccine for hepatitis A virus, produce protective immunity that is limited to the generation of antibodies and helper T cells, but they cannot induce killer T cells. Accordingly, the ability of these preparations to induce protection is limited to pathogens that can be destroyed by extracellular defenses. Unlike the live attenuated vaccines, the protective immunity induced by inactivated vaccines is normally short term and requires repeated booster injections to achieve lifetime immunity. Based on these immunological characteristics, live attenuated vaccines represent the vaccines of choice. Still, they are not without problems. For instance, there are many safety issues related to the use of live attenuated vaccines. The potential exists for the attenuated vaccine to mutate back to the original disease-causing organism through a process called reversion. Attenuated vaccines may also cause disease when inoculated into persons with weak or compromised immune systems, such as cancer patients receiving chemotherapy or AIDS patients, or in the elderly where the immune system deteriorates with age. Furthermore, live vaccines can infect individuals other than the inoculated individual and thus inadvertently expose a disease to a susceptible unknowing individual.

Even though inactivated vaccines are safer than their live attenuated counterparts, certain problems also exist with some inactivated vaccines. For instance, the whole organism used as the inactivated vaccine can be contaminated with components from cell culture that are not removed during the manufacturing process. This contaminated material may be an important factor in autoimmune disease. Additional shortcomings of inactivated vaccines include contamination by components of the pathogen that are not important in the generation of protective immunity. These components may generate immune responses that are not relevant to protective immunity. Deleterious reactions, such as inflammation and allergic reactions, may also result from vaccination with the inactivated whole organism. These concerns regarding contaminants and the safety issues related to whole organism vaccines point to the use of purified subunit component vaccines.

In these subunit vaccines, only the components of the microorganism involved in conferring protective immunity are included, while other portions of the microorganism are removed in an extensive purification process. This increases the cost of manufacturing the vaccine to improve its safety. Subunit component vaccines have an increased specificity that can target the immune response in a very effective manner; again these vaccines elicit protective immunity by the generation of antibodies and limited T-helper responses. However, if antibodies alone are insufficient to provide protective immunity against a particular pathogen, it becomes necessary to also involve the activated T-lymphocyte component of the immune response. As a need for vaccines against new pathogens emerges, safe vaccines that elicit both antibodies and activated T cells will have an advantage, particularly when the requirements for protective immunity in the host are not yet unknown. It would be a distinct advantage for vaccine development to have a technology that could induce the broad immunity normally associated with a live attenuated vaccine while exhibiting the safety and the focus of the subunit preparations. In addition, any simplification in manufacturing and increase in stability is likely to positively impact on vaccine development for the developing world.

II. DNA VACCINES

A. Concepts of DNA Vaccines

Recent work from a number of laboratories has involved injection of a DNA plasmid containing foreign genes for proteins of a pathogen or cancer antigens directly into a host. This injection results in the subsequent expression of the foreign gene in that host and the presentation of the specific encoded proteins to the immune system (Fig. 1). DNA vaccine constructs are produced as small circular vehicles or plasmids. These plasmids are constructed with a promoter site, which starts the transcription process, an antigenic DNA sequence, and a messenger RNA stop site containing the poly A tract necessary for conversion of the messenger RNA sequence into the antigen protein by the ribosomal protein manufacturing machinery (Fig. 2). The concept of genetic immunization provides that both DNA and RNA that encode specific proteins can be used to gen-

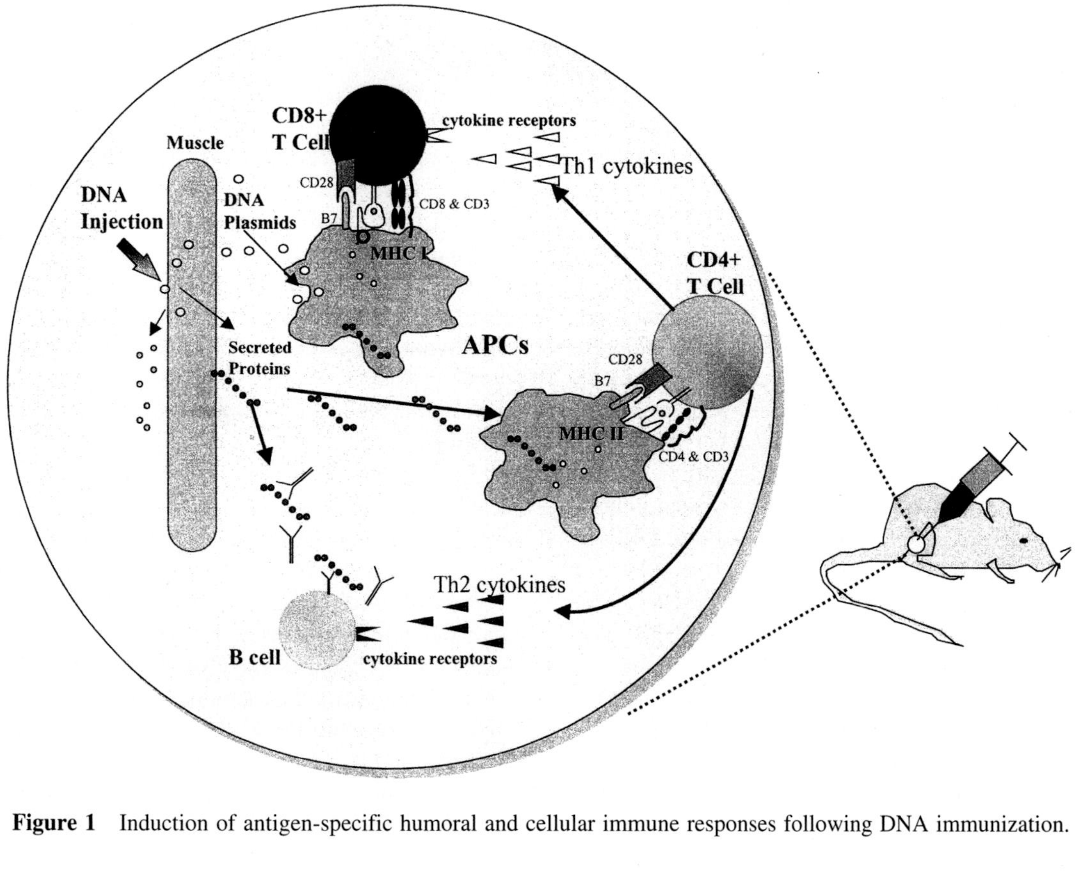

Figure 1 Induction of antigen-specific humoral and cellular immune responses following DNA immunization.

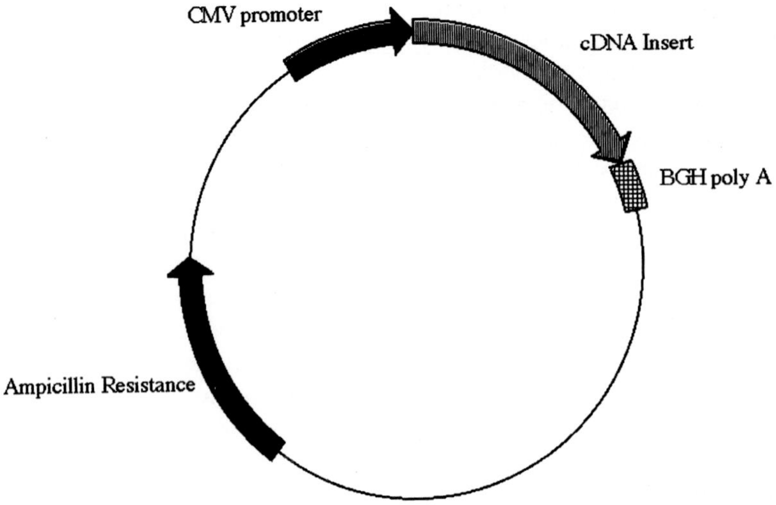

Figure 2 A diagram of a DNA vaccine construct consisting of a mammalian expression vector. The plasmids are constructed with a promoter, an antigenic DNA sequence, and a messenger RNA stop site containing the poly A tract.

erate specific immune responses. Since DNA and RNA are both nucleic acids, the term nucleic acid vaccine has also been used to describe this process.

B. History of DNA Inoculation

The ability of genetic material to deliver genes for therapeutic purposes and its use in gene therapy has been appreciated for some time. Early experiments describing DNA inoculation into living cells were DNA transfer experiments performed by a number of investigators in the 1950 and 1960s (3–5). These reports describe the ability of DNA preparations isolated from tumors or viral infections to induce tumors or virus infection following injection into animals. Importantly, many such inoculated animals developed antibody responses to the proteins encoded within the injected DNA sequences. Over the next 20 years a number of scattered reports all focusing on gene function or gene therapy techniques provided evidence that injection of viral DNA or plasmids containing foreign gene resulted in antibody production related to the DNA inoculations. Longer-term expression of foreign genes was described in 1990 by Wolff and colleagues following plasmid inoculation in vivo (6). These two separate observations demonstrated that DNA in the absence of vectors could deliver proteins that might have biological relevance. While both of these studies focused on the use of this technology for gene-replacement strategies, studies were already underway in several laboratories using this same technology for vaccine applications.

In 1992, Tang et al. reported that injection of DNA encoding human growth hormone into mice resulted in transient hormone production followed by the development of antibodies in the inoculated animals specific for the human growth hormone gene (7). This pioneering work utilized a ''genetic gun'' or gene gun to shoot gold particles covered with DNA through the skin layers of mice. While these investigators were actually studying the use of this technology for a gene-replacement strategy, they described this development of antibody responses due to this unusual immunization procedure as genetic immunization. Almost simultaneously with the above publication, a vaccine meeting held at the Cold Spring Harbor Laboratory in September 1992 described the use of DNA immunization to generate humoral and cellular immune responses against a human pathogen as well as protection from both tumors and viral challenges in animal systems. (Personal Communications).

The investigators from Merck and Vical reported on the development of immune responses to intramuscular injected plasmid-encoding pathogen proteins. They observed that both antibody responses as well as CTL responses were induced to influenza viral gene products by this immunization technique. Furthermore, vaccinated mice were able to resist lethal viral challenge. Robinson and colleagues reported on the use of the gene gun to deliver influenza virus genes in DNA plasmids and reported that both antibody and T-lymphocyte responses were produced in vaccinated mice and chickens. In challenge studies these responses were protective. The use of the gene gun allowed investigators to deliver very low (ng) amounts of DNA at the site of injection and still observe immune responses. Weiner and colleagues reported the direct injection of DNA encoding the genes for the human immunodeficiency virus (HIV). Again both antibodies and T-lymphocyte responses specific for the viral gene products were observed in experimental animals. Because HIV does not infect mice, an in vivo mouse model was used where tumor cells that are normally lethal to the mice were constructed to express HIV proteins. Animals who were vaccinated with the HIV DNA vaccine were demonstrated to be immune to these HIV antigen–expressing tumor cells. While the audience was skeptical about the ability of nonliving genetic material to produce useful immune responses, the large amount of data presented by each of these groups representing several years of successful work in diverse systems could no longer be ignored by the scientific and vaccine community. DNA vaccines were officially born.

Following these initial reports, DNA vaccination and the generation of antibody and T-lymphocyte responses as well as protective responses in a variety of animal models have been reported in the scientific literature for many human pathogens such as hepatitis B virus, rabies virus, herpes simplex virus, hepatitis C virus, human T-cell leukemia virus, human papillomavirus, and TB (8–10).

C. Potential Advantages of DNA Vaccines

As summarized in Table 1 nucleic acid immunization may afford several potential advantages over traditional vaccination strategies, such as whole killed or live attenuated virus and recombinant protein-based vaccines, without the specific shortcomings and inherent risks associated with these vaccination methods. Like inactivated or subunit vaccines, DNA vaccines appear conceptually safe since they are nonreplicating and nonlive. In contrast to inactivated or subunit vaccine, DNA vaccine cassettes produce immunological responses that are more similar to live vaccine preparations. By directly introducing DNA into the host cell, the host cell is essentially directed to produce the antigenic protein, mimicking viral replication or tumor cell marker presentation in the host. Unlike a live attenuated vaccine, conceptually there is little risk from reversion to a disease-causing pathogen from the injected DNA, and there is no risk for secondary infection as the material injected is not living and not infectious. Furthermore, multicomponent DNA vaccines can be engineered to include specific immunogens, which could optimize and amplify desirable immunological responses. This ability to target multiple antigenic components may be a particularly important characteristic of DNA vaccines, since multicomponent DNA vaccines can be engineered to include specific immunogens that could optimize and amplify desirable immunological responses.

Table 1 Potential Advantages of DNA Vaccines

Safety: little risk for reversion to a disease-causing form; no risk for secondary infection

Efficacy: induce both humoral and cellular immune responses; can be repeatedly injected without adverse reactions

Better design: DNA vaccines can be manipulated to present all or part of the genome; genes that lead to undesired immunological inhibition may be removed

Enhanced manufacturing and storage capability: beter stability and storage capability compared to traditional vaccine formulations; more simple and less expensive manufacturing process

D. Mechanism of DNA Vaccines

The exact mechanism for DNA immunization has been a subject of major debate (11–13), but is likely to be similar to traditional antigen presentation. In the body's immune system, cells need to process and present antigenic peptides to lymphocytes in order to stimulate antigen-specific immune response. Thus, antigen must be processed and presented to T lymphocytes by antigen-presenting cells (APCs) (14). Antigen presentation and recognition is a complex biological process, which involves many interactions between APCs and T cells (Fig. 3). Four primary components are critical in the professional APCs ability to present the antigen to T cells and activate them for appropriate immune responses. These components are MHC-antigen complexes, costimulatory molecules (primarily CD80 and CD86), intracellular adhesion molecules, and soluble cytokines. Naive T cells circulate through the body across lymph nodes and secondary lymphoid organs such as the spleen. Their migration is mediated, among other factors, by intercellular adhesion molecules and cytokines. As the T cells travel, they bind to and dissociate from various APCs. This action is mediated through adhesion molecules. When a naive T cell binds to an APC expressing a relevant MHC-peptide complex, the T cell expresses high levels of high-affinity IL-2 receptor. Only when this T cell receives a costimulatory signal through CD80/CD86-CD28 interaction does the T cell make soluble IL-2, which then binds to the receptors and drives the now-armed effector T cell to activate and proliferate.

Antigen is expressed at significant levels in muscle following intramuscular inoculation of plasmid DNA (6). Using reporter gene injections in mice, various investiga-

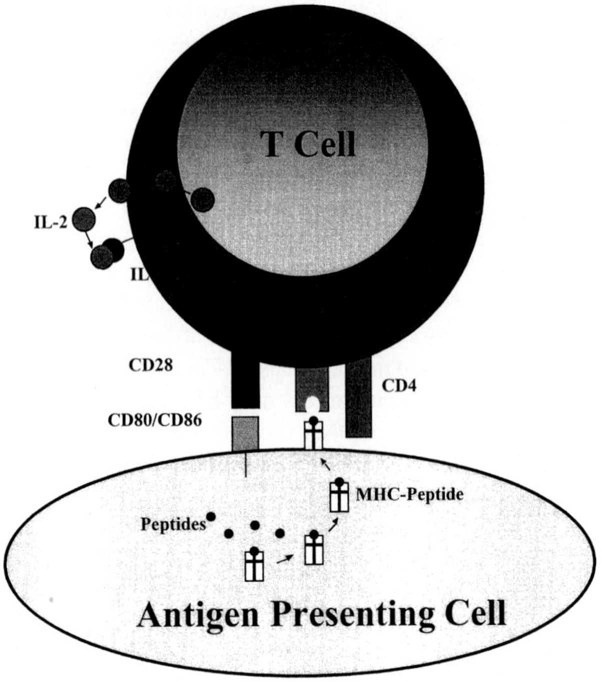

Figure 3 Effective T-cell activation by APC. The interaction between antigen-MHC and T-cell receptor leads to the expression of IL-2 receptor. This T cell proliferates when the second signal is provided from APC's costimulatory proteins. CD28-CD80/CD86 ligation initiates the production of IL-2 production and leads to the proliferation of activated T cell.

tors have reported the detection of gene expression after intramuscular (i.m.) injection of DNA expression cassettes (6). Protein expression was detected in the quadriceps muscle of mice after injecting plasmid vectors encoding chloramphenicol acetyltransferase, luciferase, and β-galactosidase reporter genes into the muscle.

Muscle cells have several structural and functional features that seem to make them well suited for DNA uptake in vivo (15). Muscle consists of multinucleated contractile muscle fibers with cylindrical shape and tapered ends. These muscle fibers have mycogenic stem cells attached to them. When the muscle fibers are damaged or stressed, the stem cells are activated. The resulting myoblasts proliferate and eventually fuse to form new muscle fibers. It is believed that this continual activation and proliferation of the myoblasts allow a more opportunistic uptake of injected DNA. Because it has been shown that the uptake of the injected DNA and the subsequent production of protein occurs in muscle cells, they have been proposed as a potential site of antigen processing and presentation. However, the myocytes that make up the muscle tissues do not express CD80 or CD86 costimulatory molecules needed for efficient presentation, although a new study has identified an additional costimulatory molecule distinct from CD80 or CD86, which can be expressed in muscle cells (16). The question of ability of muscle cells to provide costimulatory signals drives the current debate in the literature about the mechanism of antigen presentation following intramuscular DNA immunization.

One potential mechanism is that the antigens produced in muscle are secreted from transfected muscle cells or released due to cell apoptosis (11,12). Such exogenous antigen could then be taken up by professional APCs in the draining lymph nodes, where the antigen is processed via the MHC class I pathway of these cells. These APCs are then hypothesized to present the processed peptides to T cells. Recently, there have been reports that indicate that the immune system has an inherent mechanism by which exogenous antigens access MHC class I molecules. One recent report identified dendritic cells as the potent mediator of such presentation antigen derived from phagocytosed apoptotic cells (17). Immature dendritic cells engulf apoptotic cells and cross-present antigen from these sources to induce class I restricted CTLs.

Another possible mechanism is the direct transfection of professional APCs by the injected DNA. Such a mechanism may be more likely in intradermal delivery of DNA because skin is rich in professional antigen-presenting cells, especially dendritic cells. Condon et al. have reported that, through DNA immunization into skin, they were able to show expression of proteins encoded by DNA plasmids (18). On the other hand, such a mechanism is less likely within the muscle tissue, where there are significantly fewer APCs. More recently, studies have reported that direct transfection of dendritic cells can occur following intramuscular inoculation DNA vaccine constructs, albeit at a lower level (19). Another study indicates that macrophages may be a target cell for DNA transfected in vivo and that such a target might be important in driving immune responses in vivo (20). A clear understanding of the role of antigen-presenting cells in DNA vaccination could have important implications for this technology.

III. DNA VACCINES FOR HIV-1 AND CANCER

A. DNA Vaccines for HIV-1

The human immunodeficiency virus-1 (HIV-1) is a retrovirus, which preferentially infects and kills $CD4^+$ T cells and macrophages, ultimately resulting in immune system failure and multipathogen infections. Recent breakthroughs in combination therapy using three or more different antiretroviral agents have generated optimism regarding the ability to control viral replication in vivo (21). However, this therapeutic regimen is costly, and it is too early to tell whether this approach can eradicate established infection (21,22). The costs and the stringent administration regimen requirements of these pharmaceutical agents make it clear that these drugs will only be effectively utilized in a limited part of the world population. Therefore, to address the worldwide problem of HIV-1 infection, there remains a need for a prophylactic vaccination strategy designed to control the epidemic through mass immunization campaigns (23).

One of the major obstacles in the development of a vaccine against HIV-1 is uncertainty regarding the exact immune correlates of protection (24). In studies of long-term nonprogressor groups of HIV-infected individuals, evidence supports the notion that correlates of protection against HIV-1 could be provided by humoral, cellular, or even both arms of the immune response (25,26). High levels of type-specific neutralizing antibody have been observed in protected primates in some homologous challenge models (27–31). Neutralizing antibodies are susceptible to viral deception through antigenic diversity of the HIV-1 envelope, and the ability of neutralizing antibody to prevent viral pathogenesis is still under considerable investigation (32–35).

One of the hallmarks of HIV-1 disease progression is the loss of cellular immune function, and the presence of strong cellular responses in some instances can correlate with control of viral replication (9,36). In cases of acute HIV-1 infection studied by several investigators, viral clearance was associated with specific CTL activity in each case (37,38). In addition, a subset (7 of 20) of occupationally exposed health-care workers who were not infected possessed transient HIV-1–specific CTL response (39). HIV-1–specific CTLs were also found in a number of chronically exposed sex workers in Gambia who continue to resist infection with HIV-1 (40). In spite of these studies supporting the role of neutralizing antibodies and CTLs in conferring immunity to infection, some vaccinated primates exhibiting both neutralizing antibody and CTL responses were not protected from subsequent viral challenge in the pathogenic simian immunodeficiency virus (SIV) model (41). Recently, the important role of CD4 helper responses in the anti-HIV immune response has been highlighted (42). Such responses likely have importance for both humoral as well as $CD8^+$ effector responses.

The advantages of nucleic acid immunization listed above make it well suited as a potentially useful vaccination strategy against HIV-1. Within the HIV genome, there are several potential immunological targets for DNA vaccination (Fig. 4). The HIV-1 genome is organized into three major structural and enzymatic genes, two regulatory genes, and four accessory genes (43). The first major gene target is *env,* which codes for the outer viral envelope proteins. HIV enters the $CD4^+$ cells via envelope–CD4 receptor complex. Following entry of HIV viral core, synthesis of a double-stranded DNA version of the HIV genome (called DNA provirus) begins by the viral DNA polymerase reverse transcriptase (RT). The DNA provirus is then translocated to the nucleus as part of the protein-DNA preintegration complex and is integrated into the host cell genome with the help of the viral integrase (Int) enzyme. The provirus then replicates with the host DNA each time the cell divides. The gene *gag* codes for the core protein, and *pol* codes for the enzymatic proteins RT, Int, and protease (Pro). In general, these enzymatic proteins remain somewhat conserved and preserve their catalytic functions. Accordingly, these proteins may be less divergent immune targets than envelope proteins for CTL-mediated responses (44).

The regulatory genes *tat* and *rev* affect HIV-1 gene expression. Viral transcription is increased several hundred–fold by tat transactivation (43), making it an obvious target for therapeutic intervention. The rev protein increases the release of unspliced structural RNAs from the nucleus by displacing host splicing factors, which otherwise prevent RNA transport from the nucleus to the cytoplasm (45). In addition, rev is a critical component in the production of the structural proteins of HIV-1. Immune responses directed against rev could target this essential gene sequence and thus interfere with the viral life cycle.

In addition to the regulatory genes, HIV-1 carries an additional set of accessory genes, *vif* (virion infectivity factor), *vpr* (viral protein r), *vpu* (viral protein u), and *nef* (negative factor), which are potential targets for DNA immunization. These accessory genes can be deleted from the viral genome without eliminating replication in vitro, suggesting that these gene products play a secondary rather than primary role in viral infection. The vif protein is located in the plasma membrane and may be important for production of infectious virions (46). In contrast to vif, vpu seems to facilitate the degradation of intracellular CD4 molecules (46). The vpr protein is found in the viral particle in high amounts and appears to have several biological activities, including the ability to increase viral transcription as well as to reactivate virus from cellular latency and arrest host cell division (47,48). Nef has never been shown to be critical for viral infection of cell lines in vitro (49), although experiments performed with the related SIV found that rhesus macaques infected with virus having a deletion in *nef* had dramatically lower levels of viral replication (50). Developing DNA vaccine constructs directed

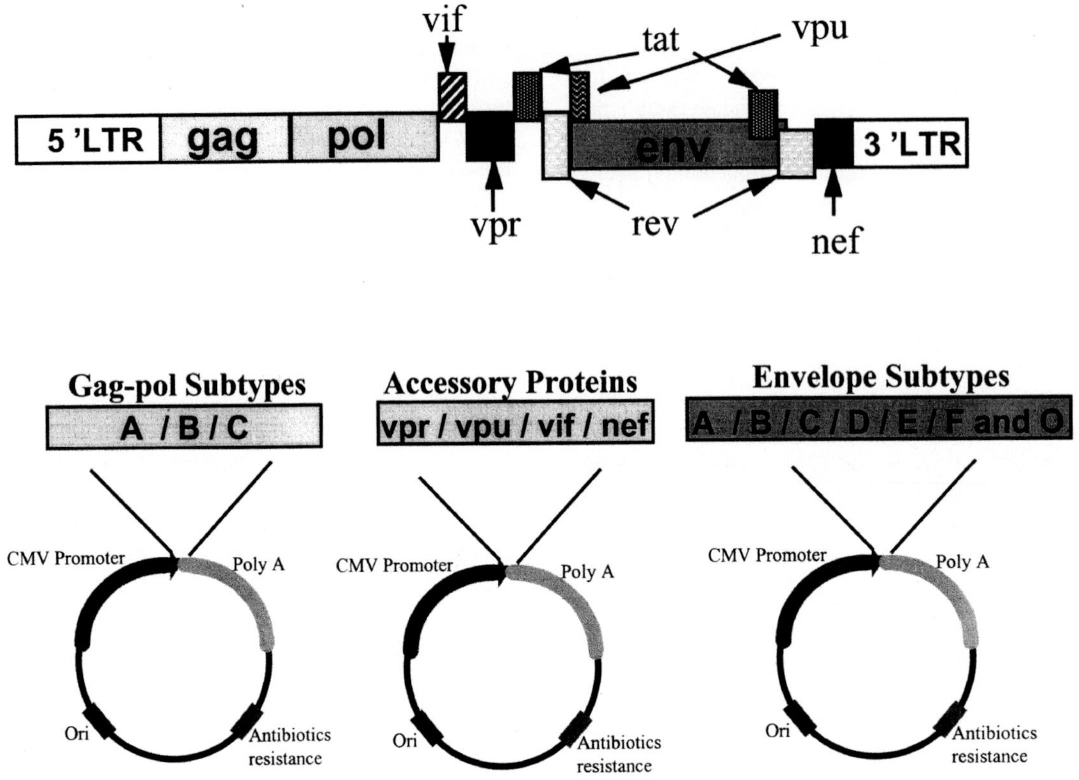

Figure 4 Potential immunological targets for DNA vaccination against HIV-1 include *env, gag,* and *pol* genes as well as the four accessory genes.

against these accessory genes could provide additional arsenal in our battle against HIV-1.

DNA expression cassettes encoding for HIV-1 envelopes (strains HXB2, -MN, and -Z6) were among the first to be analyzed for immunogenicity (Fig. 4) (51). Initial studies demonstrated that mice immunized with envelope constructs produced antibodies specific to recombinant gp160, gp120, and gp41 proteins. The antisera neutralized HIV-1 isolates in vitro at a low level (52). Neutralization of homologous isolates has also been reported after immunization with constructs based on the HIV-1 NL4-3 isolate in the presence of relatively low anti-envelope IgG titers (53). Moreover, the pM160-MN construct not only demonstrated neutralization of homologous isolates, but also showed lower, yet measurable, neutralization of the heterologous HIV-1 Z6 isolate (52). In addition to the humoral responses, cellular immune responses were observed from envelope-inoculated mice. Induction of T-helper (Th) cell proliferative response against recombinant gp120 protein was observed (51). In addition, cytotoxic T-lymphocyte responses have been observed against both targets infected with recombinant vaccinia expressing envelope protein and targets prepared with envelope peptides (51,53,54).

In contrast to the high level of sequence divergence observed in the envelope glycoproteins of HIV-1, their *gag* and *pol* gene sequences appear to be less variable immunological targets. Thus, combining env constructs with gag/pol constructs could result in a more potent vaccination program. Expression cassettes encoding for both gag- and pol-elicited antigen-specific antibody, Th, and CTL responses were observed (55). In addition to the DNA immunogen cassettes encoding env and gag/pol proteins, DNA expression cassettes targeting nef and vif accessory proteins have been developed, and they have been shown to induce both antigen-specific humoral and cellular responses in mice (56,57).

B. DNA Vaccines for Cancer

Although advances in science have led to countless theories and methods designed to combat human carcinoma, the battle is far from over. Surgical excision of tumors, drug therapies, and chemotherapy have been effective in certain cases, but in other situations, particularly when the tumor has begun to metastasize, effective treatment is far more difficult and far less potent. Thus, researchers are continually investigating novel and more effective treatment strategies for various forms of cancer. Research, in recent years, has turned toward the use of vaccines to treat cancer. To this end, several proteins produced by tumor cells became a target for vaccine development. These tumor-associated antigens are predominantly expressed in a tissue-specific manner and are expressed at greatly increased levels in affected cells. Besides being important diagnostic aids, these antigens represent appropriate targets for the development of cancer vaccines (58).

Tumor-associated antigens (TAA) are proteins produced by tumor cells that can be presented on the cell surface in the context of major histocompatibility complexes (59). Recently, these antigens have been the focus of study as a viable option for immunotherapy of various types of cancer. In this review we will examine the progress in the investigation of the immunological effects of two such TAAs: carcinoembryonic antigen (CEA) and prostate-specific antigen (PSA).

1. DNA Vaccine Strategies Using CEA

Human CEA is a 180 kDa glycoprotein expressed in elevated levels in 90% of gastrointestinal malignancies, including colon, rectal, stomach, and pancreatic tumors, 70% of lung cancers, and 50% of breast cancers (59,60). CEA is also found in human fetal digestive organ tissue, hence the name carcinoembryonic antigen (61). It has been discovered that CEA is expressed in normal adult colon epithelium as well, albeit at far lower levels (62,63). Sequencing of CEA shows that it is associated with the human immunoglobulin gene superfamily and that it may be involved in the metastasizing of tumor cells (61).

The immune response to nucleic acid vaccination using a CEA DNA construct was characterized in a murine model. The CEA insert was cloned into a vector containing the cytomegalovirus (CMV) early promoter/enhancer and injected intramuscularly. CEA specific humoral and cellular responses were detected in the immunized mice. These responses were comparable to the immune response generated by rV-CEA (62). The CEA DNA vaccine was also characterized in a canine model, where sera obtained from dogs injected intramuscularly with the construct demonstrated an increase in antibody levels (64). Cellular immune responses quantified using the lymphoblast transformation (LBT) assay also revealed proliferation of CEA-specific lymphocytes. Therefore, a CEA nucleic acid vaccine was able to induce both arms of the immune responses (64). CEA DNA vaccines are currently being investigated in humans.

2. DNA Vaccine Strategies Using PSA

Prostate cancer is the most common form of cancer and the second most common cause of cancer-related death in American men (65). The appearance of prostate cancer is much more common in men over the age of 50 (66). Three of the most widely used treatments are surgical excision of the prostate and seminal vesicles, external bean irradiation, and androgen deprivation. However, conventional therapies lose their efficacy once the tumor has metastasized, which is the case in more than half of initial diagnoses (67,68).

PSA is a serine protease and a human glandular kallikrein gene product of 240 amino acids, which is secreted by both normal and transformed epithelial cells of the prostate gland (69,70). Because cancer cells secrete much higher levels of the antigen, PSA level is a particularly reliable and effective diagnostic indicator of the presence of prostate cancer (71). PSA is also found in normal prostate epithelial tissue, and its expression is highly specific (67).

The immune responses induced by a DNA vaccine encoding for human PSA has been investigated in a murine model (72). The vaccine construct was constructed by cloning a gene for PSA into expression vectors under control of a CMV promoter. Following the injection of the PSA DNA construct (pCPSA), various assays were performed to measure both the humoral and cellular immune responses of the mice. PSA-specific immune responses induced in vivo by immunization were characterized by enzyme-linked immunosorbent assay (ELISA), T-helper proliferation cytotoxic T-lymphocyte (CTL), and flow cytometry assays. Strong and persistent antibody responses were observed against PSA for at least 180 days following immunization. In addition, a significant T-helper cell proliferation was observed against PSA protein. Immunization with pCPSA also induced MHC class I $CD8^+$ T-cell–restricted cytotoxic T-lymphocyte response against tumor cell targets expressing PSA. The induction of PSA-specific humoral and cellular immune responses following injection with pCPSA was also observed in rhesus macaques (J. Kim, unpublished data).

IV. INDUCTION OF IMMUNE RESPONSES IN PRIMATES

It would be desirable to evaluate in primates DNA vaccine constructs that induced high levels of immune responses in mice. Nonhuman primates represent the most relevant animal challenge model for HIV vaccine studies. Specifically, there are currently three different primate models for HIV vaccine studies. They include the HIV challenge model in chimpanzees and the SIV and chimeric SIV/HIV-1 (SHIV-1) challenge models in macaques. Chimpanzees can be infected by HIV isolates from humans, although they do not readily develop AIDS-like disease. On the other hand, the SIV challenge model uses the macaque SIV virus, which replicates to high levels and causes an AIDS-like disease in both cynomolgus and rhesus macaques. The chimeric SHIV viruses were constructed by replacing SIV envelope genes with specific HIV-1 envelope genes (73). The SHIV viruses replicate in macaques similarly to SIV and represent an infectious challenge model for HIV-1 envelope–based vaccines. Importantly, certain SHIV strains such as SHIV 89.6P are pathogenic.

DNA vaccination has been shown to induce both strain-specific neutralizing antibodies as well as antigen-specific T-cell responses in both macaques and chimpanzees. The ability of DNA vaccines to provide protective immunity from viral challenge in primates has had mixed results. In a chimpanzee HIV challenge model, two out of two chimpanzees inoculated with constructs encoding for HIV envelope and gag/pol proteins from strain MN were protected from an i.v. challenge with a high dose (250 chimpanzee ID_{50}) of a heterologous stock of HIV-1 SF2 (74). In an early macaque study, four cynomolgus monkeys immunized with two different HIV-1 envelope constructs (encoding subtypes B and D) resulted in an induction of antigen-specific humoral responses including neutralizing antibodies and cellular responses including proliferative and cytotoxic responses (75). On the other hand, only one of four cynomolgus macaques were protected from intravenous challenge with 50 $TCID_{50}$ of a SHIV-1 HxB2 chimeric virus stock. More recently, two of two rhesus monkeys primed with large doses of HIV-1 gp120 DNA vaccine constructs and boosted with gp160 protein were protected from an i.v. challenge with 25 $TCID_{50}$ of SHIV-1 HXB2 (76). However, protein vaccines alone can protect in this model in a type-specific fashion, and protection is based on the ability of protein to boost the type-specific neutralizing antibody response. More recently, however, priming with gp160 DNA and boosting with recombinant protein did not result in protection in the identical SHIV model (77). Thus, the effectiveness of this vaccine strategy is unclear in the macaque model. In addition to these DNA and protein prime/boost studies, other prime/boost strategies using DNA and recombinant viruses (such as recombinant poxvirus and adenovirus) are being investigated. Although cellular immune responses have been reported to enhance with such prime/boost strategies, their effects on viral protection have not been established (78).

The protective effects of DNA vaccine constructs in the SIV challenge model have been significantly less encouraging. Seven rhesus macaques were immunized with DNA vaccines encoding both envelope (four different plasmids) and gag (one plasmid) genes of SIV and were challenged with pathogenic SIV_{mac251} after their sixth immunization. Although vaccines induced positive responses, none of the vaccinated animals were protected from infection or disease (79).

More recently, we immunized rhesus macaques with DNA vaccine constructs encoding for HIV env/rev and SIV gag/pol proteins (J. Kim, unpublished submitted). Vaccinated animals were challenged intravenously with SHIV IIIB. Half of the animals in the vaccine group exhibited protection from infection based on sensitive limiting dilution co-culture, demonstrating a dramatic effect on viral replication of the vaccines tested. The protected animals were reboosted with SIV DNA vaccines and were rechallenged i.v. with pathogenic SIV_{mac239}. All vaccinated animals were negative for viral co-culture and antigenemia and remained healthy.

Whether the protection from SIV challenge is entirely due to DNA vaccines alone or due to DNA and SHIV challenge should be further studied. It is important to consider the role of SHIV challenge as a boosting agent for gag-specific cellular responses in this study. In any case, these results demonstrate that protection from pathogenic challenge can be achieved in the absence of viral replication that reaches a threshold level of replication for effective vaccination, and these findings could be important in assessing relevant multicomponent vaccination strategies for HIV.

V. SAFETY AND EFFICACY STUDIES IN HUMANS

The ultimate goal of vaccine development is to demonstrate safety and efficacy in humans. The first DNA vaccine studies to enter the clinic were DNA vaccines encoding for HIV-1 MN envelope (80). Fifteen healthy HIV-1–seropositive volunteers with >500 $CD4^+$ lymphocytes/mL were enrolled in this study. Patients in the trial received three injections, each separated by 10 weeks, with escalating dosage (3 dosage groups of 5 subjects) of envelope vaccine. Preliminary results reveal no significant clinical or laboratory adverse effects measured in any of the dosage groups (30, 100, 300 μg). More importantly, the immunized individuals developed an increase in antibody responses to envelope proteins and peptides after receiving the 100 μg dose. Some increases in cellular responses including the lymphoproliferative and CTL responses as well as β-chemokine expression were also observed (80).

These preliminary results demonstrate that the injection of even relatively low doses of a single immunogen DNA vaccine is capable of augmenting both existing humoral and cellular immune responses in humans. In addition to the initial human trials, phase I trials evaluating a gag/pol construct as a therapeutic vaccine as well as a prophylactic DNA vaccine study for HIV have been undertaken. In another clinical study, the healthy volunteers who were immunized with DNA vaccines encoding for malaria proteins developed CTL responses against the target cells prepared with malaria peptides (81). Taken together, these studies are dramatically expanding our knowledge of DNA vaccines for clinical use in humans.

VI. MOLECULAR ADJUVANTS AS AN IMMUNE-MODULATION STRATEGY

The primary goal of the first-generation DNA immunization studies were to demonstrate and evaluate the DNA vaccines' ability to elicit humoral and cellular responses in vivo in a safe and well-tolerated manner. As we explore the next generation of DNA vaccines, it would be desirable to refine current DNA vaccination strategies to elicit more clinically efficacious immune responses. In this regard, the next generation of nucleic acid vaccines may require better control of the magnitude and direction (humoral or cellular) of the immune responses induced. Such modulation of immune responses can be accomplished by the use of genetic adjuvants. Genetic or molecular adjuvants are different from the traditional adjuvants in that they are comprised of gene expression constructs encoding for immunologically important molecules. These molecules include cytokines, chemokines, and costimulatory molecules (9). These molecular adjuvant constructs could be co-administered along with immunogen constructs to modulate the magnitude and direction (humoral or cellular) of the immune responses induced by the vaccine cassettes themselves (Fig. 5). Such use of molecular adjuvant constructs results in concurrent kinetics of in vivo expression for both the adjuvant and antigen proteins. This ability to engineer targeted immune responses may be a particularly important aspect of a multicomponent DNA vaccine strategy.

A. Cytokine Molecular Adjuvants

In order to focus the immune responses induced from DNA vaccines, we and others have investigated the co-delivery of molecular adjuvants to modulate vaccine responses (55,82–90). We initially reported that co-immunization of GM-CSF cDNA with DNA vaccine constructs increases antigen-specific antibody and T-helper cell proliferation responses, while co-immunization with IL-12 cDNA results in weaker antibody responses and enhanced T-helper cell proliferation in mice (55,82). In addition, IL-12 co-immunization resulted in a significant enhancement of CTL responses. Importantly, we observed a significant enhancement of CTL response in vivo with the co-administration of murine IL-12 genes with four different HIV-1 DNA immunogens (*gag/pol, env, vif,* and *nef*), which were $CD8^+$ T-cell– and MHC class I–restricted. In contrast, almost no effect on CTL induction was observed with the genes for GM-CSF in these studies. Iwasaki et al. (88) reported a similar finding using GM-CSF and IL-12 co-delivery with DNA immunogen encoding for influenza NP.

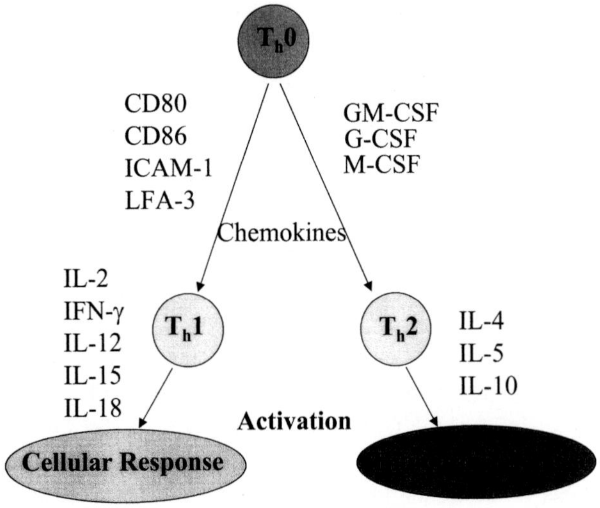

Figure 5 Cytokines, chemokines, and costimulatory molecules play critical roles in the immune and inflammatory responses. Based upon their specific function in the immune system, these cytokines could be further grouped as proinflammatory, Th1, and Th2 cytokines. Along with costimulatory molecules and chemokines, these cytokines also play important roles in the activation and proliferation of T and B cells.

More recently, we investigated the induction and regulation of immune responses from the co-delivery of proinflammatory cytokines (IL-1α, and TNF-β), Th1 cytokines (IL-2, IL-15, and IL-18), and Th2 cytokines (IL-4, IL-5, and IL-10) (83). We observed that some Th1 as well as Th2 cytokine genes increased the antibody response, specifically co-injection with IL-2, IL-4, IL-5, IL-10, and IL-18, all resulted in increased levels of antibodies. We also found that co-injection with TNF-α, TNF-β, IL-2, IL-10, and IL-18 resulted in a dramatic enhancement of T-helper proliferation response, while co-injection with IL-5 and IL-15 resulted in a more moderate increase in T-helper proliferation. Furthermore, among all co-injection combinations, we found that only TNF-α and IL-15 co-injections resulted in a high level of CTL enhancement similar to that of IL-12 co-injection. Co-injection with TNF-β, IL-2, and IL-18 resulted in a more moderate increase in CTL response over those groups immunized with only DNA immunogen. As observed with IL-12 co-injection, the en-

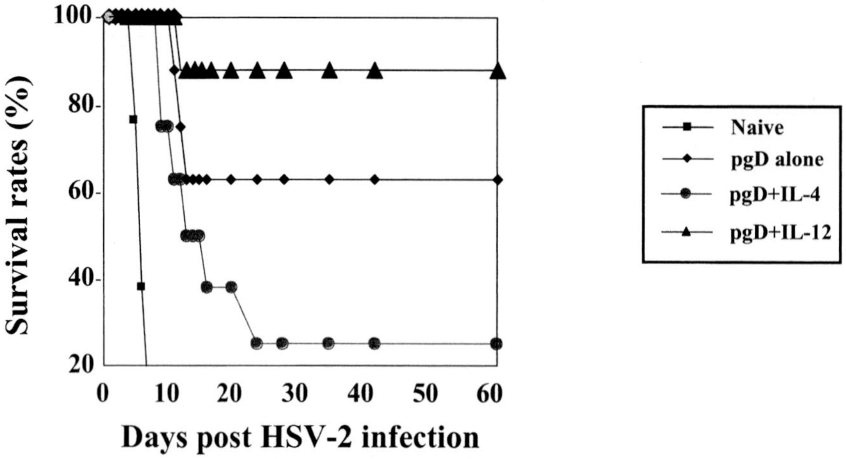

Figure 6 Protection from lethal HSV-2 challenge. Each group of mice (n = 10) was immunized with gD DNA vaccines (60 μg) and/or cytokine genes (40 μg) at 0 and 2 weeks. Three weeks after the second immunization, mice (n = 8) were challenged i.v. with $200 \times LD_{50}$ of HSV-2 strain 186 (7×10^5 pfu).

hancement of CTL responses observed from the co-injections with TNF-α and IL-15 were restricted by MHC class I and were $CD8^+$ T-cell–dependent.

We also investigated whether the Th1- or Th2-type immune response is more important for protection from HSV-2 infection (91). We co-delivered DNA expression construct encoding for HSV-2 gD protein with the gene plasmids encoding for Th1-type (IL-2, 12, 15, 18) and Th2-type (IL-4, IL-10) cytokines in an effort to drive immunity induced by vaccination. We then analyzed the vaccine modulatory effects on resulting immune phenotype and on the mortality and the morbidity of the immunized animals following HSV lethal challenge (Fig. 6). We observed that Th1 cytokine gene co-administration not only enhanced survival rate, but also reduced the frequency and severity of herpetic lesions following intravaginal HSV challenge. On the other hand, co-injection with Th2 cytokine genes increased the rate of mortality and morbidity of the challenged mice. Again, among the Th1-type cytokine genes tested, IL-12 was particularly a potent adjuvant for the gD DNA vaccination, resulting in increased survival and decreased animal morbidity.

B. Chemokine Molecular Adjuvants

Similar to cytokine gene co-delivery, we found that the co-immunization with chemokine genes along with DNA immunogen constructs can modulate the direction and magnitude of induced immune responses (85). We observed that co-immunization with IL-8 and MIP-1α genes increased the antibody response in a similar manner to IL-4 or GM-CSF co-immunization. We also found that co-injection with IL-8 and RANTES resulted in a dramatic enhancement of T-helper proliferation response. Among all co-injection combinations, we found that RANTES and MCP-1 co-injections resulted in a high level of CTL enhancement, almost as significant as IL-12, a potent CTL inducer for DNA vaccines. The use of these chemokine vaccines could be particularly important as HIV vaccine modulators of β-chemokines. In this regard, we observed that β-chemokines as vaccine adjuvants augmented β-chemokine production in a vaccine antigen-specific manner. This aspect could be especially important for a development of an HIV vaccine.

C. Costimulatory Molecule Molecular Adjuvants

Professional APCs initiate T-cell activation through binding of antigenic peptide-MHC complexes to specific T-cell receptor molecules. In addition, the APCs provide critical costimulatory signals to T cells that are required for the clonal expansion and differentiation of T cells. Among different costimulatory molecules, B7 molecules (CD80 and CD86) have been observed to provide potent immune signals (92,93). They bind to their receptors (CD28/CTLA-4) present on T cells. The CD80 and CD86 molecules are surface glycoproteins and members of immunoglobulin superfamily, which are expressed only on professional APCs (92–94). The blocking of this additional costimulatory signal leads to T-cell anergy (95).

We reported that CD86 molecules play a prominent role in the antigen-specific induction of $CD8^+$ CTLs when delivered as vaccine adjuvants (86). Co-administration of CD86 cDNA along with DNA encoding HIV-1 antigens intramuscularly dramatically increased antigen-specific T-cell responses without a significant change in the level of the humoral response. This enhancement of CTL response was both MHC class I–restricted and $CD8^+$ T-cell–dependent. Similar results have been obtained by other investigators, who also found that CD86, not CD80 co-expression results in the enhancement of T-cell–mediated immune responses (88,89).

Accordingly, we speculated that engineering of nonprofessional APCs such as muscle cells to express CD86 costimulatory molecules could empower them to prime CTL precursors. On the other hand, the enhancement effect of CD86 co-delivery could also have been mediated through the direct transfection of a small number of professional APCs residing within the muscle tissue. Subsequently, these cells could have greater expression of costimulatory molecules and could in theory become more potent. To investigate this issue we constructed a set of bone marrow chimeric animals between normal mice and mice bearing a disrupted β_2-microglobulin (β_2m) gene (96). These bone marrow chimeras could respond and develop functional CTL responses following immunization with vaccinia virus. Next we immunized chimeric animals with a DNA vaccine expressing HIV-1_{MN} envelope protein (pCEnv) and plasmids encoding CD80 or CD86 genes (pCD80 or pCD86). Using this model, we observed that in vivo transfection of only pCEnv and pCD86 could engineer non–bone marrow–derived cells, such as muscle cells, to prime and expand CTLs. This study suggests that CD86 and not CD80 plays a central role in the generation of the antigen-specific CTL responses. These results indicate that the strategy of engineering muscle cells to be more efficient APCs could be an important tool for the optimization of antigen-specific T-cell–mediated immune responses in a pursuit of more rationally designed vaccines and immune therapies through the control of MHC class I restriction. This method of engineering nonhematopoietic cells to be more efficient APCs could be especially important in cases where antigen alone fails to elicit a CTL response due to poor presentation by the host APCs.

In light of these findings, we further investigated the strategy of engineering immune responses using additional costimulatory molecules (97). We co-immunized cDNA expression cassettes encoding intracellular adhesion molecule (ICAM)-1, lymphocyte function–associated antigen (LFA)-3, and vascular cell adhesion molecule (VCAM)-1 along with DNA immunogens and analyzed the resulting antigen-specific immune responses. We observed that antigen-specific T-cell responses can be enhanced by the co-expression of DNA immunogen and adhesion molecules ICAM-1 and LFA-3. Co-expression of ICAM-1 or LFA-3 molecules along with DNA immunogens resulted in a significant enhancement of Th-cell proliferative responses. In addition, co-immunization with ICAM-1 (and more moderately with LFA-3) resulted in a dramatic enhancement of CD8-restricted CTL responses. Although VCAM-1 and ICAM-1 are similar in size, VCAM-1 co-immunization did not have any measurable effect on cell-mediated responses. Rather, these results imply that ICAM-1 and LFA-3 provide direct T-cell costimulation. These observations were further supported by the finding that co-injection with ICAM-1 dramatically enhanced the level of IFN-γ and β-chemokines MIP-1α, MIP-1β, and RANTES produced by stimulated T cells. Through comparative studies we observed that ICAM-1/LFA-1 T-cell costimulatory pathways are independent of CD86/CD28 pathways, and they may synergistically expand T-cell responses in vivo. Furthermore, these studies indicate that $CD8^+$ effector T cells at the site of inflammation can regulate the level of effector function through the expression of specific chemokines and adhesion molecules Fig. 7 (85,97). Therefore, the end-stage effector T cells in the expansion phase of an antigen-specific immune response could direct their destiny through coordinated expression and release of these molecules.

VII. USE OF MOLECULAR ADJUVANTS IN PRIMATES

We sought to evaluate whether the enhancement of immune responses observed in mice with co-immunization with cytokine genes could also be achieved in rhesus macaques. DNA vaccines for HIV env/rev and STV gag/pol alone were evaluated for their immunogenicity and compared to these vaccines, which also included IL-2 or IFN-γ (Th1) or IL-4 (Th2) cytokine cDNA constructs (J. Kim, unpublished). The cytokines dramatically enhanced seroconversion induced by the vaccines and appeared to modulate cellular responses as well, although more modestly. Vaccinated animals were challenged intravenously with SHIV IIIB. Half of the animals in the vaccine or vaccine 1 + 1 Th1 cytokine groups exhibited protection from infection based on sensitive limiting dilution co-culture, demonstrating a dramatic effect on viral replication of the vaccines tested. The protected animals were reboosted with SIV DNA vaccines (SIV and cytokine constructs) and were rechallenged i.v. with pathogenic SIV_{mac239}. All vaccinated animals were negative for viral co-culture and antigenemia. In contrast, the control animals exhibited antigenemia by 2 weeks postchallenge and exhibited greater than 10 log of virus/10^6 cells in limiting dilution co-culture. The control animal exhibited CD4 cell loss and developed SIV-

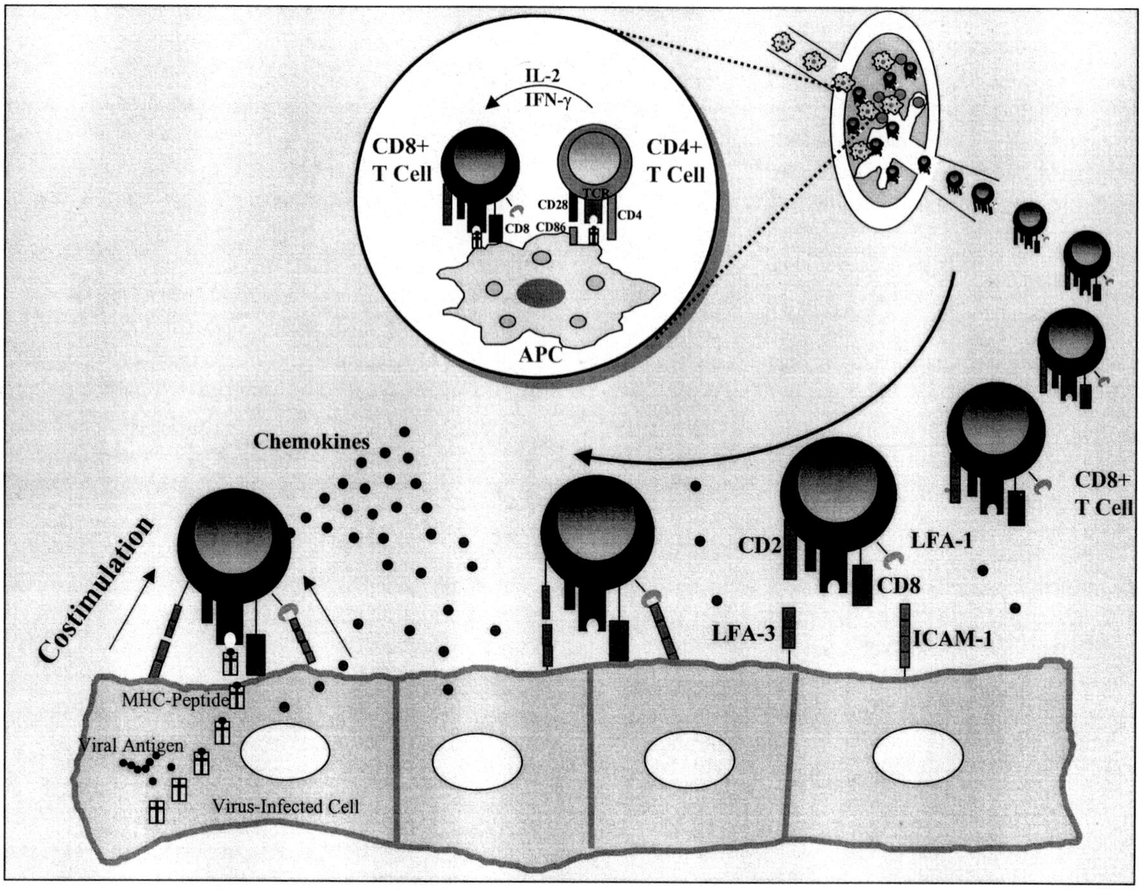

Figure 7 Regulation of CD8 + T-cell expansion by adhesion molecules and chemokines in the periphery. Specific adhesion molecules and chemokines provide modulatory signals to CD8 + T cells in effector stage. This network of cytokine, chemokine, costimulatory molecules, and adhesion molecules represents a coordinated regulation and maintenance of effector T cells in the periphery.

related wasting within 14 weeks of high viral burden and subsequently failed to thrive. Vaccinated animals were virus-negative and remained healthy. While exact correlates of protection could include cellular responses, neutralizing antibody responses do not appear to correlate with control of viral replication and infection in these studies. These studies establish that multicomponent DNA vaccines can directly impact viral replication and disease in a highly pathogenic challenge system, potentially broadening our immunological weapons against HIV.

VIII. ADVANTAGES OF USING MOLECULAR ADJUVANTS

The overall objective of any immunization strategy is to induce specific immune responses, which could protect the immunized individual from a given pathogen over his or her lifetime. One major challenge in meeting this goal is that the correlates of protection from an individual pathogen vary from one infectious agent to the next. It would be a distinct advantage to design immunization strategies, which can be ''targeted'' according to the correlates of protection known for the particular pathogen (Fig. 8). As summarized in Fig. 9 and Table 2, in this regard we observed that significant modulation was possible through the use of molecular adjuvants along with DNA vaccine constructs. This strategy of using molecular adjuvant network underscores an important level of control in the induction of specific immune responses to tailor vaccination programs more closely to the correlates of protection, which vary from disease to disease. This type of fine control of vaccine and immune therapies was previously very difficult to obtain. Controlling the magnitude and direction of the immune response could be advantageous in a wide

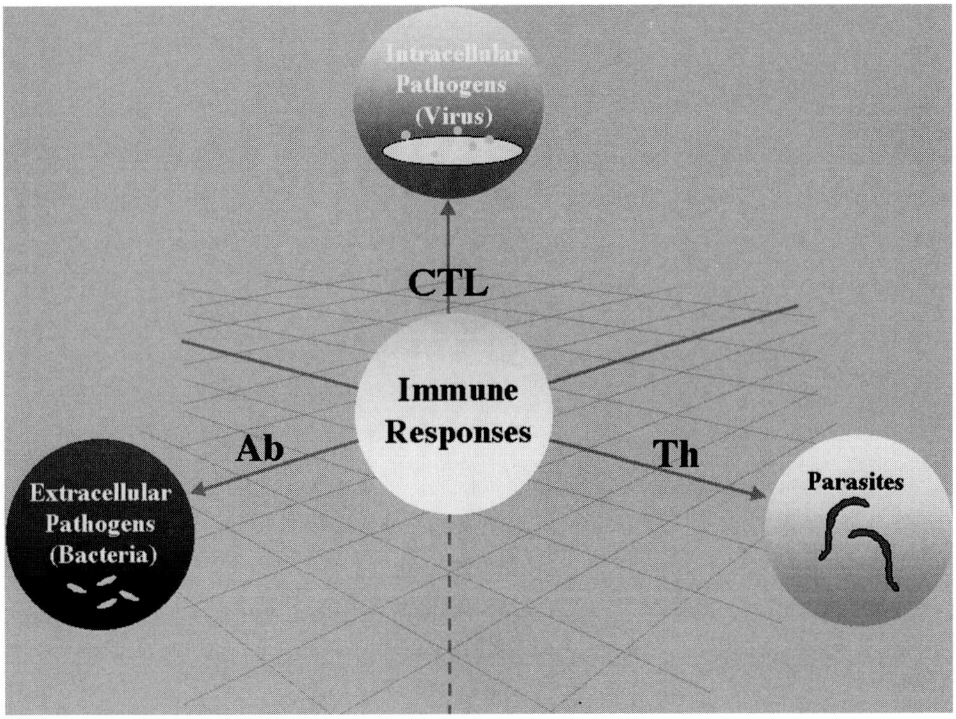

Figure 8 The potential utility of the molecular adjuvant network. Tailoring the induction of specific immune responses by vaccination programs against viral, bacterial, or parasitic diseases could be beneficial. Ab (Antibody), Th (T helper cell), CTL (cytotoxic T-lymphocyte).

Table 2 Summary of Immune Modulation by Molecular Adjuvants

	Molecular adjuvant	Immune modulation		
		Ab	Th	CTL
Pro-inflammatory cytokines	TNF-α	+++	++++	++++
	TNF-β	+	+	+
	IL-1α	+++	++	+/−
Th1 cytokines	IFN-γ	++	++++	++
	IL-2	+++	++++	+
	IL-12	−	++++	++++
	IL-15	++	++	++++
	IL-18	+++	++++	++
Th2 cytokines	IL-4	++++	+	+/−
	IL-5	++++	++	+/−
	IL-10	++++	+++	+/−
Hematopoeitic cytokines	G-CSF	+	++	+
	GM-CSF	++++	++++	+
	M-CSF	++	+	++++
Chemokines	IL-8	+++	++++	+/−
	MIP-1α	++++	++	+/−
	RANTES	+	++++	++++
	MCP-1	+/−	+	++++
Costimulatory molecules	CD80	+/−	+	+/−
	CD86	+/−	++++	++++
	ICAM-1	+/−	++++	++++
	LFA-3	+/−	+++	++

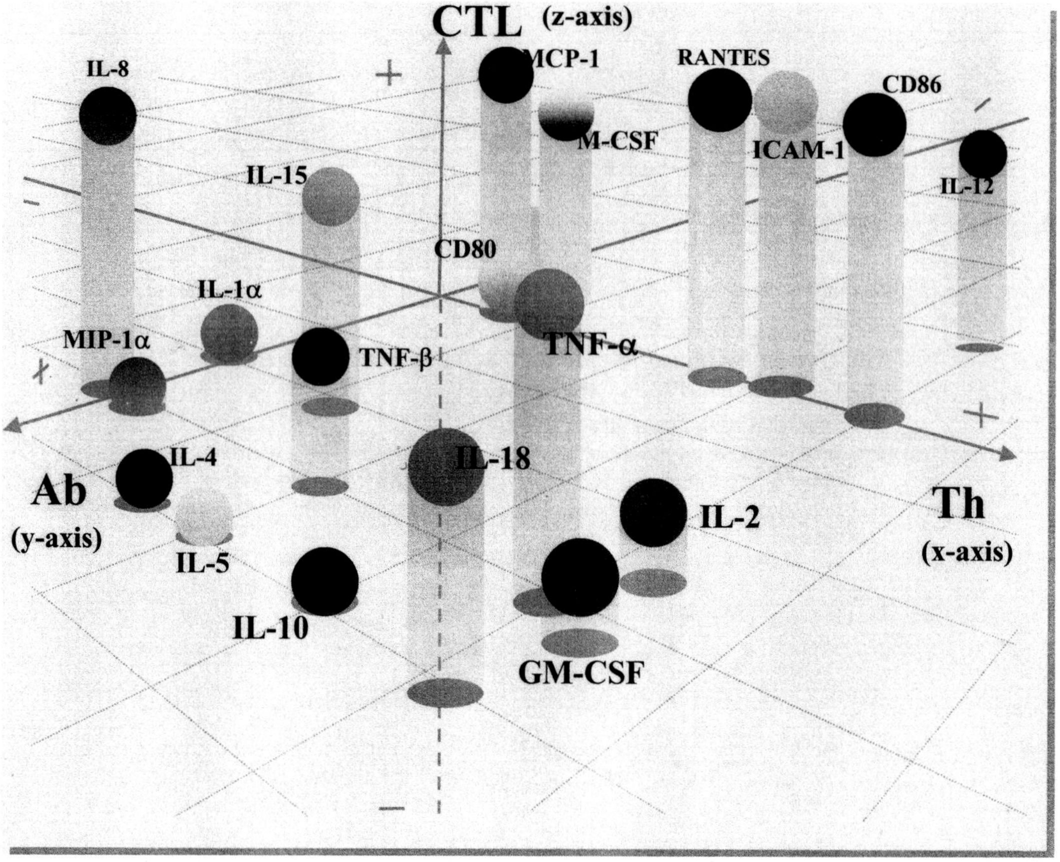

Figure 9 A summary of the molecular adjuvant co-administration effects on antibody (y-axis), T-helper (x-axis), and cytotoxic T-lymphocyte responses (z-axis). Each adjuvant is plotted on the three-dimensional axis according to its effects on the three modes of immune response.

variety of vaccine strategies, including HIV-1. A substantial number of current literature supports that T-cell–mediated responses are more critical for providing protective immunity against HIV infection (42,98,99). In such cases where T-cell–mediated response is paramount, IL-12, MCP-1, RANTES, CD86, or ICAM-1 genes could be chosen as the immune modulator to be co-delivered with a specific DNA immunogen. On the other hand, for building vaccines to target extracellular bacteria, for example, MIP-1*α*, Th2 cytokines, or GM-CSF genes could be co-injected. Additionally, in cases where both $CD4^+$ T-helper cells and antibodies play more important roles in protection, IL-2, IL-8, or GM-CSF could be co-delivered. Furthermore, these genes can be combined with one or more additional cytokine or costimulatory genes to further control the immune responses. Additional studies in higher animal models such as the primates can further address potential risks and benefits of applying this genetic adjuvant network, ultimately leading to modulation of human diseases.

IX. CONCLUSION

DNA immunization holds great promise for providing safe and inexpensive vaccines for many infectious pathogens, including HIV-1. The direct injection of foreign genes by genetic immunization has resulted in specific immune responses that exhibit characteristics of protective immunity against a number of infectious agents in a variety of animal models. Genetic vaccination cassettes targeting each of HIV-1's three major genes (*env, gag, and pol*), regulatory genes, and accessory genes have been developed and studied in small animals, primates, and humans. DNA vaccine constructs for cancer-targeting tumor-specific antigens have also been studied in a variety of animal models. Developing successful vaccines for HIV-1 or cancer will likely involve targeting multiple antigenic components to direct and empower the immune system. Such a collection of immunization cassettes should be capable of stimulating broad immunity against both humoral and cellular epitopes, thus giving a vaccine the maximum ability to deal with viral immune escape or tumor growth. DNA vaccines can be combined with other vaccines including recombinant protein, poxvirus, adenovirus, as well as others to further enhance initial immune responses. In addition, the potential of the molecular adjuvant co-administration to dramatically enhance and regulate the antigen-specific humoral and cellular immune responses induced by DNA immunogens represents an important new avenue for vaccine and immune therapeutic exploration. Although further studies are warranted, these studies collectively support that optimized combinations of DNA expression cassettes coding for env, gag/pol, accessory proteins, costimulatory molecules, cytokines, chemokines, or other vaccine modulators may provide the basis for an effective vaccination strategy against HIV-1 or cancer.

REFERENCES

1. Plotkin SA, Mortimer EA. Vaccines. Philadelphia: W.B. Saunders Co., 1988.
2. Janeway CA, Travers P. Immunobiology. Current Biology Ltd./Garland, London, 1994.
3. Stasney J, Cantarow A, Paschkis KE. Production of neoplams by injection of fractions of mammalian neoplasms. Cancer Res 1955; 11:775–782.
4. Paschkis KE, Cantarow A, Stasney J. Induction of neoplasms by injection of tumor chromatin. J Natl Cancer Inst 1955; 15:1525–1532.
5. Ito Y. A tumor-producing factor extracted by phenol from papillomatous tissue of cottontail rabbits. Virology 1960; 12:596–601.
6. Wolff JA, Malone RW, Williams P, Chong W, Acsadi G, Jani A, Felgner PL. Direct gene transfer into mouse muscle in vivo. Science 1990; 247:1465–1468.
7. Tang D, DeVit M, Johnston S. Genetic immunization is a simple method for eliciting an immune response. Nature 1992; 356:152–154.
8. Chattergoon M, Boyer J, Weiner DB. Genetic immunization: a new era in vaccines and immune therapies. FASEB J 1997; 11:753–763.
9. Kim JJ, Weiner DG. DNA/genetic vaccination for HIV. Springer Sem Immunopathol 1997; 19:174–195.
10. Donnelly JJ, Ulmer JB, Shiver JW, Liu MM. DNA vaccines. Annu Rev Immunol 1997; 15:617–648.
11. Doe B, Selby M, Barnett S, Baenzinger J, Walker CM. Induction of cytotoxic T lymphocytes by intramuscular immunization with plasmid DNA is facilitated by bone marrow-derived cells. Proc Natl Acad Sci USA 1996; 93: 8578–8583.
12. Corr M, Lee DJ, Carson DA, Tighe H. Gene vaccination with naked plasmid DNA: mechanism of CTL priming. J Exp Med 1996; 184:1555–1560.
13. Pardoll DM, Beckerleg AM. Exposing the immunology of naked DNA vaccines. Immunity 1995; 3:165–169.
14. Brodsky FM, Guagliardi LE. The cell biology of antigen processing and presentation. Ann Rev Immunol 1991; 9: 707–744.
15. Goebels N, Michaelis D, Wekerle M, Hohlfeld R. Human myoblasts as antigen-presenting cells. J Immunol 1992; 149:661–667.
16. Behrens LMK, Misgeld T, Goebels N, Wekerle H, Hohlfeld R. Human muscle cells express a functional costimulatory molecule distinct from B7.1 (CD80) and B7.2 (CD86) in vivo and in inflammatory lesions. J Immunol 1998; 161: 5943–5951.
17. Albert ML, Saulter B, Bhardwaj N. Dendritic cells acquire antigen from apoptotic cells and induce class I-restricted CTLs. Nature 1998; 392:86–89.
18. Condon C, Watkins SC, Celluzzi CM, Thompson K, Falo LD. DNA-based immunization by in vivo transfection of dendtric cells. Nature Med 1996; 10:1122–1128.
19. Casares S, Inaba K, Brumeanu TD, Steinman RM, Bona CA. Antigen presentation by dendritic cells after immunization with DNA encoding a major histocompatibility complex class II-restricted viral epitope. J Exp Med 1997; 186: 1481–1486.
20. Chattergoon MA, Robinson TA, Boyer JD, Weiner DB. Specific immune induction following DNA-based immunization through in vivo transfection and activation of macrophages. J Immunol 1998; 160:5707–5718.
21. Ho DD. Therapy of HIV infections: problems and prospects. Bull NY Acad Med 1996; 73:37–45.
22. Condra JH, Holder DJ, Schleif WA, Blahy OM, Danovich RM, Gabryelski LJ, Graham DJ, Laird D, Quintero JC, Rhodes A, Robbins HL, Roth E, Shivaprakash M, Yang T, Chodakewitz JA, Deutsch PJ, Leavitt RY, Massari FE, Mellors JW, Squires KE, Steigbigel RT, Teppler H, Emini EA. Genetic correlates of in vivo viral resistance to indinavir, a human immunodeficiency virus type 1 protease inhibitor. J Virol 1996; 70:8270–8276.
23. WorldBank. Investing in health. In: World Development Report 1993. Oxford University Press, Oxford 1993:62–63.
24. Cohen J. AIDS research: the mood is uncertain. Science 1993; 260:1254–1255.
25. Chao BH, Costopoulos DS, Curiel T, Bertonis JM, Chisholm P, Williams C, Schooley RT, Rosa JJ, Fisher RA, Maraganore JM. A 113-amino acid fragment of CD4 produced in *Eschericha coli* blocks human immunodefeciency virus-induced cell fusion. J Biol Chem 1989; 264:5812–5817.
26. Pantaleo G, Menzo S, Vaccarezza M, Graziosi C, Cohen OY, Demarest JF, Montefiori D, Orenstein JM, Fox C, Schrager LK, et al. Studies in subjects with long-term non-progressive Human immunodeficiency virus infection. N Engl J Med 1995; 332:209–216.
27. Berman P, Gregory TJ, Riddle L, Nakamura GR, Champe MA, Porter JP, Wurm FM, Hershberg RD, Cobb EK, Eichberg JW. Protection of chimpanzees from infection by HIV-1 after vaccination with recombinant glycoprotein gp120 but not gp160. Nature 1990; 345:622–625.
28. Barrett N, Eder G, Dorner F. Characterization of a vaccinia-derived recombinant HIV-1 gp160 candidate vaccine and

its immunogenicity in chimpanzees. Biotech Therapeut 1991; 2:91–106.
29. Bruck C, Thiriart C, Fabry L, et al. HIV-1 envelope elicited neutralizing antibody titres correlate with protection and virus load in chimpanzees. J Cell Biochem 1993; 17:88.
30. Girard M, Kieny MP, Pinter A, et al. Immunization of chimpanzees confers protection against challenge with human immunodeficiency virus. Proc Natl Acad Sci USA 1991; 88:542–546.
31. Marthas ML, Miller CJ, Sutjipto S, Higgins J, Torten J, Lohman BL, Unger R, Kiyono H, McGhee JB, Marx PA, Pederson NC. Efficacy of live-attenuated and whole-inactivated simian immunodeficiency virus vaccines against vaginal challenge with virulent SIV. J Med Prim 1992; 21: 99–107.
32. Montefiori DC, Reimann KA, Wyand MS, Manson K, Lewis MG, Collman RG, Sodroski JG, Bolognesi DP, Letvin NL. Neutralizing antibodies in sera from macaques infected with chimeric simian-human immunodeficiency virus containing the envelope glycoproteins of either a laboratory-adapted variant or a primary isolate of human immunodeficiency virus type 1. J Virol 1998; 72:3427–3431.
33. Burton DR, Montefiori DC. The antibody response in HIV-1 infection. AIDS 1997; 11(suppl A):587–98.
34. Moore J, Trkola A. HIV type 1 coreceptors, neutralization serotypes, and vaccine development. AIDS Res Hum Retrov 1997; 13:733–736.
35. Etemad-Moghadam B, Karlsson GB, Halloran M, Sun Y, Schenten D, Fernandes M, Letvin NL, Sodroski J. Characterization of simian-human immunodeficiency virus envelope glycoprotein epitopes recognized by neutralizing antibodies from infected monkeys. J Virol 1998; 72: 8437–8445.
36. Letvin NL. Progress in the development of an HIV-1 vaccine. Science 1998; 280:1875–1880.
37. Koup RA, Safrit JT, Cao Y, Andrews CA, McLeod G, Borkowsky W, Farthing C, Ho DD. Temporal association of cellular immune responses with the initial control of viremia in primary human immunodeficiency virus type 1 syndrome. J Virol 1994; 68:4650.
38. Borrow P, Lewicki H, Hahn H, Shaw GM, Oldstone MBA. Virus-specific CD8+ cytotoxic T lymphocyte activity associated with control of viremia in primary human immunodeficiency virus type 1 infection. J Virol 1994; 68:6103.
39. Pinto L, Sullivan J, Berzofsky JA, Clerici M, Kessler HA, Landay AL, Shearer GM. Env-specific cytotoxic T lymphocyte responses in HIV seronegative health care workers occupationally exposed to HIV-contaminated body fluids. J Clin Invest 1995; 96:867–876.
40. Rowland-Jones S, Sutton J, Ariyoshi K, Dong T, Gotch F, McAdam S, Whitby D, Sabally S, Allimore A, Corrah T, Takiguchi M, McMichael A, Whittle H. HIV-specific T-cells in HIV-exposed but uninfected Gambian women. Nat Med 1995; 1:59–64.
41. Hulskotte EG, Geretti A-M, Siebelink KH, van Amerongen G, Cranage MP, Rud EW, Norley SG, de Vries P, Osterhaus AD. Vaccine-induced virus neutralizing antibodies and cytotoxic T cells do not protect macaques from experimental infection with Simian immunodeficiency virus $SIV_{mac32H(J5)}$. J Virol 1995; 69:6289–6296.
42. Rosenberg ES, Billingsley JM, Caliendo AM, Boswell SL, Sax PE, Kalams SA, Walker BD. Vigorous HIV-1-specific CD4+ T cell responses associated with control of viremia. Science 1997; 278:1447–1450.
43. Cullen B, Greene WC. Functions of the auxiliary gene products of the human immunodeficiency virus type 1. Virology 1990; 178:1–5.
44. Nixon D, Townsend AR, Elvin JG, Rizza CR, Gallwey J, McMichael AJ. HIV-1 gag-specific cytotoxic T lymphocytes defined with recombinant vaccinia virus and synthetic peptides. Nature 1988; 336:484–487.
45. Malim M, Hauber J, Le SY, Maizel JV, Cullen BR. The HIV-1 *rev* trans-activator acts through a structured target sequence to activate a nuclear export of unspliced viral mRNA. Nature 1989; 338:254–257.
46. Strebhel K, Dauherty D, Clouse K, Cohen D, Folks T, Martin MA. The HIV ''A'' (sor) gene product is essential for virus infectivity. Nature 1987; 328:728–730.
47. Levy DN, Fernandes LS, Williams WV, Weiner DB. Induction of cell differentiation by human immunodeficiency virus 1 vpr. Cell 1993; 72:541–550.
48. Levy DN, Refaeli Y, Weiner DB. Extracellular vpr protein increases cellular permissiveness to HIV replication and reactivates virus from latency. J Virol 1994; 69:1243–1252.
49. Kim S, Ikeuchi K, Byrn R, Groopman J, Baltimore D. Lack of a negative influence on viral growth by the *nef* gene of human immunodeficiency virus type 1. Proc Natl Acad Sci USA 1989; 86:9544–9548.
50. Kestler H, Ringler DJ, Mori K, Panicalli DL, Sehgai PK, Daniel MD, Desrosiers RC. Importance of the *nef* gene for maintenance of high virus loads and for the development of AIDS. Cell 1991; 65:651–662.
51. Wang B, Ugen KE, Srikantan V, Agadjanyan MG, Dang K, Refaeli Y, Sato A, Boyer J, Williams WV, Weiner DB. Gene inoculation generates immune responses against human immunodeficiency virus type 1. Proc Natl Acad Sci USA 1993; 90:4156–4160.
52. Wang B, Boyer JD, Ugen KE, Srikantan V, Ayyavoo V, Agadjanyan MG, Williams WV, Newman M, Coney L, Carrano R, Weiner DB. Nucleic acid-based immunization against HIV-1: induction of protective in vivo immune responses. AIDS 1995; 9:S159–170.
53. Lu S, Santoro JC, Fuller DH, Haynes JR, Robinson HL. Use of DNAs expressing HIV-1 *env* and non-infectious HIV-1 particles to raise antibody responses in mice. Virology 1995; 209:147–154.
54. Haynes J, Fuller DH, Eisenbraun MD, Ford MJ, Pertmer TM. Accell® particle-mediated DNA immunization elicits humoral, cytotoxic and protective responses. AIDS Res Hum Retrovir 1994; 10:S43–45.
55. Kim JJ, Ayyvoo V, Bagarazzi ML, Chattergoon MA, Dang K, Wang B, Boyer JD, Weiner DB. In vivo engineering of

a cellular immune response by co-administration of IL-12 expression vector with a DNA immunogen. J Immunol 1997; 158:816–826.
56. Ayyavoo V, Nagashunmugam T, Boyer JD, Sundarasamy M, Fernandes LS, Le P, Lin J, Nguyen C, Chattergoon MA, Goedert JJ, Friedman H, Weiner DB. Development of genetic vaccines for pathogenic genes: construction of attenuated Vif DNA immunization cassettes. AIDS 1997; 11: 1433–1444.
57. Ayyavoo V, Nagashunmugam T, Phung T, Buckner C, Kudckodkar S, Le P, Reddy PJ, Santiago L, Patel M, Tea L, Weiner DB. Construction of attenuated HIV-1 accessory gene immunization cassettes. Vaccine 1998; 16: 1872–1879.
58. Sogn JA, Finerty JF, Heath AL, Shen GLC, Austin FC. Cancer vaccines: the perspective of the Cancer Immunology Branch, NCI. Ann NY Acad Sci 1993; 690:322–330.
59. Kelley JR, Cole DJ. Gene therapy strategies utilizing carcinoembryonic antigen as a tumor associated antigen for vaccination against solid malignancies. Gene Ther Mol Biol 1998; 2:14–30.
60. Zaremba S, Barzaga E, Zhu M, Soares N, Tsang N, Schlom J. Identification of an enhancer agonist cytotoxic T lymphocyte peptide from human carcinoembryonic antigen. Cancer Res 1997; 57:4570–4577.
61. Foon KA, Chakraborty M, John WJ, Sherratt A, Kohler H, Bhattacharya-Chatterjee M. Immune response to the carcinoembryonic antigen in patients treated with an anti-idiotype antibody vaccine. J Clin Invest 1997; 96:334–342.
62. Conry RM, LoBuglio AF, Kantor J, Schlom J, Loechel F, Moore SE, Sumerel LA, Barlow DL, Abrams S, Curiel DT. Immune response to a carcinoembryonic antigen polynucleotide vaccine. Cancer Res 1994; 54:1164–1168.
63. Conry RM, LoBuglio AF, Curiel DT. Polynucleotide-mediated immunization therapy of cancer. Semin Oncol 1996; 23:135–147.
64. Smith BF, Baker HJ, Curiel DT, Jiang W, Conry RM. Humoral and cellular immune responses of dogs immunized with a nucleic acid vaccine encoding human carcinoembryonic antigen. Gene Ther 1998; 5:865–868.
65. Boring CC, Squires TS, Tong T. Cancer statistics, 1994. CA 1994; 44:7–26.
66. Gilliland FD, Keys CR. Male genital cancers. Cancer 1995; 75:295–315.
67. Wei C, Willis RA, Tilton BR, Looney RJ, Lord EM, Barth RK, Frelinger JG. Tissue-specific expression of the human prostate-specific antigen gene in transgenic mice: Implications for tolerance and immunotherapy. Proc Natl Acad Sci USA 1997; 94:6369–6374.
68. Ko SC, Gotoh A, Thalmann GN, Zhau HE, Johnston DA, Zhang WW, Kao C, Chung LWK. Molecular therapy with recombinant p53 adenovirus in an androgen-independent, metastatic human prostate cancer model. Hum Gene Ther 1996; 7:1683–1691.
69. Wang MC, Kuriyama M, Papsidero LD, Loor RM, Valenzyela LA, Murphy LP, Chu TM. Prostate antigen of human cancer patients. Methods Cancer Res. 1982; 19:179–197.
70. Watt KWK, Lee P-J, Timkulu TM, Chan W-P, Loor R. Human prostate-specific antigen: structural and functional similarity with serine proteases. Proc Natl Acad Sci USA 1986; 83:3166–3170.
71. Labrie F, DuPont A, Suburu R, Cusan L, Tremblay M, Gomez JL, Edmond J. Serum prostate specific antigen as a pre-screening test for prostate cancer. J Urol 1992; 151: 1283–1290.
72. Kim JJ, Trivedi NN, Wilson DM, Mahalingam S, Morrison L, Tsai A, Chattergoon MA, Dang K, Patel M, Ahn L, Chalian AA, Boyer JD, Kieber-Emmons T, Agadjanyan MG, Weiner DB. Molecular and immunological analysis of genetic prostate specific antigen (PSA) vaccine. Oncogene 1998; 17:3125–3135.
73. Schultz A, Hu S. Primate models for HIV vaccines. AIDS 1993; 7:5161–5170.
74. Boyer JD, Ugen KE, Wang B, Agadjanyan MG, Gilbert L, Bagarazzi M, Chattergoon M, Frost P, Javadian A, Williams WV, Refaeli Y, Ciccarelli RB, McCallus D, Coney L, Weiner DB. Protection of chimpanzees from high-dose heterologous HIV-1 challenge by DNA vaccination. Nat Med 1997; 3:526–532.
75. Boyer JD, Wang B, Ugen K, Agadjanyan MG, Javadian MA, Frost P, Dang K, Carrano R, Ciccarelli R, Coney L, Williams WV, Weiner DB. Protective anti-HIV immune responses in non-human primates through DNA immunization. J Med Primatol 1996; 25:242–250.
76. Letvin NL, Montefiori DC, Yasutomi Y, Perry HC, Davies M-E, Lekutis C, Alroy M, Freed DC, Lord CI, Handt LK, Liu MA, Shiver JW. Potent, protective anti-HIV immune responses generated by bimodal HIV envelope DNA plus protein vaccination. Proc Natl Acad Sci USA 1997; 94: 9378–9383.
77. Putkonen P, Quesada-Rolander M, Leandersson A-C, Schwartz S, Thorstensson R, Okuda K, Wahren B, Hinkula J. Immune responses but no protection against SHIV by gene-gun delivery of HIV-1 DNA followed by recombinant subunit protein boosts. Virology 1998; 250:293–301.
78. Kent SJ, Zhao A, Best SJ, Chandler JD, Boyle DB, Ramshaw IA. Enhanced T-cell immunogenicity and protective efficacy of a human immunodeficiency virus type 1 vaccine regimen consisting of consecutive priming with DNA and boosting with recombinant fowlpox virus. J Virol 1998; 72: 10180–10188.
79. Lu S, Arthos J, Montefiori DC, Yasutomi Y, Manson K, Mustafa F, Johnson E, Santoro JC, Wissink J, Mullins JI, Haynes JR, Letvin NL, Wyand M, Robinson HL. Simian immunodeficiency virus DNA vaccine trial in macaques. J Virol 1996; 70:3978–3991.
80. MacGregor RR, Boyer N-D, Ugen KE, Lacy K, Gluckman S, Bagarazzi ML, Chattergoon M, Baine Y, Higgins TJ, Ciccarelli RB, Coney IR, Ginsberg RS, Weiner DB. First human trial of a facilitated DNA plasmid vaccine for HIV-1: safety and host response. J Infect Dis 1998; 178:92–100.
81. Wang R, Doolan DL, Le TP, Hedstrom RC, Coonan KM, Charoenvit Y, Jones TR, Hobart P, Margalith M, Ng J,

Weiss WR, Sedegah M, de Taisne C, Norman JA, Hoffman SL. Induction of antigen-specific cytotoxic T lymphocytes in humans by a malaria DNA vaccine. Science 1998; 282: 476–480.
82. Kim JJ, Ayyavoo V, Bagarazzi ML, Chattergoon M, Boyer JD, Wang B, Weiner DB. Development of a multi-component candidate vaccine for HIV-1. Vaccine 1997; 15: 879–883.
83. Kim JJ, Trivedi NN, Nottingham L, Morrison L, Tsai A, Hu Y, Mahalingam S, Dang K, Ahn L, Doyle NK, Wilson DM, Chattergoon MA, Chalian AA, Boyer JD, Agadjanyan MG, Weiner DB. Modulation of amplitude and direction of in vivo immune responses by co-administration of cytokine gene expression cassettes with DNA immunogens. Eur J Immunol 1998; 28:1089–1103.
84. Kim JJ, Maguire Jr HC, Nottingham LK, Morrison LD, Tsai A, Sin JI, Chalian AA, Weiner DB. Co-administration of IL-12 or IL-10 expression cassettes drives immune responses towards a Thl phenotype. J Interf Cyto Res 1998; 18: 537–547.
85. Kim JJ, Nottingham LK, Sin JI, Tsai A, Morrison L, Oh J, Dang K, Hu Y, Kazahaya K, Bennett M, Dentchev T, Wilson DM, Chalian AA, Boyer JD, Agadjanyan MG, Weiner DB. CD8 positive T cells controls antigen-specific immune responses through the expression of chemokines. J Clin Invest 1998; 102:1112–1124.
86. Kim JJ, Bagarazzi ML, Trivedi N, Hu Y, Chattergoon MA, Dang K, Mahalingam S, Agadjanyan MG, Boyer JD, Wang B, Weiner DB. Engineering of in vivo immune responses to DNA immunization via co-delivery of costimulatory molecule genes. Nat Biot 1997; 15:641–645.
87. Chow Y-H, Huang W-L, Chi W-K, Chu Y-D, Tao M-H. Improvement of hepatitis B virus DNA vaccines by plasmids coexpressing hepatitis B surface antigen and interleukin-2. J Virol 1997; 71:169–178.
88. Iwasaki A, Stiernholm BJ, Chan AK, Berstein NL, Barber BH. Enhanced CTL responses mediated by plasmid DNA immunogens encoding costimulatory molecules and cytokines. J Immunol 1997; 158:4591–4601.
89. Tsuji T, Hamajima K, Ishii N, Aoki I, Fukushima J, Xin KQ, Kawamoto S, Sasaki S, Matsunaga K, Ishigatsubo Y, Tani K, Okubo T, Okuda K. Immunomodulatory effects of a plasmid expressing B7-2 on humanimmunodeficiency virus-1-specific cell-mediated immunity induced by a plasmid encoding the viral antigen. Eur J Immunol 1997; 27:782–787.
90. Xiang Z, Ertl HC. Manipulation of the immune response to a plasmid-encoded viral antigen by coinoculation with plasmids expressing cytokines. Immunity 1995; 2:129–135.
91. Sin JI, Kim JJ, Boyer JD, Huggins C, Higgins T, Weiner DB. In vivo modulation of immune responses and protective immunity against herpes simplex virus-2 infection using cDNAs expressing Th1 and Th2 type cytokines in gD DNA vaccination. J Virol 1998; 73:501–509.
92. Lanier LL, O'Fallon S, Somoza C, Phillips JH, Linsley PS, Okumura K, Ito D, Azuma M. CD80 (B7) and CD86 (B70) provide similar costimulatory signals for T cell proliferation, cytokine production, and generation of CTL. J Immunol 1995; 154:97–105.
93. Linsley PS, Clark EA, Ledbetter JA. The T cell antigen, CD28, mediates adhesion with B cells by interacting with activation antigen, B7/BB-1. Proc Natl Acad Sci USA 1990; 87:5031–5035.
94. June C, Bluestone JA, Nadler LM, Thompson CB. The B7 and CD28 receptor families. Immunol Today 1994; 15: 321–333.
95. Schwartz RH. Costimulation of T lymphocytes: the role of CD29, CTLA-4, and B7/BB1 in interleukin-2 production and immunotherapy. Cell 1992; 71:1065–1068.
96. Agadjanyan MG, Kim JJ, Trivedi N, Wilson DM, Monzavi-Karbassi B, Morrison LD, Nottingham LK, Dentchev T, Tsai A, Dang K, Chalian AA, Maldonado MA, Williams WV, Weiner DB. CD86 (B7-2) can function to drive MHC-restricted antigen-specific cytotoxic T lymphocyte responses in vivo. J Immunol 1999; 162:3417–3427.
97. Kim JJ, Tsai A, Nottingham LK, Morrison L, Cunning D, Oh J, Lee DJ, Dang K, Dentchev T, Chalian AA, Agadjanyan MG, Weiner DB. Intracellular adhesion molecule-1 (ICAM-1) modulates β-chemokines and provides costimulatory signals required for T cell activation and expansion in vivo. J Clin Invest 1999; 103:869–877.
98. Ogg GS, Jin X, Bonhoeffer S, Dunbar PR, Nowak MA, Monard S, Segal JP, Cao Y, Rowland-Jones SL, Cerundolo V, Hurley A, Markowitz M, Ho DD, Nixon DF, McMichael AJ. Quantitation of HIV-1-specific cytotoxic T lymphocytes and plasma load of viral RNA. Science 1998; 279: 2103–2106.
99. Lekutis C, Shiver JW, Liu MA, Letvin NL. HIV-1 env DNA vaccine administered to rhesus monkeys elicits MHC class II-restricted CD4+ T helper cells that secrete IFN-gamma and TNF-alpha. J Immunol 1997; 158:4471–4477.

Index